Wolff's Headache and Other Head Pain

Wolff's Headache and Other Head Pain

Eighth Edition

Edited by

Stephen D. Silberstein, MD, FACP
Director, Jefferson Headache Center
Thomas Jefferson University Hospital
and
Professor of Neurology
Thomas Jefferson University
Philadelphia, Pennsylvania

Richard B. Lipton, MD
Director, Headache Unit
Montefiore Medical Center
and
Professor and Vice-Chairman, Department of Neurology
Albert Einstein College of Medicine
Bronx, New York

David W. Dodick, MD, FRCP(C), FACP
Director, Headache Program
and
Professor of Neurology
Mayo Clinic
Scottsdale, Arizona

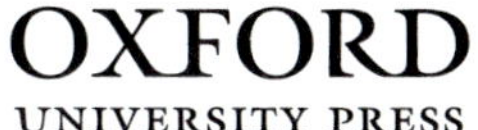

2008

OXFORD
UNIVERSITY PRESS

Oxford University Press, Inc., publishes works that further
Oxford University's objective of excellence
in research, scholarship, and education.

Oxford New York
Auckland Cape Town Dar es Salaam Hong Kong Karachi
Kuala Lumpur Madrid Melbourne Mexico City Nairobi
New Delhi Shanghai Taipei Toronto

With offices in
Argentina Austria Brazil Chile Czech Republic France Greece
Guatemala Hungary Italy Japan Poland Portugal Singapore
South Korea Switzerland Thailand Turkey Ukraine Vietnam

Published by Oxford University Press, Inc.
198 Madison Avenue, New York, New York 10016
www.oup.com

Oxford is a registered trademark of Oxford University Press

Library of Congress Cataloging-in-Publication Data

Wolff's headache and other head pain.—8th ed./[edited by]
Stephen D. Silberstein, Richard B. Lipton, David W. Dodick.
p. ; cm.
Includes bibliographical references and index.
ISBN: 978-0-19-536565-8
1. Headache.
[DNLM: 1. Headache. 2. Headache Disorders. WL 342 W856 2007] I. Title:
Headache and other head pain. II. Silberstein, Stephen D. III. Lipton,
Richard B. IV. Dodick, David. V. Wolff, Harold G. (Harold George),
1898-Wolff's headache and other head pain.
RB128.W68 2007
616.8'491—dc22 2007016231

Cover Image: fMRI activation of the ipsilateral trigeminal ganglion (left panel), ipsilateral spinal trigeminal nucleus (second panel from left), the contralateral thalamus (third panel from left), and the contralateral cortex (right panel) in response to heat stimulation of the right side of the face. (From Borsook, D., Burstein, R., and Becerra, L. Functional imaging of the human trigeminal system: Opportunities for new insights into pain processing in health and disease. J. Neurobiol. 2004; 61(1), 107-125, by permission of John Wiley & Sons.)

9 8 7 6 5 4 3 2 1
Printed in the United States of America
on acid-free paper

The Editors dedicate this edition to John Edmeads, a long-time contributor to *Wolff's Headache*, and mentor and dear friend to us all.

Acknowledgments

Stephen Silberstein would like to thank his wife of 39 years, Marsha, and his children, Joshua and Aaron, for their love, support, and a sense of sanity. He also thanks his uncle Herbert Marks for always being there when he needed him.

Richard Lipton would like to thank his wife of 30 years, Amy, and his children, Lianna and Justin, for their constant love and support.

David Dodick would like to thank his wife of 20 years, Paula, and his children, Samson and Sydney, for their unwavering love and support.

Acknowledgments

Foreword

Physicians who see headache patients will welcome this eighth edition of Harold Wolff's magnificent "Headache Bible," and those who are involved in educating students, trainees, and colleagues about headaches will especially welcome it. In my Foreword to the seventh edition, published in 2001, I outlined the history of the previous editions, starting with the first in 1948. Wolff wrote the first two editions himself, and it was the second, published in 1963, at which time I was a neurology resident, that sparked my initial interest in headaches.

Wolff died in 1962, after completing the second edition. His trainee, Don Dalessio, a leader in American headache circles, solely edited the third (1972) through the fifth editions (1986) and was then joined by Steve Silberstein for the sixth edition (1993), and Richard Lipton for the seventh. Dalessio stepped down and is replaced by the very able David Dodick for this current edition, which contains new chapters, including a history of migraine starting with Hippocrates, and Jim Lance's personal perspective of headaches in the past 50 years, during which he played a major role. Other new chapters include the Pathophysiology of Aura, Headaches in Women, Headaches in the Elderly, and Headache Emergencies Including Thunderclap Headache. Of the two new chapters on treatment, one is procedural, reviewing nerve blocks, neurostimulation, and botulinum injections; and the other reflects the personal experiences of three senior headache experts (Lipton, Saper, and Silberstein) on how to convert treatment failure into success.

This new edition remains a tribute to the great Harold Wolff, who introduced science to the study of headache. I feel privileged to be part of the Wolff legacy by again introducing a new edition of his creation.

Robert B. Daroff, MD
Cleveland, Ohio

Preface

It has been 60 years since Harold G. Wolff published the first edition of this seminal work, and 6 years since its last edition. We are confident that the authors assembled for this eighth edition will ably carry on Wolff's legacy and make previous editors and authors proud to have been a part of this important work.

Since the publication of the seventh edition, the first International Classification of Headache Disorders (ICHD-1) has been extensively revised. The basis for this revision (ICHD-2) is the tremendous advances that have occurred in the genetics, epidemiology, biology, and clinical spectrum of primary and secondary disorders, as well as the description and refinement in our understanding of new headache disorders. The evidence base for current and future treatments has also developed rapidly over the past 6 years.

This edition remains under the stewardship of Stephen Silberstein and Richard Lipton, who, with Donald Dalessio, were responsible for the acclaim and remarkable success of the seventh edition. David Dodick has joined Silberstein and Lipton as junior editor on the current edition. We have added new authors, an international faculty has been maintained, and each chapter is authored by authoritative and, in many instances, pioneering figures in their respective scientific and clinical fields.

The advances in the field of headache medicine permeate the book and are also reflected in the new chapters on *Headache in Women*, *Headache in the Elderly*, *Emergency Headaches, Including Thunderclap Headache*, and timely chapters for clinicians on *Why Treatment Fails* and *Peripheral Procedures: Nerve Blocks, Peripheral Neuro Stimulation, and Botulinum Toxin Injections.*

The scope and complexity of headache have resulted in the United Council for Neurologic Subspecialties including headache medicine as a neurologic subspecialty, allowing board certification of headache medicine specialists and accreditation of headache fellowships training programs. Our comprehensive yet easily accessible text will provide an ongoing source of information, stimulation, and inspiration for *students* at every level.

Philadelphia — Stephen D. Silberstein
Bronx — Richard B. Lipton
Scottsdale — David W. Dodick

Contents

Contributors

Avi Ashkenazi, MD
Assistant Professor of Neurology
Thomas Jefferson University
Philadelphia, Pennsylvania

Thorsten Bartsch, MD
Department of Neurology
University Hospital Schleswig-Holstein
Kiel, Germany

Marcelo E. Bigal, MD, PhD
Department of Neurology
Albert Einstein College of Medicine
Bronx, New York
and
Director of Research
The New England Center for Headache
Stamford, Connecticut

Christopher J. Boes, MD
Consultant, Department of Neurology Mayo Clinic
Assistant Professor of Neurology
Mayo Clinic College of Medicine
Rochester, Minnesota

Nikolai Bogduk, MD, PhD, DSc, M Med, Dip Anat, FFPM (ANZCA), FAFRM, FAFMM
Professor of Pain Medicine
University of Newcastle
and
Director, Department of Clinical Research
Newcastle Bone and Joint Institute
Royal Newcastle Centre
Newcastle, New South Wales
Australia

Paul W. Brazis, MD
Professor of Neurology
Consultant in Neurology and Neuro-Ophthalmology
Mayo Clinic - Jacksonville
Jacksonville, Florida

Rami Burstein, PhD
Associate Professor
Vice Chairman, Research Department of Anesthesia and Critical Care
Beth Israel Deaconess Medical Center
Department of Neurobiology
Harvard Medical School
Boston, Massachusetts

Dawn C. Buse, PhD
Department of Neurology
Albert Einstein College of Medicine of Yeshiva University
Assistant Professor, Clinical Health Psychology Doctoral Program
Ferkauf Graduate School of Psychology of Yeshiva University
Director of Psychology
Montefiore Headache Center
Bronx, New York

David J. Capobianco, MD
Department of Neurology
Mayo Clinic College of Medicine
Jacksonville, Florida

James J. Corbett, MD
McCarty Professor and Chairman for Neurology
University of Mississippi Medical center
Jackson, Mississippi

Donald J. Dalessio, MD
Consultant in Neurology
Scripps Clinic and Research Foundation
La Jolla, California

Prof. Dr. med. Martin Dichgans
Neurology Klinikum
Ludwig-Maximilians-Universität München
München, Germany

Hans-Christoph Diener, MD
Professor and Chairman, Department of Neurology
University Essen
Essen, Germany

David W. Dodick, MD
Professor of Neurology
Mayo Medical School
Scottsdale, Arizona

Anne Ducros MD, PhD
Emergency Headache Department
Hôpital Lariboisière
Paris, France

Katharina Eikermann-Haerter, MD
Stroke and Neurovascular Regulation Laboratory
Department of Radiology
Massachusetts General Hospital and Harvard Medical School
Charlestown, Massachusetts

Randolph W. Evans, MD
Clinical Professor of Neurology
Baylor College of Medicine
Houston, Texas

Stefan Evers, MD, PhD
Department of Neurology
University of Münster
Münster, Germany

Michel D. Ferrari, MD, PhD
Department of Neurology
Leiden University Medical Centre
Leiden, The Netherlands

Frederick G. Freitag, DO
Diamond Headache Clinic
Chicago, Illinois

Deborah I. Friedman, MD, FAAN
Departments of Ophthalmology and Neurology
University of Rochester School of Medicine and Dentistry
Rochester, New York

Jonathan P. Gladstone, MD
Gladstone Headache Clinic
Sunnybrook Health Sciences
The Hospital for Sick Children
University of Toronto
Toronto, Ontario, Canada

Peter J. Goadsby, MD PhD DSc FRACP FRCP
Institute of Neurology
London, United Kingdom
and
Department of Neurology
University of California, San Francisco
San Francisco, California

Steven B. Graff-Radford, DDS
Co-Director, the Pain Center
Cedars-Sinai Medical Center
Adjunct Professor, UCLA School of Dentistry
and
Clinical Professor, USC School of Dentistry
Los Angeles California

Brian M. Grosberg, MD
Montefiore Headache Unit
Albert Einstein College of Medicine
Bronx, New York

Steven R. Hahn, MD
Professor of Clinical Medicine
Instructor in Psychiatry
Albert Einstein College of Medicine
and
Adult Primary Care Service
Jacobi Medical Center
Bronx, New York

Sandra W. Hamelsky, PhD, MPH
Department of Neurology
Albert Einstein College of Medicine
Marlboro, New Jersey

Andrew D. Hershey, MD, PhD
Associate Professor of Pediatrics and Neurology
University of Cincinnati
and
Director, Headache Center
Associate Director, Neurology Research
Children's Hospital Medical Center
Cincinnati, Ohio

Kenneth A. Holroyd, PhD
Edwin & Ruth Kennedy Distinguished Professor of Psychology
Psychology Department
Ohio University
Athens, Ohio

Gene G. Hunder, MD
Professor of Medicine
Division of Rheumatology
Mayo Clinic
Rochester, Minnesota

Zaza Katsarava, MD, PhD, MSc
Department of Neurology
University of Essen Germany

James W. Lance MD, Hon DSc, FRCP[Lond], FRACP
Professor Emeritus of Neurology
University of New South Wales

Sydney
and
Honorary Consultant Neurologist
Prince of Wales Hospital
Sydney, Australia

Marc E. Lenaerts, MD
Headache Section
Department of Neurology
Oklahoma University Health Sciences Center
Oklahoma City, Oklahoma

Morris Levin, MD
Associate Professor of Medicine (Neurology)
Associate Professor of Psychiatry
Dartmouth Medical School
Co-director, Dartmouth Headache Center
Director, Dartmouth Neurology Residency Training Program
Hanover, New Hampshire

Zhicheng Li, MD
Instructor, Department of Neurology
Montefiore Headache Center
Albert Einstein College of Medicine
Bronx, New York

Gay L. Lipchik, PhD
Director, Saint Vincent Health Psychology Services
Erie, Pennsylvania

Richard B. Lipton, MD
Director, Headache Unit
Montefiore Medical Center
and
Professor and Vice-Chairman
Department of Neurology
Albert Einstein College of Medicine
Bronx, New York

Elizabeth Loder, MD
Chief, Division of Headache and Pain
Department of Neurology
Brigham and Women's/ Faulkner Hospitals
Boston, Massachusetts

Manjit Matharu, BSc, MBChB, PhD, MRCP
Senior Lecturer and Honorary Consultant Neurologist
Headache Group
Institute of Neurology
London, United Kingdom

Laszlo Mechtler, MD
Director, Dent Headache Center
Dent Neurologic Institute
Clinical Associate Professor of Neurology and Neuroimaging
State University of New York at Buffalo
Amherst, New York

Karl Messlinger
Institute of Physiology and Pathophysiology
University of Erlangen-Nuernberg
Erlangen, Germany

Bahram Mokri, MD
Professor of Neurology
Mayo Clinic
Rochester, Minnesota

Michael A. Moskowitz, MD
Professor of Neurology
Massachusetts General Hospital
Harvard Medical School
Affiliate Member of the Faculty Harvard-MIT Division of Health & Science Technology
Department of Radiology Stroke and Neurovascular Regulation Laboratory
Charlestown, Massachusetts

Alan C. Newman, DDS
Cedars-Sinai Medical Center
Adjunct Professor, UCLA School of Dentistry
Los Angeles, California

Lawrence C. Newman, MD
Director, The Headache Institute
Saint Luke's—Roosevelt Hospital Center
New York, New York

Michael L. Oshinsky, PhD
Assistant Professor, Department of Neurology
Thomas Jefferson University
Philadelphia, Pennsylvania

Russell C. Packard, MD, FACP
Vice Chair, Psychiatry
Professor of Neuropsychiatry
University of North Texas
Health Sciences Center
Fort Worth, Texas

Donald B. Penzien, PhD
Professor of Psychiatry and Human Behavior
Director, Head Pain Center
University of Mississippi Medical Center
Jackson, Mississippi

Jeanetta C. Rains, PhD
Center for Sleep Evaluation
Elliot Hospital
Manchester, New Hampshire

Todd D. Rozen, MD
Michigan Head-Pain and Neurological Institute
Ann Arbor, Michigan
and
Clinical Associate Professor of Neurology
Wayne State University
Detroit, Michigan

Joel R. Saper, MD
Founder and Director of Michigan Head Pain and Neurological Institute
Ann Arbor, Michigan

Ann I. Scher, PhD
Department of Preventive Medicine and Biometrics
Uniformed Services University
Bethesda, Maryland

Wouter I. Schievink, MD
Department of Neurosurgery
Cedars-Sinai Medical Center
Los Angeles, California

Todd J. Schwedt, MD
Assistant Professor of Neurology
Washington University School of Medicine
Washington University Headache Center
St. Louis, Missouri

Stephen D. Silberstein, MD
Professor of Neurology
Thomas Jefferson University
Director, Jefferson Headache Center
Thomas Jefferson University Hospital
Philadelphia, Pennsylvania

Walter "Buzz" Stewart, PhD, MPH
Associate Chief Research Officer
Geisinger Center for Health Research
Geisinger Health System
Danville, Pennsylvania

Andrew M. Strassman, PhD
Department of Anesthesia/Critical Care, DA 717
Beth Israel Deaconess Medical Center
Boston, Massachusetts

Jerry W. Swanson, MD, FACP
Professor of Neurology
Mayo Clinic College of Medicine
Chair, Division of Headache
Mayo Clinic
Rochester, Minnesota

Michael Wall, MD
Departments of Neurology
University of Iowa College of Medicine
Veterans Administration Medical Center
Iowa City, Iowa

Eelco FM. Wijdicks, MD
Professor of Neurology
Chair, Division of Critical Care Neurology
Mayo Clinic College of Medicine
Rochester, Minnesota
and
Consultant, Neurological-Neurosurgical Intensive Care Unit
St. Marys Hospital

Thomas O. Willcox, Jr. MD
Department of Otolaryngology-Head and Neck Surgery
Thomas Jefferson University
Philadelphia, Pennsylvania

Paul Winner, DO, FAAN
Director Palm Beach Headache Center
Director Premiere Research Institute @ Palm Beach Neurology
Clinical Professor of Neurology at Nova Southeastern University
Ft. Lauderdale, Florida

William B. Young, MD
Associate Professor
Director, Inpatient Program
Jefferson Headache Center
Thomas Jefferson University Hospital
Philadelphia, Pennsylvania

I General Consideration: Classification, Epidemiology and Mechanisms

1 The History of Migraine from Hippocrates to Harold Wolff

Christopher J. Boes, MD and Donald J. Dalessio, MD

INTRODUCTION

In his superb monograph on migraine published in 1932, Henry Alsop Riley wrote (Riley, 1932):

> If one should search for the human ill which has manifested itself most widely during all times and among all people, there can be but little doubt that headache would attain this unenviable distinction. It is not surprising, therefore, that one form of this disorder, migraine, perhaps the most baffling and dramatic form of pain in the head should have acquired recognition as a definite symptom-complex early in medical history. (p. 429)

A student of the history of medicine quickly realizes that much has been written about migraine over the centuries, partly because many physicians and scientists have suffered from the ailment. For example, John Hughlings Jackson, considered the father of English neurology, once told a younger colleague who had approached him: "Stop! I am just observing my migraine" (Critchley and Critchley, 1998). In 1940, Samuel Alexander Kinnier Wilson wrote, "migraine has been portrayed by its victims in medicine and science more fully than any other malady, not excluding gout" (Wilson, 1940). Ralph Waldo Emerson wrote, "all history becomes subjective; in other words there is properly no history, only biography" (Emerson, 1990). We have indeed been subjective in choosing which authors to focus on. We will stop our review at approximately 1950 as the history of migraine in the last 50 years is described in Chapter 2 by Professor James W. Lance.

HIPPOCRATES (c.460–c.370 BC)

There are references to sick-headedness and head pain in Sumerian poems and Egyptian papyri, but we will begin our discussion of migraine with Hippocrates (Fig. 1–1). Hippocrates and his Greek followers emphasized clinical observation, and he "was first to emancipate medicine from trammels of superstition and delusions of philosophy" (Bender, 1966). The "Father of Medicine's" observations on migraine were concise (Critchley, 1967):

> Most of the time he seemed to see something shining before him like a light, usually in part of the right eye; at the end of a moment, a violent pain supervened in the right temple, then in all the head and neck, where the head is attached to the spine . . . vomiting, when it became possible, was able to divert the pain and rend it more moderate. (pp. 28–29)

In Isler's opinion, the writings of Hippocrates have been misinterpreted as migraine with aura because of the suggestive visual symptoms (Isler, 1987). Isler feels that the authors of the Hippocratic corpus (collection) were mainly writing about secondary and not primary headaches (Isler, 1987).

ARETAEUS (AD 81–?)

Aretaeus (Fig. 1–2) was born in Cappadocia (modern Turkey), and later lived in Alexandria and Rome (Critchley, 1967). His classic description has "caused him ordinarily to be regarded as the discoverer of migraine" (Critchley, 1967). Aretaeus was a splitter, and divided headache

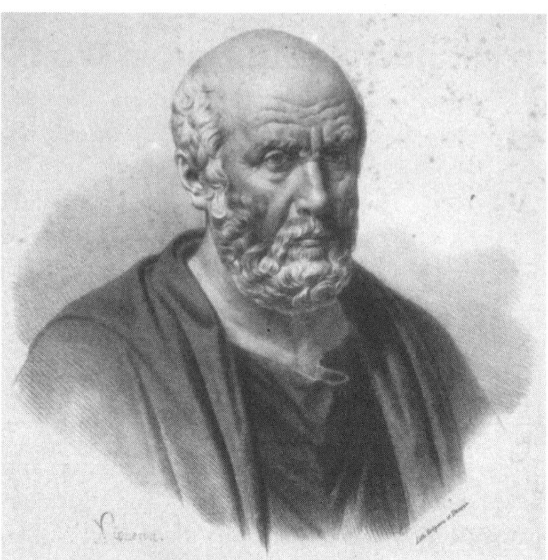

Figure 1–1 Hippocrates. (Courtesy of the National Library of Medicine.)

into cephalalgia (mild, infrequent, short-lasting headache), cephalea (more severe and longer-lasting headache), and heterocrania (migraine) (Isler, 1987). Isler and Koehler write that cephalalgia and cephalea represent tension-type headaches (Isler and Koehler, 2006), whereas Schiller comments that cephalea refers to headache with an underlying structural cause (Schiller, 1975). All authors agree that Aretaeus was describing migraine when he wrote about heterocrania (Aretaeus, 1856):

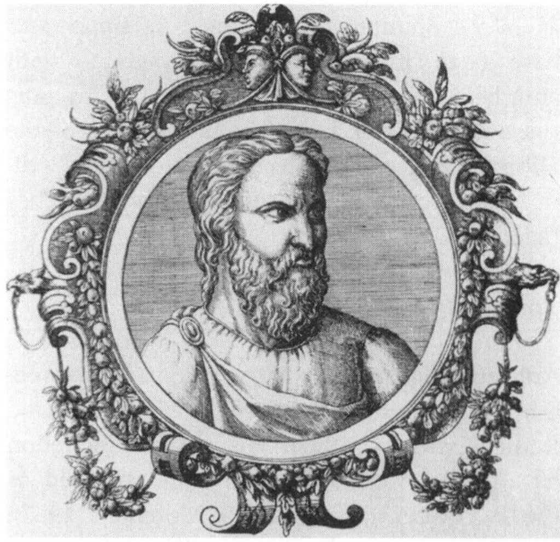

Figure 1–2 Aretaeus. (Courtesy of the National Library of Medicine.)

> In certain cases, the parts on the right side, or those on the left solely, so far that a separate temple, or ear, or one eyebrow, or one eye, or the nose which divides the face into two equal parts; and the pain does not pass this limit, but remains in the half of the head. This is called Heterocrania, an illness by no means mild, even though it intermits, and although it appears to be slight. For if at any time it set in acutely, it occasions unseemly and dreadful symptoms . . . nausea; vomiting of bilious matters; collapse of the patient; but if the affection be protracted, the patient will die; or if more light and not deadly, it becomes chronic; there is much torpor, heaviness of the head, anxiety and ennui. For they flee the light; the darkness soothes their disease: nor can they bear readily to look upon or hear anything disagreeable; their sense of smell is vitiated, neither does anything agreeable to smell delight them, and they have also an aversion to fetid things: the patients, moreover, are weary of life, and wish to die. (pp. 294–295)

Of course, patient death during a migraine is unusual, and Critchley has written that Aretaeus had probably observed patients with periodic headaches culminating in aneurysmal subarachnoid hemorrhage (Critchley, 1967).

GALEN (AD 131–201)

Galen (Fig. 1–3) was born in Pergamon (modern Turkey) and later worked in Alexandria and Rome. As is well known, he was a proponent of the humoral theory, and felt that imbalances of the four essential humors (blood, phlegm, yellow bile, and black bile) lead to disease. His teachings were accepted as dogmas for 1500 years, until they were challenged by Vesalius and Harvey (Bender, 1966). Galen called unilateral headache “hemicrania,” which over time became known as “megrim” or “migraine” (Critchley, 1967). Galen wrote (Critchley, 1967):

> Hemicrania is a painful disorder affecting approximately one half of the head, either

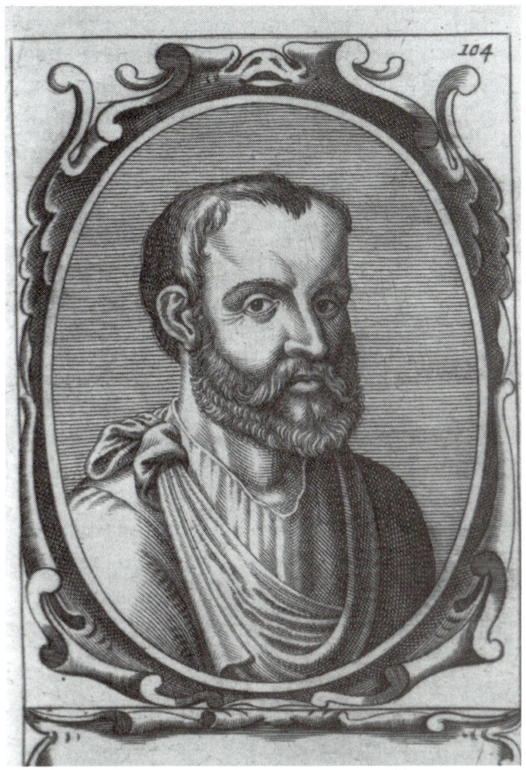

Figure 1–3 Galen. (Courtesy of the National Library of Medicine.)

> the right or left side, and which extends along the length of the longitudinal suture . . . It is caused by the ascent of vapours, either excessive in amount, or too hot, or too cold. (p. 30)

THOMAS WILLIS (1621–1675)

Thomas Willis (Fig. 1–4) was a seventeenth century English anatomist and physician who introduced the word "neurology" and whose name is immortalized in the eponym for the circle of arteries at the base of the brain. In 1672, Willis published *Two Discourses of the Soul of Brutes Which is the Vital and Sensitive (Soul) of Man* in which he "directed attention to what he called habitual headache, of which there were two types, namely the continual and the intermitting, the latter being more common" (Critchley, 1967). In the text, he described a particular female patient with migraine. The following translation from the Latin

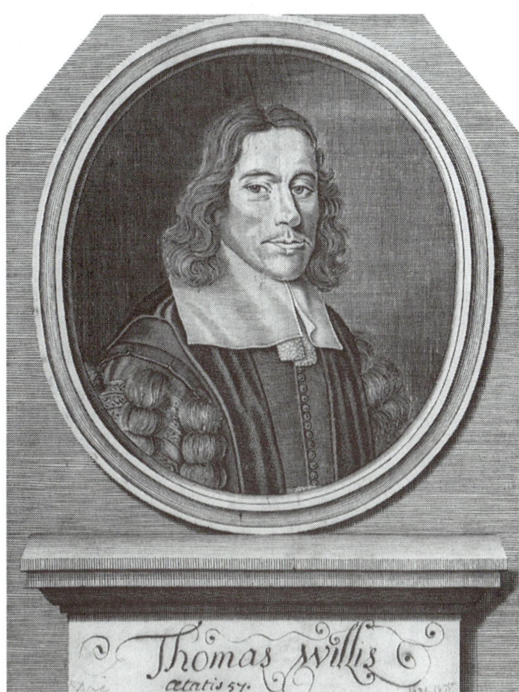

Figure 1–4 Thomas Willis. (Courtesy of the National Library of Medicine.)

text is from an article written by Macdonald Critchley in 1937 (Critchley, 1937):

> Some years since, I was sent for to visit a most noble Lady, for above twenty years sick with almost a continual Headach, at first intermitting . . . Growing well of a Feavour before she was twelve years old, she became obnoxious to pains in the Head, which were wont to arise, sometimes of their own accord, and more often upon every light occasion. This sickness being limited to no one place of the Head, troubled her sometimes on one side, sometimes on the other, and often thorow the whole compass of the Head. During the fit (which rarely ended under a day and a night's space, and often held for two, three, or four days) she was impatient of light, speaking, noise, or of any motion, sitting upright in her Bed, the Chamber made dark, she would talk to no body, nor take any sleep, or sustenance. At length about the declination of the fit, she was wont to lye down with a heavy and disturbed sleep, from which awaking she found herself better, and so by degrees grew

> well, and continued indifferently well till the time of the intermission. Formerly, the fits came not but occasionally, and seldom under twenty days of a month, but afterwards they came more often: and lately she was seldom free. Moreover, upon sundry occasions, or evident causes (such as the change of the Air, or the year, the great Aspects of the Sun and Moon, violent passions, and errors in diet) she was more cruelly tormented with them. But although this Distemper most grievously afflicting this noble Lady, above twenty years (when I saw her) having pitched its tents near the confines of the Brain, had so long besieged its regal tower, yet it had not taken it: for the sick Lady, being free from a Vertigo, swimming in the Head, Convulsive Distempers, and any Soporiferous symptom, found the chief faculties of her soul sound enough. (p. 44)

The patient here was Anne, Countess of Conway, a noted English philosopher. Anne's headaches began at age 12, occurred intermittently for a period of time, and then became continuous. She died at age 48 of unclear causes (Critchley, 1937). Her refractory headaches were also treated by William Harvey, Robert Boyle, and others (Critchley, 1937). About Willis' description of Anne's headaches, Critchley wrote (Critchley, 1937):

> We may pause for a while to ask ourselves what diagnosis would probably be made to-day in Lady Conway's case. Intractable and prostrating headaches, appearing first at puberty and persisting for thirty-six years, intermittent at first, almost certainly indicate a severe and chronic form of migraine. Their association with vomiting (mentioned in a letter from her brother), their frequent unilateral situation, their appearance "upon every light occasion," the concomitant photophobia and intolerance to noise, their duration of thirty-six hours to four days, their conclusion in a heavy and disturbed sleep, are all strongly confirmatory. The absence of intellectual change, of epileptiform seizures, and of somnolence furthermore confirm the diagnosis of migraine and serve to exclude the grosser intracranial disorders such as tumour, aneurysm or hydrocephalus. (p. 47)

This is probably the first patient described with chronic migraine (Boes and Capobianco, 2005). Aretaeus mentioned that if the attack was lighter and not deadly it became chronic, but he did not clarify what he meant by chronic, and thus priority should go to Willis.

Willis also reported premonitory symptoms in migraine (Critchley, 1967):

> A beautiful and young woman, indued with a slender habit of body, and an hot blood, being obnoxious to an hereditary headach was wont to be afflicted with frequent and wandering fits of it, to wit, some upon every light occasion, and some of their own accord; that is, arising without any evident cause. On the day before the coming of the spontaneous fit of this disease, growing very hungry in the evening, she eat a most plentiful supper, with an hungry, I may say a greedy appetite; presaging by this sign, that the pain of the head would most certainly follow the next morning; and the event never failed this augury. For as soon as she awaked, being afflicted by a most sharp torment, thorow the whole forepart of her head, she was troubled also with vomiting, sometimes of an acid, and as it were a vitriolock, humor, and some times of a cholerick and highly bitterish: hence according to this sign this headach is thought to arise from the vice of the stomach. (p. 34)

Le Pois had previously described premonitory features in 1618 (Lane and Davies, 2006).

Willis embraced polypharmacy for headaches (Lance and Goadsby, 2005), and to the modern reader the wisest advice offered is coffee (Willis, 1685). Willis mentioned an interesting treatment: "the use of Millepedes ought not here to be omitted, or set lightly by, in regard that their express'd Juice, distill'd Water, and also the Powder prepar'd of them, often contribute egregiously to the Cure of ancient and obstinate Head-achs" (Willis, 1685). Such therapy seems tolerable compared to the therapeutic advice of Ali ibn Isa, who in approximately AD 1000 recommended that "for the effective treatment of long-standing headache the patient may bind over his head a mole long dead and putrid" (Ali ibn Isa and Wood, 1936) or to the approximately AD 800 recommendations of medieval physicians concerning the efficacy of vulture (Edmeads, 1991):

> The bones from its head wrapped in deer skin will cure any pain and headache; its brain, mixed with the best of oil and put in the nose, will expel all ailments of the head. (p. 2)

For the treatment of cephalea and heterocrania, Aretaeus recommended inducing sneezing by placing testicle-of-beaver powder intranasally to "bring off phlegm" (Aretaeus, 1856). All these remedies seem to be worse than the disease (Ali ibn Isa and Wood, 1936)!

SAMUEL AUGUSTE ANDRE DAVID TISSOT (1728–1797)

Tissot (Fig. 1–5) was a Swiss physician who devoted over 80 pages to migraine in his late eighteenth century book entitled *Treatise on the Nerves and Their Disorders* (Pearce, 2003). He felt that migraine was generally due to a gastric disorder. Although his gastric theory has not stood the test of time, his clinical descriptions are classic (Pearce, 2003):

> Migraine is distinguished by the severity of the pain, by a kind of periodical return, by the similarity of different attacks . . . the pain, however, does not set in at first in its full severity, which it does not usually attain for an hour and a half, and then remains at the same intensity for some hours . . . After the headache vomiting frequently sets in, which is attended by relief; the pain diminishes, and the patient sometimes falls into a tranquil sleep for some hours, and awakes feeling quite well. (p. 171)

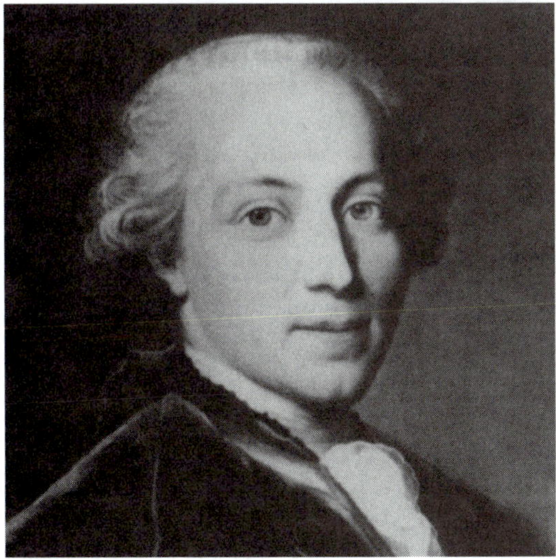

Figure 1–5 Samuel Auguste Tissot. (Courtesy of the University of Lausanne.)

Tissot also described the spectrum of aura in one sufferer (Liveing, 1873):

> I was consulted by an officer in the Austrian service, thirty-two years of age, whose migraine was of a well-marked nervous type. "I have suffered from the age of nine years," these are his words, "from migraine which, at its commencement, seized me about every two months, sometimes oftener; I have also been more than a year without it. It begins in the eyes; when I least expect it my sight becomes suddenly disordered, but more on one side than the other, like that of a person who has looked at the sun. This lasts about ten minutes; afterwards an arm and a leg of the same side, one time one side and one another, go to sleep. I feel a tingling as if ants were on them; I have the same feeling in the mouth and tongue, and further, during this period, I have the greatest difficulty in speaking. This lasts about half a quarter of an hour; afterwards, the pains in the head commence, but only in the temples, where they persist with great severity during seven or eight hours. When I can be sick, I get relief. (p. 64)"

HUBERT AIRY (1838–1903) AND OTHERS ON VISUAL AURA

Although not the first to describe visual aura, Airy's account and his plate depicting his own visual changes are superb (Fig. 1–6). In 1870, Airy published the article, "On a distinct form of transient hemiopsia" in *Philosophical Transactions of the Royal Society of London*. The paper starts with Airy citing reports of visual aura by Wollaston, Arago, Brewster, Herschel, Wheatstone, Dufour, Fothergill, Parry, and his father, George Airy.

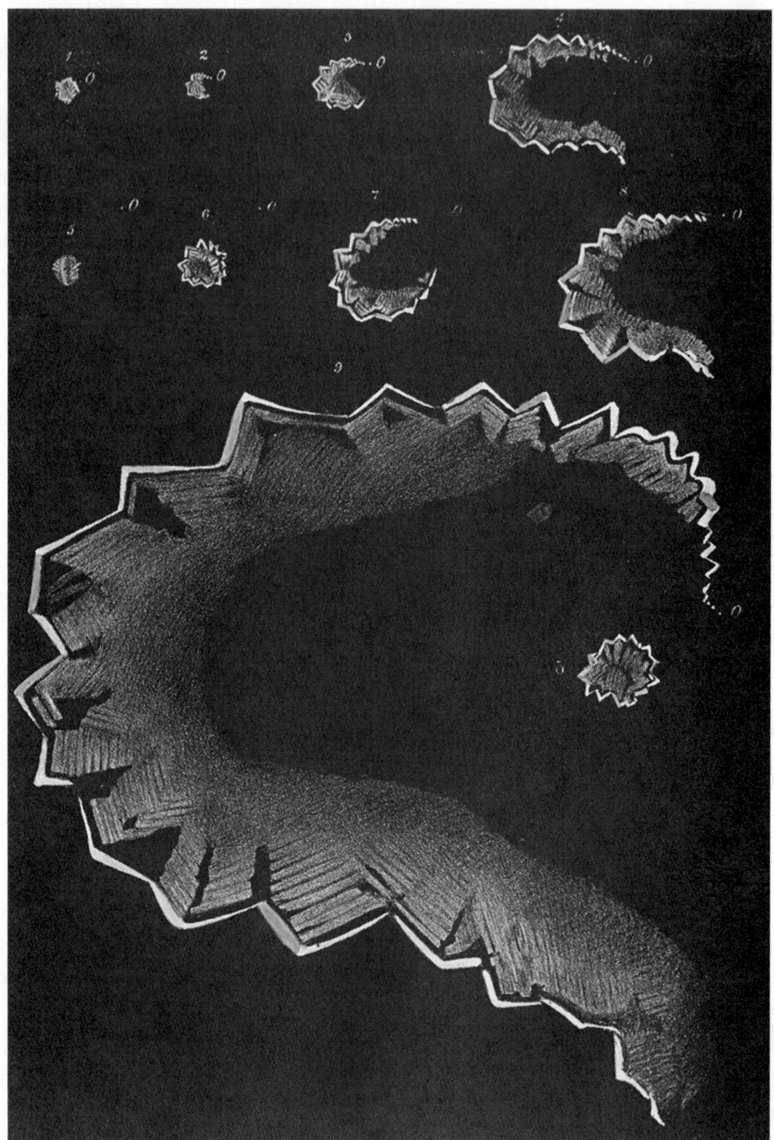

Figure 1–6 Airy's Sinistral (left-sided) Teichopsia. The letter O marks the fixation point in every illustration. Numbers 1–4 refer to the early stages of a visual aura that began close to the fixation point, as seen in the dark. The increasing numbers represent progression in time. Numbers 5–8 refer to a similar series of the early stages of a left-sided teichopsia beginning a few degrees below and to the left of the fixation point. Number 9 shows a fully developed sinistral teichopsia. The δ marks the beginning of a second attack, beginning nearly where the first began. This fresh attack never attains full development, "unless it arise on the opposite side, when I have known a second attack develop itself immediately after the first" (Airy, 1870). [From Airy, H. (1870). On a distinct form of transient hemiopsia. *Philosophical Transactions of the Royal Society of London,* 160:247–264.]

Airy coined the term teichopsia, which means town-wall vision, to represent the "bastioned form of transient hemiopsia which I have been describing" (Airy, 1870). He outlined the main characteristics (Airy, 1870):

1. Dependence on mental anxiety, bodily exhaustion, overwork to the eyes, gastric derangement, want of exercise.

2. Origin from a small spot near the centre of vision.
3. Orderly outward spread from the original spot.
4. Blindness to boundaries, but not to general impressions of light and colour.
5. Luminosity in the dark.
6. Bright bastioned margin, with gleams of various colours.
7. Tremor and "boiling."
8. Gradual occupation of one (lateral) half of the field of view.
9. Gradual recovery of clear vision in rear of the outward-spreading cloud.
10. Disappearance of the phenomenon in about half an hour.
11. Sequelae: headache and nausea, and sometimes affection of speech and hearing, and even an approach to hemiplegia. (p. 262)

Airy commented, "[the] main division into dextral and sinistral teichopsia will correspond then to the distinction between right and left permanent hemiopsia, and will depend upon temporary affection of the left or right optic tract, or its origin in the corresponding optic thalamus" (Airy, 1870).

In the 1880s, the occipital cortex was given as the seat of the visual derangement in migraine visual aura (Schiller, 1975). In 1941, Karl Lashley (Fig. 1–7) extensively investigated his own auras (Fig. 1–8) and concluded the following (Lashley, 1941):

> Maps of the scotomas of ophthalmic migraine sketched at brief intervals during an attack suggest that a wave of intense excitation is propagated at a rate of about 3 mm. per minute across the visual cortex. This wave is followed by complete inhibition of activity, with recovery progressing at the same rate. Sometimes the inhibition spreads without the preceding excitatory wave. (p. 339)

Coincidentally and serendipitously, Aristides Leao (Fig. 1–9) observed the following while doing research at Harvard University (Leao, 1944):

> Early in the development of the study an interesting response, elicited by electrical stimulation, was noticed in the cortex of rabbits. The distinctive feature of this response was a marked, enduring reduction of the "spontaneous" electrical activity of the cortex... Simultaneous records from several pairs of electrodes showed that the depression spread out, slowly in all directions, from the region stimulated... Spreading depression of the electrical activity could also be elicited by mechanical stimulation of the cerebral cortex... Recovery of the initial pattern of spontaneous activity... requires 5 to 10 minutes at each region... Only with supraminimal stimulation does the depression spread to the opposite hemisphere... Specific activity, different from the spontaneous, often develops during the period of depression of a region. (pp. 359–361, 363, 388)

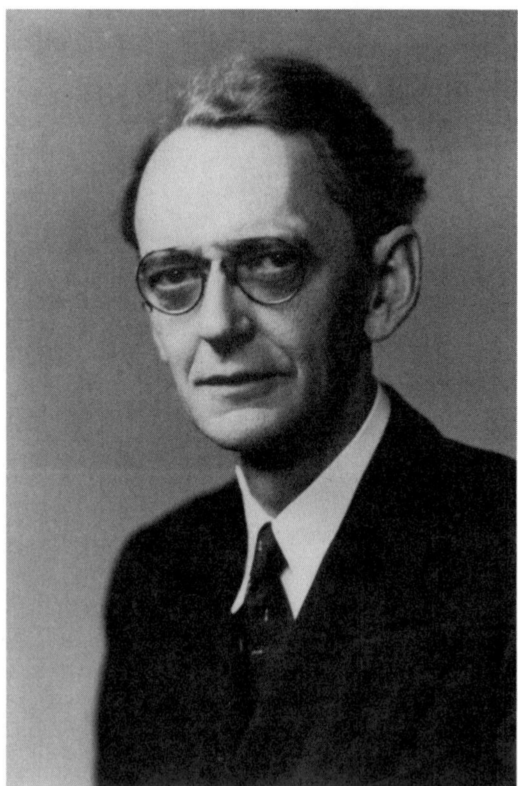

Figure 1–7 Karl Lashley. (Reproduced with permission from the Karl S. Lashley Papers, 1923–1958, Department of Special and Area Studies Collections, George A. Smathers Libraries, University of Florida.)

The speed of the spread was in the order of 3 mm/min, exactly the rate reported by Lashley (Teive et al.,

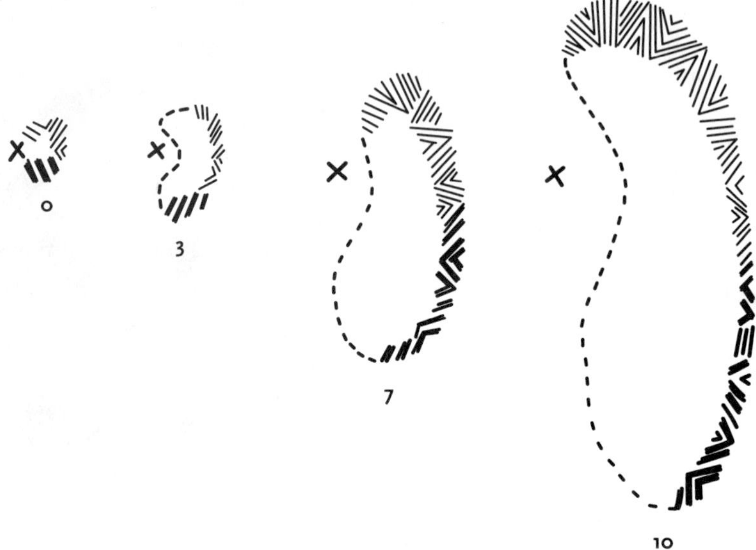

Figure 1–8 Lashley's depiction of his own right-sided visual aura. The X in each case indicates the fixation point. The numbers refer to the number of minutes elapsed after the visual aura was first noted. The scintillations occur along the advancing margin, which is made up of a network of intersecting lines and angles. This positive phenomenon is followed by a negative scotoma. [Reproduced with permission from Lashley, KS. (1941). Patterns of cerebral integration indicated by the scotomas of migraine. *Arch Neurol Psychiatr,* 46:331–339. Copyright © 1941 American Medical Association.]

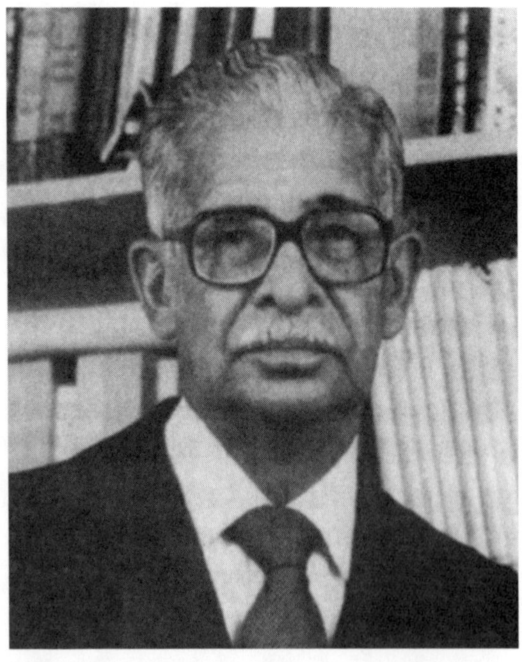

Figure 1–9 Aristides Leao. (Courtesy of the Brazilian Academy of Sciences Memory Project.)

2005). Thus cortical spreading depression was summarized as a wave of short-lasting neuronal excitation, followed by prolonged depression of cortical neuronal activity (Teive et al., 2005). An association with the positive and negative aspects of migraine visual aura was suspected (Lane and Davies, 2006). In another paper on spreading depression in 1945, Leao commented (Leao and Morison, 1945):

> Much has been written about vascular phenomena both in clinical epilepsy and the presumably related condition of migraine. The latter disease with the marked dilatation of major blood vessels and the slow march of scotomata in the visual or sensory sphere is suggestively similar to the experimental phenomenon here described, in spite of the fact that known scotomata are still felt to be vasoconstrictor in nature. (p. 44)

Leao was unaware of Lashley's article on migraine aura when he made this observation (Teive et al., 2005).

VASCULAR VERSUS NEUROGENIC THEORISTS (LATHAM VERSUS LIVEING)

The two main theories of migraine causation, a little over 125 years ago, were vascular and neurogenic, for "pain and aura make of migraine a perennial see-saw problem" (Schiller, 1975). Two British physicians with opposing viewpoints on the cause of migraine were Peter Wallwork Latham (1832–1923) and Edward Liveing (1832–1919). We have chosen these among many candidates as the prototypical vascular and neurogenic theorists. Latham published a two-part article supporting his theory in the *British Medical Journal* in March of 1872, and Liveing published his migraine causation article in the same journal the following month. "It seems as if an aroused Liveing had submitted his paper as soon as he had seen Latham's" (Schiller, 1975).

Peter Wallwork Latham (Fig. 1–10) was Deputy Professor of Medicine at Addenbrooke's, the university hospital at Cambridge (Schiller, 1975). His vasomotor hypothesis was as follows (Latham, 1872):

> First of all . . . we have contraction of the vessels of the brain, and so a diminished supply of blood produced by excited action of the sympathetic; and . . . the exhaustion of the sympathetic following on this excitement causes the dilatation of the vessels and the headache. (p. 306)

Latham explained that vasoconstriction caused the aura symptoms and vasodilatation the headache (Latham, 1872):

> This disturbance of vision . . . is due to defective supply of blood to one side of the brain from the contraction of the cerebral arteries. . . [later] the resistance of the arteries is overcome, the action of the sympathetic is exhausted, and the same condition results as is observed after section of this nerve. The vessels become distended, the head throbs and aches. (p. 336)

He comments that his theory "is advanced not as certain and proved, but only as possibly true" (Latham, 1872).

Edward Liveing (Fig. 1–11) was assistant physician to King's College Hospital in London. In addition to his 1872 *British Medical Journal* article, Liveing published *On Megrim, Sick-headache, and Some Allied Disorders: A Contribution to the Pathology of Nerve-storms* in 1873 (Liveing, 1873). *On Megrim* is considered the first major treatise devoted to the subject of migraine, unquestionably regarded as a minor classic (Critchley, 1967), and unsurpassed as a historical survey (Schiller, 1975). Liveing emphasized the protean symptoms of migraine. Sacks comments that "almost every phenomenon of migraine, however rare or strange, was noticed and noted by him" (Sacks, 1997). Liveing believed that headache may be secondary to dilatation, but he did not feel that the vascular theory explained aura, the vegetative symptoms throughout the body, and the changes in patterns of attacks (Pearce, 2003). He commented that "I am not at all disposed to deny that disorders of local circulation occur in the course of megrim, and that the implication of the sympathetic may play an important part in their production; but I regard them among the least constant and regular

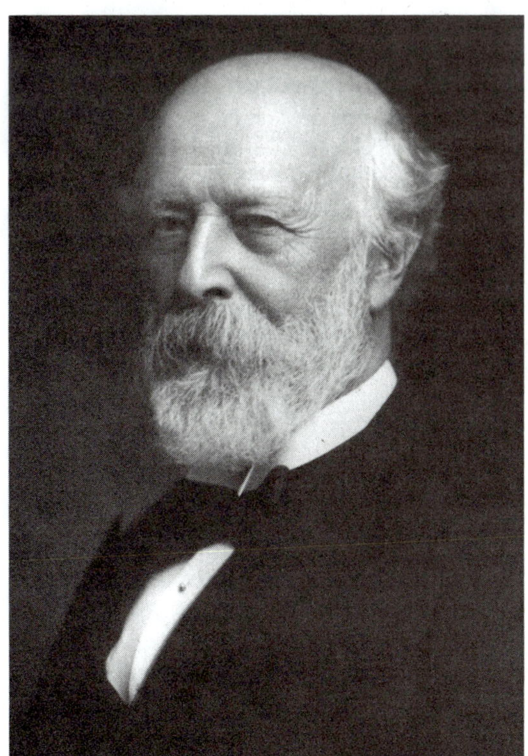

Figure 1–10 Peter Wallwork Latham. (Courtesy of the Addenbrooke's Hospital Archives.)

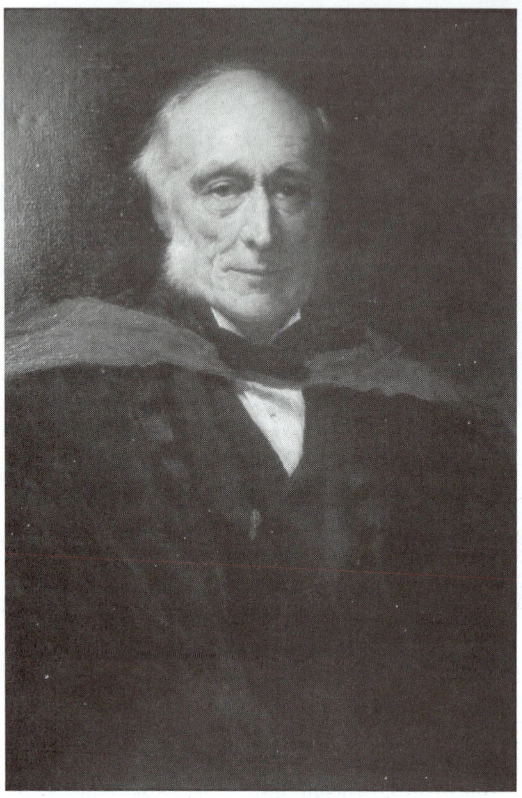

Figure 1–11 Edward Liveing. (Courtesy of The Royal College of Physicians of London.)

of the phenomena, and certainly not as essential and as the cause of the rest" (Liveing, 1872). Liveing commented that "the malady is essentially one of the nervous system, mostly hereditary, and of which the paroxysms may be described as nerve-storms" (Liveing, 1872). He felt that "the cause must be of a kind to explain both the interruption of the ordinary transmission of objective impressions and their replacement by subjective ones" (Liveing, 1872). He proposed that "no hypothesis seemed to me so well adapted to explain the phenomena as that of a nerve-storm traversing more or less of the sensory tract from the optic thalami to the ganglia of the vagus, or else radiating in the same tract from a focus in the neighbourhood of the quadrigeminal bodies" (Liveing, 1872). Sacks described Liveing's nerve-storm as, "a form of centrencephalic seizure, the activity of which is projected rostrally upon the cerebral hemispheres, and peripherally via the ramifications of the autonomic nervous system" (Sacks, 1970).

The vascular versus neurogenic debate continues even today. Edmeads stated in 1989 that "if we swing between vascular and neurogenic views of migraine, it is probably because both vascular and neurogenic mechanisms for migraine exist and are important" (Edmeads, 1989).

EDWARD WOAKES (1837–1912) AND THE STORY OF ERGOT

Ergot is produced by the fungus *Claviceps purpurea* which grows in ears of rye (Koehler and Isler, 2002). The term "ergot" is derived from the French word "argot," which means "rooster's spur" (Silberstein et al., 2002). The banana-shaped sclerotium, which is the resting stage of the fungus, looks like a rooster's bony leg-spur. Epidemics of ergotism have been reported for centuries. Victims of gangrenous ergotism prayed to saints for help, especially St. Anthony (Koehler and Isler, 2002). Gangrenous ergotism was eventually called "St. Anthony's fire." Roosters use their spurs as weapons, and likewise physicians over the years added ergot to their therapeutic armamentarium. Ergot was initially used to hasten childbirth. In 1842 Bonjean prepared an aqueous extract which he called "ergotine," and this was later injected subcutaneously (Koehler and Isler, 2002). This form of ergot was not therapeutically reliable, as the quality and quantity of the contents varied. Edward Woakes (Fig. 1–12), an English physician, is credited with being the first to report the efficacy of ergot of rye in treating migraine (Woakes, 1868; Koehler and Isler, 2002). His patient John Gray is described (Woakes, 1868):

> Case IV. Hemicrania—John Gray, aged about 35, has been repeatedly under treatment for that form of neuralgia known as brow ague. His attacks . . . sometimes they are very severe . . . He was last seen in May 1868, when he had a very sharp attack of neuralgia of the right temple. He was ordered to take, every four hours, an ounce of a mixture of two drachms of liquid extract of ergot in six ounces of infusion of ergot. After taking this for two or three days, he was cured more satisfactorily and quickly than in his former attacks. (p. 361)

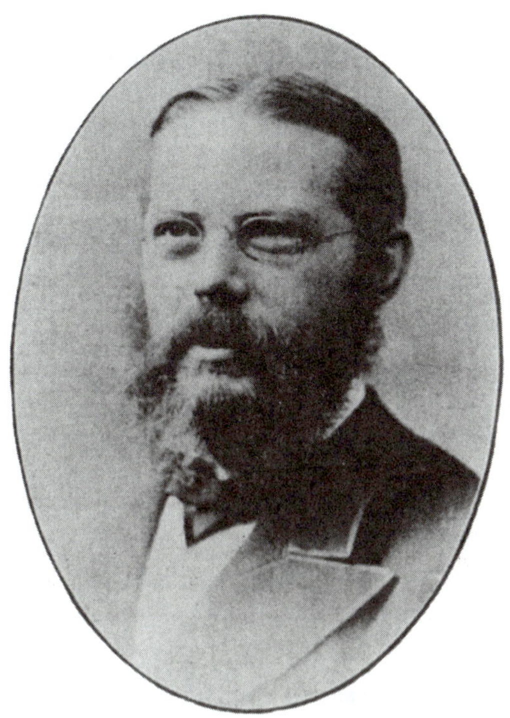

Figure 1–12 Edward Woakes. [Reproduced with permission from Wentges, RTR. (1972). Edward Woakes: the history of an eponym. *J Laryngol Otol,* 86:501–512.]

At the time, the term "brow ague" was used for hemicrania lasting from 6 to 24 hours (Koehler and Isler, 2002).

In 1918, Stoll isolated the alkaloid ergotamine, which provided predictable pharmacological effects (Koehler and Isler, 2002). Maier reported a successful trial in migraine in 1926 (Lance and Goadsby, 2005), which was confirmed by Trautmann using placebo in 1928 (Isler and Koehler, 2006). Critchley comments that ergotamine was "introduced somewhat gradually into neurological practice and it is difficult to assign credit to any particular pioneer, though [William G.] Lennox in the States was an early advocate of this drug" (Critchley, 1967). Wolff's important ergotamine research is mentioned later in this chapter. Dihydroergotamine was synthesized in 1943, and Bayard Horton and colleagues published the first report of its efficacy in treating migraine in 1945 (Horton et al., 1945). Horton also published the first controlled study of the use of the combination of 1 mg of ergotamine and 100 mg of caffeine in the treatment of migraine (Horton et al., 1948). Peters and Horton were the first to clearly identify ergotamine-overuse headache in their classic paper of 1951 (Peters and Horton, 1951).

WILLIAM GOWERS (1845–1915) AND JOHN HUGHLINGS JACKSON (1835–1911)

Sir William Gowers has been described as the greatest clinical neurologist of all time (Critchley, 1949). One of his mentors at National Hospital for the Paralyzed and Epileptic, Queen Square, London UK, was John Hughlings Jackson. Philosophy was the attribute brought to the study of nervous disorders by Jackson (Critchley, 1964). "They make a perfect and harmonious pair, Jackson's vision dovetailing into Gowers' superlative gifts at the bedside; the one a thinker and speculator, the other a diagnostician and teacher" (Critchley, 1964). Both thought the seat of migraine was the brain.

Jackson (Fig. 1–13) classified migraine as an epilepsy in the generic sense because underlying it was a "discharging lesion" (Jackson, 1958). He stated, "it seems to me that all clinical evidence

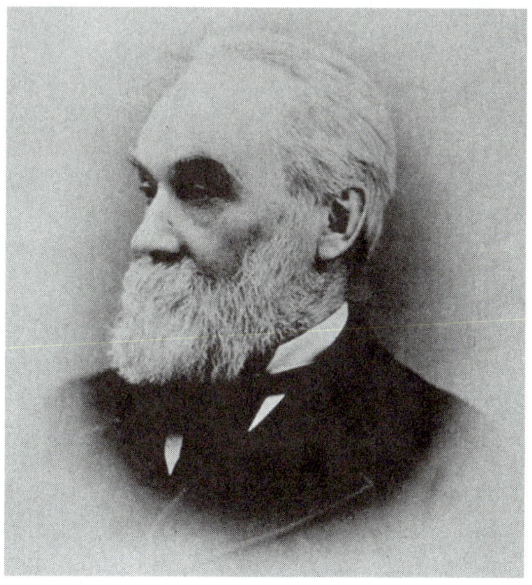

Figure 1–13 John Hughlings Jackson. (Courtesy of the National Library of Medicine.)

points to the region of the optic thalamus as the seat of the discharging lesion in cases of migraine with visual phenomena" (Jackson, 1958). He clarified that the discharge was in the "convolutions in connection with the thalamus opticus" (Jackson, 1958). He felt that the headache was a post-ictal phenomenon, commenting, "some of the symptoms of migraine, the headache among others, are, I think, after-effects of the discharge producing the paroxysm" (Jackson, 1958).

Gowers (Fig. 1–14) doubted the vasomotor hypothesis, and felt the seat of migraine aura was in the cortex (Gowers, 1888):

> The sensory symptoms must depend on deranged action of the sensory centres in some part of the brain. They indicate a combination of arrest of action and of over-action in the nerve cells concerned . . . To explain them on the vasomotor hypothesis we must assume, first, an initial spasm of the arteries in a small region of the brain; secondly, that the contraction always begins at the same place; and, thirdly, that it can give rise to a definite, uniform, and very peculiar disturbance of function. There is no evidence of the truth of any one of these assumptions . . . It is at least as easy to conceive that the vascular changes are the result of the disturbance in the sensory centres, or are the effect of associated derangement of vasomotor centres, as it is to consider that the vascular condition is the primary change . . . Thus the sensory symptoms are probably due to a peculiar kind of functional disturbance in some of the nerve cells of the cerebral cortex. At the same time it is possible that the peculiar disturbance may spread to cells of lower centres. (pp. 1184–1185)

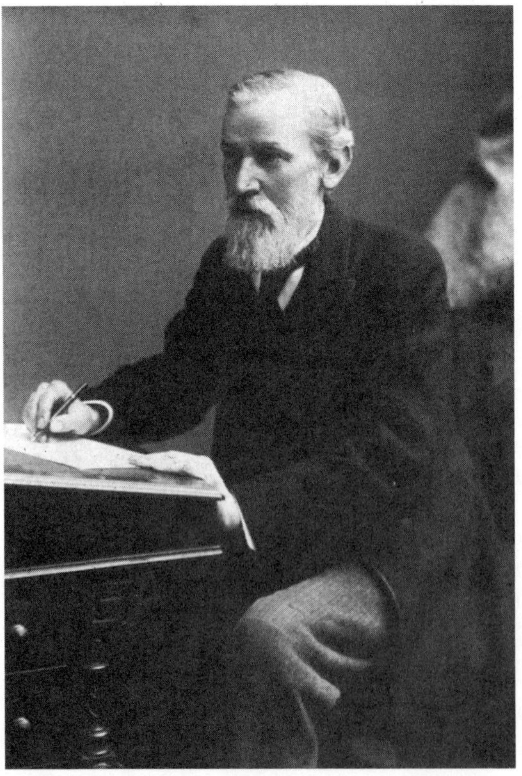

Figure 1–14 William Gowers. (Courtesy of the National Library of Medicine.)

He was less sure of the cause of the headache (Gowers, 1888):

> The cause of the headache is obscure . . . When the pain is opposite in side to the sensory symptoms we are obliged to assume that its seat is the cerebral hemisphere that is deranged, or the membranes covering the hemisphere. When it is local in situation—as at a point in one temple—and is on the same side as the sensory symptoms, it appears to be neuralgic in character, the result of some central disturbance referred to the periphery, and not necessarily corresponding in side to the morbid process causing it . . . the first kind of pain may be the result of vascular conditions . . . it is probable that vascular derangement may intensify symptoms which it does not cause, and most nerve pains are rendered more intense by arterial pulsation . . . Du Bois Reymond suggested that the pain is actually felt in the arteries, and is due to the spasmodic contraction of their walls; but until some other evidence is forthcoming of the occurrence of arterial pain, the theory can scarcely be regarded as admissible. (p. 1185)

Gowers was one of the first to divide migraine treatment into preventive and acute therapy (Gowers, 1888; Edmeads, 1991):

> The special treatment consists first in the continuous administration of drugs, with

> the object of rendering the attacks less frequent and less severe, and, secondly, the treatment of the attacks themselves. (p. 1187)

His Gowers' mixture, which included nitroglycerine, was a favored migraine preventive for decades (Pearce, 2003).

HAROLD G. WOLFF (1898–1962)

Harold Wolff (Fig. 1–15) was born in New York City, and subsequently attended Harvard College and Harvard Medical School (DeJong, 1982; Dalessio, 2001). At Harvard, he was influenced by the famous neurologist Stanley Cobb. He did his clinical training at the Roosevelt Hospital and Cornell Clinic in New York City, and then returned to Harvard to do research on the cerebral circulation under Henry Forbes (DeJong, 1982). Wolff also did research with Adolf Meyer, leading to his unified concept of the mind–body relationship. In addition, he studied neurohumoral transmission with Loewi in Austria and the conditioned reflex with Pavlov in Leningrad. When the New York Hospital–Cornell Medical Center opened in 1932, Wolff was made head of neurology (Dalessio, 2001). He became Professor of Medicine in Neurology in the 1940s at Cornell Medical College. In the 1950s, a grateful patient of his endowed a chair at Cornell, and Wolff was named the Anne Parrish Titzell Professor of Medicine in Neurology. For several years, he edited the *Archives of Neurology*, and he was president of the American Neurological Association. He published 539 papers and 14 books and monographs, including the first edition of *Headache and Other Head Pain* in 1948. This book became known as the "Headache Bible" (Daroff, 2001).

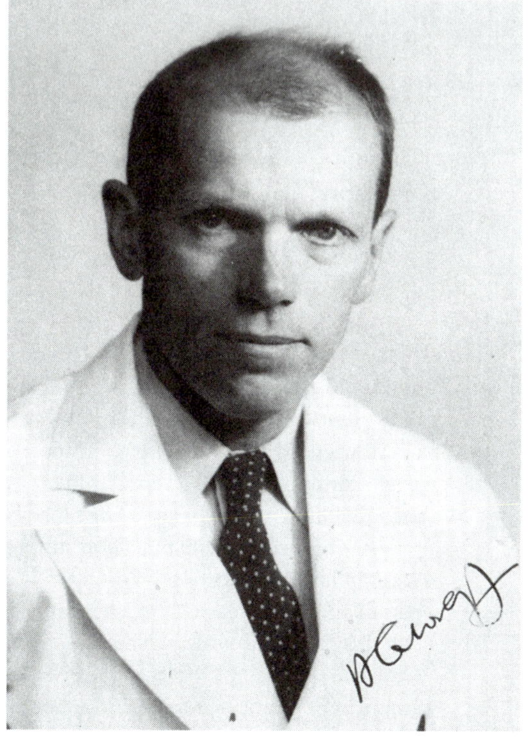

Figure 1–15 Harold Wolff. (Courtesy of the National Library of Medicine.)

Wolff's "attempts to understand the relationship of the network of nerves surrounding the cerebral blood vessels led to his exhaustive study of headache and head pain" (DeJong, 1982). Wolff, himself a migraineur, is credited with being one of the first to experimentally study migraine and other headaches. Dalessio, one of his students, wrote (Dalessio, 2001):

> For Harold Wolff, there was no day without its experiment. He spent long hours in his laboratories on the sixth floor, well known as the testing ground where pain might be induced, headache brought about, hypnotic suggestions used, anger aroused, or situations of frustration created for the sake of observation. The laboratories were themselves simple ... for they were made to study people, not animals or molecules or other subunits but functioning human beings. (p. 4)

In a landmark study, Ray and Wolff identified the pain-sensitive intracranial structures by evaluating neurosurgical patients under local anesthesia (Ray and Wolff, 1940). These included the venous sinuses and their tributaries, parts of the dura at the base, and the dural arteries and the cerebral arteries at the base of the brain. The cranium and brain parenchyma were not sensitive to pain.

In a classic 1938 paper, Graham and Wolff placed tambours over the branches of the external carotid artery to demonstrate that factors that decreased the amplitude of pulsation decreased the intensity of headache and vice versa (Fig. 1–16) (Graham and Wolff, 1938). Factors that decreased the pulsation amplitude included intravenous ergotamine and manual compression of the temporal and occipital arteries. The authors concluded that "these data lend support to the postulate that the head pain of the migraine attack is produced by distension of cranial arteries and that termination of the headache by ergotamine tartrate is due to the capacity of this agent to constrict these cranial arteries and thus reduce the amplitude of their pulsations" (Graham and Wolff, 1938). The patients in this 1938 study were examined after the aura phase. Wolff subsequently studied the effect of amyl nitrite on migraine visual aura (Wolff, 1948):

> It is apparent from these experiments that cranial vasodilatation associated with a sustained normal level of blood pressure caused symptoms to disappear, whereas a procedure that decreased cranial blood flow caused the

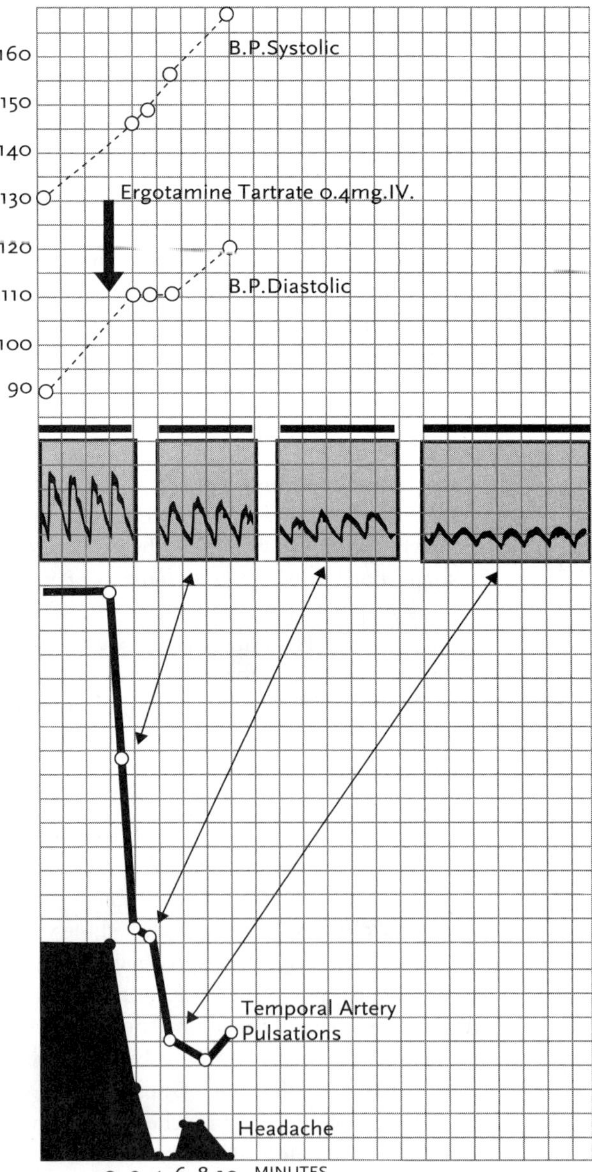

Figure 1–16 Figure from 1938 Graham and Wolff paper showing the relationship of the amplitude of pulsations in the temporal artery to the intensity of headache after administration of ergotamine, as recorded by tambours placed over the arteries. The decrease in pulsation amplitude following injection of ergotamine paralleled the decrease in headache intensity. [Reproduced with permission from Graham, JR, and HG Wolff. (1938). Mechanism of migraine headache and action of ergotamine tartrate. *Arch Neurol Psychiatr*, 39:737–763. Copyright © 1938 American Medical Association.]

> symptom to become worse. From this it may be deduced that cranial vasoconstriction was responsible for the visual defect in this patient with migraine ... it is also likely that the cause of the visual defect was ... within the cranial cavity ... Hence it is inferred that visual preheadache phenomena result from dysfunction of cerebral vessels, in contrast to headache phenomena, which result mainly from dilatation of extracerebral vessels ... It is of interest that the preheadache visual phenomena seldom overlap the headache phenomena. This indicates that cerebral vasoconstriction has terminated before extracerebral vasodilatation has begun. It is probable that there is also dilatation of cerebral vessels following the vasoconstriction, but it is likely that such cerebral vasodilatation plays a minor part in the headache. (pp. 263–264)

This was Wolff's hypothesis concerning visual aura, not his dogma, as is made clear in the second edition of his textbook (Wolff, 1963):

> This evidence supporting the view that the occipital lobe may be implicated in some patients with scotoma as a part of the migraine attack and that the defect is due to the cerebral ischemia secondary to vasoconstriction is not conclusive. (p. 239)

In the second edition of his book, he updated his proposed pathophysiology of vascular headache (Wolff, 1963):

> At the onset of headache there is concomitant dilatation of the large arteries, arterioles, and metarterioles. The dilatation of the arterioles and metarterioles increases the capillary hydrostatic pressure. The elevated... pressure favors the accumulation of pain-threshold-lowering material in the subcutaneous tissue of the scalp. There is thus present in the tissue in greater amounts than normal a substance, postulated as "headache stuff" ... The pain of vascular headache of the migraine type can be seen as the outcome of combined effects of large artery dilatation plus the action of pain-threshold-lowering substances accumulating in the blood vessel walls and perivascular tissue ... the result is a sterile inflammatory reaction, neurogenically induced. (pp. 289, 326)

On the most basic level, the Wolff vascular theory of migraine was similar to the hypothesis offered by Latham in 1872. The Wolff–Latham theory dominated headache research for several years (Sacks, 1970). Lane and Davies comment, "although subsequent discoveries have negated some of his conclusions, Harold Wolff's influence and contributions to the furtherance of the scientific evaluation of headache in the early part of the twentieth century cannot be overstated" (Lane and Davies, 2006).

References

Airy, H. (1870). On a distinct form of transient hemiopsia. *Philos Trans R Soc Lond*, 160:247–264.

Ali ibn Isa and Wood, CA (1936). *Memorandum Book of a Tenth-century Oculist for the Use of Modern Ophthalmologists: A Translation of the Tadhkirat of Ali Ibn Isa of Baghdad (cir. 940–1010 AD.). The Most Complete, Practical and Original of All the Early Textbooks on the Eye and Its Diseases*. Northwestern University, Chicago.

Aretaeus. (1856). *The Extant Works of Aretaeus, the Cappadocian* (F. Adams, ed.). Sydenham Society, London.

Bender, GA (1966). *Great Moments in Medicine*. Northwood Institute Press, Detroit.

Boes, CJ and Capobianco, DJ (2005). Chronic migraine and medication-overuse headache through the ages. *Cephalalgia*, 25:378–390.

Critchley, M (1937). The malady of Anne, Countess Conway: a case for commentary. *King's College Hospital Gazette*, 17:44–49.

Critchley, M (1949). *Sir William Gowers, 1845–1915: A Biographical Appreciation*. William Heinemann, London.

Critchley, M (1964). William Gowers, 1845–1915. In *The Black Hole and Other Essays*, pp. 108–114. Pitman, London.

Critchley, M (1967). Migraine: from Cappadocia to Queen Square. In *Background to Migraine* (R Smith, ed.), pp. 28–38. Springer-Verlag, New York.

Critchley, M and Critchley, EA (1998). *John Hughlings Jackson: Father of English Neurology*. Oxford University Press, New York.

Dalessio, DJ (2001). Remembrances of Dr. Harold G. Wolff. In *Wolff's Headache and Other Head Pain* (7th edn.) (SD Silberstein, RB Lipton, and DJ Dalessio, eds.), pp. 3–5. Oxford University Press, New York.

Daroff, RB (2001). Foreword. In *Wolff's Headache and Other Head Pain* (7th edn.) (SD Silberstein, RB Lipton, and DJ Dalessio, eds.), pp. vii–viii. Oxford University Press, New York.

DeJong, R (1982). *A History of American Neurology*. Raven Press, New York.

Edmeads, J (1989). Migraine—resuscitation of the vascular theory. *Headache,* 29:55–56.

Edmeads, J (1991). The treatment of headache: a historical perspective. In *Drug Therapy for Headache* (RM Gallagher, ed.), pp. 1–8. Marcel Dekker, Inc., New York.

Emerson, RW (1990). History. In *Ralph Waldo Emerson: Selected Essays, Lectures, and Poems* (RD Richardson, Jr. ed.), p. 131. Bantam Books, New York.

Gowers, WR (1888). *A Manual of Diseases of the Nervous System.* P. Blakiston, Son, and Company, Philadelphia.

Graham, JR and Wolff, HG (1938). Mechanism of migraine headache and action of ergotamine tartrate. *Arch Neurol Psychiatr,* 39:737–763.

Horton, BT, Peters, GA, and Blumenthal, LS (1945). A new product in the treatment of migraine: a preliminary report. *Proc Staff Meet Mayo Clin,* 20:241–248.

Horton, BT, Ryan, R, and Reynolds, JL (1948). Clinical observations on the use of E.C. 110, a new agent for the treatment of headache. *Proc Staff Meet Mayo Clin,* 23:105–108.

Isler, H (1987). Retrospect: the history of thought about migraine form Aretaeus to 1920. In *Migraine: Clinical and Research Aspects* (JN Blau, ed.), pp. 659–674. Johns Hopkins University Press, Baltimore.

Isler, H and PJ Koehler (2006). History of the headache. In *The Headaches* (3rd edn). (J Olesen, PJ Goadsby, NM Ramadan, P Tfelt-Hansen, and KMA Welch, eds.), pp. 1–7. Lippincott Williams and Wilkins, Philadelphia.

Jackson, JH (1958). In *Selected Writings of John Hughlings Jackson,* Vol. 2. (J. Taylor, ed.), pp. 312, 371. Basic Books, New York.

Koehler, PJ and Isler, H (2002). The early use of ergotamine in migraine. Edward Woakes' report of 1868, its theoretical and practical background and its international reception. *Cephalalgia,* 22:686–691.

Lance, JW and Goadsby, PJ (2005). The history of headache. In *Mechanism and Management of Headache* (7th edn.), pp. 1–8. Elsevier Butterworth Heinemann, Philadelphia.

Lane, R and Davies, P (2006). A brief history of migraine. In *Migraine,* pp. 1–40. Taylor and Francis Group, New York.

Lashley, KS (1941). Patterns of cerebral integration indicated by the scotomas of migraine. *Arch Neurol Psychiatr,* 46:331–339.

Latham, PW (1872). Clinical lecture on nervous or sick-headaches. *Brit Med J,* I: 305–306, 336–337.

Leao, AAP (1944). Spreading depression of activity in the cerebral cortex. *J Neurophysiol,* 7:359–390.

Leao, AAP and Morison, RS (1945). Propagation of spreading cortical depression. *J Neurophysiol,* 8:33–45.

Liveing, E (1872). Observations on megrim or sick-headache. *Brit Med J,* I: 364–366.

Liveing, E (1873). *On Megrim, Sick-Headache, and Some Allied Disorders: A Contribution to the Pathology of Nerve-storms.* J. and A. Churchill, London.

Pearce, JMS (2003). *Fragments of Neurological History.* Imperial College Press, London.

Peters, GA and Horton, BT (1951). Headache: with special reference to the excessive use of ergotamine preparations and withdrawal effects. *Proc Staff Meet Mayo Clin,* 26:153–161.

Ray, BS and Wolff, HG (1940). Experimental studies on headache: pain-sensitive structures of the head and their significance in headache. *Arch Surg,* 41:813–856.

Riley, HA (1932). Migraine. *Bull Neurol Inst NY,* 2:429–544.

Sacks, OW (1970). *Migraine: The Evolution of a Common Disorder.* University of California Press, Berkeley.

Sacks, OW (1997). Introduction. In *Edward Liveing on Megrim, Sick-headache, and Some Allied Disorders: A Contribution to the Pathology of Nerve-storms,* pp. IX–XXVIII. Arts and Boeve, Nijmegen.

Schiller, F (1975). The migraine tradition. *Bull Hist Med,* 49:1–19.

Silberstein, SD, Lipton, RB, and Goadsby, PJ (2002). Historical introduction. In *Headache in Clinical Practice* (2nd edn), pp. 1–8. Martin Dunitz, London.

Teive, H.A.G, Kowacs, PA, Maranhao Filho, P, Piovesan, EJ, and Werneck, LC (2005). Leao's cortical spreading depression: from experimental "artifact" to physiological principle. *Neurology,* 65:1455–1459.

Willis, T (1685). *The London Practice of Physick: or the Whole Practical Part of Physick Contained in the Works of Dr. Willis. Faithfully Made English, and Printed Together for the Publick Good.* Thomas Basset and William Crooke, London.

Wilson, SAK (1940). Migraine. In *Neurology* (AN Bruce, ed.), pp. 1570–1594. Edward Arnold and Co., London.

Woakes, E (1868). On ergot of rye in the treatment of neuralgia. *Brit Med J,* II:360–361.

Wolff, HG (1948). Headache in the migraine syndrome. In *Headache and Other Head Pain,* pp. 255–318. Oxford University Press, New York.

Wolff, HG (1963). Headache in the migraine syndrome. In *Headache and Other Head Pain* (2nd edn), pp. 227–385. Oxford University Press, New York.

2 The Last 50 Years of Headache History: A Personal Perspective

James W Lance

When we encountered a suspicious headache history in the 1950s, how did we investigate it? The first step was to obtain a plain X-ray of the skull to look at the pituitary fossa, auditory meatus, and position of the calcified pineal gland—perhaps even using Chamberlain's line or Bull's angle to eliminate platybasia.

Next, an electroencephalogram was used as a screening test to check for focal changes. If a focal abnormality were found, or if there were lateralizing symptoms or signs on examination, a direct puncture arteriogram was next on the list, often performed by neurologists or neurosurgeons, as neuroradiologists were thin on the ground in those days.

If suspicions remained, and there were no signs of raised intracranial pressure, a pneumoencephalogram was undertaken, a diabolical test in which air was trickled into the lumbar sac with the patient sitting and head flexed so that the passage of air through the ventricular system could be visualized radiologically—at the expense of a splitting headache in the recipient.

In the event of a myelogram becoming necessary,the operator had to don red goggles half an hour before the investigation to adapt his eyes to the dark as there were no image intensifiers. One then observed a black eel-like image slide slowly through a dark-green sea,to show the outline of the cervical spinal cord.

How we welcomed the advent of radioactive isotope scanning and then, in the 1970s, the miraculous invention by EMI engineers in England of the "EMI scan" now known as Computerized Axial Tomography, CT, or CAT scanning.

The use of magnetic resonance imaging (MRI) was still well in the future.

THE FIFTIES AND SIXTIES

In the 1950s, headache was not a particularly popular topic. Harold G Wolff died in 1962 at the age of 64, shortly after completing the manuscript of the second edition of his monograph, *Headache and Other Head Pain.*

I had the pleasure of meeting him and Helen Goodell on my way to work in Boston in 1960.

Wolff attended the last meeting of the Ad Hoc Committee on Headache Classification, which was convened in 1960 with its conclusion being published in 1962.

Ostfeld (1993) recalls that the chairman of the ad hoc committee, Arnold Friedman, provided each committee member with exactly 25 sheets of paper and 4 pencils, sharpened to exactly the same length. The other members of the committee were A M Ostfeld, John R Graham, E Charles Kunkle, and K H Finkley. The committee could meet only on Sundays but, "fortuitously, the Sunday cold buffet at the Harvard Club was excellent." Their classification made sense and was a valuable contribution although limited by the frequent use of qualifying adjectives such as "commonly" and "usually."

The American Association for Study of Headache (now the American Headache Society) was founded in the same year, 1962.

Friedman published extensively on clinical topics, an early example of which is the study of 2000 cases of migraine and tension headache (Friedman et al., 1954). He later became interested in serotonin, and was a co-author in a seminal paper demonstrating that the infusion of serotonin intravenously would ease migraine headaches (Kimball et al., 1960). He and Macdonald Critchley of London became the *Grand Old Men of Headache* in the English-speaking world of those days, attending every seminar and forming the Headache Research Committee of the World Federation of Neurology. Critchley later became President of the WFN.

Macdonald Critchley was a tall imposing figure, one of the foremost English neurologists of the twentieth century. Apart from his lifelong interest in headache, for he was a migraine sufferer himself, he wrote a classic treatise on the parietal lobes, published in 1953, and biographies of James Parkinson, Sir William Gowers, and Hughlings Jackson, the last of which he completed shortly before his death in 1997. He was a keen student of the unusual or bizarre and wrote books and essays such as *The Black Hole* and *The Divine Banquet of the Brain*.

He started headache clinics at Kings College Hospital and the National Hospital, Queen Square, London in 1955. He was one of the founders of the British Migraine Trust in 1965 with Lord Brain as Chairman, and delivered a paper at the first British Migraine Symposium on "Migraine From Cappadocia to Queen Square" in 1966. I remember one meeting in Italy when he was repeatedly referred to as Lord Critchley, a title that I think would have suited him.

He started the headache tradition in the United Kingdom that was continued with Dr. Marcia Wilkinson, Dr. K J Zilkha, Dr. J N Blau, and later, Dr. Ann Macgregor at the City of London Migraine Clinic and Dr. Frank Clifford Rose and Dr. Richard Peatfield at the Princess Margaret Migraine Clinic at Charing Cross Hospital. Dr. Clifford Rose went on to play a major role in the British Migraine Trust and the World Federation of Neurology, as well as being an author and editor of many texts on headache.

In the Netherlands, George Bruyn, scholar and classicist, was the mentor for Michel Ferrari and his colleagues, the next generation of research workers. He made notable contributions to headache and cranial neuralgias in *Handbook of Clinical Neurology* of which he was an editor.

Enrico Greppi (1899–1969) founded the first headache center in Europe, in 1954. Although his primary fields were hematology and gerontology, Greppi had a philosophical view of headache, "as a relatively autonomous illness." He had the foresight to set up specialized departments for various disciplines within medicine, in his Department of Internal Medicine in Florence and inspired Federigo Sicuteri, who became the first director of the headache center at the age of 34. The Italian Society for the Study of Headache created the Greppi Award in 1983 to be awarded annually for the best original paper on headache or its related studies. This and the Harold G Wolff Memorial Award of the American Headache Society have provided a stimulus to research work from then until the present day.

Professor Sicuteri and Professor Marcello Fanciullacci established Florence as a world center for headache research. The former's view that headaches had a central origin and were related to a deficiency of brain serotonin still guides much of our thought today. He founded the Italian Society for the Study of Headache in 1976, and the Italian contribution to headache research has been consistent since then. He organized successful world congresses, *Headache 80* and *Florence Headache 87*.

The European Federation of Headache Societies was created in Venice, in 1990, but its publication *The Journal of Headache and Pain* is under the aegis of the Italian Society.

Sicuteri's paper on the prophylactic and therapeutic properties of UML-491 (methysergide) in migraine was the start of the serotonin story (Sicuteri 1959). Here was an apparent antagonist of serotonin that really worked in preventing migraine. With his colleagues, he followed this trail to show that the breakdown product of serotonin, 5-hydroxyindoleacetic acid (5-HIAA) was excreted excessively in urine during migraine headache (Sicuteri et al., 1961).

These papers and the observations of Dalessio et al. (1961) and Kimball et al. (1960) fired our enthusiasm in Sydney. We already had a strong clinical interest in migraine (Selby and Lance, 1960). We resolved to carry the story forward by analyzing the platelet content of serotonin during migraine headache. We then confirmed that 5-HIAA excretion was increased and demonstrated that the platelet content of serotonin [5-hydroxytryptamine (5-HT)] was low during migraine headache (Curran et al., 1965) and that blood platelets discharged their 5-HT at the onset of headache, whether spontaneous or induced by reserpine (Anthony et al., 1967).

The infusion of 5-HT 2.0–7.5 mg intravenously, eased spontaneous or induced migraine headaches but caused unpleasant side effects such as tightness in the chest, faintness, flushing, and paraesthesiae, which made it impractical as a treatment for acute attacks. These observations came to the attention of Patrick Humphrey at the Glaxo Laboratories in England who set out to develop a drug that had the beneficial effects of serotonin without such marked side effects.

Leaping ahead some 20 years, Ferrari et al. (1989) reported that the platelet release of 5-HT was limited to migraine without aura; nevertheless, they found that the level of plasma 5-HT increased by more than 100% during migraine headache whether it was preceded by an aura or not.

At first, there were only two receptors (labelled M and D for their affinity for morphine and dibenzyline) known for serotonin but, as the story unravelled, the number of receptors grew (Saxena and Ferrari, 1992). Humphrey exploited their characteristics, finding an agent that had specific effects on the B and D sub-types of the 5-HT$_1$ receptor, designated GR43175, later known as sumatriptan (Humphrey et al., 1990).

In Germany, on the basis of arteriovenous oxygen differences in blood taken from external jugular vein in patients with and without migraine, Heyck (1969) put forward the theory that arteriovenous shunts opened in migraine, diverting blood away from the cerebral cortex.

The hypothesis was that ergotamine cured migraine by constricting arteriovenous shunts, a point of view that received support from Pramod Saxena's work later on which described the effect of ergotamine and sumatriptan on arteriovenous shunts in the pig cerebral circulation (Saxena, 1978).

The emphasis, in the 1950s and 1960s, remained on the vascular component of migraine headache. In the 1950s, Dalsgaard Neilsen in Denmark had studied the susceptibility of migraine sufferers to develop a headache more readily than control subjects with a nitroglycerin patch applied to the skin (Tfelt-Hansen, 2001). Axel Klee (1968) analyzed the symptoms of severe migraine attacks with particular reference to aura symptoms and regarded migraine as a disorder of the hind-brain circulation. It was fortunate that Neils Lassen was pioneering methods of measuring cerebral blood flow in Denmark (Lassen and Ingvar, 1961) with techniques that were brilliantly exploited in the 1970s and 1980s by the Copenhagen Group. The Danish Migraine Society was started in 1968.

TREATMENT IN THE 1960s

How did we treat migraine in the 1960s?

The mainstay of acute treatment was ergotamine, given by mouth, alone or in combination with caffeine and an anti-emetic, or by medihaler, suppository or injection. Sir Charles Symonds had advocated a nocturnal injection of dihydroergotamine as a preventative measure for cluster headache (Symonds, 1956).

A favourite prophylactic agent for migraine was "Bellergal," a combination of ergotamine tartrate 0.3 mg, phenobarbitone 20 mg, and belladonna alkaloids 0.1 mg, given three times daily. Over a six-month open trial period, we found substantial improvement in patients treated with methysergide (64%), cyproheptadine (46%), "Bellergal" (34%), and placebo (20%). Of the 320 patients treated with methysergide, 32 withdrew because of side effects (Curran and Lance, 1964).

We also studied the medications available for the treatment of chronic tension headache in 280 patients, 239 of whom had headaches every day. When amitriptyline proved superior to other agents in an open trial, we undertook a double-blind crossover trial with placebo in 27 new patients, confirming the efficacy of amitriptyline (Lance and Curran, 1964), which has remained the mainstay of treatment to the present day.

In 1968, pizotifen (then code-named BC-105) became available with results roughly comparable with cyproheptadine. For recalcitrant patients who had not responded to conventional medications, we undertook an open trial of the monoamine oxidase inhibitor phenelzine 15 mg, three times daily for up to 2 years in 25 patients, 20 of whom responded with reduction in headache frequency to half or less (Anthony and Lance, 1969). The next advance in prophylactic therapy had to await the introduction of noradrenergic β-blocking agents (Weber and Reinmuth, 1971).

SEVENTIES AND EIGHTIES

In the next two decades, the Viking invasion from Norway, Sweden, and Denmark gathered pace. Erik Skinhój (1973) demonstrated that regional cerebral blood flow was diminished during migraine aura although cerebral angiography appeared normal. This was the beginning of a series of studies that burst upon the headache world, clearly documenting for the first time blood flow changes of spreading depression in the aura phase of migraine that had only been suspected clinically before (Olesen et al., 1981, 1990).

The Copenhagen School used epidemiological, clinical, and laboratory investigations to study the whole spectrum of headache. Work began on a classification of headache under the chairmanship of Jes Olesen, published in 1988 and since revised in 2004. In *Basic Mechanisms of Headache,* published in 1988, 16 of the 40 chapters came from the Danish School. Clinical trials were put on a firm basis by Peer Tfelt-Hansen who also summarized the history of headache research in Denmark (Tfelt-Hansen, 2001).

The International Headache Society was founded in 1982 as a result of the work of a committee comprising Ottar Sjaastad, (Norway), Desmond Carroll (UK), Robert Kunkel (USA), Edgard Raffaelli (Brazil), and Federigo Sicuteri (Italy). The First International Headache Congress was held in Munich in 1983 with Dieter Soyka of Kiel, West Germany, as the President. Congresses have been held every second year since (see Box 2–1).

Otto Sjaastad, in Norway, was a prime mover in the formation of the International Headache Society and later became the foundation editor of *Cephalalgia* which he started in 1981. He described Chronic Paroxysmal Hemicrania (Sjaastad and Dale, 1974), Hemicrania Continua (Sjaastad and Spierings, 1984), SUNCT (shortlasting unilateral neuralgiform headache attacks with conjunctival injection and tearing) syndrome (Sjaastad et al., 1989), and the "Jabs and Jolts" syndrome in 1992; probably, the same indomethacin responsive entity was described with vascular headaches as *Cluster Headache Variant* by Medina and Diamond (1981). His views on cluster headache and other trigeminal autonomic cephalgias were summarized in a monograph (Sjaastad, 1992). He influenced many neurologists, notably Edgard Raffaeli and Maurice Vincent from Brazil. Raffaeli started the Brazilian Headache Society, in 1979. Sjaastad had an abiding interest in cervicogenic headache (Sjaastad et al., 1990). Pain referred from the neck was placed on a firm anatomical basis by Bogduk et al. (1985).

The effectiveness of lithium in cyclic psychiatric disorders led Karl Ekbom (1977) to try this agent in the treatment of chronic cluster headache, causing immediate partial remission and leading to lithium becoming standard therapy for

Box 2–1 IHS Congresses.

Year	Place	Organisers
1983	Munich, Germany	Volker Pfaffenrath
1985	Copenhagen, Denmark	Jes Olesen
1987	Florence, Italy	Frederigo Sicuteri
1989	Sydney, Australia	James Lance
1991	Washington DC, USA	Ninan T. Mathew
1993	Paris, France	Marie-Germaine Bousser
1995	Toronto, Canada	Marek Gawel
1997	Amsterdam, The Netherlands	Michel D. Ferrari; Jean Schoenen
1999	Barcelona, Spain	Miguel J.A. Láinez
2001	New York, USA	Fred Sheftell
2003	Rome, Italy	Giuseppi Nappi; Virgilio Gallai
2005	Kyoto, Japan	Fumihiko Sakai
2007	Stockholm, Sweden	Carl G.H.; Dahlöf Lars Edvinsson

this condition. Also in Sweden, Bo Bille continued a study of migrainous school children starting in the 1950s. He published a 40-year follow-up (Bille, 1997) showing that more than 50% of children were still subject to migraine between the ages of 47 and 53 years. Lars Edvinsson in Lund began a lasting collaboration with Peter Goadsby, then in Sydney, studying the release of vasoactive peptides after thermocoagulation of the trigeminal ganglion and during cluster headache and migraine (Goadsby et al., 1988, 1990). Carl Dahlof and Lars Edvinsson were chairmen of the Organizing Committee for the Thirteenth Congress of the International Headache Society held in Stockholm, in 2007.

Leaving Scandinavia for the USA, but continuing a theme of therapy for cluster headache, Kudrow (1980) consolidated the evidence for the use of oxygen inhalation in curtailing the pain of cluster headaches. Verapamil was first reported as being an effective preventative treatment by Meyer and Hardenberg (1983). Cluster headaches, migraine, and tension headaches may be associated with stabbing pains described as "ice-pick" pains by Raskin and Schwartz (1980) and later called primary stabbing headaches.

Hypnic headaches were also first reported from San Francisco by Raskin (1988). Day and Raskin (1986) described "thunderclap headaches" which have recently been shown by Marie-Germaine Bousser and her colleagues in Paris to be associated with reversible angiopathy (segmental vasoconstriction of the cerebral circulation) (Ducros et al., 2005). The Paris group have played a leading role in the study of menstrual migraine and the relationship between headache and cerebral vascular disease, including thrombosis of the cerebral veins and venous sinuses (Bousser et al., 1985).

Numbness or a sense of movement in one half of the tongue accompanying occipital pain on sudden neck movement was described as the neck–tongue syndrome by Lance and Anthony (1980) and the anatomical basis clarified by Bogduk (1981). Anthony (1985) reported that steroid injections into the region of the occipital nerve could abort a bout of cluster headaches.

Olesen and his colleagues had established the likelihood of cortical spreading depression as the basis of the migraine aura. In Houston, Sakai and Meyer (1978) demonstrated that cerebral perfusion increased during migraine headaches and that this persisted, even when headache abated after the administration of codeine. On the other hand, headache persisted in some patients, even when the superficial temporal or common carotid artery was compressed (Drummond and Lance, 1983). On clinical grounds, migraine appeared to be a primary disturbance of the brain with secondary vascular features but the physiological link between the two had not been clarified. Laboratory experiments in cat and monkey by Goadsby, Lambert, and our other colleagues in Sydney found such a link by showing that the cerebral circulation could be controlled by the parasympathetic outflow in the greater superficial petrosal branch of the facial nerve from the brainstem (Lance et al., 1983). Moskowitz (1984) in Boston described an experimental model using antidromic activation of the trigeminal nerve of the rat, producing plasma extraversation from cerebral vessels as a potential source of vascular pain.

Stimulation of the trigeminal nerve in cats and radiofrequency lesions of that nerve in humans were shown to cause an increase in calcitonin gene-related peptide (CGRP) and substance P in the cranial venous outflow (Goadsby et al., 1988). More specific stimulation of pain-producing structures, such as the superior sagittal sinus in cats, also released CGRP (Zagami et al., 1990), which was found to be the case in human patients with migraine (Goadsby et al., 1990). The interpretation of these studies was that vasoactive peptides play a part in the vasodilatation, and possibly the pain, of migraine headaches.

THE NINETIES AND BEYOND

It is probable that individuals vary in their susceptibility to migraine, a "migrainous threshold," determined by excitatory aminoacids, monoamines, opioids, and other factors. In the USA, Michael Welch's group used nuclear resonance spectroscopy to examine the chemical shift properties of 31p resonance signals and deduced that magnesium ion concentration was lower during migraine headache (Ramadan et al., 1989) which could increase excitatory aminoacid activation at *N*-methyl-D-aspartic acid (NMDA) receptors (Welch and Ramadan, 1995).

Physiological changes have also been demonstrated in the migrainous brain. The primary response in the visual cortex is sometimes enhanced in migrainous subjects and fails to habituate with repeated stimulation (Olesen et al., 2006), which could underlie the sensitivity of patients to flickering light and glare.

Migraine headache may increase in frequency until it recurs almost daily under the influence of anxiety, depression, or analgesic abuse, although retaining some of the characteristics of migraine. Mathew (1987) coined the term, "transformed migraine," to cover this common sequence. The frequent use of triptans or ergotamines as well as analgesics was reported to lead to chronic daily headaches in Germany (Limmroth et al., 2002). Young and Silberstein (2001) in the USA reported that abstinence from analgesics reduced headache frequency to half or less, thus opening up a new approach to chronic daily headache.

The genetic basis of migraine has attracted increasing scrutiny. Twin studies have shown that approximately half the susceptibility to migraine is of genetic origin and the other half is determined by environmental influences. First-degree relatives of patients suffering from migraine with aura have nearly four times the risk of developing the same condition (Russell and Olesen, 1995). Genes for Familial Hemiplegic Migraine have been found on chromosome 19 in approximately 55% of cases and chromosome 1 in 15%, with 30% still undetermined. In this volume, Ferrari has summarized the history and complexity of the modern approach to genetics.

Perhaps the most remarkable revelations about functional changes in migraine have come about through positron emission tomography (PET) and MRI scanning. Woods et al. (1994) discovered diminished cerebral blood flow in a patient who developed migraine headache with some blurring of vision but not traditional aura symptoms, starting in the occipital cortex and moving anteriorly, in a manner mimicking cortical spreading depression, previously demonstrated by Olesen and his colleagues during typical auras. Supporting evidence came from Denuelle et al. (2005a) who noted a patchy cortical hypoperfusion in seven patients during migraine headaches without aura. If this phenomenon is widespread, it could well account for the blurred vision, lack of concentration, and confusion commonly encountered in migraine without aura.

Advances in headache imaging have taken place in Britain and Germany, much of it in collaboration, and recently, in France. PET scanning has demonstrated activation in the region of the periaqueductal gray matter (PAG) contralateral to migraine headache (Weiller et al., 1995) and in the ipsilateral pons near the locus ceruleus (Bahra et al., 2001), both areas of interest in the endogenous pain-control system. Increased metabolism in the hypothalamus as well as mid-brain and pons, during migraine headache, has been described by Denuelle et al. (2005b). Hypothalamic activation has also been described in cluster headache (May et al., 1998), SUNCT (May, Bahra, et al., 1999), hemicrania continua (Matharu et al., 2004), and chronic paroxysmal hemicrania (Matharu et al., 2005)

Studies at Harvard on functional imaging of the trigeminal nerve and its central pathways promises to add to our knowledge of facial pain and headache (Borsook et al., 2006).

Structural changes have been discovered in the area of activity in the posterior hypothalamus in cluster headache patients (May, Ashburner, et al., 1999), and stimulation of this area has been shown to relieve chronic cluster headaches (Leone et al., 2001) and SUNCT (Leone et al., 2005).

Stimulation of the PAG in patients to relieve severe bodily pain has been reported to initiate migraine-like headaches (Raskin et al., 1987; Veloso and Kumar, 1996), indicating that the endogenous pain-control system can be switched on or off selectively by the PAG. These clinical observations have been supported by animal experiments. Knight and Goadsby (2001) found that stimulation of the PAG in cats blocked trigemino-vascular input into the spinal nucleus of the trigeminal nerve at the second cervical segment reversibly. Calcium channel blockade in the PAG facilitated trigeminal nociception (Knight et al., 2002) whereas activation of 5-HT $_{1B/D}$ receptors in the PAG inhibited nociception (Bartsch et al., 2004). In a similar cat model, Lambert et al. (2006) demonstrated that the second-order trigeminal neurons in nucleus caudalis were inhibited by stimulation of the serotonergic Nucleus Raphe Magnus. This inhibitory process was switched-off by cortical spreading depression or by repetitive photic stimulation, thus providing a neat analogy with the migrainous process. It was partly suppressed by the iontophoretic application of a 5-$HT_{1B/D}$ antagonist. These experimental findings fit well with the general clinical concept of changes in cortex or hypothalamus suppressing the endogenous pain-control system, thus permitting an inflow of painful impulses from the periphery, the development of sensitization of central trigeminal pathways (Burstein et al., 2000) and dilatation of cranial arteries with the development of pulsatile headache. It remains to be seen whether these advances in knowledge of mechanisms and neurotransmitters translates into treatments that can be readily available and affordable. Already, a CGRP antagonist has proven an effective agent in the acute treatment of migraine (Olesen et al., 2004).

HOW FAR HAVE WE COME IN 50 YEARS?

In parallel with increasing interest in research and clinical aspects of headache, headache clinics and societies have sprung up worldwide. At the last count, there were 43 national headache societies. This is a refreshing change that surely augurs well for future advances and the wise application of those remedies that we already possess. Headache medicine has now been accepted as a board-certified sub-specialty in the USA.

The International Headache Society, its Classification Subcommittee, the advice for regulation of clinical trials, and the proliferation of specialist journals and electronic media have placed the subject on a rational basis. I can recall a conference in the early anecdotal days when a surgeon told the audience that his nasal operation had cured all but three of the 100 cases of migraine that he had treated. "What a coincidence," the doctor sitting next to me said, "They must be the three patients that I sent him."

In the early 1950s, only one central neurotransmitter was known—acetylcholine at the Renshaw cell in the spinal cord. We were bold enough to hypothesize that serotonin and noradrenaline could eventually prove to have some central function. The rate of increase of scientific knowledge and the technology of imaging has been truly amazing since then. On the clinical front, the description of new syndromes and causes of headache has widened our horizons.

Improvements in treatment have been less dramatic. Since the excitement of the triptans, there has been little to stir the blood. There was a long hiatus in prophylaxis of migraine between the noradrenergic beta blockers and the introduction of valproate, (Silberstein, 1996). The demonstration that propranolol can modulate transmission of trigeminovascular impulses at the thalamic level (Shields and Goadsby, 2005) may be a pointer to possible sites of central action of anti-epileptic drugs. With the exception of topiramate which as been accepted as a prophylactic agent for migraine, the newer anticonvulsants and peptide-blocking agents have yet to find a definitive place in management.

The history of headache now merges with the present. I am aware that I have not mentioned many people, countries, and themes though I would like to have done so, and apologize for sins of omission and commission. This, after all, is a personal perspective. Many of the gaps will be filled by present clinicians and laboratory workers, including the editors and authors of this volume, in whose hands and brains the next 50 years of headache history rests.

References

Anthony, M (1985). Arrest of attacks of cluster headaches by local steroid injection of the occipital nerve. In *Migraine: Clinical and Research Advances* (F Clifford Rose, ed.), pp. 169–173. Karger, Basel.

Anthony, M, Hinterberger, H, and Lance, JW (1967). Plasma serotonin in migraine and stress. *Arch Neurol,* 16:544–552.

Anthony, M and Lance, JW (1969). Monamine oxidase inhibition in the treatment of migraine. *Arch Neurol,* 21:263–268.

Bahra, A, Mathuru, MS, Buchel, C et al. (2001). Brainstem activation specific to migraine headache. *Lancet,* 357:1016–1017.

Bartsch, T, Knight, YE, and Goadsby, PJ (2004). Activation of 5-HT $_{1B/D}$ receptors in the periaqueductal grey inhibits meningeal nociception. *Ann Neurol,* 56:371–381.

Bille, B (1997). A 40-year follow-up of school children with migraine. *Cephalalgia,* 17:488–491.

Bogduk, N (1981). An anatomical basis for the neck-tongue syndrome. *J Neurol Neurosurg Psychiat,* 44:202–208.

Bogduk, N, Corrigan, B, Kelly, P et al. (1985). Cervical headache. *Med J Aust,* 143:202, 206–207.

Borsook, D, Burstein, R, Moulton, E et al. (2006). Functional imaging of the trigeminal system: applications to migraine pathophysiology. *Headache*, 46(Suppl. 1): S32–S38.

Bousser, MG, Chiras, J, Bories, J et al. (1985). Cerebral venous thrombosis—a review of 35 cases. *Stroke*, 16:199–213.

Burstein, R, Cutrer, MF, and Yarnitsky, D (2000). The development of cutaneous allodynia during a migraine attack. *Brain*, 123:1703–1709.

Curran, DA, Hinterberger, H, and Lance, JW (1965). Total plasma serotonin, 5-hydroxyindoleacetic acid and p-hydroxy-m-methoxymandelic acid excretion in normal and migrainous subjects. *Brain*, 88:997–1010.

Curran, DA and Lance, JW (1964). Clinical trial of methysergide and other preparations in the management of migraine. *J Neurol Neurosurg Psychiat*, 27:463–469.

Dalessio, DJ, Camp, WA, Goodell, H et al. (1961). Studies on headache. The mode of action of UML-491 and its relevance to vascular headache of the migraine type. *Arch Neurol*, 4:235–240.

Day, JW and Raskin, NH (1986). Thunderclap headache. Symptoms of unruptured cerebral aneurysm. *Lancet*, II:1247–1248.

Denuelle, M, Fabre, N, Payoux, P et al. (2005a). Posterior cortical hypoperfusion during spontaneous attacks of migraine without aura: a PET study. *Cephalalgia*, 25:859.

Denuelle, M, Fabre, N, Payoux, P et al. (2005b). Hypothalamic activation in spontaneous migraine attacks: a PET study. *Cephalalgia*, 25:858.

Drummond, PD and Lance, JW (1983). Extracranial vascular changes and the source of pain in migraine headache. *Ann Neurol*, 13:32–37.

Ducros, A, Sarov, M, Roos, C et al. (2005). Recurrent thunderclap headaches revealing reversible angiopathy of the central nervous system. *Cephalalgia*, 25:859.

Ekbom, K (1977). Lithium in the treatment of chronic cluster headache. *Headache*, 17:39–40.

Ferrari, MD, Odink, J, Tapparelli, C et al. (1989). Serotonin metabolism in migraine. *Neurology*, 39:1239–1242.

Friedman, AP, Von Storch, TJC, and Merritt, HJ (1954). Migraine and tension headaches: a clinical study of 2000 cases. *Neurology*, 4:773–788.

Goadsby, PJ, Edvinsson, L, and Ekman, R (1988). Release of vasoactive peptides in the extracerebral circulation of man and the cat during activation of the trigeminal system. *Ann Neurol*, 23:193–196.

Goadsby, PJ, Edvinsson, L, and Ekman, R (1990). Vasoactive peptide release in the extracerebral circulation of humans during migraine headache. *Ann Neurol*, 28:183–187.

Heyck, H (1969). Pathogenesis of migraine. *Res clin Stud Headache*, 2:1–28.

Humphrey, PPA, Feniuk, W, Perren, MJ et al. (1990). Serotonin and migraine *Ann NY Acad Sci*, 600:587–598.

Kimball, RW, Friedman, AP, and Vallejo, E (1960). Effect of serotonin in migraine patients. *Neurology*, 10:107–111.

Klee, A (1968). A clinical study of migraine with particular reference to the most severe cases. Thesis. Munksgaard, Copenhagen.

Knight, YE, Bartsch, T, Kaube, H et al. (2002). P/Q-type calcium channel blockade in the PAG facilitates trigeminal nociception: a functional genetic link for migraine? *J Neurosci*, 22:1–6.

Knight, YE and Goadsby, PJ (2001). The periaqueductal grey matter modulates trigeminovascular input: a role in migraine? *Neuroscience*, 106:793–800.

Kudrow, L (1980). *Cluster Headache: Mechanism and Management*. Oxford University Press, Oxford.

Lambert, GA, Hoskin, K, and Zagami, AS (2006). A cortical cause for migraine? *Cephalalgia*, 26:1386.

Lance, JW and Anthony, M (1980). Neck-tongue syndrome on sudden turning of the head. *J Neurol Neurosurg Psychiat*, 43:97–101.

Lance, JW and Curran, DA (1964). Treatment of chronic tension headache. *Lancet* I:1236–1239.

Lance, JW, Lambert, GA, Goadsby, PJ et al. (1983). Brainstem influences on the cephalic circulation. Experimental data from cat and monkey of relevance to the mechanism of migraine. *Headache*, 23:258–265.

Lassen, NA and Ingvar, DH (1961). The blood flow of the cerebral cortex determined by radio-active Krypton-85. *Experientia*, 17:42–45.

Leone, M, Franzini, A, D'andrea, G, et al. (2005). Deep brain stimulation to relieve drug-resistant SUNCT. *Ann Neurol* 57:924–927.

Leone, M, Franzini, A, and Bussone, G (2001). Stereotactic stimulation of the posterior hypothalamic grey matter in a patient with intractable cluster headache. *N Engl J Med*, 345:1428–1429.

Limmroth, V, Katsarava, Z, Fritsche, G et al. (2002). Features of medication overuse headache following overuse of different acute headache drugs. *Neurology*, 59:1011–1014.

Matharu, MS, Cohen, AS, Frackowiak, RSJ et al. (2005). Posterior hypothalamic activation in paroxysmal hemicrania using PET. *Cephalalgia*, 25:858.

Matharu, MS, Cohen, AS, McGonigle, DJ et al. (2004). Posterior hypothalamic and brainstem activation in hemicrania continua. *Headache*, 44:747–761.

Mathew, NT (1987). Transformed or evolutional migraine. *Headache*, 27:305–306.

May, A, Ashburner, J, Buchel, C et al. (1999). Correlation between structural and functional changes in brain in an idiopathic headache syndrome. *Nat Med*, 5:836–838.

May, A, Bahra, A, Buchel, C et al. (1998). Hypothalamic activation in cluster headache attacks. *Lancet*, 352:275–278.

May, A, Bahra, A, Buchel, C et al. (1999). Functional MRI in spontaneous attacks of SUNCT: short lasting neuralgiform headache with conjunctival injection and tearing. *Ann Neurol*, 46:791–793.

Medina, TL and Diamond, S (1981). Cluster headache variant. Spectrum of a new headache syndrome. *Arch Neurol*, 38:705–709.

Meyer, JS and Hardenberg, J (1983). Clinical effectiveness of calcium entry blockers in prophylactic treatment of migraine and cluster headache. *Headache*, 23:266–277.

Moskowitz, MA (1984). The neurobiology of vascular head pain. *Ann Neurol*, 16:157–168.

Olesen, J, Diener, H-C, Husstedt, I-W et al. (2004). Calcitonin gene-related peptide (CGRP) receptor antagonist BIBN 4096 BS is effective in the treatment of migraine attacks. *New Engl J Med*, 350:1104–1110.

Olesen, J, Friberg, L, Olsen, TS et al. (1990). Timing and topography of cerebral blood flow, aura and headache during migraine attacks. *Ann Neurol*, 28:791–798.

Olesen, J, Larsen, B, and Lauritzen, M (1981). Focal hyperemia followed by spreading oligemia and impaired activation of rCBF in classic migraine. *Ann Neurol* 9:344–352.

Olesen, J, Tfelt-Hansen, P, Welch, KM et al. (2006). Neurophysiology of migraines. In *The Headaches* (3rd edn), pp. 369–376. Lippincott, Williams and Wilkins, Philadelphia.

Ostfeld, AM (1993). The ad hoc committee on headache classification. *Cephalalgia*, 13(Suppl. 12):11–12.

Ramadan, NM, Halvorson, H, Vande-Linde, A et al. (1989). Low brain magnesium in migraine. *Headache*, 29:416–419.

Raskin, NH (1988). The hypnic headache syndrome. *Headache*, 28:534–536.

Raskin, NH, Hosobuchi, Y, and Lamb, S (1987). Headache may arise from perturbation of the brain. *Headache*, 27:416–420.

Raskin, NH and Schwartz, RK (1980). Ice-pick-like pains. *Neurology*, 30:203–305.

Russell, MB and Olesen, J (1995). Increased familial risk and evidence of genetic factor in migraine. *Brit Med J*, 311:541–544.

Sakai, F and Meyer, JS (1978). Regional cerebral hemodynamics during migraine and cluster headache measured by the 133 Xe inhalation method. *Headache*, 18:122–132.

Saxena, PR (1978). Arteriovenous shunting and migraine. *Res Clin Stud Headache*, 6:89–102.

Saxena, PR and Ferrari, MD (1992). From serotonin receptor classification to the anti-migraine drug sumatriptan. *Cephalalgia*, 12:187–196.

Selby, G and Lance, JW (1960). Observations on 500 cases of migraine and allied vascular headache. *J Neurol Neurosurg Psychiat*, 23:23–32.

Shields, KG and Goadsby, PJ (2005). Propranolol modulates trigeminovascular responses in thalamic ventroposteromedial nucleus: a role in migraine? *Brain*, 128:86–97.

Sicuteri, F (1959). Prophylactic and therapeutic properties of UML-491 in migraine. *Int Arch Allergy*, 15:300–307.

Sicuteri, F, Testi, A, and Anselmi, B (1961). Biochemical investigations in headache: increase in hydroxyindoleacetic acid during migraine attacks. *Int Arch Allergy*, 19:55–58.

Silberstein, SD (1996). Divalproex sodium in headache. Literature review and clinical guidelines. *Headache*, 36:547–555.

Sjaastad, O (1992). *Cluster Headache Syndrome*. W.B. Saunders, London.

Sjaastad, O and Dale, I (1974). Evidence for a new (?) treatable headache entity. *Headache*, 14:105–108.

Sjaastad, O, Fredrickson, TA, and Pfaffenrath, V (1990). Cervicogenic headache: diagnostic criteria. *Headache*, 30:725–726.

Sjaastad, O, Saunte, C, Salvesan, R et al. (1989). Short-lasting unilateral neuralgiform headache attacks with conjunctival injection, tearing, sweating and diarrhea. *Cephalalgia*, 9:147–156.

Sjaastad, O and Spierings, EL (1984). Hemicrania continua: another headache absolutely responsive to indomethacin. *Cephalalgia*, 4:65–70.

Skinhój, E (1973). Haemodynamic changes within the brain during migraine. *Arch Neurol*, 29:95–98.

Symonds, CP (1956). A particular variety of headache. *Brain*, 79:217–232.

Tfelt-Hansen, P (2001). History of headache research in Denmark. *Cephalalgia*, 21:748–752.

Veloso, F and Kumar, K (1996). Deep brain implant migraine. *J Neurol Neurosurg Psychiat*, 46(Suppl. 7): A168–A169.

Weber, RB and Reinmuth, OM (1971). The treatment of migraine with propranolol. *Neurology*, 21:404–405.

Weiller, C, May, A, Limroth, V et al. (1995). Brain stem activation in spontaneous human migraine attacks. *Nat Med*, I:658–660.

Welch, KM and Ramadan, NM (1995). Mitochondria, magnesium and migraine. *J Neurol Sci*, 134:9–14.

Woods, RP, Iacoboni, M, and Mazziotta, JC (1994). Bilateral spreading hypoperfusion during spontaneous migraine headache. *N Engl J Med*, 331:1689–1692.

Young, WB and Silberstein, SD (2001). Long term follow-up of patients treated for chronic headache with analgesic overuse. *Cephalalgia*, 21:873.

Zagami, AS, Goadsby, PJ, and Edvinsson, L (1990). Stimulation of the superior sagittal sinus in the cat causes release of vasoactive peptides. *Neuropeptides*, 16:69–75.

3 Overview of Diagnosis and Classification

Richard B Lipton, Stephen D Silberstein, and David Dodick

INTRODUCTION

Headache is a leading reason for medical consultation and particularly for neurological consultation (Linet et al., 1991; Pascual et al., 1995). A tremendous range of disorders can present with headache. A systematic approach to headache classification and diagnosis is therefore essential both for clinical management and research.

It is useful to distinguish headache classification from headache diagnosis. Classification refers to the orderly arrangement of various headache disorders and their diagnostic criteria. Diagnosis refers to the application of these criteria to individual patients. The International Classification of Headache Disorders-1 (ICHD-1), brought out in 1988 by the International Headache Society (IHS) (Headache Classification Committee of the International Headache Society, 1988), created the accepted standard for headache diagnosis, establishing both uniform terminology and consistent operational diagnostic criteria for the entire range of headache disorders. Translated into 22 languages, the ICHD-1 facilitated clinical practice, epidemiological studies, and multinational clinical trials for many years (Tfelt-Hansen et al., 2000). Published in January of 2004, the second edition of *The International Classification of Headache Disorders* (*ICHD-2*) (Headache Classification Committee of the International Headache Society, 2004) sets a new standard for diagnosis and research. Though the basic structure of the classification is preserved, there were many changes that will influence headache treatment. These changes include a restructuring of the criteria for migraine, new sub-classification of tension-type headache (TTH), introduction of the concept of trigeminal autonomic cephalgias (TACs), and addition of several previously unclassified types of primary headache. The revised classification was developed by a consensus of headache experts and a literature review. Though based on relevant literature, the classification represents a clinical consensus based on data, experience, judgment, and compromise. Nonetheless, the classification has provided a new foundation for clinical practice and research, and has already been revised.

In this chapter, we present an overview of the ICHD-2 classification (Headache Classification Committee of the International Headache Society, 2004), highlighting the primary headache disorders and their diagnostic criteria. We offer an algorithmic approach to primary headache diagnosis based on attack frequency and duration, using the second edition of the ICHD-2 classification.

THE REVISED IHS CLASSIFICATION—AN OVERVIEW

The ICHD-2 classifies headache disorders into three major categories: primary headaches, secondary headaches, and cranial neuralgias; central and primary facial pain; and other headaches (Table 3–1). The primary headaches include four categories: migraine, TTH, TACs, and other primary headaches. There are also eight categories of secondary headache (Table 3–1). The criteria for the primary headaches are clinical and descriptive and, with a few exceptions (i.e., familial hemiplegic migraine) are based on headache features and the exclusion of other disorders, not etiology. In contrast, secondary headaches are classified based on etiology and are attributed to another disorder.

TABLE 3–1 First Level of the International Classification of Headache Disorders, 2nd Edition.

Part one: The primary headaches
1. Migraine
2. Tension-type headache
3. Cluster headache and other trigeminal autonomic cephalgias
4. Other primary headaches

Part two: The secondary headaches
5. Headache attributed to head and/or neck trauma
6. Headache attributed to cranial or cervical vascular disorder
7. Headache attributed to non-vascular intracranial disorder
8. Headache attributed to a substance or its withdrawal
9. Headache attributed to infection
10. Headache attributed to disorder of homoeostasis
11. Headache or facial pain attributed to disorder of cranium, neck, eyes, ears, nose, sinuses, teeth, mouth, or other facial or cranial structures
12. Headache attributed to psychiatric disorder

Part three: Cranial neuralgias, central and primary facial pain, and other headaches
13. Cranial neuralgias and central causes of facial pain
14. Other headaches, cranial neuralgia, and central or primary facial pain

The ICHD-2 provides operational rules for the classification that are summarized below (Headache Classification Committee of the International Headache Society, 2004):

1. The classification is hierarchical, allowing diagnoses with varying degrees of specificity, using up to four digits for coding at subordinate levels. The first digit specifies the major diagnostic type, for example, *Migraine* (1.) or *Tension-type headache* (2.0). The second digit indicates a sub-type within the category, for example, *Migraine with aura* (1.2) (Table 3–1). Subsequent digits permit more specific diagnosis for some sub-types of headache: according to circumstantial requirements, familial hemiplegic migraine, for example, could be coded as *Migraine* (1), *Migraine with aura* (1.2) or, most precisely, as *Familial hemiplegic migraine* (1.2.4).
2. In clinical practice, patients should receive a diagnosis for each headache type or sub-type they have experienced within the last year. For example, the same patient may have and should be coded for all of *Medication overuse headache* (8.2), *Migraine without aura* (1.1), and *Frequent episodic tension-type headache* (2.2). Multiple diagnostic codes should be listed in the order of importance of the headache disorder to the patient.
3. For headaches that meet all but one of a set of diagnostic criteria, without fulfilling those of another headache disorder, there are "probable" sub-categories: for example, *Probable migraine* (1.6).
4. Primary headache disorders are both diagnoses of inclusion, in that certain features must be present, and diagnoses of exclusion, in that other disorders that might be the cause of the headache must be included. This means that (1) the history and physical and neurological examinations do not suggest any of the disorders classified as secondary headaches; (2) these suggest such a disorder but it is ruled out by investigations; or (3) such disorder is present, but the headache does not occur for the first time in close temporal relation to it.
5. Secondary headache diagnoses are applied when a patient develops a new type of headache for the first time in close temporal relation to onset of another disorder known to cause headache; the headache is categorized as "attributed to" that disorder.
6. Diagnosis of secondary headache in a patient with a preexisting primary headache can be challenging. When headache worsens in the presence of another disorder known to cause headache, there are two possibilities. First, worsening may represent exacerbation of the preexisting primary headache. Second, it may represent onset (and superimposition upon the primary headache) of a new, secondary headache.

Onset of a secondary headache is more likely when (1) there is a very close temporal relation to onset of the potentially causative disorder; (2) exacerbation of the headache is marked, or differs in pattern from the pre-existing disorder; (3) other evidence is strong that the potentially causative disorder can cause headache of the type experienced; or (4) there is improvement or disappearance of headache, or return to the earlier pattern, after relief from the potentially causative disorder.

MIGRAINE (ICHD-2: 1.0)

Migraine is classified into five major categories, the most important two of which are *Migraine without aura* (1.1) and *Migraine with aura* (1.2). This is unchanged from 1988 but, in comparison with the 1988 system, there is a restructuring of the criteria for migraine with aura. *Chronic migraine* (1.5.1) has been added and the criteria have been revised (Olesen et al., 2006). Ophthalmoplegic "migraine," now considered a cranial neuralgia, has been moved to item 13 (*Cranial neuralgias and central causes of facial pain*). When a patient fulfils criteria for more than one type of migraine, each type should be diagnosed and coded. Since chronic migraine usually develops from episodic migraine, a patient coded 1.5.1 will usually have an additional code for the antecedent disorder (usually 1.1).

Overall, migraine is an extraordinarily common disorder affecting approximately 12% of Western populations (see Chapter 3). Prevalence is higher in females (18%) than males (6%) and varies inversely with socioeconomic status. Herein, we will briefly review the sub-types of migraine. They are discussed in more detail in Chapter 10.

Migraine Without Aura

Relative to ICHD-1, the diagnostic criteria for *Migraine without aura* (1.1) in ICHD-2 are only slightly modified (Table 3–2). They require at least five lifetime attacks, lasting 4–72 hours, with at least two of four pain features and at least one of two sets of associated symptoms. In children, attacks may be shorter, 1–72 hours, and in young children, photophobia and phonophobia may be inferred from behavior rather than reported. In addition, when attacks occur at a frequency ⩾15 days per month the diagnoses are *Chronic migraine* (1.5.1) plus *Migraine without aura* (1.1).

As before, criteria for migraine without aura are met by various combinations of features. With regard to pain, unilateral, pulsating headache meets the criteria but so does bilateral, pressing headache if it is moderate or severe in intensity and aggravated by routine physical activity. With regard to associated features, a patient without nausea or vomiting but with both photophobia and phonophobia may fulfil the criteria (Table 3–2). Like the other primary headache disorders, secondary headache must be excluded.

Migraine with Aura

The criteria for *Migraine with aura* (1.2) were substantially revised. The typical aura of migraine is characterized by focal neurological features that usually precede migrainous headache but may accompany it or occur in the absence of the headache (Table 3–3) (Olesen et al., 1990). Typical aura symptoms develop over ⩾5 minutes and last no

Table 3–2 ICHD-2 Criteria for 1.1 Migraine without Aura.

A. At least five attacks fulfilling criteria B–D
B. Headache attacks last 4–72 hours (untreated or unsuccessfully treated)
C. Headache has at least two of the following characteristics:
   1. Unilateral location
   2. Pulsating quality
   3. Moderate or severe pain intensity
   4. Aggravation by, or causing avoidance of, routine physical activity (e.g., walking or climbing stairs)
D. During the headache attack, at least one of the following:
   1. Nausea and/or vomiting
   2. Photophobia and phonophobia
E. Symptoms not attributed to another disorder

TABLE 3–3 Revised ICHD-2 Criteria for 1.2.1 Typical Aura with Migraine Headache.

A. At least two attacks fulfilling criteria B–D
B. Aura consisting of at least one of the following, but no motor weakness:
    1. Fully reversible visual symptoms including positive features (e.g., flickering lights, spots or lines) and/or negative features (i.e., loss of vision)
    2. Fully reversible sensory symptoms including positive features (i.e., pins and needles) and/or negative features (i.e., numbness)
    3. Fully reversible dysphasic speech disturbance
C. At least two of the following:
    1. Homonymous visual symptoms and/or unilateral sensory symptoms
    2. At least one aura symptom develops gradually over ⩾5 minutes and/or different aura symptoms occur in succession over ⩾5 minutes
    3. Each symptom lasts ⩾5 and ⩽60 minutes
D. Headache fulfilling criteria B–D for 1.1 *Migraine without aura* begins during the aura or follows the aura within 60 minutes
E. Symptoms not attributed to another disorder

more than 60 minutes, and visual aura is overwhelmingly the most common (Jensen et al., 1986). Typical visual aura is homonymous, often having a hemianopic distribution and expanding in the shape of a crescent with a bright, ragged edge, which scintillates. Scotoma, photopsia, or phosphenes and other visual manifestations may occur. Visual distortions such as metamorphopsia, micropsia, and macropsia are more common in children (Lippman, 1952; Klee and Willanger, 1966; Silberstein and Young, 1995).

Sensory symptoms occur in about one-third of patients who have migraine with aura (Manzoni et al., 1985). Typical sensory aura consists of numbness (negative symptom) *and* tingling or paresthesia (positive symptoms). The distribution is often cheiro-oral (face and hand). Dysphasia may be part of typical aura but motor weakness, symptoms of brain-stem dysfunction, and changes in level of consciousness, all of which may occur (Russel and Olesen, 1996), signal particular sub-types of migraine with aura (hemiplegic, and basilar-type).

Recently, typical migraine aura has been noted to occur with non-migrainous headache (i.e., headache not fulfilling the criteria of 1.1). Such cases are coded *Typical aura with non-migraine headache* (1.2.2). Reports have associated apparently typical aura with cluster headache (CH), chronic paroxysmal hemicrania, and hemicrania continua (HC) (Silberstein et al., 2000; Matharu and Goadsby, 2001; Peres et al., 2002). These cases are classified according to both disorders [e.g., *Cluster headache* (3.1) plus *Typical aura with non-migraine headache* (1.2.2)].

Typical aura occurring in the absence of any headache (Whitty, 1967; Willey, 1979; Ziegler and Hanassein, 1990) is coded *Typical aura without headache* (1.2.3), a disorder most often reported by middle-aged men (Staehelin-Jensen et al., 1981). Differentiating this benign disorder from transient ischemic attack (TIA), a medical emergency, may require investigation, especially when it first occurs after age 40, when negative features (i.e., hemianopia) are predominant or when the aura is of atypical duration (Fisher, 1980).

Familial hemiplegic migraine (1.2.4, FHM) is the first migraine syndrome to be linked to a specific set of genetic polymorphisms (Haan et al., 1997; Carrera et al., 2001; Ducros, 2001; De Fusco et al., 2003). The criteria for this disorder (Klee and Willanger, 1966) include those of *Migraine with aura* (1.2) except that aura includes some degree of motor weakness (hemiparesis) and may be more prolonged than 60 minutes (up to 24 hours); additionally, at least one first-degree relative must have had similar attacks (also meeting these criteria). Cerebellar ataxia may occur in 20% of FHM sufferers. The onset of weakness may be abrupt, but usually lasts less than 1 hour (Staehelin-Jensen et al., 1981). A person with FHM may develop migraine with aura when an adult, and migraine without aura later in life (Staehelin-Jensen et al., 1981).

The three known loci for FHM are on chromosomes 1, 2 and 19, but some families do not link to either of these, indicating that there is at least one additional locus (Ophoff et al., 1996, 1997).

Patients otherwise meeting these criteria but who have no family history of this disorder are classified as having *sporadic hemiplegic migraine* (SHM, 1.2.5), a disorder new to the revised classification (Thomsen et al., 2003).

Basilar-type migraine (1.2.6) is a new term, replacing "basilar migraine." The change is intended to remove the implication that the basilar artery (or, necessarily, its territory) is involved. The distinguishing feature of basilar-type migraine is a symptom profile that suggests posterior fossa involvement (Kuhn et al., 1997). Diagnosis requires at least two of the following aura symptoms, all fully reversible: dysarthria, vertigo, tinnitus, decreased hearing, double vision, visual symptoms simultaneously in both temporal and nasal fields of both eyes, ataxia, decreased level of consciousness, and simultaneously bilateral paresthesias. Basilar-type migraine should be diagnosed only when weakness is absent, because 60% of patients with FHM have basilar-type symptoms. The headache meets criteria for 1.1 *Migraine without aura* (Table 3–2).

Childhood Periodic Syndromes That Are Common Precursors of Migraine

A number of more or less well-described disorders are classified under this heading (Hosking, 1988). *Cyclical vomiting* (1.3.1) occurs in up to 2.5% of schoolchildren (Withers, et al., 1998; Fleisher, 1999; Li, 2001). The hallmark of this disorder is recurrent and stereotyped episodes of intense but otherwise unexplained nausea and vomiting which last 1 hour to 5 days in children free of symptoms interictally. Vomiting occurs at least four times in an hour, and no signs of gastrointestinal disease can be found.

Abdominal migraine (1.3.2) afflicts up to 12% of schoolchildren with recurrent attacks of abdominal pain associated with anorexia, nausea, and sometimes vomiting (Abu-Arafeh and Russel, 1995; Al-Twaijri and Shevell, 2002). The abdominal pain has all of the following characteristics: midline location, periumbilical or poorly localized; dull or "just sore" quality; moderate or severe intensity. During the attack, there are at least two of anorexia, nausea, vomiting and/or pallor. Physical examination and investigations exclude other causes of these symptoms.

Benign paroxysmal vertigo (1.3.3) is a disorder characterized by recurrent (at least five) attacks, each of multiple episodes of severe vertigo resolving spontaneously after minutes to hours (Drigo et al., 2001). Neurological examination and audiometric and vestibular functions are all normal between attacks, and the electroencephalogram is also normal.

Retinal Migraine

This disorder is rare. Recurrent attacks (at least two) of fully reversible scintillations, scotomata, or blindness, affecting one eye only, are accompanied or followed within 1 hour by migrainous headache (fulfilling criteria for 1.1). Other causes of monocular visual loss, including TIA, optic neuropathy, and retinal detachment must be ruled out by appropriate investigation (Troost and Zagami, 2000). A review suggests that many patients with monocular "aura" experience retinal infarction of migrainous origin (Solomon and Grosberg, 2003). These patients should be coded as having *Migrainous infarction* (1.5.4) in the current version of ICHD-2.

Complications of Migraine

Chronic migraine (1.5.1) (see controversies in the classification of chronic daily headache, below) was initially defined by the headache meeting criteria for migraine without aura on ⩾15 days per month for ⩾3 months, in the absence of medication overuse. Most cases of chronic migraine, following this approach, evolve from episodic migraine, often from migraine without aura (Silberstein and Lipton, 2001). As a consequence, chronic migraine is considered a complication of migraine. When medication overuse is present (Katsarava et al., 2001) (acute anti-migraine drugs and/or opioids or combination analgesics taken on ⩾10 days per month, or simple analgesics on ⩾15 days per month), it is a likely cause of chronic headache. Neither *Chronic migraine* (1.5.1) nor *Medication-overuse headache* (8.2) can be diagnosed with confidence until the overused medication has been withdrawn: improvement within 2 months is expected if the latter diagnosis is correct (and is necessary to confirm it), not if the former is present. Meanwhile, the codes to be assigned are that of the antecedent migraine (usually *Migraine without aura,* 1.1) plus *Probable medication-overuse headache* (8.2.7) plus *Probable chronic migraine* (1.6.5).

These criteria faced several challenges. First, patients with frequent migraine often take medications and find it difficult to discontinue them. As a consequence, using the original criteria, medication overuse could not be diagnosed. Second, many patients treat migraine while pain is mild, before full-blown migraine attacks develop. As a consequence, an attack may be relieved before diagnostic criteria for migraine are met. For these and other reasons, in field tests, a minority of patients with transformed migraine met criteria for chronic migraine.

In response to these difficulties, Olesen et al. (1996) proposed revised criteria for chronic migraine and medication-overuse headache (Tables 3–4 and 3–5). The revised chronic migraine criteria require 15 days of headache per month and a link to migraine on 8 of the days. Links include meeting criteria for migraine without aura or treating with a migraine-specific medication.

The revised definition of medication overuse headache specifies a requisite frequency of treatment but relief with medication withdrawal (Table 3–5).

Status migrainosus (1.5.2) refers to an attack of migraine with a headache phase lasting >72 hours (Bento and Esperanca, 2000). The pain is severe (a diagnostic criterion) and debilitating. Non-debilitating attacks lasting more than 72 hours are coded as *Probable migraine without aura* (1.6.1).

Persistent aura without infarction (1.5.13 is diagnosed when aura symptoms, otherwise typical of past attacks, persist for >1 week. Investigation shows no evidence of infarction: it is an unusual but well-documented complication of migraine that is now being introduced into the IHS classification (Bento and Esperanca, 2000). If aura symptoms last more than 1 hour (typical aura), but less than 1 week (persistent aura without infarction), a code of 1.6.2 (probable migraine with aura), specifying the atypical feature (prolonged aura), should be assigned.

TABLE 3–4 ICHD-2 Criteria for Chronic Migraine.

A 1.5.1 Chronic migraine

- A. Headache (tension-type and/or migraine) on 15 or more days per month for at least 3 months[a]
- B. Occurring in a patient who has had at least five attacks fulfilling criteria B–D for 1.1 *Migraine without aura*
- C. On 8 or more days per month, for at least 3 months, the headache has fulfilled C1 and/or C2 below, that is, has fulfilled criteria for pain and associated symptoms of migraine without aura
  1. At least two of a–d
     - a. Unilateral location
     - b. Pulsating quality
     - c. Moderate or severe pain intensity
     - d. Aggravation by or causing avoidance of routine physical activity (e.g., walking or climbing stairs)

     and at least one of a or b
     - a. Nausea and/or vomiting
     - b. Photophobia and phonophobia
  2. Treated and relieved by triptan(s) or ergot before the expected development of C1 above
- D. Symptoms not a result of medication overuse[b] and not attributed to another causative disorder[c]

[a]Characterization of frequently recurring headache generally requires a headache diary to record information on pain and associated symptoms day-by-day for at least 1 month. Sample diaries are available at www.i-h-s.org.

[b]Medication overuse as defined under 8.2 *Medication overuse headache.*

[c]History and physical and neurological examinations either do not suggest any of the disorders listed in groups 5–12 or they do suggest such disorder but it is ruled out by appropriate investigations, or such disorder is present but headache does not develop in close temporal relation to the disorder.

Migrainous infarction (1.5.4) is an uncommon occurrence. One or more otherwise typical aura symptoms persist beyond 1 hour and neuroimaging confirms ischemic infarction. Strictly applied, these criteria distinguish this disorder from other causes of stroke, which must be excluded (Rothrock et al., 1988): the neurological deficit develops during the course of an apparently

TABLE 3–5 Revised ICHD-2 Criteria for Medication Overuse Headache.

A 8.2 Medication overuse headache
Diagnostic criteria:

A. Headache present on ⩾15 days/month
B. Regular overuse for ⩾3 months of one or more acute/symptomatic treatment drugs as defined under sub forms of 8.2
   1. Ergotamine, triptans, opioids, **or** combination analgesic medications on ⩾10 days/month on a regular basis for > 3 months
   2. Simple analgesics **or** any combination of ergotamine, triptans, analgesics, or opioids on ⩾15 days/month on a regular basis for > 3 months without overuse of any single class alone
C. Headache has developed or markedly worsened during medication overuse

typical attack of migraine with aura, and exactly mimics the aura of previous attacks.

Migraine and epilepsy are comorbid disorders (Rains et al., 2001). Headaches are common in the post-ictal period, but epilepsy can be triggered by migraine (migralepsy). The criteria for *Migraine-triggered seizure* (1.5.5) require that a seizure fulfilling diagnostic criteria for one type of epileptic attack occurs during or within 1 hour after a migraine aura.

Probable Migraine

Between 10% and 45% of patients with features of migraine fail to meet all criteria for migraine (or any of its sub-types) (Rains et al., 2001). If a single criterion is missing (and the full set of criteria for another disorder are not met), the applicable code is *Probable migraine* (1.6). Epidemiologic studies demonstrate that probable migraine is common and associated with temporary disability and reduction in the health-related quality of life (Patel et al., 2003).

TENSION-TYPE HEADACHE (ICHD-2: 2.0)

TTH is the most common type of primary headache, with one-year-period prevalence ranging from 31% to 74% (Schwartz et al., 1998). The 1988 classification distinguished two sub-types, episodic TTH (<15 attacks per month) and chronic TTH (⩾15 attacks per month) (Headache Classification Committee of the International Headache Society, 1988). The revised classification distinguishes three sub-types: ***Infrequent episodic TTH*** (2.1) (headache episodes on <1 day per month), ***Frequent episodic TTH*** (2.2) (headache episodes on 1–14 days per month) and ***Chronic TTH*** (2.3) (headache on ⩾15 days per month, perhaps without recognizable episodes) (Klee and Willanger, 1966).

The diagnostic criteria for TTH are presented in Table 3–6. In contrast to migraine, the main pain features of TTH are bilateral location, non-pulsating quality, mild-to-moderate intensity and lack of aggravation by routine physical activity. The pain is not accompanied by nausea, though just one of photo- or phonophobia does not exclude the diagnosis.

Chronic TTH evolves from episodic TTH in most cases. This feature of evolution is described in the notes but is not part of the formal criteria. Like chronic migraine, chronic TTH cannot be diagnosed in patients overusing acute medication (see *Controversies in the classification of chronic daily headache*, below). Such patients often meet criteria for and, in fact, have *Medication-overuse headache* (8.2), although withdrawal of the medication is required to confirm this diagnosis. A recently recognized disorder that phenotypically resembles chronic TTH, but is nosologically distinct from it (as far as is known), does not evolve from an episodic headache but is daily and unremitting from onset or within three days of onset. This condition is separately classified as *New daily-persistent headache* (4.8).

Probable TTH

This code is used when headache fulfils all but one of the criteria for TTH and does not fulfil criteria for migraine without aura.

CLUSTER HEADACHE AND OTHER TACS (ICHD-2: 3.0)

The addition of the term TACs to the classification reflects the observation that CH is one of a group of primary headache disorders characterized by

Table 3–6 Revised IHS Diagnostic Criteria for Episodic Tension-type Headache (TTH).

2.1 *Infrequent episodic TTH*

- A. At least 10 episodes occurring on < 1 day per month on average (<12 days per year) and fulfilling criteria B–D
- B. Headache lasting from 30 minutes to 7 days
- C. Headache has at least two of the following characteristics:
  1. Bilateral location
  2. Pressing/tightening (non-pulsating) quality
  3. Mild or moderate intensity
  4. It is not aggravated by routine physical activity, such as walking or climbing stairs
- D. Both of the following:
  1. No nausea or vomiting (anorexia may occur)
  2. No more than one of the following: photophobia and phonophobia
- E. Not attributed to another disorder

2.2 *Frequent episodic TTH*

- A. At least 10 episodes occurring on ⩾1 but < 15 days per month for at least 3 months (⩾12 and < 180 days per year) and fulfilling criteria B–D

B–E: As 2.1

2.X.1 *Infrequent/frequent episodic TTH associated with pericranial tenderness*

- A. Episodes fulfilling criteria A–E for 2.X
- B. Increased pericranial tenderness on manual palpation

2.X.2 *Infrequent/frequent episodic TTH not associated with pericranial tenderness*

- A. Episodes fulfilling criteria A–E for 2.X
- B. No increased pericranial tenderness

(where X is 1 for infrequent episodic TTH and 2 for frequent episodic TTH).

trigeminal activation coupled with parasympathetic activation. Clinically these disorders are characterized by pain in and around one eye with ipsilateral autonomic features. ICHD-2 includes several disorders not quoted in the previous edition.

Cluster Headache

The diagnostic criteria for CH have not substantially changed. This disorder manifests as intermittent, short-lived, and excruciating unilateral head pain accompanied by autonomic dysfunction. The pain of CH is described variously as sharp, boring, drilling, knife-like, piercing, or stabbing, in contrast to the pulsating pain of migraine. It usually peaks in 10–15 minutes but remains excruciatingly intense for an average of 1 hour within a duration range of 15–180 minutes. During this pain, patients find it difficult to lie still, exhibiting often marked agitation and restlessness, and autonomic signs are usually obvious. After an attack, the patient remains exhausted for some time (Dodick et al., 2000).

CH is classified into two sub-types. Attacks of *Episodic cluster headache* (3.1.1) occur in cluster periods lasting from 7 days to 1 year separated by attack-free intervals of 1 month or more. Approximately 85% of CH patients have the episodic subtype. In chronic CH (3.1.2), attacks recur for >1 year without remission, or with remissions lasting <1 month. Chronic CH can evolve from episodic CH, or develop de novo (Dodick et al., 2000) and may revert to episodic CH.

Patients have been described who have both CH and trigeminal neuralgia, and received the denomination of cluster-tic syndrome (Goadsby and Lipton, 1997). In the IHS scheme they should receive both diagnoses.

Paroxysmal Hemicrania

As a group, the paroxysmal hemicranias have three main features: (1) at least 20 frequent (more than five per day) attacks of short-lived (2–30 minutes), severe, and strictly unilateral orbital, supraorbital, or temporal pain; (2) symptoms of parasympathetic activation ipsilateral to the pain (as in CH); and (3) absolute response to therapeutic doses of indomethacin (Sjaastad and Dale, 1974; Antonaci and Sjaastad, 1989).

The 1988 classification included chronic paroxysmal hemicrania only. The revised classification includes *Episodic paroxysmal hemicrania* (3.2.1) and *Chronic paroxysmal hemicrania* (3.2.2, CPH). Like CH, these disorders are distinguished by the presence or absence of attack-free intervals lasting 1 month or more.

Some patients with both CPH and trigeminal neuralgia have been described (CPH-tic syndrome) (Monzillo et al., 2000); they should receive both diagnoses.

Short-lived Unilateral Neuralgiform Headache Attacks with Conjunctival Injection and Tearing

The short-lived unilateral neuralgiform headache attacks with conjunctival injection and tearing (SUNCT) syndrome (3.3) is a very rare primary headache. The diagnostic criteria require at least 20 high-frequency attacks (3–200 per day) of unilateral orbital, supraorbital, or temporal stabbing or pulsating pain, lasting 5–240 seconds and accompanied by ipsilateral conjunctival injection and lacrimation. The attacks are characteristically dramatic, with moderately severe pain peaking in intensity within 3 seconds and prominent tearing (Pareja and Sjaastad, 1997; Goadsby et al., 2001).

Probable Trigeminal Autonomic Cephalalgia

Headache attacks believed to be a sub-type of TAC but fulfilling all but one of the diagnostic criteria for it are diagnosed as probable TAC.

OTHER PRIMARY HEADACHES (ICHD-2: 4.0)

This group of miscellaneous primary headache disorders includes some mimics of potentially serious secondary headaches, which need to be carefully evaluated by imaging or other appropriate tests. Some, like hypnic headache, primary thunderclap headache, HC and new daily-persistent headache (NDPH) were not included in the first IHS classification.

Primary Stabbing Headache

Episodic localized stabs of head pain occurring spontaneously in the absence of any structural cause (formerly referred to as "jabs and jolts") are diagnosed as *Primary stabbing headache* (4.1). Pain is exclusively or predominantly in the distribution of the first division of the trigeminal nerve (orbit, temple, and parietal area). It lasts for up to a few seconds and recurs at irregular intervals with a frequency ranging from one to many per day. Other features such as autonomic signs are lacking (Dangond and Spierings, 1993; Sjaastad et al., 2003).

Primary Cough Headache

This headache is brought on suddenly by coughing, straining, or Valsalva maneuver, and not otherwise, in the absence of any underlying disorder such as cerebral aneurysm or, especially, Arnold–-Chiari malformation (Pascual et al., 1996). Diagnostic neuroimaging, with special attention to the posterior fossa and base of the skull, is mandatory to differentiate secondary and primary forms of cough headache (Calandre et al., 1996).

Primary Exertional Headache

This disorder is triggered by physical exercise, and not otherwise, and is distinguished from *Primary cough headache* (4.2) (above) and *Headache associated with sexual activity* (4.4) (below). Primary exertional headache is pulsating and lasts from 5 minutes to 48 hours. After the first occurrence of any exertional headache of sudden onset, appropriate investigations must exclude subarachnoid hemorrhage and arterial dissection (Green, 2001).

Primary Headache Associated with Sexual Activity

Headache precipitated by sexual activity usually begins as a dull bilateral ache as sexual excitement increases, and suddenly becomes intense at orgasm (Lance, 1976). Two sub-types are classified: *Pre-orgasmic headache* (4.4.1), a dull ache in the head and neck, and *Orgasmic headache* (4.4.2), explosive and severe and occurring with orgasm. Diagnosis of the latter requires exclusion of subarachnoid hemorrhage and arterial dissection (D'Andrea et al., 2002).

Hypnic Headache

This primary headache disorder of the elderly (Newman et al., 1990) is characterized by short-lived attacks (typically 30 minutes) of nocturnal head pain that awakens the patient at a constant time each night, in many cases on more nights than not. It does not occur outside sleep. Hypnic headache is usually bilateral [though unilaterality does not exclude the diagnosis (Dodick et al., 1998)] and usually mild to moderate, very different from the unilateral orbital or periorbital knife-like intense pain of CH. Autonomic features are absent.

Primary Thunderclap Headache

Severe headache of abrupt onset, which mimics the pain of a ruptured cerebral aneurysm, is classified as *Primary thunderclap headache* (4.6), although this code is not applied to thunderclap headache meeting the criteria for 4.2, 4.3, or 4.4 (above). Intensity peaks in less than 1 minute. Pain lasts from 1 hour to 10 days and may recur within the first week after onset but not regularly over subsequent weeks or months (Dodick et al., 1999). This diagnosis can be established only after excluding subarachnoid hemorrhage.

Hemicrania Continua

This daily and continuous strictly unilateral headache is defined by its absolute response to therapeutic doses of indomethacin. Pain is moderate, with exacerbations of severe pain, and autonomic symptoms accompany these exacerbations although less prominently than in CH and chronic paroxysmal hemicrania (Sjaastad and Spierings, 1984; Bordini et al., 1991). Some bilateral or alternating-side cases have been reported (Rapoport and Bigal, 2003).

New Daily-Persistent Headache (See Controversies in the Classification of Chronic Daily Headaches, Below)

The essence of this headache, which otherwise resembles *Chronic tension-type headache* (2.3), is that it is daily and unremitting from or very soon (<3 days) after onset. There is no history of evolution from episodic headache (Silberstein and Lipton, 2001). Diagnosis is not confirmed until it has been present for >3 months, and cannot be made if this manner of onset is not clearly recalled by the patient. Nor can it made in the presence of medication overuse. NDPH is typically bilateral, pressing or tightening in quality, of mild-to-moderate intensity and unaffected by routine physical activity, although the diagnostic criteria require only any two of these features. There may be any but not more than one of photophobia, phonophobia, or mild nausea. In practice, many patients

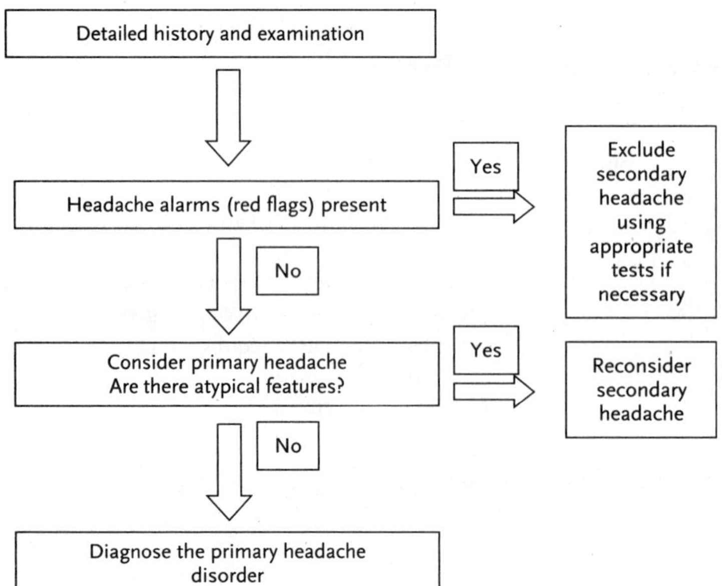

Figure 3–1 Algorithm for headache diagnosis.

with the temporal profile of NDPH have migraine features.

HEADACHE DIAGNOSIS

Headache diagnosis using the revised ICHD-2 criteria should proceed in an orderly fashion. In this discussion, we assume one headache disorder is present. If multiple headache disorders occur together, the conceptual process needs to be repeated for each.

First, one needs to distinguish primary from secondary headaches. The approach is to search for "red flags" that suggest the possibility of secondary headache (Fig. 3–1), to conduct the work-up indicated by those red flags (Table 3–7) and thereby to diagnose any secondary headache disorder that is present (Silberstein et al., 2001).

TABLE 3–7 Red Flags in the Diagnosis of Headache (Modified from Evans et al. 2001).

Red Flag	*Consider*	*Possible Investigation(s)*
Sudden-onset headache	Subarachnoid hemorrhage, bleed into a mass or AVM, mass lesion (especially posterior fossa)	Neuroimaging Lumbar puncture (after neuroimaging evaluation)
Worsening-pattern headache	Mass lesion, subdural hematoma, medication overuse	Neuroimaging
Headache with systemic illness (fever, neck stiffness, cutaneous rash)	Meningitis, encephalitis, Lyme disease, systemic infection, collagen vascular disease, arteritis	Neuroimaging Lumbar puncture Biopsy Blood tests
Focal neurologic signs, or symptoms other than typical visual or sensory aura	Mass lesion, AVM, collagen vascular disease	Neuroimaging Collagen vascular evaluation
Papilledema	Mass lesion, pseudotumor, encephalitis, meningitis	Neuroimaging Lumbar puncture (after neuroimaging evaluation)
Triggered by cough, exertion or Valsalva	Subarachnoid hemorrhage, mass lesion	Neuroimaging Considerer lumbar puncture
Headache during pregnancy or post-partum	Cortical vein/Cranial sinus thrombosis Carotid dissection Pituitary apoplexy	Neuroimaging
New headache type in a patient with		
Cancer	Metastasis	Neuroimaging, Lumbar puncture
Lyme disease	Meningoencephalitis	Neuroimaging, Lumbar puncture
HIV	Opportunistic infection, tumor	Neuroimaging, Lumbar puncture

Abbreviations: AVM, arteriovenous malformation; HIV; human immunodeficiency virus.

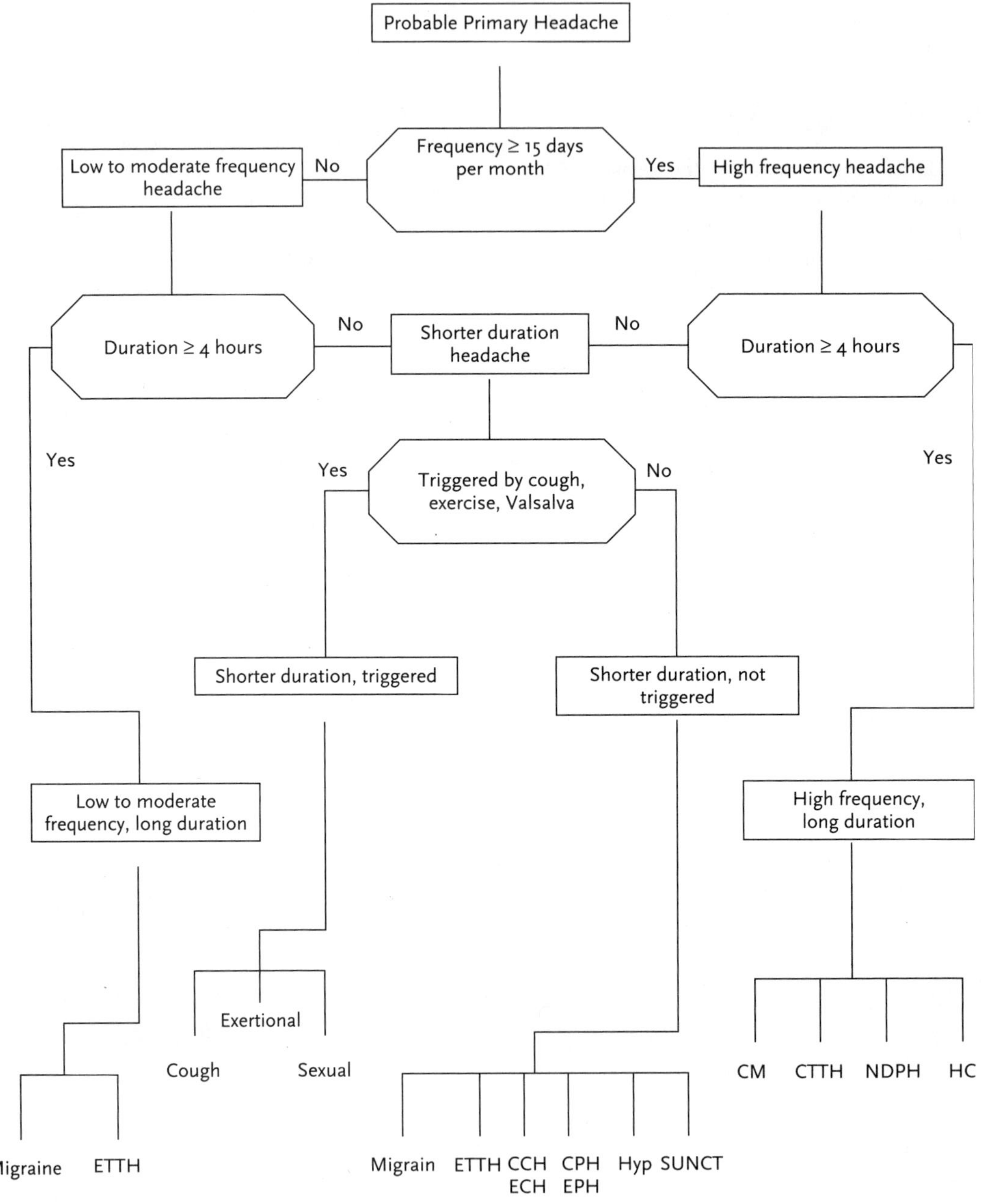

Figure 3–2 Algorithm for primary headache diagnosis. *Abbreviations*: CCH, chronic cluster headache; CM, chronic migraine; CPH, chronic paroxysmal hemicrania; CTTH, chronic tension-type headache; ECH, episodic cluster headache; EPH, episodic paroxysmal hemicrania; ETTH, episodic tension-type headache; HC, hemicrania continua; NDPH, new daily persistent headache; PSH, primary stabbing headache.

In the absence of secondary headache, the clinician proceeds to diagnosing a primary headache disorder. If headache is atypical or difficult to classify, the possibility of secondary headache should be reconsidered, although the modifying effect of any treatment being taken should be kept in mind. We propose the approach to differential diagnosis based on Figure 3–2 (see Appendix 1).

The first step is to divide primary headaches, based on average monthly frequency of the headaches, into those of low-to-moderate frequency (<15 headache days per month), or those of high frequency (⩾15 headache days per month). Second, based on average duration, classify the headache as one of shorter-duration (<4 hours a day) or longer-duration (⩾4 hours). Low-to-moderate frequency headaches of long duration include migraine and episodic TTH; high-frequency headaches of long duration include chronic migraine, chronic TTH, NDPH, and HC.

Third, for shorter-duration headache of low or high frequency, consider whether it is triggered or not by coughing, straining or Valsalva maneuver or by exertion or sexual activity. High-frequency, short-duration headaches not triggered by these include episodic and chronic CH, episodic and chronic paroxysmal hemicrania, hypnic headache, and SUNCT syndrome. Headaches triggered by cough, exertion, and sexual activity include the disorders named for these triggers.

The approach to differential diagnosis and the precise criteria for each disorder are presented elsewhere (Silberstein et al., 2001; Headache Classification Committee of the International Headache Society, 2004). These algorithms should help neurologists generate differential diagnoses based on the second edition of the IHS criteria.

References

Abu-Arafeh, I and Russel, G (1995). Prevalence and clinical features of abdominal migraine compared with those of migraine headache. *Arch Dis Child*, 72:413–417.

Al-Twaijri, WA and Shevell, MI (2002). Pediatric migraine equivalents: occurrence and clinical features in practice. *Pediatr Neurol*, 26:365–368.

Antonaci, F and Sjaastad, O (1989). Chronic paroxysmal hemicrania (CPH): a review of the clinical manifestations. *Headache*, 29:648–656.

Bento, MS and Esperanca, P (2000). Migraine with prolonged aura. *Headache*, 40:52–53.

Bordini, C, Antonaci, F, Stovner, LJ et al. (1991). "Hemicrania continua": a clinical review. *Headache*, 31:20–26.

Calandre, L, Hernandez-Lain, A, Lopez-Valdes, E (1996). Benign Valsalva's maneuver-related headache: an MRI study of six cases. *Headache*, 36:251–253.

Carrera, P, Stenirri, S, Ferrari, M et al. (2001). Familial hemiplegic migraine: a ion channel disorder. *Brain Res Bull*, 56:239–241.

D'Andrea, G, Granella, F, and Verdelli, F (2002). Migraine with aura triggered by orgasm. *Cephalalgia*, 22:485–486.

Dangond, F and Spierings, EL (1993). Idiopathic stabbing headaches lasting a few seconds. *Headache*, 33:257–258.

De Fusco, M, Marconi, R, Silvestri, L et al. (2003). Haploinsufficiency of ATP1A2 encoding the Na/K pump a2 subunit associated with familial hemiplegic migraine type 2. *Nat Genet*, 33, 193–196.

Dodick, DW, Mosek, AC, and Campbell, IK (1998). The hypnic ("alarm clock") headache syndrome. *Cephalalgia*, 18:152–156.

Dodick, DW, Brown, RD, Britton, JW et al. (1999). Nonaneurysmal thunderclap headache with diffuse, multifocal, segmental and reversible vasospasm. *Cephalalgia*, 19:118–123.

Dodick, DW, Rozen, TD, Goadsby, PJ et al. (2000). Cluster headache. *Cephalalgia*, 20:787–803.

Ducros, A, Denier, C, Joutel, A, et al. (2001). The clinical spectrum of familial hemiplegic migraine associated with mutations in a neuronal calcium channel. *N Engl J Med*, 345:17–24.

Drigo, P, Carli, G, and Laverda, AM (2001). Benign paroxysmal vertigo of childhood. *Brain Dev*, 23:38–41.

Evans, RW, Rozen, TD, and Adelman, JU (2001). Neuroimaging and Other Diagnostic Testing in Headache. In *Wolff's Headache and Other Facial Pain* (SD Silberstein, RB Lipton, and DJ Dalessio, eds.), pp. 3–49. Oxford, New York.

Fisher, CM (1980). Late-life migraine accompaniments as a cause of unexplained transient ischemic attacks. *Can J Neurol Sci*, 7:9–17.

Fleisher, DR (1999). Cyclic vomiting syndrome and migraine. *J Pediatr*, 134:533–535.

Goadsby, PJ and Lipton, RB (1997). A review of paroxysmal hemicranias, SUNCT syndrome and other short-lasting headaches with autonomic features, including new cases. *Brain*, 120:193–209.

Goadsby, PJ, Matharu, MS, and Boes, CJ (2001). SUNCT syndrome or trigeminal neuralgia with lacrimation. *Cephalalgia*, 21:82–83.

Green, MW (2001). A spectrum of exertional headaches. *Headache*, 4:1085–1092.

Haan, J, Terwindt, GM, and Ferrari, MD (1997). Genetics of migraine. *Neurol Clin*, 15:43–60.

Headache Classification Committee of the International Headache Society (1988). Classification and diagnostic criteria for headache disorders, cranial neuralgias and facial pain. *Cephalalgia*, 8(Suppl. 7):1–96.

Headache Classification Committee of the International Headache Society (2004). The International Classification of Headache Disorders. *Cephalalgia*, 24:1–160.

Headache Classification Committee of the International Headache Society (2006).

Headache Classification Committee of the International Headache Society (2006). New appendix criteria open for a broader concept of chronic migraine. *Cephalalgia*, 26:469–470.

Hosking, G (1988). Special forms: variants of migraine in childhood. In *Migraine in Childhood* (JM Hockaday, ed.), pp. 35–53. Butterworths, Boston.

Jensen, K, Tfelt-Hansen, P, Lauritzen, M et al. (1986). Classic migraine, a prospective recording of symptoms. *Acta Neurol Scand*, 73:359–362.

Katsarava, Z, Fritsche, G, Muessig, M et al. (2001). Clinical features of withdrawn headache following overuse of triptans and other headache drugs. *Neurology*, 57:1694–1698.

Klee, A and Willanger, R (1966). Disturbances of visual perception in migraine. *Acta Neurol Scand*, 42:400–414.

Kuhn, WF, Kuhn, SC, and Daylida, L (1997). Basilar migraine. *Eur J Emerg Med*, 4:33–38.

Lance, JW (1976). Headaches related to sexual activity. *J Neurol Neurosurg Psychiat*, 39:1226–1230.

Li, BU (2001). Cyclic vomiting syndrome: age-old syndrome and new insights. *Semin Pediatr Neurol*, 8:13–21.

Linet, MS, Celentano, DD, and Stewart, WF (1991). Headache characteristics associated with physician consultation: a population-based survey. *Am J Prev Med*, 7:40–46.

Lippman, CV (1952). Certain hallucinations peculiar to migraine. *J Nerv Ment Dis*, 116:346.

Manzoni, G, Farina, S, Lanfranchi, M et al. (1985). Classic migraine: clinical findings in 164 patients. *Eur Neurol*, 24:163–169.

Matharu, MJ and Goadsby, PJ (2001). Post-traumatic chronic paroxysmal hemicrania (CPH) with aura. *Neurology*, 56:273–275.

Monzillo, PH, Sanvito, WL, and Da Costa, AR (2000). Cluster-tic syndrome: report of five new cases. *Arq Neuropsiquiatr*, 58(2B):518–521.

Newman, LC, Lipton, RB, and Solomon, S (1990). The hypnic headache syndrome: a benign headache disorder of the elderly. *Neurology*, 40:1904–1905

Olesen, J, Friberg, L, Olsen, TS et al. (1990). Timing and topography of cerebral blood flow, aura, and headache during migraine attacks. *Ann Neurol*, 28:791–798.

Ophoff, RA, Terwindt, GM, Vergouwe, MN et al. (1996). Familial hemiplegic migraine and episodic ataxia type-2 are caused by mutations in the $Ca_2{}^+$ channel gene CACNL1A4. *Cell*, 87:543–552.

Ophoff, RA, Terwindt, GM, Vergouwe, MN et al. (1997). Wolff Award 1997. Involvement of a Ca2+ channel gene in familial hemiplegic migraine and migraine with and without aura. Dutch Migraine Genetics Research Group. *Headache*, 37:479–485.

Pareja, JA and Sjaastad, O (1997). SUNCT syndrome. A clinical review. *Headache*, 37:195–202.

Pascual, J, Combarros, O, Leno, C et al. (1995). Distribution of headache by diagnosis as the reason for neurologic consultation. *Med Clin*, 104:161–164.

Pascual, J, Iglesias, F, Oterino, A et al. (1996). Cough, exertional, and sexual headaches: an analysis of 72 benign and symptomatic cases. *Neurology*, 46:1520–1524.

Patel, N, Bigal, ME, Kolodner, K et al. (2003). Disability and health-related quality of life in strict migraine vs probable migraine (migrainous headache) and control subjects within a health plan. *Cephalalgia* (in press).

Patel, N, Bigal, ME, Kolodner, KB, et al. (2004). Prevalence and impact of migraine and probable migraine in a health plan. *Neurology*, 63:1432–1438.

Peres, MF, Siow, HC, and Rozen, TD (2002). Hemicrania continua with aura. *Cephalalgia*, 22:246–248.

Rains, JC, Penzien, DB, Lipchik, GL et al. (2001). Diagnosis of migraine: empirical analysis of a large clinical sample of atypical migraine (IHS 1.7) patients and proposed revision of the IHS criteria. *Cephalalgia*, 21:584–595.

Rapoport, AM and Bigal, ME (2003). Hemicrania continua: clinical and nosographic update. *Neurol Sci*, 24 (Suppl. 2):S118–S121.

Rothrock, JF, Walicke, P, Swenson, MR et al. (1988). Migrainous stroke. *Arch Neurol*, 45:63–67.

Russel, MB and Olesen, J (1996). A nosographic analysis of the migraine aura in a general population. *Brain*, 119:355–361.

Schwartz, BS, Stewart, WF, Simon, D et al. (1998). Epidemiology of tension-type headache. *JAMA*, 279(5):381–383.

Silberstein, SD and Young, WB (1995). Migraine aura and prodrome. *Seminars Neurol*, 45:175–182.

Silberstein, SD, Niknam, R, Rozen, TD et al. (2000). Cluster headache with aura. *Neurology*, 54:219–221.

Silberstein, SD and Lipton, RB (2001). Chronic daily headache, including transformed migraine, chronic tension-type headache, and medication overuse. In *Wolff's Headache and Other Head Pain* (SD Silberstein, RB Lipton, and Dalessio DJ, eds.), pp. 247–282. Oxford University Press, New York.

Silberstein, SD, Lipton, RB, and Dalessio, DJ (2001). Overview, diagnosis and classification of headache. In *Wolff's Headache and Other Facial Pain* (SD Silberstein, RB Lipton, and DJ Dalessio, eds.), pp. 6–26. Oxford, New York.

Sjaastad, O and Dale, I (1974). Evidence for a new (?) treatable headache entity. *Headache*,14:105–108.

Sjaastad, O and Spierings, EL (1984). Hemicrania continua: another headache absolutely responsive to indomethacin. *Cephalalgia*, 4:65–70.

Sjaastad, O, Pettersen, H, and Bakketeig, LS (2003). Extracephalic jabs/idiopathic stabs. Vaga study of headache epidemiology.*Cephalalgia*, 23(1):50–54.

Solomon, S and Grosberg, BM (2003). Retinal migraine (abstract). *Headache*, 43:510.

Staehelin-Jensen, T, Olivarius, B, Kraft, M et al. (1981). Familial hemiplegic migraine. A reappraisal and long-term follow-up study. *Cephalalgia*, 1:33–39.

Tfelt-Hansen, P, Block, G, Dahlof, C et al. (2000). Guidelines for controlled trials of drugs in migraine: second edition. *Cephalalgia*, 20(9):765–786.

Thomsen, LL, Ostergaard, E, Olesen, J et al. (2003). Evidence for a separate type of migraine with aura: sporadic hemiplegic migraine. *Neurology*, 60:595–601.

Troost, T and Zagami, AS (2000). Ophthalmoplegic migraine and retinal migraine. In *The Headaches* (J Olesen, P Tfelt-Hansen, and KMA Welch, eds.), pp. 511–516. Lippincott Willians & Wilkins, Philadelphia.

Whitty, CVM (1967). Migraine without headache. *Lancet*, ii:283–285.

Willey, RG (1979). The scintillating scotoma without headache. *Ann Ophthalmol*, 11:581–585.

Withers, GD, Silburn, SR, and Forbes, DA (1998). Precipitants and aetiology of cyclic vomiting syndrome. *Acta Paediatr*, 87(3):272–277.

Ziegler, DK and Hanassein, RS (1990). Specific headache phenomena: their frequency and coincidence. *Headache*, 30:152–160.

4 Headache: Epidemiology and Impact

Richard B Lipton, Marcelo E Bigal, Sandra Hamelsky, and Ann I Scher

INTRODUCTION

Recurrent headache disorders impose a substantial burden on individual headache sufferers, on their families, and on society (Stovner, 2007). As noted in Chapter 3, headache disorders are divided into secondary disorders, attributable to an underlying condition, and primary disorders, such as migraine, trigeminal autonomic cephalalgias, and tension type headache, where there is no underlying cause. The epidemiology of secondary headache is largely determined by the epidemiology of the underlying cause. Therefore, in this chapter, we will focus on the epidemiology of primary headache disorders.

Epidemiology is the study of diseases, their risk factors, causes, natural history, and burden in the population. While epidemiologic studies are often population-based, this is particularly important for headache because the disorder is so often underascertained in the health care system. Accordingly, we will focus herein on population studies that measure the frequency, distribution, and burden of disease in the population (Scher et al., 1999; Lipton, Diamond, et al., 2001; Lipton, Stewart, et al., 2001, Lipton et al., 2007; Stovner et al., 2007). Widely used measures of disease frequency include incidence and prevalence. Incidence quantifies the number of new events or cases of a disease that develop in a defined population over a defined period of time. Prevalence refers to the proportion of a population that has the disease over a given period of time and is an important measure of the burden of disease (Scher et al., 1999). In headache, other widely used measures of burden include lost workday equivalents and disability-adjusted life years (DALYs).

As part of the "Global Campaign to Reduce the Burden of Headache," organized by World Health Organization (WHO) Stovner et al. (2007) recently reviewed population studies and calculated DALYs for migraine, tension-type headache (TTH) and chronic daily headache (CDH). They estimated that the worldwide prevalences were 47% for current headache, 10% for current migraine, 38% for current TTH, and 3% for current CDH. They also found that lifetime prevalences were somewhat higher for headache (66%), migraine (14%), and TTH (46%). Reliable lifetime estimates for CDH are not available.

Herein, we emphasize the epidemiology of and risk factors for migraine, as well as the impact the disease has on the individual and society. We also highlight risk factors for migraine progression and briefly review the epidemiology of tension-type headache. Studies that used standard case definitions as provided by the *International Classification of Headache Disorders* (*ICHD*) (Headache Classification Subcommittee of the International Headache Society, 2004) will be emphasized. The comorbidity of migraine is discussed in Chapter 10.

EPIDEMIOLOGY OF MIGRAINE

Overview

In this section, we will first consider the prevalence and distribution of migraine and then discuss its incidence. We will then consider measures of the burden of migraine on individual sufferers, their families, and society.

Prevalence

The prevalence of migraine has been assessed in numerous studies using a variety of case definitions and methods. Estimates became much less variable once standard diagnostic criteria were developed and applied. Most large studies generate estimates in the 15%–20% range for females and 4%–7% range for men. In the United States, there have been three large-scale studies in nationally representative samples of the US population conducted in 1989 (American Migraine Study 1—AMS-1; Stewart et al., 1992), in 1999 (American Migraine Study 2—AMS-2; Lipton, Diamond, et al., 2001; Lipton, Stewart, et al., 2001) and in 2004 (American Migraine Prevalence and Prevention Study—AMPPS; Lipton et al., 2007).

In AMS-1, 15,000 households received mailed questionnaires, and each household member who had severe headache was asked to respond to detailed questions about symptoms, frequency, and severity of the headaches. After a single mailing, 20,468 subjects between 12 and 80 years of age responded to the survey. The prevalence of migraine was 17.6% in females and 5.7% in males (Fig. 4–1). To identify shifting patterns in epidemiology, 10 years later, the same research team conducted a study that was methodologically identical.. In this study, AMS-2, validated questionnaires were mailed to 20,000 households, generating responses from about 30,000 individuals respondents (Lipton, Diamond, et al., 2001; Lipton, Stewart, et al., 2001). Results were virtually identical to the previous study in terms of prevalence, though rates of diagnosis and treatment had improved.

In 2004, the largest migraine epidemiology study, the American Migraine Prevalence and Prevention Study (AMPPS), was conducted. It provided results identical to the previous two, indicating that the prevalence of migraine has been stable in the United States at least over the last 15 years (Lipton et al., 2007). The prevalence of migraine has been recently reviewed (Stovner, 2007).

Prevalence by Age and Gender

Most studies of migraine report that prevalence is higher in females at all post-pubertal ages and that it also varies according to age. These patterns are exemplified by the data from the AMPPS shown in Fig. 4–2; migraine prevalence is highest between 25 and 55 years of age, typically the peak productive years of life (Lipton, Diamond, et al., 2001; Lipton, Stewart, et al., 2001; Lipton et al., 2002, 2007). This may help explain the sizeable impact of migraine on both absenteeism and attendance, as discussed below.

Prior to puberty, the prevalence of migraine is slightly higher in boys than girls (Bille, 1989; Abu-Arefeh and Russell, 1994). For example, Mortimer and colleagues (1992) reported that migraine prevalence was greater in boys between 3 and 5 years of age and also 5 and 7 years of age. For the ages between 7 and 11 years, prevalence was approximately equal between the genders. However, as adolescence approaches, migraine prevalence accelerates in females. After age 11, prevalence is often higher in girls than boys (Mortimer et al., 1992; Raieli et al., 1995) and remains so for the rest of the lifespan (Stovner et al., 2007).

In the adult population, in every region of the world, and in every racial and ethnic group

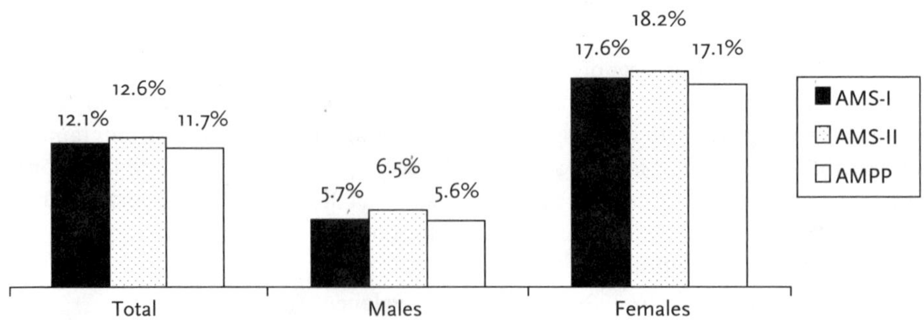

Figure 4–1 One-year period prevalence of migraine by sex in three large U.S. studies.

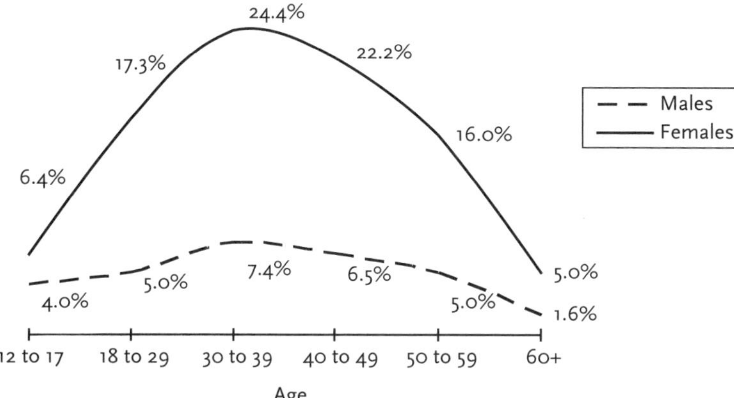

Figure 4–2 Migraine prevalence by age and sex. Data from the AMPPS.

studied, migraine is two to three times more common among females than males (Lipton et al., 1998, Lipton, Stewart, et al., 1999; Lipton, Stewart, et al., 2001, Lipton et al., 2005). In the AMS-1 and 2, as well as in the AMPPS, the average female-to-male migraine prevalence ratio is around 2.8, with a peak of 3.3 between ages 40 and 45 years. The ratio remains above 2.0 even after the age of menopause.

Prevalence by Race and Geographical Region

The available evidence suggests that migraine prevalence varies by race and geographical region. Stewart and colleagues (1996) conducted a population-based study in the United States and reported that the lowest prevalence was observed among Asian Americans, intermediate estimates were reported in African–Americans, and the highest prevalence estimates were observed among whites, before and after adjusting for demographic covariates. A more recent meta-analysis confirmed these findings: prevalence was lowest in Africa and Asia and higher in Europe, Central America and South America. The highest estimates were found in North America (Scher et al., 1999). Fig. 4–3 presents a figure of the age-adjusted migraine prevalence by geographical region.

Since migraine prevalence is low in Africa and Asia, and remains low among African–Americans and Asians in the United States, it has been hypothesized that there are race-related differences in genetic susceptibility to migraine. However, since prevalence in Asia is even lower than in the United States, other variables such as environmental risk factors or culturally determined differences in symptom-reporting may further explain the international variation.

Prevalence by Socioeconomic Status

In the United States, several population-based studies have demonstrated that in the community, migraine prevalence is inversely related to household income (Lipton et al., 1998; Lipton, Stewart, et al., 1999; Lipton, Stewart, et al., 2001; Lipton et al., 2005). As income or education increased, migraine prevalence declined.

The National Health Interview Survey also demonstrated lower prevalence in the low-income compared with middle-income group; however, prevalence was highest among the highest-income group (Stang and Osterhaus, 1993). Since this study relied on self-reported medical diagnosis of migraine, and medical diagnosis of migraine rises with income, differential ascertainment by income may explain the association in the highest-income group. Studies conducted outside the United States have not consistently supported the inverse relationship between migraine prevalence and household income.

Migraine is more common in people from low-income households but less common in

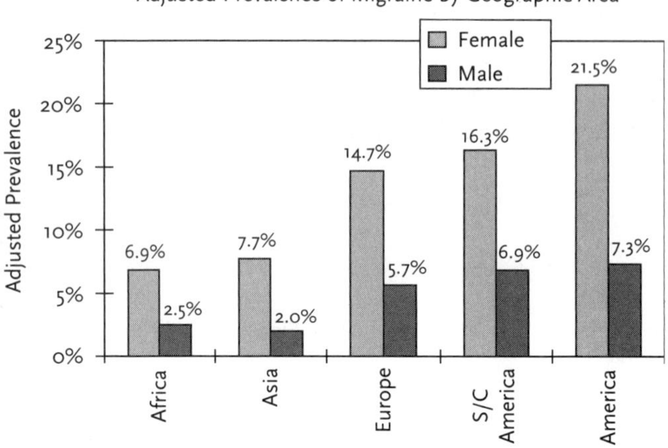

Figure 4–3 Adjusted prevalence of migraine by geographic area and gender in a meta-analysis of studies using IHS criteria. (From Scher et al., 2001.)

African–Americans and Asians in the United States. These patterns of prevalence by race are also reflected in international studies as migraine is most common in North America and Europe and less so in Africa and Asia.

Association exists between migraine and socioeconomic status (SES) (Launer et al., 1999). In addition, in a population-based study conducted in England, no association was found between migraine and SES (Steiner et al., 2003). The reasons for the international variation are unclear.

The influence of income in migraine prevalence, as evidenced by population studies in the United States (Lipton, Diamond et al., 2001; Lipton, Stewart, et al., 2001; Lipton et al., 2007), has been the subject of much debate with two major alternative explanations. According to the social causation hypothesis, factors associated with low SES, such as stress, poor diet, or limited access to medical care, act to increase disease prevalence. The opposing social selection hypothesis suggests that disease-related dysfunction interferes with educational and occupational functioning, which in turn would lead to low income. To further explore the influence of income on migraine prevalence, we conducted a large population study on adolescents, since this group makes no more than a modest contribution to family income. We found that in adolescents with family history of migraine, household income does not have a significant effect, probably because of the higher biological predisposition or due to a common stressor even. In those without a strong predisposition, household income is associated with prevalence (Bigal, Lipton, et al., 2007).

Incidence

Migraine incidence is best studied in longitudinal studies of people at risk for the disease. However, few such studies have been reported. The studies that have been published report varying results, probably because of differences in study populations (e.g., age, geographical area) as well as study methodology.

Breslau and colleagues (1996) estimated the incidence of migraine in a random sample of members of a large health maintenance organization who were in the age group 21–30 years. A total of 1007 participants were initially interviewed. The 5-year incidence of migraine was estimated among the 848 people who did not meet the criteria for migraine at baseline. A total of 71 (8.4%) cases of migraine were identified [female 60 (12.0%); male 11 (3.2%)]. This study likely underestimated the incidence of migraine because it included subjects from a very narrow age range, older than the age of suspected peak risk for incident migraine.

Stewart and colleagues (1991) reported a higher incidence based on results from a population-based study that used the reported age of onset to estimate the incidence of migraine. Telephone interviews were conducted among 10,169 residents of Washington County, Maryland, who were between the ages of 12 and 29. In total, 392 males and 1018 females were identified as migraine sufferers. While this study included a broader age range than that of Breslau and colleagues, the generalizability of the results are also limited because only individuals between the ages of 12 and 29 years were interviewed.

Below the age of 10, the incidence of migraine, especially migraine without aura, was higher among males than females. For example, among females of age between 6 and 7 years, the incidence rate was 6.3 per 1000 person years for migraine with aura and 5.4 per 1000 person years for migraine without aura. For males in the same age group, the incidence rate for migraine with aura was 5.6 per 1000 and migraine without aura was 8.3 per 1000. However, during the adolescent years, the incidence of migraine is higher in females than males. For example, among females between 12 and 13 years old, the incidence rate was 14.1 for migraine with aura and 17.3 for migraine without aura per 1000. The corresponding percentages for males were 3.5 and 9.9 per 1000. Most of the new-onset cases among females were cases of migraine without aura. In addition, the peak incidence of migraine per 1000 was higher among females (migraine without aura: females 18.9, males 10.1; migraine with aura: females 14.1, males 6.6) but occurred earlier in males (migraine without aura: females 14–17 years old, males 10–11 years old; migraine with aura: females 12–13 years old, males 4–5 years old).

Stang and colleagues (1992) used linked medical records to estimate the incidence of migraine in Olmstead County, Minnesota. Of the 6400 patient records reviewed, 629 fulfilled the International Headache Society (IHS) criteria for migraine. Among females, the incidence of migraine peaked between 20 and 24 years, at 6.9 per 1000 person years. In males, the highest incidence rate, 2.5 per 1000 person years, occurred between 10 and 14 years. The decreased incidence rates and later peaks in incidence relative to Stewart and colleagues (1991) and Breslau and colleagues (1996) may have occurred because only individuals who consulted a health care provider for headache were identified.

More recently, Lyngberg and colleagues (2003) published a population-based study of the incidence of migraine in a Danish population. This study was a follow-up to a cross-sectional epidemiology study from 1989. Of the 453 subjects ranging in age from 25 to 64 years who did not have migraine in 1989, 42 developed migraine during the study period, resulting in an annual incidence of 0.8%. The annual incidence in females was 1.5% and in males 0.3%. The study was too small to provide age-specific estimates of incidence.

INDIVIDUAL IMPACT OF MIGRAINE

Individual Impact

Attack characteristics. The individual impact of migraine can be measured in many ways. It is important to assess the pattern of symptoms as well as the frequency and severity of attacks. Factors such as the level of pain intensity, the presence and severity of associated symptoms (nausea, vomiting, photophobia, phonophobia), and attack duration are important determinants of the severity of an individual attack. However, migraine also has a cumulative impact over time. Quality-of-life studies help quantify the impact of individual attacks as well as quality of life between episodes. Several studies indicate that most migraine sufferers report severe pain and the presence of associated symptoms with their migraine attacks.

In a study of migraine sufferers in the United States, 80% reported pain that was severe or very severe. The remaining subjects reported mild-to-moderate pain. In addition to pain, associated symptoms were common. More than half of the subjects reported photophobia (81.9%) and phonophobia (77.9%). Approximately 60% reported that nausea accompanied their migraine headache more than half of the time. Vomiting was uncommon (Lipton, Stewart, et al., 2001).

The overall impact of the illness is determined not just by attack characteristics, but also by attack frequency. On average, migraine sufferers report one to two migraine attacks per month. The duration of an untreated attack varies by gender. Among females, approximately 71% of attacks last longer than 24 hours. In contrast, 48% of males reported attacks that lasted longer than 24 hours. These findings are similar to those reported in other studies (Stewart et al., 1992).

Health-related quality of life. Health-related quality of life (HRQoL) studies are generally considered a more qualitative assessment of the burden of migraine. They measure the individual impact of a disease in the following domains: physical, psychological, social, spiritual and role-functioning, and general well being. Both generic and disease-specific measures have been used to evaluate quality of life among migraine sufferers. While generic quality-of-life instruments are designed to measure the impact of a range of illnesses using a common scale, disease-specific measures contain questions that address the quality-of-life impact of a specific illness.

Several studies based on population in the United States and Europe have evaluated HRQoL among migraine sufferers and a control population (Gobel et al., 1994; Launer et al., 1999; Lipton, Liberman et al., 1999; Tekle Haimanot et al., 1995). All of these studies included a contemporaneous nonmigraine sufferer control population. HRQoL scores in the migraine population were significantly lower than those in the control population. These studies described the relationships between HRQoL, migraine frequency, disability, and depression. As migraine frequency and disability increased, HRQoL decreased. These studies also confirmed that migraine and depression are comorbid. Furthermore, they found that migraine status was associated with decreased HRQoL scores, even after controlling for depression.

THE IMPACT OF MIGRAINE ON THE FAMILY

Because migraine affects women more often than men and is most common between ages 25 and 55, the years of child rearing, a substantial impact on family life might be expected. However, of the many studies focusing on the burdens of migraine, relatively few have examined its impact on the families of those directly affected. A Canadian study reported that 90% of people with migraine reported postponing their household work because of headaches, 30% had canceled family and social activities during their last migraine attack, and 66% feared letting others down because of their headaches (Edmeads et al., 1993). Other studies (Kryst and Scherl, 1994; Smith, 1998; Holmes et al., 2001) found that migraine attacks brought significant disruption to family life, with impact on spouses, children, and friends.

In an epidemiological study conducted in the United Kingdom and the United States, the impact of migraine on family life was assessed both from the perspective of those with migraine and from the perspective of their partners (Lipton et al., 2003). A validated computer-assisted telephone interview identified 574 people with migraine from a population sample of 4007 in mainland England, and 568 from a sample of 4376 in Philadelphia County in the United States. In a follow-up interview, questions were asked of the proband about the impact of migraine. Similar questions were also asked of the proband's partner regarding the impact of the proband's migraine on their participation in social, family, and leisure activities and on family relationships. Of 389 people with migraine living with a household partner, 85% reported substantial reductions in their ability to do household work and chores, 45% missed family, social, and leisure activities, and 32% avoided making plans for fear of having to cancel them due to headaches. One-half believed that because of their migraine they were more likely to argue with their partners (50%) and children (52%), while the majority (52%–73%) reported other adverse consequences for their relationships with their partner and children, and at work. About one-third (36%) believed they would be better partners but for their headaches. Participating partners ($n = 100$) partly confirmed these findings: 29% felt that arguments were more common because of headaches, and 20%–60% reported other negative effects on relationships at home. When compared with subjects who did not have migraine, a statistically significant higher proportion of migraine partners were unsatisfied with work demands placed on them ($p = 0.02$), with their level or responsibilities and duties ($p = 0.02$), and with their ability to perform ($p = 0.001$). These results suggest that the impact of migraine extends to household partners and other family members.

Symptom profile and disability related to migraine vary substantially, both within and among individuals. The disability of migraine can be severe and has a substantial impact on society, as well as the individual, his or her family, and society. The societal impact of migraine is usually measured in economic terms. Direct costs consist primarily of health care utilization. Indirect costs include missed work (i.e.,absenteeism) and reduced productivity while at work (attendance) due to migraine. The individual impact is often measured by examining attack frequency and severity, as well as the global impact of repeated attacks. Studies of the family members of migraine sufferers provide insight into how the disease affects those around them.

Societal Impact

Direct costs. Direct costs include all of the costs of diagnosing and treating a particular disorder. In the case of migraine, this includes health care utilization figures such as rates of outpatient visits, hospitalization, the use of emergency department services, and costs of prescriptions.

Studies have reported that patients with migraine have higher direct medical costs than the general population, primarily due to greater frequency of physician and emergency department visits (Clouse and Osterhaus, 1994; Edmeads and Mackell, 2002). To assess health care resource use associated with migraine, Clouse and Osterhaus conducted a study among 1336 migraine sufferers enrolled in a United HealthCare affiliated plan (Clouse and Osterhaus, 1994). Subjects were eligible for consideration if they had been enrolled in the plan for at least one year, had a medical claim for migraine, and had a pharmacy claim for medication potentially used for migraine treatment. During an 18-month follow-up period, the consultation rates of migraine sufferers ($n = 1336$) were compared with nonmigraine sufferers ($n = 1336$) matched on the basis of age, sex, duration of enrollment, and subscriber/dependent status. Migraine sufferers made 2616 visits for migraine, and 19,971 visits for reasons other than migraine. In contrast, nonmigraine sufferers made a total of 13,072 visits during the same period. Interestingly, a small proportion of migraine sufferers accounted for the majority of physician visits. While most migraine sufferers reported one-to-four physician visits per year, only a small proportion (7.6%) reported more than 12 visits. An important limitation of this study is the selected study population: only migraine sufferers who sought treatment were included.

In another population-based study, individuals with migraine were matched with a migraine-free control group on the basis of age, sex, employment status, and several comorbidities such as heart attack, angina, stroke, cancer, diabetes, and asthma (Edmeads and Mackell, 2002). Both the frequency and quantity of health care utilization were greater for the migraine group than the control group. Migraine sufferers were significantly ($p < 0.001$) more likely to report having visited a general practitioner, psychiatrist, or other medical specialist. In addition, while 24% of migraine sufferers reported an emergency department visit during the previous 6 months, only 15% of the comparison group reported a visit ($p < 0.001$). Migraine sufferers also reported significantly more frequent physician visits (3.5 versus 2.8, $p < 0.001$) and emergency department visits (0.4 versus 0.2, $p < 0.001$) than the control population.

This study has two important limitations. First, it included only self-reported migraine sufferers, although 60% reported that they had been diagnosed by a physician. Secondly, because of the study methodology, it was not possible to distinguish between migraine-related visits and those related to comorbid conditions. However, matching the migraine sufferers with a control population based on five comorbidities should have minimized the extent to which comorbidities confound the results.

Studies conducted in the United States show that although physician consultation among migraine sufferers increased over the last 15 years, migraine remains substantially underdiagnosed and undertreated (Lipton et al., 1998; Lipton, Stewart, et al., 1999; Lipton, Stewart, et al., 2001; Lipton et al., 2005). Consultation is more common among females than males and with increase in age. In addition, more severe attacks, reflected by higher pain intensity, the number of migraine symptoms, attack duration, and disability are all associated with an increased likelihood of physician consultation.

Two population-based studies have translated health care use into direct costs (Hu et al., 1999; Edmeads and Mackell, 2002). Hu and colleagues (1999) reported the direct costs of migraine by analyzing a US population–based sample. In this study, the annual treatment costs of migraine were estimated to be over $1 billion, about $100 per migraine sufferer per year.

The costs of diagnosing and treating migraine (direct costs) are far less than the costs of productivity losses due to migraine. As a consequence, improving health care delivery for migraine could be cost-effective from a societal perspective.

Physician visits (60%) and prescription drugs (30%) accounted for the majority of treatment-related costs. Emergency department visits accounted for a small proportion of total costs (1%).

Edmeads and Mackell (2002) estimated direct medical costs among self-identified migraine sufferers compared with a matched control group. Over a 6-month period, total direct medical costs including physician visits, emergency department visits, and hospitalization were significantly higher ($p < 0.039$) in the migraine group ($522) than the control population ($415). The costs of physician and emergency department visits were strong drivers behind the significant difference in total direct medical costs. The cost of outpatient physician visits was $221 for the migraine group and $177 for the comparison group ($p < 0.001$). Emergency department visits were also significantly higher ($p < 0.001$) in the migraine group ($33) versus the control population ($18). The direct costs in this study are underestimated because they do not include the cost of prescription medication.

Headache severity is related to the direct costs. In one study (Osterhaus et al., 1992), a four-point grading system that scaled pain and disability was used to classify subjects. According to the results of this scale, Grade 1 patients are defined by relatively low or moderate pain intensity without activity limitations. Grade 2 patients are defined by high pain intensity without activity limitations. Grade 3 patients are defined by moderate activity limitations. Grade 4 patients are defined by severe activity limitations. Using data collected in a self-administered questionnaire, the investigators classified members of the managed care organization, Group Health of Puget Sound, into the grading system and then followed the patients for 2 years. Claims data for these patients indicated that as the grade of headache severity increased, so did headache treatment costs. Among Grade 1 patients, treatment costs were $200 per patient per year. In contrast, Grade 4 patients had headache treatment costs that were $800 per patient per year.

Edmeads and Mackell (2002) compared the direct medical costs among a population-based sample of self-identified moderate and severe migraine sufferers. The average number of physician and emergency department visits were significantly higher for the severe group compared with the moderate group ($p < 0.004$). Total medical costs were higher in the severe group ($605.38) than the moderate group ($471.96). The difference was not statistically significant.

Indirect costs. While the direct costs of migraine are substantial, the indirect costs are even greater. Indirect costs include the aggregate effects of migraine on productivity at work, at home, and in other roles. Many migraine sufferers miss work because of their headaches, and reduced productivity as a result of working during a migraine is common. Since it is important to measure absenteeism as well as work loss due to reduced productivity, many studies examine actual days of missed work, time at work with headache, and percent effectiveness while at work with a headache. The components are sometimes combined in an index termed lost workday equivalents (LWDEs), which equals actual days of missed work plus days at work with headache times 1 minus percent effectiveness while at work with headache (Osterhaus et al., 1992).

Several studies have been conducted in population-based samples of migraine sufferers, and two used daily disability diaries to minimize recall bias.

Von Korff and colleagues (1998) estimated the number of lost workdays and LWDEs in a population-based sample of employed migraine sufferers who completed a daily diary for 3 months. A daily diary was used to improve the accuracy of the work loss data. During the 3-month period, migraine sufferers missed an average of 1.1 days due to headache. Subjects who continued to work during a headache attack reported work effectiveness that was reduced by 41%. Migraine sufferers reported an average of three LWDEs.

Michel and colleagues (1999) conducted a 3-month prospective daily diary study examining work loss data among 231 migraine sufferers and 188 nonheadache-prone subjects. Participants used a daily diary to record the presence or absence of headache and the work situation that day (unemployment, holiday, weekend, medical reason, nonmedical reason). Absenteeism was classified into two groups: sickness-related absenteeism (i.e., number of workdays missed or interrupted for medical reasons) and headache-related absenteeism (i.e., number of workdays missed or interrupted on days with headache). In this study, migraine sufferers reported an average of 1.45 missed days due to medical reasons, 0.25 of which were due to headache. Sickness-related absenteeism was statistically higher in migraine sufferers than nonheadache-prone subjects. The control population, on the other hand, reported 0.96 sickness-related days, 0.7 of which were due to headache. The difference was due to higher absenteeism related to comorbid medical conditions, not headache reasons.

While most studies have reported time lost from work due to a migraine, few studies have recorded the number of days missed from household activities. Edmeads and Mackell (2002), however, calculated the number of days missed from both employment and household activities over a 6-month period. Among full-time and part-time workers, the migraine sufferers missed 5 days of work, while the control group missed only 3 days ($p < 0.001$). The migraine sufferers who were not employed missed more days of household duties ($n = 18$ days) than their counterparts ($n = 14$ days). However, the difference was not statistically significant ($p = 0.177$).

Since migraine sufferers avoid sick leave for headache, it is important to measure time lost due to reduced productivity while working with a headache. The amount of lost work time due to LWDEs is significant. In one study, migraine sufferers lost only 1.1 days due to headache over a 3-month period, but lost three days due to headache-related reduced productivity (Von Korff et al., 1998).

The indirect costs of migraine in a population-based sample of migraine sufferers was estimated using prevalence estimates derived from two existing population-based databases. Assuming that the percentage of people working for pay among migraine sufferers is the same as the general population (i.e., 73% of males and 57% of females), lost productivity costs per year are $690 for males and $1127 for females (Stewart et al., 2003).

Other studies reported the indirect costs of migraine in population-based samples but reported much lower cost estimates. In one study, the total indirect costs were $240 per migraine sufferer per year (Michel et al., 1999). The estimate was lower probably because the number of lost workdays reported by this population was on the low end, and the investigators did not account for LWDEs that would have further increased the estimate. Furthermore, the scale upon which the wages were calculated was not specified. However, since this was a French study, the wages may be different than that used for the studies conducted in the United States.

A second study calculated the cost of lost workdays and household days among a population-based sample of migraine sufferers and a control population. The cost of time missed from paid employment was significantly higher ($p = 0.018$) in the migraine-sufferer group ($477.47) than the control group ($309.90). Among migraine sufferers who were not employed, the average lost productivity cost was $1214.44. In the control population, however, the average lost productivity cost was lower ($912.48). This difference was not statistically significant ($p = 0.174$).

Stewart and colleagues (2003) used data from the American Productivity Audit to estimate the pain-related lost productive time and the associated costs due to headache and other conditions in the US workforce. Overall, 5.4% of the workforce reported lost productive time due to headache (pain in the past 2 weeks). The mean lost productive time for headache was 3.5 hours per week. Lost productive time due to headache was much more common than absenteeism. The cost of lost productive time due to headache is substantial: the total cost of lost productive time due to headache in the US workforce is $20 billion per year, most of which is in the form of reduced productivity while at work (Stewart et al., 2003). For migraine, the total cost of lost productivity is about $13 per year (Hu et al., 1999).

TENSION-TYPE HEADACHE

Overview

In this section we review the prevalence and burden of TTH. Detailed summary tables for prevalence are provided by Stovner et al. (2007).

Prevalence

Estimates for the 1-year period prevalence of TTH vary widely, ranging from 14.3 (Lavados and Tenhamm, 1998) to 93.0 (Rasmussen et al., 1991) for episodic tension-type headache (ETTH) and 0.0 (Tekle Haimanot, et al., 1995; Lavados and Tenhamm, 1998) to 8.1 (Tekle Haimanot et al., 1995) for chronic tension-type headache (CTTH) (Table 4–1). Lifetime prevalences are higher than 1-year period prevalences. Like migraine, variation in prevalence estimates may be due to differences in study methods, case definition and demographic factors, particularly age. While the contribution of these factors to variation in case definition has been studied for migraine, it has not been well studied for TTH.

Rasmussen et al. (1991) conducted the first population study to examine the prevalence of TTH. Potential participants were identified from the Danish National Central Person Registry, and invited to a general health examination, with an emphasis on headache. In this study of 740 subjects, the 1-year period prevalence of ETTH was 74.0%. Since potential subjects were invited to a health exam with an emphasis on headache, this may represent an overestimate. In the United States, Schwartz et al. (1998) examined the epidemiology of ETTH and CTTH based on telephone interview surveys of 13,345 residents of Baltimore County, Maryland. The 1-year period prevalence of ETTH was 38.3%, substantially lower than the Danish study (Rasmussen et al., 1991; Rasmussen, 1992).

In Santiago, Chile, Lavados and Tenhamm (1998) conducted in-person interviews in a representative sample of 1385 adults. Subjects reported details about the type of headache that they suffered from most often. The 1-year prevalence of ETTH was 24.3%. The lower prevalence in this study compared with the US-based study (Schwartz et al., 1998) may be explained by differences in case definition. In Santiago, only the most common type of headache was eligible for classification. In the US-based study, classification based on a single headache type yielded lower prevalence estimates than classification regarding all headache types.

The prevalence of CTTH is markedly lower than that of ETTH. Across studies, 1-year period prevalence estimates range from 1.7% to 2.2% (Rasmussen et al., 1991; Tekle Haimanot, et al., 1995; Lavados and Tenhamm, 1998; Schwartz et al., 1998; Castillo et al., 1999). Overall, 4%–5% of the population report headaches on 15 or more days per month (Rasmussen et al., 1991; Tekle Haimanot et al., 1995; Lavados and Tenhamm, 1998; Schwartz et al., 1998; Castillo et al., 1999).

Prevalence by Gender and Age

The prevalence of ETTH and CTTH varies with gender and age. TTH is slightly more common among women than men. For example, in the United States, 42% of women and 36% of men have ETTH, yielding an overall gender prevalence ratio of 1.16 (Schwartz et al., 1998). Female preponderance occurred at all ages, races, and educational levels. Most studies report a higher prevalence of TTH among women (Rasmussen et al.,1991; Pryse-Phillips et al., 1992; Wong et al., 1995; Barea et al., 1996; Wang et al., 1997; Lavados and Tenhamm, 1998), with female-to-male gender ratios ranging from 1.16 (Schwartz et al., 1998) to 1.9 (Lavados and Tenhamm, 1998).

Female preponderance for CTTH is substantially greater than that of ETTH. For example, in the United States, the prevalence of CTTH was 2.8 in women and 1.4 in men, with an overall gender prevalence ratio of 2.0 (Schwartz et al., 1998). Other studies also report female preponderance in CTTH (Tekle Haimonot et al., 1995; Lavados and Tenhamm, 1998; Castillo et al., 1999). Schwartz et al. (1998) noted that female preponderance in CTTH falls between that of ETTH and migraine and suggested that the gender ratio may imply a biological link to migraine.

The prevalence of TTH may vary by age, although results are inconsistent across studies. Several studies show that prevalence peaks in the 30s and 40s, with a decline thereafter (Pryse-Phillips et al., 1992; Wong et al., 1995; Lavados and Tenhamm, 1998; Schwartz et al., 1998). One study suggested that prevalence decreases with age (Rasmussen et al., 1991). Gobel et al. found no difference in prevalence according to age. The lack of association with age in the study by conducted Gobel et al. (1994) may be attributed to the use of very wide age intervals—in most studies, age is

TABLE 4–1 Prevalence of Very Frequent Headache in Adult Populations (Ordered by date of Publication)

Author (Year of Publication)	*Country*	*N*	*Case Definition*	*Age Range*	*Prevalence (%)*			*F:M*	*Analgesic Overuse (%)*
					Total	*CTTH*	**CM**		
Scher et al. (1998)[23]	US	13,343	15+/month	18–65	4.1	2.2	1.3	1.8	
Castillo et al. (1999)[39]	Spain	1883	15+/month, 4+hours/day	14+	4.7	2.2	2.4	8.7	25
Wang (2000)[22]	China	1533	15+/month, 6+ months	65+	3.9	2.7	1.0	3.1	25
Hagen (2000)[40]	Norway	51,383	15+/month	20+	2.4			1.6	
Ho (2001)[43]	Singapore	2096	>180/year	12+	3.3				
Lu et al. (2001)[26]	Taiwan	3377	15+/month, 4+hours/day	15+	3.2	1.4	1.7	2.3	34
Prencipe (2001)[42]	Italy	833	15+/month	65+	4.4	2.5	1.6	2.4	38
Lantéri-Minet (2003)[41]	France	10,585	Daily	15+	3.0			2.6	
Takeshima (2004)[44]	Japan	5758	CTTH only	20+		2.1			

Abbreviations: CM, chronic migraine (transformed migraine); CTTH, chronic tension-type headache; F:M, female to male prevalence ratio.

Analgesic overuse based on Silberstein[45] criteria.

categorized into 10-year intervals (Rasmussen et al., 1991; Pryse-Phillips et al., 1992; Wong et al., 1995; Lavados and Tenhamm, 1998; Schwartz et al., 1998)—20-year age groupings in this study may have attenuated the relationship to age.

Several authors report that the prevalence of CTTH increases with age (Tekle Haimanot et al., 1995; Lavados and Tenhamm, 1998; Schwartz et al., 1998;). Some individuals may begin with ETTH; headaches may gradually increase over time until criteria for CTTH are met (Merikangas and Frances, 1993; Langemark et al., 1988).

Prevalence by Race and Geographic Region

Geographic and racial differences may account for part of the variation in the prevalence of TTH among studies. Studies have shown prevalence to be highest in the Western Hemisphere (Rasmussen et al., 1991; Pryse-Phillips et al., 1992; Lavados and Tenhamm, 1998; Schwartz et al., 1998) and lowest in Asian countries (Wong et al., 1995).

A US-based study examined TTH prevalence by race (Schwartz et al., 1998). The prevalence of ETTH was found to be significantly higher in Caucasians than in African–Americans in both men (40.1% versus 22.8%) and women (46.8% versus 30.9%). The prevalence of CTTH by race paralleled the observations for ETTH: prevalence was higher in Caucasians than in African–Americans in both men (1.6% versus 1.0%) and women (3.0% versus 2.2%). The explanation for these racial patterns remains uncertain.

Prevalence by SES

The relationship between SES and TTH prevalence varies among studies. Schwartz et al. (1998) used educational level as a measure of SES. ETTH prevalence was directly related to education, peaking in individuals who had a graduate level education (men, 48.5%; women, 48.9%). Similarly, Lavados and Tenhamm (1998) found a direct relation between ETTH prevalence and SES. Other studies, including a German study that used only two educational categories (i.e., basic and secondary) (Gobel et al., 1994), have not found this direct association (Pryse-Phillips et al., 1992; Gobel et al., 1994). Perhaps their analysis lacked sensitivity because they used only two categories. The influence of SES may also vary by country. While migraine prevalence declines with SES, the prevalence of ETTH increases, at least in the United States. These discrepant epidemiologic patterns support the view that migraine and ETTH are nosologically distinct.

CTTH shows a different relationship to SES than ETTH. Two studies reported that the prevalence of CTTH declines with increasing educational level, especially among women (Lavados and Tenhamm, 1998; Schwartz et al., 1998). Though one study found no association (Gobel et al., 1994), this pattern of an inverse relationship is similar to findings in migraine, not ETTH. Schwartz et al. (1998) point out that CTTH, with its higher risk in women and strong relationship to SES, has an epidemiologic profile intermediate between that of ETTH and migraine.

Headache Characteristics by Demographics

The clinical characteristics of TTH are described in Chapter 10. The clinical profile of TTH varies by gender and the most important features will be highlighted herein. Overall, bilateral pain occurs in the majority of TTH sufferers, but it occurs with greater frequency in women than men (Lavados and Tenhamm, 1998). Throbbing pain is common in men (66.4%) and women (56.8%) with ETTH; this feature, often viewed as a hallmark of migraine, poorly discriminates the two disorders. Pressing pain is also frequently reported. Many subjects with TTH report that pain is exacerbated with movement (men 69.8%, women, 75.5%; $p = 0.4$), which is surprising, since pain that is exacerbated by movement is normally associated with migraine rather than TTH. Photophobia or phonophobia is common, especially in women. If both features are present, the diagnosis is not possible, but each feature occurred in isolation with surprising frequency.

Economic Impact

The first population-based study to examine work-loss data in ETTH was reported by Rasmussen et al. (1992) in Denmark. Twelve percent of employed participants were absent from work at least once during the previous year because of ETTH. The majority of those who missed work (68%) were absent for 1–7 days during the previous year. Twenty-five percent were absent between 8 and 14 days during the year, and only 16% were absent more than 14 days during the previous year.

Schwartz et al. (1997, 1998) also measured the impact of headache in the workplace in a study conducted in Baltimore County, Maryland. Inability to function (actual missed work) and reduced ability to function were measured separately. Of the lost work time associated with headache, 19% of missed workdays and 22% of the reduced - effectiveness days were specifically due to ETTH (Schwartz et al., 1997). Among subjects with ETTH, 8.3% reported missed workdays (absenteeism), while 43.6% reported reduced effectiveness days at work due to headache. Among those with missed workdays, an average of 8.9 missed workdays were reported while subjects with reduced effectiveness days reported approximately 5.0 reduced effectiveness days per person. Lavados and Tenhaman (1998) found higher levels of missed work among their sample of TTH sufferers: 25% of men and 38.9% of women reported missed work due to their headaches.

The proportions of subjects with CTTH and ETTH who reported lost and reduced effectiveness days were similar: 11.8% of CTTH sufferers reported lost workdays and 46.5% reported reduced effectiveness days (Schwartz et al., 1997). CTTH sufferers reported lost workdays and reduced effectiveness days more frequently than ETTH sufferers. Subjects with lost workdays reported an average of 27.4 lost workdays per person; subjects with reduced effectiveness days reported approximately 20.4 reduced effectiveness days per person.

EPIDEMIOLOGY OF CDH

The prevalence of CDH has been surprisingly consistent at about 4% of the adult and elderly population. In children, epidemiologic data is limited and case definitions are variable, but the prevalence of very frequent headache in late childhood and adolescence may approach levels seen in adults (Fig. 4–4). In adulthood, CDH is about twice as common in women as compared to men, even in elderly populations.

CDH sub-types. Nomenclature for CDH subtypes is in flux. While recent changes in headache nomenclature have been implemented (Headache Classification Committee of the International Headache Society, 2004, 2006), continuing uncertainty about the role of medication-overuse in the etiology of CDH as well as diagnostic (and possibly etiologic) overlap between the CDH subtypes continues to make definition and application of standardized nomenclature of these disorders difficult. In this chapter, we will use Silberstein–Lipton criteria because most published studies use variants of these criteria (Silberstein et al., 1996). Fortunately, agreement between Silberstein–Lipton criteria and the new chronic migraine criteria is high.

Most people with CDH have either chronic tension-type or transformed migraine headaches, but this term also includes rare headache syndromes including hemicrania continua as well as new daily persistent headache (NDPH) and chronic disorders of short duration. In population studies, chronic TTH and CDH with migrainous features are equally common (Fig. 4–5). In contrast, the vast majority of CDH patients in subspecialty care begins with a history of migraine or continue to have migraine features; this has lead to the perception that CDH is a complication (e.g., mediated through medication overuse) or natural progression of episodic migraine (Mathew et al., 1982, 1987).

Socioeconomic status. CDH appears to be more common in individuals with low SES (Scher, Stewart et al., 1998; Wang et al., 2000; Lu, et al., 2001; Scher, Stewart et al., 2003). In a US-based case–control study, the risk of CDH was elevated in those with less than high school education relative to those with graduate-level education [OR = 3.35 (2.1–5.3)] (Scher, Stewart et al., 2003). In a Norwegian population study, Hagen et al. found that the risk of CDH for those with low education (<10 years) was elevated relative to those with high education (13+ years of education) for both women [relative risk (RR) = 2.4 (1.1–4.9)] and men [RR = 1.6 (1.1–2.1)]. Similar results were seen for low social class, for women [RR = 2.6 (1.5–4.6)] and men [RR = 1.4 (1.0–2.0)], and for low income, for men [RR = 1.8 (1.2–2.7)] but not for women [RR = 0.9 (0.6–1.4)].

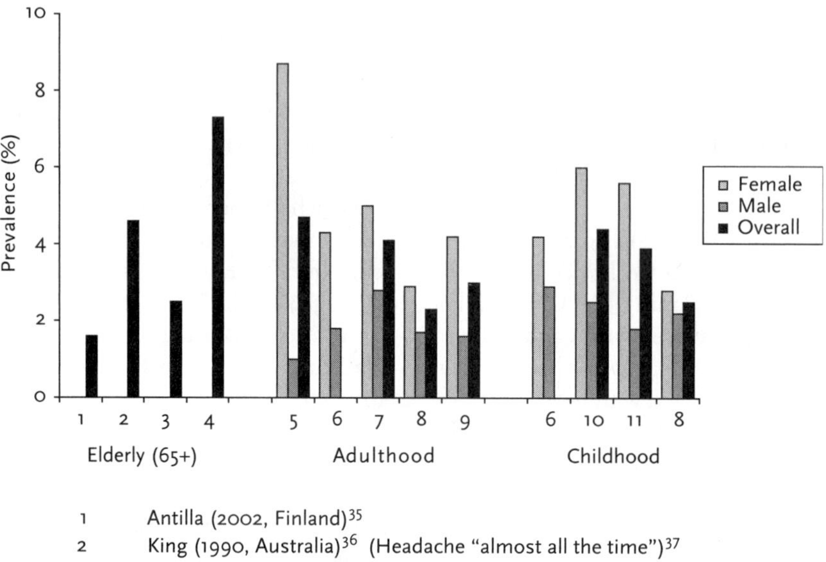

1 Antilla (2002, Finland)[35]
2 King (1990, Australia)[36] (Headache "almost all the time")[37]
3 Kristánsdóttir (1993, Iceland) (Headache "almost daily or daily")
4 Rhee (2000, US)[38] (Headache "Almost every day" or "every day")
5 Castillo (1999, Spain)[39]
6 Lu (2001, Taiwan)[26]
7 Scher (1998, US)[23]
8 Hagen (2000, Norway)[40] (Data extracted)
9 Lanteri-Minet (2003, France)[41]
10 Prencipe (2001, Italy)[42]
11 Wang (1999, Kinmen Island)[22]

Figure 4–4 Prevalence of chronic daily headache or frequent headache in population studies by age. 1, Antilla (2002, Finland); 2, King (1990, Australia) (Headache "almost all the time"); 3, Kristánsdóttir (1993, Iceland) (Headache "almost daily or daily"); 4, Rhee (2000, US) (Headache "Almost every day" or "every day"); 5, Castillo (1999, Spain); 6, Lu (2001, Taiwan); 7, Scher et al. (1998, US); 8, Hagen (2000, Norway) (Data extracted); 9, Lanteri-Minet (2003, France); 10, Prencipe (2001, Italy); 11, Wang (2000, Kinmen Island).

Sleep apnea has long been viewed as a headache-aggravating factor. This is supported by a case–control study showing that CDH cases were more likely to be habitual (daily) snorers than episodic headache controls (Scher et al., 2003). CDH cases were also more likely to report sleep problems and to be either short or long sleepers [unpublished data from (Scher et al., 2003)]. This association between CDH and habitual snoring was neither explained by cardiovascular factors associated with sleep-disordered breathing [e.g., increasing age, male gender, hypertension, body-mass index (BMI)], nor was it explained by potential confounders such as caffeine consumption, hypertension, or depression.

Stressful life eventswere found to be associated with CDH onset in a case–control study (Stewart et al., 2001). Cases and controls were interviewed about the occurrence of specific life events (moves, job changes, child-related changes, changes in marital status, deaths in the family or of close friends, and ongoing "extremely stressful" life events) in the time before CDH onset up to the present time. Events were divided into pre-CDH events and post-CDH events, with a randomly generated year corresponding to CDH onset for the cases used for the controls. Overall, cases reported more pre-CDH events than the controls (2.7 versus 2.0, $p < 0.001$, rank-sum test). No difference was found for post-CDH events, strengthening a causal interpretation.

A large study based on adolescent students from Taiwan measured the presence of childhood stressors (e.g., parental divorce, child abuse, etc.)

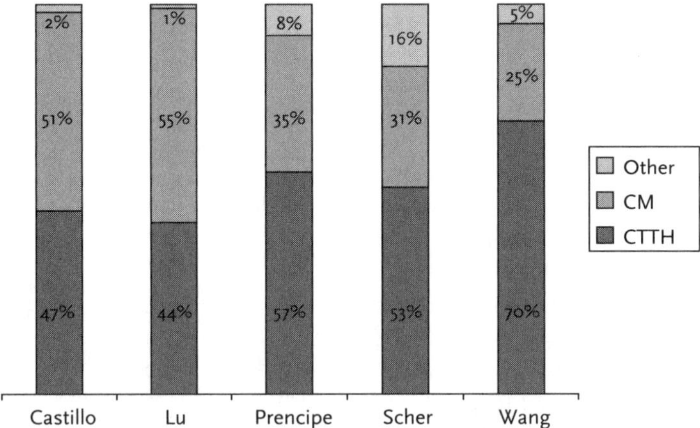

Tension-Type Headache, and Other Chronic Daily Headache

Figure 4–5 Proportion of chronic daily headache sufferers with chronic migraine, chronic tension-type headache, and other chronic daily headache. CM, chronic migraine (transformed migraine); CTTH, chronic tension-type headache.

using the Global Family Environment Scale and compared scores between students with CDH and a control group (Juang et al., 2004). They found that the CDH students had about a 10% higher score on this scale—suggesting that the presence of these negative life events might be involved in the onset of adolescent CDH. In addition, head and neck injury and high headache frequency have been associated with progression to CDH (Scher et al., 2003; Couch et al., 2007).

Prognosis and Natural History

Results from three population-based studies suggest that rates of remission are high in CDH. In a US-based population sample, more than one-half (60%) of CDH cases at baseline had remitted to less than 180 headache days per year at follow-up, although remission to a more "normal" headache frequency, of <1 headache per week, was much less common (16%) (Scher et al., 2003). Individuals with more frequent headaches at baseline were at higher risk of incident CDH at follow-up, and individuals with less frequent CDH had a higher likelihood of remission at follow-up. While this finding is somewhat tautologic (because those with more frequent headache are closer to being cases than those with infrequent headaches), it may be that higher vigilance is warranted to prevent headache progression in those who are already headache-prone. A similar remission rate was reported in Taiwan (65% remitted to fewer than 15 headaches per month after 2 years) (Lu et al., 2001), although remission was lower in an elderly Chinese population (33% had remitted over a 4-year period) (Wang et al., 2000). A German clinic-based study of migraine sufferers found a 1 year incidence rate for CDH of 14% (Katsarava et al., 2004). Estimates may be higher than in the US-based study because the clinic-based sample has more severe disease, or because migraine itself is a risk factor.

Other prognostic factors were associated with an increased risk of CDH and a reduced risk of remission. In the US-based study, women, whites, those of lower levels of educational achievement, and the previously married (e.g., widowed, divorced, or separated) were at increased risk of CDH at baseline and at reduced risk of remission at follow-up (Scher et al., 2003). Obesity, defined as a BMI ⩾30, was predictive of 1-year CDH incidence in this population. The reason why obesity would predispose individuals to headache progression is uncertain. Subsequent studies have shown that obesity is associated with increased frequency of attacks among migraine sufferers (Bigal et al., 2006), that the prevalence of transformed migraine increases with BMI (Bigal and Lipton, 2006), and that the link is between obesity and migraine progression and not with headaches overall (Bigal, Tsang, et al., 2007).

Medication use as a prognostic factor: two prospective studies from Asia show that CDH sufferers with medication overuse had a worse prognosis at follow-up than CDH sufferers without medication overuse. Lu et al. followed 106 CDH sufferers for 2 years. Of these, 36 (34%) overused medication at baseline. After 2 years of follow-up, 18/36 (50%) of those who overused medication had persistent CDH versus 19/70 (27%) of the nonusers (RR = 1.8, 95% confidence interval (CI): 1.1–3.1). Among 60 elderly CDH sufferers studied, 15 (25%) overused medication. At follow-up at least 2 years later, 14/15 (93%) of overusers and 21/37 (57%) of nonoverusers had persistent CDH (RR = 1.6, 95% CI: 1.2–2.3). In the clinic-based German study, medication overuse predicted incident CDH in episodic migraine specialty patients, even after adjusting for baseline headache frequency (Katsarava et al., 2004). In effect, these studies suggest that medication overuse is associated witha worse prognosis. They did not distinguish between medication overuse as a cause of CDH or a marker for headache intractability.

Zwart et al. interviewed a large population-based sample twice over a 10-year period. Individuals who used analgesics daily or weekly at baseline were more likely to have chronic pain at follow-up compared to individuals who used analgesics less than once a week. Reasons for medication use at baseline were not assessed. Headache frequency at baseline (and the "at-risk" population for CDH) was also not assessed. These interesting results do not support the hypothesis that CDH sufferers overusing medication have a worse prognosis than CDH sufferers not habituated to medication overuse, since individuals with CDH were not identified in the baseline survey.

References

Abu-Arefeh, I and Russell, G (1994). Prevalence of headache and migraine in schoolchildren. *BMJ*, 309:765–769.

Anttila, P, Metashonkala, L, Aromma, M, et al. (2002). Determinants of tension-type headache in children. *Cephalalgia*, 22;401–408.

Barea, LM, Tannhauser, M, Rotta, NT (1996). An epidemiologic study of headache among children and adolescents of southern Brazil. *Cephalalgia*, 8;545–549.

Bigal, ME, Liberman, JN, and Lipton, RB (2006). Obesity and migraine: a population study. *Neurology*, 66 (4):545–550.

Bigal, ME and Lipton, RB (2006). Obesity is a risk factor for transformed migraine but not for chronic tension-type headache. *Neurology*, 67:252–257.

Bigal, ME, Lipton, RB, Winner, P, et al. (2007). Epidemiology, burden, and patterns of treatment for adolescents in the United States. *Neurology*, 69;16–25.

Bigal, ME, Tsang, A, Loder, E, et al. (2007). Body mass index and primary headaches. The AMPP study. *Arch Intern Med* (in press).

Bigal, ME, Lipton, RB, Winner, P, Reed, ML, Diamond, S, Stewart, WF (2007). Migraine in adolescents: association with socioeconomic status and family history. *Neurology*, 69;16–25.

Bille, B (1989). Migraine in children: prevalence, clinical features, and a 30-year follow up. In *Migraine and Other Headaches* (MD Ferrari and X Lataste, eds.), pp. 29–38. Parthenon, Carnforth, UK.

Breslau, N, Chilcoat, HD, and Andreski, P (1996). Further evidence on the link between migraine and neuroticism. *Neurology*, 47:663–667.

Castillo, J, Munoz, P, Guitera, V, Pascual, J (1999). Epidemiology of chronic daily headache in the general population. *Headache*, 39;190–196.

Castillo, J, Munoz, P, Guitera, V, Pascual, J (1999). Kaplan Award 1998: Epidemiology of headache in the general population. *Headache*, 39;190–196.

Clouse, JC and Osterhaus, JT (1994). Healthcare resource use and costs associated with migraine in a managed healthcare setting. *Ann Pharmacother*, 28:659–664.

Couch, JR, Lipton, RB, Stewart, WF, Scher, AI (2007). Head and neck injury (HANI) as a risk factor for developement of chronic daily headache (CDH): a population-based study. *Neurology*, 68;A89.

Edmeads, J, Findlay, H, Tugwell, P, et al. (1993). Impact of migraine and tension-type headache on life-style, consulting behaviour, and medication use: a Canadian population survey. *Can J Neurol Sci*, 20:131–137.

Edmeads, J and Mackell, JA (2002). The economic impact of migraine: an analysis of direct and indirect costs. *Headache*, 42:501–509.

Gobel, H, Petersen-Braun, M, and Soyka, D (1994). The epidemiology of headache in Germany: a nationwide survey of a representative sample on the basis of the headache classification of the International Headache Society. *Cephalalgia*, 14:97–106.

Hagen, Z, Zwart, JA, Vatten, L, Stovner, LJ, Bovim, G (2000). Prevalence of migraine and non-migrainous headache–head-HUNT: a large population-based study. *Cephalalgia*, 20;900–906.

Headache Classification Subcommittee of the International Headache Society (2004). Classification of headache disorders: 2nd edition. *Cephalalgia*, 24:9–150.

Headache Classification Committee; Olesen, J, Bousser, MG, Diener, HC (2006). New appendix criteria open for a broader concept of chronic migraine. *Cephalalgia*, 26(6):742–746.

Ho, KH, Ong, BK (2001). Headache characteristics and race in Singapors: results of a randomized national survey. *Headache*, 41;279–284.

Holmes, WF, MacGregor, EA, and Dodick, D (2001). Migraine-related disability: impact and implications for sufferers' lives and clinical issues. *Neurology*, 56: S13–S19.

Hu, XH, Markson, LE, Lipton, RB, et al. (1999). Burden of migraine in the United States: disability and economic costs. *Arch Intern Med*, 159:813–818.

Juang, KD, Wang, SJ, Fuh, JL et al. (2004). Association between adolescent chronic daily headache and childhood adversity: a community-based study. *Cephalalgia*, 24:54–59.

Katsarava, Z, Schneeweiss, S, Kurth, T, et al. (2004). Incidence and predictors for chronicity of headache in patients with episodic migraine. *Neurology*, 62 (5):788–790.

King, NJ, Sharpley, CF (1990). Headache activity in children and adolescents. *J Paediatr Child Health*, 26;50–54.

Kristansdottir, G, Wahlberg, V (1993). Sociodemographic differences in the prevalence of self-reported headache in Icelandic school-children. *Headache*, 33;376–380.

Kryst, S and Scherl, ER (1994). Social and personal impact of headache in Kentucky. In *Headache Classification and Epidemiology* (J Olesen, ed.), pp. 345–350. Raven Press, New York.

Langemark, M, Olesen, J, Poulsen, DL, Bech, P (1998). Clinical characterization of patients with chronic tension headache. *Headache*, 28;590–596.

Lanteri-Minet, M, Auray, JP, El Hasnaoui, A, Dartigues, JF, Duru, G, Henry, P, Lucas, C, Pradalier, A, Chazot, G, Gaudin, AF (2003). Prevalence and description of chronic daily headache in the general population in France. *Pain*, 102;143–149.

Launer, LJ, Terwindt, GM, and Ferrari MD (1999). The prevalence and characteristics of migraine in a population-based cohort: the GEM study. *Neurology*, 53:537–542.

Lavados, PM, Tenham, E (1998). Epidemiology of tension-type headache in Santiago, Chile: a prevalence study. *Cephalalgia*, 8;552–558.

Lipton, RB, Bigal, ME, Kolodner, K, et al. (2003). The family impact of migraine: population-based studies in the USA and UK. *Cephalalgia*, 23:429–440.

Lipton, RB, Diamond, D, Freitag, F, et al. (2005). Migraine prevention patterns in a community sample. Results from the American Migraine Prevalence and Prevention (AMPP) study. *Headache*, 45:792.

Lipton, RB, Liberman, JN, Kolodner, KB, et al. (1999). Migraine headache disability and quality of life: a population-based case-control study. *Headache*, 39:365.

Lipton, RB, Diamond, S, Reed, M, et al. (2001). Migraine diagnosis and treatment: results from the American Migraine Study II. *Headache*, 41(7):638–645.

Lipton, RB, Stewart, WF, Diamond, S, et al. (2001). Prevalence and burden of migraine in the United States: data from the American Migraine Study II. *Headache*, 41:646–657.

Lipton, RB, Scher, AI, Kolodner, K, et al. (2002). Migraine in the United States: epidemiology and patterns of health care use. *Neurology*, 58:885–894.

Lipton, RB, Stewart, WF, Kolodner, K, et al. (1999). Epidemiology and patterns of healthcare use for migraine in the United States. *Headache*, 39:363–364.

Lipton, RB, Stewart, WF, and Simon, D (1998). Medical consultation for migraine: results of the American Migraine Study. *Headache*, 38:87–96.

Lipton, RB, Bigal, ME, Diamond, M, et al.; AMPP Advisory Group (2007). Migraine prevalence, disease burden, and the need for preventive therapy. *Neurology*, 68 (5):343–349.

Lu, SR, Fuh, JL, Chen, WT, et al. (2001). Chronic daily headache in Taipei, Taiwan: prevalence, follow-up and outcome predictors. *Cephalalgia*, 21(10):980–986.

Lyngberg, A, Jensen, R, Rasmussen, BK, et al. (2003). Incidence of migraine in a Danish population-based follow-up study [abstract]. *Cephalalgia*, 23:596.

Mathew, NT, Stubits, E, and Nigam, MP (1982). Transformation of episodic migraine into daily headache: analysis of factors. *Headache*, 22(2):66–68.

Mathew, NT, Reuveni, U, and Perez, F (1987). Transformed or evolutive migraine. *Headache*, 27(2):102–106.

Merikangas, KR, Frances, A (1993). Development of diagnostic criteria for headache syndromes: lessons from psychiatry. *Cephalalgia*, 13;34–38.

Michel, P, Dartigues, JF, Duru, G, et al. (1999). Incremental absenteeism due to headache in migraine: results from the Mig-Access French national cohort. *Cephalalgia*, 19:503–510.

Mortimer, MJ, Kay, J, and Jaron, A (1992). Epidemiology of headache and childhood migraine in an urban general practice using Ad Hoc, Vahlquist and IHS criteria. *Dev Med Child Neurol*, 34:1095–1101.

Osterhaus, JT, Gutterman, DL, and Plachetka, JR (1992). Healthcare resource and lost labour costs of migraine headache in the US. *Pharmacoeconomics*, 2:67–76.

Prencipe, M, Casini, AR, Ferretti, C et al. (2001). Prevalence of headache in an elderly population: attack frequency, disability, and use of medication. *J Neurol Neurosurg Psychiat*, 70;377–381.

Pryse-Phillips, W, Findlay, H, Tugwell, P, Edmeads, J, Nelson, RF (1992). *J Neurol Sci*, 19;333–339.

Raieli, V, Raimondo, D, Cammalleri, R, et al. (1995). Migraine headaches in adolescents: a student population-based study in Montreale. *Cephalalgia*, 15:5–12.

Rasmussen, B, Jensen, R, Olesen, J (1991). A population-based analysis of the diagnostic criteria of the International Headache Society. *Cephalalgia*, 11;129.

Rasmussen, B (1992). Migraine and tension-type headache in a general population: sychosocial factors. *Int J Epidemiol*, 21;1138–1143.

Rhee, H (2000). Prevalence and predictors of headaches in US adolescents. *Headache*, 40;528–538.

Scher, AI, Stewart, WF, Liberman, J, et al. (1998). Wolff Award 1998. Prevalence of frequent headache in a population sample. *Headache*, 38:497–506.

Scher, AI, Stewart, WF, and Lipton, RB (1999). Migraine and headache: a meta-analytic approach. In

Epidemiology of Pain (IK Crombie, PR Croft, and SJ Linton, eds.), pp. 159–170. IASP Press, Seattle.

Scher, AI, Liptonm, RB, and Stewart, WF (2003). Habitual snoring as a risk factor for chronic daily headache. *Neurology*, 60(8):1366.

Scher, AI, Stewart, WF, Ricci, JA, et al. (2003). Factors associated with the onset and remission of chronic daily headache in a population-based study. *Pain*, 106 (1–2):81–89.

Schwartz, BS, Stewart, WF, Lipton, RB (1997). Lost workdays and decreased work effectiveness associated with headache in the workplace. *J Occup Environ Med*, 32;320–327.

Schwartz, BS, Stewart, WF, Simon, D, et al. (1998). The epidemiology of tension type headache. *JAMA*, 279:381–383.

Silberstein, SD, Lipton, RB, and Sliwinski, M (1996). Classification of daily and near-daily headaches: field trial of revised IHS criteria. *Neurology*, 47(4):871–875.

Smith, R (1998). Impact of migraine on the family. *Headache*, 38:423–426.

Stang, PE and Osterhaus, JT (1993). Impact of migraine in the United States: data from the National Health Interview Survey. *Headache*, 33:29–35.

Stang, PE, Yanagihara, PA, Swanson, JW, et al. (1992). Incidence of migraine headache: a population-based study in Olmstead County, Minnesota. *Neurology*, 42:1657–1662.

Steiner, TJ, Scher, AI, Stewart, WF, et al. (2003). The prevalence and disability burden of adult migraine in England and their relationships to age, gender and ethnicity. *Cephalalgia*, 23:519–527.

Stewart, WF, Linet, MS, Celentano, DD, et al. (1991). Age- and sex-specific incidence rates of migraine with and without visual aura. *Am J Epidemiol*, 134:1111–1120.

Stewart, WF, Lipton, RB, Celentano, DD, et al. (1992). Prevalence of migraine headache in the United States. Relation to age, income, race, and other sociodemographic factors. *JAMA*, 267:64–69.

Stewart, WF, Lipton, RB, and Liberman, J (1996). Variation in migraine prevalence by race. *Neurology*, 47:52–59.

Stewart, WF, Scher, AI, and Lipton, RB (2001). The Frequent Headache Epidemiology study (FrHE): stressful life events and risk of chronic daily headache. *Neurology*, 56(8):A138–A139.

Stewart, WF, Ricci, JA, Chee, E, et al. (2003). Lost productive time and cost due to common pain conditions in the US workforce. *JAMA*, 290:2443–2454.

Stovner, LJ, Hagen, K, Jensen, R, Katsarava, Z, Lipton, R, Scher, A, Steiner, T, Zwart, JA (2007). The global burden of headache: a documentation of headache prevalence and disability worldwide. *Cephalalgia*, 27:193–210.

Takeshima, T, Tshizaki, K, Fukuhara, Y, Ijiri, T, Kusumi, M, et al. (2004). Population-based door-to-door survey of migraine in Japan: the Daisen study. *Headache*, 44:18–19.

Tekle Haimanot, R, Seraw, B, Forsgren, L, et al. (1995). Migraine, chronic tension-type headache, and cluster headache in an Ethiopian rural community. *Cephalalgia*, 15:482–488.

Von Korff, M, Stewart, WF, and Lipton, RB (1994). Assessing headache severity. New directions. *Neurology*, 44: S40–S46.

Von Korff, M, Stewart, WF, Simon, DJ, et al. (1998). Migraine and reduced work performance: a population-based diary study. *Neurology*, 50:1741–1745.

Wang, SJ, Fuh, JL, Lu, SR, Liu, CY, Hsu, LC, Wang, PN, Liu, HC (1997). *Neurology*, 49; 195–200.

Wang, SJ, Fuh, JL, Lu, SR, et al. (2000). Chronic daily headache in Chinese elderly: Prevalence, risk factors, and biannual follow-up. *Neurology*, 54:314–319.

Wong, TW, Wong, KS, Yu, TS, Kay, R (1995). Prevalence of migraine and other headaches in Hong Kong. *Neuroepidemiology*, 14;82–91.

5 Neuroimaging and Other Diagnostic Testing in Headache

Randolph W Evans, Todd D Rozen, and Laszlo Mechtler

Most patients with headache can be diagnosed simply from a good history and general and neurologic examinations. In some cases, however, diagnostic testing is necessary to distinguish primary causes from secondary ones which may share similar features. The differential diagnosis of headache is one of the longest in all of medicine with more than 300 different types and causes. In this chapter, we discuss the reasons for diagnostic testing, indications for neuroimaging, electroencephalography (EEG), lumbar puncture (LP), and clinical laboratory studies. We also review diagnostic testing in adults and children with a normal neurologic examination, migraine, first or worst headaches, and those over the age of 50.

REASONS FOR DIAGNOSTIC TESTING

Authorities differ over general indications for diagnostic testing. According to Saper and colleagues, "In general, we believe that most patients with recurring, frequent headache will require some neurodiagnostic testing" (Saper et al., 1999). According to Lance and Goadsby, "Only a few headache patients require investigation beyond a careful history and physical examination" (Lance and Goadsby, 2005). The indications for diagnostic testing are variable and the neurologist must make decisions on a case-by-case basis. Clinical situations where neurologists consider diagnostic testing are listed in Table 5–1.

There are many other reasons why neurologists recommend diagnostic testing: "our stubborn quest for diagnostic certainty" (Kassirer, 1989); faulty cognitive reasoning; the medical decision rule where it is better to impute disease than to risk overlooking it; busy practice conditions where tests are ordered as a shortcut; patient expectations; financial incentives; professional peer pressure where recommendations for routine and esoteric tests are expected as a demonstration of competence; and medico-legal issues (Woolf and Kamerow, 1990; Beresford, 1999). The attitudes and demands of patients and families and the practice of defensive medicine are especially important reasons in the case of headaches. In the era of managed care, equally compelling reasons for not ordering diagnostic studies include physician fears of de-selection and capitation. Lack of funds and underinsurance continue to be barriers for appropriate diagnostic testing for many patients.

DIAGNOSTIC TESTING OPTIONS

Brain CT Versus MRI

Computerized tomography (CT) will detect most abnormalities that may cause headaches. CT is generally preferred over magnetic resonance imagery (MRI) for the evaluation of acute subarachnoid hemorrhage (SAH), acute head trauma, and bony abnormalities; however, there are a number of disorders that may be missed on routine CT of the head including vascular disease, neoplastic disease, cervico-medullary lesions, and infections (Table 5–2). MRI is more sensitive than CT in the detection of posterior fossa and cervicomedullary lesions, ischemia, white matter abnormalities (WMAs), cerebral venous thrombosis (CVT), subdural and epidural hematomas, neoplasms (especially in the posterior fossa), meningeal disease [such as carcinomatosis, diffuse meningeal enhancement in low cerebrospinal fluid (CSF) pressure syndrome, and sarcoid], and cerebritis and brain abscess,

Table 5–1 Reasons to Consider Neuroimaging for Headaches.

Temporal profile and headache features
1. The "first or worst" headache
2. Subacute headaches with increasing frequency or severity
3. A progressive or new daily persistent headache
4. Chronic daily headache
5. Headaches always on the same side
6. Headaches not responding to treatment

Demographics
7. New onset headaches in patients who have cancer or who test positive for HIV infection
8. New onset headaches after age 50
9. Patients with headaches and seizures

Associated symptoms and signs
10. Headaches associated with symptoms and signs such as fever, stiff neck, nausea, and vomiting
11. Headaches other than migraine with aura associated with focal neurologic symptoms or signs
12. Headaches associated with papilledema, cognitive impairment, or personality change

Source: With permission from Evans, RW (1999). Headaches. In *Diagnostic Testing in Neurology* (RW Evans, ed.), p. 2. WB Saunders, Philadelphia.

Table 5–2 Causes of Headache that can be Missed on Routine CT Scan of the Head.

Vascular disease
- Saccular aneurysms
- Arteriovenous malformations (especially posterior fossa)
- Subarachnoid hemorrhage
- Carotid or vertebral artery dissections
- Infarcts
- Cerebral venous thrombosis
- Vasculitis
- White matter abnormalities
- Subdural and epidural hematomas

Neoplastic disease
- Neoplasms (especially in the posterior fossa)
- Meningeal carcinomatosis
- Pituitary tumor and hemorrhage

Cervicomedullary lesions
- Chiari malformations
- Foramen magnum meningioma

Infections
- Paranasal sinusitis
- Meningoencephalitis
- Cerebritis and brain abscess

Other
- Low cerebrospinal fluid pressure syndrome
- Idiopathic hypertrophic pachymeningitis

Source: Modified with permission from Evans, RW (1999). Headaches. In *Diagnostic Testing in Neurology* (RW Evans, ed.), p. 3. WB Saunders, Philadelphia.

and low-pressure headache from a CSF leak. Pituitary pathology is more likely to be detected on MRI of the brain than a CT.

As the cost of MRI has decreased, MRI is generally preferred over CT for the evaluation of headaches. The yield of MRI may vary depending on the field strength of the magnetic, the use of paramagnetic contrast, the selection of acquisition sequences, and the use of magnetic resonance angiography (as discussed later in this chapter) and venography. However, MRI may be contraindicated (e.g., the presence of an aneurysm clip or pacemaker). In addition, about 8% of patients are claustrophobic, and of this group, about 2% are unable to tolerate the study.

Neuroimaging During Pregnancy

When there are appropriate indications, neuroimaging should be performed during pregnancy. With the use of lead shielding, a standard CT scan of the head exposes the uterus to less than 1 mrad. A radiation dose of 15 rad is necessary to cause deformities that might justify pregnancy termination. MRI is more sensitive to rare disorders that may occur during pregnancy such as pituitary apoplexy (Fig. 5–1), cerebral venous sinus thrombosis (with the addition of MR venography), and metastatic choriocarcinoma. There is no known risk of MRI during pregnancy but there is some controversy because the magnets induce an electric field and slightly raise the core temperature (<1°C.). A survey of pregnant MRI workers found no adverse fetal outcome (Kanal et al., 1993); no adverse fetal effects from MRI have been documented to date. It is generally accepted that MRI, like all imaging techniques, should be used judiciously in pregnant patients when benefits outweigh risks (Birchard et al., 2005). Although there is no known risk of intravenous contrast for CT scan or gadolinium for MRI, contrast and gadolinium should be avoided if possible. The radiation dose for a typical cervical or intracranial arteriogram is less than 1 mrad. The American College of Obstetricians and Gynecologists' guidelines on the use of diagnostic imaging modalities during pregnancy state that MRI is not associated with known adverse fetal defects; however, they recommend avoiding use of contrast agents unless medically necessary for the mother (see Fig. 5–1).

Electroencephalography

The EEG was a standard test for the evaluation of headaches in the pre-CT era. Gronseth and Greenberg (1995) reviewed the literature from 1941 to 1994 on the utility of EEG in the evaluation of patients with headache. Most of the articles had serious methodologic flaws. The only significant abnormality reported in studies with a reasonable design was prominent driving in response to photic stimulation ("The H-response") in migraineurs with sensitivity ranging from 26% (Rowan, 1974) to 100% (Simon, 1982) and specificity from 80% (Smyth, 1964) to 91% (Simon, 1982). This finding, while interesting, is not necessary for the clinical diagnosis of migraine. If the purpose of the EEG is to exclude an underlying structural lesion such as a neoplasm, CT or MRI imaging is far superior.

The report of the Quality Standards Subcommittee of the AAN suggests the following practice parameter: "The electroencephalogram (EEG) is not useful in the routine evaluation of patients with headache. This does not exclude the use of EEG to evaluate headache patients with associated symptoms suggesting a seizure disorder such as atypical migrainous aura or episodic loss of consciousness. Assuming head imaging capabilities are readily available, EEG is not recommended to exclude a structural cause for headache" (American Academy of Neurology, 1995).

A report of the Quality Standards Subcommittee of the American Academy of Neurology and the Practice Committee of the Child Neurology Society (Lewis et al., 2002) makes the following pediatric recommendations: "EEG is not recommended in the routine evaluation of a child with recurrent headaches, as it is unlikely to provide an etiology, improve diagnostic yield, or distinguish migraine from other types of headache (Level C; class II and class III evidence)."

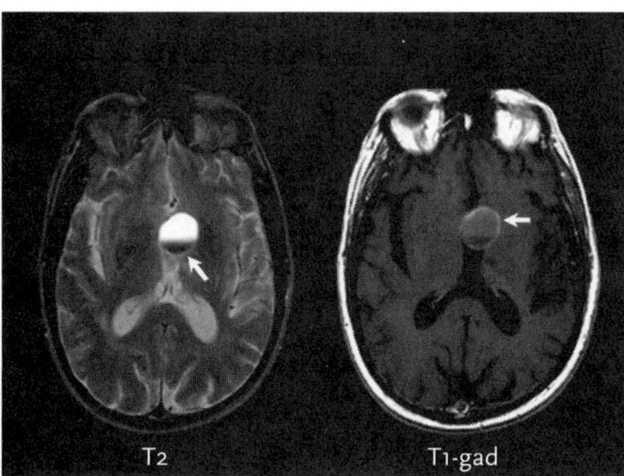

Figure 5–1 Pituitary apoplexy in the third trimester of a 34-year-old woman with acute onset of the worst headache of her life.

Lumbar Puncture

MRI or CT scan is always performed before a LP for the evaluation of headaches except in some cases where acute meningitis is suspected. LP can be diagnostic for meningitis or encephalitis, meningeal carcinomatosis or lymphomatosis, SAH, and high (e.g., idiopathic intracranial hypertension/pseudotumor cerebri) or low CSF pressure. In cases of blood dyscrasias, the platelet count should be 50,000 or greater before safely performing the LP and the INR should be less than 1.7 in patients using warfarin. The CSF opening pressure should always be measured when investigating headaches. When measuring the opening pressure, it is important for the patient to be in a lateral decubitus position, relaxed and have the head and legs at least partially extended to avoid recording a falsely elevated pressure.

After neuroimaging, as discussed, examples where LP is often indicated include the following: the first or worst headache; headache with fever or other symptoms or signs suggesting an infectious cause; a subacute or progressive headache [e.g., a human immunodeficiency virus (HIV) positive patient or a person with carcinoma]; an atypical chronic headache (e.g., to rule out pseudotumor cerebri in an obese woman without papilledema); and a headache that has not responded to typical medication regimes.

There are numerous potential complications of LP, the most common being low CSF pressure headache, which occurs in about 30% of cases when the conventional bevel-tipped or Quincke needle is used (Evans, 2006). The risk of headache can be dramatically reduced to about 5%–10% by using an atraumatic needle such as the Sprotte or Whitacre and replacing the stylet before withdrawing the needle (Armon and Evans, 2005).

Blood Tests

Blood tests are generally not helpful for the diagnosis of headaches; however, there are numerous indications where blood tests may strongly support a clinical diagnosis, including the following: erythrocyte sedimentation rate or C-reactive protein to consider the possibility of giant cell arteritis; erthyrocyte sedimentation rate, rheumatoid factor, and antinuclear antibody in a patient with headache and arthralgias to evaluate for possible collagen vascular diseases such as lupus (Amit et al., 1999); a monospot in a teenager with headaches, sore throat, and cervical adenopathy; a complete blood count (CBC), liver function tests, HIV test, or Lyme antibody in some patients with a suspected infectious cause for headache; an anticardiolipin antibody and lupus anticoagulant in a migraineur with extensive WMAs on MRI; a thyroid-stimulating hormone (TSH), since headache may be a symptom in 14% of cases of hypothyroidism; and hyperthyroidism is a contraindication to ergotamine therapy. Tests may include a CBC, since headache may be a symptom when the hemoglobin concentration is reduced by one-half or more; blood urea nitrogen and creatinine to exclude renal failure which can cause headache; serum calcium, since hypercalcemia can be associated with headaches; CBC and platelets, because thrombotic thrombocytopenic purpura can cause headaches; and endocrine studies, in a patient with headaches and a pituitary tumor. Coagulopathy testing should always be considered in headache patients who develop stroke-like spells along with their pain or who have prolonged aura. Testing should include the following: lupus anticoagulant, anticardiolipin antibodies, Protein C and S, antithrombin III, factor V Leiden, prothrombin gene 20210 mutation analysis, activated protein C resistance, homocysteine, and polymorphisms of methylenetetrahydrofolate reductase Additionally, blood tests may be indicated as a baseline and for monitoring for certain medications such as valproic acid for migraine prophylaxis, carbamazepine for trigeminal neuralgia, and lithium for chronic cluster headaches.

Blood or urine toxicology screens should be completed in patients who present on multiple medications including opioids or butalbital-containing compounds or in those who have seen multiple physicians for their headaches. Sadly, some chronic headache patients do not divulge their entire medication list or if they are using illicit substances.

HEADACHES AND A NORMAL NEUROLOGIC EXAMINATION

Neuroimaging Studies in Adults

The yield of abnormal neuroimaging in studies of patients with headaches as the only neurologic symptom and normal neurologic examinations depends upon a number of factors including the duration of the headache, study design (prospective versus retrospective), who orders the scan, and the type of scan performed (Frishberg, 1994). The percentage of abnormal scans is higher when ordered by neurologists (Baker, 1983) or a tertiary care center (Laffey, 1978) compared with primary care physicians and represents case selection bias. In reported computerized axial tomography (CT scan) series, the yield may vary depending upon the generation of scanner and whether iodinated contrast was used. The yield of MRI may vary depending upon the field strength of the magnet, the use of paramagnetic contrast, the selection of acquisition sequences, and the use of magnetic resonance angiography.

Frishberg (1994) reviewed eight CT scan studies of 1825 patients with unspecified headache types and varying durations of headache (Carrera et al., 1977; Laffey et al., 1978; Russell et al., 1978; Sargent et al., 1979; Larson et al., 1980; Baker, 1983; Weingarten et al., 1992; Mitchell et al., 1993). The summarized findings from these studies is combined with four additional studies of 1566 CT scans in patients with headache and normal neurologic examinations (Sotaniemi et al., 1991; Dumas et al., 1994; Akpek et al., 1995; Demaerel et al., 1996) for a total of 3389 scans. The overall percentages of various pathologies are as follows: brain tumors, 1%; arteriovenous malformations (AVMs), 0.2%; hydrocephalus, 0.3%; aneurysm, 0.1%; subdural hematoma, 0.2%; and strokes (including chronic ischemic process), 1.1%.

There are four studies of patients with chronic headaches and a normal neurologic examination. Combining three of these studies with 1282 patients, the only clinically significant pathology was one low-grade glioma and one saccular aneurysm (Weingarten et al., 1992; Dumas et al., 1994; Akpek et al., 1995); however, a fourth study of 363 consecutive CT scans found significant pathology in 11 (3%) including 2 with intraventricular cysts, 4 with meningiomas, and 5 with malignant neoplasms (Demaerel et al., 1996).

Weingarten et al. (1992) extrapolated various types of data from a health maintenance organization of 100,800 adult patients. The estimated prevalence (in patients with chronic headache and a normal neurologic examination) of a CAT scan demonstrating an abnormality requiring neurosurgical intervention may have been as low as 0.01%. It is not certain whether detection of additional pathology on MRI scan would change this percentage. For example, complaints of headache with a normal neurologic examination may be seen in patients with type I Chiari malformation, which is easily detected on MRI but not CT scans (Arnett, 2004). Pituitary hemorrhage can produce a migraine-like acute headache with a normal neurologic examination (Evans, 1997). Pituitary infarction, with severe headache, photophobia, and CSF pleocytosis, can initially be quite similar to aseptic meningitis or meningoencephalitis (Embil, 1997). Pituitary pathology is more likely to be detected on a routine MRI than CT scan.

Wang et al. (2001) retrospectively reviewed the medical records and MRI images of 402 adult patients (286 women and 116 men) who had been evaluated by the neurology service with a primary complaint of chronic headache (a duration of 3 months or more) and no other neurologic symptoms or findings. Major abnormalities (a mass, caused mass effect, or was believed to be the likely cause of the patient's headache) were found in 15 patients (3.7%) including a glioma, meningioma, metastases, subdural hematoma, and AVM, 3 presented with hydrocephalus, and 2 with Chiari I malformations. They were found in 0.6% of patients with migraine, 1.4% of those with tension headaches, 14.1% of those with atypical headaches, and 3.8% of those with other types of headache.

Tsushimo and Endo (2005) retrospectively reviewed the clinical data and MR studies of 306 adult patients (136 men and 170 woman) all of whom were referred for MRI evaluation of chronic or recurrent headache with a duration of 1 month or, no other neurologic symptoms or focal findings at physical examination, and no prior head surgery, head trauma, or seizure. In this study, 55.2% had no abnormalities, 44.1% had minor abnormalities, and 0.7% (2) had clinically significant abnormalities (pituitary macroadenoma and subdural hematoma). Neither contrast material enhancement ($n = 195$) nor repeated MR imaging ($n = 23$) contributed to the diagnosis.

Sempere and colleagues (2005) reported a study of 1876 consecutive patients (1243 females, 633 males) aged 15 years or older, with a mean age of 38 years, with headaches that had an onset at least 4 weeks previously who were referred to two neurology clinics in Spain. One-third of the headaches were new onset, and two-thirds had been present for more than 1 year. Subjects had the following types of headache: migraine (49%), tension-type (35.4%), cluster (1.1%), posttraumatic (3.7%), and indeterminate (10.8%). Normal neurological examinations were found in 99.2% of the patients. CT scan was performed in 1432 patients and MRI in 580; 136 patients underwent both studies.

Neuroimaging studies detected significant lesions in 22 patients (1.2%) of whom 17 had a normal neurological examination. The only variable or "red flag" associated with a higher probability of intracranial abnormalities was an abnormal neurological examination with a likelihood ratio of 42. The diagnoses in these 17 patients were pituitary adenoma ($n = 3$), large arachnoid cyst ($n = 2$), meningioma ($n = 2$), hydrocephalus ($n = 2$), Arnold–Chiari type I malformation, ischemic stroke, cavernous angioma, AVM, low-grade astrocytoma, brain stem glioma, colloid cyst, posterior fossa papilloma (one of each). Of these 17 patients, 8 were treated surgically: hydrocephalus ($n = 2$), pituitary adenoma, large arachnoid cyst, meningioma, AVM, colloid cyst, and papilloma (one of each) (see Fig. 5–2).

The rate of significant intracranial abnormalities in patients with headache and normal neurological examination was 0.9%. Neuroimaging studies discovered incidental findings in 14 patients (75%): three pineal cysts, three intracranial lipomas, and eight arachnoid cysts. The yield of neuroimaging studies was higher in the group with indeterminate headache (3.7%) than in the migraine (0.4%) or tension-type headache (0.8%) groups. The study does not provide information on WMAs in migraineurs. MRI performed in 119 patients with normal CT revealed significant lesions in two cases: a small meningioma and an acoustic neurinoma. No saccular aneurysms were detected; MR angiography was not obtained.

The studies do not give information about the detection of paranasal sinus disease, however, which may be the cause of headache. For example, sphenoid sinusitis may cause a severe, intractable, new-onset headache that interferes with sleep and is not relieved by simple analgesics. There may be associated pain or paraesthesias in the distribution of the fifth cranial nerve and photophobia or eye tearing with or without fever or nasal drainage. The headache may mimic other causes such as migraine or meningitis (Silberstein, 2004).

American Academy of Neurology Practice Parameter

A report of the Quality Standards Subcommittee of the American Academy of Neurology

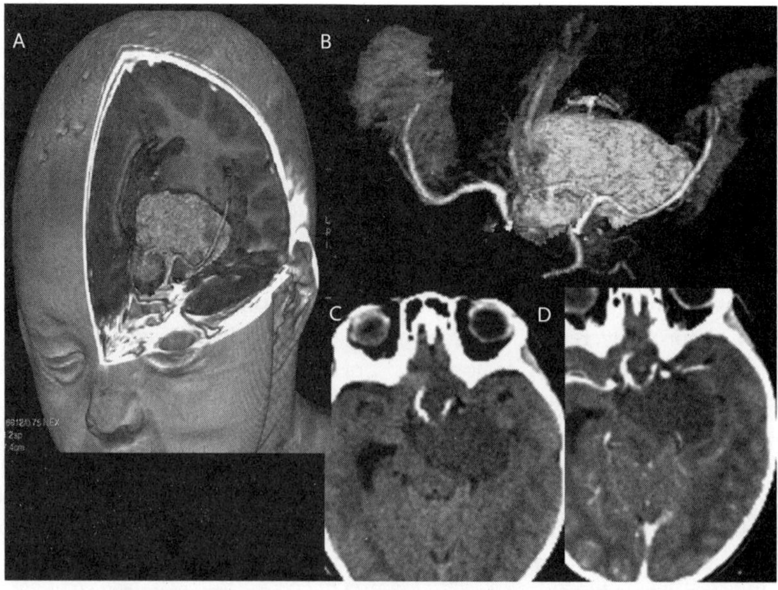

Figure 5–2 A 4-year-old with progressive headaches, papilledema and and obstructive hydrocephalus. (A) and (B) shows a 3-D reconstruction of a craniopharyngioma: green representing tumor, blue represents calcification and red is the surrounding vasculature. (C) and (D) demonstrates contrast CT of a suprasellar hypodensity as well as a right temporal horn enlargement. Reproduced with kind permission of Ron Alberico MD.

(Silberstein, 2000) makes the following recommendations for nonacute headache:

> The following symptoms significantly increased the odds of finding a significant abnormality on neuroimaging in patients with nonacute headache: rapidly increasing headache frequency; history of lack of coordination; history of localized neurologic signs or a history such as subjective numbness or tingling ; and history of headache causing awakening from sleep (although this can occur with migraine and cluster headache). The absence of these symptoms did not significantly lower the odds of finding a significant abnormality on neuroimaging.
>
> *Consider neuroimaging in patients with an unexplained abnormal finding on the neurologic examination (Grade B).*
> *Consider neuroimaging in patients with atypical headache features or headaches that do not fulfill the strict definition of migraine or other primary headache disorder (or have some additional risk factor, such as immune deficiency), when a lower threshold for neuroimaging may be applied (Grade C).*

No evidence-based recommendations are established for the following: presence or absence of neurologic symptoms (Grade C); tension-type headache (Grade C); and relative sensitivity of MRI as compared with CT in the evaluation of migraine or other nonacute headache (Grade C)."

Neuroimaging in Children

A number of studies have investigated the findings of neuroimaging in children with headaches. Dooley et al. reported the retrospective findings on CT scans of 41 children with headaches and normal neurologic examinations referred to a secondary or tertiary care facility (Dooley, 1990). Only one scan was abnormal, demonstrating a choroid plexus papilloma. Chu and Shinnar (1992) obtained brain-imaging studies in 30 children, ages 7 or younger, with headaches referred to pediatric neurologists. The studies were normal except for five with incidental findings.

Maytal et al. (1996) obtained MRI or CT scans or both in 78 children, ages 3–18 years, with headaches. With the exception of six patients, the neurologic examinations were normal. The studies were normal except for incidental cerebral abnormalities in four and mucoperiosteal thickening of the paranasal sinuses in seven. Wöber-Bingöl et al. (1996) prospectively obtained MRI scans in 96 children, ages 5–18 years, with headaches and normal neurologic examinations who were referred to an outpatient headache clinic. The studies were normal except for 17 (17.7%) with incidental findings.

Medina et al. (1997) retrospectively reported MRI findings in 315 children, ages 3–20 years (mean 11 years), with headaches. The neurologic examinations were abnormal in 89 patients. Thirteen (4%) had surgical space-occupying lesions. After analyzing risk factors for these lesions as well as the prior literature, Medina and colleagues suggest guidelines for neuroimaging in children with headache (Table 5–3).

Lewis and Dorbad (2000) retrospectively reviewed records of children aged 6–18 years with migraine and chronic daily headache with normal examinations. Of 54 patients with migraine who underwent either CT (42) or MRI

TABLE 5–3 Reasons to Consider Neuroimaging for Children with Headaches.

1. Persistent headaches of less than 6 months duration that do not respond to medical treatment
2. Headache associated with abnormal neurologic findings, especially if accompanied by papilledema, nystagmus, or gait or motor abnormalities
3. Persistent headaches associated with an absent family history of migraine
4. Persistent headache associated with substantial episodes of confusion, disorientation, or emesis
5. Headaches that awaken a child repeatedly from sleep or occur immediately on awakening
6. Family history or medical history of disorders that may predispose one to central nervous system lesions and clinical or laboratory findings suggestive of central nervous system involvement

Source: From Medina, S, Pinter JD, Zurakowski, D et al. (1997). Children with headache: clinical predictors of surgical space-occupying lesions and the role of neuroimaging. *Radiology*, 202:819–824.

(12) scans, the yield of abnormalities was 3.7%, none clinically relevant. Of 25 patients with chronic daily headache who underwent either CT (17) or MRI (8) scans, the yield of abnormalities was 16%, none clinically relevant.

Carlos et al. (2000), in a retrospective chart review, identified all pediatric migraine patients who had a CT or MRI to investigate their headaches. Ages ranged from 3 to 18 years. Of the 93 patients, 35 had CT, 14 had MRI, and 9 had both. Twenty-two had abnormalities but none of these abnormalities were felt to be related to the patients' headaches. Alehan (2002) prospectively obtained neuroimaging (49 MRI scans, 11 CT scans) in 60 out of 72 consecutive children diagnosed with migraine or tension-type headaches. Ten percent of scans had findings related to their headache with no neoplasms and none of the patients requiring surgery.

Mazzotta et al. (2004) performed a prospective study at multiple pediatric headache centers in which 6535 first-time referrals up to the age of 18 were studied. Based on the indications of the diagnostic flow-chart, 1485 underwent neuroimaging testing. Incidental findings were observed in 138 (9.3%) subjects. Abnormal results were observed in 273 (18.5%) subjects. Findings that led to the diagnosis of secondary headache were observed in 135 (9.1%) including sinusitis in 57% and intracranial space-occupying lesions in 17.4% (see Fig. 5–3).

A report of the Quality Standards Subcommittee of the American Academy of Neurology and the Practice Committee of the Child Neurology Society (Lewis et al., 2002) makes the following recommendations:

1. Obtaining a neuroimaging study on a routine basis is not indicated in children with recurrent headaches and a normal neurologic examination (Level B; class II and class III evidence).
2. Neuroimaging should be considered in children with an abnormal neurologic examination (e.g., focal findings, signs of increased intracranial pressure, significant alteration

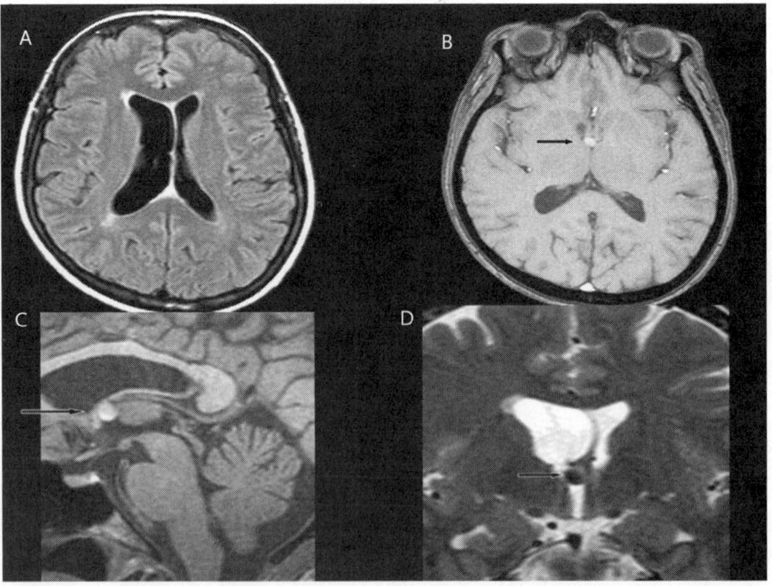

Figure 5–3 60-year-old with episodic headaches and syncope. A. FLAIR axial image showing a right lateral ventriculomegaly and early transependymal CSF flow. B.T1W fat saturation axial image confirms an ovoid mass adjacent to the right foramen of Monro. C. Sagittal T1W images show the colloid cyst as a mass that shortens the T1W (hyperintense) consistent with proteinacious material. D. The T2W image shows the short T2 (hypointense)cyst enlarging and partially obstructing the intraventricular foramen with transependymal CSF leak adjacent to the frontal pole.

of consciousness) or the coexistence of seizures, or both (Level B; class II and class III evidence).

3. Neuroimaging should be considered in children in whom there are historical features to suggest the recent onset of severe headache, change in the type of headache, or if there are associated features that suggest neurologic dysfunction (Level B; class II and class III evidence).

Risk/benefit and Cost/benefit of Neuroimaging

Table 5–4 summarizes the estimated risks and benefits of neuroimaging in patients with headaches and normal neurologic examinations. Although, for many patients, the scan helps to relieve anxiety, for others, the scan may produce anxiety when nonspecific abnormalities are found such as incidental anatomical variants or white matter lesions. We suspect that many neurologists have seen patients with isolated headaches referred by primary care physicians with a request to rule out multiple sclerosis when white matter lesions are detected.

Although the cost of finding significant pathology is quite high, the cost of neuroimaging is significantly decreasing under some managed-care contracts. Cost/benefit estimates should also include the cost to the physician of malpractice suits filed when patients with significant

Table 5–4 Balance Sheet.

	CT	*MRI*	*No test*
Health outcomes			
Benefits			
Discovery of potentially treatable lesions			
(1) Migraine	0.3%	0.4%	0
(2) Any headache	2.4%	2.4%	0
Relief of anxiety	30%	30%	0
Harms			
Iodine reaction			
Mild	10%		
Moderate	1%		
Severe	0.01%		
Death	0.002%		
Claustrophobia			
Mild	5%	15%	0
Moderate (needs sedation)	1%	5–10%	
Severe (unable to comply)	1–2%		
False-positive studies	No data	No data	
Cost (charges)	Varies widely depending upon the payor		

CT or MRI in Patients with Headache and Normal Neurologic Examinations. Technology: CT with intravenous contrast or MRI without contrast. Indications: (1) migraine and (2) any headache.

Source: Modified with permission from Frishberg, BM (1994). The utility of neuroimaging in the evaluation of headache in patients with normal neurologic examinations. *Neurology*, 44:1196.

pathology do not have neuroimaging and the cost to the patient and society of premature death and disability of undetected treatable lesions.

NEUROIMAGING IN MIGRAINE

Incidence of Pathology

Frishberg (1994) reviewed four CT scan studies (Cala and Mastaglia, 1976; Hungerford et al., 1976; Masland et al., 1978; Cuetter and Aita, 1983), four MRI scan studies (Soges et al., 1988; Jacome and Leborgne, 1990; Igarashi et al., 1991; Osborn et al., 1991), and one combined MRI and CT scan study (Kuhn and Sheklar, 1990) of 897 scans of patients with migraine. These findings are combined with more recent reports of one CT scan study of 284 patients (Dumas et al., 1994) and six studies of MRI scans of 444 patients (Pavese et al., 1991; Ziegler et al., 1991; Fazekas et al., 1992; Robbins and Friedman, 1992; de Benedittis et al., 1995; Cooney et al., 1996) for a total of 1625 scans of patients with various types of migraine. Other than WMAs, the studies showed no significant pathology except for four brain tumors (three of which were incidental findings) and one AVM (in a patient with migraine and a seizure disorder). Sempere et al. (2005) found a similarly low yield of 0.4%.

White Matter Abnormalities and Subclinical Infarcts

Fourteen MRI studies have investigated WMAs on scans of migraine patients. WMAs are foci of hyperintensity on both proton density and T2-weighted images in the deep and periventricular white matter due to either interstitial edema or perivascular demyelination. WMAs are easily detected on MRI but are not seen on CAT scan (Kuhn and Shekar, 1990).

The percentages of WMAs for all types of migraine range from 12% (Osborn et al., 1991) to 46% (Soges et al., 1988). WMAs have been reported to be both more frequent in the frontal region of the centrum semiovale (Igarashi et al., 1991; De Benedittis et al., 1995) and no more frequent (Pavese et al., 1994) than in the white matter of the parietal, temporal, and occipital lobes. Six out of the eight studies using controls found a higher incidence of WMAs in migraineurs. The incidence of WMAs in controls ranged from 0% (Rovaris et al., 2001) to 14% (Fazekas et al., 1992). One small study reported a similar incidence of WMAs in patients with tension-type headaches (34.3%) as compared with those with migraine (32.1%) and this was greater than the 7.4% observed in controls (De Benedittis et al., 1995)

Four studies found similar percentages of WMAs comparing migraine with aura to migraine without aura (Prager et al., 1991; Pavese et al., 1994; DeBenedittis et al., 1995; Cooney et al., 1996) while two others reported a higher percentage in migraine with aura (Igarashi et al., 1991; Fazekas et al., 1992). Out of three small studies of basilar migraine, two found WMAs in 17% of cases studied (Jacome and Leborgne, 1990; Cooney et al., 1996) and one found 38% (Fazekas et al., 1992). WMAs are variably reported as more often present in adult migraineurs more than 40 years old and less than 60 (Prager et al., 1991; Cooney et al., 1996) and equally present (Fazekas et al., 1992) compared to those 40 or younger. Cooney et al. (1996) found an increased frequency of WMAs associated with age over 50 and with medical risk factors (hypertension, atherosclerotic heart disease, diabetic mellitus, autoimmune disorder, or demyelinating disease) but not with gender, migraine subtype, or duration of migraine symptoms.

In a series of 16 consecutive migraineurs (14 without aura and 2 with aura), Rovaris et al. (2001) found white matter lesions in 5 (31%). The pattern of MRI lesions fulfilled diagnostic criteria suggestive of multiple sclerosis (MS) in four—none of the patients had any other neurological symptoms or signs. Cervical spine MRI studies were obtained in all subjects as well as in 17 age- and gender-matched controls with the detection of no cord lesions.

Kruit et al. (2004) obtained MRI scans on a population-based sample of Dutch adults of ages 30–60 years suffering from migraine with aura (n = 161), migraine without aura (n = 134), and well-matched controls (n = 140) (see Fig. 5–4). No participants reported a history of stroke or transient ischemic attack or had relevant abnormalities at standard neurological examination. There

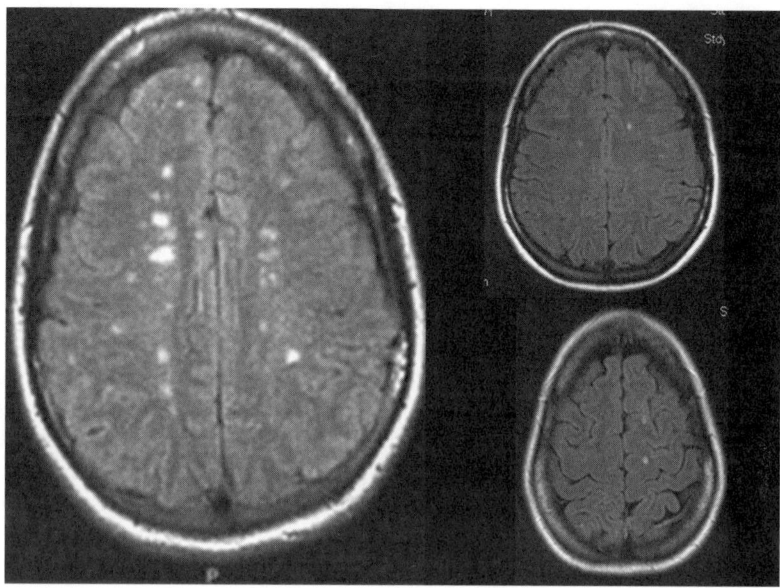

Figure 5–4 Patient is a 27-year-old female with migraines with aura. No other cerebrovascular risk factors. Exam normal.

was no significant difference between patients with migraine and controls in overall infarct prevalence (8.1% versus 5.0%); however, in the cerebellar region of the posterior circulation territory, patients with migraine had a higher prevalence of infarct than controls (5.4% versus 0.7%). The adjusted odds ratio (OR) for posterior infarct varied by migraine subtype and attack frequency. The adjusted OR was 13.7 for patients with migraine with aura compared with controls. In patients with migraine with a frequency of attacks of one or more per month, the adjusted OR was 9.3. The highest risk was in patients with migraine with aura with one attack or more per month (OR, 15.8). Kruit et al. (2005) hypothesize that focal (possibly migraine-related) hypoperfusion, rather than microembolic occlusion, is responsible for most of the cerebellar infarcts.

Thirty-eight percent of the subjects in both the migraine and control groups had at least one medium-size deep white matter lesion (DWML). Among women, the risk for high DWML load was increased in patients with migraine compared with controls (OR, 2.1); this risk increased with attack frequency (highest in those with one attack per month: OR, 2.6) but was similar in patients with migraine with or without aura. In men, controls and patients with migraine did not differ in the prevalence of DWMLs. There was no association between severity of periventricular white matter lesions (PVWMLs) and migraine, irrespective of sex, migraine attack frequency, or subtype. There were no differences in the distributions and the mean values of grades of severity of PVWMLs between patients with migraine and controls. These results did not vary by sex, migraine subtype, and/or migraine attack frequency.

Kruit et al. (2006) further reported the brainstem and cerebellar hyperintense lesions found in their same migraine population. Infratentorial hyperintensities were identified in 13 of 295 (4.4%) migraineurs and in 1 of 140 (0.7%) controls. Twelve cases had hyperintensities, mostly bilaterally, in the dorsal basis pontis (described for the first time in migraine). Those with infratentorial hyperintensities also had supratentorial white matter lesions more often. The cause may be small-vessel disease (arteriosclerosis), repetitive perfusion deficits, or both.

While the cause of WMAs in migraine is not certain, various hypotheses have been advanced including increased platelet aggregability with microemboli, abnormal cerebrovascular regulation, and repeated attacks of hypoperfusion during the aura (Igarashi et al., 1991; Pavese et al., 1994; De Benedittis et al., 1995; Kruit et al., 2004). The presence of antiphospholipid antibodies might be another risk factor for WMAs in migraine (Tietjen, 1992). The reported incidence of antiphospholipid antibodies in migraine ranges from 0% (Hering et al., 1991) to 24% (Robbins, 1991). In one MRI study, however, the presence of WMAs showed no correlation with the presence of anticardiolipin antibodies (Igarashi et al., 1991). The presence of anticardiolipin antibodies is not an additional risk factor for stroke in migraineurs (Daras et al., 1995). Tietjen et al. (1998) found that, compared to control subjects, there was no increase in frequency of anticardiolipin positivity in adults under 60 years of age with transient focal neurologic events, or in those with migraine with or without aura. In migraine patients with white matter lesions (Initso et al., 2006), antiphospholipid antibodies were not detected and serum levels of antithrombin III and proteins C and S were normal. The potential role of patent foramen ovale as a source or conduit for microemboli and WMAs or posterior infarctions is unclear, but the higher prevalence of patent foramen ovale (PFO) in migraineurs with aura raises this association as a possibility (Anzola, 1999). PFO may be detected using a variety of techniques including bubble-contrast trans-thoracic echocardiography, trans-esophageal echocardiology, or bubble-contrast transcranial Doppler, (see Fig. 5–5) although the latter does not distinguish a shunt at the atria from one at the pulmonary level (Spencer, 2004).

A subgroup of migraineurs may have a genetic predisposition for white matter lesions on MRI scans. Cerebral autosomal dominant arteriopathy with subcortical infarcts and leukoencephalopathy (CADASIL) is a familial genetic disease with migraine as a common symptom and severe WMAs on MRI as a consistent neuroimaging finding even prior to the development of any clinical symptoms (Fig. 5–4). Chabriat et al. (1995) described several members of a family with an autosomal dominant illness manifested by migraine attacks and a significant leukoencephalopathy on MRI but without other specific manifestations of CADASIL. Mourad et al. (2006) also describe four patients over the age of 60 with typical Notch3 mutations leading to CADASIL who did not have dementia or disability but had extensive WMA on

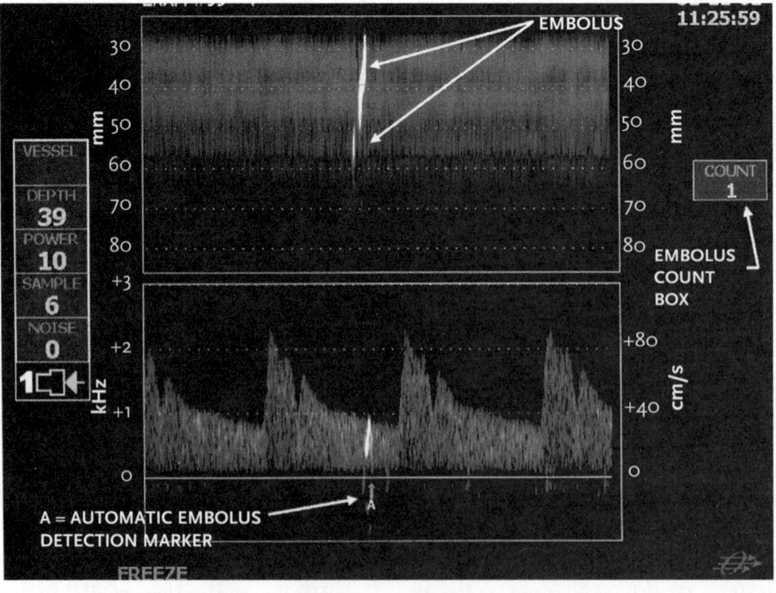

Figure 5–5 A 40-year-old female with migraine with aura and white matter lesions on MRI. Transcranial Doppler (TCD) bubble test with agitated saline and valsalva maneuver detects emboli. Subsequent Transesophageal Echocardiogram confirms the presence of a Patent Foramen Ovale (PFO).

MRI. It is possible that there is a specific gene locus for migraine with white matter changes. Variable gene penetrance could result in CADASIL at one extreme and individuals with tiny T2 hyperintense white matter foci and migraine alone at the other extreme.

MELAS is the term used for the syndrome clinically characterized by mitochondrial myopathy, encephalopathy, lactic acidosis, and stroke. MRI findings include abnormal signal intensity in the basal ganglia and infarctions. In patients with this disorder, magnetic resonance spectroscopy (MRS) shows an elevation of lactate and may be more sensitive than MRI in the detection of MELAS-associated abnormalities. Clinically, migraine is part of the clinicalspectrum of MELAS with over 70% of these patients having a history of migraine. MELAS can begin with typical migraine, progressing to hemiplegic migraine, and then to ischemic stroke. MRS potentially may be used as a screening device for mitochondrial cytopathy and as a tool to follow response to treatment (Iizuka and Sakai, 2005) (see Fig. 5–6).

Arteriovenous malformations, brainstem vascular malformations, and migraine

The prevalence of AVMs is about 0.5% in postmortem studies (Brown et al., 1988). In contrast to saccular aneurysms, upto 50% of patients studied present with symptoms or signs other than hemorrhage. Headache without distinctive features (such as frequency, duration, or severity) is the presenting symptom in up to 48% of cases (The Arteriovenous Malformation Study Group, 1999) (see Figs. 5–7 and 5–8).

Migraine-like headaches, with and without visual symptoms, can be associated with AVMs especially those in the occipital lobe which is the predominant location of about 20% of parenchymal AVMs (Kupersmith et al., 1996; Frishberg, 1997). Although headaches that always occur on the same side (side-locked) are present in 95% of those with AVMs (Bruyn, 1984), 17% of those with migraine without aura and 15% of patients with migraine with aura have side-locked headaches (Leone et al., 1993).

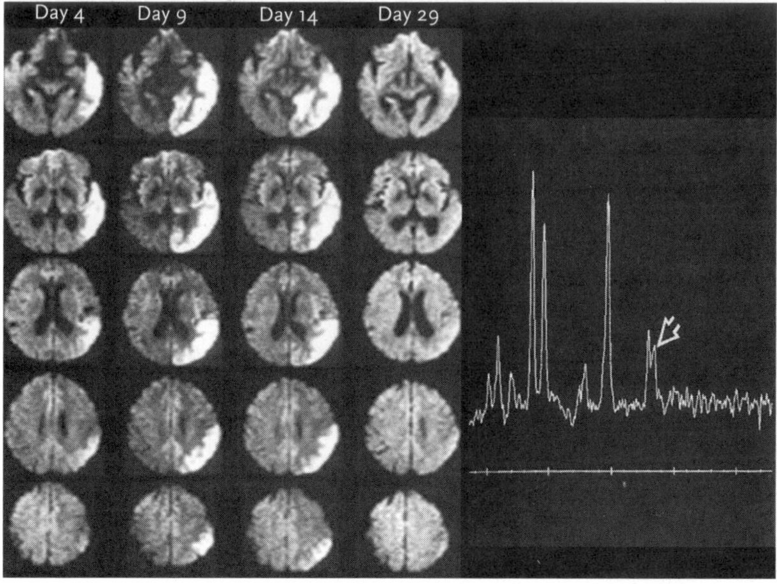

Figure 5–6 47-year-old with migrainous headache followed by aphasia and psychosis, then developed GM sz on day 8. Diagnosis is MELAS A. Diffusion weighted imaging (DWI) shows extensive changes on the left in a non- vascular pattern resolving by Day 29. MRS shows a characteristic pattern in 65 % of cases, a lactate doublet peak at 1.3ppm. (arrow). Approximately 80% of patients with the clinical characteristics of MELAS have a heteroplasmic A-to-G point mutation in the dihydrouridine loop of the tRNALeu (UUR) gene at base pair 3243 (ie, A3243G mutation). Iizuka et al. Current Neurovascular research, 2005

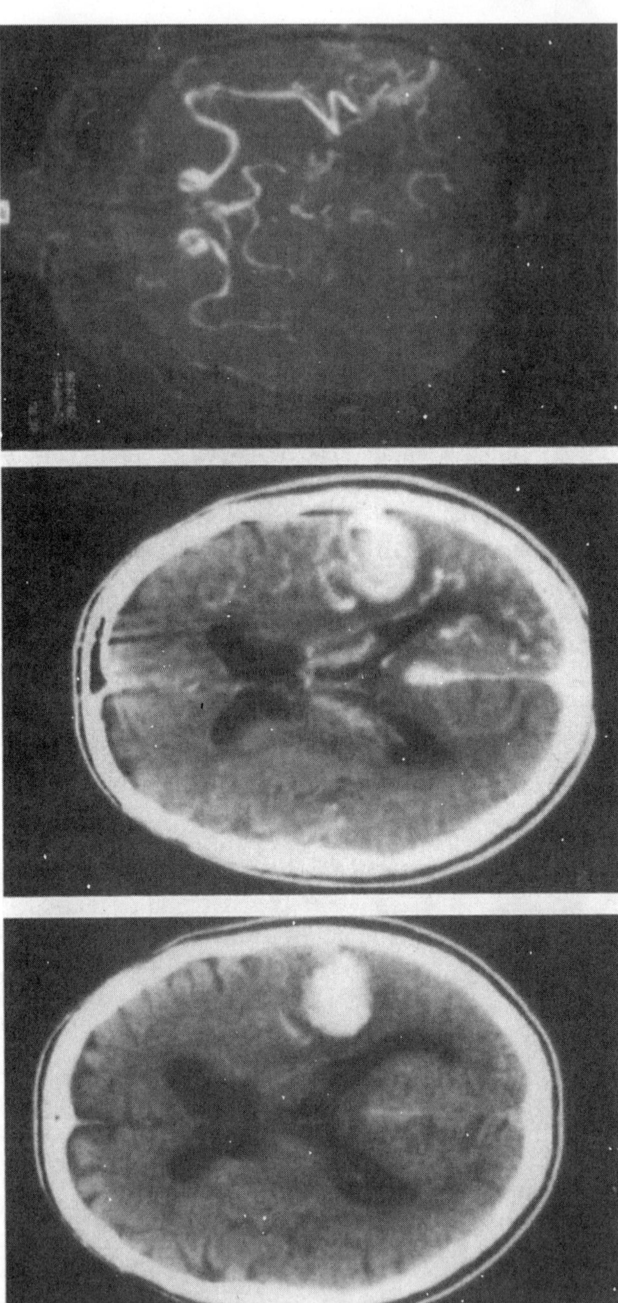

Figure 5–7 Arteriovenous malformation (reprinted with permission from Rozen, T.D., Silberstein, S.D., and D. Friedman (1999). Neuroimaging of Headache. In Neuroimaging (J. O. Greenberg, ed.), pp. 89–106, McGraw-Hill, New York.

Migraine due to an AVM is usually atypical and rarely meets the International Headache Society criteria for migraine. In a series of 109 patients with headache and AVMs, Ghossoub et al. (2001) reported the following features: nonpulsating, 95%; nausea, vomiting, light, or noise sensitivity, 4.1%; unilateral and homolateral to the AVM, 70%; duration less than 3 hours, 77%; 1–2 per month, 82.5%; and usually mild responding to simple analgesics. Bruyn (1984) reported the following features in patients with migraine-like symptoms and AVM: unusual associated signs (papilledema, field cut, bruit), 65%; short duration of headache attacks, 20%; brief scintillating scotoma, 10%; absent family history, 15%; atypical sequence of aura, headache, and vomiting, 10%; and seizures, 25%.

The following brainstem vascular malformations have been associated with migraine meeting criteria established by the International Headache Society: a hemorrhagic midbrain cavernoma resulting in a contralateral headache(Goadsby, 2002); a pontine bleed from a cavernous angioma with initially ipsilateral headache then bilateral with aura (Afridi and Goadsby, 2003); pontine capillary telangiectasia with signs of residual hemorrhage with bilateral headaches initially with aura (Obermann et al., 2006); and a midbrain/upper-pons hemorrhagic AVM/cavernous malformation resulting in a contralateral headache with aura (Malik and Young, 2006). These cases provide evidence for the involvement of the brainstem in the initiation of migraine.

American Academy of Neurology Practice Parameter

- A report of the Quality Standards Subcommittee of the American Academy of Neurology (Silberstein, 2000) makes the following recommendation: "Neuroimaging is not usually warranted in patients with migraine and a normal neurologic examination (Grade B)."

ACUTE SEVERE NEW ONSET HEADACHES ("FIRST OR WORST")

Differential Diagnosis

Perhaps 1% of patients presenting to the emergency room have headache often of acute onset as their chief complaint (Morgenstern et al., 2001). Table 5–5 lists the extensive list of possible causes of the acute severe new onset headache (the "first or worst") (Davenport, 2002). About 12%–25% of patients presenting to the emergency department with a sudden-onset severe headache described as the worst headache of their life have a SAH (de Falco, 2004). A prospective study of 148 patients with acute severe headaches seen by general practitioners in the Netherlands found SAH to be the cause in 25% (Linn et al., 1994).

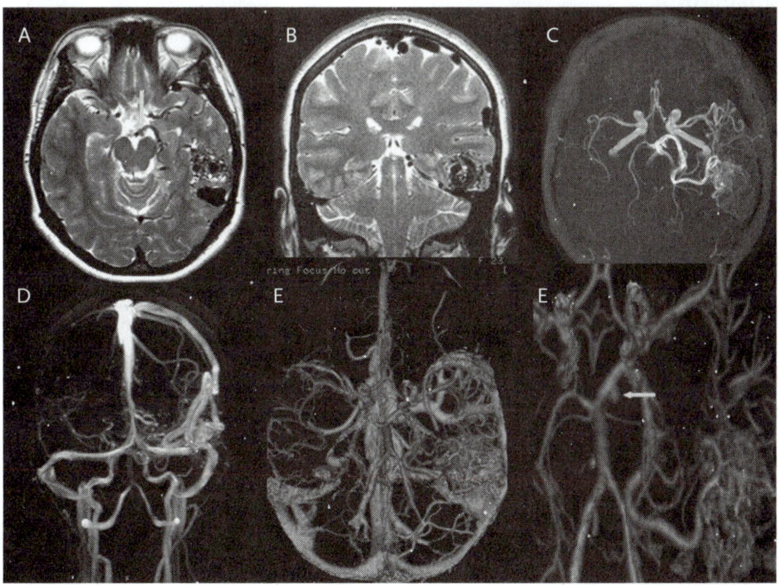

Figure 5–8 A 30-year-old with progressive daily headaches and normal exam. A - B On T2W axial and coronal images a large AVM involving the left temporal lobe with massive draining veins are seen. In addition a left PCA aneurysm was found (yellow arrow). C Axial MRA and MRV confirm the large AVM. Finally E and F are computerized tomography angiograms (CTA) showing the delicate detail between arterial and venous circulation, as well as the PCA aneurysm (yellow arrow).

TABLE 5–5 Differential Diagnosis of the Acute Severe New Onset Headache ("First or Worst").

- Crash migraine
- Cluster headache
- Miscellaneous
  - Primary exertional headache
  - Primary orgasmic cephalgia
- Posttraumatic
  - Associated with vascular disorders
    - Acute ischemic cerebrovascular disease
    - Subdural and epidural hematomas
    - Parenchymal hemorrhage
    - Unruptured saccular aneurysm
    - Subarachnoid hemorrhage
    - Systemic lupus erythematosis
    - Temporal arteritis
    - Internal carotid and vertebral artery dissection
    - Cerebral venous thrombosis
    - Acute hypertension
      - Pressor response
      - Pheochromocytoma
      - Pre-eclampsia
  - Associated with nonvascular intracranial disorders
    - Intermittent hydrocephalus
    - Benign intracranial hypertension
    - Post lumbar puncture
    - Related to intrathecal injections
    - Intracranial neoplasm
    - Pituitary apoplexy
- Acute intoxications
  - Associated with noncephalic infection
    - Acute febrile illness
    - Acute pyelonephritis
- Cephalic infection
    - Meningoencephalitis
    - Acute sinusitis
  - Acute mountain sickness
  - Disorders of eyes
    - Acute optic neuritis
    - Acute glaucoma
  - Cervicogenic
    - Greater occipital neuralgia
    - Cervical myositis
    - Cervical facet and root syndromes
  - Trigeminal neuralgia

Source: With permission from Evans, RW (1999). Headaches. In *Diagnostic Testing in Neurology* (RW Evans, ed.), p. 7. WB Saunders, Philadelphia.

There are many causes of SAH (Table 5–6). About 80% of SAH are due to ruptured intracranial aneurysms (Al-Shahi et al., 2006; Suarez et al., 2006) and 5% are due to rupture of intracranial AVMs. In about 15% of cases, an arteriogram does not demonstrate the cause of the bleeding. In about 50% of these arteriogram negative cases, the CT scan reveals blood confined to the cisterns around the midbrain, perimesencephalic hemorrhage, which may be caused by a ruptured prepontine or interpeduncular cistern-dilated vein or venous malformation. Other causes of arteriogram negative SAH are listed in Table 5–7.

Over 30,000 people per year in the United States have a SAH from a ruptured saccular aneurysm, resulting in over 18,000 deaths (Raps et al., 1994; Suarez, 2006). Based upon a meta-analysis, the prevalence of saccular aneurysms in the general population is about 2%, with 93% < 10 mm of aneurysms (Rinkel et al., 1998). Perhaps 50% of SAHs will present with a Hunt and Hess grade I (no symptoms or minimal headache, slight nuchal rigidity) or II (moderate-to-severe headache, no

TABLE 5–6 Causes of Nontraumatic Subarachnoid Hemorrhage.

- 80% Intracranial saccular aneurysm
- 5% Intracranial arteriovenous malformation
- 15% Negative arteriogram
- 50% Benign perimesencephalic (pretruncal) hemorrhage
- 50% Other causes
  - Occult aneurysm
  - Mycotic aneurysm
  - Vertebral or carotid artery dissection
  - Dural arteriovenous malformation
  - Spinal arteriovenous malformation
  - Sickle cell anemia
  - Coagulation disorders
  - Drug abuse (cocaine and methamphetamine)
  - Primary or metastatic intracranial tumors (e.g., pituitary, melanoma)
  - Primary or metastatic cervical tumors
  - CNS infection (e.g., herpes encephalitis)
  - CNS vasculitides

Source: With permission from Evans, RW (1999). Headaches. In *Diagnostic Testing in Neurology* (RW Evans, ed.), p. 7. WB Saunders, Philadelphia.

TABLE 5–7 Approximate Probability of Recognizing an Aneurysmal Subarachnoid Hemorrhage on CT Scan After the Initial Event

Time	*Probability (%)*
Day 0	95
Day 3	74
1 week	50
2 weeks	30
3 weeks	almost 0

Source: With permission from Evans, RW (1999). Headaches. In *Diagnostic Testing in Neurology* (RW Evans, ed.), p. 9. W.B. Saunders, Philadelphia.

neurodeficit other than cranial nerve palsy). Although most patients with headache due to SAH will have the worst headache of their life with maximum intensity within 5 minutes (Linn et al., 1998), SAH can be easily overlooked (Johnston and Robinson, 1998). Ten percent of patients have no headache at onset and 8% describe a mild, gradually increasing headache (Weir, 1994). A stiff neck is absent in 36% of patients (Kassell et al., 1990). Ten percent to forty three percent of patients with SAH have a sentinel headache (Polmear, 2003). Aware of the diverse presentations of SAH, how should you exclude aneurysmal SAH?

CT and MRI Scans and Aneurysmal SAH

A CT scan without contrast is the neuroimaging study of choice in the detection of acute SAH with a high initial sensitivity (Table 5–7). In a cooperative series of 3521 patients, findings on the first CT scan after rupture of a saccular aneurysm were as follows: normal, 8.3%; decreased density, 1.1%; mass effect, 6.1%; aneurysm, 5%; hydrocephalus, 15.2%; intraventricular hematoma, 16.7%; intracerebral hematoma, 17.4%; subdural hematoma, 1.3%; and SAH, 85.2% (Kassell et al., 1990). CT scan detected aneurysmal SAH in 92% of patients on day 0 decreasing to 58% on day 5. The percentage of scans which were normal on day 0 was 3.3%; day 1, 7.2%; and day 5, 27.3%. False positives can occur from mistaking calcification such as of the falx cerebri for blood or anoxic encephalopathy as diffuse subarchnoid hemorrhage (al-Yamany et al., 1999).

Van der Wee et al. (1995) performed a prospective series of 175 consecutive patients with sudden headache and a normal neurologic examination. CT scans performed within the first 12 hours detected SAH in 117 for a detection rate of 98%. In the remaining 58 patients, LP was performed 12 or more hours after the onset of the headache. Two out of the fifty-eight were found to have xanthochromic CSF by spectrophotometric analysis. Both of these patients were found to have aneurysms.

Based upon a prospective study of 100 patients, the probability of recognizing an aneurysmal hemorrhage on CT scan is 50% after 1 week, 30% after 2 weeks (mostly patients with hematomas), and almost nil after 3 weeks (van Gijn and van Dongen, 1982). The increased attenuation values in the basal cisterns and fissures usually disappeared by day 5–9. Most hematomas resolved between days 14 and 22.

The pattern of hemorrhage in the absence of an intracerebral hematoma helps to suggest the location of the ruptured saccular aneurysm (Table 5–8) (Ghoshhajra et al., 1979; Wang et al., 1995). CT is the most sensitive and specific test for diagnosing a ruptured anterior cerebral artery aneurysm or anterior communicating artery aneurysm (van der Jagt et al., 1999). SAH only in the prepontine cistern or interpeduncular fossa may indicate a venous or capillary rupture (Yuichi,

TABLE 5–8 Aneurysm Sites Suggested by the Location of SAH

Site of Aneurysm	*Predominant Location of SAH*
Anterior communicating artery	Interhemispheric fissure and/or septum pellucidum
Middle cerebral artery	Sylvian fissure cistern
Posterior communicating artery	Suprasellar cistern
Infratentorial arteries	Posterior fossa cistern
Unknown origin	Diffuse, symmetrical cisterns

Source: With permission from Evans, RW (1999). Headaches. In *Diagnostic Testing in Neurology* (RW Evans, ed.), p. 9. W.B. Saunders, Philadelphia.

1981; Rinkel et al., 1991) although, about 5% of the time, a basilar artery aneurysm is responsible (Rinkel et al., 1991).

CT scan without contrast is preferred over MRI in the acute setting for the evaluation of possible SAH because of the wide availability of CT scans, lower expense, and faster scanning time. However, fluid-attenuated inversion recovery (FLAIR) MR imaging can detect SAH that may not be apparent on CT scans but may be revealed by LP (see Fig. 5–9). In a small acute series, FLAIR MRI on a 1.5-T unit was positive in only 16.7% (2/12 cases) (Mohamed et al., 2004). False-positives for SAH can also occur for a variety of reasons, such as patients with strokes who had previously undergone contrast-enhanced perfusion studies, renal failure, active seizures, inspired oxygen, and various artifacts. MRI using a gradient echo T2 sequence is more sensitive than CT between 4 and 14 days (100% versus 75%) (Mitchell et al., 2001) and between 6 and 30 days (100% versus 45.5%) (Yuan et al., 2005) after the ictus.

Lumbar Puncture and SAH

A LP should be performed in all patients with a new onset headache suspicious for SAH who have normal CT scans. Since LP can result in clinical deterioration and death after SAH, a CT scan should be performed first with the exception of certain cases where acute meningitis is suspected (Duffy, 1982; van Gijn, 1992).

CSF Examination and Xanthochromia

Red blood cells (RBCs) are present in the CSF in virtually all cases of SAH and clear in a variable period of time from about 6 to 30 days (Tourtellotte et al., 1964). However, distinguishing a traumatic LP from a SAH can be highly problematic. Although a decrease in RBCs from the first to the third test tube can be seen after a traumatic tap (Fishman, 1992), a similar decrease can be seen after a previous bleed (Buruma, 1981).

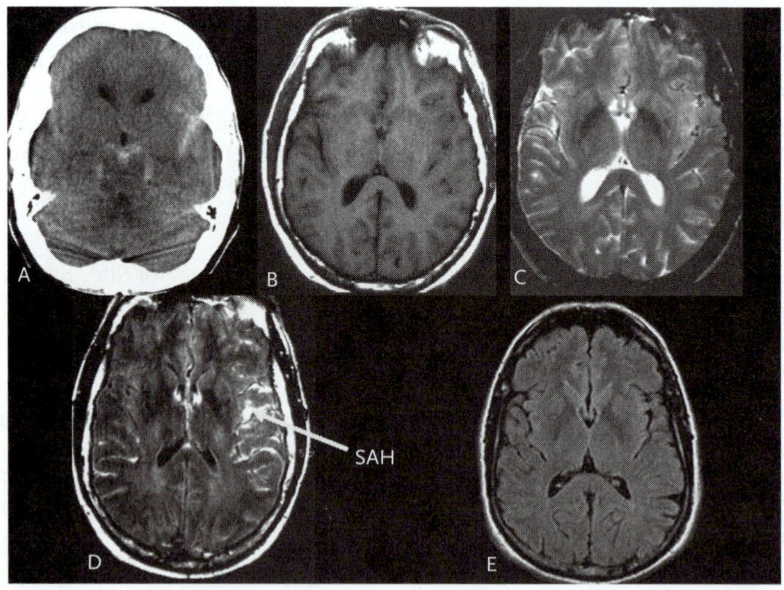

Figure 5–9 A 30-year-old male experiencing the worst headache of his life was found to have subarachnoid hemorrhage (SAH) due to a left middle cerebral aneurysm rupture. CT (A) is the study of choice within 24 hours of acute onset of symptoms when compared to MRI specifically T1(B) and T2(C)-weighted images. Red arrow points to hyperdensity within the Sylvian fissure representing blood. Fluid Attenuated Inversion Recovery (FLAIR) sequence (E) is as sensitive as CT between 24–72 hours and more sensitive after 72 hours. Yellow arrow points to subarachnoid hyperintensity representing blood. A normal FLAIR (F) image is shown for comparison. FLAIR imaging is especially useful when SAH patients have symptoms 7 days prior to presenting to the emergency room or a physician. Reproduced with kind permission of Rohit Bakshi MD.

A 25% reduction between the first and third tubes can be seen in cases of ruptured aneurysms (Heasley et al., 2005). Heasley et al. (2005) also contrast how few RBCs may be present in SAH, comparing two cases of aneurysmal SAH documented on arteriogram with a negative CT that had only 69 and 80 RBCs/mm^3, respectively, compared with a patient with no pathology whose CSF revealed 414,750 RBCs/mm^3. After a traumatic tap, the number of RBCs may stay constant in all three tubes (Vermeulen, 1989). Since crenation occurs very soon after RBCs enter CSF, the presence of crenated RBCs is not a reliable sign of SAH (Vermeulen and van Gijn, 1990).

Xanthochromia may be helpful in the detection of SAH. When RBCs break down in CSF, they release oxyhemoglobin which is degraded by macrophages and other cells in the leptomeninges to bilirubin by the third-to-fourth day (Barrows et al., 1955). These two pigments are responsible for xanthochromia (literally "yellow color" but refers to a colored supernatant) after SAH. The CSF supernatant is pink or pink–orange due to oxyhemoglobin, yellow due to bilirubin, and an intermediate color if both are present. Methemoglobin, a reduction product of hemoglobin, is found in encapsulated subdural hematomas and in old loculated intracerebral hemorrhages (Fishman, 1992).

Although oxyhemoglobin can be detected as early as 2 hours after entry of RBCs into CSF, xanthochromia is not present in all cases until after 12 hours (Vermeulen et al., 1989). Therefore, to avoid confusing blood-stained CSF from a traumatic LP with a SAH, a suggestion has been made to delay LP until 12 hours after the ictus (Vermeulen and van Gijn, 1990; Al-Shahi et al., 2006); however, this is not always practical when many evaluations for patients with severe headaches and a normal examination are done as outpatients or in the emergency room.

Unfortunately, the presence of xanthochromia assessed by spectrophotometry cannot absolutely distinguish between SAH and a traumatic LP. Because oxyhemoglobin can form in vivo, false-positives for SAH can occur from traumatic taps with even a small number of RBCs (Morgenstern et al., 1998); however, bilirubin and methemoglobin form in vitro only. Based upon a model of adding blood to clear CSF, Graves and Sidman (2004) concluded that CSF xanthochromia assessed by spectrophotometry may be observed within 2 hours after traumatic LP and sooner in samples with greater than 10,000 RBCs/mm^3. Conversely, xanthochromia in traumatic LP with less than 5000 RBCs warrants further investigation for SAH. When the CSF RBC count is elevated above 10,000 RBCs/mm^3, or the time between sample acquisition and analysis is prolonged, the clinician should not rely on xanthochromia to confirm SAH.

Xanthochromia is best detected by spectrophotometry since the naked eye can only detect xanthochromia about half the time (Vermeulin and van Gijn, 1990; Petzold et al., 2006). Absorption spectrophotometry, which is a measurement of the light intensity in different regions of the visible spectrum (400–700 nm) after its transmission through an absorbing medium, can detect oxyhemoglobin and bilirubin by their characteristic maximum absorption bands of 415 and 455 nm, respectively (Vermeulen and van Gijn, 1990; Weir, 1994). The probability of detecting xanthochromia by spectrophotometry at various times after SAH is shown in Table 5–9 (Vermeulen et al., 1989); however, a false negative case at 7 days has been reported (McCarron and Choudhari, 2005). In addition, spectrophotometry has limited availability in emergency departments and is available in only perhaps 0.3% of hospital laboratories in the United States (Edlow et al., 2002).

The clinical utility of spectrophotometry is somewhat debatable because of false positives. Wood et al. (2005), in a prospective study of 253

TABLE 5–9 The Probability of Detecting Xanthochromia with Spectrophotometry in the Cerebrospinal Fluid at Various Times After a Subarachnoid Hemorrhage

Time	*Probability (%)*
12 Hours	100
1 Week	100
2 Weeks	100
3 Weeks	Over 70
4 Weeks	Over 40

Source: Vermeulen, M, Hasan, D, Blijenberg, BG et al. (1989). Xanthochromia after subarachnoid haemorrhage needs no revisitation. *J Neurol Neurosurg Psychiatr*, 52:826–828.

patients, found that spectrophotometry has limited clinical utility. Although the sensitivity was 100%, the specificity was only 75.2% with a positive predictive value as an indicator of SAH of 3.3%. Similarly, based upon a prospective series of emergency room patients, Perry et al. (2006) also found only moderate-to-poor specificity of spectrophotometry when used for the diagnosis of SAH. Conversely, Gunawardena et al. (2004) reported that CSF spectrophotometry resulted in the diagnosis of an intracranial aneurysm in 2% (9/463) of patients with CT-negative suspected SAH and nonfocal neurological examinations when the LP was performed more than 12 hours and less than 2 weeks after the ictus. Less than 1% of patients with oxyhemoglobin alone had aneurysms diagnosed, while 21% of patients with bilirubin had an aneurysm.

Other causes of xanthochromia include the following: jaundice, usually with a total plasma bilirubin of 10–15 mg/dl; CSF protein greater than 150 mg/dl; dietary hypercarotenemia; malignant melanomatosis; oral intake of rifampin; and traumatic LPs (Fishman, 1992).

Cerebral Angiography, Magnetic Resonance Angiography, and Spiral CT Angiography

After SAH, a neurovascular study should be performed, since about 20% of patients have multiple aneurysms. Although saccular aneurysms are usually detected on an initial digital subtraction (DS) angiogram, false negatives can occur in 6% (Urbach et al., 1998) to 16% (Iwanaga et al., 1990), often missing an anterior communicating artery aneurysm. Potential reasons for false negatives include vasospasm, thrombosis of the aneurysm, observer error, and technical factors such as inadequate oblique views (Iwanaga, 1990; Wolpert and Caplan, 1992). A repeat DS angiography (DSA) should be repeated after 2 weeks in the following circumstances: findings of vasospasm; an incomplete or inadequate study; an aneurysmal pattern of blood on the initial CAT scan (Rinkel et al., 1992) and when a CAT scan performed within 4 days after the SAH shows thin or thick subarachnoid blood, particularly with a lot of blood in the basal frontal inter-hemispheric fissure (Iwanaga, 1990). Occasionally, a third DSA may be necessary to demonstrate an aneurysm (Mehdorn et al., 1992).

Neurologic complications occasionally occur due to cerebral angiography. A prospective study of 1000 consecutive cerebral arteriograms from the Barrow Neurological Institute reported a 1% overall incidence of neurologic deficit and a 0.5% incidence of persistent deficit. All the complications occurred in patients being evaluated for a history of stroke, transient ischemic event, or carotid bruit, with an average age of 73 years (Heiserman et al., 1994). Although there were none in the 137 studies performed for SAH, complications associated with vasospasm can certainly occur. In a retrospective study of 483 cerebral angiographic examinations in 454 patients using the DSA technique, the frequency of all neurologic complications was 2.3%, with persistent neurologic deficits in 0.4% (Leffers and Wagner, 2000). A higher incidence of complications may occur in departments with a low volume of studies or when performed by inexperienced physicians (Gabrielsen, 1994).

MR angiography is useful but not as sensitive as DSA in the detection of saccular aneurysms (see Fig. 5–10). MR angiography with 3D time-of-flight sequences has a sensitivity of about 90% for intracranial aneurysms of 3 mm or greater as compared with DSA (Okahara et al., 2002). Contrast-enhanced MR angiography may increase the yield. Okahara et al. (2002) found significant inter-observer variability in detection of aneurysms on MR angiography studies as follows: 79% for neuroradiologists, 75% for neurosurgeons, 63% for general radiologists, and 60% for radiology residents.

Spiral (helical) CT angiography is very promising. CT angiography with a 16-detector row machine with 3D interpretation on workstations may detect intracranial saccular aneurysms with equivalent accuracy to DSA (Tipper et al., 2005); however, Dammert et al. (2004) found less accuracy for multi-slice CTA especially for aneurysms smaller than 4 mm (83%). In addition, older-generation four-slice scanners with interpretation of hard-copy films may have a lower yield of 85%–93% and may miss smaller aneurysms of diameter less than 3 mm (Strayle-Batra et al., 1998).

Spiral CT can be very useful instead of, or as an alternative to, MR angiography for patients with

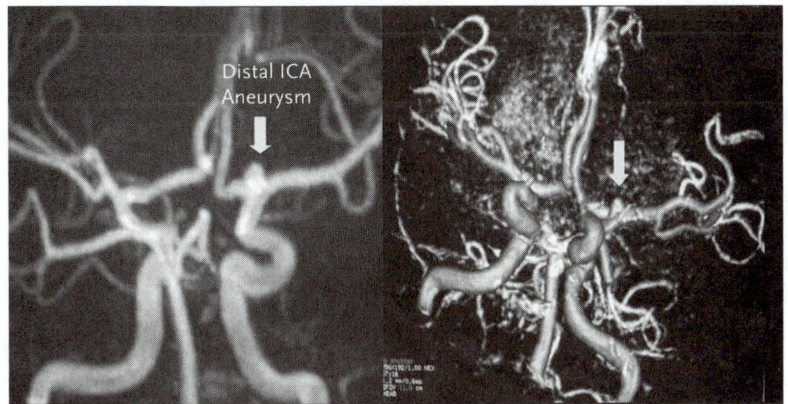

Figure 5–10 A 35-year-old women presents with a severe throbbing left frontal headache associated with nausea and photophobia. Although the headache was characteristic of a migraine, an MRA was ordered because of a family history of cerebral aneurysm. A distal left internal carotid aneurysm was found (arrow) and eventually clipped. Headaches resolved.

contraindications to MRI such as pacemakers, intracranial ferromagnetic clips, and severe claustrophobia; however, in addition to contrast allergy, there is additional risk of intravenous contrast in patients with renal insufficiency, dehydration, and diabetes. In practice, MR and CT angiography are both limited by the quality of the equipment, the images, and the ability of the interpreting physician.

NEW DAILY HEADACHES

Table 5–10 lists some of the causes for daily headaches that have been present for more than 3 months. New daily persistent headache (NDPH) is unique in that it starts daily from onset, and is a diagnosis of exclusion. Some secondary disorders can be present, such as a thunderclap headache, whereas others may develop gradually over 1–3 days. New daily headaches with a normal neurological examination could be due to various causes particularly when seen within the first 2 months after onset, including postmeningitis headache, chronic meningitis, brain tumors, leptomeningeal metastasis, temporal arteritis, chronic subdural hematomas, posttraumatic headaches, sphenoid sinusitis, and hypertension (see Fig. 5–11). When the headaches have been present for more than 3 months with a normal neurological examination, the yield of testing is low. A few additional examples will be discussed.

TABLE 5–10 Differential Diagnosis of Daily Headaches for More Than 3 Months

Primary headaches
- New daily persistent headache
- Chronic migraine
- Chronic tension type
- Chronic cluster headache
- Hemicrania continua

Secondary headaches may mimic new daily persistent headache
- Postmeningitis headache
- Chronic meningitis
- Primary with medication rebound
- Neoplasms
- Chronic subdural hematoma
- Posttraumatic headaches
- Sphenoid sinusitis
- Hypertension
- Low cerebrospinal fluid pressure syndrome
- Cervical artery dissections
- Pseudotumor cerebri (idiopathic and secondary intracranial hypertension)
- Cerebral venous thrombosis
- Arteriovenous malformation
- Chiari malformation
- Temporal arteritis
- Cervicogenic
- Temporomandibular joint dysfunction

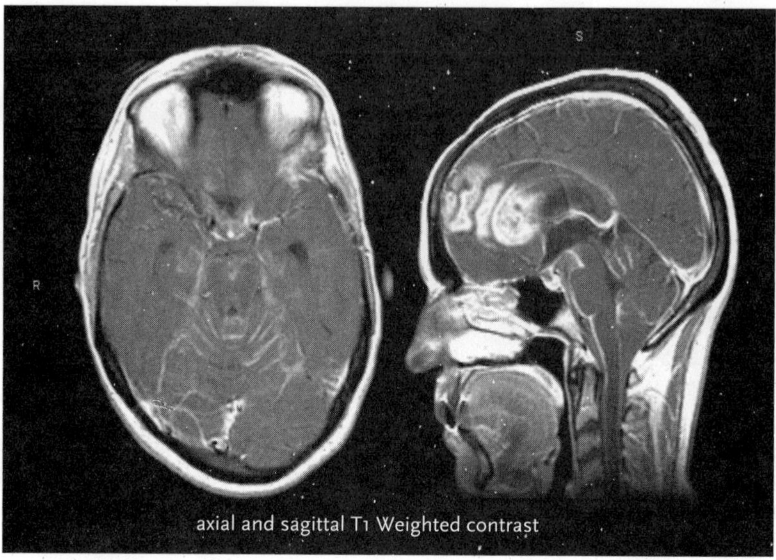

Figure 5–11 A 65-year-old male with a 2-year history of bronchogenic carcinoma who now presents with continuous progressive occipital headache that was unresponsive to medication. Axial and sagittal T1-weighted contrast MRI studies confirmed leptomeningeal enhancement within the sulci and leptomeninges. The sugar coating of the brainstem, cerebellum, falx, and spinal cord is characteristic of leptomeningeal disease. In a patient with a known history of cancer, further studies i.e. lumbar puncture, may not be needed for appropriate treatment.

Spontaneous intracranial hypotension (SIH) syndrome often presents with a headache that is present when a patient is upright but is relieved by lying down, thus an orthostatic headache; however, as SIH syndrome persists, a chronic daily headache may be present without orthostatic features. SIH syndrome may also present with other types of headaches, including exertional without any orthostatic features, acute thunderclap onset, paradoxical orthostatic headaches (present in recumbency and relieved when upright), intermittent headaches due to intermittent leaks, and the acephalgic form with no headaches at all (Mokri, 2004). Neck or interscapular pain may precede the onset of headache in some cases by days or weeks. MRI abnormalities of the brain and spine are variably present in perhaps 90% of cases. An MRI scan of the brain may reveal diffuse pachymeningeal (dural) enhancement with gadolinium without leptomeningeal (arachnoid and pial) involvement and, in some cases, subdural fluid collections, which return to normal with resolution of the headache (Mokri, 2004; Schievink, 2006) (see Fig. 5–12). Other MRI findings in SIH include: an enlarged pituitary gland, descent of the cerebellar tonsils, crowding of the posterior fossa, flattening of the optic chiasm, enlarged cerebral venous sinuses and reduction in size of the subarachnoid cisterns (Mokri, 2004).

Cervical artery dissections, which can present with headache or neck pain alone (Arnold et al., 2006), can be a rare cause of new daily headaches (Mokri, 2002). Occasionally, the headaches can persist intermittently for months, and even years, and can lead to a pattern of chronic daily headaches especially after cervical carotid artery dissection.

Headache is present in up to 90% of cases of CVT and is often the initial symptom and occasionally the only symptom (Cumurciuc et al., 2005). The headache can be unilateral or bilateral in any location, mild-to-severe, and intermittent or constant. The onset is usually subacute but can be sudden or thunderclap. The headache is almost always associated with other neurological signs such as papilledema, focal deficits, seizures, disorders of consciousness, or cranial nerve palsies.

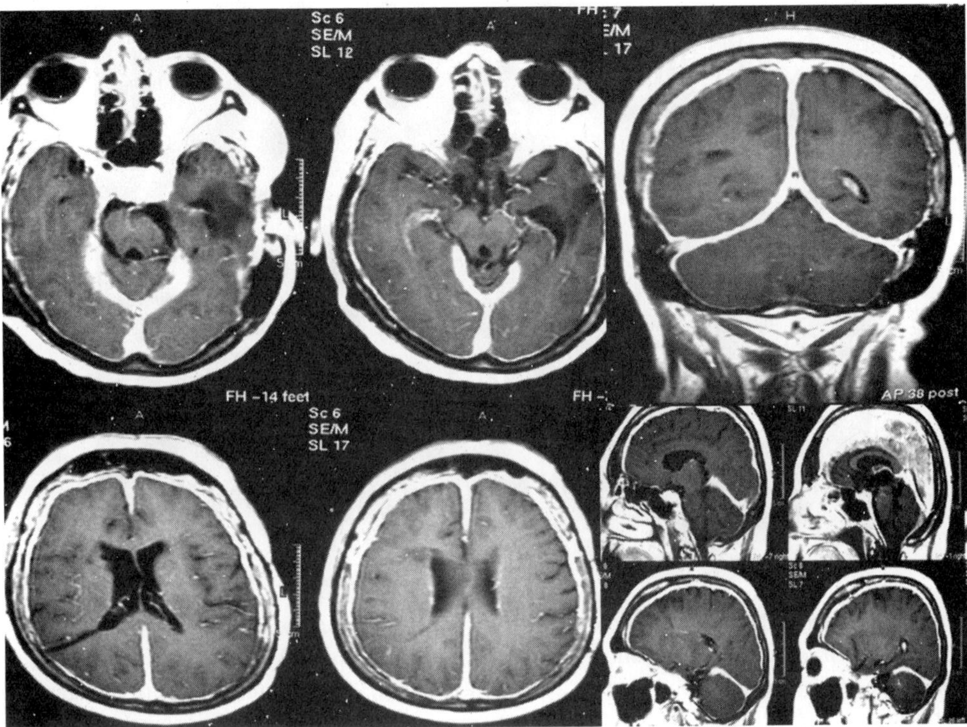

Figure 5–12 Gadolinium contrast MR images in the axial, coronal and sagittal plane demonstrating diffuse pachymeningeal thickening and enhancement. Patient is a 40 year-old male complaining of postural headaches after resection of left middle fossa meningioma. In patients with positional or exertional headaches contrast studies may be diagnostic in Intracranial hypotension.

CVT can be a mimic of idiopathic intracranial hypertension.

Neuroimaging studies have variable sensitivities in diagnosing CVT. CT only diagnoses about 20% of cases of CVT when demonstrating the hyperdensity of the thrombosed sinus on plain images and the delta sign seen with superior sagittal sinus thrombosis after contrast administration. Helical CT venography is a very sensitive diagnostic method. CVT may be missed on routine MRI imaging of the brain although echo-planar T2*-weighted MRI may increase the sensitivity (Selim et al., 2002). Magnetic resonance venography (MRV) increases the sensitivity of MR especially within the first 5 days of onset or after 6 weeks. CVT can also be demonstrated, of course, on DS venography (see Fig. 5–13).

Chiari I malformation is a typically congenital malformation of cerebellar tonsillar herniation at least 3–5 cm below the foramen magnum associated with crowding of the craniocervical junction, obstructive hydrocephalus, and syringomyelia. In an imaging study of children with headaches aged 2–18 (Schwedt et al., 2006), Chiari type I malformation was identified in 14 of 241 (5.8%) patients. Five of fourteen (35.7%) patients with Chiari I malformation in this had headaches secondary to their malformation. Three patients had surgical decompression with significant headache relief in 2. The other nine patients were diagnosed with migraine (35.7%) and tension-type (28.6%) headaches. Although headache is the most commonly presenting complaint of Chiari I malformation, the malformation is typically an incidental

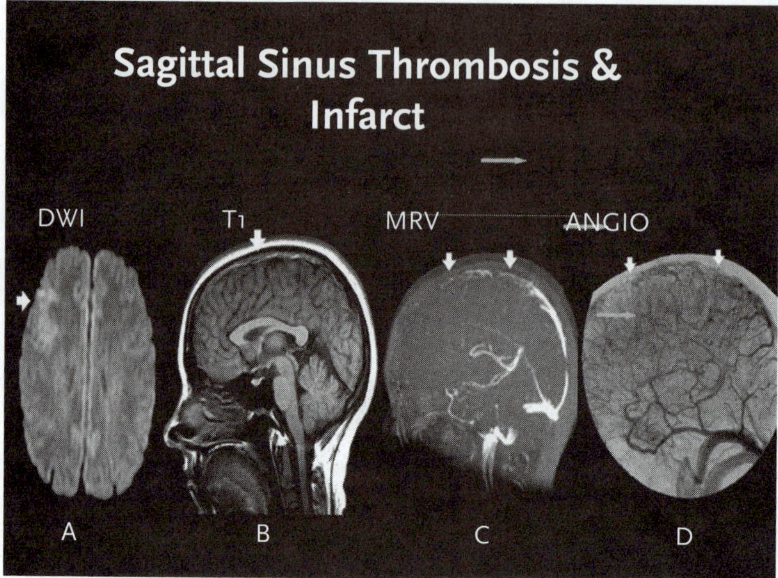

Figure 5–13 A 32-year-old women who presented with a severe headache and seizure. Diffusion weighted images (A) confirm an acute right frontal lobe infarct not in the typical arterial distribution. T1 and T2 weighted images were normal within the first 24 h of presentation. T1-weighted sagittal (B) images showed a increased signal representing a thrombus within the superior sagittal sinus. MR venogram (C) and venous phase angiogram (D) support the diagnosis of superior sagittal thrombosis. Risk factors for venous thrombosis include: dehydration, pregnancy, oral contraceptives, trauma, DIC, neoplasms, hypercoagable states, infections and idiopathic. Reproduced with kind permission of Rohit Bakshi.

finding on MRI studies done for primary headaches.

NEW ONSET HEADACHES IN PATIENTS OVER THE AGE OF 50

When new onset headaches begin in patients over the age of 50, the physician should consider the various primary headache disorders as well as the multiplicity of secondary headaches (Table 5–11). While new onset tension-type headaches are rather common, migraine and cluster-type headaches uncommonly begin after age 50 (in about 2% and 13%, respectively). Obtaining an MRI scan in late-onset cluster (possibly for all cluster headache patients) might be considered, especially if atypical features are present. Secondary causes of cluster headache include: internal carotid artery dissection; pseudoaneurysm of intracavernous carotid artery; aneurysm of the anterior communicating, carotid, or basilar artery; AVM of the middle cerebral territory or occipital lobe; high cervical meningioma; unilateral cervical cord or

TABLE 5–11 Common Causes of Headache Beginning in Late Life

Secondary headache disorders
Mass lesions
Temporal arteritis
Medication-related headache
Trigeminal neuralgia
Postherpetic neuralgia
Systemic disease
Disease of the cranium, neck, eyes, ears, and nose
Cerebrovascular disease
Parkinson's disease
Primary headache disorders
Migraine
Tension-type headache
Cluster headache
Hypnic headache

Source: With permission from Lipton, RB, Pfeffer, D, Newman, LC et al. (1993). Headaches in the elderly. *J Pain Symptom Manage*, 8:88.

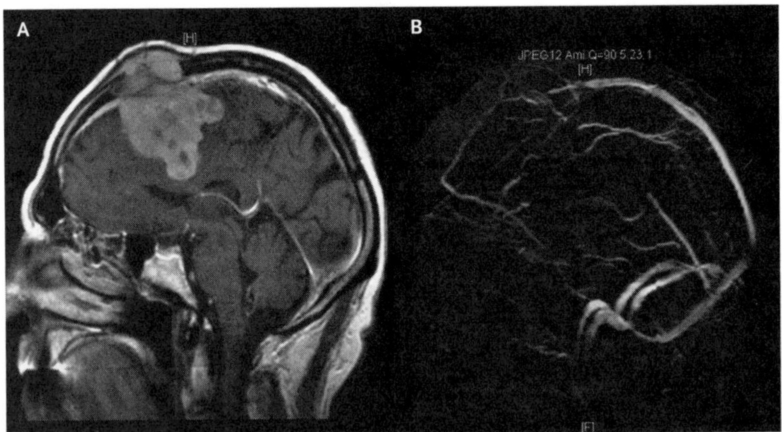

Figure 5–14 60-year-old man with a chronic frontal headache and growing bump on his forehead. T1W contrast images show a large enhancing frontal mass that erodes the calvarium and uplifts the scalp. B. The MRV confirms infiltration and occlusion of the superior sagittal sinus. Headaches resolved after resection of a menigioma.

lateral medullary infarction; pituitary adenoma; meningioma of the lesser wing of the sphenoid; maxillary sinus foreign body; orbitosphenoidal aspergillosis; CVT; and orbital myositis.

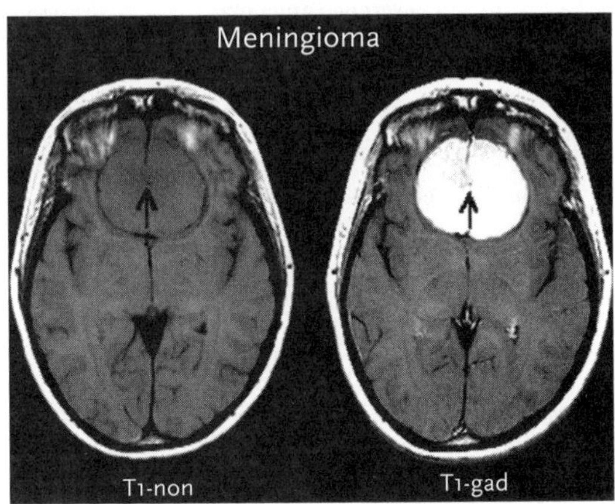

Figure 5–15 Typical olfactory meningioma in a 56 year-old female presenting with bifrontal headaches and cognitive changes. A. Non-contrast T1 weighted axial MR image shows an isointense large extra-axial mass distorting the frontal lobe. B. With gadolinium contrast there is homogenous enhancement. Postoperatively, headaches and dementia completely resolved.

Hypnic headaches present as headaches awakening the patient from sleep at a consistent time almost nightly, in those usually age 40 or older. The pain, which lasts from 15 minutes to 6 hours, can be unilateral or bilateral and throbbing or nonthrobbing (Evers and Goadsby, 2003). Rarely, the autonomic symptoms so prevalent in cluster headache are seen in hypnic headache. The diagnosis is one of exclusion, since secondary causes of nocturnal headaches include drug withdrawal, temporal arteritis, sleep apnea, nocturnal hypertension-headache syndrome, oxygen desaturation, pheochromocytomas, primary and secondary neoplasms, communicating hydrocephalus, subdural hematomas, subacute angle-closure glaucoma, and vascular lesions (Peres, 2007).

The common causes of secondary headache disorders beginning in later life include the following: mass lesions such as subdural hematomas and neoplasm; temporal arteritis; medication-related headaches including headaches caused by specific medications as well as medication rebound or withdrawal headaches; trigeminal neuralgia; postherpetic neuralgia; systemic disease such as infections, acute hypertension, hypoxia or hypercarbia, and other metabolic abnormalities such as hypercalcemia or severe anemia; headaches associated with disorders of the cranium, neck, eyes, ears, and nose including cervicogenic

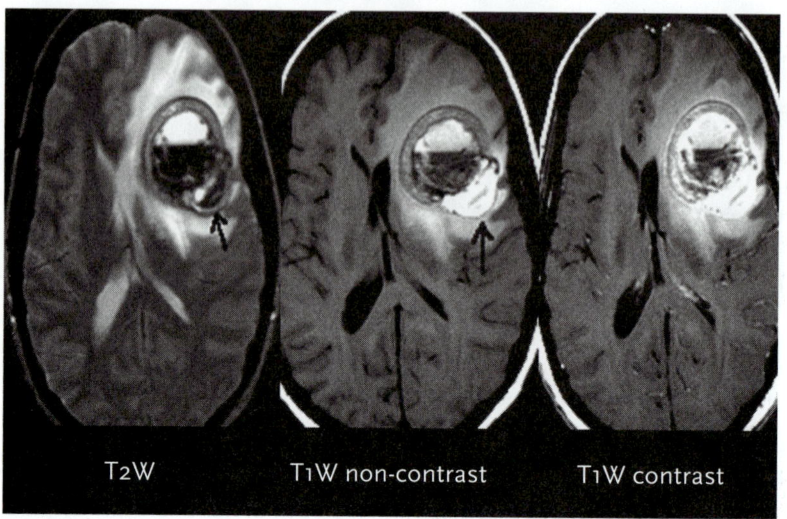

Figure 5–16 Axial MRI study shows an encapsulated single hemorrhagic metastasis within the left frontal lobe that is associated with vasogenic edema, ventricular and sulcal effacement, as well as early midline shift. Patient is a 36-year-old female who presented with severe throbbing left frontal headache with nausea that was acute in onset. Past medical history is significant for cutaneous melanoma resected 5 years ago. Patient's headaches resolved after complete resection of this metastatic melanoma followed by external beam radiation.

headache, glaucoma, otitis, sinusitis, and dental infections; cerebrovascular disease; and the one-third of patients with Parkinson's disease who report headaches (Lipton et al., 1993; Edmeads, 1997) (see Fig. 5–14, 15, and 16).

Pascual and Berciano (1994) performed a study of 193 patients age 65 and over seen by the neurology service in the past 15 years with de novo headache as their initial and main symptom. The most frequent diagnoses were tension-type headaches in 43% and trigeminal neuralgia in 19%. Only one patient met migraine criteria. Fifteen percent had a secondary headache disorder due to conditions such as stroke, temporal arteritis, or intracranial neoplasm. Although the incidence of patients with de novo headaches attending a general hospital decreased with age, the risk of headache due to serious conditions increased 10 times after age 65.

References

ACOG Committee on Obstetric Practice (2004). ACOG Committee Opinion. Number 299, September, 2004 (replaces No. 158, September, 1995). Guidelines for diagnostic imaging during pregnancy. *Obstet Gynecol*, 104:647–651.

Afridi, S and Goadsby, PJ (2003). New onset migraine with a brain stem cavernous angioma. *J Neurol Neurosurg Psychiatr*, 74:680–682.

Akpek, S, Arac, M, Atilla, S et al. (1995). Cost effectiveness of computed tomography in the evaluation of patients with headache. *Headache*, 35:228–230.

Al-Shahi, R, White, PM, Davenport, RJ et al. (2006). Subarachnoid haemorrhage. *BMJ*, 333:235–240.

Al-Yamany, M, Deck, J, Bernstein, M (1999). Pseudo-subarachnoid hemorrhage: a rare neuroimaging pitfall. *Can J Neurol Sci*, 26:57–59.

American Academy of Neurology (1994). The utility of neuroimaging in the evaluation of headache in patients with normal neurologic examinations. *Neurology*, 44:1353–1354.

American Academy of Neurology (1995). Practice parameter: the electroencephalogram in the evaluation of headache. *Neurology*, 45:1411–1413.

Amit, M, Molad, Y, Levy, O (1999). Headache and systemic lupus erythematosis and its relation to other disease manifestations. *Clin Exp Rheumatol*, 17:467–470.

Anzola, GP, Magoni, M, Guindani, M et al. (1999). Potential source of cerebral embolism in migraine with aura: a trans cranial Doppler study. *Neurology*, 52:1622–1625.

Armon, C and Evans, RW (2005). Addendum to assessment: prevention of post-lumbar puncture headaches:

report of the Therapeutics and Technology Assessment Subcommittee of the American Academy of Neurology. *Neurology*, 65:510–512.

Arnett, BC (2004). Tonsillar ectopia and headaches. *Neurol Clin*, 22:229–236.

Arnold, M, Cumurciuc, R, Stapf, C et al. (2006). Pain as the only symptom of cervical artery dissection. *J Neurol Neurosurg Psychiatr*, 77(9):1021–1024.

The Arteriovenous Malformation Study Group (1999). Arteriovenous malformations of the brain in adults. *New England J Med*, 340:1812–1818.

Baker, H (1983). Cranial CT in the investigation of headache: cost effectiveness for brain tumors. *J Neuroradiol*, 10:112–116.

Barrows, LJ, Hunter, FT, and Banker, BQ (1955). The nature and clinical significance of pigments in the cerebrospinal fluid. *Brain*, 78:59–80.

Beetham, R, Fahie-Wilson, MN, and Park, D (1998). What is the role of spectrophotometry in the diagnosis of subarachnoid haemorrhage? *Ann Clin Biochem*, 35:1–4.

Beresford, HR (1999). Medicolegal aspects. In *Diagnostic Testing in Neurology* (RW Evans, ed.), pp. 479–488. W. B. Saunders, Philadelphia.

Birchard, KR, Brown, MA, Hyslop, WB et al. (2005). MRI of acute abdominal and pelvic pain in pregnant patients. *AJR Am J Roentgenol*, 184:452–458.

Brown, RD, Wiebers, DO, Forbes, G et al. (1988). The natural history of unruptured intracranial arteriovenous malformations. *J Neurosurg*, 68:352–357.

Bruyn, GW (1984). Intracranial arteriovenous malformation and migraine. *Cephalalgia*, 4:191–207.

Buruma, OJ, Janson, HL, Den Bergh, FA, Bots, GT (1981). Blood-stained cerebrospinal fluid: traumatic puncture or haemorrhage? *J Neurol Neurosurg Psychiatr*, 44:144–147,

Cala, L and Mastaglia, F (1976). Computerized axial tomography findings in a group of patients with migrainous headaches. *Proc Aust Acad Neurol*, 13:35–41.

Carlos, RA, Santos, CS, Kumar, S et al. (2000). Neuroimaging studies in pediatric migraine headaches. *Headache*, 40:404.

Carrera, G, Gerson, D, Schnur, J et al. (1977). Computerized tomography of the brain in patients with headache or temporal lobe epilepsy: findings and cost effectiveness. *J Comput Assist Tomogr*, 1:200–203.

Chu, ML and Shinnar, S (1992). Headaches in children younger than 7 years of age. *Arch Neurol*, 49:79–82.

Cooney, BS, Grossman, RI, Farber, RE et al. (1996). Frequency of magnetic resonance imaging abnormalities in patients with migraine. *Headache*, 36:616–621.

Cuetter, A and Aita, J (1983). CT scanning in classic migraine [letter]. *Headache*, 23:195.

Cumurciuc, R, Crassard, I, Sarov, M et al. (2005). Headache as the only neurological sign of cerebral venous thrombosis: a series of 17 cases. *J Neurol Neurosurg Psychiatr*, 76:1084–1087.

Dammert, S, Krings, T, Moller-Hartmann, W et al. (2004). Detection of intracranial aneurysms with multislice CT: comparison with conventional angiography. *Neuroradiology*, 46:427–434.

Daras, M, Koppel, B, Leyfermann, M et al. (1995). Anticardiolipin antibodies in migraine patients: an additional risk factor for stroke? *Neurology*, 45(Suppl. 4): A367–A368.

Davenport, R (2002). Acute headache in the emergency department. *J Neurol Neurosurg Psychiatr*, 72:ii33–ii37.

De Benedittis, G, Lorenzetti, A, Sina, C et al. (1995). Magnetic resonance imaging in migraine and tension-type headache. *Headache*, 35:264–268.

de Falco, FA (2004). Sentinel headache. *Neurol Sci*, 25: S215–S217.

Demaerel, P, Boelaert, I, Wilms, G et al. (1996). The role of cranial computed tomography in the diagnostic work-up of headache. *Headache*, 36:347–348.

Dooley, JM, Camfield, PR, O'Neill M et al. (1990). The value of CT scans for children with headaches. *Can J Neurol Sci*, 17:309–310.

du Boulay, GH and Ruiz, JS (1983). CT changes associated with migraine. *AJNR Am J Neuroradiol*, 4:472–473.

Duffy, GP (1982). Lumbar puncture in spontaneous subarachnoid haemorrhage. *BMJ*, 285:1163–1164.

Dumas, MD, Pexman, W, and Kreeft, JH (1994). Computed tomography evaluation of patients with chronic headache. *Can Med Assoc J*, 151:1447–1452.

Edlow, JA, Bruner, KS, Horowitz, GL (2002). Xanthochromia. *Arch Pathol Lab Med*, 126:413–415.

Edmeads, J (1997). Headaches in older people. How are they different in this age-group? *Postgrad Med*, 101:91–94, 98, 100.

Embil, JM, Kramer, M, Kinnear, S et al. (1997). A blinding headache. *Lancet*, 349:182.

Evans, RW (1997). Migrainelike headaches in pituitary apoplexy. *Headache*, 37:455–456.

Evans, RW (2003). New daily persistent headache. *Curr Pain Headache Rep*, 7:303–307.

Evans EW (2006). Complications of lumbar puncture. In *Neurology and trauma* (2nd edn) Evans, RW (ed.), pp. 697–715, Oxford University Press, New York.

Evans, RW (1999). Headaches. In *Diagnostic Testing in Neurology* (RW Evans, ed.), pp. 1–19. W.B. Saunders, Philadelphia.

Evers, S and Goadsby, PJ (2003). Hypnic headache: clinical features, pathophysiology, and treatment. *Neurology*, 60:905–909.

Fazekas, F, Koch, M, Schmidt, R et al. (1992). The prevalence of cerebral damage varies with migraine type: a MRI study. *Headache*, 32:287–291.

Fisher, CM (1984). Painful states: a neurological commentary. *Clin Neurosurg*, 31:32–53.

Fishman, RA (1992). Chapter 7. Examination of the cerebrospinal fluid: techniques and complications. In *Cerebrospinal Fluid in Diseases of the Nervous System* (FA Fisherman, ed.) pp. 183–252. W.B. Saunders, Philadelphia.

Frishberg, BM (1994). The utility of neuroimaging in the evaluation of headache in patients with normal neurologic examination. *Neurology*, 44:1191–1197.

Frishberg, BM (1997). Neuroimaging in presumed primary headache disorders. *Semin Neurol*, 17:373–382.

Gabrielsen, TO (1994). Neurologic complications of cerebral angiography. *AJNR*, 15:1408–1411.

Ghoshhajra, K, Scotti, L, Marasco, J et al. (1979). CT detection of intracranial aneurysm in subarachnoid hemorrhage. *AJR Am J Roentgenol*, 132:613–616.

Ghossoub, M, Nataf, F, Merienne, L et al. (2001). Characteristics of headache associated with cerebral arteriovenous malformations. *Neurochirurgie*, 47(2–3 Pt 2):177–183.

Goadsby, PJ (2002). Neurovascular headache and a midbrain vascular malformation: evidence for a role of the brainstem in chronic migraine. *Cephalalgia*, 22:107–111.

Goadsby, PJ (2007). Cluster headache. In *MedLink Neurology* (S Gilman, ed.). Arbor, San Diego. Available at www.medlink.com

Graves, P and Sidman, R (2004). Xanthochromia is not pathognomonic for subarachnoid hemorrhage. *Acad Emerg Med*, 11:131–135.

Gronseth, GS and Greenberg, MK (1995). The utility of electroencephalogram in the evaluation of patients presenting with headache: a review of the literature. *Neurology* 45:1263–1267.

Gunawardena, H, Beetham, R, Scolding, N et al. (2004). Is cerebrospinal fluid spectrophotometry useful in CT scan-negative suspected subarachnoid haemorrhage? *Eur Neurol*, 52:226–229.

Heasley, DC, Mohamed, MA, and Yousem, DM (2005). Clearing of red blood cells in lumbar puncture does not rule out ruptured aneurysm in patients with suspected subarachnoid hemorrhage but negative head CT findings. *ANJR Am J Neuroradiol*, 26:820–824.

Heiserman, JE, Dean, BL, Hodak, JA et al. (1994). Neurologic complications of cerebral angiography. *AJNR*, 15:1401–1407.

Hering, R, Couturier, EGM, Steiner, TJ et al. (1991). Anticardiolipin antibodies in migraine. *Cephalalgia*, 11:19–21.

Hungerford, G. duBoulay, G, and Zilkha, K (1976). Computerized axial tomography in patientswith severe migraine: a preliminary report. *J Neurol Neurosurg Psychiatr*, 39:990–994.

Igarashi, H, Sakai, F, Kan, S et al. (1991). Magnetic resonance imaging of the brain in patients with migraine. *Cephalalgia*, 11:69–74.

Iizuka, T and Sakai, F (2005), Pathogenesis of stroke-like episodes in MELAS: analysis of neurovascular cellular mechanisms. *Curr Neurovasc Res*, 2(1):29–45.

Initso D, Di Renzo F, Rinaldi G et al. Brain MRI white matter lesions in migraine patients: is there a relationship with antiphospholipid antibodies and coagulation parameters? *Eur J Neurol* 2006, 13:1364–1369

Iwanaga, H, Wakai, S, Ochiai, C et al. (1990). Ruptured cerebral aneurysms missed by initial angiographic study. *Neurosurg*, 27:45–51.

Jacome, DE and Leborgne, J (1990). MRI studies in basilar artery migraine. *Headache* 30:88–90.

Johnston, SD and Robinson, TJ (1998). Subarchnoid haemorrhage: difficulties in diagnosis and treatment. *Postgrad Med*, 74:743–748.

Kanal, E, Gillen, J, Evans, JA et al. (1993). Survey of reproductive health among female MR workers. *Radiology*, 187:395–399.

Kassell, NF, Torner, JC, Haley, EC et al. (1990). The international cooperative study on the timing of aneurysm surgery. Part I: Overall management results. *J Neurosurg*, 73:18–36.

Kassirer, JP (1989). Our stubborn quest for diagnostic certainty. A cause of excessive testing. *N Engl J Med*, 320:1489–1491.

Kaufmann, P, Shungu, DC, Sano, MC et al. (2004). Cerebral lactic acidosis correlates with neurological impairment in MELAS. *Neurology*, 62:1297–1302.

Kruit, MC, van Buchem, MA, Hofman, PA et al. (2004). Migraine as a risk factor for subclinical brain lesions. *J Am Med Assoc*, 291:427–434.

Kruit, MC, Launer, LJ, Ferrari, MD et al. (2005). Infarcts in the posterior circulation territory in migraine. The population-based MRI CAMERA study. *Brain*, 128(Pt 9):2068–2077.

Kruit, MC, Launer, LJ, Ferrari, MD et al. (2006). Brain stem and cerebellar hyperintense lesions in migraine. *Stroke*, 37(4):1109–1112.

Kuhn, MJ and Shekar, PC (1990). A comparative study of magnetic resonance imaging and computed tomography in the evaluation of migraine. *Comput Med Imaging Graph*, 14:149–152.

Kupersmith, MJ, Vargas, ME, Yashar, A et al. (1996). Occipital arteriovenous malformations: visual disturbances and presentation. *Neurology*, 46:953–957.

Laffey, P, Oaks, W, Sawmi, R et al. (1978). *Computerized Tomography in Clinical Medicine: Data Supplement.* Philadelphia: Medical Directions.

Lance, JW and Goadsby, PJ (2005). *Mechanism and Management of Headache* (8th Edn). Elsevier, Philadelphia, p. 359.

Larson, E, Omenn, G, and Lewis, H (1980). Diagnostic evaluation of headache: impact of computerized tomography and cost effectiveness. *JAMA*, 243:359–362.

Leffers, AM and Wagner, A (2000). Neurologic complications of cerebral angiography. A retrospective study of complication rate and patient risk factors. *Acta Radiol*, 41:204–210.

Leone, M, D'Amico, D, Frediani, F et al. (1993). Clinical considerations on side-locked unilaterality in long lasting primary headaches. *Headache*, 33:381–384.

Lewis, DW, Ashwal, S, Dahl, G et al. (2002). Practice parameter: evaluation of children and adolescents with recurrent headaches: report of the Quality Standards Subcommittee of the American Academy of

Neurology and the Practice Committee of the Child Neurology Society. *Neurology*, 59:490–498.

Linn, FH, Wijdicks, EF, van der Graaf, Y et al. (1994). Prospective study of sentinel headache in aneurysmal subarachnoid haemorrhage. *Lancet*, 344:590–593.

Linn, FHH, Rinkel, GJE, Algra, A et al. (1998). Headache characteristics in subarachnoid haemorrhage and benign thunderclap headache. *J Neurol Neurosurg Psychiatr*, 65:791–793.

Lipton, RB, Pfeffer, D, Newman, LC et al. (1993). Headaches in the elderly. *J Pain Symptom Manage*, 8:87–97.

Malik, SN and Young, WB (2006). Midbrain cavernous malformation causing migraine-like headache. *Cephalalgia*, 26:1016–1019.

Masland, W, Friedman, A, and Buchsbaum, H (1978). Computerized axial tomography of migraine. *Res Clin Stud Headache*, 6:136–140.

Maytal, J, Bienkowski, RS, Patel, M et al. (1996). The value of brain imaging in children with headaches. *Pediatrics*, 96:413–416.

Mazzotta, G, Floridi, F, Mattioni, A et al. (2004). The role of neuroimaging in the diagnosis of headache in childhood and adolescence: a multicentre study. *Neurol Sci*, 25(Suppl. 3):S265–S266.

McCarron, MO and Choudhari, KA (2005). Aneurysmal subarachnoid leak with normal CT and CSF spectrophotometry. *Neurology*, 64:923.

Medina, S, Pinter, JD, Zurakowski, D et al. (1997). Children with headache: clinical predictors of surgical space-occupying lesions and the role of neuroimaging. *Radiology*, 202:819–824.

Mehdorn, HM, Dietrich, V, Kalff, R et al. (1992). Subarachnoid hemorrhage of unknown etiology: long-term prognosis. *Neurosurg Rev*, 15:27–31.

Mitchell, P, Wilkinson, ID, Hoggard, N et al. (2001). Detection of subarachnoid haemorrhage with magnetic resonance imaging. *J Neurol Neurosurg Psychiatr*, 70:205–211.

Mitchell, C, Osborn, R, and Grosskreutz, S (1993). Computerized tomography in the headache patient: is routine evaluation really necessary? *Headache*, 33:82–86.

Mohamed, M, Heasly, DC, Yagmurlu, B et al. (2004). Fluid-attenuated inversion recovery MR imaging and subarachnoid hemorrhage: not a panacea. *AJNR Am J Neuroradiol*, 25:545–550.

Mokri, B (1997). Headache in spontaneous carotid and vertebral artery dissections. In *Headache* (PJ Goadsby and SD Silberstein, eds.), pp. 327–353. Butterworth-Heinemann, Boston.

Mokri, B (2002). Headache in cervical artery dissections. *Curr Pain Headache Rep*, 6:209–216.

Mokri, B (2004). Low cerebrospinal fluid pressure syndromes. *Neurol Clin*, 22:55–74.

Morgenstern, LB, Luna-Gonzales, H, Huber, JC et al. (1998). Worst headache and subarachnoid hemorrhage: prospective, modern computed tomography and spinal fluid analysis. *Ann Emerg Med*, 32:297–304.

Morgenstern, LB, Huber, JC, Luna-Gonzales, H et al. (2001). Headache in the emergency department. *Headache*, 41:537–541.

Mourad, A, Levasseur, M, Bousser, MG et al. (2006). [CADASIL with minimal symptoms after 60 years] *Rev Neurol (Paris)*, 162(8–9):827–831.

Obermann, M, Gizewski, ER, Limmroth, V et al. (2006). Symptomatic migraine and pontine vascular malformation: evidence for a key role of the brainstem in the pathophysiology of chronic migraine. *Cephalalgia*, 26:763–766.

Okahara, M, Kiyosue, H, Yamashita, M et al. (2002). Diagnostic accuracy of magnetic resonance angiography for cerebral aneurysms in correlation with 3D-digital subtraction angiographic images: a study of 133 aneurysms. *Stroke*, 33:1803–1808.

Osborn, RE, Alder, DC, and Mitchell, CS (1991). MR imaging of the brain in patients with migraine headaches. *AJNR*, 12:521–524.

Pascual, J and Berciano J (1994). Experience in the diagnosis of headaches that start in elderly people. *J Neurol Neurosurg Psychiatr*, 57:1255–1257.

Pascual-Leone, A and Pascual, APL (1992). Occipital neuralgia: another benign cause of "thunderclap headache." *J Neurol Neurosurg Psychiatr*, 55:411.

Pavese, N, Canapicchi, R, Nuti, A et al. (1994). White matter MRI hyperintensities in a hundred and twenty-nine consecutive migraine patients. *Cephalalgia*, 14:342–345.

Peres, MFP (2007). Sleep disorders associated with headaches. In *MedLink Neurology* (S Gilman, ed.). MedLink Corp, San Diego. Available at www.medlink.com

Perry, JJ, Sivilotti, ML, Stiell, IG et al. (2006). Should spectrophotometry be used to identify xanthochromia in the cerebrospinal fluid of alert patients suspected of having subarachnoid hemorrhage? *Stroke*, 37:2467–2472.

Petzold, A, Sharpe, LT, and Keir, G (2006). Spectrophotometry for cerebrospinal fluid pigment analysis. *Neurocrit Care*, 4:153–162.

Polmear, A (2003). Sentinel headaches in aneurysmal subarachnoid haemorrhage: what is the true incidence? A systematic review. *Cephalalgia*, 23:935–941.

Raps, EC, Galetta, SL, Rogers, J et al. (1994). Unruptured aneurysms and headache. *Arch Neurol*, 51:447–448.

Rinkel, GJE, Wijdicks, EFM, Hasan, D et al. (1991). Outcome in patients with subarachnoid haemorrhage and negative angiography according to pattern of haemorrhage on computed tomography. *Lancet*, 338:964–968.

Rinkel, GJE, Wijdicks, EFM, Vermeulen, M et al. (1991). Nonaneurysmal perimesencephalic subarachnoid hemorrhage: CT and MR patterns that differ from aneurysmal rupture. *Am J Neuroradiol*, 12:829–834.

Rinkel, GJE, Djibuti, M, Algra, A et al. (1998). Prevalence and risk of rupture of intracranial aneurysms. A systematic review. *Stroke*, 29:251–256.

Robbins, L et al. (1991). Migraine and anticardiolipin antibodies-case reports of 13 patients and the prevalence of antiphospholipid antibodies in migraineurs. *Headache*, 31:537–539.

Robbins, L and Friedman, H (1992). MRI in migraineurs. *Headache*, 32:507–508.

Rocca, MA, Ceccarelli, A, Falini, A et al. (2006). Diffusion tensor magnetic resonance imaging at 3.0 tesla shows subtle cerebral grey matter abnormalities in patients with migraine. *J Neurol Neurosurg Psychiatr*, 77:686–689.

Rovaris, M, Bozzali, M, Rocca, MA et al. (2001). An MR study of tissue damage in the cervical cord of patients with migraine. *J Neurol Sci*, 183:43–46.

Rowan, AJ (1974). The electroencephalographic characteristics of migraine. *Arch Neurol*, 37:95–99.

Russell, D, Nakstad, P, and Sjaastad, O (1978). Cluster headache: pneumoencephalographic and cerebral computerized axial tomographic findings. *Headache*, 18:272–273.

Saper, JR, Silberstein, S, Gordon, CD et al. (1999). *Handbook of Headache Management* (2nd Edn). Lippincott Williams and Wilkins, Philadelphia , p. 20.

Sargent, J, Lawson, C, Solbach, P ct al. (1979). Use of CT scans in an outpatient headache population: an evaluation. *Headache*, 19:388–390.

Schievink, WI (2006). Spontaneous spinal cerebrospinal fluid leaks and intracranial hypotension. *JAMA*, 295:2286–2296.

Schwedt, TJ, Guo, Y, and Rothner, AD (2006). "Benign" imaging abnormalities in children and adolescents with headache. *Headache*, 46(3):387–398.

Selim, M, Fink, J, Linfante, I et al. (2002). Diagnosis of cerebral venous thrombosis with echo-planar T2*-weighted magnetic resonance imaging. *Arch Neurol*, 59(6):1021–1026.

Sempere, AP, Porta-Etessam, J, Medrano, V et al. (2005). Neuroimaging in the evaluation of patients with non-acute headache. *Cephalalgia*, 25:30–35.

Silberstein, SD (2000). Practice parameter: evidence-based guidelines for migraine headache (an evidence-based review): report of the Quality Standards Subcommittee of the American Academy of Neurology. *Neurology*, 55 (6):754–762.

Silberstein, SD, Lipton, RB, and Goadsby, PJ (2002). *Headache in Clinical Practice*. Martin Dunitz, London.

Silberstein, SD (2004). Headaches due to nasal and paranasal sinus disease. *Neurol Clin*, 22:1–19.

Simon, RH, Zimmerman, AW, Tasman, A et al. (1982). Spectral analysis of photic stimulation in migraine. *Electroenceph Clin Neurophysiol*, 53:270–276.

Smyth, VOG and Winter, AL (1964). The EEG in migraine. *Electroenceph Clin Neurophysiol*, 16:194.

Soges, LJ, Cacayorin, ED, Petro, GR et al. (1988). Migraine: evaluation by MR. *AJNR*, 9:425–429.

Sotaniemi, KA, Rantala, M, Pyhtinen, J et al. (1991). Clinical and CT correlates in the diagnosis of intracranial tumours. *J Neurol Neurosurg Psychiatr*, 54:645–647.

Spencer, MP, Moehring, M, Jersurm, J et al. (2004). Power m-mode tran cranial Doppler for diagnosis of patient foramen ovale and assessing trans catheter closure. *J Neuroimaging*, 14:342–349.

Strayle-Batra, M, Skalej, M, Wakhloo, AK et al. (1998). Three-dimensional spiral CT angiography in the detection of cerebral aneurysm. *Acta Radiol*, 39:233–238.

Suarez, JI, Tarr, RW, and Selman, WR (2006). Aneurysmal subarachnoid hemorrhage. *N Engl J Med*, 354:387–396.

Swartz, RH and Kern, RZ (2004). Migraine is associated with magnetic resonance imaging white matter abnormalities: a meta-analysis. *Arch Neurol*, 61:1366–1368.

Tietjen, GE (1992). Migraine and antiphospholipid antibodies. *Cephalalgia*, 12:69–74.

Tietjen, GE, Day, M, Norris, L et al. (1998). Role of anticardiolipin antibodies in young persons with migraine and transient focal neurologic events. A prospective study. *Neurology*, 50:1433–1440.

Tourtellotte, WW, Metz, LN, Bryan, ER et al. (1964). Spontaneous subarachnoid hemorrhage. Factors affecting the rate of clearing of the cerebrospinal fluid. *Neurology*, 14:301–306.

Tsushima, Y and Endo, K (2005). MR imaging in the evaluation of chronic or recurrent headache. *Radiology*, 235:575–579.

Urbach, H, Zentner, J, and Solymosi, L (1998). The need for repeat angiography in subarachnoid haemorrhage. *Neuroradiology*, 40:6–10.

van der Jagt, M, Hasan, D, Bijvoet, HW et al. (1999). Validity of prediction of the site of ruptured intracranial aneurysms with CT. *Neurology*, 52:34–39.

van der Wee, N, Rinkel, GJE, Hasan, D et al. (1995). Detection of subarachnoid haemorrhage on early CT: is lumbar puncture still needed after a negative scan? *J Neurol Neurosurg Psychiatr*, 58:357–359.

van Gijn, J (1992). Subarachnoid hemorrhage. *Lancet*, 339:653–655.

van Gijn, J and van Dongen, KJ (1982). The time course of aneurysmal haemorrhage on computed tomograms. *Neuroradiology*, 23:153–156.

Vermeulen, M, Hasan, D, Blijenberg, BG et al. (1989). Xanthochromia after subarachnoid haemorrhage needs no revisitation. *J Neurol Neurosurg Psychiatr*, 52:826–828.

Vermeulen, M and van Gijn, J (1990). The diagnosis of subarachnoid haemorrhage. *J Neurol Neurosurg Psychiatr*, 53:365–372.

Wang, AM, Bisese, JH, and Jackson, CTL (1995). Computed tomography of cerebrovascular disease. In *Cerebrovascular Disease. Imaging and Interventional Treatment Options* (CL Rumbaugh, AM Wang, and FY Tsai, eds), pp. 153–187. Igaku-Shoin, New York.

Wang, HZ, Simonson, TM, Greco, WR et al. (2001). Brain MR imaging in the evaluation of chronic headache in patients without other neurologic symptoms. *Acad Radiol*, 8:405–408.

Weingarten, S, Kleinman, M, Elperin, L et al. (1992). The effectiveness of cerebral imaging in the diagnosis of chronic headache: a reappraisal. *Arch Intern Med*, 152:2457–2462.

Weir, B (1994). Headaches from aneurysms. *Cephalalgia*, 14:79–87.

Wöber-Bingöl, C, Wöber, C, Prayer, D et al. (1996). Magnetic resonance imaging for recurrent headache in childhood and adolescence. *Headache*, 36:83–90.

Wolpert, SM and Caplan, LR (1992). Current role of cerebral angiography in the diagnosis of cerebrovascular diseases. *AJR Am J Roentgenol*, 159:191–197.

Wood, MJ, Dimeski, G, and Nowitzke, AM (2005). CSF spectrophotometry in the diagnosis and exclusion of spontaneous subarachnoid haemorrhage. *J Clin Neurosci*, 12:142–146.

Woolf, SH and Kamerow, DB (1990). Testing for uncommon conditions. The heroic search for positive test results. *Arch Intern Med*, 15:2451–2458.

Yuan, MK, Lai, PH, Chen, JY et al. (2005). Detection of subarachnoid hemorrhage at acute and subacute/chronic stages: comparison of four magnetic resonance imaging pulse sequences and computed tomography. *J Chin Med Assoc*, 68:131–137.

Yuichi, I, Shigeo, S, Takeshi, M et al. (1981). Postcontrast computed tomography in subarachnoid hemorrhage from ruptured aneurysms. *J Comput Assist Tomogr*, 5:341–344.

Ziegler, DK, Batnitzky, S, Barter, R et al. (1991). Magnetic resonance image abnormality in migraine with aura. *Cephalalgia*, 11:147–150.

6 Anatomy and Physiology of Pain-sensitive Cranial Structures

Karl Messlinger, Andrew M Strassman, and Rami Burstein

INNERVATION OF THE MENINGES

The dura mater encephali is innervated by sensory, sympathetic, and parasympathetic nerve fibers. Cell somas of meningeal afferents supplying the medial meningeal artery are located predominantly within the ophthalmic division (V1) of the ipsilateral trigeminal ganglion and, to a minor extent, within the maxillary (V2) and mandibular (V3) divisions (Mayberg et al., 1984). Cell somas of meningeal afferents supplying the middle cranial fossa are found mainly in V3 (Steiger et al., 1982). Cell somas of meningeal afferents supplying basal intracranial arteries as well as the superior sagittal sinus are found not only in the trigeminal ganglion but also in the first and second cervical root ganglia (Arbab et al., 1986; Liu et al., 2004). Cell somas of sympathetic fibers are found predominantly in the ipsilateral superior cervical ganglion (Edvinsson and Uddman, 1981; Keller et al., 1989; Uddman et al., 1989). Cell somas of parasympathetic fibers are found in the sphenopalatine and otic ganglia and in ganglia associated with the internal carotid artery (Amenta et al., 1980; Edvinsson and Uddman, 1981; Edvinsson et al., 1989; Suzuki et al., 1989; Hardebo et al., 1991; Suzuki and Hardebo, 1991). Anatomical classification of nerve fibers in dural and pial blood vessels is based on their peptidergic content (Liu-Chen et al., 1986; Edvinsson et al., 1988, 1989; von During et al., 1990; Keller and Marfurt, 1991). Meningeal nerve fibers containing calcitonin gene-related peptide (CGRP), substance P (SP), and neurokinin A (NKA) are thought to belong to the sensory system. Together, they form a dense network of fibers around blood vessels as well as in nonvascular regions (Keller and Marfurt, 1991; Messlinger et al., 1993; Strassman et al., 2004). Meningeal nerve fibers containing neuropeptide Y (NPY) are most likely of sympathetic origin, whereas those containing vasoactive intestinal polypeptide (VIP) are of parasympathetic origin (Suzuki et al., 1989; Keller and Marfurt, 1991).

In the context of vascular headache, it has been proposed that meningeal sensory fibers can be stimulated to release neuropeptides from their peripheral endings, where they can evoke components of neurogenic inflammation, including SP-mediated dural plasma extravasation and CGRP-mediated dural and pial vasodilation (McCulloch et al., 1986; Edvinsson et al., 1987; Markowitz et al., 1987; Shepheard et al., 1993; Kurosawa et al., 1995; Carmody et al., 1996).

RESPONSE PROPERTIES OF MENINGEAL NOCICEPTORS

Anatomic and physiologic studies suggest that the majority of meningeal sensory fibers are unmyelinated C-units or thinly myelinated Aδ-units (Dostrovsky et al., 1991; Strassman et al., 1996; Bove and Moskowitz, 1997), although a substantial number of Aδ fibers are also present (Liu-Chen et al., 1986; Levy and Strassman, 2002b; Strassman et al., 2004). These sensory fibers could be activated by mechanical and thermal stimulation (Dostrovsky et al., 1991; Bove and Moskowitz, 1997), as well as by chemical stimuli such as hypertonic saline, potassium chloride, capsaicin, buffer solutions of low or high osmolarity, or a mixture of inflammatory mediators (Strassman et al., 1996). Applying inflammatory agents such as bradykinin, prostaglandin E2 (PGE2), serotonin, and histamine to the dura produce not only activation but also sensitization of meningeal nociceptors (Strassman et al., 1996; Levy and Strassman, 2002a). Clinical manifestations of sensitization of meningeal nociceptors during migraine include throbbing of the headache and its exacerbation during routine physical activities such as coughing, sneezing, bending over, rapid head shaking, breath holding, climbing stairs, or walking (Blau and Dexter, 1981; Rasmussen et al., 1991). Accordingly, fluctuations in intracranial pressure (Daley et al., 1995) associated with normal vascular pulsation (4–10 mmHg), as well as those associated with bending over or coughing (4–25 mmHg), could activate meningeal nociceptors when they are sensitized in the presence of migraine but not when they are not sensitized in the absence of migraine.

THE TRIGEMINAL BRAINSTEM NUCLEAR COMPLEX

The central processes of trigeminal primary afferents terminate in several sensory nuclei, which as a whole are called the trigeminal brain stem nuclear complex (TBNC). The TBNC is composed of the principal sensory nucleus (Vp) and the spinal trigeminal nucleus (Vsp). The spinal trigeminal nucleus is subdivided into three subnuclei (Olzewski, 1950): a rostral subnucleus oralis (Vo), a middle subnucleus interpolaris (Vi), and a caudal subnucleus caudalis (Vc). The subnucleus caudalis is often termed the medullary dorsal horn (MDH) because of its anatomic and physiologic similarities to the spinal dorsal horn. Histologically, it consists of three distinct regions (Olzewski, 1950): an outer marginal region (lamina I), the substantia gelatinosa (lamina II), and a deep magnocellular region (Laminae III–V). Lamina V merges with the medullary reticular formation (Nord and Kyler, 1968), thus making the ventral boundary of the MDH unclear.

All subnuclei of the TBNC are somatotopically organized from dorsal to ventral (Hayashi et al., 1984; Shigenaga et al., 1986; Strassman and Vos, 1993). Mandibular afferents terminate preferentially in the dorsal region (dorsomedial in the MDH), ophthalmic afferents terminate in the ventral region (ventrolateral in MDH), and maxillary terminals are interposed. The rostrocaudal organization of the TBNC is less clear, except in Vc, where the rostrocaudal axis of the face is represented from rostral to caudal (Yokota and Nishikawa, 1980).

On the basis of clinical observations and animal studies, it has been recognized that Vc is primarily responsible for processing nociceptive and temperature information from the face and head, whereas Vp is involved in processing tactile information. Isolated lesions of Vc ipsilaterally caused complete or partial loss of pain and temperature sensation, whereas tactile sensations remained nearly intact (Lisney, 1983). Nevertheless, evidence supports a role of Vi, Vo, and Vp in trigeminal nociception as well (Kunc, 1970; Young, 1982; Broton et al., 1988; Graham et al., 1988).

CENTRAL TERMINATIONS OF SENSORY FIBERS IN THE TBNC

The distribution of nociceptive afferent terminals in the trigeminal brain stem has been studied by axonal tracing combined with immunohistochemistry and intracellular injections of physiologically identified axons. Somatic high-threshold mechanoreceptive (nociceptive) Aδ-units form extensive terminal arbors in lamina I and outer lamina II of Vc (Hayashi, 1985) and to a lesser extent in the superficial region of Vi. A second termination area is localized in laminae III–V of Vc (Jacquin et al., 1986, 1988). Corneal primary afferent fibers, which are thought to be mainly nociceptive, terminate largely in the outer laminae of Vc (Panneton and Burton, 1981) and sparingly in Vp and Vo (Panneton and Burton, 1981). SP- and CGRP-positive (peptidergic markers of nociceptors) nerve fibers of peripheral origin are abundant in the outer layer of Vc and the transition zone between Vi and Vc (Vi/Vc) (Amano et al., 1986; Pearson and Jennes, 1988; Tashiro et al., 1991; Boissonade et al., 1993; Henry et al., 1996). Unmyelinated meningeal fibers supplying the superior sagittal sinus terminate in the ventrolateral region of laminae I–II of the upper cervical spinal cord (C1–3), Vc, and Vi/Vc transition zone but not in the rostral subnuclei (Liu et al., 2004). Myelinated meningeal fibers of superior sagittal sinus origin terminate exclusively in laminae III–IV at C1–3 (Liu et al., 2004).

RESPONSE PROPERTIES OF TBNC NEURONS

According to their preferred modality of stimulation, neurons in Vc and C1–2 are classified as low-threshold mechanoreceptive (LTM), innocuous thermoreceptive, wide-dynamic-range (WDR), and nociceptive-specific (NS) (Mosso and Kruger, 1973; Price et al., 1976; Hu et al., 1981; Hu, 1990). NS neurons respond solely to noxious stimulus intensities, whereas WDR neurons are more responsive to noxious than to innocuous stimuli (Price et al., 1976; Yokota and Nishikawa, 1980; Hu, et al., 1981; McHaffie et al., 1994). Both WDR and NS neurons receive primary afferent input from slowly conducting fibers (Aδ alone or Aδ plus C), whereas WDR neurons also receive input from Aβ fibers, accounting for their tactile sensitivity. The majority of WDR and NS neurons also respond to noxious heat applied to their cutaneous receptive field. A somewhat smaller proportion also respond to noxious cold stimuli (McHaffie et al., 1994). A distinct group of nociceptive specific neurons, responding to heat, pinch, and cold, has been described in lamina I of the spinal cord and Vc (Craig and Dostrovsky, 2001; Craig, 2003). Within Vc, LTM neurons are found mainly in the deep laminae (III–IV and V), thermoreceptive neurons in the superficial laminae (I–II), WDR neurons primarily in lamina V, and NS neurons preferentially in laminae I–II but also in V (Price et al., 1976; Yokota and Nishikawa, 1980; Hu et al., 1981; Amano et al., 1986; Craig and Dostrovsky, 1991; Burstein et al., 1998; Malick et al., 2000; Craig, 2003).

Nociceptive neurons in Vc and C1–2 also respond to stimulation of muscles, temporomandibular joint, intranasal mucosa, cornea, tooth pulp, and blood vessels of the intracranial dura (Nagano et al., 1975; Amano et al., 1986; Sessle et al., 1986; Broton et al., 1988; Dostrovsky et al., 1991; Malick et al., 2000). The convergence of afferent input from superficial and deep tissues has been postulated as the basis for the clinical phenomenon of referred pain of deep or visceral origin.

DURA-SENSITIVE NEURONS IN THE TBNC

Dura-sensitive neurons are found in Vc (Burstein et al., 1998), Vi (Davis and Dostrovsky, 1988c), Vo (Davis and Dostrovsky, 1988c), the upper cervical cord (Lambert et al., 1991; Burstein et al., 1998; Burstein and Jakubowski, 2004), and the lateral cervical nucleus (Lambert et al., 1991; Angus-Leppan et al., 1994). Rostrocaudally, the majority of these neurons are located in caudal Vc/rostral C1 and within the Vi/Vc transition zone (Schepelmann et al., 1999). In humans, stimulation of supratentorial dural structures elicits pain in the periorbital, frontal, or parietal regions of the head (Ray and Wolff, 1940). Similarly, in the cat and the rat, Vc trigeminovascular neurons exhibit receptive fields in the same regions of the head (Davis and Dostrovsky, 1988c; Schepelmann et al., 1999). In the rat, Vc trigeminovascular neurons often exhibit large receptive fields extending over maxillary and mandibular areas (Burstein et al., 1998). In addition to dural shock, dura-sensitive neurons in Vc could also be activated by traction of dural blood vessels (Davis and Dostrovsky, 1988c), heat applied to the dural surface (Fischer et al., 2005), and topical or subarachnoid infusion or intrasinus injection of bradykinin and other algesic or inflammatory agents (Davis and Dostrovsky, 1988a; Ebersberger et al., 1997; Burstein et al., 1998; Schepelmann et al., 1999). Application of inflammatory agents in the dura can produce not only activation but also sensitization of trigeminovascular neurons in Vc and C1–2 (Burstein et al., 1998; Yamamura et al., 1999).

Among the common symptoms of *central* sensitization during migraine is the phenomenon of allodynia, wherein patients become irritated by mundane mechanical and thermal stimulation of the scalp and facial skin (Living, 1873; Wolff et al., 1953; Selby and Lance, 1960; Burstein et al., 2000). This hypersensitivity is manifested in response to activities such as combing; shaving; breathing cold air; and wearing eyeglasses, contact lenses, earrings, or necklaces.

NOCICEPTIVE PROJECTIONS FROM VC AND C1–2 TO THE THALAMUS AND OTHER SUB-CORTICAL NUCLEI

The major thalamic projection related to pain and temperature perception arises from neurons in Vc that reach the thalamus via a crossed pathway that joins the contralateral spinothalamic tract. These trigeminothalamic neurons are located primarily in laminae I and V of Vc and C1–2. Lamina V cells have a major projection to the ventral posteromedial thalamic nucleus (VPM), whereas those in lamina I terminate in several other distinct regions that are species dependent. In the monkey, there is a prominent projection from lamina I of Vc to the posterior ventromedial nucleus (VMpo) as well as to the ventrocaudal medialis dorsalis (MDvc) but only a sparse projection to VPM (Craig, 2004). In the rat, Vc lamina I neurons project largely to VPM, the posterior nucleus (PO), the posterior triangular nucleus, and the nucleus submedius (Yoshida et al., 1991; Iwata et al., 1992; Jasmin et al., 2004). However, neurons in lamina I and V of Vc and C1–2 that are specifically dura-sensitive project to VPM, PO, and the parafascicular nucleus (Burstein et al., 1998).

In addition to the thalamus, TBNC neurons also project to a number of diencephalic and brain stem areas involved in regulation of autonomic, endocrine, affective, and motor functions. For example, all TBNC subnuclei contain neurons that project directly to the hypothalamus (Malick and Burstein, 1998). The majority of these neurons are found bilaterally in laminae I, II, and V of C1–2 and Vc, in the transition zone between Vc and Vi, and in the paratrigeminal nucleus, thus suggesting a role in nociception. In fact, trigeminohypothalamic tract neurons in C1–2 and Vc respond preferentially or exclusively to noxious mechanical and thermal stimulation of the facial skin and to electrical, mechanical, and chemical stimulation of the dura (Burstein et al., 1998; Malick et al., 2000). Within the hypothalamus, these ascending neurons project to the lateral preoptic, anterior, lateral, perifornical, and caudal nuclei. Because neurons in these hypothalamic nuclei integrate complex physiologic functions and behaviors, and because disruption of emotional, endocrine, autonomic, and other physiologic functions are frequently associated with migraine attacks, trigeminohypothalamic tract neurons may provide the afferent limb for the initiation of these symptoms.

Important bilateral projections from the TBNC to the parabrachial and Kölliker-Fuse nuclei also have been identified (Bernard et al., 1989; Hayashi and Tabata, 1990; Fujino et al., 1996). Neurons in the caudal spinal trigeminal complex, including those in the superficial laminae of the MDH, send axons to the external portion of the lateral parabrachial area. A large percentage of somatosensory neurons in the parabrachial nuclei respond exclusively to noxious stimuli (Hayashi and Tabata, 1990). It has been postulated that this projection is part of a trigemino(ponto)amygdaloid pathway that may be involved in the affective, behavioral, and autonomic reactions to noxious events (Bernard et al., 1989), which also may apply to severe headaches such as migraine.

Tract tracing studies have demonstrated trigeminal afferent and TBNC projections to a number of other brain stem nuclei, including the nucleus of the solitary tract (Marfurt and Rajchert, 1991), superior colliculus (Bruce et al., 1987), cerebellum (Mantle-St John and Tracey, 1987), and inferior olive (Jacquin et al., 1989). These pathways may be involved in mediating nonperceptual somatic and visceral reflexes.

Nociceptive trigeminal neurons undoubtedly also activate other structures in the brain stem, including the periaqueductal gray, nucleus raphe magnus, reticular formation, and various brain stem autonomic nuclei (Keay and Bandler, 1998; Hoskin et al., 2001).

THALAMIC PROCESSING OF NOCICEPTIVE INFORMATION

Nociceptive information arising from craniofacial structures is mediated primarily by ascending projections that relay in the thalamus and terminate in the cortex. Existence of nociceptive pathways that bypass the thalamus and project directly (Burstein and Potrebic, 1993) and indirectly (Bernard and Besson, 1990) to cortical areas such as the amygdala and orbitofrontal cortex suggests that some aspects of pain sensation could arise without relay in the thalamus.

Lateral and medial thalamic regions have been implicated in nociception. The lateral region includes the ventrobasal complex (VBC) and an area ventroposterior to it. The VBC contains somatotopically organized neurons that relay tactile information from the face and mouth and the rest of the body to the primary somatosensory cortex. Most of the neurons in this region are non-nociceptive and respond to low threshold mechanical stimuli. Neurons in VPM (the medial portion of VBC) have orofacial receptive fields (Dubner et al., 1978; Guilbaud et al., 1994). In the rat and primate, only 10% of the VBC neurons are nociceptive and they are scattered throughout the nucleus; in the cat, nociceptive neurons are found only on the perimeter of VBC (Yokota et al., 1986; Guilbaud et al., 1994; Willis, 1997). NS neurons have also been reported in the ventroposterior inferior (VPI) and VMpo thalamic nuclei (Apkarian and Shi, 1994; Craig et al., 1994). VPI neurons project to the secondary somatosensory cortex (SII), whereas VMpo neurons project to SI and insular cortex (Craig and Dostrovsky, 1997); both regions have been implicated in nociception in recent imaging studies.

The medial thalamus is a complex collection of separate nuclei whose role in nociception is poorly understood. These nuclei generally have widespread and diffuse inputs and projections. They receive inputs from nociceptive neurons in the spinal cord, Vc, and the reticular formation (Craig and Dostrovsky, 1997; Willis, 1997) and project to widespread cortical areas, and their receptive fields extend over large orofacial and body regions. This feature has given rise to the view that the medial thalamus mediates the affective-motivational aspects of pain.

Studies in the cat have identified dura-sensitive neurons in VPM and PO with cutaneous receptive fields around the periorbital area (Davis and Dostrovsky, 1988b; Davis and Dostrovsky, 1988c; Zagami and Lambert, 1990; Zagami and Lambert, 1991; Angus-Leppan et al., 1995). About 50% of the neurons were nociceptive, responding to algogenic chemical stimuli of the dura. The relay of somatosensory information by VPM versus PO varies with (1) the physiologic properties of their neurons, (2) the input they receive from the dorsal horn, and (3) their projections to the somatosensory cortex. Most nociceptive neurons in VPM exhibit small receptive fields confined to the contralateral face (Davis and Dostrovsky, 1988b; Chiaia et al., 1991; Diamond et al., 1992; Bushnell et al., 1993; Duncan et al., 1993; Tremblay et al., 1993; Koyama et al., 1998). Nociceptive neurons in PO exhibit large receptive fields that span unilaterally or bilaterally across large areas of the body (Poggio and Mountcastle, 1960; Poggio and Mountcastle, 1963; Curry, 1972; Brinkhus et al., 1979; Chiaia et al., 1991; Diamond et al., 1992; Apkarian and Shi, 1994; Gauriau and Bernard, 2004). The VPM receives direct input from MDH laminae containing nociceptive neurons (Burton and Craig, 1979; Burton et al., 1979; Berkley, 1980; Hu et al., 1981; Yasui et al., 1983; Albe-Fessard et al., 1985; Cliffer et al., 1991; Gauriau and Bernard, 2004).The PO receives direct input not only from nociceptive neurons in the MDH but also from the spinal cord (Jones and Burton, 1974; Berkley, 1980; Cliffer et al., 1991; Fabri and Burton, 1991; Gauriau and Bernard, 2004). VPM neurons project mainly to S1 (Herkenham, 1980; Jensen and Killackey, 1987; Chmielowska et al., 1989; Lu and Lin, 1993; Gauriau and Bernard, 2004). PO neurons project to S1 and granular insular (GI) cortex (Burton and Jones, 1976; Carvell and Simons, 1987; Koralek et al., 1988; Lu and Lin, 1993; Gauriau and Bernard, 2004).

CORTICAL PROCESSING OF NOCICEPTIVE INFORMATION

Direct nociceptive projections from the thalamus to S1 and GI, together with electrophysiological evidence for nociceptive neurons in S1 (Kenshalo and Isensee, 1983; Lamour, Guilbaud, et al., 1983; Lamour, Willer, et al., 1983; Kenshalo et al., 1988; Chudler et al., 1990; Vin-Christian et al., 1992) suggest that the cortex plays a role in processing and modulating pain perception. Current understanding of the role of S1 and GI in pain perception relies mostly on imaging studies in humans (Bushnell et al., 1999; Treede et al., 1999, 2000). These imaging studies have suggested that S1 is involved primarily in sensory discrimination aspects of pain perception, whereas GI is involved primarily in affective and perhaps autonomic responses to pain.

References

Albe-Fessard, D, Berkley, KJ, Kruger, L, et al. (1985). Diencephalic mechanisms of pain sensation. *Brain Res*, 356:217–296.

Amano, N, Hu, JW, and Sessle, BJ (1986). Responses of neurons in feline trigeminal subnucleus caudalis (medullary dorsal horn) to cutaneous, intraoral, and muscle afferent stimuli. *J Neurophysiol*, 55:227–243.

Amenta, F, Sancesario, G, Ferrante, F, et al. (1980). Acetylcholinesterase-containing nerve fibers in the dura mater of guinea pig, mouse, and rat. *J Neural Transm*, 47:237–242.

Angus-Leppan, H, Olausson, B, Boers, P, et al. (1994). Convergence of afferents from superior sagittal sinus and tooth pulp on cells in the upper cervical spinal cord of the cat. *Neurosci Lett*, 182:275–278.

Angus-Leppan, H, Olausson, B, Boers, P, et al. (1995). Convergence of afferents from superior sagittal sinus and tooth pulp on cells in the thalamus of the cat. *Cephalalgia*, 15:191–199.

Apkarian, AV and Shi, T (1994). Squirrel monkey lateral thalamus. I. Somatic nociresponsive neurons and their relation to spinothalamic terminals. *J Neurosci*, 14:6779–6795.

Arbab, MA, Wiklund, L, and Svendgaard, NA (1986). Origin and distribution of cerebral vascular innervation from superior cervical, trigeminal and spinal ganglia investigated with retrograde and anterograde WGA-HRP tracing in the rat. *Neuroscience*, 19:695–708.

Berkley, KJ (1980). Spatial relationships between the terminations of somatic sensory and motor pathways in the rostral brainstem of cats and monkeys. I. Ascending somatic sensory inputs to lateral diencephalon. *J Comp Neurol*, 193:283–317.

Bernard, JF and Besson, JM (1990). The spino(trigemino) pontoamygdaloid pathway: electrophysiological evidence for an involvement in pain processes. *J Neurophysiol*, 63:473–490.

Bernard, JF, Peschanski, M, and Besson, JM (1989). A possible spino (trigemino)-ponto-amygdaloid pathway for pain. *Neurosci Lett*, 100:83–88.

Blau, JN and Dexter, SL (1981). The site of pain origin during migraine attacks. *Cephalalgia*, 1:143–147.

Boissonade, FM, Sharkey, KA, and Lucier, GE (1993). Trigeminal nuclear complex of the ferret: anatomical and immunohistochemical studies. *J Comp Neurol*, 329:291–312.

Bove, GM and Moskowitz, MA (1997). Primary afferent neurons innervating guinea pig dura. *J Neurophysiol*, 77:299–308.

Brinkhus, HB, Carstens, E, and Zimmermann, M (1979). Encoding of graded noxious skin heating by neurons in posterior thalamus and adjacent areas in the cat. *Neurosci Lett*, 15:37–42.

Broton, JG, Hu, JW, and Sessle, BJ (1988). Effects of temporomandibular joint stimulation on nociceptive and nonnociceptive neurons of the cat's trigeminal subnucleus caudalis (medullary dorsal horn). *J Neurophysiol*, 59:1575–1589.

Bruce, LL, McHaffie, JG, and Stein, BE (1987). The organization of trigeminotectal and trigeminothalamic neurons in rodents: a double-labeling study with fluorescent dyes. *J Comp Neurol*, 262:315–330.

Burstein, R and Jakubowski, M (2004). Analgesic triptan action in an animal model of intracranial pain: a race against the development of central sensitization. *Ann Neurol*, 55:27–36.

Burstein, R and Potrebic, S (1993). Retrograde labeling of neurons in the spinal cord that project directly to the amygdala or the orbital cortex in the rat. *J Comp Neurol*, 335:469–485.

Burstein, R, Yamamura, H, Malick, A, et al. (1998). Chemical stimulation of the intracranial dura induces enhanced responses to facial stimulation in brain stem trigeminal neurons. *J Neurophysiol*, 79:964–982.

Burstein, R, Yarnitsky, D, Goor-Aryeh, I, et al. (2000). An association between migraine and cutaneous allodynia. *Annals Neurol*, 47:614–624.

Burton, H and Craig, AD Jr. (1979). Distribution of trigeminothalamic projection cells in cat and monkey. *Brain Res*, 161:515–521.

Burton, H, Craig, ADJ, Poulos, DA, et al. (1979). Efferent projections from temperature sensitive recording loci within the marginal zone of the nucleus caudalis of the spinal trigeminal complex in the cat. *J Comp Neurol*, 183:753–778.

Burton, H and Jones, EG (1976). The posterior thalamic region and its cortical projection in New World and Old World monkeys. *J Comp Neurol*, 168:249–301.

Bushnell, MC, Duncan, GH, Hofbauer, RK, et al. (1999). Pain perception: is there a role for primary somatosensory cortex? *Proc Natl Acad Sci USA*, 96:7705–7709.

Bushnell, MC, Duncan, GH, and Tremblay, N (1993). Thalamic VPM nucleus in the behaving monkey. I. Multimodal and discriminative properties of thermosensitive neurons. *J Neurophysiol*, 69:739–752.

Carmody, J, Pawlak, M, and Messlinger, K (1996). Lack of a role for substance P in the control of dural arterial flow. *Exp Brain Res*, 111:424–428.

Carvell, GE and Simons, DJ (1987). Thalamic and corticocortical connections of the second somatic sensory area of the mouse. *J Comp Neurol*, 265:409–427.

Chiaia, NL, Rhoades, RW, Fish, SE, et al. (1991). Thalamic processing of vibrissal information in the rat: II. Morphological and functional properties of medial ventral posterior nucleus and posterior nucleus neurons, *J Comp Neurol*, 314:217–236.

Chmielowska, J, Carvell, GE, and Simons, DJ (1989). Spatial organization of thalamocortical and corticothalamic projection systems in the rat SmI barrel cortex. *J Comp Neurol*, 285:325–338.

Chudler, EH, Anton, F, Dubner, R, et al. (1990). Responses of nociceptive SI neurons in monkeys and pain sensation in humans elicited by noxious thermal stimulation: effect of interstimulus interval. *J Neurophysiol*, 63:559–569.

Cliffer, KD, Burstein, R, and Giesler, GJ Jr. (1991). Distributions of spinothalamic, spinohypothalamic, and spinotelencephalic fibers revealed by anterograde transport of PHA-L in rats. *J Neurosci*, 11:852–868.

Craig, AD (2003). Pain mechanisms: labeled lines versus convergence in central processing. *Annu Rev Neurosci*, 26:1–30.

Craig, AD (2004). Distribution of trigeminothalamic and spinothalamic lamina I terminations in the macaque monkey. *J Comp Neurol*, 477:119–148.

Craig, AD, Bushnell, MC, Zhang, ET (1994). A thalamic nucleus specific for pain and temperature sensation. *Nature*, 372:770–773.

Craig, AD and Dostrovsky, J (1997). Processing of nociceptive information at supraspinal levels. In *Anesthesia: Biologic foundations* (TL Yaksh, ed.), pp. 625-642. Lippincott-Raven Publishers, Philadelphia.

Craig, AD and Dostrovsky, JO (1991). Thermoreceptive lamina I trigeminothalamic neurons project to the nucleus submedius in the cat. *Exp Brain Res*, 85:470–474.

Craig, AD and Dostrovsky, JO (2001). Differential projections of thermoreceptive and nociceptive lamina I trigeminothalamic and spinothalamic neurons in the cat. *Journal of Neurophysiology*, 86:856–870.

Curry, MJ (1972). The exteroceptive properties of neurones in the somatic part of the posterior group (PO). *Brain Res*, 44:439–462.

Daley, ML, Pasupathy, H, Griffith, M, et al. (1995). Detection of loss of cerebral vascular tone by correlation of arterial and intracranial pressure signals. *IEEE Trans Biomed Eng*, 42:420–424.

Davis, KD and Dostrovsky, JO (1988a). Cerebrovascular application of bradykinin excites central sensory neurons. *Brain Res*, 446:401–406.

Davis, KD and Dostrovsky, JO (1988b). Properties of feline thalamic neurons activated by stimulation of the middle meningeal artery and sagittal sinus. *Brain Res*, 454:89–100.

Davis, KD and Dostrovsky, JO (1988c). Responses of feline trigeminal spinal tract nucleus neurons to stimulation of the middle meningeal artery and sagittal sinus. *J Neurophysiol*, 59:648–666.

Diamond, ME, Armstrong-James, M, Budway, MJ, et al. (1992). Somatic sensory responses in the rostral sector of the posterior group (POm) and in the ventral posterior medial nucleus (VPM) of the rat thalamus: dependence on the barrel field cortex. *J Comp Neurol*, 319:66–84.

Dostrovsky, JO, Davis, KD, and Kawakita, K (1991). Central mechanisms of vascular headaches. *Can J Physiol Pharmacol*, 69:652–658.

Dubner, R, Sessle, BJ, and Storey, AT (1978). *The Neural Basis of Oral and Facial Function*. Plenum, New York.

Duncan, GH, Bushnell, MC, Oliveras, JL, et al. (1993). Thalamic VPM nucleus in the behaving monkey. III. Effects of reversible inactivation by lidocaine on thermal and mechanical discrimination. *J Neurophysiol*, 70:2086–2096.

Ebersberger, A, Ringkamp, M, Reeh, PW, et al. (1997). Recordings from brain stem neurons responding to chemical stimulation of the subarachnoid space. *J Neurophysiol*, 77:3122–3133.

Edvinsson, L, Brodin, E, Jansen, I, et al. (1988). Neurokinin A in cerebral vessels: characterization, localization and effects in vitro. *Regul Pept*, 20:181–197.

Edvinsson, L, Ekman, R, Jansen, I, et al. (1987). Calcitonin gene-related peptide and cerebral blood vessels: distribution and vasomotor effects. *J Cereb Blood Flow Metab*, 7:720–728.

Edvinsson, L, Hara, H, and Uddman R (1989). Retrograde tracing of nerve fibers to the rat middle cerebral artery with true blue: colocalization with different peptides. *J Cereb Blood Flow Metab*, 9:212–218.

Edvinsson, L and Uddman, R (1981). Adrenergic, cholinergic and peptidergic nerve fibres in dura mater– involvement in headache? *Cephalalgia*, 1:175–179.

Fabri, M and Burton, H (1991). Topography of connections between primary somatosensory cortex and posterior complex in rat: a multiple fluorescent tracer study. *Brain Res*, 538:351–357.

Fischer, MJC, Koulchitsky, S, and Messlinger, K (2005). The nonpeptide calcitonin gene-related peptide receptor antagonist BIBN4096BS lowers the activity of neurons with meningeal input in the rat spinal trigeminal nucleus. *J Neurosci*, 25:5877–5883.

Fujino, Y, Koyama, N, and Yokota, T (1996). Differential distribution of three types of nociceptive neurons within the caudal bulbar reticular formation in the cat. *Brain Res*, 715:225–229.

Gauriau, C and Bernard, JF (2004). A comparative reappraisal of projections from the superficial laminae of the dorsal horn in the rat: the forebrain. *J Comp Neurol*, 468:24–56.

Graham, SH, Sharp, FR, and Dillon, W (1988). Intraoral sensation in patients with brainstem lesions: role of the rostral spinal trigeminal nuclei in pons. *Neurology*, 38:1529–1533.

Guilbaud, G, Bernard, JF, and Besson, JM (1994). Brain areas involved in nociception and pain. In *Textbook of Pain*, Vol. 3. (P. Wall and R Melzack, eds.), pp. 113–128. Churchill-Livingston, Edinburgh.

Hardebo, JE, Arbab, M, Suzuki, N, et al. (1991). Pathways of parasympathetic and sensory cerebrovascular nerves in monkeys. *Stroke*, 22:331–342.

Hayashi, H (1985). Morphology of terminations of small and large myelinated trigeminal primary afferent fibers in the cat. *J Comp Neurol*, 240:71–89.

Hayashi, H, Sumino, R, and Sessle, BJ (1984). Functional organization of trigeminal subnucleus interpolaris: nociceptive and innocuous afferent inputs, projections to thalamus, cerebellum, and spinal cord, and descending modulation from periaqueductal gray. *J Neurophysiol*, 51:890–905.

Hayashi, H and Tabata, T (1990). Pulpal and cutaneous inputs to somatosensory neurons in the parabrachial area of the cat. *Brain Res*, 511:177–179.

Henry, MA, Johnson, LR, Nousek-Goebl, N, et al. (1996). Light microscopic localization of calcitonin gene-related peptide in the normal feline trigeminal system and following retrogasserian rhizotomy. *J Comp Neurol*, 365:526–540.

Herkenham, M (1980). Laminar organization of thalamic projections to the rat neocortex. *Science*, 207:532–535.

Hoskin, KL, Bulmer, DCE, Lasalandra, M, et al. (2001). Fos expression in the midbrain periaqueductal grey after trigeminovascular stimulation. *J Anat*, 198:29–35.

Hu, JW (1990). Response properties of nociceptive and non-nociceptive neurons in the rat's trigeminal subnucleus caudalis (medullary dorsal horn) related to cutaneous and deep craniofacial afferent stimulation and modulation by diffuse noxious inhibitory controls. *Pain*, 41:331–345.

Hu, JW, Dostrovsky, JO, and Sessle, BJ (1981). Functional properties of neurons in cat trigeminal subnucleus caudalis (medullary dorsal horn). I. Responses to oral-facial noxious and nonnoxious stimuli and projections to thalamus and subnucleus oralis. *J Neurophysiol*, 45:173–192.

Iwata, K, Kenshalo, DR Jr., Dubner, R, et al. (1992). Diencephalic projections from the superficial and deep laminae of the medullary dorsal horn in the rat. *J Comp Neurol*, 321:404–420.

Jacquin, MF, Barcia, M, and Rhoades, RW (1989). Structure-function relationships in rat brainstem subnucleus interpolaris: IV. Projection neurons. *J Comp Neurol*, 282:45–62.

Jacquin, MF, Renehan, WE, Mooney, RD, et al. (1986). Structure-function relationships in rat medullary and cervical dorsal horns. I. Trigeminal primary afferents. *J Neurophysiol*, 55:1153–1186.

Jacquin, MF, Stennett, RA, Renehan, WE, et al. (1988). Structure-function relationships in the rat brainstem subnucleus interpolaris: II. Low and high threshold trigeminal primary afferents. *J Comp Neurol*, 267:107–130.

Jasmin, L, Burkey, AR, Granato, A, et al. (2004). Rostral agranular insular cortex and pain areas of the central nervous system: a tract-tracing study in the rat. *J Comp Neurol*, 468:425–440.

Jensen, KF and Killackey, HP (1987). Terminal arbors of axons projecting to the somatosensory cortex of the adult rat. I. The normal morphology of specific thalamocortical afferents. *J Neurosci*, 7:3529–3543.

Jones, EG and Burton, H (1974). Cytoarchitecture and somatic sensory connectivity of thalamic nuclei other than the ventrobasal complex in the cat. *J Comp Neurol*, 154:395–432.

Keay, KA and Bandler, R (1998). Vascular head pain selectively activates ventrolateral periaqueductal gray in the cat. *Neurosci Lett*, 245:58–60.

Keller, JT and Marfurt, CF (1991). Peptidergic and serotoninergic innervation of the rat dura mater. *J Comp Neurol*, 309:515–534.

Keller, JT, Marfurt, CF, Dimlich, RV, et al. (1989). Sympathetic innervation of the supratentorial dura mater of the rat. *J Comp Neurol*, 290:310–321.

Kenshalo, DR Jr., Chudler, EH, Anton, F, et al. (1988). SI nociceptive neurons participate in the encoding process by which monkeys perceive the intensity of noxious thermal stimulation. *Brain Res*, 454:378–382.

Kenshalo, DR Jr. and Isensee, O (1983). Responses of primate SI cortical neurons to noxious stimuli. *J Neurophysiol*, 50:1479–1496.

Koralek, KA, Jensen, KF, and Killackey, HP (1988). Evidence for two complementary patterns of thalamic input to the rat somatosensory cortex. *Brain Res*, 463:346–351.

Koyama, N, Nishikawa, Y, and Yokota, T (1998). Distribution of nociceptive neurons in the ventrobasal complex of macaque thalamus. *Neurosci Res*, 31:39–51.

Kunc, Z (1970). Significant factors pertaining to the results of trigeminal tractotomy. In *Trigeminal Neuralgia* (R Hassler and AE Walker eds.), pp. 90–98. W.B. Saunders, Philadelphia.

Kurosawa, M, Messlinger, K, Pawlak, M, et al. (1995). Increase of meningeal blood flow after electrical stimulation of rat dura mater encephali: mediation by calcitonin gene-related peptide. *Br J Pharmacol*, 114:1397–1402.

Lambert, GA, Zagami, AS, Bogduk, N, et al. (1991). Cervical spinal cord neurons receiving sensory input from the cranial vasculature. *Cephalalgia*, 11:75–85.

Lamour, Y, Guilbaud, G, and Willer, JC (1983). Rat somatosensory (SmI) cortex: II. Laminar and columnar organization of noxious and non-noxious inputs. *Exp Brain Res*, 49:46–54.

Lamour, Y, Willer, JC, and Guilbaud, G (1983). Rat somatosensory (SmI) cortex: I. Characteristics of neuronal responses to noxious stimulation and comparison with responses to non- noxious stimulation. *Exp Brain Res*, 49:35–45.

Levy, D and Strassman, AM (2002a). Distinct sensitizing effects of the cAMP-PKA second messenger cascade on rat dural mechanonociceptors. *J Physiol*, 538:483–493.

Levy, D and Strassman, AM (2002b). Mechanical response properties of A and C primary afferent neurons innervating the rat intracranial dura. *J Neurophysiol*, 88:3021–3031.

Lisney, SJ (1983). Some current topics of interest in the physiology of trigeminal pain: a review. *J R Soc Med*, 76:292–296.

Liu, Y, Broman, J, and Edvinsson, L (2004). Central projections of sensory innervation of the rat superior sagittal sinus. *Neuroscience*, 129:431–437.

Liu-Chen, LY, Liszczak, TM, King, JC, et al. (1986). Immunoelectron microscopic study of substance P-containing fibers in feline cerebral arteries. *Brain Res*, 369:12–20.

Liveing, E (1873). *On Megrim, Sick Headache*. Arts & Boeve Publishers, Nijmegen.

Lu, SM and Lin, RC (1993). Thalamic afferents of the rat barrel cortex: a light- and electron-microscopic study using Phaseolus vulgaris leucoagglutinin as an anterograde tracer. *Somatosens Mot Res*, 10:1–16.

Malick, A and Burstein, R (1998). Cells of origin of the trigeminohypothalamic tract in the rat. *J Comp Neurol*, 400:125–144.

Malick, A, Strassman, AM, and Burstein, R (2000). Trigeminohypothalamic and reticulohypothalamic tract neurons in the upper cervical spinal cord and caudal medulla of the rat. *J Neurophysiol*, 84:2078–2112.

Mantle-St John, LA and Tracey, DJ (1987). Somatosensory nuclei in the brainstem of the rat: independent projections to the thalamus and cerebellum. *J Comp Neurol*, 255:259–271.

Marfurt, CF and Rajchert, DM (1991). Trigeminal primary afferent projections to "non-trigeminal" areas of the rat central nervous system. *J Comp Neurol*, 303:489–511.

Markowitz, S, Saito, K, and Moskowitz, MA (1987). Neurogenically mediated leakage of plasma protein occurs from blood vessels in dura mater but not brain. *J Neurosci*, 7:4129–4136.

Mayberg, MR, Zervas, NT, and Moskowitz, MA (1984). Trigeminal projections to supratentorial pial and dural blood vessels in cats demonstrated by horseradish peroxidase histochemistry. *J Comp Neurol*, 223:46–56.

McCulloch, J, Uddman, R, Kingman, TA, et al. (1986). Calcitonin gene-related peptide: functional role in cerebrovascular regulation. *Proc Natl Acad Sci USA*, 83:5731–5735.

McHaffie, JG, Larson, MA, and Stein, BE (1994). Response properties of nociceptive and low-treshold neurons in rat trigeminal pars caudalis. *J Comp Neurol*, 347:409–425.

Messlinger, K, Hanesch, U, Baumgartel, M, et al. (1993). Innervation of the dura mater encephali of cat and rat: ultrastructure and calcitonin gene-related peptide-like and substance P-like immunoreactivity. *Anat Embryol*, 188:219–237.

Mosso, JA and Kruger, L (1973). Receptor categories represented in spinal trigeminal nucleus caudalis. *J Neurophysiol*, 36:472–488.

Nagano, S, Myers, JA, and Hall, RD (1975). Representation of the cornea in the brain stem of the rat. *Exp Neurol*, 49:653–670.

Nord, SG and Kyler, HJ (1968). A single unit analysis of trigeminal projections to bulbar reticular nuclei of the rat. *J Comp Neurol*, 134:485–494.

Olzewski, J (1950). On the anatomical and functional organization of the spinal trigeminal nucleus. *J Comp Neurol*, 92:401–413.

Panneton, WM and Burton, H (1981). Corneal and periocular representation within the trigeminal sensory complex in the cat studied with transganglionc transport of horseradish peroxidase. *J Comp Neurol*, 199:327–344.

Pearson, JC and Jennes, L (1988). Localization of serotonin- and substance P-like immunofluorescence in the caudal spinal trigeminal nucleus of the rat. *Neurosci Lett*, 88:151–156.

Poggio, GF and Mountcastle, VB (1960). A study of the functional contributions of the lemniscal and spinothalamic systems to somatic sensibility. Central nervous mechanisms in pain. *Bull Johns Hopkins Hosp*, 106:266–316.

Poggio, GF and Mountcastle, VB (1963). The functional properties of ventrobasal thalamic neuronsstudied in unanesthetized monkeys. *J Neurophysiol*, 26:775–806.

Price, DD, Dubner, R, and Hu, JW (1976). Trigeminothalamic neurons in nucleus caudalis responsive to tactile, thermal, and nociceptive stimulation of monkey's face. J *Neurophysiol*, 39:936–953.

Rasmussen, BK, Jensen, R, and Olesen, J (1991). A population-based analysis of the diagnostic criteria of the International Headache Society. *Cephalalgia*, 11:129–134.

Ray, BS and Wolff, HG (1940). Experimental studies on headache. Pain-sensitive structures of the head and their significance in headache. *Arch Surg*, 41:813–856.

Schepelmann, K, Ebersberger, A, Pawlak, M, et al. (1999). Response properties of trigeminal brain stem neurons with input from dura mater encephali in the rat. *Neuroscience*, 90:543–554.

Selby, G and Lance, JW (1960). Observations on 500 cases of migraine and allied vascular headache. *J Neurol Neurosurg Psychiatr*, 23:23–32.

Sessle, BJ, Hu, JW, Amano, N, et al. (1986). Convergence of cutaneous, tooth pulp, visceral, neck and muscle afferents onto nociceptive and non-nociceptive neurones in trigeminal subnucleus caudalis (medullary dorsal horn) and its implications for referred pain. *Pain*, 27:219–235.

Shepheard, SL, Williamson, DJ, Hill, RG, et al. (1993). The non-peptide neurokinin1 receptor antagonist, RP 67580, blocks neurogenic plasma extravasation in the dura mater of rats. *Br J Pharmacol*, 108:11–12.

Shigenaga, Y, Okamoto, T, Nishimori, T, et al. (1986). Oral and facial representation in the trigeminal principal and rostral spinal nuclei of the cat. *J Comp Neurol*, 244:1–18.

Steiger, HJ, Tew, JM Jr., and Keller, JT (1982). The sensory representation of the dura mater in the trigeminal ganglion of the cat. *Neurosci Lett*, 31:231–236.

Strassman, AM, Raymond, SA, and Burstein, R (1996). Sensitization of meningeal sensory neurons and the origin of headaches. *Nature*, 384:560–564.

Strassman, AM and Vos, BP (1993). Somatotopic and laminar organization of fos-like immunoreactivity in the medullary and upper cervical dorsal horn induced by noxious facial stimulation in the rat. *J Comp Neurol*, 331:495–516.

Strassman, AM, Weissner, W, Williams, M, et al. (2004). Axon diameters and intradural trajectories of the dural innervation in the rat. *J Comp Neurol*, 473:364–376.

Suzuki, N and Hardebo, JE (1991). Anatomical basis for a parasympathetic and sensory innervation of the intracranial segment of the internal carotid artery in man. Possible implication for vascular headache. *J Neurol Sci*, 104:19–31.

Suzuki, N, Hardebo, JE, and Owman, C (1989). Origins and pathways of cerebrovascular nerves storing substance P and calcitonin gene-related peptide in rat. *Neuroscience*, 31:427–438.

Tashiro, T, Takahashi, O, Satoda, T, et al. (1991). Distribution of axons showing calcitonin gene-related peptide- and/or substance P-like immunoreactivity in the sensory trigeminal nuclei of the cat. *Neurosci Res*, 11:119–133.

Treede, RD, Apkarian, AV, Bromm, B, et al. (2000). Cortical representation of pain: functional characterization of nociceptive areas near the lateral sulcus. *Pain*, 87:113–119.

Treede, RD, Kenshalo, DR, Gracely, RH, et al. (1999). The cortical representation of pain. *Pain*, 79:105–111.

Tremblay, N, Bushnell, MC, and Duncan, GH (1993). Thalamic VPM nucleus in the behaving monkey. II. Response to air-puff stimulation during discrimination and attention tasks. *J Neurophysiol*, 69:753–763.

Uddman, R, Hara, H, and Edvinsson, L (1989). Neuronal pathways to the rat middle meningeal artery revealed by retrograde tracing and immunocytochemistry. *J Auton Nerv Syst*, 26:69–75.

Vin-Christian, K, Benoist, JM, Gautron, M, et al. (1992). Further evidence for the involvement of SmI cortical neurons in nociception: modifications of their responsiveness over the early stage of a carrageenin-induced inflammation in the rat. *Somatosens Mot Res*, 9:245–261.

von During, M, Bauersachs, M, Bohmer, B, et al. (1990). Neuropeptide Y- and substance P-like immunoreactive nerve fibers in the rat dura mater encephali. *Anat Embryol (Berl)*, 182:363–373.

Willis, WD (1997). Nociceptive functions of thalamic neurons. *In Thalamus, Volume II Experimental and Clinical Aspects* Vol. 2, (M Steriade and EG Jones. eds.), pp. 373–424. Elsevier Science Ltd., Oxford UK.

Wolff, HG, Tunis, MM, and Goodell, H (1953). Studies on migraine. *Arch. Internal Med*, 92:478–484.

Yamamura, H, Malick, A, Chamberlin, NL, et al. (1999). Cardiovascular and neuronal responses to head stimulation reflect central sensitization and cutaneous allodynia in a rat model of migraine. *J Neurophysiol*, 81:479–493.

Yasui, Y, Itoh, K, Mizuno, N, et al. (1983). The posteromedial ventral nucleus of the thalamus (VPM) of the cat: direct ascending projections to the cytoarchitectonic subdivisions. *J Comp Neurol*, 220:219–228.

Yokota, T and Nishikawa, N (1980). Reappraisal of somatotopic tactile representation within trigeminal subnucleus caudalis. *J Neurophysiol*, 43:700–712.

Yokota, T, Nishikawa, Y, and Koyama, N (1986). Tooth pulp input to the shell region of nucleus ventralis posteromedialis of the cat thalamus. *J Neurophysiol*, 56:80–98.

Yoshida, A, Dostrovsky, JO, Sessle, BJ, et al. (1991). Trigeminal projections to the nucleus submedius of the thalamus in the rat. *J Comp Neurol*, 307:609–625.

Young, RF (1982). Effect of trigeminal tractotomy on dental sensation in humans. *J Neurosurg*, 56:812–818.

Zagami, AS and Lambert, GA (1990). Stimulation of cranial vessels excites nociceptive neurones in several thalamic nuclei of the cat. *Exp Brain Res*, 81:552–566.

Zagami, AS and Lambert, GA (1991). Craniovascular application of capsaicin activates nociceptive thalamic neurones in the cat. *Neurosci Lett*, 121:187–190.

7 Pathophysiology of Headache

Peter J Goadsby and Michael L Oshinsky

INTRODUCTION

Migraine is the most common form of disabling primary headache that afflicts our patients (see Chapter 3, this volume) so its pathophysiology deserves particular attention. Moreover, the explosion of knowledge on the primary headaches (Lance and Goadsby, 2005) since the last edition of this volume makes a chapter on generic headache pathophysiology no longer practical, or indeed sensible, as it once seemed (Goadsby, 2001b). Certainly the pain-producing structures in the head are generic and their anatomy and physiology is addressed elsewhere (see Chapter 6, this volume). Here, we attempt to integrate what is known of the anatomy and physiology of the pain structures with the possible brain mechanisms that may underpin migraines by dissecting the pathophysiology from a clinical viewpoint. Patients and physicians alike value an understanding of the condition as a prelude to, indeed pivotal to, its management. This chapter attempts to provide that background.

Migraine—Explaining the Clinical Features

Migraine is in essence a familial episodic disorder whose key marker is headache with certain associated features (Headache Classification Committee of the International Headache Society, 2004). It is these features that give clues to its pathophysiology and will ultimately provide insights leading to new treatments.

The essential elements to be integrated are as follows:

- Genetics of migraine (Chapter 9);
- Physiological basis for the aura (Chapter 8);
- Anatomy of head pain, particularly that of the trigeminovascular system (Chapter 6);
- Physiology and pharmacology of activation of the peripheral branches of the ophthalmic branch of the trigeminal nerve;
- Physiology and pharmacology of the trigeminal nucleus, in particular its most caudal part, the trigeminocervical complex;
- Brainstem and diencephalic modulatory systems that influence trigeminal pain transmission and other sensory modality processing (Fig. 7–1).

Migraine is a form of sensory processing disturbance with wide ramifications within the central nervous system, although we will use pain pathways as an example, it is useful to remember that migraine is not simply a pain problem. Some of these issues are dealt with in greater detail in the chapters indicated and we will only outline them here for integration.

Genetics of Migraine

One of the most important aspects of the pathophysiology of migraine is the inherited nature of the disorder. It is clear from clinical practice that many patients have first degree relatives who also suffer from migraine (Silberstein et al., 2002; Lance and Goadsby, 2005). Transmission of migraine from parents to children has been reported as early as the seventeenth century (Willis, 1682), and numerous published studies have reported a positive family history (Russell, 1997). Elsewhere (Chapter 9, this volume) a detailed case for migraine being essentially an autosomal dominant condition are made. One important form of migraine, familial hemiplegic migraine (FHM), is briefly discussed because of the generic principle of an ionopathic disturbance that it suggests (Goadsby and Kullmann, 2005).

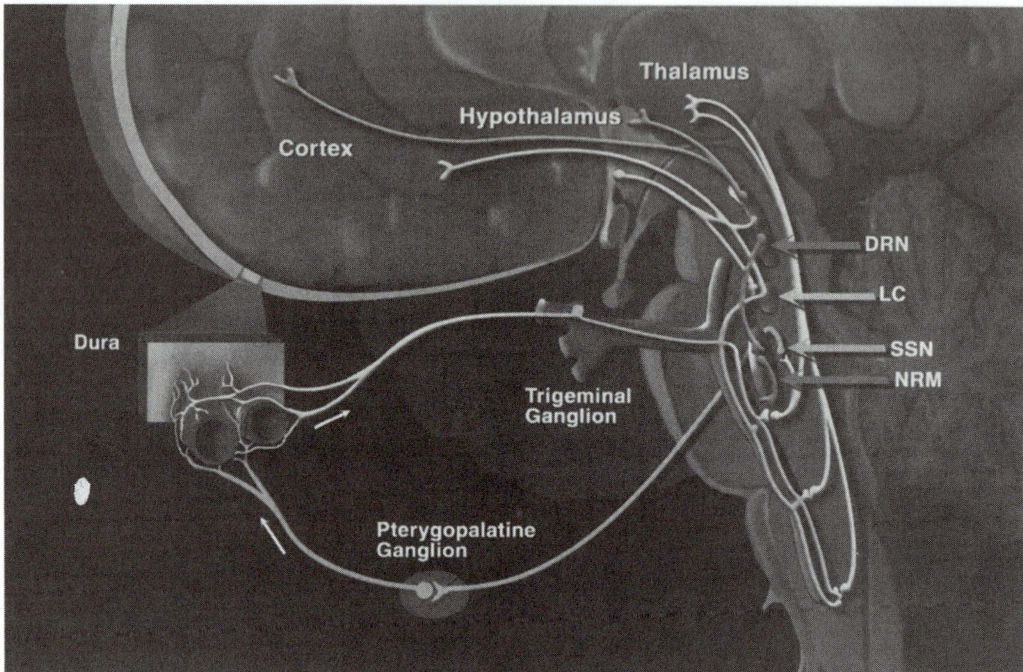

Figure 7–1 Illustration of some elements of migraine biology. Patients inherit a dysfunction in brain control systems for pain and other afferent stimuli, which can be triggered and are in turn capable of activating the trigeminovascular system as the initiating event in a positive feedback of neurally-driven vasodilatation. Pain from cervical inputs that terminates in the trigeminocervical complex accounts for the nontrigeminal distribution of pain in many patients. Migraine has thus a pain system for its expression and brain centers modulatory systems, that define the associated symptoms and periodicity of the clinical syndrome.

Familial Hemiplegic Migraine

FMH is an autosomal dominant disorder characterized by neurologic disturbance including hemiparesis during the aura phase. In approximately 50% of the reported families, FHM has been assigned to chromosome 19p13 (Joutel et al., 1994; Ophoff et al., 1994). Few clinical differences have been found between chromosome 19-linked and unlinked FHM families (Ducros et al., 2001), except for cerebellar ataxia, which occurs in approximately 50% of the chromosome 19-linked but in none of the unlinked families (Joutel et al., 1993; Haan et al., 1994; Joutel et al., 1994; Ophoff et al., 1994; Teh et al., 1995). Another less striking difference includes the fact that patients from chromosome 19-linked families are more likely to have attacks that can be triggered by minor head trauma and are accompanied by coma (Terwindt et al., 1996).

The biological basis for the linkage to chromosome 19 is mutations (Ophoff et al., 1996) involving the $Ca_v2.1$ (P/Q) type voltage-gated calcium channel (Ertel et al., 2000) *CACNA1A* gene, now known as FHM-I. Mutations in the *ATP1A2* gene (De Fusco et al., 2003; Marconi et al., 2003) have been identified to be responsible for about 20% of FHM families. The gene codes for a Na^+/K^+ ATPase and the mutation results in a smaller electrochemical gradient for Na^+. One effect of this change is to reduce or inactivate astrocytic glutamate transporters leading to a build up of synaptic glutamate, which is important for sensitization of the trigeminal nucleus caudalis (Oshinsky and Luo, 2006). Most recently the gene for FHM-III has been identified as a mutation in a sodium channel gene *SCN1A* (Dichgans et al., 2005). This mutation would facilitate repetitive high-frequency discharges which might, again, increase synaptic glutamate levels.

Taken together, the known mutations suggest that migraine or at least the neurological manifestations currently called the aura are caused by a channelopathy (Goadsby and Ferrari, 2001). Linking the channel disturbance for the first time to the aura process has demonstrated that human mutations expressed in a knockin mouse produce a reduced threshold for cortical spreading depression (CSD) (van den Maagdenberg et al., 2004), which has some profound implications for understanding that process (Goadsby, 2004).

Migraine Aura

Migraine aura is defined as a focal neurological disturbance manifest as visual, sensory, or motor symptoms (Headache Classification Committee of the International Headache Society, 2004). It is seen in about 30% of patients (Rasmussen and Olesen, 1992), and it is clearly neurally driven (Olesen et al., 1990; Cutrer et al., 1998). The case for the aura being the human equivalent of the CSD of Leao (1944a, 1944b) has been well made (Lauritzen, 1994) and is detailed elsewhere in this volume (Chapter 8).

What remains in question is whether aura is indeed pain-producing (Goadsby, 2001a).

Several arguments have been advanced as to whether the aura process is capable of directly exciting nociceptive afferents. It has been suggested that the production of plasma protein extravasation (PPE) by aura supports this position (Bolay et al., 2002), although there seems now overwhelming evidence from clinical trials that PPE is not pivotal in migraine (Peroutka, 2005). Similarly, it has been contended that effects of migraine preventives in aura provide evidence for a broader role of aura in migraine (Ayata et al., 2006). On the other hand, topiramate, a proven preventive agent in migraine (Brandes et al., 2004; Diener et al., 2004; Silberstein et al., 2004), also inhibits CSD in cats and rats acutely (Akerman and Goadsby, 2004). Although topiramate also inhibits trigeminal neurons activated by nociceptive intracranial afferents (Storer and Goadsby, 2004) but not by a mechanism local to the trigeminocervical complex (Storer and Goadsby, 2005). The mechanism for the preventive effect of topiramate in migraine therefore remains unclear.

Last, there are several clinical questions that are unanswered or pose a conundrum for the aura migraine-pain hypothesis

- Aura is clearly not present by clinical criteria in most patients, perhaps it is silent, but it must be very quiet to have avoided detection for four millennia;
- Aura can be seen during or even after pain, or most important in the absence of pain (Goadsby, 2002b);
- Aura can be aborted by ketamine without an effect on headache (Kaube et al., 2000);
- Aura is not specific to migraine because it is also seen in cluster headache (Silberstein et al., 2000; Bahra et al., 2002; Langedijk et al., 2005), paroxysmal hemicrania (Matharu and Goadsby, 2001), short-lasting unilateral neuralgiform headache attacks with conjunctival injection and tearing (SUNCT) (Cohen and Goadsby, 2006), tension-type headache (Peres and Viera, 2006), and hemicrania continua (Peres et al., 2002).

The issue seems far from resolved.

Headache—Anatomy

The Trigeminal Innervation of Pain-producing Intracranial Structures

Surrounding the large cerebral vessels, pial vessels, large venous sinuses, and dura mater is a plexus of largely unmyelinated fibers that arise from the ophthalmic division of the trigeminal ganglion (Liu-Chen et al., 1984) and in the posterior fossa from the upper cervical dorsal roots (Arbab et al., 1986). Trigeminal nociceptive fibers innervating cerebral vessels arise from neurons in the trigeminal ganglion that contain substance P, calcitonin gene-related peptide (CGRP) (Uddman et al., 1985), which are released when the trigeminal ganglion is stimulated either in humans or cats (Goadsby et al., 1988). Although not demonstrated specifically for dural nociceptors, other trigeminal nociceptors on the muscles and face of humans and rats also release glutamate, which significantly potentiates their physiology (Carlton, 2001). Stimulation of the cranial vessels, such as the superior sagittal sinus (SSS), is certainly painful in humans (Wolff, 1948; Feindel et al., 1960). Human dural nerves that innervate the cranial vessels largely consist of small diameter myelinated and unmyelinated fibers (Penfield and McNaughton, 1940) that almost certainly subserve a nociceptive function. Further detail of the anatomy of this innervation is to be found in Chapter 6 of this volume (Table 7–1).

Headache Physiology—Peripheral Activation

PPE

Neurogenic plasma extravasation is seen following electrical stimulation of the trigeminal ganglion in rats (Markowitz et al., 1987). Plasma extravasation can be blocked by ergot alkaloids, indomethacin, acetylsalicylic acid, and the serotonin-$5HT_{1B/1D}$ agonist, sumatriptan (Moskowitz and Cutrer, 1993). Structural changes in the dura mater including mast cell degranulation and changes in postcapillary venules including platelet aggregation (Dimitriadou et al., 1991, 1992), are well described with this stimulus. Although it is generally accepted that such changes, and particularly the initiation of a sterile inflammatory response, would cause pain (Strassman et al., 1996; Burstein et al., 1998), it is not clear whether this is sufficient of itself or requires other stimulators or promoters, particularly whether it occurs in migraine patients. Preclinical studies suggest that CSD may be a sufficient stimulus to activate trigeminal neurons (Bolay et al., 2002), although this has been a controversial area (Moskowitz et al., 1993; Ingvardsen et al., 1997, 1998; Ebersberger et al., 2001; Goadsby, 2001a).

Although plasma extravasation in the retina, which is blocked by Sumatriptan, can be seen after trigeminal ganglion stimulation in experimental animals, no changes are seen with retinal angiography during acute attacks of migraine or cluster headache (May, Shepheard, et al., 1998). A limitation of this study was the probable sampling of both retina and choroids elements in rats, given that choroidal vessels have fenestrated capillaries (Steuer et al., 2004). Clearly, however, blockade of neurogenic PPE is not completely predictive of antimigraine efficacy in humans as evidenced by the failure in clinical trials of substance P, neurokinin-1 antagonists (Goldstein et al., 1997; Connor et al., 1998; Norman et al., 1998; Diener and The RPR100893 Study Group, 2003), specific PPE blockers, CP122,288 (Roon et al.,

Table 7–1 Neuroanatomical Processing of Vascular Head Pain.

	Structure	*Comments*
Target innervation • Cranial vessels • Dura mater	Ophthalmic branch of trigeminal nerve	
1st	Trigeminal ganglion	Middle cranial fossa
2nd	Trigeminal nucleus *(quintothalamic tract)*	Trigeminal n. caudalis and C_1/C_2 dorsal horns
3rd	Thalamus	Ventrobasal complex Medial n. of posterior group Intralaminar complex
Modulatory	Midbrain Hypothalamus	Periaqueductal grey matter?
Final • Insulae • Frontal cortex • Anterior cingulate cortex • Basal ganglia	Cortex	

1997), and 4991w93 (Earl et al., 1999), an endothelin antagonist (May et al., 1996) and a neurosteriod (Data et al., 1998). A more detailed account of these failed developments is available elsewhere (Peroutka, 2005).

Sensitisation and Migraine Although it is unclear that there is a significant sterile inflammatory response in the dura mater during migraine, it is obvious that some form of sensitisation takes place during migraine, because allodynia is common and has been recognised for many years (Gowers, 1888). About two thirds of patients complain of pain from nonnoxious stimuli, allodynia (Selby and Lance, 1960; Burstein, Cutrer, et al., 2000; Burstein, Yarnitsky, et al., 2000). A particularly interesting aspect is the demonstration of allodynia in the upper limbs ipsilateral and contralateral to the pain. This finding is consistent with at least third order neuronal sensitisation, such as sensitisation of thalamic neurons and firmly places the pathophysiololgy within the central nervous system. Sensitisation in migraine may also be peripheral with local release of inflammatory markers, which would certainly activate trigeminal nociceptors (Strassman et al., 1996). More likely, migraine is a form of central sensitisation, which may be classical central sensitisation (Burstein et al., 1998), or a form of disinhibitory sensitisation with dysfunction of descending modulatory pathways (Knight et al., 2002; Bartsch et al., 2004). Just as dihydroergotamine (DHE) can block trigeminovascular nociceptive transmission (Hoskin et al., 1996), probably at least by a local effect in the trigeminocervical complex (Lambert et al., 1992; Storer and Goadsby, 1997), it can also reverse central sensitisation associated with dural stimulation by an inflammatory soup (Pozo-Rosich and Oshinsky, 2005).

Neuropeptide Studies

Electrical stimulation of the trigeminal ganglion in both humans and cats leads to increases in extracerebral blood flow and local release of both CGRP and SP (Goadsby et al., 1988). In cats, trigeminal ganglion stimulation also increases cerebral blood flow by a pathway traversing the greater superficial petrosal branch of the facial nerve (Goadsby and Duckworth, 1987) again releasing a powerful vasodilator peptide, vasoactive intestinal polypeptide (VIP) (Goadsby and Macdonald, 1985; May and Goadsby, 1999). Interestingly, the VIPergic innervation of the cerebral vessels is predominantly anterior rather than posterior (Matsuyama et al., 1983), and this may contribute to this regions vulnerability to spreading depression, explaining why the aura is so very often seen to commence posteriorly. Stimulation of the more specifically vascular pain-producing SSS increases cerebral blood flow (Lambert et al., 1988) and jugular vein CGRP levels (Zagami et al., 1990). Human evidence that CGRP is elevated in the headache phase of migraine (Goadsby et al., 1990; Gallai et al., 1995), cluster headache (Goadsby and Edvinsson, 1994; Fanciullacci et al., 1995), and chronic paroxysmal hemicrania (Goadsby and Edvinsson, 1996) supports the view that the trigeminovascular system may be activated in a protective role in these conditions. Recent work suggests in what seems like less affected patients indicates these changes are not seen (Tvedskov et al., 2005), although it is clear that the earlier studies were done in the substantially pretriptan era on patients with advanced attacks attending emergency rooms for treatment. Moreover, NO-donor triggered migraine, which is in essence typical migraine (Iversen et al., 1989; Afridi et al., 2004), also results in increased CGRP levels (Juhasz et al., 2003) that can be blocked by sumatriptan (Juhasz et al., 2005), just as in spontaneous migraine (Goadsby and Edvinsson, 1993). It is of interest in this regard that compounds which have not shown activity in migraine (Earl et al., 1999; Roon et al., 2000), notably the conformationally restricted analogue of sumatriptan, CP122,288 (Knight et al., 1999), and the conformationally restricted analogue of zolmitriptan, 4991w93 (Knight et al., 2001), were both ineffective inhibitors of CGRP release after SSS stimulation in the cat. The recent development of a highly specific CGRP antagonist (Doods et al., 2000) without vascular effects (Petersen et al., 2004; Petersen et al., 2005), and the announcement of proof-of-concept for a CGRP antagonist in acute migraine (Olesen, Diener, Husstedt, et al., 2004), firmly establishes this as a novel and important new emerging principle for acute migraine. At the same time the lack of any effect of CGRP blockers on PPE, explains in some part why that model has proved inadequate at translation into human therapeutic approaches.

Headache Physiology—Central Activation

The Trigeminocervical Complex

Fos immunohistochemistry is a method for labelling activated neurons (Morgan and Curran, 1991). After meningeal irritation with blood, Fos expression is noted in the trigeminal nucleus caudalis (Nozaki et al., 1992), whereas after stimulation of the SSS Fos-like immunoreactivity is seen in the trigeminal nucleus caudalis and in the dorsal horn at the C_1 and C_2 levels in cats (Kaube, Keay, et al., 1993) and monkeys (Goadsby and Hoskin, 1997; Hoskin et al., 1999). These latter findings are in accord with similar data using 2-deoxyglucose measurements with SSS stimulation (Goadsby and Zagami, 1991). Similarly, stimulation of a branch of C_2, the greater occipital nerve, increases metabolic activity in the same regions, that is, trigeminal nucleus caudalis and $C_{1/2}$ dorsal horn (Goadsby et al., 1997). In experimental animals one can record directly from trigeminal neurons with both supratentorial trigeminal input and input from the greater occipital nerve, a branch of the C_2 dorsal root (Bartsch and Goadsby, 2002). Stimulation of the greater occipital nerve for 5 minutes results in substantial increases in responses to supratentorial dural stimulation, which can last for over an hour (Bartsch and Goadsby, 2002). Conversely, stimulation of the middle meningeal artery dura mater with the C-fiber irritant mustard oil sensitises responses to occipital muscle stimulation (Bartsch and Goadsby, 2003). Taken together, these data suggest convergence of cervical and ophthalmic inputs at the level of the second order neuron. Moreover, stimulation of a lateralised structure, the middle meningeal artery, produces Fos expression bilaterally in both cat and monkey brain (Hoskin et al., 1999). This group of neurons from the superficial laminae of trigeminal nucleus caudalis and $C_{1/2}$ dorsal horns should be regarded functionally as the *trigeminocervical* complex.

These data demonstrate that trigeminovascular nociceptive information comes by way of the most caudal cells. This concept provides an anatomical explanation for the referral of pain to the back of the head in migraine. Moreover, experimental pharmacological evidence suggests that some abortive antimigraine drugs, such as, ergot derivatives (Lambert et al., 1992; Hoskin et al., 1996), acetylsalicylic acid (Kaube et al., 1993b), sumatriptan (Kaube et al., 1993a; Levy et al., 2004), eletriptan (Goadsby and Hoskin, 1999; Lambert et al., 2002), naratriptan (Goadsby and Knight, 1997; Cumberbatch et al., 1998), rizatriptan, (Cumberbatch et al., 1997) and zolmitriptan (Goadsby and Hoskin, 1996) can have actions at these second order neurons that reduce cell activity and suggest a further possible site for therapeutic intervention in migraine. This action can be dissected out to involve each of the 5-HT_{1B}, 5-HT_{1D}, and 5-HT_{1F} receptor subtypes (Goadsby and Classey, 2003), and are consistent with the localization of these receptors on peptidergic nociceptors (Potrebic et al., 2003). Interestingly, triptans also influence the CGRP promoter (Durham et al., 1997), and regulate CGRP secretion from neurons in culture (Durham and Russo, 1999), as does nitric oxide (Bellamy et al., 2006). Furthermore, the demonstration that some part of this action is postsynaptic with either 5-HT_{1B} or 5-HT_{1D} receptors located *non*presynatically (Goadsby et al., 2001; Maneesi et al., 2004) offers a prospect of highly anatomically localised treatment options. Although data that suggest externalisation of 5-HT_{1D} receptors with stimulation (Ahn and Basbaum, 2006) may provide an interesting way to understand the challenge of why sumatriptan given by injection (Bates et al., 1994) or oral zolmitriptan (Dowson, 1996), and eletriptan (Olesen, Diener, Schoenen, et al., 2004) during migraine aura did not prevent head pain.

Higher Order Processing

Following transmission in the caudal brain stem and high cervical spinal cord information is relayed rostrally.

Thalamus Processing of vascular nociceptive signals in the thalamus occurs in the ventroposteromedial (VPM) thalamus, medial nucleus of the posterior complex and in the intralaminar thalamus (Zagami and Goadsby, 1991). Zagami (1991) has shown by application of capsaicin to the SSS that trigeminal projections with a high degree of nociceptive input are processed in neurons particularly in the VPM thalamus and in its ventral periphery. These neurons in the VPM can be modulated by activation of $GABA_A$ inhibitory receptors (Shields et al., 2003) and perhaps of more direct clinical relevance by propranolol though a β_1-adrenoceptor mechanism (Shields and Goadsby, 2005). Remarkably, triptans through $5\text{-}HT_{1B/1D}$ mechanisms can also inhibit VPM neurons locally, as demonstrated by microiontophoretic application (Shields and Goadsby, 2006), suggesting a hitherto unconsidered locus of action for triptans in acute migraine. Human imaging studies have confirmed activation of thalamus contralateral to pain in acute migraine (Bahra et al., 2001; Afridi, Giffin, et al., 2005), cluster headache (May, Bahra, et al., 1998), and in SUNCT (May et al., 1999; Cohen et al., 2006).

Activation of Modulatory Regions Stimulation of nociceptive afferents by stimulation of the SSS in cats activates neurons in the ventrolateral periaqueductal grey matter (PAG) (Hoskin et al., 2001). PAG activation in turn feeds back to the trigeminocervical complex with an inhibitory influence (Knight and Goadsby, 2001; Knight et al., 2003). PAG is clearly included in the area of activation seen in PET studies in migraineurs (Weiller et al., 1995). This typical negative feedback system will be further considered below as a possible mechanism for the symptomatic manifestations of migraine.

Another potentially modulatory region activated by stimulation of nociceptive trigeminovascular input is the posterior hypothalamic grey (Benjamin et al., 2004). This area is crucially involved in several primary headaches, notably cluster headache (Goadsby, 2002c), SUNCT (May et al., 1999), paroxysmal hemicrania (Matharu et al., 2005), and hemicrania continua (Matharu, Cohen, et al., 2004). Moreover, the clinical features of the premonitory phase (Giffin et al., 2003), and other features of the disorder (Bes et al., 1982; Peroutka, 1997), suggest dopamine neuron involvement. Recently, it has been shown that dopamine, probably through predominantly D_2 receptor-mediated mechanisms, can inhibit trigeminocervical transmission (Bergerot et al., 2007). Orexin A and B are hypothalamic neuropeptides that bind to two G-protein coupled receptors termed: OX_1 and OX_2 (Sakurai et al., 1998). Orexins are involved in feeding, sleep/wake cycle, and hormone regulation (de Lecea and Sutcliffe, 1999; Beuckmann and Yanagisawa, 2002) and have been linked to the modulation of nociceptive processing (Bingham et al., 2001; Grudt et al., 2002; Yamamoto et al., 2002). Orexin A inhibits neurogenic dural vasodilation (Holland et al., 2005) and trigeminocervical neuronal activation from stimulation of trigeminovascular nociceptive afferents (Holland et al., 2006). Orexinergic neurons in the posterior hypothalamus can be both pro and antinociceptive (Bartsch et al., 2004), offering a further possible region whose dysfunction might involve promotion of the perception of head pain.

Central Modulation of Trigeminal Pain

Brain Imaging in Humans

Functional brain imaging with positron emission tomography (PET) has demonstrated activation of the dorsal midbrain, including the PAG, and in the dorsal pons, near the locus coeruleus, in studies during migraine without aura (Weiller et al., 1995). Dorsolateral pontine activation is seen with PET in spontaneous episodic (Afridi, Giffin, et al., 2005) and chronic migraine (Matharu, Bartsch, et al., 2004) and with nitrogylcerin-triggered attacks (Bahra et al., 2001; Afridi, Matharu, et al., 2005). These areas are active immediately after successful treatment of the headache but are not active interictally. The activation corresponds with the brain region that Raskin (1987) initially reported, and Veloso confirmed (Veloso et al., 1998), to cause migraine-like headache when stimulated in patients with electrodes implanted for pain control. Similarly, Welch et al. (2001) have noted excess iron in the PAG of patients with episodic and chronic migraine, and chronic migraine can develop after a bleed into a cavernoma in the region of the PAG (Goadsby, 2002a) or with a lesion of the pons (Afridi and Goadsby, 2003; Obermann et al., 2007).

Animal Studies of Sensory Modulation

It has been shown in animals that stimulation of nucleus locus coeruleus, the main central noradrenergic nucleus, reduces cerebral blood flow in a frequency-dependent manner (Goadsby et al., 1982) through an α_2-adrenoceptor-linked mechanism (Goadsby et al., 1985). This reduction is maximal in the occipital cortex (Goadsby and Duckworth, 1989). Although a 25% overall reduction in cerebral blood flow is seen, extracerebral vasodilatation occurs in parallel (Goadsby et al., 1982). The locus coeruleus receives important inputs from orexinergic neurons in the hypothalamus (Horvath et al., 1999; Ivanov and Aston-Jones, 2000), and can affect arousal by altering locus coeruleus neuronal activity (Hagan et al., 1999). Indeed it is well recognised that locus coeruleus neurons modulate arousal states in at least behaving primates (Foote et al., 1980, 1991). In addition the main serotonin-containing nucleus in the brain stem, the midbrain dorsal raphe nucleus, can increase cerebral blood flow when activated (Goadsby et al., 1991). Furthermore, stimulation of PAG will inhibit sagittal sinus evoked trigeminal neuronal activity in cats (Knight and Goadsby, 2001), whereas blockade of P/Q-type voltage-gated Ca^{2+} channels in the PAG facilitates trigeminovascular nociceptive processing (Knight et al., 2002) with the local GABAergic system in the PAG still intact (Knight et al., 2003).

Electrophysiology of Migraine in Humans

Studies of evoked potentials and event-related potentials provide some link between animal studies and human functional imaging (Kaube and Giffin, 2002). Authors have shown changes in neurophysiological measures of brain activation but there is much discussion as to how to interpret such changes (Schoenen et al., 2003). Perhaps the most reliable theme is that the migrainous brain does not habituate to signals in a normal way (Schoenen et al., 1995; Proietti-Cecchini et al., 1997; Wang and Schoenen, 1998; Afra et al., 2000). Similarly, contingent negative variation (CNV), an event related potential, is abnormal in migraineurs compared to controls (Schoenen and Timsit-Berthier, 1993). Changes in CNV predict attacks (Kropp and Gerber, 1998) and preventive therapies alter, normalise, such changes (Maertens de Noordhout et al., 1985). Attempts to correlate clinical phenotypes with electrophysiological changes (Gantenbein et al., 2004), may enhance further studies in this area.

What is Migraine?

Migraine is an inherited, episodic disorder involving sensory sensitivity. Patients complain of pain in the head that is throbbing, but there is no reliable relationship between vessel diameter and the pain (Olesen et al., 1990; Kruuse et al., 2003) or its treatment (Limmroth et al., 1996). They complain of discomfort from normal lights and the unpleasantness of routine sounds. Some report otherwise pleasant odours are unpleasant. Normal movement of the head causes pain, and many mention a sense of unsteadiness as if they have just stepped off a boat, having been nowhere near the water. How can the perception of so many sensory modalities be so wrong?

Migraine aura cannot be the trigger, there is no evidence at all after 4000 years that it occurs in more than 30% of migraine patients; aura can be experienced without pain at all, and is seen in the other primary headaches. There is not a photon of extra light that migraine patients receive over others, so for that symptom and phonophobia and osmophobia, the basis of the problem must be abnormal central processing of a normal signal. Perhaps electrophysiological changes in the brain have been mislabeled as *hyperexcitability* whereas dyshabituation might be a simpler explanation. If migraine was basically a sensory attentional problem with changes in cortical synchronisation (Niebur et al., 2002), *hypersynchronisation* (Angelini et al., 2004), all its manifestations could be accounted for in a single overarching pathophysiological hypothesis of a disturbance of subcortical sensory modulation systems (Goadsby, 2003). Although it seems likely that the trigeminovascular system, and its cranial autonomic reflex connections, the trigeminal-autonomic reflex (May and Goadsby, 1999), act as a feed-forward system to facilitate the acute attack, the fundamental problem in migraine is in the brain. Unravelling its basis will deliver great benefits to patients and considerable understanding of some very fundamental neurobiological processes.

References

Afra, J, Sandor, P, and Schoenen, J (2000). Habituation of visual and intensity dependence of cortical auditory evoked potentials tend to normalise just before and during migraine attacks. *Cephalalgia*, 20:347.

Afridi, S, Giffin, NJ, Kaube, H, et al. (2005). A PET study in spontaneous migraine. *Arch Neurol*, 62:1270–1275.

Afridi, S and Goadsby PJ (2003). New onset migraine with a brainstem cavernous angioma. *J Neurol, Neurosurg Psychiatr*, 74:680–682.

Afridi, S, Kaube, H, and Goadsby, PJ (2004). Glyceryl trinitrate triggers premonitory symptoms in migraineurs. *Pain*, 110:675–680.

Afridi, S, Matharu, MS, Lee, L, et al. (2005). A PET study exploring the laterality of brainstem activation in migraine using glyceryl trinitrate. *Brain*, 128:932–939.

Ahn, AH and Basbaum, AI (2006). Tissue injury regulates serotonin 1D receptor expression: implications for the control of migraine and inflammatory pain. *J Neurosci*, 26:8332–8338.

Akerman, S and Goadsby, PJ (2004). Topiramate inhibits cortical spreading depression in rat and cat: a possible contribution to its preventive effect in migraine. *Cephalalgia*, 24:783–784.

Angelini, L, de Tommaso, M, Guido, M, et al. (2004). Steady-state visual evoked potentials and phase synchronization in migraine patients. *Phys Rev Lett*, 93:038103-1-038103-4.

Arbab, MA, Wiklund, L, and Svendgaard, NA (1986). Origin and distribution of cerebral vascular innervation from superior cervical, trigeminal and spinal ganglia investigated with retrograde and anterograde WGA-HRP tracing in the rat. *Neuroscience*, 19:695–708.

Ayata, C, Jin, H, Kudo, C, et al. (2006). Suppression of cortical spreading depression in migraine prophylaxis. *Ann Neurol*, 59:652–661.

Bahra, A, Matharu, MS, Buchel, C, et al. (2001). Brainstem activation specific to migraine headache. *Lancet*, 357:1016–1017.

Bahra, A, May, A, and Goadsby, PJ (2002). Cluster headache: a prospective clinical study in 230 patients with diagnostic implications. *Neurology*, 58:354–361.

Bartsch, T and Goadsby, PJ (2002). Stimulation of the greater occipital nerve induces increased central excitability of dural afferent input. *Brain*, 125:1496–1509.

Bartsch, T and Goadsby, PJ (2003). Increased responses in trigeminocervical nociceptive neurones to cervical input after stimulation of the dura mater. *Brain*, 126:1801–1813.

Bartsch, T, Levy, MJ, Knight, YE, et al. (2004). Differential modulation of nociceptive dural input to [hypocretin] Orexin A and B receptor activation in the posterior hypothalamic area. *Pain*, 109:367–378.

Bates, D, Ashford, E, Dawson, R, et al. (1994). Subcutaneous sumatriptan during the migraine aura. *Neurology*, 44:1587–1592.

Bellamy, J, Bowen, EJ, Russo, AF, et al. (2006). Nitric oxide regulation of calcitonin gene-related peptide gene expression in rat trigeminal ganglia neurons. *Eur J Neurosci*, 23:2057–2066.

Benjamin, L, Levy, MJ, Lasalandra, MP, et al. (2004). Hypothalamic activation after stimulation of the superior sagittal sinus in the cat: a Fos study. *Neurobiol Dis*, 16:500–505.

Bergerot, A, Storer, RJ, and Goadsby, PJ (2007). Dopamine inhibits trigeminovascular transmission in the rat. *Ann Neurol*, 61:251–262.

Bes, A, Geraud, A, Guell, A, et al. (1982). Dopaminergic hypersensitivity in migraine: a diagnostic test? *Nouv Presse Med*, 11:1475–1478.

Beuckmann, CT and Yanagisawa, M (2002). Orexins: from neuropeptides to energy homeostasis and sleep/wake regulation. *J Mol Med*, 80:329–342.

Bingham, S, Davey, PT, Babbs, AJ, et al. (2001). Orexin-A, an hypothalamic peptide with analgesic properties. *Pain*, 92:81–90.

Bolay, H, Reuter, U, Dunn, AK, et al. (2002). Intrinsic brain activity triggers trigeminal meningeal afferents in a migraine model. *Nat Med*, 8:136–142.

Brandes, JL, Saper, JR, Diamond, M, et al. (2004). Topiramate for migraine prevention: a randomized controlled trial. *JAMA*, 291:965–973.

Burstein, R, Cutrer, MF, and Yarnitsky, D (2000). The development of cutaneous allodynia during a migraine attack. *Brain*, 123:1703–1709.

Burstein, R, Yamamura, H, Malick, A, et al. (1998). Chemical stimulation of the intracranial dura induces enhanced responses to facial stimulation in brain stem trigeminal neurons. *J Neurophysiol*, 79:964–982.

Burstein, R, Yarnitsky, D, Goor-Aryeh, I, et al. (2000). An association between migraine and cutaneous allodynia. *Ann Neurol*, 47:614–624.

Carlton, SM (2001). Peripheral excitatory amino acids. *Curr Opin Pharmacol*, 1:52–56.

Cohen, AS and Goadsby, PJ (2006). Short-lasting unilateral neuralgiform headache attacks with conjunctival injection and tearing (SUNCT) or cranial Autonomic features (SUNA). A prospective clinical study of SUNCT and SUNA. *Brain*, 129:2746–2760.

Cohen, AS, Matharu, MS, Kalisch, et al. (2006). Functional MRI in SUNCT (short-lasting unilateral neuralgiform headache attacks with conjunctival injection and tearing) and SUNA (short-lasting unilateral neuralgiform headache attacks with cranial autonomic symptoms) shows differential hypothalamic activation with increasing pain. *Cephalalgia*, 26:1402–1403.

Connor, HE, Bertin, L, Gillies, S, et al. (1998). The GR205171 Clinical Study Group. Clinical evaluation of a novel, potent, CNS penetrating NK_1 receptor antagonist in the acute treatment of migraine. *Cephalalgia*, 18:392.

Cumberbatch, MJ, Hill, RG, and Hargreaves, RJ (1997). Rizatriptan has central antinociceptive effects against durally evoked responses. *Eur J Pharmacol*, 328:37–40.

Cumberbatch, MJ, Hill, RG, and Hargreaves, RJ (1998). Differential effects of the $5HT_{1B/1D}$ receptor agonist naratriptan on trigeminal versus spinal nociceptive responses. *Cephalalgia*, 18:659–664.

Cutrer, FM, Sorensen, AG, Weisskoff, RM, et al. (1998). Perfusion-weighted imaging defects during spontaneous migrainous aura. *Ann Neurol*, 43:25–31.

Data, J, Britch, K, Westergaard, N, et al. (1998). A double-blind study of ganaxolone in the acute treatment of migraine headaches with or without an aura in premenopausal females. *Headache*, 38:380.

De Fusco, M, Marconi, R, Silvestri, L, et al. (2003). Haploinsufficiency of ATP1A2 encoding the Na^+/K^+ pump $\alpha 2$ subunit associated with familial hemiplegic migraine type 2. *Nat Genet*, 33:192–196.

de Lecea, L and Sutcliffe, JG (1999). The hypocretins/orexins: novel hypothalamic neuropeptides involved in different physiological systems. *Cell Mol Life Sci*, 56:473–480.

Dichgans, M, Freilinger, T, Eckstein, G, et al. (2005). Mutation in the neuronal voltage-gated sodium channel *SCN1A* causes familial hemiplegic migraine. *Lancet*, 366:371–377.

Diener, HC, Tfelt-Hansen, P, Dahlof, C, et al. (2004). Topiramate in migraine prophylaxis—results from a placebo-controlled trial with propranolol as an active control. *J Neurol*, 251:943–950.

Diener, H-C and The RPR100893 Study Group (2003). RPR100893, a substance-P antagonist, is not effective in the treatment of migraine attacks. *Cephalalgia*, 23:183–185.

Dimitriadou, V, Buzzi, MG, Moskowitz, MA (1991). Trigeminal sensory fiber stimulation induces morphological changes reflecting secretion in rat dura mater mast cells. *Neuroscience*, 44:97–112.

Dimitriadou, V, Buzzi, MG, Theoharides, TC, et al. (1992). Ultrastructural evidence for neurogenically mediated changes in blood vessels of the rat dura mater and tongue following antidromic trigeminal stimulation. *Neuroscience*, 48:187–203.

Doods, H, Hallermayer, G, Wu, D, et al. (2000). Pharmacological profile of BIBN4096BS, the first selective small molecule CGRP antagonist. *Br J Pharmacol*, 129:420–423.

Dowson, A (1996). Can oral 311C90, a novel 5-HT1D agonist, prevent migraine headache when taken during an aura? *Eur Neurol*, 36:28–31.

Ducros, A, Denier, C, Joutel, A, et al. (2001). The clinical spectrum of familial hemiplegic migraine associated with mutations in a neuronal calcium channel. *N Engl J Med*, 345:17–24.

Durham, PL and Russo, AF (1999). Regulation of calcitonin gene-related peptide secretion by a serotonergic antimigraine drug. *J Neurosci*, 19:3423–3429.

Durham, PL, Sharma, RV, and Russo, AF (1997). Repression of the calcitonin gene-related peptide promoter by 5-HT1 receptor activation. *J Neurosci*, 17:9545–9553.

Earl, NL, McDonald, SA, Lowy, MT, et al. (1999). Efficacy and tolerability of the neurogenic inflammation inhibitor, 4991W93, in the acute treatment of migraine. *Cephalalgia*, 19:357.

Ebersberger, A, Schaible, H-G, Averbeck, B, et al. (2001). Is there a correlation between spreading depression, neurogenic inflammation, and nociception that might cause migraine headache? *Ann Neurol*, 41:7–13.

Ertel, EA, Campbell, KP, Harpold, MM, et al. (2000). Nomenclature of voltage-gated calcium channels. *Neuron*, 25:533–535.

Fanciullacci, M, Alessandri, M, Figini, M, et al. (1995). Increase in plasma calcitonin gene-related peptide from extracerebral circulation during nitroglycerin-induced cluster headache attack. *Pain*, 60:119–123.

Feindel, W, Penfield, W, and McNaughton, F (1960). The tentorial nerves and localization of intracranial pain in man. *Neurology*, 10:555–563.

Foote, SL, Aston-Jones, G, and Bloom, FE (1980). Impulse activity of locus coeruleus neurons in awake rats and monkeys is a function of sensory stimulation and arousal. *Proc Natl Acad Sci USA*, 77:3033–3037.

Foote, SL, Berridge, CW, Adams, LM, et al. (1991). Electrophysiological evidence for the involvement of the locus coeruleus in alerting, orienting, and attending. *Prog Brain Res*, 88:521–32.

Gallai, V, Sarchielli, P, Floridi, A, et al. (1995). Vasoactive peptides levels in the plasma of young migraine patients with and without aura assessed both interictally and ictally. *Cephalalgia*, 15:384–390.

Gantenbein, A, Goadsby, PJ, and Kaube, H (2004). Introduction of a clinical scoring system for migraine research applied to electrophysiological studies. *Cephalalgia*, 24:1095–1096.

Giffin, NJ, Ruggiero, L, Lipton, RB, et al. (2003). Premonitory symptoms in migraine: an electronic diary study. *Neurology*, 60:935–940.

Goadsby, PJ (2001a). Migraine, aura and cortical spreading depression: why are we still talking about it? *Ann Neurol*, 49:4–6.

Goadsby, PJ (2001b). The pathophysiology of headache. In *Wolff's Headache and Other Head Pain* (SD Silberstein, RB Lipton, and S Solomon, ed.), pp. 57–72. Oxford University Press, Oxford.

Goadsby, PJ (2002a). Neurovascular headache and a midbrain vascular malformation- evidence for a role of the brainstem in chronic migraine. *Cephalalgia*, 22:107–111.

Goadsby, PJ (2002b). Parallel concept of migraine pathogensis. *Ann Neurol*, 51:140.

Goadsby, PJ (2002c). Pathophysiology of cluster headache: a trigeminal autonomic cephalgia. *Lancet Neurol*, 1:37–43.

Goadsby, PJ (2003). Migraine pathophysiology: the brainstem governs the cortex. *Cephalalgia*, 23:565–566.

Goadsby, PJ (2004). Migraine aura: a knock-in mouse with a knock-out message. *Neuron*, 41:679–680.

Goadsby, PJ, Akerman, S, and Storer, RJ (2001). Evidence for postjunctional serotonin ($5\text{-}HT_1$) receptors in the trigeminocervical complex. *Ann Neurol*, 50:804–807.

Goadsby, PJ and Classey, JD (2003). Evidence for $5\text{-}HT_{1B}$, $5\text{-}HT_{1D}$ and $5\text{-}HT_{1F}$ receptor inhibitory effects on trigeminal neurons with craniovascular input. *Neuroscience*, 122:491–498.

Goadsby, PJ and Duckworth, JW (1987). Effect of stimulation of trigeminal ganglion on regional cerebral blood flow in cats. *Am J Physiol*, 253:R270–R274.

Goadsby, PJ and Duckworth JW (1989). Low frequency stimulation of the locus coeruleus reduces regional

cerebral blood flow in the spinalized cat. *Brain Res*, 476:71–77.
Goadsby, PJ and Edvinsson, L (1993). The trigeminovascular system and migraine: studies characterizing cerebrovascular and neuropeptide changes seen in humans and cats. *Ann Neurol*, 33:48–56.
Goadsby, PJ and Edvinsson, L (1994). Human *in vivo* evidence for trigeminovascular activation in cluster headache. *Brain*, 117:427–434.
Goadsby, PJ and Edvinsson, L (1996). Neuropeptide changes in a case of chronic paroxysmal hemicrania-evidence for trigemino-parasympathetic activation. *Cephalalgia*, 16:448–450.
Goadsby, PJ, Edvinsson, L, and Ekman, R (1988). Release of vasoactive peptides in the extracerebral circulation of man and the cat during activation of the trigeminovascular system. *Ann Neurol*, 23:193–196.
Goadsby, PJ, Edvinsson, L, and Ekman, R (1990). Vasoactive peptide release in the extracerebral circulation of humans during migraine headache. *Ann Neurol*, 28:183–187.
Goadsby, PJ and Ferrari, MD (2001). Migraine: a multifactorial, episodic neurovascular channelopathy? In Channelopaties of the Nervous System (MR Rose and Griggs RC, ed.), pp. 274–292. Butterworth Heinemann, Oxford.
Goadsby, PJ and Hoskin, KL (1996). Inhibition of trigeminal neurons by intravenous administration of the serotonin $(5HT)_{1B/D}$ receptor agonist zolmitriptan (311C90): are brain stem sites a therapeutic target in migraine? *Pain*, 67:355–359.
Goadsby, PJ and Hoskin, KL (1997). The distribution of trigeminovascular afferents in the nonhuman primate brain *Macaca nemestrina*: a c-fos immunocytochemical study. *J Anat*, 190:367–375.
Goadsby, PJ and Hoskin, KL (1999). Differential effects of low dose CP122,288 and eletriptan on fos expression due to stimulation of the superior sagittal sinus in cat. *Pain*, 82:15–22.
Goadsby, PJ, Hoskin, KL, and Knight, YE (1997). Stimulation of the greater occipital nerve increases metabolic activity in the trigeminal nucleus caudalis and cervical dorsal horn of the cat. *Pain*, 73:23–28.
Goadsby, PJ and Knight, YE (1997). Inhibition of trigeminal neurons after intravenous administration of naratriptan through an action at the serotonin $(5HT_{1B/1D})$ receptors. *Br J Pharmacol*, 122:918–922.
Goadsby, PJ and Kullmann, DK (2005). Another migraine gene - further opportunities to understand an important disorder. *Lancet*, 366:345–346.
Goadsby, PJ, Lambert, GA, and Lance, JW (1982). Differential effects on the internal and external carotid circulation of the monkey evoked by locus coeruleus stimulation. *Brain Res*, 249:247–254.
Goadsby, PJ, Lambert, GA, and Lance JW (1985). The mechanism of cerebrovascular vasoconstriction in response to locus coeruleus stimulation. *Brain Res*, 326:213–217.
Goadsby, PJ and Macdonald, GJ (1985). Extracranial vasodilatation mediated by VIP (Vasoactive Intestinal Polypeptide). *Brain Res*, 329:285–288.
Goadsby, PJ and Zagami, AS (1991). Stimulation of the superior sagittal sinus increases metabolic activity and blood flow in certain regions of the brainstem and upper cervical spinal cord of the cat. *Brain*, 114:1001–1011.
Goadsby, PJ, Zagami, AS, and Lambert, GA (1991). Neural processing of craniovascular pain: a synthesis of the central structures involved in migraine. *Headache*, 31:365–371.
Goldstein, DJ, Wang, O, Saper, JR, et al. (1997). Ineffectiveness of neurokinin-1 antagonist in acute migraine: a crossover study. *Cephalalgia*, 17:785–790.
Gowers, WR (1888). *A Manual of Diseases of the Nervous System*. P. Blakiston, Son & Co, Philadelphia.
Grudt, TJ, van den Pol, AN, and Perl, ER (2002). Hypocretin-2 (orexin-B) modulation of superficial dorsal horn activity in rat. *J Physiol*, 538:517–525.
Haan, J, Terwindt, GM, Bos, PL, et al. (1994). Familial hemiplegic migraine in The Netherlands. *Clin Neurol Neurosurg*, 96:244–249.
Hagan, JJ, Leslie, RA, Patel, S, et al. (1999). Orexin A activates locus coeruleus cell firing and increases arousal in the rat. *Proc Natl Acad Sci USA*, 96:10911–10916.
Headache Classification Committee of the International Headache Society. (2004). The International Classification of Headache Disorders (second edition). *Cephalalgia*, 24:1–160.
Holland, PR, Akerman, S, and Goadsby, PJ (2005). Orexin 1 receptor activation attenuates neurogenic dural vasodilation in an animal model of trigeminovascular nociception. *J Pharmacol Exp Ther*, 315:1380–1385.
Holland, PR, Akerman, S, and Goadsby, PJ (2006). Modulation of nociceptive dural input to the trigeminal nucleus caudalis via activation of the orexin 1 receptor in the rat. *Eur J Neurosci*, 24:2825–2833.
Horvath, TL, Peyron, C, Diano, S, et al. (1999). Hypocretin (orexin) activation and synaptic innervation of the locus coeruleus noradrenergic system. *J Comp Neurol*, 415:145–159.
Hoskin, KL, Bulmer, DCE, Lasalandra, M, et al. (2001). Fos expression in the midbrain periaqueductal grey after trigeminovascular stimulation. *J Anat*, 197:29–35.
Hoskin, KL, Kaube, H, and Goadsby, PJ (1996). Central activation of the trigeminovascular pathway in the cat is inhibited by dihydroergotamine. A c-Fos and electrophysiology study. *Brain*, 119:249–256.
Hoskin, KL, Zagami, A, and Goadsby, PJ (1999). Stimulation of the middle meningeal artery leads to Fos expression in the trigeminocervical nucleus: a comparative study of monkey and cat. *J Anat*, 194:579–588.
Ingvardsen, BK, Laursen, H, Olsen, UB, et al. (1997). Possible mechanism of c-fos expression in trigeminal

nucleus caudalis following spreading depression. *Pain*, 72:407–415.

Ingvardsen, BK, Laursen, H, Olsen, UB, et al. (1998). Comment on Ingvardsen, BK, Laursen, H, Olsen, UB, et al. (1997). Possible mechanism of c-fos expression in trigeminal nucleus caudalis following cortical spreading depression. *Pain*, 72:407–415. Reply to Moskowitz, MA and Kraig, R. *Pain*, 76:265–267.

Ivanov, A and Aston-Jones, G (2000). Hypocretin/orexin depolarizes and decreases potassium conductance in locus coeruleus neurons. *Neuroreport*, 11:1755–1758.

Iversen, HK, Olesen, J, and Tfelt-Hansen, P (1989). Intravenous nitroglycerin as an experimental headache model. Basic characteristics. *Pain*, 38:17–24.

Joutel, A, Bousser, MG, Biousse, V, et al. (1993). A gene for familial hemiplegic migraine maps to chromosome 19. *Nat Genet*, 5:40–45.

Joutel, A, Ducros, A, Vahedi, K, et al. (1994). Genetic heterogeneity of familial hemiplegic migraine. *Am J Hum Genet*, 55:1166–1172.

Juhasz, G, Zsombok, T, Jakab, B, et al. (2005). Sumatriptan causes parallel decrease in plasma calcitonin gene-related peptide (CGRP) concentration and migraine headache during nitroglycerin induced migraine attack. *Cephalalgia*, 25:179–183.

Juhasz, G, Zsombok, T, Modos, EA, et al. (2003). NO-induced migraine attack: strong increase in plasma calcitonin gene-related peptide (CGRP) concentration and negative correlation with platelet serotonin release. *Pain*, 106:461–470.

Kaube, H and Giffin, NJ (2002). The electrophysiology of migraine. *Curr Opin Neurol*, 15:303–309.

Kaube, H, Herzog, J, Kaufer, T, et al. (2000). Aura in some patients with familial hemiplegic migraine can be stopped by intranasal ketamine. *Neurology*, 55:139–141.

Kaube, H, Hoskin, KL, and Goadsby, PJ (1993a). Inhibition by sumatriptan of central trigeminal neurones only after blood-brain barrier disruption. *Br J Pharmacol*, 109:788–792.

Kaube, H, Hoskin, KL, and Goadsby, PJ (1993b). Intravenous acetylsalicylic acid inhibits central trigeminal neurons in the dorsal horn of the upper cervical spinal cord in the cat. *Headache*, 33:541–550.

Kaube, H, Keay, KA, Hoskin, KL, et al. (1993). Expression of c-*Fos*-like immunoreactivity in the caudal medulla and upper cervical cord following stimulation of the superior sagittal sinus in the cat. *Brain Res*, 629:95–102.

Knight, YE, Bartsch, T, and Goadsby, PJ (2003). Trigeminal antinociception induced by bicuculline in the periaqueductal grey (PAG) is not affected by PAG P/Q-type calcium channel blockade in rat. *Neurosci Lett*, 336:113–116.

Knight, YE, Bartsch, T, Kaube, H, et al. (2002). P/Q-type calcium channel blockade in the PAG facilitates trigeminal nociception: a functional genetic link for migraine? *J Neurosci*, 22:1–6.

Knight, YE, Edvinsson, L, and Goadsby, PJ (1999). Blockade of CGRP release after superior sagittal sinus stimulation in cat: a comparison of avitriptan and CP122,288. *Neuropeptides*, 33:41–46.

Knight, YE, Edvinsson, L, and Goadsby, PJ (2001). 4991W93 inhibits release of calcitonin gene-related peptide in the cat but only at doses with $5HT_{1B/1D}$ receptor agonist activity. *Neuropharmacology*, 40:520–525.

Knight, YE and Goadsby, PJ (2001). The periaqueductal gray matter modulates trigeminovascular input: a role in migraine? *Neuroscience*, 106:793–800.

Kropp, P and Gerber, WD (1998). Prediction of migraine attacks using a slow cortical potential, the contingent negative variation. *Neurosci Lett*, 257:73–76.

Kruuse, C, Thomsen, LL, Birk, S, et al. (2003). Migraine can be induced by sildenafil without changes in middle cerebral artery diameter. *Brain*, 126:241–247.

Lambert, GA, Boers, PM, Hoskin, KL, et al. (2002). Suppression by eletriptan of the activation of trigeminovascular sensory neurons by glyceryl trinitrate. *Brain Res*, 953:181–188.

Lambert, GA, Goadsby, PJ, Zagami, AS, et al. (1988). Comparative effects of stimulation of the trigeminal ganglion and the superior sagittal sinus on cerebral blood flow and evoked potentials in the cat. *Brain Res*, 453:143–149.

Lambert, GA, Lowy, AJ, Boers, P, et al. (1992). The spinal cord processing of input from the superior sagittal sinus: pathway and modulation by ergot alkaloids. *Brain Res*, 597:321–330.

Lance, JW and Goadsby, PJ (2005). *Mechanism and Management of Headache*. Elsevier, New York.

Langedijk, M, van der Naalt, J, Luijckx, GJ, et al. (2005). Cluster-like headache aura status. *Headache*, 45:80–81.

Lauritzen, M (1994). Pathophysiology of the migraine aura. The spreading depression theory. *Brain*, 117:199–210.

Leao, AAP (1944a). Pial circulation and spreading activity in the cerebral cortex. *J Neurophysiol*, 7:391–396.

Leao, AAP (1944b). Spreading depression of activity in cerebral cortex. *J Neurophysiol*, 7:359–390.

Levy, D, Jakubowski, M, and Burstein, R (2004). Disruption of communication between peripheral and central trigeminovascular neurons mediates the antimigraine action of 5HT 1B/1D receptor agonists. *Proc Natl Acad Sci USA*, 101:4274–4279.

Limmroth, V, May, A, Auerbach, P, et al. (1996). Changes in cerebral blood flow velocity after treatment with sumatriptan or placebo and implications for the pathophysiology of migraine. *J Neurol Sci*, 138:60–65.

Liu-Chen, L-Y, Gillespie, SA, Norregaard, TV, et al. (1984). Co-localization of retrogradely transported wheat germ agglutinin and the putative neurotransmitter substance P within trigeminal ganglion cells projecting to cat middle cerebral. *J Comp Neurol*, 225:187–192.

Maertens de Noordhout, A, Timsit-Berthier, M, and Schoenen, J (1985). Contingent negative variation

(CNV) in migraineurs before and during prophylactic treatment with beta-blockers. *Cephalalgia*, 5:34–35.

Maneesi, S, Akerman, S, Lasalandra, MP, et al. (2004). Electron microsopic demonstration of pre- and post-synaptic 5-HT_{1D} and 5-HT_{1F} receptor immunoreactivity (IR) in the rat trigeminocervical complex (TCC) new therapeutic possibilities for the triptans. *Cephalalgia*, 24:148.

Marconi, R, De Fusco, M, Aridon, P, et al. (2003). Familial hemiplegic migraine type 2 is linked to 0.9Mb region on chromosome 1q23. *Ann Neurol*, 53:376–381.

Markowitz, S, Saito, K, and Moskowitz, MA (1987). Neurogenically mediated leakage of plasma proteins occurs from blood vessels in dura mater but not brain. *J Neurosci*, 7:4129–4136.

Matharu, MS, Bartsch, T, Ward, N, et al. (2004). Central neuromodulation in chronic migraine patients with suboccipital stimulators: a PET study. *Brain*, 127:220–230.

Matharu, MS, Cohen, AS, Frackowiak, RSJ, et al. (2005). Posterior hypothalamic activation in paroxysmal hemicrania using PET. *Cephalalgia*, 25:859.

Matharu, MS, Cohen, AS, McGonigle, DJ, et al. (2004). Posterior hypothalamic and brainstem activation in hemicrania continua. *Headache*, 44:462–463.

Matharu, MS and Goadsby, PJ (2001). Post-traumatic chronic paroxysmal hemicrania (CPH) with aura. *Neurology*, 56:273–275.

Matsuyama, T, Shiosaka, S, Matsumoto, M, et al. (1983). Overall distribution of vasoactive intestinal polypeptide-containing nerves on the wall of the cerebral arteries: an immunohistochemical study using whole-mounts. *Neuroscience*, 10:89–96.

May, A, Bahra, A, Buchel, C, et al. (1998). Involvement of the hypothalamic grey in cluster headache: a positron emission tomography (PET) study. *Eur J Neurol*, 5:S7–S8.

May, A, Bahra, A, Buchel, C, et al. (1999). Functional MRI in spontaneous attacks of SUNCT: short-lasting neuralgiform headache with conjunctival injection and tearing. *Ann Neurol*, 46:791–793.

May, A, Gijsman, HJ, Wallnoefer, A, et al. (1996). Endothelin antagonist bosentan blocks neurogenic inflammation, but is not effective in aborting migraine attacks. *Pain*, 67:375–378.

May, A and Goadsby, PJ (1999). The trigeminovascular system in humans: pathophysiological implications for primary headache syndromes of the neural influences on the cerebral circulation. *J Cereb Blood Flow Metab*, 19:115–127.

May, A, Shepheard, S, Wessing, A, et al. (1998). Retinal plasma extravasation can be evoked by trigeminal stimulation in rat but does not occur during migraine attacks. *Brain*, 121:1231–1237.

Morgan, JI and Curran, T (1991). Stimulus-transcription coupling in the nervous system: involvement of the inducible proto-oncogenes fos and jun. *Annu Rev Neurosci*, 14:421–451.

Moskowitz, MA and Cutrer, FM (1993). SUMATRIPTAN: a receptor-targeted treatment for migraine. Annu Rev Med, 44:145–154.

Moskowitz, MA, Nozaki, K, and Kraig, RP (1993). Neocortical spreading depression provokes the expression of C-fos protein-like immunoreactivity within the trigeminal nucleus caudalis via trigeminovascular mechanisms. *J Neurosci*, 13:1167–1177.

Niebur, E, Hsiao, SS, and Johnson, KO (2002). Synchrony: a neural mechanism for attentional selection? *Curr Opin Neurobiol*, 12:190–194.

Norman, B, Panebianco, D, and Block, GA (1998). A placebo-controlled, in-clinic study to explore the preliminary safety and efficacy of intravenous L-758,298 (a prodrug of the NK1 receptor antagonist L-754,030) in the acute treatment of migraine. *Cephalalgia*, 18:407.

Nozaki, K, Boccalini, P, and Moskowitz, MA (1992). Expression of c-fos-like immunoreactivity in brainstem after meningeal irritation by blood in the subarachnoid space. *Neuroscience*, 49:669–680.

Obermann, M, Gizewski, ER, Limmroth, V, et al. (2007). Symptomatic migraine and pontine vascular malformation: evidence for a key role of the brainstem in the pathophysiology of chronic migraine. *Cephalalgia*, 26:763–766.

Olesen, J, Diener, H-C, Husstedt, I-W, et al. (2004). Calcitonin gene-related peptide (CGRP) receptor antagonist BIBN4096BS is effective in the treatment of migraine attacks. *N Engl J Med*, 350:1104–1110.

Olesen, J, Diener, HC, Schoenen, J, et al. (2004). No effect of eletriptan administration during the aura phase of migraine. *Eur J Neurol*, 11:671–677.

Olesen, J, Friberg, L, Skyhoj-Olsen, T, et al. (1990). Timing and topography of cerebral blood flow, aura, and headache during migraine attacks. *Ann Neurol*, 28:791–798.

Ophoff, RA, van Eijk, R, Sandkuijl, LA, et al. (1994). Genetic heterogeneity of familial hemiplegic migraine. *Genomics*, ; 22:21–26.

Ophoff, RA, Terwindt, GM, Vergouwe, MN, et al. (1996). Familial hemiplegic migraine and episodic ataxia type-2 are caused by mutations in the Ca^{2+} channel gene CACNL1A4. *Cell*, 87:543–552.

Oshinsky, ML and Luo, J (2006). Neurochemistry of trigeminal activation in an animal model of migraine. *Headache*, 46:S39–S44.

Penfield, W and McNaughton, FL (1940). Dural headache and the innervation of the dura mater. *Arch Neurol Psychiatr*, 44:43–75.

Peres, MF and Viera, DS (2006). Tension-type headache with aura. *Cephalalgia*, 26:349–350.

Peres, MFP, Siow, HC, and Rozen, TD (2002). Hemicrania continua with aura. *Cephalalgia*, 22:246–248.

Peroutka, SJ (1997). Dopamine and migraine. *Neurology*, 49:650–656.

Peroutka, SJ (2005). Neurogenic inflammation and migraine: implications for therapeutics. *Mol Interv*, 5:306–313.

Petersen, KA, Birk, S, Doods, H, et al. (2004). Inhibitory effect of BIBN4096BS on cephalic vasodilatation induced by CGRP or transcranial electrical stimulation in the rat. *Br J Pharmacol*, 143:697–704.

Petersen, KA, Birk, S, Lassen, LH, et al. (2005). The CGRP-antagonist, BIBN4096BS does not affect cerebral or systemic haemodynamics in healthy volunteers. *Cephalalgia*, 25:139–147.

Potrebic, S, Ahn, AH, Skinner, K, et al. (2003). Peptidergic nociceptors of both trigeminal and dorsal root ganglia express serotonin 1D receptors: implications for the selective antimigraine action of triptans. *J Neurosci*, 23:10988–10997.

Pozo-Rosich, P and Oshinsky, M (2005). Effect of dihydroergotamine (DHE) on central sensitisation of neurons in the trigeminal nucleus caudalis. *Neurology*, 64: A151.

Proietti-Cecchini, A, Afra, J, and Schoenen, J (1997). Intensity dependence of the cortical auditory evoked potentials as a surrogate marker of central nervous system serotonin transmission in man: demonstration of a central effect for the 5HT1B/1D agonist zolmitriptan (311C90, Zomig). *Cephalalgia*, 17:849–854.

Raskin, NH, Hosobuchi, Y, and Lamb, S (1987). Headache may arise from perturbation of brain. *Headache*, 27:416–420.

Rasmussen, BK and Olesen, J (1992). Migraine with aura and migraine without aura: an epidemiological study. *Cephalalgia*, 12:221–228.

Roon, K, Diener, HC, Ellis, P, et al. (1997). CP-122,288 blocks neurogenic inflammation, but is not effective in aborting migraine attacks: results of two controlled clinical studies. *Cephalalgia*, 17:245.

Roon, KI, Olesen, J, Diener, HC, et al. (2000). No acute antimigraine efficacy of CP-122,288, a highly potent inhibitor of neurogenic inflammation: results of two randomized double-blind placebo-controlled clinical trials. *Ann Neurol*, 47:238–241.

Russell, MB (1997). Genetic epidemiology of migraine and cluster headache. *Cephalalgia*, 17:683–701.

Sakurai, T, Amemiya, A, Ishii, M, et al. (1998). Orexins and orexin receptors: a family of hypothalamic neuropeptides and G protein-coupled receptors that regulate feeding behavior. *Cell*, 92:696–697.

Schoenen, J, Ambrosini, A, Sandor, PS, et al. (2003). Evoked potentials and transcranial magnetic stimulation in migraine: published data and viewpoint on their pathophysiologic significance. *Clin Neurophysiol*, 114:955–972.

Schoenen, J and Timsit-Berthier, M (1993). Contingent negative variation: methods and potential interest in headache. *Cephalalgia*, 13:28–32.

Schoenen, J, Wang, W, Albert, A, et al. (1995). Potentiation instead of habituation characterizes visual evoked potentials in migraine patients between attacks. *Eur J Neurol*, 2:115–122.

Selby, G and Lance, JW (1960). Observations on 500 cases of migraine and allied vascular headache. *J Neurol, Neurosurg Psychiatr*, 23:23–32.

Shields, KG and Goadsby, PJ (2005). Propranolol modulates trigeminovascular responses in thalamic ventroposteromedial nucleus: a role in migraine? *Brain*, 128:86–97.

Shields, KG and Goadsby, PJ (2006). Serotonin receptors modulate trigeminovascular responses in ventroposteromedial nucleus of thalamus: a migraine target? *Neurobiol Dis*, 23:491–501.

Shields, KG, Kaube, H, and Goadsby, PJ (2003). GABA receptors modulate trigeminovascular nociceptive transmission in the ventroposteromedial (VPM) thalamic nucleus of the rat. *Cephalalgia*, 23:728.

Silberstein, SD, Lipton, RB, and Goadsby, PJ (2002). *Headache in Clinical Practice*. Martin Dunitz, London.

Silberstein, SD, Neto, W, Schmitt, J, et al. (2004). Topiramate in migraine prevention: results of a large controlled trial. *Arch Neurol*, 61:490–495.

Silberstein, SD, Niknam, R, Rozen, TD, et al. (2000). Cluster headache with aura. *Neurology*, 54:219–221.

Steuer, H, Jaworski, A, Stoll, D, et al. (2004). In vitro model of the outer blood-retina barrier. *Brain Res Brain Res Protoc*, 13:26–36.

Storer, RJ and Goadsby, PJ (1997). Microiontophoretic application of serotonin $(5HT)_{1B/1D}$ agonists inhibits trigeminal cell firing in the cat. *Brain*, 120:2171–2177.

Storer, RJ and Goadsby, PJ (2004). Topiramate inhibits trigeminovascular neurons in the cat. *Cephalalgia*, 24:1049–1056.

Storer, RJ and Goadsby, PJ (2005). Topiramate has a locus of action outside of the trigeminocervical complex. *Neurology*, 64:A150–A151.

Strassman, AM, Raymond, SA, and Burstein, R (1996). Sensitization of meningeal sensory neurons and the origin of headaches. *Nature*, 384:560–563.

Teh, BT, Silburn, P, Lindblad, K, et al. (1995). Familial cerebellar periodic ataxia without myokymia maps to a 19-cM region on 19p13. *Am J Hum Genet*, 56:1443–1449.

Terwindt, GM, Ophoff, RA, Haan, J, et al. (1996). Familial hemiplegic migraine: a clinical comparison of families linked and unlinked to chromosome 19. *Cephalalgia*, 16:153–155.

Tvedskov, JF, Lipka, K, Ashina, M, et al. (2005). No increase of calcitonin gene-related peptide in jugular blood during migraine. *Ann Neurol*, 58:561–568.

Uddman, R, Edvinsson, L, Ekman, R, et al. (1985). Innervation of the feline cerebral vasculature by nerve fibers containing calcitonin gene-related peptide: trigeminal origin and co-existence with substance P. *Neurosci Lett*, 62:131–136.

van den Maagdenberg, AM, Pietrobon D, Pizzorusso, T, et al. (2004). A Cacna1a knock-in migraine mouse model with increased susceptibility to cortical spreading depression. *Neuron*, 41:701–710.

Veloso, F, Kumar, K, and Toth, C (1998). Headache secondary to deep brain implantation. *Headache,* 38:507–515.

Wang, W and Schoenen, J (1998). Interictal potentiation of passive "oddball" auditory event-related potentials in migraine. *Cephalalgia,* 18:261–265.

Weiller, C, May, A, Limmroth, V, et al. (1995). Brain stem activation in spontaneous human migraine attacks. *Nat Med,* 1:658–660.

Welch, KM, Nagesh, V, Aurora, S, et al. (2001). Periaqueductal grey matter dysfunction in migraine: cause or the burden of illness? *Headache,* 41:629–637.

Willis, T (1682). *Opera Omnia.* Henricum Wetstenium, Amstelaedami.

Wolff, HG (1948). *Headache and Other Head Pain.* Oxford University Press, New York.

Yamamoto, T, Nozaki-Taguchi, N, and Chiba, T (2002). Analgesic effect of intrathecally administered orexin-A in the rat formalin test and in the rat hot plate test. *Br J Pharmacol,* 137:170–176.

Zagami, AS and Goadsby, PJ (1991). Stimulation of the superior sagittal sinus increases metabolic activity in cat thalamus. In *New Advances in Headache Research: 2* (FC Rose, ed.), pp. 169–171. Smith-Gordon and Co Ltd, London.

Zagami, AS, Goadsby, PJ, and Edvinsson, L (1990). Stimulation of the superior sagittal sinus in the cat causes release of vasoactive peptides. *Neuropeptides,* 16:69–75.

Zagami, AS and Lambert, GA (1991). Craniovascular application of capsaicin activates nociceptive thalamic neurons in the cat. *Neurosci Lett,* 121:187–190.

8 Pathophysiology of Aura

Katharina Eikermann-Haerter and Michael Moskowitz

Among the more typical forms of migraine headache, migraine with aura is the best studied and arguably the best understood. Migraine aura is common, affecting up to 5% of the adult population (Agostoni and Aliprandi, 2006). Migraine aura is associated with neurologic symptoms that often spread over a characteristic time frame and in most cases precede the development of a migraine-like headache. Ninety-nine percent of aura patients experience visual phenomenon in at least some attacks, whereas 54% and 32% describe sensory and/or aphasic aura, respectively (Kirchmann, 2006). If more than a single symptom develops, the auras tend to occur in succession; almost all individuals describe symptoms of visual aura. Positive symptoms (shimmering lights, zigzagging line, or paresthesia) are sometimes followed by negative symptoms, such as a scotoma or numbness.

According to the International Classification of Headache Disorders (ICHD-2), diagnosis of migraine with aura (ICHD-2 codes 1.2.1-6) requires specific clinical features as well as the absence of other causative diseases. The following three major subtypes of migraine with aura are distinguished (more than one subtype may occur in the same person):

1. Typical (nonhemiplegic) aura (a) with migraine headache, (b) with nonmigraine headache, or (c) without headache. To meet the criteria for diagnosis of typical (nonhemiplegic) aura, symptoms must be either visual, sensory, or speech related, and the first two should be one-sided. Propagation is a key feature, as is duration (5–60 minutes). Since pathogenesis of nonhemiplegic migraine with aura is multifactorial, and the disease is genetically heterogeneous with a complex mode of inheritance, the classification of subtypes relies exclusively on clinical data.
2. Hemiplegic migraine is subdivided into familial and sporadic hemiplegic migraine. In addition to the typical aura, these forms are characterized by motor weakness. Often, patients report two or three additional aura symptoms besides the motor weakness, including fully reversible visual, and sensory symptoms or dysphasic speech disturbances (Eri.ksen et al., 2006).
3. Basilar-type migraine is characterized by auras clearly originating either from brain stem or from both hemispheres (Headache Classification Subcommittee of the International Headache Society, 2004). Symptoms include dysarthria, vertigo, diplopia, ataxia, or a decrease in the level of consciousness; bilateral paresthesias are sometimes experienced.

THE PHENOMENON OF CORTICAL SPREADING DEPRESSION

There is growing evidence that cortical spreading depression (CSD) underlies the typical forms of migraine aura (Lauritzen, 1994). CSD, originally described by Leao (Leao, 1944), is an intense depolarization of neuronal and glial membranes accompanied by a massive disruption of ionic gradients, and loss of membrane resistance. It is characterized by cessation of spontaneous or evoked synaptic activity, and massive glutamate and K^+ release, causing extracellular K^+ concentrations ($[K^+]_e$) to rise above 50 mM. The marked decrease in membrane resistance also results in an increase in intracellular Na^+ and Ca^{2+}, and may cause the typical electrocortical recordable DC potential shifts. Elevated $[K^+]_e$ is a strong depolarizing stimulus that promotes the contiguous spread of a depolarization wave across neural tissue. Large unregulated release of excitatory amino acids like glutamate and direct intercellular transfer of ions and small molecules through gap junctions facilitate the spread.

Although little is known about initiation of spontaneous attacks in humans, CSD can be evoked by depolarization of a minimum volume of brain tissue, such as during cerebral ischemia and cortical trauma, or direct cortical application of excitatory amino acids, Na^+/K^+-pump inhibitors or K^+ in both lissencephalic (Leao, 1944) or folded cortex (James et al., 1999). In experimental paradigms, the CSD threshold is exceeded when local physiologic K^+ concentrations build up (for reasons outlined below) (see Fig. 8–1).

Triggering CSD requires activation of the N-methyl-D-aspartate (NMDA) receptor subtype in rat cerebral cortex (Gorelova et al., 1987) and in human neocortical tissues (Gorji et al., 2001). In turn, CSD induces the release of glutamate from the cortex (Van Harreveld, 1959), and levels are increased in cerebrospinal fluid (CSF) (Martinez et al., 1993). Once triggered, CSD slowly propagates (2–5 mm/minute) to adjacent tissues without regard to functional cortical divisions or arterial territories but does not propagate across major sulci (Somjen, 2001).

CSD in cerebral cortex is associated with characteristic blood flow fluctuations in cerebral cortex: an initial, small, brief, species-dependent reduction in cerebral blood flow is followed by a profound hyperemia, reaching up to 200% of baseline, and then by a long-lasting oligemia (60%–90% of baseline), which usually lasts up to an hour, although oligemia for as long as 3 days has been reported (Otori et al., 2003). CSD may exert multiple effects on blood vessel tone that go beyond a direct and immediate effect on vasomotion, probably by inducing significant changes in second messenger cascades (Read et al., 2001),

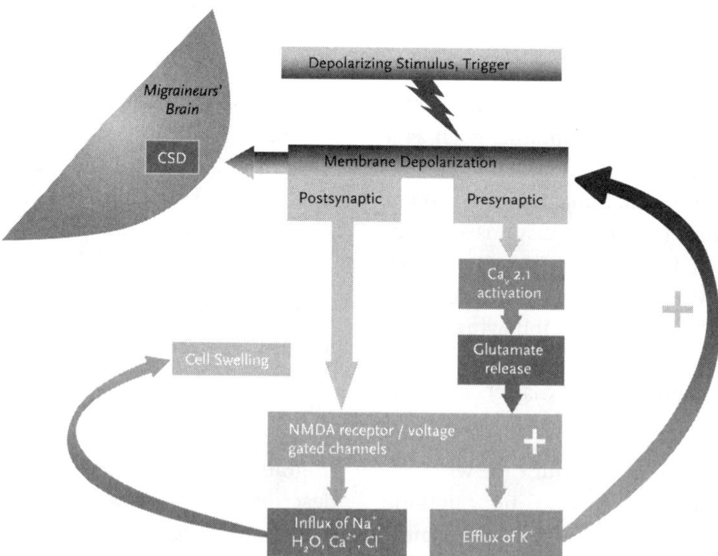

Figure 8–1 Presumptive mechanism of CSD induction and perpetuation. CSD can be evoked by depolarization of a minimum "critical" volume of brain tissue to increase extracellular K^+ concentration ($[K^+]_{ec}$) over a threshold concentration that exceeds tissue buffering mechanisms. This increase in $[K^+]_{ec}$ then depolarizes adjacent brain tissue to initiate the self-sustaining spread. Membrane depolarization activates voltage gated channels, and an increased Ca^{2+} influx via $Ca_v2.1$ activation (presynaptic effects) with subsequent activation of NMDA receptors by glutamate release. $[K^+]_{ec}$ further increases after swelling of astrocytes and decreased exracellular space. [Modified from Pietrobon, D (2005). Migraine: new molecular mechanisms. *Neuroscientist,* 11:373–386.]

immediate early genes, growth factors, neurotransmitter and neuromodulatory systems, as well as inflammatory mediators, such as interleukin-1β or tumor necrosis factor-α (Kunkler and Kraig, 1998). Interestingly, CSD does not cause injury or cell death in normal brain (Somjen, 2001). However, under conditions of energy compromise (e.g., stroke), anoxic depolarization, and periinfarct, spreading depolarizations are associated with a reduction in tissue adenosine triphosphate (ATP), oxygen, and pH (Somjen, 2001), in addition to massive redistribution of ions across membranes as mentioned above. Ischemic depolarizing events increase the metabolic burden and exacerbate the energy deficit thereby expanding infarct size (Selman et al., 2004).

CSD has been investigated in experimental animals, in vivo and in vitro for over five decades (Leao, 1944; Bures et al., 1974; Kruger et al., 1999; Somjen, 2001), and in human neocortical and hippocampal tissue in vitro (Sramka et al., 1977; Avoli et al., 1991). Direct and indirect evidence supporting CSD in human brain in situ has only recently been obtained using functional magnetic resonance imaging (MRI) (Hadjikhani et al., 2001), epidural electrophysiological recordings (Strong, 2003; Strong et al., 2002; Fabricius et al., 2006), and intracortical multiparametric electrodes (Mayevsky et al., 1996).

Published experimental as well as human data strongly suggest that CSD is the pathophysiologic trigger for both migraine aura and headache (Bolay et al., 2002; Haerter, 2005; Dalkara et al., 2006;). Bolay showed that intrinsic brain activity triggers trigeminal meningeal afferents in a migraine model. Although the mechanism of activation remains unstudied, it has been assumed that H^+, K^+, NO and other agents released into the extracellular space depolarize adjacent perivascular trigeminal axons surrounding local blood vessels, but more work is needed to clarify this point. These events are facilitated by CSD-induced activation of matrix metalloproteinases (MMPs) and mild disruption of the blood–brain barrier (BBB) (Gursoy-Ozdemir et al., 2004). MMPs belong to a superfamily of endopeptidases involved in processes such as opening of the BBB (Aoki et al., 2002), edema formation (Rosenberg et al., 2001), invasion of neural tissue by blood-derived immune cells (Leppert et al., 1995), and shedding of cytokines and cytokine receptors (Chandler et al., 1997). NFκB, and proinflammatory cytokines like tumor necrosis factor-α (TNF-α) and interleukin-1β (IL-1β) (Jander et al., 2001), which are elevated after CSD, bind to the promoter region of the *MMP-9* gene (Yong et al., 2001). The data are consistent with the formulation that intense neuro-glial depolarisation facilitates the access of hydrophilic molecules to approximate and discharge meningeal trigeminovascular afferents.

CSD UNDERLIES MIGRAINE AURA: CLINICAL EVIDENCE

Since its discovery, CSD has been a prime candidate to explain the event underlying migraine aura (Leao, 1944): In 1958, Milner (Milner, 1958) pointed out the similarity between the velocity of CSD propagation and the march visual aura reported by Lashley (1941). The velocity of spread is approximately 3 mm/minute, consistent with the speed of CSD in mammalian cortex. Also, the spread of oligemia, estimated during a migraine attack, exhibits a similar velocity. The observed time course suggests that the focal symptoms are not secondary to oligemia, because initially the tissue appears well arteriolized and spreading oligemia is a secondary event and tends to be mild [25%–35% below baseline in average (Olesen et al., 1981; Lauritzen et al., 1983)]. Focal symptoms and blood flow changes are thought to be secondary to electrophysiological changes caused by spreading depression (Lauritzen et al., 1983). Nevertheless, severe hypoxia or ischemia can trigger CSD.

Indeed, cerebral ischemia is one of the known experimental triggers of CSD, and migraine is associated with an increased risk of stroke, especially in younger patients (Kruit et al., 2004) with a remarkable increase in women suffering from migraine with aura (Bousser and Welch, 2005). This relationship is particularly strong in the posterior circulation, as evidenced by a 15-fold increased risk in cerebellar lesions in migraine patients both with and without aura (Kruit et al., 2005). Recent data in patients with patent foramen ovale (PFO) or atrial septal defects suggest that not only stroke but also migraine headache may be induced by small microthromboemboli. Furthermore, PFO are more common in migraineurs with aura, and migraine with aura is more prevalent in patients with PFO (Schwedt and Dodick, 2006). Cardiac or pulmonary arterial defects with right to left shunts may increase the risk of cryptogenic stroke and are also associated with a higher incidence of migraine. Furthermore, closure of such defects significantly reduces the frequency of migraine attacks in many patients, and reportedly abolishes migraine headache in some patients (Spies and Schrader, 2006). These findings suggest that subclinical cerebral ischemia due to paradoxical embolism may trigger a migraine attack, probably by evoking CSD in a susceptible person (Anzola et al., 2000; Wilmshurst and Nightingale, 2001; Morandi et al., 2003; Schwerzmann et al., 2004; Wilmshurst et al., 2004; 2004b; Azarbal et al., 2005; Reisman et al., 2005). However, more controlled prospective clinical trials will be required to clarify and solidify this association.

CSD UNDERLIES MIGRAINE AURA: EVIDENCE FROM RADIOLOGY

Neuroimaging studies including single photon emission computed tomography (SPECT), positron emission tomography (PET) and MRI provided indirect evidence linking CSD and migraine. The evidence from MR is the most technically advanced and convincing. For example, blood oxygen level-dependent (BOLD) MRI detects the ratio of nonparamagnetic oxygenated hemoglobin to paramagnetic deoxyhemoglobin and is roughly a measure of oxygen delivery minus consumption. BOLD, the basis for functional imaging, is influenced by neuronal activity, including flow, volume, and oxygen consumption (D'Esposito et al., 2003; Kim et al., 2007). Recently, BOLD imaging detected a focal increase in blood flow during migraine visual aura. The increased BOLD signal spread within occipital cortex at a rate of 3.5 mm/minute and was retinotopically congruent with the patient's aura (Hadjikhani et al., 2001) (see Fig. 8–2). This initial increased BOLD signal was followed minutes later by a decrease, suggesting a rise and then a fall in cerebral blood flow. Further evidence that CSD underlies visual aura comes from experiments using magnetencephalography (MEG). The DC MEG field shifts measured during patients' spontaneous or visually triggered visual aura resembled those previously measured during CSD spreading across a sulcus in gyrencephalic animal models (Bowyer et al., 1999).

CSD UNDERLIES MIGRAINE AURA: EVIDENCE FOR AN INCREASED CORTICAL EXCITABILITY IN MIGRAINEURS

Preliminary evidence suggests that patients suffering from migraine with aura have a reduced threshold of cortical depolarization. For example, migraineurs exhibit a reduced threshold to evoke phosphenes (bright scintillations) after transcranial magnetic stimulation. Patients with probable chronic migraine (PCM) reportedly show increased stimulus-induced excitability, which may correlate with the frequency of their migraine attacks (Aurora et al., 2005).

More mechanistic insights come from studies in patients and animal models of autosomal dominant familial hemiplegic migraine (FHM) syndromes. Patients experience episodes of prolonged but reversible unilateral motor deficits accompanying migraine headache, and as noted above, more than 60% of these patients also suffer from migraine attacks with typical aura or even without aura.

Biophysical studies revealed that FHM1 mutations produce gain-of-function at the single PQ-type $Ca_v2.1$ channel level and, as a consequence, increased calcium entry and $Ca_v2.1$-dependent neurotransmitter release from cortical neurons. $Ca_v2.1$ channels are expressed on presynaptic terminals and somatodendritic membranes in brain structures implicated in migraine pathogenesis and central control of nociception, including the cerebral cortex, the trigeminal ganglia, and brainstem nuclei (Pietrobon and Striessnig, 2003). These channels play a prominent role in controlling neurotransmitter release, particularly at central excitatory synapses (Pietrobon, 2005a), and also might have additional postsynaptic functions, for example, in neural excitability. Mutations in the *CACNA1A* gene on chromosome 19p13, which encodes the $\alpha1$ pore-forming subunit of PQ-type Ca^{2+} channels, account for 50% of FHM families and are responsible for the FHM1 phenotype (Ophoff et al., 1996). Seventeen different missense mutations within *CACNA1A* have been linked to FHM1 so far, producing substitutions of conserved amino acids in important

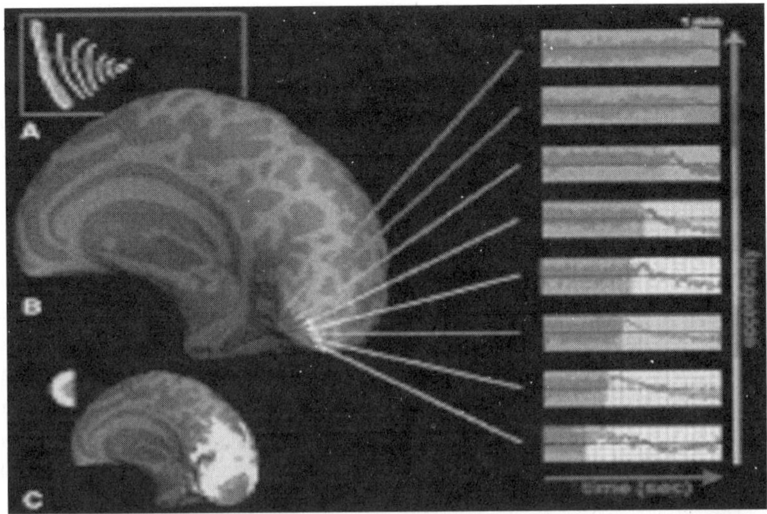

Figure 8–2 Spreading suppression of cortical activation during migraine aura. (*A*) A patient's drawing showing the progression of the scintillations and the visual aura affecting the left hemifield over a duration of 20 minutes. The fixation point appears as a small white cross. The red line shows the overall direction of progression of the visual percept. (*B*) A computer generated reconstruction shows a hyperinflated midsagittal view of the patient's brain based on anatomical MR data. The posterior medial aspect of occipital lobe is shown. In this format, the cortical sulci and gyri appear in darker and lighter gray, respectively, on a computationally inflated surface. MR signal changes over time are shown to the right. Each time course was recorded from one in a sequence of voxels that were sampled along the calcarine sulcus, in the primary visual cortex (V1), from the posterior pole to more anterior location, as indicated by arrowheads. A similar BOLD response was found within all of the voxels, differing only in the time of onset of the MR perturbation. The perturbations developed earlier in the foveal area, compared with more eccentric representations of retinotopic visual cortex. This finding was consistent with the progression of the aura from central to peripheral eccentricities in the corresponding visual field (*A* and *C*). (*C*) The MR maps of retinotopic eccentricity from this same subject, acquired during interictal scans. As shown in the logo chart on the right in the upper left, voxels that show retinotopically specific activation in the fovea are coded in red (centered at 1.5° eccentricity). Parafoveal eccentricities are shown in blue, and more peripheral eccentricities are shown in green (centered at 3.8° and 10.3°, respectively). [From Hadjikhani, N, Sanchez Del Rio, M, Wu, O, et al. (2001). Mechanisms of migrane aura revealed by functional MRI in human visual cortex. *Proc Natl Acad Sci USA*, 98:4687–4692.]

functional domains of the protein, including the pore lining and the voltage sensing element (Pietrobon, 2005b).

FHM2 mutations produce loss of function of the α2 Na^+/K^+ ATPase, which is a P-type ion pump that uses ATP to actively countertransport Na^+ and K^+ ions. Twenty-three different missense mutations in the ATP1A2 gene on chromosome 1q23 have been described (Vanmolkot et al., 2006) to date. These point mutations produce substitutions of conserved amino acids in important functional regions, such as the intracellular four to five loop, which contains the nucleotide-binding domain, and the extracellular seven to eight loop, which is responsible for β subunit binding (Jorgensen et al., 2003). The Na^+/K^+ ATPase generates the ion gradients that maintain resting membrane potential and cell volume, providing the driving force for nutrient and neurotransmitter uptake, as well as clearance of K^+ from the extracellular space during neuronal activity (D'Ambrosio et al., 2002).

The FHM3 mutation accelerates recovery from fast inactivation of $Na_v1.5$ and possibly $Na_v1.1$

channels, an effect that is predicted to increase neuronal firing rates. SCN1A was identified as the mutated gene on chromosome 2q24 encoding the α1-subunit of $Na_v1.1$ channels (Dichgans et al., 2005). This Gln1489Lys missense mutation is located in a cytoplasmatic segment of somatodendrites, implying that $Na_v1.1$ channels may play a key role in mediating dendritic excitability, an important component of synaptic signal processing (Johnston et al., 1996). Experiments with $scn1a^{-/-}$ and $scn1a^{-/+}$ mice revealed a reduction of GABA-ergic interneuron excitability, a finding that might underlie the epileptic phenotype observed in these mice (Yu et al., 2006). Because of its association with FHM3, enhanced susceptibility to CSD may contribute to its phenotype. As a consequence of overactivity at mutated Na^+ channels that recover more rapidly from fast inactivation, a relatively weak depolarizing stimulus (perhaps without consequences in healthy individuals) may cause excessive neuronal firing that increases extracellular K^+ above the critical value that triggers CSD in mutated channels.

Mutations in genes encoding proteins expressed by neurons and glia have implicated the excitatory amino acid glutamate in a pivotal role modulating CSD threshold, and a critical involvement of cortical hyperexcitability in the pathophysiology of migraine. FHM is characterized by an increase in the concentration of glutamate via enhanced synaptic release from neurons as a result of higher Ca^{2+}-influx into presynaptic terminals (FHM 1) or as a consequence of decreased removal of K^+ and glutamate from the synaptic cleft (FHM 2). In patients with FHM3, extracellular K^+ might be increased as a result of excessive firing of neurons expressing mutant $Na_V1.1$ Gln1489Lys channels. High extracellular glutamate and K^+-concentration decrease CSD threshold in mice (Ayata et al., 2000; van den Maagdenberg et al., 2004), which may explain susceptibility to both CSD and aura (motor, visual, somatosensory) and the high incidence of migraine headache in FHM patients (Moskowitz et al., 2004) (see Fig. 8–3).

CSD UNDERLIES MIGRAINE AURA: LABORATORY EVIDENCE

Experiments using genetically-engineered mice have revealed mechanistic insights into causes and consequences of CSD relevant to migraine. For example, spontaneous mutations within the orthologous FHM-1 gene show marked elevations in CSD threshold. The *tottering* mutation (a proline to leucine substitution in the S5–S6 linker region of repeat domain II of α-1 subunit in P/Q-type Ca^{++} channel) causes impaired presynaptic Ca^{++} influx (i.e., loss of function), and reduced neurotransmitter release, mainly inhibiting excitatory neurotransmission (Fletcher et al., 1996; Doyle et al., 1997; Caddick et al., 1999; Plomp et al., 2000; Qian and Noebels, 2000). *Tottering* and *leaner* mice also show a 10-fold resistance to CSD, with a slower CSD propagation speed and failure to sustain regenerative spread of the depolarization wave, especially present in the leaner mutation (Ayata et al., 2000). In vitro, selective blockade of voltage-gated Ca^{++} channels (P/Q-type) (Westenbroek et al., 1995) decreased neurotransmitter release (particularly glutamate) (Dunlap et al., 1995), and played a major role in suppressing KCl-induced CSD (Richter et al., 2002).

Knockin mice expressing the human mutation (R192Q) in the *CACNA1A* gene encoding the α1-poreforming subunit of P/Q-type Ca^{++} ($Ca_v2.1$) channels show increased susceptibility to CSD (van den Maagdenberg et al., 2004). This point mutation linked to FHM-1 alters channel kinetics so that Ca^{++} influx is enhanced through single $Ca_v2.1$ channels under depolarizing conditions (Tottene et al., 2002). As a result, mutated Ca^{++} channels open at lower depolarizing voltages and neurotransmitter release is presumably increased. Because the control of transmitter release by $Ca_v2.1$ channels is much more prevalent in excitatory (e.g., glutamate) than inhibitory (e.g., GABA) synapses (Caddick et al., 1999; Ayata et al., 2000), FHM-1 gain-of-function mutations may increase neuronal excitability and by doing so lower CSD threshold. Increased cortical excitability is even more pronounced in knockin mice carrying the S218L mutation in the IS4–IS5 loop of the $Ca_v2.1$ α1-subunit. In patients expressing these mutations, typical FHM attacks can be triggered by minor head trauma and are frequently followed by deep coma or stupor, and long-lasting, severe cerebral edema (Kors et al., 2001). Interestingly, female mice expressing the R192Q mutation exhibit a significantly more pronounced head and face grooming behavior (Chanda, 2006), as

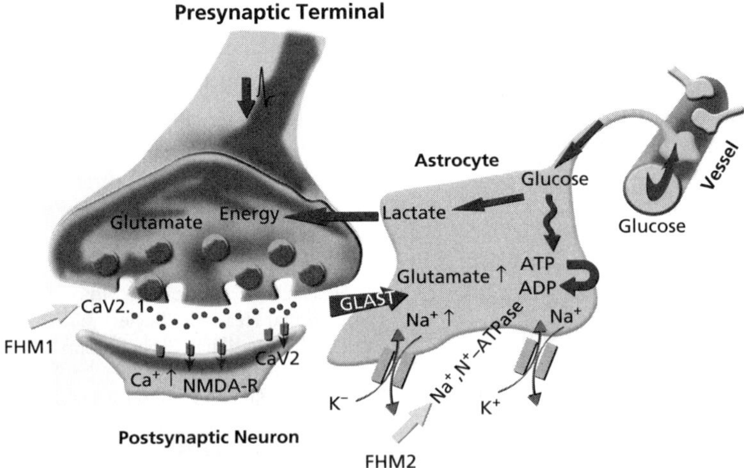

Figure 8–3 This schematic illustrates several mechanisms by which cortical excitability becomes enhanced in familial hemiplegic migraine, an autosomal dominant subtype with prolonged motor, sensory and visual auras. Families with FHM type 1 express point mutations in voltage gated Ca-channels expressed on presynaptic nerve endings. Cav2.1 channels regulate postsynaptic excitability as well as neurotransmitter release, especially of glutamate. The gain of function mutation of Cav2.1 channels in FHM-l patients is hypothesized to increase glutamate release as a consequence of increased Ca++-influx over a wide range of voltages.

FHM-2 expresses mutations in the alpha subunit of the Na+/K+-ATPase expressed on astrocytes resulting in a loss of pump function. As a consequence, Ke increases, and the Na-gradient diminishes, thereby reducing the activity of GLAST, the astrocytic glutamate uptake transporter. Decrease in transporter function leads to an increase in synaptic glutamate concentration. Changes in Ke and synaptic glutamate concentration enhance neuronal network excitability.

Taken together, FHM mutations render the brain more susceptible to electrophysiological phenomenons like cortical spreading depression.

Source: [From Moskowitz, MA, Bolay, H, and Dalkara, T (2004). Deciphering migraine mechanisms: clues from familial migraine genotypes. Ann Neurol. 55:276-280.]

well as a higher susceptibility toward CSD than male mice. The latter was completely abrogated by ovariectomy (Haerter, 2006). This observation is consistent with a higher prevalence of affected females in FHM (5:2; see Thomsen et al., 2002; Eriksen et al., 2006) and suggests that sex steroids may modulate CSD susceptibility.

Interestingly, Eriksen et al. (2006) also describe a female preponderance in nonhemiplegic migraine with aura (2.7:1), and in sporadic hemiplegic migraine, the ratio is 4.25 females:1 male. These findings suggest that genetic variations modulate both CSD as well as migraine susceptibility, and that nongenetic factors may serve as triggering or modulating events. In women, the sex steroid hormone profile may be important. Recently, Gorji's group showed in vitro that estrogen enhanced the repetition rate as well as the amplitude of spreading depression in neocortical slices (Sachs et al., 2007). Furthermore, administration of estrogen enhances glutamatergic effects on Purkinje cells (Smith et al., 1987; Smith, 1989, 1994). Estrogen and progesterone reportedly evoke changes in excitability during transcranial magnetic stimulation (Smith et al., 2002). The precise mechanism linking sex steroids to migraine remains for further study. Other factors, such as changes in physiological state (sleep, exercise, hunger, stress), or environmental factors (diet, light) have also been implicated in triggering migraine but are even less well understood as modulators of cortical excitability.

CSD UNDERLIES MIGRAINE AURA: PHARMACOLOGICAL EVIDENCE

Drugs that are effective in treating migraine *prophylactically* also decrease incidence and severity of CSD (Ayata et al., 2006). Long-term administration of valproate, topiramate, amitryptiline, propranolol, and methysergide block CSD evoked by chemical or electrical stimulation after chronic administration despite distinct chemistry and pharmacology. The effects were enantiomer-specific (i.e., DL-propranolol suppressed CSD whereas the D-isomer was ineffective in the model and clinically), as well as time- and dose-dependent.

When given *acutely*, intranasal application of the noncompetitive NMDA receptor antagonist ketamine reduces both the severity and duration of the neurological deficit in FHM (Kaube and Goadsby, 1994), and subcutaneous administration decreases pain as an acute and prophylactic treatment (Nicolodi and Sicuteri, 1995). In rats, the NMDA receptor antagonist MK-801 reduces the frequency of KCl-induced CSD (van der Hel et al., 1998) as well as capsaicin-induced c-fos expression within trigeminal nucleus caudalis due to a decrease in trigeminovascular activation from meningeal afferents (Mitsikostas and Sanchez del Rio, 2001). The nonselective AMPA/KA receptor LY293558 antagonist was superior to placebo on all efficacy measures in a multicenter randomized controlled trial (Sang et al., 2004), and also demonstrated preclinical efficacy in models of pain (Simmons et al., 1998). Furthermore, this drug was effective in the rat "plasma protein extravasation model" and in the "c-fos inhibition model" of migraine; other α-amino-3-hydroxy-5-methylisoxazole-4-propionic acid (AMPA) receptor antagonists inhibited the induction of spreading depression in the chicken retina (Kertesz et al., 2004). Moreover, Mg^{++} both blocks NMDA receptor-coupled cation channels (Mayer et al., 1984) and significantly reduces the frequency of KCl-induced CSD in rats (van der Hel et al., 1998). It may thereby lead to a rapid and sustained relief of an attack in patients (Mauskop and Altura, 1998). Thus, the effects of NMDA receptor agonists and antagonists on CSD and migraine aura/headache further suggest that NMDA receptors and glutamate play a key role in migraine pathophysiology, probably by modulating neuronal network excitability.

Bibliography

Headache Classification Subcommittee of the International Headache Society (2004).

The International Classification of Headache Disorders: 2nd edition. *Cephalalgia*, 24(Suppl. 1):9–160.

Horton, SC and Bunch, TJ (2004). Migraine Epidemiology, Clinical Presentations, and Comorbidity. *Headache*, 44:734–735.

Agostoni, E and Aliprandi, A (2006). The complications of migraine with aura. *Neurol Sci*, 27(Suppl. 2):S91–S95.

Anzola, GP, Del Sette, M, Rozzini, L, et al. (2000). The migraine-PFO connection is independent of sex. *Cerebrovasc Dis*, 10:163.

Aoki, T, Sumii, T, Mori, T, et al. (2002). Blood-brain barrier disruption and matrix metalloproteinase-9 expression during reperfusion injury: mechanical versus embolic focal ischemia in spontaneously hypertensive rats. *Stroke*, 33:2711–2717.

Aurora, SK, Barrodale, P, Chronicle, EP, et al. (2005). Cortical inhibition is reduced in chronic and episodic migraine and demonstrates a spectrum of illness. *Headache*, 45:546–552.

Avoli, M, Drapeau, C, Louvel, J, et al. (1991). Epileptiform activity induced by low extracellular magnesium in the human cortex maintained in vitro. *Ann Neurol*, 30:589–596.

Ayata, C, Jin, H, Kudo, C, et al. (2006). Suppression of cortical spreading depression in migraine prophylaxis. *Ann Neurol*, 59:652–661.

Ayata, C, Shimizu-Sasamata, M, Lo, EH, et al. (2000). Impaired neurotransmitter release and elevated threshold for cortical spreading depression in mice with mutations in the alpha1A subunit of P/Q type calcium channels. *Neuroscience*, 95:639–645.

Azarbal, B, Tobis, J, Suh, W, et al. (2005). Association of interatrial shunts and migraine headaches: impact of transcatheter closure. *J Am Coll Cardiol*, 45:489–492.

Bolay, H, Reuter, U, Dunn, AK, et al. (2002). Intrinsic brain activity triggers trigeminal meningeal afferents in a migraine model. *Nat Med*, 8:136–142.

Bousser, MG and Welch, KM (2005). Relation between migraine and stroke. *Lancet Neurol*, 4:533–542.

Bowyer, SM, Okada, YC, Papuashvili, N, et al. (1999). Analysis of MEG signals of spreading cortical depression with propagation constrained to a rectangular cortical strip. I. Lissencephalic rabbit model. *Brain Res*, 843:71–78.

Bures, J, Buresova, O, and Krivanek, J (1974). *The Mechanism and Applications of Leao's Spreading Depression of Electroencephalographic Activity*. Academic Press, New York.

Caddick, SJ, Wang, C, Fletcher, CF, et al. (1999). Excitatory but not inhibitory synaptic transmission is reduced in lethargic (Cacnb4(lh)) and tottering (Cacna1atg) mouse thalami. *J Neurophysiol*, 81:2066–2074.

Chanda, ML Baran, I, Levenstadt, JS, et al. (2006). Behavioral evidence of photophobia and light-induced head pain in familial hemiplegic migraine type 1 (FHM-1) R192Q Cacna1a knockin mice. *Soc. Neurosci. Abstr.*

Chandler, S, Miller, KM, Clements, JM, et al. (1997). Matrix metalloproteinases, tumor necrosis factor and multiple sclerosis: an overview. *J Neuroimmunol*, 72:155–161.

Dalkara, T, Zervas, NT, and Moskowitz, MA (2006). From spreading depression to the trigeminovascular system. *Neurol Sci*, 27(Suppl. 2):S86–S90.

D'Ambrosio, R, Gordon, DS, and Winn, HR (2002). Differential role of KIR channel and Na(+)/K(+)-pump in the regulation of extracellular K(+) in rat hippocampus. *J Neurophysiol*, 87:87–102.

D'Esposito, M, Deouell, LY, and Gazzaley, A (2003). Alterations in the BOLD fMRI signal with ageing and disease: a challenge for neuroimaging. *Nat Rev Neurosci*, 4:863–872.

Dichgans, M, Freilinger, T, Eckstein, G, et al. (2005). Mutation in the neuronal voltage-gated sodium channel SCN1A in familial hemiplegic migraine. *Lancet*, 366:371–377.

Doyle, J, Ren, X, Lennon, G, et al. (1997). Mutations in the Cacnl1a4 calcium channel gene are associated with seizures, cerebellar degeneration, and ataxia in tottering and leaner mutant mice. *Mamm Genome*, 8:113–120.

Dunlap, K, Luebke, JI, and Turner, TJ (1995). Exocytotic Ca2+ channels in mammalian central neurons. *Trends Neurosci*, 18:89–98.

Eriksen, MK, Thomsen, LL, and Olesen, J (2006). Implications of clinical subtypes of migraine with aura. *Headache*, 46:286–297.

Fabricius, M, Fuhr, S, Bhatia, R, et al. (2006). Cortical spreading depression and peri-infarct depolarization in acutely injured human cerebral cortex. *Brain*, 129:778–790.

Fletcher, CF, Lutz, CM, O'Sullivan, TN, et al. (1996). Absence epilepsy in tottering mutant mice is associated with calcium channel defects. *Cell*, 87:607–617.

Gorelova, NA, Koroleva, VI, Amemori, T, et al. (1987). Ketamine blockade of cortical spreading depression in rats. *Electroencephalogr Clin Neurophysiol*, 66:440–447.

Gorji, A, Scheller, D, Straub, H, et al. (2001). Spreading depression in human neocortical slices. *Brain Res*, 906:74–83.

Gursoy-Ozdemir, Y, Qiu, J, Matsuoka, N, et al. (2004). Cortical spreading depression activates and upregulates MMP-9. *J Clin Invest*, 113:1447–1455.

Hadjikhani, N, Sanchez Del Rio, M, Wu, O, et al. (2001). Mechanisms of migraine aura revealed by functional MRI in human visual cortex. *Proc Natl Acad Sci USA*, 98:4687–4692.

Haerter, K, Ayata, C, Moskowitz, MA. (2005). Cortical spreading depression: a model for understanding migraine biology and future drug targets. *Headache Curr*, 2:97–103.

Haerter, K, Kudo, C, Ferrari, MD, et al. (2006). Susceptibility to cortical spreading depression in Familial Hemiplegic Migraine-1 (R192Q) knockin mice: gene-dosage relationship and modulation by female sex. 2006 Neuroscience Meeting, Program # 502.5.

James, MF, Smith, MI, Bockhorst, KH, et al. (1999). Cortical spreading depression in the gyrencephalic feline brain studied by magnetic resonance imaging. *J Physiol*, 519(Pt 2):415–425.

Jander, S, Schroeter, M, Peters, O, et al. (2001). Cortical spreading depression induces proinflammatory cytokine gene expression in the rat brain. *J Cereb Blood Flow Metab*, 21:218–225.

Johnston, D, Magee, JC, Colbert, CM,, et al. (1996). Active properties of neuronal dendrites. *Annu Rev Neurosci*, 19:165–186.

Jorgensen, PL, Hakansson, KO, and Karlish, SJ (2003). Structure and mechanism of Na,K-ATPase: functional sites and their interactions. *Annu Rev Physiol*, 65:817–849.

Kaube, H and Goadsby, PJ (1994). Anti-migraine compounds fail to modulate the propagation of cortical spreading depression in the cat. *Eur Neurol*, 34:30–35.

Kertesz, S, Kapus, G, and Levay, G (2004). Interactions of allosteric modulators of AMPA/kainate receptors on spreading depression in the chicken retina. *Brain Res*, 1025:123–129.

Kim, YR, van Meer, MP, Mandeville, JB, et al. (2007). fMRI of delayed albumin treatment during stroke recovery in rats: implication for fast neuronal habituation in recovering brains. *J Cereb Blood Flow Metab*, 27:142–153.

Kirchmann, M (2006). Migraine with aura: new understanding from clinical epidemiologic studies. *Curr Opin Neurol*, 19:286–293.

Kors, EE, Terwindt, GM, Vermeulen, FL, et al. (2001). Delayed cerebral edema and fatal coma after minor head trauma: role of the CACNA1A calcium channel subunit gene and relationship with familial hemiplegic migraine. *Ann Neurol*, 49:753–760.

Kruger, H, Heinemann, U, and Luhmann, HJ (1999). Effects of ionotropic glutamate receptor blockade and 5-HT1A receptor activation on spreading depression in rat neocortical slices. *Neuroreport*, 10:2651–2656.

Kruit, MC, Launer, LJ, van Buchem, MA, et al. (2005). MRI findings in migraine. *Rev Neurol (Paris)*, 161:661–665.

Kruit, MC, van Buchem, MA, Hofman, PAM, et al. (2004). Migraine as a risk factor for subclinical brain lesions. *JAMA*, 291:427–434.

Kunkler, PE and Kraig, RP (1998). Calcium waves precede electrophysiological changes of spreading depression in hippocampal organ cultures. *J Neurosci*, 18:3416–3425.

Lashley, K (1941). Patterns of cerebral integration indicated by the scotomas of migraine. *Arch Neurol Psychiatr*, 46:331–339.

Lauritzen, M (1994). Pathophysiology of the migraine aura. The spreading depression theory. *Brain*, 117(Pt 1):199–210.

Lauritzen, M, Skyhoj Olsen, T, Lassen, NA, et al. (1983). Changes in regional cerebral blood flow during the course of classic migraine attacks. *Ann Neurol*, 13:633–641.

Leao, AAP (1944). Spreading depression of activity in cerebral cortex. *J Neurophysiol*, 7:359–390.

Leppert, D, Waubant, E, Galardy, R, et al. (1995). T cell gelatinases mediate basement membrane transmigration in vitro. *J Immunol*, 154:4379–4389.

Martinez, F, Castillo, J, Rodriguez, JR, et al. (1993). Neuroexcitatory amino acid levels in plasma and cerebrospinal fluid during migraine attacks. *Cephalalgia*, 13:89–93.

Mauskop, A and Altura, BM (1998). Role of magnesium in the pathogenesis and treatment of migraines. *Clin Neurosci*, 5:24–27.

Mayer, ML, Westbrook, GL, and Guthrie, PB (1984). Voltage-dependent block by Mg^{2+} of NMDA responses in spinal cord neurones. *Nature*, 309:261–263.

Mayevsky, A, Doron, A, Manor, T, et al. (1996). Cortical spreading depression recorded from the human brain using a multiparametric monitoring system. *Brain Res*, 740:268–274.

Milner, PM (1958). Note on a possible correspondence between the scotomas of migraine and spreading depression of Leao. *Electroencephalogr Clin Neurophysiol Suppl*, 10:705.

Mitsikostas, DD and Sanchez del Rio, M (2001). Receptor systems mediating c-fos expression within trigeminal nucleus caudalis in animal models of migraine. *Brain Res Brain Res Rev*, 35:20–35.

Morandi, E, Anzola, GP, Angeli, S, et al. (2003). Transcatheter closure of patent foramen ovale: a new migraine treatment? *J Interv Cardiol*, 16:39–42.

Moskowitz, MA, Bolay, H, and Dalkara, T (2004). Deciphering migraine mechanisms: clues from familial hemiplegic migraine genotypes. *Ann Neurol*, 55:276–280.

Nicolodi, M and Sicuteri, F (1995). Exploration of NMDA receptors in migraine: therapeutic and theoretic implications. *Int J Clin Pharmacol Res*, 15:181–189.

Olesen, J, Larsen, B, and Lauritzen, M (1981). Focal hyperemia followed by spreading oligemia and impaired activation of rCBF in classic migraine. *Ann Neurol*, 9:344–352.

Ophoff, RA, Terwindt, GM, Vergouwe, MN, et al. (1996). Familial hemiplegic migraine and episodic ataxia type-2 are caused by mutations in the Ca2+ channel gene CACNL1A4. *Cell*, 87:543–552.

Otori, T, Greenberg, JH, and Welsh, FA (2003). Cortical spreading depression causes a long-lasting decrease in cerebral blood flow and induces tolerance to permanent focal ischemia in rat brain. *J Cereb Blood Flow Metab*, 23:43–50.

Pietrobon, D (2005a). Function and dysfunction of synaptic calcium channels: insights from mouse models. *Curr Opin Neurobiol*, 15:257–265.

Pietrobon, D (2005b). Migraine: new molecular mechanisms. *Neuroscientist*, 11:373–386.

Pietrobon, D and Striessnig, J (2003). Neurobiology of migraine. *Nat Rev Neurosci*, 4:386–398.

Plomp, JJ, Vergouwe, MN, Van den Maagdenberg, AM, et al. (2000). Abnormal transmitter release at neuromuscular junctions of mice carrying the tottering alpha(1A) Ca(2+) channel mutation. *Brain*, 123 (Pt 3):463–471.

Qian, J and Noebels, JL (2000). Presynaptic Ca(2+) influx at a mouse central synapse with Ca(2+) channel subunit mutations. *J Neurosci*, 20:163–170.

Read, SJ, Hirst, WD, Upton, N, et al. (2001). Cortical spreading depression produces increased cGMP levels in cortex and brain stem that is inhibited by tonabersat (SB-220453) but not sumatriptan. *Brain Res*, 891:69–77.

Reisman, M, Christofferson, RD, Jesurum, J, et al. (2005). Migraine headache relief after transcatheter closure of patent foramen ovale. *J Am Coll Cardiol*, 45:493–495.

Richter, F, Ebersberger, A, and Schaible, HG (2002). Blockade of voltage-gated calcium channels in rat inhibits repetitive cortical spreading depression. *Neurosci Lett*, 334:123–126.

Rosenberg, GA, Cunningham, LA, Wallace, J, et al. (2001). Immunohistochemistry of matrix metalloproteinases in reperfusion injury to rat brain: activation of MMP-9 linked to stromelysin-1 and microglia in cell cultures. *Brain Res*, 893:104–112.

Sachs, M, Pape, HC, Speckmann, EJ, et al. (2007). The effect of estrogen and progesterone on spreading depression in rat neocortical tissues. *Neurobiol Dis*, 25:27–34.

Sang, CN, Ramadan, NM, Wallihan, RG, et al. (2004). LY293558, a novel AMPA/GluR5 antagonist, is efficacious and well-tolerated in acute migraine. *Cephalalgia*, 24:596–602.

Schwedt, TJ and Dodick, DW (2006). Patent foramen ovale and migraine—bringing closure to the subject. *Headache*, 46:663–671.

Schwerzmann, M, Wiher, S, Nedeltchev, K, et al. (2004). Percutaneous closure of patent foramen ovale reduces the frequency of migraine attacks. *Neurology*, 62:1399–1401.

Selman, WR, Lust, WD, Pundik, S, et al. (2004). Compromised metabolic recovery following spontaneous spreading depression in the penumbra. *Brain Res*, 999:167–174.

Simmons, RM, Li, DL, Hoo, KH, et al. (1998). Kainate GluR5 receptor subtype mediates the nociceptive response to formalin in the rat. *Neuropharmacology*, 37:25–36.

Smith, MJ, Adams, LF, Schmidt, PJ, et al. (2002). Effects of ovarian hormones on human cortical excitability. *Ann Neurol*, 51:599–603.

Smith, SS (1989). Estrogen administration increases neuronal responses to excitatory amino acids as a long-term effect. *Brain Res*, 503:354–357.

Smith, SS (1994). Female sex steroid hormones: from receptors to networks to performance—actions on the sensorimotor system. *Prog Neurobiol*, 44:55–86.

Smith, SS, Waterhouse, BD, and Woodward, DJ (1987). Sex steroid effects on extrahypothalamic CNS. I. Estrogen augments neuronal responsiveness to iontophoretically applied glutamate in the cerebellum. *Brain Res*, 422:40–51.

Somjen, GG (2001). Mechanisms of spreading depression and hypoxic spreading depression-like depolarization. *Physiol Rev*, 81:1065–1096.

Spies, C and Schrader, R (2006). Transcatheter closure of patent foramen ovale in patients with migraine headache. *J Interv Cardiol*, 19:552–557.

Sramka, M, Brozek, G, Bures, J, et al. (1977). Functional ablation by spreading depression: possible use in human stereotactic neurosurgery. *Appl Neurophysiol*, 40:48–61.

Strong, AJ (2003). Detecting and characterizing spreading depression in the injured human brain. *J Cereb Blood Flow Metab*, 23:748.

Strong, AJ, Fabricius, M, Boutelle, MG, et al. (2002). Spreading and synchronous depressions of cortical activity in acutely injured human brain. *Stroke*, 33:2738–2743.

Thomsen, LL, Eriksen, MK, Roemer, SF, et al. (2002). A population-based study of familial hemiplegic migraine suggests revised diagnostic criteria. *Brain*, 125:1379–1391.

Tottene, A, Fellin, T, Pagnutti, S, et al. (2002). Familial hemiplegic migraine mutations increase Ca(2+) influx through single human CaV2.1 channels and decrease maximal CaV2.1 current density in neurons. *Proc Natl Acad Sci USA*, 99:13284–13289.

van den Maagdenberg, AM, Pietrobon, D, Pizzorusso, T, et al. (2004). A Cacna1a knockin migraine mouse model with increased susceptibility to cortical spreading depression. *Neuron*, 41:701–710.

van der Hel, WS, van den Bergh, WM, Nicolay, K, et al. (1998). Suppression of cortical spreading depressions after magnesium treatment in the rat. *Neuroreport*, 9:2179–2182.

Van Harreveld, A (1959). Compounds in brain extracts causing spreading depression of cerebral cortical activity and contraction of crustacean muscle. *J Neurochem*, 3:300–315.

Vanmolkot, KR, Kors, EE, Turk, U, et al. (2006). Two de novo mutations in the Na,K-ATPase gene ATP1A2 associated with pure familial hemiplegic migraine. *Eur J Hum Genet*, 14:555–560.

Westenbroek, RE, Sakurai, T, Elliott, EM, et al. (1995). Immunochemical identification and subcellular distribution of the alpha 1A subunits of brain calcium channels. *J Neurosci*, 15:6403–6418.

Wilmshurst, P and Nightingale, S (2001). Relationship between migraine and cardiac and pulmonary right-to-left shunts. *Clin Sci (Lond)*, 100:215–220.

Wilmshurst, PT, Pearson, MJ, Nightingale, S, et al. (2004). Inheritance of persistent foramen ovale and atrial septal defects and the relation to familial migraine with aura. *Heart*, 90:1315–1320.

Yong, VW, Power, C, Forsyth, P, et al. (2001). Metalloproteinases in biology and pathology of the nervous system. *Nat Rev Neurosci*, 2:502–511.

Yu, FH, Mantegazza, M, Westenbroek, RE, et al. (2006). Reduced sodium current in GABAergic interneurons in a mouse model of severe myoclonic epilepsy in infancy. *Nat Neurosci*, 9:1142–1149.

9 Genetics of Primary Headache

Michel D Ferrari and Martin Dichgans

INTRODUCTION

Recent advances in genetics have started to transform our understanding of primary headaches. There is increasing evidence for a genetic component to cluster headache (CH) and tension-type headache (TTH). However, the greatest breakthroughs have occurred in the area of migraine, a dynamic field in which data are rapidly accumulating. In this chapter, we discuss key findings and recent developments in genetic epidemiology, monogenic disorders, knock-in mouse models, and complex multifactorial genetics.

MIGRAINE

Genetic Epidemiology

Migraine often runs in families (Kors et al., 2004). Population-based studies have confirmed that the risk of migraine in first-degree relatives is increased 1.5–4-fold. The familial risk appeared greatest for patients with migraine with aura, with a young age at onset, and a high attack severity and disease disability (Russell and Olesen, 1995; Stewart et al., 1997; Stewart et al., 2006).

Some authors concluded, on the basis of different heritability estimates, that migraine with and without aura are different entities (Russell and Olesen, 1995; Russell et al., 2002; Ludvigsson et al., 2006). In view of various clinical and genetic arguments, it seems very unlikely that migraine itself differs; rather the aura component may have some heritable biological distinction. Main arguments include the high comorbidity of attacks with and without aura within migraineurs and the remarkable intrapersonal variability of the disease presentation in the various stages of life, for example, with aura as a child, without aura as a young adult, and aura without headache after age 50. Furthermore, *latent class analysis* on International Headache Society (IHS) migraine characteristics (unilateral location, pulsating quality, nausea/vomiting etc.), in two large populations from Australia and the Netherlands, did not support the hypothesis that migraine with and without aura are distinct disorders (Nyholt et al., 2004; Ligthart et al., 2006). A Finnish study of more than 200 migraine families suggested that there is a continuum from pure migraine with aura at the neural end of the spectrum to pure migraine without aura at the headache end of the spectrum, and migraine both with and without aura in between (Kallela et al., 2001). In conclusion, the different migraine subtypes appear to be different clinical expressions of the same disorder.

Twin studies are the classical method used to investigate the relative importance of genetic and environmental factors. In twin pairs drawn from the general population, the pair-wise concordance rates for migraine were significantly higher among monozygotic than among dizygotic twin pairs, indicating that genetic factors are important in the susceptibility to migraine. However, as concordance rates never reached 100%, environmental factors must be involved as well, making migraine a true multifactorial disorder (Honkasalo et al., 1995; Gervil et al., 1999; Ulrich et al., 1999; Mulder et al., 2003). The relative importance of genetic factors can be estimated from a large population-based twin study investigating 30,000 twin pairs from six countries (Mulder et al., 2003). The heritability was 40%–50%, and shared environmental factors were considered to have a minor effect on the susceptibility to migraine.

This finding is in accord with that of a comparison between twins raised together and raised apart (Ziegler et al., 1998; Svensson et al., 2003).

Strategies to Identify Genes for Migraine

The identification of genes for multifactorial disorders like migraine is hampered by a number of complicating factors. Multiple genes contribute to the susceptibility; most contributing genes display low penetrance; and the phenotypic expression is modulated by endogenous and exogenous nongenetic factors. Furthermore, complex disorders are usually very prevalent and may start at a high age, complicating a reliable distinction between affected and nonaffected populations. A problem in migraine is the paucity of clinically useful biomarkers and the difficulty in some cases to reliably distinguish between migraine with aura and migraine without aura.

Several genetic approaches have been used to identify genes for migraine. The first, and thus far most successful approach, has been the identification of genes in families with rare monogenic subtypes of migraine. This has been done by using traditional linkage analysis (testing several hundreds to thousands of genetic markers spread over all chromosomes and selecting those markers, i.e., the chromosomal region best segregated with the disease), positional cloning techniques, and mutation analysis. This approach is based on the hypothesis that rare monogenic subtypes and common multifactorial types of migraine share common genes and related biochemical pathways for the trigger threshold and initiation mechanisms of attacks. Thus, the rare monogenic variant may serve as a genetic and/or functional model for the common complex forms. In the latter case, the *functional* changes caused by the causative gene mutations are more relevant than the genes themselves, as they might hint at shared pathogenic pathways. So far, genes have been identified for the following monogenic conditions: familial hemiplegic migraine (FHM) and its sporadic variant, sporadic hemiplegic migraine (SHM); cerebral autosomal dominant arteriopathy with subcortical infarcts and leukoencephalopathy (CADASIL), a complex syndrome with migraine as part of the phenotypic spectrum; and other hereditary angiopathies. The details of these findings, and the implications for the common forms of migraine, will be discussed shortly.

A second linkage analysis approach that is often used in complex traits is affected sib-pair analysis. With this approach, chromosomal areas that are shared by affected siblings with a probability higher than by chance alone are identified. This is then followed by case-control association studies testing single nucleotide polymorphisms (SNPs) in candidate genes in the shared regions. The goal is to identify SNPs, and thus gene alleles, that statistically differ in frequency between cases and controls and cause increased susceptibility to the disease. A third, hypothesis-driven, approach is direct testing of candidate genes in case-control association studies. A promising extension of this approach is the possibility of nonhypothesis-driven testing for genome-wide association by scanning hundreds of thousands of SNPs in extended and clinically homogenous populations (Hirschhorn and Daly, 2005; Duerr et al., 2006).

Familial Hemiplegic Migraine

FHM is a rare, severe, monogenic subtype of migraine with aura, characterized by at least some degree of hemiparesis during the aura (Ferrari, 1998). The hemiparesis may last from minutes to several hours or even days. Patients are frequently initially misdiagnosed with epilepsy. Apart from the hemiparesis, the other headache and aura features of the FHM attack are identical to those of attacks of the common types of migraine. In addition to attacks with hemiparesis, the majority of FHM patients also experience attacks of "normal" migraine with or without aura (Terwindt et al., 1998b; Ducros et al., 2001; Thomsen et al., 2003).

As in the common forms of migraine, attacks of FHM may be triggered by mild head trauma. Thus, from a clinical point of view, FHM seems a valid model for the common forms of migraine (Ferrari, 1998). Major clinical differences, apart from the hemiparesis, include that 20% of FHM cases may also be associated with cerebellar ataxia and other neurologic symptoms such as epilepsy, mental retardation, brain edema, and (fatal) coma. Thus far, three genes for FHM have been published, but based on unpublished linkage results in several families, there are more to come.

CACNA1A (FHM1)

The first gene identified for FHM is the *CACNA1A* gene on chromosome 19p13. It is responsible for approximately 50% of all FHM families and encodes the ion-conducting, pore-forming α_{1A} subunit of $Ca_v2.1$ (P/Q-type) voltage-gated neuronal calcium channels (Ophoff et al., 1996) (Fig. 9–1). The main function of neuronal P/Q-type calcium channels is to modulate release of neurotransmitters, both at peripheral neuromuscular junctions and central synapses, mainly within the cerebellum, brainstem, and cerebral cortex (Catterall, 1998). More than 50 *CACNA1A* mutations have been associated with a wide range of clinical phenotypes (Fig. 9–1 and (Haan et al., 2005)). These include pure forms of FHM (Ophoff et al., 1996), combinations of FHM with various degrees of cerebellar ataxia (Ophoff et al., 1996; Ducros et al., 2001), or fatal coma due to excessive cerebral edema (Kors et al., 2001), and disorders not associated with FHM such as episodic ataxia type 2 (Ophoff et al., 1996; Jen et al., 2004), progressive ataxia (Yue et al., 1997), spinocerebellar ataxia type 6 (Zhuchenko et al., 1997), and absence (Imbrici et al., 2004) and generalized epilepsy (Jouvenceau et al., 2001; Haan et al., 2005). All FHM1 mutations identified thus far are missense mutations. The T666M and R583Q mutation are particularly frequent, and some mutations, including T666M, are associated with permanent cerebellar signs (Ducros et al., 2001). Interestingly, in several FHM families, *CACNA1A* mutations were also found in individuals who only had "normal" nonparetic migraine but no FHM. This suggests that FHM1 mutations may also be implicated in the common forms of migraine, probably due to genetic and nongenetic modulating factors.

ATP1A2 (FHM2)

The *ATP1A2* FHM2 gene on chromosome 1q23 encodes the α_2 subunit of a Na^+/K^+ ATPase

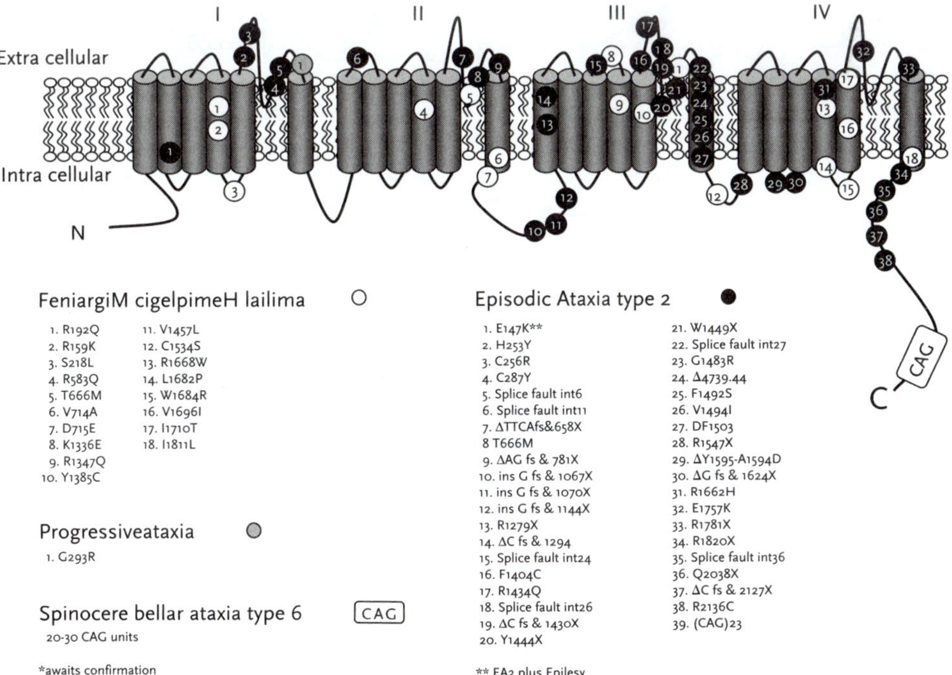

Figure 9–1 Distribution of familial hemiplegic migraine 1(FHM1) mutations in $Ca_v2.1$: The pore-forming subunit of the P/Q-type voltage-gated neuronal calcium channel contains four repeated domains each encompassing six transmembrane segments. Positions of mutations and associated clinical phenotypes are illustrated by different symbols (*CACNA1A* ref. seq.: GenBank accession number X99897).

(De Fusco et al., 2003; Marconi et al., 2003). The Na^+/K^+-ATPase utilizes the free energy of adenosine triphosphate (ATP) hydrolysis to export 3 Na^+ ions and import 2 K^+ ions per ATP molecule, thereby generating net current and maintaining the electrochemical gradients of Na^+ and K^+ across the plasma membrane (Kaplan, 2002; Jørgensen et al., 2003). A whole series of transport processes mediated by secondary active cotransporters or ion channels is coupled to these gradients. The steep Na^+ gradient is essential for the transport of glutamate and Ca^{2+}. *ATP1A2* is predominantly expressed in neurons at neonatal age and in glial cells at adult age (De Fusco et al., 2003; Moseley et al., 2003; Vanmolkot et al., 2003). In adults, an important function of this specific ATPase is to modulate the re-uptake of potassium and glutamate from the synaptic cleft into the glial cell. Mutations in the *ATP1A2* gene are responsible for at least 20% of FHM cases (Fig. 9–2) and have been associated with pure FHM (De Fusco et al., 2003; Riant et al., 2005; Vanmolkot et al., 2006) and FHM in combinations with cerebellar ataxia (Spadaro et al., 2004), mental retardation (Jurkat-Rott et al., 2004; Vanmolkot, Stroink, et al., 2006), alternating hemiplegia of childhood (Bassi et al., 2004; Swoboda et al., 2004), benign focal infantile convulsions (Vanmolkot et al., 2003), and other forms of epilepsy (Haan et al., 2005). In an Italian family, a variant in the *ATP1A2* gene segregated with basilar migraine, a subtype of migraine with aura characterized by aura symptoms attributable to the brainstem and both occipital lobes (Ambrosini et al., 2005). Unfortunately, no functional studies were reported, precluding a definite conclusion as to whether this gene variation is also *causally* linked to basilar migraine. Of note, *ATP1A2* variants were identified in two non-FHM

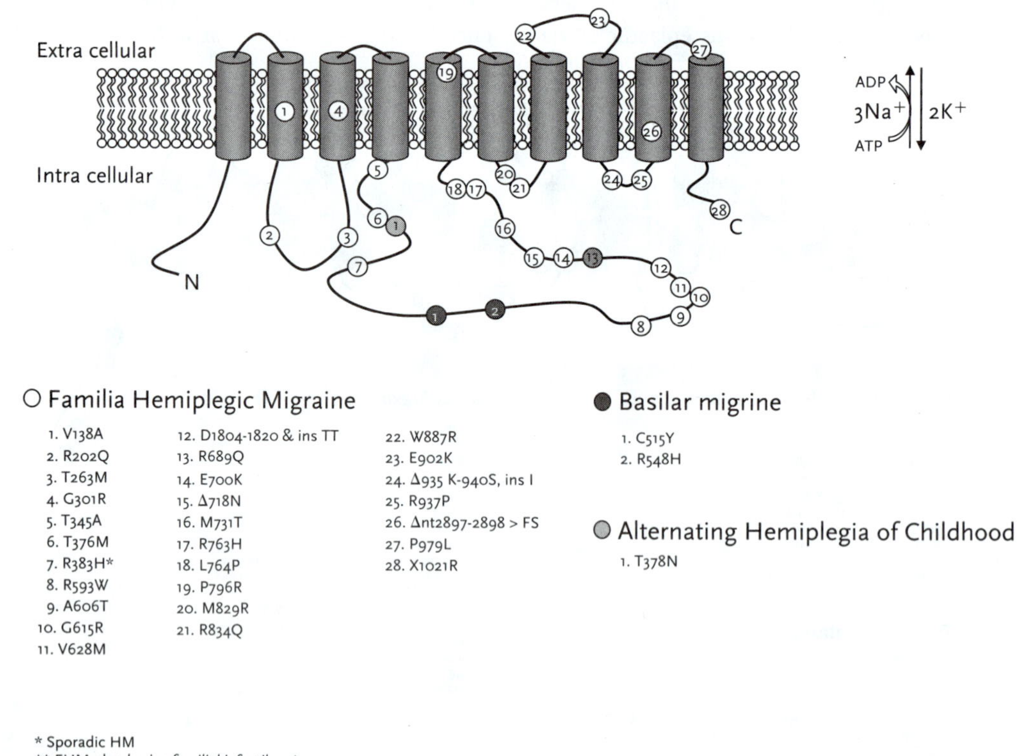

Figure 9–2 Distribution of familial hemiplegic migraine 2 (FHM2) mutations in the sodium-potassium ATPase: The α_2 subunit of sodium potassium pumps is located in the plasma membrane and contains ten transmembrane segments. Positions of mutations and associated clinical phenotypes are indicated in the schematic drawing of the protein (*ATP1A2* ref. seq.: GenBank accession number NM_000702).

migraine families, suggesting that this gene may be involved in the susceptibility to common forms of migraine (Todt et al., 2005).

SCN1A (FHM3)

The *SCN1A* gene on chromosome 2q24 encodes the α_1 subunit of a neuronal voltage-gated sodium ($Na_v1.1$) channel. The $Na_v1.1$ channel is critical for the generation and propagation of action potentials in the brain. A wide range of mutations in this gene is known to be associated with childhood epilepsy and febrile seizures (for review, Meisler and Kearney, 2005), and migraine has not been reported as part of the spectrum of these disorders. Thus, the identification of a novel Q1489K mutation in three German FHM families came to some surprise (2005) (Fig. 9–3). The three families share a common haplotype suggesting a common ancestry. Recently, the same authors identified another mutation (L1649Q) in a North-American family confirming the relationship between *SCNA1* and FHM (Vanmolkot et al., 2007). However, screening of a large number of FHM families suggests that the *SCN1A* gene is a rare cause of FHM (unpublished observations).

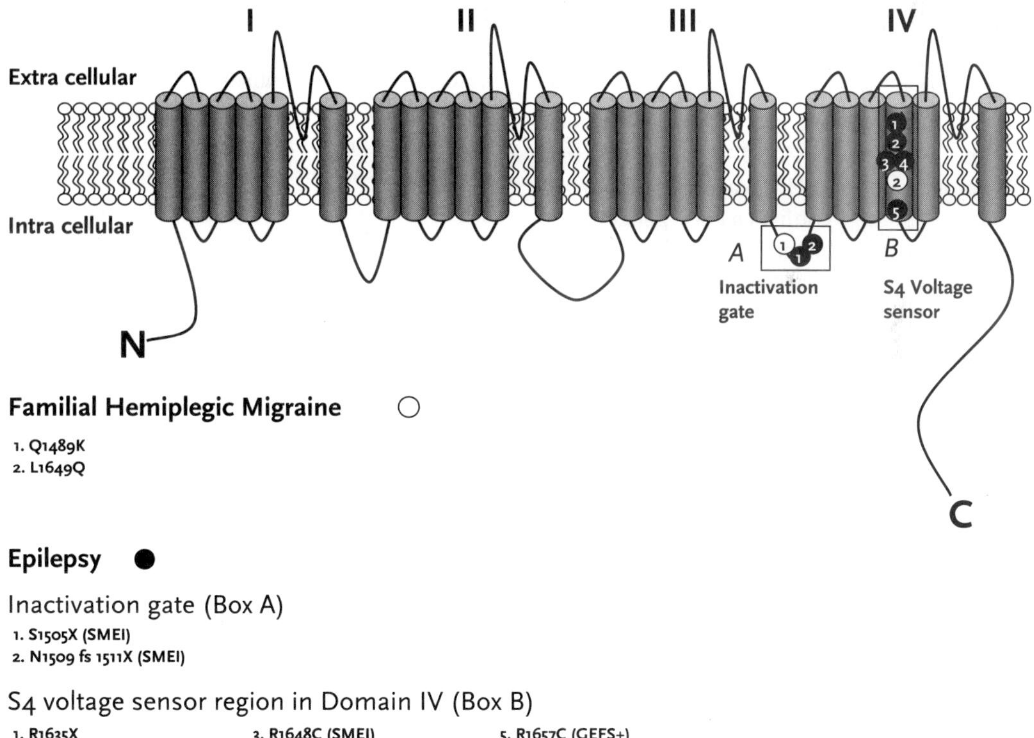

Figure 9–3 Distribution of familial hemiplegic migraine 3 (FHM3) mutations in neuronal voltage-gated sodium ($Na_v1.1$): The pore-forming α_1 subunit of the neuronal voltage-gated sodium channel is located in the plasma membrane and contains four repetitive domains, each encompassing six transmembrane segments. The two FHM3 mutations identified thus far are located in the inactivation gate (Q1489K) and D4/S4 voltage sensor (L1649Q). A variety of $Na_v1.1$ mutations has previously been described in patients with childhood epilepsy (severe myoclonic epilepsy in infancy and generalized epilepsy with febrile seizures plus reviewed in Kanai et al., 2004; Meisler and Kearney, 2005). For illustrative reasons severe myoclonic epilepsy in infancy and generalized epilepsy with febrile seizures plus mutations located next to the FHM3 mutations are displayed (*SCN1A* ref. seq.: GenBank accession number NM_006920).

Sporadic Hemiplegic Migraine

Patients with hemiplegic migraine are not always clustered in families. Singleton cases, without affected family members, are quite frequent and may sometimes represent the first "FHM patient" (de novo mutation) in a family (Thomsen et al., 2003a; Vanmolkot et al., 2006). Apart from sharing the clinical phenotype with the common forms of migraine, SHM and common migraine also show a remarkable genetic epidemiological relationship. SHM patients have a highly increased risk of suffering from typical migraine with aura, and their first-degree relatives have a highly increased risk of migraine both with and without aura (Thomsen et al., 2003b). In an initial study, only 2 of 27 SHM patients were found to carry *CACNA1A* mutations (Terwindt et al., 2002). However, a more recent study found FHM gene mutations, in particular ATP1A2 mutations, in a larger proportion of SHM cases (unpublished data). These findings confirm a close genetic relationship between FHM and SHM and have implications for genetic testing and counseling.

Functional Consequences of FHM Gene Mutations

Understanding the functional consequences of gene mutations is crucial to understanding the disease pathways. For the FHM genes, this has been studied in cellular models, in transgenic knock-in mouse models carrying a human pathogenic mutation (FHM1), and in knock-out mouse models (FHM2).

Cellular Models for FHM1 CACNA1A Mutations

Several FHM1 and episodic ataxia type 2 mutations have been analyzed with electrophysiological techniques in neuronal and nonneuronal cell models (Kraus et al., 1998; Hans et al., 1999; Kraus et al., 2000; Jouvenceau et al., 2001; Tottene et al., 2002; Cao et al., 2004; Imbrici et al., 2004;). While episodic ataxia type 2 *CACNA1A* mutations all show a dramatic decrease or even complete loss of current density (Guida et al., 2001; Jen et al., 2001; Jouvenceau et al., 2001; Wappl et al., 2002; Imbrici et al., 2004; Spacey et al., 2004; Wan et al., 2005; Jeng et al., 2006), FHM1 mutations cause different effects on channel conductance, kinetics, and/or expression in transfected cells (Kraus et al., 1998; Hans et al., 1999; Kraus et al., 2000; Tottene et al., 2002; Cao et al., 2004; Tottene et al., 2005). The most consistent change found with FHM1 mutations, when tested in a *single channel configuration*, was a hyperpolarizing shift of about 10 mV of the activation voltage (Kraus et al., 1998; Hans et al., 1999; Tottene et al., 2005). The change in calcium influx could, however, alter during high neuronal activity. Mutant T666M and V714A channels have a low conductance mode that may sometimes switch to the wild type state (Hans et al., 1999). For other FHM mutations, like R583Q and D715E, accumulation of inactivated channels was observed during repetitive stimulation (Kraus et al., 2000). Such phenomena could contribute to the paroxysmal presentation of symptoms.

The gain-of-function effects found in *single channel* test models, *in theory*, will lead to an easier opening of channels in neurons. The overall change in calcium influx is, however, difficult to predict and seem to depend, at least partly, on the model that is being used. For instance, Cao et al. (2004) found evidence for *reduced* calcium influx at the *whole cell* level in transfections of *cultured* mouse hippocampal neurons. The in vivo consequences are determined by the delicate interplay between the functional effects of a particular mutation, the channel properties and density, the different channel subunits, and the cellular environment. The observation that different auxiliary beta-subunits of calcium channels can modulate the consequence of FHM mutations certainly adds to the complexity of predicting calcium channel functioning (Mullner et al., 2004). Therefore, in vivo data from animal models remain essential in understanding the consequences of disease-causing mutations (see below).

Naturally Occurring Cacna1a Mouse Mutants

Naturally occurring mouse mutants with *Cacna1a* missense mutations (Tottering, Rocker, Rolling Nagoya) or *Cacna1a* truncation mutations (Leaner) display different combinations and severities of various types of epilepsy and ataxia (Pietrobon, 2005). A reduction in calcium's current density appears to be the main effect of these mutated

P/Q-type channels (Dove et al., 1998; Lorenzon et al., 1998; Wakamori et al., 1998; Mori et al., 2000), with a change in channel kinetics for the Leaner and Rolling Nagoya mutants (Dove et al., 1998; Lorenzon et al., 1998; Mori et al., 2000). Two *Cacna1a*-null (knock-out) mouse models were generated showing ataxia, dystonia, and lethality at a young age (Jun et al., 1999; Fletcher et al., 2001). The total Ca^{2+} influx in cerebellar cells and neurotransmission at the neuromuscular junction was reduced in these mice. Loss of P/Q-type channels could be partly compensated for by N-, R-, and L-type channels. Moreover, Leaner mice showed an increased threshold for cortical spreading depression (CSD), a reduced release of cortical glutamate (Ayata et al., 2000), and reduced transmitter release at the neuromuscular junction (Kaja et al., 2007).

FHM1 Cacna1a Knock-in Mouse Mutants

Unlike the naturally occurring *Cacna1a* mouse mutants, transgenic knock-in mice carrying the human FHM1 R192Q mutation exhibit no overt clinical phenotype or structural abnormalities (van den Maagdenberg et al., 2004). This is very similar to the human situation: the R192Q mutation causes mild FHM attacks, very similar to the common forms of migraine, albeit with hemiparesis, without permanent (interictal) neurologic signs. Extensive functional analysis revealed multiple gain-of-function effects. These include increased Ca^{2+} influx in cerebellar neurons, increased release of neurotransmitters at the neuromuscular junction, both spontaneously and, upon stimulation, at low Ca^{2+}, and, in in vivo experiments, a reduced trigger-threshold for CSD that propagates with increased velocity. It seems that whole-animal studies may be better suited to dissect the effects of mutations and to understand the integrated physiology of the disease. Other studies aiming at functional changes within the brain stem are underway and will shed more light on the important question of whether migraine-related mechanisms within the trigeminocervical complex are also affected.

Cellular Models for FHM2 ATP1A2 Mutations

To date, more than 20 mutations in the *ATP1A2* gene have been associated with FHM. Yet, few of them have been studied for their functional consequences on the molecular level. Mutations L764P and W887R resulted in nonfunctional proteins (Capendeguy and Horisberger, 2004; Koenderink et al., 2005) whereas others showed partially active enzymes with decreased (T345M) or increased (R689Q, M731T) K^+ affinities or reduced turnover rates (R689Q,M731T) (Segall et al., 2004; Segall et al., 2005). These initial findings suggest that FHM2 associated mutations of *ATP1A2* may have diverse functional consequences. Overall, however, FHM2 mutations seem to result in a loss of function of the enzyme and thus reduce uptake of K^+ and glutamate into glial cells.

Atp1a2 Knock-out Mouse Models

α_2-Subunit deficient (*Atp1a2*-null) mice, which had been generated prior to the identification of ATP1A2 mutations in FHM2 (James et al., 1999; Ikeda et al., 2004), died immediately after birth because of severe motor deficits and absent respiration (James et al., 1999; Ikeda et al., 2003). *Atp1a2*-null fetuses of 18.5 days exhibited selective neuronal apoptosis in the amygdala and piriform cortex in response to neural hyperactivity (Ikeda et al., 2003). When kept on a 129sv genetic background *Atp1a2*-null mice displayed frequent generalized seizures and died within 24 hours after birth (Ikeda et al., 2004). The occurrence of seizures is remarkable since epilepsy is also part of the clinical phenotype in FHM2 ATP1A2 mutation carriers. Heterozygous *Atp1a2*$^{+/-}$ mice are viable and show a cardiac phenotype. Their heart shows a hypercontractile state with positive inotropic response and resembles what is typically seen after the administration of cardiac glycosides (James et al., 1999). In addition, these animals reveal enhanced fear and anxiety following conditioned fear stimuli probably because of neuronal hyperactivity in the amygdala and piriform cortex (Ikeda et al., 2003). However, it is currently unknown, whether heterozygous *Atp1a2*$^{+/-}$ mice represent a valid model for FHM2. Until now, there are no *Atp1a2* knock-in models available.

Cellular Models for FHM3 SCN1A Mutations

Both the Q1489K and L1649Q SCN1A mutation have been studied for their functional effects in tsA201 cells using the highly homologous SCN5A channel. Both mutations were found to interfere with fast inactivation of the channel, which is remarkable since the two mutations are located in very different domains of the protein. Q1489K is located in the cytoplasmic linker between domains III and IV, which is critical for fast inactivation (Fig. 9–3) (Dichgans et al., 2005; Vanmolkot et al. 2007). In contrast, L1649Q localizes to the S4 segment of domain 4. This domain acts as a voltage sensor and is implicated in channel gating. Q1489K causes a two- to four-fold faster recovery from fast inactivation (Dichgans et al., 2005), whereas L1636Q results in an overall slower inactivation of the channel; a depolarizing shift by approximately 10 mV in the voltage dependence of steady state inactivation; and an accelerated recovery from fast inactivation. These findings still await confirmation using the original SCN1A channel but suggest a "gain-of-function" mechanism in FHM3, with enhanced neuronal excitability and release of neurotransmitters. A SCN1A knock-out mouse model for epilepsy has recently been published (Yu et al., 2006), whereas there is no knock-in mouse model for FHM3.

A Common Mechanism for FHM Attacks

How can the findings on CACNA1A, ATP1A2, and SCN1A be integrated into one common pathway? CSD is an obvious candidate (Moskowitz et al., 2004). FHM1 mutations in the $Ca_v2.1$ calcium channel cause increased neurotransmitter release, including glutamate (Pietrobon, D et al., unpublished data), which can induce, maintain, and propagate CSD. FHM2 mutations in the sodium-potassium pump cause reduced glial uptake of K^+ and glutamate from the synaptic cleft. FHM3 mutations in the $Na_v1.1$ sodium channel result in hyperexcitability and most likely enhanced neurotransmitter release. The consequence is increased levels of glutamate and K^+ in the synaptic cleft, causing an increased propensity for CSD in FHM1, FHM2, and FHM3. The propensity for CSD could well explain the aura phase of migraine attacks. However, whether the enhanced tendency for CSD might also be responsible for triggering the headache phase is controversial. Also, the mechanisms triggering FHM attacks are still poorly understood. This is one of the areas where transgenic mouse models might be exceptionally valuable. The identification of additional FHM genes will likely provide further insights.

The Glutamate Transporter Gene *SLC1A3* and Hemiplegic Migraine

Recently, Jen et al. (2005) reported on a heterozygous mutation in the *SLC1A3* gene in a 10-year-old boy with a complex phenotype of episodic ataxia, hemiplegic migraine, and seizures. *SLC1A3* encodes the excitatory amino acid transporter 1 (EAAT1), which removes glutamate from the synaptic cleft. The mutation was not present in his asymptomatic parents and controls and was shown to cause a markedly reduced uptake of glutamate in cell culture experiments. The glutamate transporter genes are definitely good candidates for migraine. However, because of the occurrence in a singleton case, the obervations on EAAT1 require confirmation in other patients.

Migraine: An Ion Translocation Disorder?

Growing evidence exists that a dysfunction of ion flux or transportation is involved in the pathogenesis of the common forms of migraine. Converging arguments for a disturbance in ion translocation come from genetic, clinical neurophysiological, and neuropharmacological studies.

First, migraine, in particular migraine with aura, shares strikingly similar clinical characteristics not only with established channelopathies, such as FHM and SHM (see above), but also with episodic neuromuscular disorders, such as myotonia and periodic paralysis (Ferrari and Goadsby, 2006). These include the episodic presentation of the symptoms, a similar distribution in terms of duration and frequency of the attacks, similar trigger factors for attacks such as emotion, stress, food, alcohol and weather changes, and a similar gender-related expression, with an onset of attacks mostly around puberty and amelioration after age 40.

Second, *CACNA1A* and *ATP1A2* gene mutations have been found in patients with only the common forms of migraine, without the FHM phenotype. Furthermore, some (but not all) linkage and association studies suggest a role of FHM genes in common migraine (Terwindt et al., 2001; Haan et al., 2005). Size and homogeneity of the study populations in such studies are clearly important complicating factors.

A third line of evidence comes from clinical neurophysiologal studies in migraineurs. Ambrosini et al. (2005) found single fibre abnormalities, suggesting an altered release of acetylcholine at the neuromuscular junction, which is mainly controlled by P/Q-type $Ca_V2.1$ channels. However, these findings were not replicated in FHM1 patients with documented mutations (Terwind et al. 2004). Sandor et al. (2001) found evidence of subclinical cerebellar dysfunction. A higher proportion of migraine patients than healthy controls showed hypermetria and other subtle cerebellar signs when subjected to an automated sensitive test for cerebellar arm coordination. As P/Q-type $Ca_V2.1$ channels are highly expressed in cerebellar Purkinje cells, this finding might indicate a dysfunction of $Ca_V2.1$ channels in Purkinje cells of migraineurs, although studies on oculomotor function have produced inconsistent results (Harno et al., 2003; Wieser et al., 2004; Wilkinson et al., 2006).

Finally, neuropharmacologic animal experiments suggest that applying selective blockers of P/Q-type $Ca_V2.1$ channels within areas of the brainstem that have been associated with important migraine mechanisms can modulate these mechanisms. These include inhibition of the release of calcitonin gene-related peptide and neurogenic inflammation (Asakura et al., 2000), facilitation of trigeminal firing (Knight et al., 2002), and modulation of nociceptive transmission in the trigeminocervical complex (Shields et al., 2005).

Migraine and Hereditary Angiopathies

CADASIL

CADASIL is a nonamyloid arteriopathy caused by mutations in the *NOTCH3* gene (Joutel et al., 1996). The syndrome is characterized by recurrent subcortical infarcts, progressive white matter lesions, accumulating cognitive deficits, and stroke-related disability. Most relevant here, up to 40% of mutation carriers have migraine with aura (Chabriat et al., 1995; Dichgans et al., 1998). Migraine is among the main presenting symptoms. The *NOTCH3* gene is primarily expressed in vascular smooth muscle cells and regulates arterial differentiation during embryonic development (Domenga et al., 2004). Why mutations in this gene would cause migraine is unclear. There is no evidence for a primary neuronal effect. However, it might be that secondary neurononal damage and ischemia facilitate the occurrence of CSD and migraine attacks. The high prevalence of aura symptoms would aggre with this concept. Alternatively, there might be a primary vascular mechanism. Hemodynamic studies in transgenic mice have demonstrated an abnormal vasomotor response and disturbed autoregulation, and similar findings have been obtained in humans (Pfefferkorn et al., 2001; Lacombe et al., 2005). Studying neuronal and vascular changes in parallel in CADASIL transgenic animals may prove invaluable in dissecting the triggering mechanisms for migraine attacks.

Other Angiopathies

A rare syndrome, clinically characterized by a combination of cerebroretinal vasculopathy, Raynaud phenomenon, migraine, pseudotumor cerebri, and variable other forms of vascular dysfunction, has been linked to chromosome 3p21 in three families (Terwindt et al., 1998a; Ophoff et al., 2001). Migraine is clearly part of the syndrome (Hottenga et al., 2005). Identification of the responsible gene for this neurovascular syndrome will be important for a wide range of vascular disorders, including the pathogenesis of migraine.

An increased prevalence of migraine, in particular migraine with aura, has further been reported in another rare angiopathy (Vahedi et al., 2003). The gene for this syndrome, which is associated with porencephaly, infantile hemiparesis, and stroke has recently been identified: *COL4A1* encodes type IV collagen, an integral component of the vascular basement membrane (Gould et al., 2006). The association between migraine and several early-onset angiopathies is remarkable, but the mechanisms underlying this association are still poorly understood (Dichgans, 2003).

Mitochondrial DNA-polymerase-γ and Migraine

Evidence from various sources suggests that mitochondrial dysfunction might contribute to the occurrence of migraine (Sparaco et al., 2006). Against this background the occurrence of migraine in *POLG* mutation carriers is of interest (Winterthun et al., 2005; Hudson and Chinnery, 2006; Tzoulis et al., 2006). The nuclear *POLG* gene encodes polymerase-γ, which is essential for maintenance of mitochondrial DNA. *POLG* mutations have been associated with a variety of other phenotypes, including epilepsy (Hudson and Chinnery, 2006).

Gene Loci and Genes Implicated in Common Forms for Migraine

Linkage Studies

Genome-wide linkage studies have identified several gene regions with significant or suggestive linkage for nonhemiplegic migraine, two of which have been replicated in independent samples (Table 9–1). Linkage to chromosome 6p12.2-p21.1 in a large family with migraine with and without aura from northern Sweden (Carlsson et al., 2002) was confirmed in Australian patients (Nyholt et al., 2005), albeit with low statistic evidence for linkage (see below). Linkage to 4q24 in 50 Finnish families with migraine with aura (Wessman et al., 2002) was confirmed in a study in 289 Icelandic patients with migraine without aura (Bjornsson et al., 2003). However, both the Finnish and Icelandic populations are considered genetic isolates. Additional loci that have been mapped but not yet replicated are listed in the table. The variety reported is probably a reflection of the genetic heterogeneity of migraine.

Linkage Studies Using Quantitative Trait and Trait Component Analyses

Nyholt et al. (Lea et al., 2005a; Nyholt et al., 2005) performed a quantitative trait linkage analysis in 790 independent sib-pairs, selected from a large Australian sample of 12,245 twins. By applying latent-class analysis—a categorical analog of factor analysis for finding subtypes of related cases—they found significant linkage on chromosome 5q21 for a severe migraine phenotype with pulsating headache. They further identified potential gene loci for phonophobia (Chrs.1q21-q23 and 10), activity-prohibiting headache, and photophobia (Chrs. 6p12.2.-p21.1., 10, and 13), and nausea/vomiting (Chr 8), but with low evidence for linkage.

A Finnish study used the individual clinical symptoms of migraine (trait component analysis) to determine affection status in genome-wide linkage analysis of 50 migraine families (Anttila et al., 2006). The previously identified chromosome 4q24 locus (Wessman et al., 2002) was now found to link to several traits. Novel loci were identified for pulsation trait on 17p13, an age-at-onset trait on 4q28, and a trait combination phenotype (full IHS criteria) on 18q12. Furthermore, suggestive or nearly suggestive evidence of linkage was observed for phonophobia and aggravation by physical exercise. The use of symptoms of migraine rather than the full end diagnosis is a promising novel approach to stratify samples for genetic studies.

How relevant linkage findings for individual symptoms are, however, remains to be proven. It is reasonable to suggest that such findings might only reflect general sensitivities rather than migraine-specific relationships. That is, patients showing linkage, for example, to the photophobia gene locus might develop photophobia under a variety of conditions, such as influenza or stomach pain. A critical point is that migraine patients usually show a variable and changing pattern of symptoms over time. For instance, they may have severe nausea and vomiting together with aura as part of their migraine attacks at young age, may "lose" the aura and vomiting in their twenties to have attacks of migraine without aura, and may end up with attacks of isolated auras without headache or other associated symptoms. It seems that the presence of individual clinical characteristics are "time-locked" rather than "gene-locked," and that asking the patient for their symptoms may give different answers when asked at different stages in life.

Association Studies

In complex multifactorial disease, multiple genes likely interact with environmental factors, while

TABLE 9–1 Gene Loci for Common Forms of Migraine.

Phenotype	*Sample*	*Method*	*Chromosomal region*	*Reference*
Migraine with aura	50 families	Linkage (genome-wide)	4q24	Wessman, 2002
	43 families	Linkage (genome-wide)	11q24	Cader, 2003
	10 families	Linkage (candidate gene region)	15q11–13	Russo, 2005
Migraine without aura	1 family	Linkage (genome-wide)	14q21.2–22.3	Soragna, 2003
	289 subjects	Linkage (genome-wide)	4q21	Björnsson, 2003
Migraine with and without aura	2 families	Linkage (X-chromosomal)	Xq24–28	Nyholt, 2000
	1 family	Linkage (genome-wide)	6p12.2–21.1	Carlsson, 2002
	83 families	Linkage (candidate gene region)	1q31	Lea, 2002
Migraine (special aspects)	92 families	Linkage (genome-wide)	18p11[a]	Lea, 2005
	790 sib pairs	Linkage (genome-wide)	5q21[b]	Nyholt, 2005

[a] Severe form of migraine.

[b] Latent Class analysis: Linkage for "Migrainous Headache" Phenotype.

the effect sizes attributable to individual genetic variants are likely to be weak. Finding such genes by using the classical linkage approach in family material with common forms of migraine may be difficult. Association-based methods are a powerful instrument to identify small relative risks. In this respect they are particularly suited to address common multifactorial migraine. However, there are a number of important pitfalls when conducting such studies. Critical issues include the sample size, the definition of patients, adequate control samples, and, most importantly, replication in other populations. Montagna et al. (2005) provided an excellent overview of the many candidate gene association studies that have been done on the relationship between migraine and genes for dopamine receptors as well as genes implicated in the metabolism and transportation of serotonin (5-HT). None of the associations has been convincingly replicated. Here, we shall briefly discuss those associations that have been replicated at least once.

The enzyme 5,10-methylenetetrahydrofolate reductase (MTHFR) plays a role in maintaining homocysteine levels. An association between the C677T variant in the MTHFR gene and migraine with aura has been found in some (but not all) clinic-based (and therefore selected) study populations (Kowa et al., 2000; Kara et al., 2003; Lea et al., 2004; Oterino et al., 2004; Todt et al., 2006), but also, and most importantly, in a large sample taken from the general population (Scher et al., 2006). This makes MTHFR the first migraine-risk gene at the population level. The association was found to be enhanced in the presence of another variant (A1298C) in the same gene (Kara et al., 2003), and in combination with an angiotensin I-converting enzyme (ACE) DD/ID genotype (Lea et al., 2005b). If replicated, this would indicate the first gene–gene interaction to be involved in modulating the risk for migraine. Other replicated associations, but only in selected clinic-based samples, include associations with: a progesterone receptor (PGR) *Alu* insertion in two independent populations (Colson et al., 2005); the estrogen receptor 1 (ESR1) in two independent populations for the G594A polymorphism (Colson et al., 2005), although Oterino et al. (2006) found an association for the G325C polymorphism (three-fold increased risk), but not for the G594A polymorphism; the tumor necrosis factor gene in two separate studies (Trabace et al., 2002; Rainero et al., 2004); and variants in the ACE (Paterna et al., 2000; Kowa et al., 2005; Lea et al., 2005b). Remarkably, in one study, the ACE-DD variant seemed to have a slight protective effect against migraine in male patients (Lin et al., 2005). Also for ESR1 and PGR variants a synergistical effect increasing the risk for migraine has been observed (Colson et al., 2005).

CLUSTER HEADACHE

Twin and family history studies suggest that there is a significant genetic contribution to CH. There have been several descriptions of CH in concordant monozygotic twins (reviewed in Russell, 2004), although data from large registries have been less conclusive (Svensson et al., 2003). First-degree relatives of patients with CH have a 5–18 times higher risk—and second-degree relatives a 1–3 times higher risk—of CH than the general population (reviewed in Russell, 2004). These numbers are based on an estimated prevalence of CH of 1 per 500. The role of atypical CH is still a matter of debate, but the high prevalence of atypical CH in 21 Swedish families with typical CH might indicate shared genetic influences (Sjostrand et al., 2005). In most families the pattern of inheritance seems to be autosomal dominant with low penetrance (Russell et al., 1995). However, other patterns of inheritance have been described (De Simone et al., 2003; Russell, 2004).

A recent candidate gene association study in 109 Italian patients found an association between a polymorphism (G1246A) in the hypocretin receptor 2 (*HCRTR2*) gene and CH. This finding has been replicated in a large German cohort of CH patients (Schurks et al., 2006). However, another large study including 258 patients found no evidence for a role of the G1246A (c.922G>A [rs2653349]) polymorphism or other *HCRTR2* sequence variants in CH. (Baumber et al., 2006). A recent genome-wide linkage analysis in five Danish kindreds identified several chromosomal areas that might contribute to CH (Baumber et al., 2006), but the signals were weak, illustrating the need for large carefully selected samples and collaborative multicentre studies.

OTHER TYPES OF HEADACHES

Genetic factors seem to be further involved in TTH (Ulrich et al., 2004; Russell et al., 2006). A study involving 11,199 twin pairs from Denmark found that both the "no-TTH" and "frequent-TTH" phenotype have a genetic component, whereas "infrequent TTH" is caused primarily by environmental factors. Data regarding "chronic TTH" were inconclusive (Russell et al., 2006).

The literature includes several descriptions of families with trigeminal neuralgia and an apparent autosomal dominant mode of inheritance (Smyth et al., 2003). However, in the majority of cases family history is definitely negative. To date, no molecular genetic clues have been identified for TTH and trigeminal neuralgia

References

Akerman, S and Goadsby, PJ (2005). Topiramate inhibits cortical spreading depression in rat and cat: impact in migraine aura. *Neuroreport*, 16:1383–1387.

Ambrosini, A, D'Onofrio, M, Grieco, GS, et al. (2005). A new mutation on the ATPA2 gene in one Italian family with basilar-type migraine linked to the FHM2 locus. *Neurology*, 64: A132.

Anttila, V, Kallela, M, Oswell, G, et al. (2006). Trait components provide tools to dissect the genetic susceptibility of migraine. *Am J Hum Genet*, 79:85–99.

Asakura, K, Kanemasa, T, Minagawa, K, et al. (2000). α-Eudesmol, a P/Q-type Ca^{2+} channel blocker, inhibits neurogenic vasodilation and extravasation following electrical stimulation of trigeminal ganglion. *Brain Res*, 873:94–101.

Ayata, C, Shimizu-Sasamata, M, Lo, EH, et al. (2000). Impaired neurotransmitter release and elevated threshold for cortical spreading depression in mice with mutations in the alpha 1A subunit of P/Q type calcium channels. *Neuroscience*, 95:639–645.

Bassi, MT, Bresolin, N, Tonelli, A, et al. (2004). A novel mutation in the ATP1A2 gene causes alternating hemiplegia of childhood. *J Med Genet*, 41:621–628.

Baumber, L, Sjostrand, C, Leone, M, et al. (2006). A genome-wide scan and HCRTR2 candidate gene analysis in a European cluster headache cohort. *Neurology*, 27:1888–1893.

Bjornsson, A, Gudmundsson, G, Gudfinnsson, E, et al. (2003). Localization of a gene for migraine without aura to chromosome 4q21. *Am J Hum Genet*, 73:986–993.

Cader, ZM, Noble-Topham, S, Dyment, DA, et al. (2003). Significant linkage to migraine with aura on chromosome 11q24. *Hum Mol Genet*, 12:2511–2517.

Cao, YQ, Piedras-Renteria, ES, Smith, GB, et al. (2004). Presynaptic Ca^{2+} channels compete for channel type-preferring slots in altered neurotransmission arising from Ca^{2+} channelopathy. *Neuron*, 43:387–400.

Capendeguy, O and Horisberger, JD (2004). Functional effects of Na^{+}, K^{+}-ATPase gene mutations linked to familial hemiplegic migraine. *Neuromolecular Med*, 6:105–116.

Carlsson, A, Forsgren, L, Nylander, PO, et al. (2002). Identification of a susceptibility locus for migraine with and without aura on 6p12.2-p21.1. *Neurology*, 59:1804–1807.

Catterall, WA (1998). Structure and function of neuronal $Ca2^{+}$ channels and their role in neurotransmitter release. *Cell Calcium*, 24:307–323.

Chabriat, H, Vahedi, K, Iba-Zizen, MT, et al. (1995). Clinical spectrum of CADASIL: a study of 7 families. Cerebral autosomal dominant arteriopathy with subcortical infarcts and leukoencephalopathy. *Lancet*, 7:934–939.

Colson, NJ, Lea, RA, Quinlan, S, et al. (2005). Investigation of hormone receptor genes in migraine. *Neurogenetics*, 6:17–23.

De Fusco, M, Marconi, R, Silvestri, L, et al. (2003). Haploinsufficiency of ATP1A2 encoding the Na^{+}/K^{+} pump α_2 subunit associated with familial hemiplegic migraine type 2. *Nat Genet*, 33:192–196.

De Simone, R, Fiorillo, C, Bonuso, S, et al. (2003). A cluster headache family with possible autosomal recessive inheritance. *Neurology*, 26:578–579.

Dichgans, M (2003). A new cause of hereditary small vessel disease: angiopathy of retina and brain. *Neurology*, 14:8–9.

Dichgans, M, Freilinger, T, Eckstein, G, et al. (2005). Mutation in the neuronal voltage-gated sodium channel *SCN1A* causes familial hemiplegic migraine. *Lancet*, 366:371–377.

Dichgans, M, Mayer, M, Uttner, I, et al. (1998). The phenotypic spectrum of CADASIL: clinical findings in 102 cases. *Ann Neurol*, 44:731–739.

Domenga, V, Fardoux, P, Lacombe, P, et al. (2004). Notch3 is required for arterial identity and maturation of vascular smooth muscle cells. *Genes Dev*, 18:2730–2735.

Doods, H, Hallermayer, G, Wu, D, et al. (2000). Pharmacological profile of BIBN4096BS, the first selective small molecule CGRP antagonist. *Br J Pharmacol*, 129:420–423.

Dove, LS, Abbott, LC, and Griffit, WH (1998). Whole-cell and single-channel analysis of P-type calcium currents in cerebellar purkinje cells of leaner mutant mice. *J Neurosci*, 18:7687–7699.

Ducros, A, Denier, C, Joutel, A, et al. (2001). The clinical spectrum of familial hemiplegic migraine associated with mutations in a neuronal calcium channel. *N Engl J Med*, 345:17–24.

Duerr, RH, Taylor, KD, Brant, SR, et al. (2006). A genome-wide association study identifies IL23R as an inflammatory bowel disease gene. *Science*, 1:1461–1463.

Ferrari, MD (1998). Migraine. *Lancet*, 351:1043–1051.

Ferrari, MD and Goadsby, PJ (2006). Migraine as a cerebral ionopathy with abnormal central sensory processing. In *Neurobiology of Disease* (S Gilman and T Pedley, eds.), Elsevier, New York (in press).

Fletcher, CF, Tottene, A, Lennon, VA, et al. (2001). Dystonia and cerebellar atrophy in CACNA1A null mice lacking P/Q calcium channel activity. *FASEB J*, 15:1288–1290.

Gervil, M, Ulrich, V, Kaprio, J, et al. (1999). The relative role of genetic and environmental factors in migraine without aura. *Neurology*, 53:995–999.

Gould, DB, Phalan, FC, van Mil, SE, et al. (2006). Role of COL4A1 in small-vessel disease and hemorrhagic stroke. *N Engl J Med*, 6:1489–1496.

Guida, S, Trettel, F, Pagnutti, S, et al. (2001). Complete loss of P/Q calcium channel activity caused by a CACNA1A missense mutation carried by patients with episodic ataxia type 2. *Am J Hum Genet*, 68:759–764.

Haan, J, Kors, EE, Vanmolkot, KR, et al. (2005). Migraine genetics: an update. *Curr Pain Headache Rep*, 9:213–220.

Hans, M, Luvisetto, S, Williams, ME, et al. (1999). Functional consequences of mutations in the human alpha (1A) calcium channel subunit linked to familial hemiplegic migraine. *J Neurosci*, 19:1610–1619.

Harno, H, Hirvonen, T, Kaunisto, MA et al. (2003). Subclinical vestibulocerebellar dysfunction in migraine with and without aura. *Neurology*, 23:1748–1752.

Hirschhorn, JN and Daly, MJ (2005). Genome-wide association studies for common diseases and complex traits. *Nat Rev Genet*, 6:95–108.

Honkasalo, M-L, Kaprio, J, Winter, T et al. (1995). Migraine and concomitant symptoms among 8167 adult twin pairs. *Headache*, 35:70–78.

Hoskin, KL, Bulmer, DCE, Lasalandra, M, et al. (2001). Fos expression in the midbrain periaqueductal grey after trigeminovascular stimulation. *J Anat*, 197:29–34

Hottenga, JJ, Vanmolkot, KR, Kors, EE, et al. (2005). The 3p21.1-p21.3 hereditary vascular retinopathy locus increases the risk for Raynaud's phenomenon and migraine. *Cephalalgia*, 25:1168–1172.

Hudson, G and Chinnery, PF (2006). Mitochondrial DNA polymerase-gamma and human disease. *Hum Mol Genet*, 15: R244–R252.

Ikeda, K, Onaka, T, Yamakado, M, et al. (2003). Degeneration of the amygdala/piriform cortex and enhanced fear/anxiety behaviors in sodium pump alpha2 subunit (Atp1a2)-deficient mice. *J Neurosci*, 23:4667–4676.

Ikeda, K, Onimaru, H, Yamada, J, et al. (2004). Malfunction of respiratory-related neuronal activity in Na^+, K^+-ATPase alpha2 subunit-deficient mice is attributable to abnormal Cl- homeostasis in brainstem neurons. *J Neurosci*, 24:10693–10701.

Imbrici, P, Jaffe, SL, Eunson, LH, et al. (2004). Dysfunction of the brain calcium channel $Ca_V2.1$ in absence epilepsy and episodic ataxia. *Brain*, 127:2682–2692.

James, PF, Grupp, IL, Grupp, G, et al. (1999). Identification of a specific role for the Na,K-ATPase alpha 2 isoform as a regulator of calcium in the heart. *Mol Cell*, 3:555–563.

Jen, JC, Kim, GW, and Baloh, RW (2004). Clinical spectrum of episodic ataxia type 2. *Neurology*, 62:17–22.

Jen, JC, Wan, J, Graves, M, et al. (2001). Loss-of-function EA2 mutations are associated with impaired neuromuscular transmission. *Neurology*, 57:1843–1848.

Jen, JC, Wan, J, Palos, TP, et al. (2005). Mutation in the glutamate transporter EAAT1 causes episodic ataxia, hemiplegia, and seizures. *Neurology*, 23:529–534.

Jeng, CJ, Chen, YT, Chen, YW, et al. (2006). Dominant-negative effects of human P/Q-type $Ca2^+$ channel mutations associated with episodic ataxia type 2. *Am J Physiol Cell Physiol*, 290:1209–1220.

Jorgensen, PL, Hakansson, KO and Karlish, SJ (2003). Structure and mechanism of Na,K-ATPase: functional sites and their interactions. *Annu Rev Physiol*, 65:817–849.

Joutel, A, Corpechot, C, Ducros, A, et al. (1996). Notch3 mutations in CADASIL, a hereditary adult-onset condition causing stroke and dementia. *Nature*, 383:707–710.

Jouvenceau, A, Eunson, LH, Spauschus, A, et al. (2001). Human epilepsy associated with dysfunction of the brain P/Q-type calcium channel. *Lancet*, 358:801–807.

Jun, K, Piedras-Renteria, ES, Smith, SM, et al. (1999). Ablation of P/Q-type $Ca2^+$ channel currents, altered synaptic transmission, and progressive ataxia in mice lacking the alpha(1A)-subunit. *Proc Natl Acad Sci USA*, 96:15245–15250.

Jurkat-Rott, K, Freilinger, T, Dreier, JP, et al. (2004).Variability of familial hemiplegic migraine with novel A1A2 Na^+/K^+-ATPase variants. *Neurology*, 25:1857–1861.

Kaja, S, van d Ven, RC, Broos, LA, et al. (2007). Characterization of acetylcholine release and the compensatory contribution of non-$Ca_v2.1$ channels at motor nerve terminals of leaner $Ca_v2.1$-mutant mice. *Neuroscience*, 144:1278–1287.

Kallela, M, Wessman, M, Havanka, H, et al. (2001). Familial migraine with and without aura: clinical characteristics and co-occurence. *Eur J Neurosci*, 8:441–449.

Kanai, K, Hirose, S, Oguni, H, et al. (2004). Effect of localization of missense mutations in SCN1A on epilepsy phenotype severity. *Neurology*, 63:329–334.

Kaplan, JH (2002). Biochemistry of Na,K-ATPase. *Annu Rev Biochem*, 71:511–535.

Kara, I, Sazci, A, Ergul, E, et al. (2003). Association of the C677T and A1298C polymorphisms in the 5,10 methylenetetrahydrofolate reductase gene in patients with migraine risk. *Brain Res Mol Brain Res*, 111:84–90.

Knight, YE, Bartsch, T, Kaube, H, et al. (2002). P/Q-type calcium channel blockade in the PAG facilitates trigeminal nociception: a functional genetic link for migraine? *J Neurosci*, 22:1–6.

Koenderink, JB, Zifarelli, G, Qiu, LY, et al. (2005). Na, K-ATPase mutations in familial hemiplegic migraine lead to functional inactivation. *Biochim Biophys Acta*, 15:61–68.

Kors, EE, Terwindt, GM, Vermeulen, FL, et al. (2001). Delayed cerebral edema and fatal coma after minor head trauma: role of CACNA1A calcium channel subunit gene and relationship with familial hemiplegic migraine. *Ann Neurol*, 49:753–760.

Kors, EE, Vanmolkot, KR, Haan, J, et al. (2004). Recent findings in headache genetics. *Curr Opin Neurol*, 17:283–288.

Kowa, H, Fusayasu, E, Ijiri, T, et al. (2005). Association of the insertion/deletion polymorphism of the angiotensin I-converting enzyme gene in patients of migraine with aura. *Neurosci Lett*, 374:129–131.

Kowa, H, Yasui, K, Takeshima, T, et al. (2000). The homozygous C677T mutation in the methylenetetrahydrofolate reductase gene is a genetic risk factor for migraine. *Am J Med Genet*, 96:762–764.

Kraus, RL, Sinnegger, MJ, Glossmann, H, et al. (1998). Familial hemiplegic migraine mutations change alpha (1A) Ca^{2+} channel kinetics. *J Biol Chem*, 273:5586–5590.

Kraus, RL, Sinnegger, MJ, Koschak, A, et al. (2000). Three new familial hemiplegic migraine mutants affect P/Q-type $Ca2^+$ channel kinetics. *J Biol Chem*, 275:9239–9243.

Lacombe, P, Oligo, C, Domenga, V, et al. (2005) Impaired cerebral vasoreactivity in a transgenic mouse model of cerebral autosomal dominant arteriopathy with subcortical infarcts and leukoencephalopathy arteriopathy. *Stroke*, 36:1053–1058.

Lea, RA, Nyholt, DR, Curtain, RP, et al. (2005a). A genome-wide scan provides evidence for loci influencing a severe heritable form of common migraine. *Neurogenetics*, 6:67–72.

Lea, RA, Ovcaric, M, Sundholm, J, et al. (2004). The methylenetetrahydrofolate reductase gene variant C677T influences susceptibility to migraine with aura. *BMC Med*, 2:3.

Lea, RA, Ovcaric, M, Sundholm, J, et al. (2005b). Genetic variants of angiotensin converting enzyme and methylenetetrahydrofolate reductase may act in combination to increase migraine susceptibility. *Brain Res Mol Brain Res*, 136:112–117.

Ligthart L, Boomsma DI, Martin NG, et al. (2006). Migraine with aura and migraine without aura are not distinct entities: further evidence from a large Dutch population study. *Twin Res Hum Genet*, 9:54–63.

Lin, JJ, Wang, PJ, Chen, CH, et al. (2005). Homozygous deletion genotype of angiotensin converting enzyme confers protection against migraine in man. *Acta Neurol Taiwan*, 14:120–125.

Lorenzon, NM, Lutz, CM, Frankel, WN, et al. (1998). Altered calcium channel currents in purkinje cells of neurological mutant mouse leaner. *J Neurosci*, 18:4482–4489.

Ludvigsson, P, Hesdorffer, D, Olafsson, E, et al. (2006). Migraine with aura is a risk factor for unprovoked seizures in children. *Ann Neurol*, 59:210–213.

Marconi, R, De Fusco, M, Aridon, P, et al. (2003). Familial hemiplegic migraine type 2 is linked to 0.9Mb region on chromosome 1q23. *Ann Neurol*, 53:376–381.

Matharu, MS, Bartsch, T, Ward, N, et al. (2004). Central neuromodulation in chronic migraine patients with suboccipital stimulators: a PET study. *Brain*, 127:220–230.

Meisler, MH and Kearney, JA (2005). Sodium channel mutations in epilepsy and other neurological disorders. *J Clin Invest*, 115:2010–2017.

Montagna, P, Pierangeli, G, Cevoli, S, et al. (2005). Pharmacogenetics of headache treatment. *Neurol Sci*, 26: S143–S147.

Mori, Y, Wakamori, M, Oda, S, et al. (2000). Reduced voltage sensitivity of activation of P/Q-type Ca^{2+} channels is associated with the ataxic mouse mutation rolling Nagoya (tg(rol)). *J Neurosci*, 20:5654–5662.

Moseley, AE, Lieske, SP, Wetzel, RK, et al. (2003). The Na, K-ATPase alpha 2 isoform is expressed in neurons, and its absence disrupts neuronal activity in newborn mice. *J Biol Chem*, 14:5317–5324.

Moskowitz, MA, Bolay, H, and Dalkara, T (2004). Deciphering migraine mechanisms: clues from familial hemiplegic migraine genotypes. *Ann Neurol*, 55:276–280.

Mulder, EJ, Van Baal, C, Gaist, D, et al. (2003). Genetic and environmental influences on migraine: a twin study across six countries. *Twin Res*, 6:422–431.

Mullner, C, Broos, LA, van den Maagdenberg, AM, et al. (2004). Familial hemiplegic migraine type 1 mutations K1336E, W1684R, and V1696I alter $Ca_v2.1$ $Ca2^+$ channel gating: evidence for beta-subunit isoform-specific effects. *J Biol Chem*, 279:51844–51850.

Nyholt, DR, Gillespie, NG, Heath, AC, et al. (2004). Latent class and genetic analysis does not support migraine with aura and migraine without aura as separate entities. *Genet Epidemiol*, 26:231–244.

Nyholt, DR, Morley, KI, Ferreira, MA, et al. (2005). Genomewide significant linkage to migrainous headache on chromosome 5q21. *Am J Hum Genet*, 77:500–512.

Ophoff, RA, DeYoung, J, Service, SK, et al. (2001). Hereditary vascular retinopathy, cerebroretinal vasculopathy, and hereditary endotheliopathy with retinopathy, nephropathy and stroke map to a single locus on chromosome 3p21.1-p21.3. *Am J Hum Genet*, 69:447–453.

Ophoff, RA, Terwindt, GM, Vergouwe, MN, et al. (1996). Familial hemiplegic migraine and episodic ataxia type-2 are caused by mutations in the Ca^{2+} channel gene CACNL1A4. *Cell*, 87:543–552.

Oterino, A, Pascual, J, Ruiz de Alegria, C, et al. (2006). Association of migraine and ESR1 G325C polymorphism. *Neuroreport*, 17:61–64.

Oterino, A, Valle, N, Bravo, Y, et al. (2004). MTHFR T677 homozygosis influences the presence of aura in migraineurs. *Cephalalgia*, 24:491–494.

Paterna, S, Di Pasquale, P, D'Angelo, A, et al. (2000). Angiotensin-converting enzyme gene deletion polymorphism determines an increase in frequency of migraine attacks in patients suffering from migraine without aura. *Eur Neurol*, 43:133–136.

Pfefferkorn, T, von Stuckrad-Barre, S, Herzog, J, et al. (2001). Reduced cerebrovascular CO(2) reactivity in CADASIL: A transcranial Doppler sonography study. *Stroke*, 32, 17–21.

Pietrobon, D (2005). Function and dysfunction of synaptic calcium channels: insights from mouse models. *Curr Opin Neurobiol*, 15:257–265.

Rainero, I, Grimaldi, LM, Salani, G, et al. (2004). Association between the tumor necrosis factor-alpha-308 G/A gene polymorphism and migraine. *Neurology*, 62:141–143.

Riant, F, De Fusco, M, Aridon, P, et al. (2005). ATP1A2 mutations in 11 families with familial hemiplegic migraine. *Hum Mutat*, 26:281.

Russell, MB (2004). Epidemiology and genetics of cluster headache. *Lancet Neurol*, 3:279–283.

Russell, MB, Andersson, PG, Thomsen, LL, et al. (1995). Cluster headache is an autosomal dominantly inherited disorder in some families: a complex segregation analysis. *J Med Genet*, 32:954–956.

Russell, MB and Olesen, J (1995). Increased familial risk and evidence of genetic factor in migraine. *Br Med J*, 311:541–544.

Russell, MB, Saltyte-Benth, J, and Levi, N (2006). Are infrequent episodic, frequent episodic and chronic tension-type headache inherited? A population-based study of 11 199 twin pairs. *J Headache Pain*, 7:119–126.

Russell, MB, Ulrich, V, Gervil, M, et al. (2002). Migraine without aura and migraine with aura are distinct disorders. A population-based twin survey. *Headache*, 42:332–336.

Russo, L, Mariotti, P, Sangiorgi, E, et al. (2005). A new susceptibility locus for migraine with aura in the 15q11-q13 genomic region containing three GABA-A receptor genes. *Am J Hum Genet*, 76:327–333.

Sandor, PS, Mascia, A, Seidel, L, et al. (2001). Subclinical cerebellar impairment in the common types of migraine: a three-dimensional analysis of reaching movements. *Ann Neurol*, 49:668–672.

Scher, AI, Terwindt, GM, Verschuren, WM, et al. (2006). Migraine and MTHFR C677T genotype in a population-based sample. *Ann Neurol*, 59:372–375.

Schoenen, J, Ambrosini, A, Sandor, PS, et al. (2003). Evoked potentials and transcranial magnetic stimulation in migraine: published data and viewpoint on their pathophysiologic significance. *Clin Neurophysiol*, 114:955–972.

Schurks, M, Kurth, T, Geissler, I, et al. (2006). Cluster headache is associated with the G1246A polymorphism in the hypocretin receptor 2 gene. *Neurology*, 27:1917–1919.

Segall, L, Mezzetti, A, Scanzano, R, et al. (2005). Alterations in the alpha2 isoform of Na,K-ATPase associated with familial hemiplegic migraine type 2. *Proc Natl Acad Sci USA*, 102:11106–11111.

Segall, L, Scanzano, R, Kaunisto, MA, et al. (2004). Kinetic alterations due to a missense mutation in the Na, K-ATPase alpha2 subunit cause familial hemiplegic migraine type 2. *J Biol Chem*, 15:43692–43696.

Shields, KG, Storer, RJ, Akerman, S, et al. (2005). Calcium channels modulate nociceptive transmission in the trigeminal nucleus of the cat. *Neuroscience*, 135:203–212.

Sjostrand, C, Russell, MB, Ekbom, K, et al. (2005). Familial cluster headache. Is atypical cluster headache in family members part of the clinical spectrum? *Cephalalgia*, 25:1068–1077.

Smyth, P, Greenough, G, and Stommel, E (2003). Familial trigeminal neuralgia: case reports and review of the literature. *Headache*, 43:910–915.

Soragna, D, Vettori, A, Carraro, G, et al. (2003). A locus for migraine without aura maps on chromosome 14q21.2-q22.3. *Am J Hum Genet*, 72:161–167.

Spacey, SD, Hildebrand, ME, Materek, LA, et al. (2004). Functional implications of a novel EA2 mutation in the P/Q-type calcium channel. *Ann Neurol*, 56:213–220.

Spadaro, M, Ursu, S, Lehmann-Horn, et al. (2004). A G301R Na^+/K^+-ATPase mutation causes familial hemiplegic migraine type 2 with cerebellar signs. *Neurogenetics*, 5:177–185.

Sparaco, M, Feleppa, M, Lipton, RB, et al. (2006). Mitochondrial dysfunction and migraine: evidence and hypotheses. *Cephalalgia*, 26:361–372.

Stewart, WF, Bigal, ME, Kolodner, K, et al. (2006). Familial risk of migraine: variation by proband age at onset and headache severity. *Neurology*, 66:344–348.

Stewart, WF, Staffa, J, Lipton, RB, et al. (1997). Familial risk of migraine: a population-based study. *Ann Neurol*, 41:166–172.

Svensson, DA, Larsson, B, Waldenlind, E, et al. (2003). Shared rearing environment in migraine: results from twins reared apart and twins reared together. *Headache*, 43:235–244.

Svensson, D, Ekbom, K, Pedersen, NL, et al. (2003). A note on cluster headache in a population-based twin register. *Cephalalgia*, 23, 376–380.

Swoboda, KJ, Kanavakis, E, Xaidara, A, et al. (2004). Alternating hemiplegia of childhood or familial hemiplegic migraine?: a novel ATP1A2 mutation. *Ann Neurol*, 55:884–887.

Terwindt, GM, Haan, J, Ophoff, RA, et al. (1998a). Clinical and genetic analysis of a large Dutch family with autosomal dominant vascular retinopathy, migraine and Raynaud's phenomenon. *Brain*, 121:303–316.

Terwindt, GM, Kors, E, Haan, J, et al. (2002). Mutation analysis of the CACNA1A calcium channel subunit gene in 27 patients with sporadic hemiplegic migraine. *Arch Neurol*, 59:1016–1018.

Terwindt, GM, Kors, EE, Vein, AA, et al. (2004). Single-fiber EMG in familial hemiplegic migraine. *Neurology*, 63:1942–1943.

Terwindt, GM, Ophoff, RA, Haan, J, et al. (1998b). Variable clinical expression of mutations in the P/Q-type calcium channel gene in familial hemiplegic migraine. *Neurology*, 50:1105–1110.

Terwindt, GM, Ophoff, RA, van Eijk, R, et al. (2001). Involvement of the CACNA1A gene containing region on 19p13 in migraine with and without aura. *Neurology*, 24:1028–1032.

Thomsen, LL, Olesen, J, and Russell, MB (2003). Increased risk of migraine with typical aura in probands with familial hemiplegic migraine and their relatives. *Eur J Neurol*, 10:421–427.

Thomsen, LL, Ostergaard, E, Olesen, J, et al. (2003a). Evidence for a separate type of migraine with aura: sporadic hemiplegic migraine. *Neurology*, 60:595–601.

Thomsen, LL, Ostergaard, E, Romer, SF, et al. (2003b). Sporadic hemiplegic migraine is an aetiologically heterogeneous disorder. *Cephalalgia*, 23:921–928.

Todt, U, Dichgans, M, Jurkat-Rott, et al. (2005). Rare missense variants in ATP1A2 in families with clustering of common forms of migraine. *Hum Mutat*, 26:315–321.

Todt, U, Freudenberg, J, Goebel, I, et al. (2006).MTHFR C677T polymorphism and migraine with aura. *Ann Neurol*, 60:621–622.

Tottene, A, Pivotto, F, Fellin, T, et al. (2005). Specific kinetic alterations of human $Ca_V2.1$ calcium channels produced by mutation S218L causing familial hemiplegic migraine and delayed cerebral edema and coma after minor head trauma. *J Biol Chem*, 280:17678–17686.

Tottene, A, Tottene, A, Fellin, T, et al. (2002). Familial hemiplegic migraine mutations increase Ca^{2+} influx through single human $Ca_V2.1$ channels and decrease maximal $Ca_V2.1$ current density in neurons. *Proc Natl Acad Sci USA*, 99:13284–13289.

Trabace, S, Brioli, G, Lulli, P, et al. (2002). Tumor necrosis factor gene polymorphism in migraine. *Headache*, 42:341–345.

Tzoulis, C, Engelsen, BA, Telstad, W, et al. (2006). The spectrum of clinical disease caused by the A467T and W748S POLG mutations: a study of 26 cases. *Brain*, 129:1685–1692.

Ulrich, V, Gervil, M, Kyvik, KO, et al. (1999). Evidence of a genetic factor in migraine with aura: a population-based Danish twin study. *Ann Neurol*, 45:242–246.

Ulrich, V, Gervil, M, and Olesen, J (2004). The relative influence of environment and genes in episodic tension-type headache. *Neurology*, 8:2065–2069.

Vahedi, K, Massin, P, Guichard, JP, et al. (2003). Hereditary infantile hemiparesis, retinal arteriolar tortuosity, and leukoencephalopathy. *Neurology*, 14:57–63.

van den Maagdenberg, AMJM, Pietrobon, D, Pizzorusso, T, et al. (2004). A Cacna1a knock-in migraine mouse model with increased susceptibility to cortical spreading depression. *Neuron*, 41:701–710.

Vanmolkot, KRJ, Babini, E, de Vries, B, et al. (2006). The Novel p.L1649Q mutation in the *SCN1A* epilepsy gene is associated with familial hemiplegic migraine: genetic and functional studies. *Hum Mutat*, 28:522.

Vanmolkot KRJ, Babini E, de VB, Stam Freilinger T, Terwindt GM, et al. (2007). The noval p.L1649Q mutation in the *SCN1A* epilepsy gene is associated with familial hemiplagic migraine: genetic and functional studies. Mutation in brief 957. Online. Hum Mutat 2007 May; 28(5):522.

Vanmolkot, KRJ, Kors, EE, Hottenga, JJ, et al. (2003). Novel mutations in the Na^+,K^+-ATPase pump gene ATP1A2 associated with familial hemiplegic migraine and benign familial infantile convulsions. *Ann Neurol*, 54:360–366.

Vanmolkot, KRJ, Kors, EE, Turk, U, et al. (2006). Two de novo mutations in the Na,K-ATPase gene ATP1A2 associated with pure familial hemiplegic migraine. *Eur J Hum Genet*, 14:555–560.

Vanmolkot, KRJ, Stroink, H, Koenderink, JB, et al. (2006). Severe episodic neurological deficits and permanent mental retardation in a child with a novel FHM2 ATP1A2 mutation. *Ann Neurol*, 59:310–314.

Wakamori, M, Yamazaki, K, Matsunodaira, H, et al. (1998). Single tottering mutations responsible for the neuropathic phenotype of the P-Type calcium channel. *J Biol Chem*, 273:34857–34867.

Wan, J, Khanna, R, Sandusky, M, et al. (2005). CACNA1A mutations causing episodic and progressive ataxia alter channel trafficking and kinetics. *Neurology*, 64:2090–2097.

Wappl, E, Koschak, A, Poteser, M, et al. (2002). Functional consequences of P/Q-type $Ca2^+$ channel $Ca_v2.1$ missense mutations associated with episodic ataxia type 2 and progressive ataxia. *J Biol Chem*, 277:6960–6966.

Welch, KM, Nagesh, V, Aurora, S, et al. (2001). Periaqueductal grey matter dysfunction in migraine: cause or the burden of illness? *Headache*, 41:629–637.

Welch, KM (2005). Brain hyperexcitability: the basis for antiepileptic drugs in migraine prevention. *Headache*, 45: S25–S32.

Wessman, M, Kallela, M, Kaunisto, MA, et al. (2002). A susceptibility locus for migraine with aura, on chromosome 4q24. *Am J Hum Genet*, 70:652–662.

Wieser, T, Wolff, R, Hoffmann, KP, et al. (2004). Persistent ocular motor disturbances in migraine without aura. *Neurol Sci*, 25:8–12.

Wilkinson, F, Karanovic, O, Ross, EC, et al. (2006). Ocular motor measures in migraine with and without aura. *Cephalalgia*, 26:660–671.

Winterthun, S, Ferrari, G, He, L, et al. (2005). Autosomal recessive mitochondrial ataxic syndrome due to mitochondrial polymerase gamma mutations. *Neurology*, 12:1204–1208.

Yu, FH, Mantegazza, M, Westenbroek, RE, et al. (2006). Reduced sodium current in GABAergic interneurons in a mouse model of severe myoclonic epilepsy in infancy. *Nat Neurosci*, 9:1142–1149.

Yue, Q, Jen, JC, Nelson, SF, et al. (1997). Progressive ataxia due to a missense mutation in a calcium-channel gene. *Am J Hum Genet*, 61:1078–1087.

Zhuchenko, O, Bailey, J, Donnen, P, et al. (1997). Autosomal dominant cerebellar ataxia (SCA6) associated with small polyglutamine expansions in the α_1A-voltage-dependent calcium channel. *Nat Genet*, 15:62–69.

Ziegler, DK, Hur, YM, Bouchard, TJ, et al. (1998). Migraine in twins raised together and apart. *Headache*, 38:417–422.

II Diagnosis and Treatment of Primary Headache Disorders and Their Complications

10 Migraine Diagnosis and Comorbidity

Richard B Lipton, Ann I Scher, Stephen D Silberstein, and Marcelo E Bigal

INTRODUCTION

Migraine is a very common neurologic disorder, characterized by recurrent attacks of severe headache, autonomic nervous system dysfunction and in some patients, by aura (Headache Classification Committee, 1988, 2004). The diagnosis of migraine has been facilitated by the development and publication of the International Classification of Headache Disorders (ICHD-1 and ICHD-2) (Headache Classification Committee, 1988, 2004). The therapeutic options for migraine have greatly expanded in recent years for both acute and preventive treatments (Goadsby et al., 2002). On the acute treatment side, advances in neuroscience have led to the development of a novel class of selective serotonin (5-hydroxytryptamine), 5-$HT_{1B/1D}$ receptor agonists, known as the triptans (Ferrari et al., 2001). These agents have changed the lives of countless migraine sufferers. On the prevention side, neuromodulators such as divalproex sodium and topiramate play an expanding role in migraine management (Silberstein, 2005). Despite the availability of new and more effective treatment options, migraine remains under-diagnosed, and available therapies are not used optimally (Diamond et al., 2007; Lipton et al., 2007).

Migraine is comorbid with a number of disorders (Lipton and Silberstein, 1994; Scher, Bigal, et al., 2006). Having diagnosed migraine, comorbidity means that other disorders are more likely (Lipton and Silberstein, 1994). Comorbidity therefore mandates a need for a heightened index of diagnostic suspicion. In addition, comorbidity is an important factor that informs treatment. In this chapter, we will first review the clinical features of migraine followed by a discussion of classification and diagnosis. We will then focus on the comorbidities of migraine.

Phases and Clinical Features of Migraine

The migraine attack can be divided into four phases: the premonitory phase or prodrome occurs hours or days before the headache; the aura, neurologic symptoms that usually immediately precede the headache; the headache phase, comprised of headache and associated symptoms; and the postdrome (Table 10–1). No single phase is necessary to make a diagnosis of migraine and most patients do not have all four phases. Migraine without aura consists of at least the headache phase and perhaps the premonitory phase, the postdrome, or both. Migraine with aura consists of at least the aura and the headache and may also include premonitory and postdromal phases. If aura occurs in the absence of headache, the disorder is termed migraine aura without headache. Both may be associated with premonitory symptoms (Olesen and Lipton, 1994; Headache Classification Committee, 2004).

Premonitory Phase (Prodrome)

Premonitory phenomena occur hours to days before headache onset in about 60% of migraineurs; it consists of psychological, neurologic, or general (constitutional, autonomic) symptoms in various combinations (Blau,1980; Isler, 1986; Giffin et al., 2003; Schoonman et al., 2006) (Table 10–2). Psychological symptoms include depression, euphoria, irritability, restlessness, mental slowness, hyperactivity, fatigue, and drowsiness. Neurologic phenomena include photophobia, phonophobia, and hyperosmia among others. General symptoms include a stiff neck, a cold feeling, sluggishness, increased thirst, increased urination, anorexia, diarrhea, constipation, fluid retention,

Table 10–1 Phases of the Migraine Attack.

I. Premonitory phase
II. Aura
III. Headache
IV. Postdrome

and food cravings (Giffin et al., 2003; Kelman, 2004b). Evolutive and nonevolutive premonitory features are sometimes distinguished. The evolutive features start approximately 6 hours before the attack, gradually increasing in intensity, often culminating in the attack; a dopaminergic mechanism has been suggested (Amery, Waelkens, and Caers, 1986; Amery, Waelkens, and Van den Bergh, 1986). Nonevolutive features precede the attack and evolutive features by up to 48 hours.

Aura

The migraine aura is comprised of focal neurologic phenomena that precede or accompany an attack (Headache Classification Committee, 2004). Most aura symptoms develop slowly over 5–20 minutes and usually last less than 60 minutes. Though usually visual, the aura of migraine can be characterized by sensory or motor phenomena and language or brain stem disturbances (Table 10–3). The headache may begin before or simultaneously with the aura, or the aura may occur in isolation. Headache follows aura 80% of the time (Jensen et al., 1986) and usually begins within 60 minutes of the end of the aura. From the end of the aura to the onset of headache, patients experience symptoms including anxiety or fears, other alterations in mood, disturbances of speech or thought, or detachment from the environment or from other people. Rarely, auras may occur repeatedly, up to many times an hour for months at a time. This phenomenon has been termed "migraine aura status," a diagnosis which requires the exclusion of secondary causes (Silberstein and Young, 1995). Sacks described two variants of aura status: one characterized by recurring visual scotomata and the other characterized by repetitive sensory auras (Sacks, 1985).

Visual aura is the most common of the neurologic events; it occurs in 99% of patients who have an aura and often has a hemianopic distribution (Russell and Olesen, 1996, Kelman, 2004a). The aura may consist of photopsia (the sensation of unformed flashes of light before the eyes) or scotoma (partial loss of sight) (Lance and Anthony, 1966; Wilkinson, 1986; Hupp et al., 1989; Hachinski et al., 1973) or the almost diagnostic aura of migraine, the fortification spectrum (Hachinski et al., 1973; Wilkinson, 1986).

Visual auras vary in their complexity. Elementary visual disturbances include scotomata, simple flashes (phosphenes), specks, or geometric forms. They may move across the visual field, sometimes crossing the midline. Shimmering or undulations in the visual field may also occur and may be described by patients as "heat waves." These "minor visual disorders" are more likely to occur during than before the headache (Selby and Lance, 1960). Because they are bilateral, they are believed to arise from the occipital cortex. More complicated auras include teichopsia (Greek: town wall and vision) or fortification spectrum, the most characteristic visual aura of migraine. An arc of

Table 10–2 Premonitory Features of Migraine (Prodrome).

Psychological	*Neurological*	*General*
Depression	Photophobia	Stiff neck
Hyperactivity	Difficulty concentrating	Food cravings
Euphoria	Phonophobia	Cold feeling
Talkativeness	Dysphasia	Anorexia
Irritability	Hyperosmia	Sluggish
Drowsiness	Yawning	Diarrhea or constipation
Restlessness		Thirst
		Urination
		Fluid retention

TABLE 10–3 Aura.

Visual: scotoma; photopsia or phosphenes; geometric forms; fortification spectra; objects may rotate, oscillate, or shimmer; brightness appears often very bright

Visual Hallucinations or Distortions: metamorphopsia; macropsia; zoom or mosaic vision

Sensory: paresthesias, often migrating, often lasting for minutes (cheiro-oral), and can become bilateral

Olfactory hallucinations

Motor: weakness or ataxia

Language: dysarthria or aphasia

Delusions and Disturbed Consciousness: déjà vu, multiple conscious trance-like states

scintillating lights, usually but not always beginning near the point of fixation, may form into a herringbone-like pattern that expands to encompass an increasing portion of a visual hemifield. It migrates across the visual field with a scintillating edge of often zigzag, flashing, or occasionally colored phenomena. The visions of Hildegard of Bingen, an eleventh Century Abbess, have been attributed in part to her migrainous auras. Characteristic of the visions that she and other visionary prophets, including Ezekiel, experienced were working, boiling, or fermenting lights.

Visual distortions and hallucinations, speculated to represent Lewis Carroll's descriptions in Alice in Wonderland, can occur. These phenomena are more common in children, are usually followed by a headache, and are characterized by a complex disorder of visual perception that may include metamorphopsia, micropsia, macropsia, zoom, or mosaic vision (Sacks, 1985; Hosking, 1988). Non-visual symptoms can occur and include complex difficulties in the perception and use of the body (apraxia and agnosia); speech and language disturbances; states of double or multiple consciousness associated with deja vu or jamais vu; and elaborate dreamy, nightmarish, trance-like, or delirious states. Olfactory hallucinations may also occur (Diamond et al., 1985).

Paresthesias characterize the second most common aura and occur in about one-third of migraineurs with aura. They are typically cheiro-oral, with numbness starting in the hand, migrating up the arm, and then jumping to involve the face, lips, and tongue (Russell and Olesen, 1996). The leg is occasionally involved (Manzoni et al., 1985). As with visual auras (with positive, followed by negative, symptoms), paresthesias may be followed by numbness and, in a few cases, loss of position sense. Paresthesias begin bilaterally or become bilateral in half of patients. Sensory auras rarely occur in isolation and usually follow a visual aura (Silberstein and Lipton, 1994; Silberstein and Young, 1995). Patients may experience more than one type of aura, with a progression from one symptom to another. Most patients with a sensory aura also have a visual aura (Ziegler and Hassanein, 1990) (Figure 10–1).

Motor symptoms may occur in up to 18% of patients, often in association with sensory symptoms (Jensen et al., 1986); however, true weakness is rare and is always unilateral (Manzoni et al., 1985). Sensory ataxia is often reported as weakness (Manzoni et al., 1985); hyperkinetic movement disorders, including chorea, have been reported (Silberstein and Young, 1995). Aphasic auras have been reported in 17%–20% of patients (Manzoni et al., 1985; Jensen et al., 1986). However, since patients are rarely examined during an aura, many of the reported cases may be dysarthria and not aphasia (Manzoni et al., 1985).

Headache

A migraine headache is typically unilateral, throbbing, moderate to marked in severity, and aggravated by routine physical activity (Headache Classification Committee, 2004). The headache of migraine can occur at any time of day or night, but occurs most frequently on rising in the morning (Selby and Lance, 1960). The onset is usually gradual; the pain peaks and then subsides, and usually lasts less than 24 hours, with a range of 4–72 hours in adults and 2–48 hours in children (Headache Classification Committee of the International Headache Society, 1988). The headache is bilateral in 40% and unilateral in 60% of cases; it consistently occurs on the same side in 20% of patients (Selby and Lance, 1960). Migraineurs whose headaches alternate sides do not develop more

Figure 1: ***MIDAS Questionnaire**

INSTRUCTIONS: Please answer the following questions about ALL your headaches you have had over the last 3 months. Write your answer in the box next to each question. Write zero if you did not do the activity in the last 3 months (Please refer to the calendar below, if necessary)

1. On how many days in the last 3 months did you miss work or school because of your headaches ? .... |__|__| days
2. How many days in the last 3 months was your productivity at work or school reduced by half or more because of your headaches *(Do not include days you counted in question 1 where you missed work or school)* ? .... |__|__| days
3. On how many days in the last 3 months did you **not** do household work because of your headaches? .... |__|__| days
4. How many days in the last 3 months was your productivity in household work reduced by half or more because of your headaches *(Donot include days you counted in question3 where youdid not do household work)* ? .... |__|__| days
5. On how many days in the last 3 months did you miss family, social, or leisure activities because of your headaches? .... |__|__| days

A. On how many days in the last 3 months did you have a headache ? (If a headache lasted more than one day, count each day) .... |__|__| days

B. On a scale of 0 - 10, on average how painful were these headaches? *(where 0 = no pain at all, and 10 = pain as bad as it can be)* .... |__|__|

Version 3.0 © Innovative Medical Research 1997
*Migraine Disability Assessment Score

Figure 10–1 Migraine Disability Assessment Score (MIDAS) Questionnaire.

consistently lateralized headache with the passage of time.

The pain varies greatly in intensity, ranging from annoying to incapacitating, although most migraineurs report at least moderate pain for attacks that go untreated (Stewart et al., 1994). The pain has a throbbing quality, particularly when severe, but can be tight or bandlike (Selby and Lance, 1960). During an attack, pain may move from one part of the head to another and may radiate down the neck into the shoulder. The pain is commonly aggravated by physical activity or simple head movement. Patients prefer to lie down in a dark, quiet room. Scalp tenderness occurs in many patients during or after the headache. This tenderness may involve the head and neck and prevent the patient from lying on the affected side (Drummond, 1987).

Many migraineurs have headache profiles that do not meet the ICHD-2 criteria for migraine (Olesen, 1978). Some have probable migraine (1.6), missing one criterion, others have shorter and less severe headache and may meet the criteria for episodic tension-type headache (TTH). Some patients note that their headache begins as a TTH and builds into a "migraine" (Olesen, 1978; Drummond and Lance, 1984). We believe these phenomenologic TTHs in migraineurs often represent a forme fruste of migraine. TTH in migraine sufferers have been shown to respond to migraine specific medications, triptans, while tension-type headache in the absence of migraine does not. (Cady et al., 1997; Lipton, Stewart et al., 2000; Bigal Liberman, et al., 2006).

Migraineurs may also experience short-lived jabs of pain, lasting for seconds, occurring between more characteristic migraine attacks (known as idiopathic stabbing headache). The pain is described as an "ice pick," "needle," "nail," "jabs and jolts," or "pinprick" headache, and occurs in about 40% of migraineurs (Raskin and Schwartz, 1980).

Associated Phenomena

Migraine attacks are characteristically accompanied by other associated symptoms that often contribute to migraine-related disability. Their type and prevalence are detailed in Table 10–4. Gastrointestinal disturbances are often the most distressing symptom other than pain. Anorexia is common, but food cravings can occur; nausea occurs in 90% of patients and vomiting in about one-third (Selby and Lance, 1960; Olesen, 1978; Silberstein, 1995; Lipton Diamond, et al., 2001; Lipton et al., 2007). Gastroparesis contributes to gastrointestinal distress and poor absorption of oral medication (Volans, 1978; Saper, 1983; Boyle et al., 1990). Diarrhea occurs in about 16% of patients (Selby and Lance, 1960; Olesen, 1978; Rasmussen et al., 1991; Russell et al., 1992; Anthony and Rasmussen, 1993). Many migraineurs have enhanced sensory perception or sensitivity manifested as photophobia, phonophobia, and osmophobia, and seek a dark, quiet room (Selby and Lance, 1960; Drummond, 1986). Others will have lightheadedness and vertigo (Kuritzky et al., 1981). Premonitory symptoms, such as exhilaration, agitation, fatigue, lethargy, disorientation, hypomania, anger, rage, or depression, can continue into the headache. Constitutional, mood, and mental changes are almost universal. Blurry vision, nasal stuffiness, pallor or redness, and sensations of heat, cold, or sweating may occur. Fluid retention can develop hours to days before the headache. Frank edema may precede, accompany, or follow the headache, with resolution of the fluid retention occurring after the headache subsides (Dalessio, 1980).

The prevalence of associated symptoms is observed to be higher in clinic-based than population-based studies, probably because more effective interviewing techniques and more definitive criteria are used in the clinic. In addition, a selection bias toward patients with more severe headache may result in more symptoms being reported (Silberstein, 1995). Studies that graded the severity of nausea, photophobia, and phonophobia improved the differentiation of migraine from TTH; by definition, these symptoms were more prevalent and more severe in migraineurs (Silberstein, 1995).

Celentano et al. (1990), using a population-based telephone interview, estimated the prevalence of severe headaches in adolescents and young adults. Symptoms usually considered diagnostic of migraine (nausea and/or vomiting, visual disturbances, and photophobia) were significantly associated with prolonged and more severe pain. Although these symptoms were reported relatively infrequently in the study population, they were associated with headaches that caused the greatest impairment (Silberstein, 1995). We found similar results in a large-population study (Bigal et al., 2006).

The prevalence of migraine-associated symptoms, particularly nausea and vomiting, has also been estimated by placebo-controlled drug studies (Friedman et al., 1989; Cady et al., 1991; Ferrari et al., 2001). Forty-five percent to one hundred percent of patients had nausea prior to treatment, which was similar to prevalence rates observed in other studies of adult migraineurs. The prevalence of vomiting was much lower, but varied dramatically from study to study, as might be anticipated as a result of treatment of the acute migraine attack. Photophobia, when analyzed, occurred in 86%–97% of patients, while phonophobia was rarely analyzed (Silberstein, 1995).

Silberstein performed a telephone interview survey of 500 self-reported migraine sufferers in 1994. The most common reported symptoms associated with migraine, in addition to pain, were nausea, visual problems, and vomiting. Nausea occurred in more than 90% of all migraineurs; nearly one-third of these experienced nausea during every attack. Vomiting occurred in almost 70% of all migraineurs; nearly one-third of these vomited in the majority of attacks. Of those who experienced nausea 30.5% and of those who experienced vomiting 42.2% indicated that the symptom interfered with their ability to take

TABLE 10–4 Prevalence of Associated Symptoms in the Migraine Attack.

Reference	Study type	No. of patients	Nausea	Vomiting	Photophobia	Phonophobia	Visual disturbances	Dizziness
Selby and Lance, 1960	C	500	87	55	82	NR	41	72
Lance and Anthony, 1966	C	500	93	55	49	NR	33	NR
Olesen, 1978	C	750	86	47	NR	NR	20	NR
Iversen et al., 1990	C	30	90	NR	95	97	NR	NR
Davies et al., 1991	C	354 w/o aura w/aura	8985	6060	NRNR	NRNR	NRNR	NRNR
Rasmussen et al., 1991	P	740	82	50	83	86	NR	NR
Lipton et al., 1992	P	2479 (physician diagnosed) (nonphysician diagnosed)	74 (F) 66 (M) 60 (F) 49 (M)	39 (F) 63 (M) 18 (F) 18 (M)	72 (F) 63 (M) 63 (F) 61 (M)	68 (F) 61 (M) 65 (F) 63 (M)	56 (F) 45 (M) 30 (F) 29 (M)	NRNR
Rasmussen and Olesen, 1992a	P	58	95	62	95	98	NR	NR
Russell et al., 1992	C	61 (clinical interview) w/o auraw/aura 61 (headache diary) w/o aura w/aura	85 100 80 53	NR NR NR NR	98 100 82 68	82 100 75 60	NR NR NR NR	NR NR NR NR

their oral migraine medication. Visual problems and vomiting were also reported to occur in most attacks by 70% and 32% of respondents respectively. The only other symptom that occurred in more than 20% of respondents in a majority of attacks was sound sensitivity or auditory problems. Some symptoms that were reported by 10% or less of respondents (light sensitivity, dizziness, neck pain) occurred in a high percentage of their attacks, suggesting that these symptoms may be specific but not sensitive indicators of migraine. Most of the commonly associated symptoms were most often rated as moderate to severe, consistent with the increased severity that would be expected with the more severe headaches in this study (as a result of selection criteria) (Silberstein, 1995).

Nausea and/or vomiting, photophobia, and phonophobia are important criteria for migraine diagnosis, particularly if the headache is not accompanied by aura. Nausea and vomiting also interfere with medication ingestion and were among the principal reasons for a patient discontinuing a specific migraine medication. Gastric emptying can be delayed and oral drug absorption impaired during an attack of migraine (Volans, 1978; Boyle et al., 1990), and vomiting may result in drug loss, thereby compromising the therapeutic effectiveness of orally administered drugs (Silberstein, 1995).

Recent studies indicate that atypical symptoms are common in migraine. These include neck pain/discomfort (59%–61%), as well as sinus pain/pressure (39%–44%) (Dodick et al., 2007). In addition, osmophobia and menstrual exacerbation are associated with migraine.

Postdrome

Following the headache, the patient may have impaired concentration or may feel tired, washed out, irritable, and listless. Some people feel unusually refreshed or euphoric after an attack. Muscle weakness and aching and anorexia or food cravings can occur (Blau, 1982).

The Classification of Migraine

In the ICHD-2, migraine is divided into five categories, the two most important of which are migraine without aura (ICHD-2: 1.1) and migraine with aura (ICHD-2: 1.2). Other major categories include childhood periodic syndromes (ICHD-2: 1.3), retinal migraine (ICHD-2: 1.4), and migraine with complications.

Migraine without Aura

The diagnostic criteria for *Migraine without aura* (1.1) in ICHD-2 published in 2004 are little changed from those published in 1988. They require at least five lifetime attacks, lasting 4–72 hours. In children, attacks may be shorter, 1–72 hours, and in young children photophobia and phonophobia may be inferred from behavior rather than reported (Headache Classification Committee, 2004).

As before, criteria for migraine without aura are met by various combinations of features. Two of four features are required (Table 10–5). Typical unilateral, pulsating headache meets the criteria but so does bilateral, pressing headache if it is moderate or severe in intensity and aggravated by routine physical activity. Associated features include nausea, with or without vomiting, or both photophobia and phonophobia. In addition, neck pain, sinus pain, osmophobia, movement sensitivity, and menstrual exacerbation are part of migraine although not among ICHD-2 defining features.

TABLE 10–5 ICHD-2 Diagnostic Criteria for 1.1 *Migraine without aura.*

A. At least five attacks fulfilling criteria B–D
B. Headache attacks lasting 4–72 hours (untreated or unsuccessfully treated)
C. Headache has at least two of the following characteristics:
   1. Unilateral location
   2. Pulsating quality
   3. Moderate or severe pain intensity
   4. Aggravation by or causing avoidance of routine physical activity (e.g., walking or climbing stairs)
D. During headache at least one of the following:
   1. Nausea and/or vomiting
   2. Photophobia and phonophobia
E. Not attributed to another disorder

Migraine Aura without Headache

Periodic neurologic phenomena, which may be the aura of migraine, can occur in isolation without the headache (Whitty, 1967). These phenomena (scintillating scotoma, recurrent sensory, motor, and mental phenomena) must be differentiated from transient ischemic attacks (TIAs) and focal seizures, and are diagnosed as migraine only after full investigation and reasonable follow-up. Transient visual disturbances (TVDs), with flickering or scintillating phenomena, also occur with numerous other conditions, including blood cell diseases, retinal detachment, cluster headaches, trauma, and syncope, but are not generally associated with cerebrovascular embolic or thrombotic disease (Mattsson and Lundberg, 1999). Headache occurring in association with the symptoms of aura will help confirm the diagnosis but it does not exclude TIA. Ziegler and Hassanein (1990) reported that 44% of their patients who had headache with aura had aura without headache at some time.

Levy (1988) found that 32% of Cornell neurologists had a history of transient neurologic loss; most commonly visual (field cuts, obscurations, scotomata) and less commonly nonvisual symptoms (hemiparesis, clumsiness, paresthesias, dysarthria). Migraine was reported in 29%, occurring in 44% of those reporting and 22% of those not reporting transient central nervous system (CNS) dysfunction. None developed any residual deficit or chronic neurologic disorder at 5-year follow-up, suggesting that these are benign migrainous accompaniments.

Fisher (1980) described transient neurologic phenomena as characteristically not associated with headache (late-life migrainous accompaniments or transient migrainous accompaniments) in 188 patients over the age of 40; 60% were men and 57% had a history of recurrent headache. The attacks of episodic neurologic dysfunction lasted from 1 minute to 72 hours and had variable recurrence rates (1 attack 27%, 2–10 attacks 45%, more than 10 attacks 28%). Scintillating scotoma was considered to be diagnostic of migraine even when it occurred in isolation, whereas other episodic neurologic symptoms (paresthesias, aphasia, and sensory and motor symptoms) needed more careful evaluation (Table 10–6).

Table 10–6 Migraine Equivalents.

Scintillating scotoma
Paresthesias
Aphasia
Dysarthria
Hemiplegia
Blindness
Blurring of vision
Hemianopia
Transient monocular blindness
Ophthalmoplegia
Oculosympathetic palsy
Mydriasis
Confusion-stupor
Cyclical vomiting
Seizures
Diplopia
Deafness
Recurrence stroke deficit
Chorea

Wijman et al. (1998) determined the frequency, characteristics, and stroke outcome of subjects with migrainous visual symptoms in the Framingham study. Visual symptoms occurred in 186 subjects. Visual symptoms that corresponded to the visual aura of migraine were reported by 26 of 186 subjects (14%), with a prevalence of 1.23% overall (1.33% in women and 1.08% in men). The number of occurences ranged from 1 to 500 (10 or more in 69% of subjects) and lasted 15 to 60 minutes in 50% of subjects. In 65% of subjects the episodes were stereotypical. They began after the age of 50 in 77%. The pattern of visual manifestations varied widely among subjects. The episodes were never accompanied by headaches in 58%, and 42% had no headache history. Only in 19% of subjects did the migrainous visual episodes meet the International Headache Society (IHS) criteria for migraine aura, usually because one of the criteria ("at least one aura symptom develops gradually over more than four minutes") could not be reliably ascertained.

Three of twenty-six subjects (11.5%) had a stroke 1 or more years later; one had a subarachnoid hemorrhage (SAH) 1 year later; one had a brainstem infarct 3 years later; and one had a cardioembolic stroke secondary to atrial fibrillation 27 years later. This stroke incidence rate of 11.5% was significantly lower than the stroke incidence rate of 33.3% in subjects with TIAs in the same cohort ($p = 0.030$) (these usually occurred within 6 months) and did not differ from the stroke incidence rate of 13.6% of those without migrainous phenomena or TIAs.

O'Connor and Tredici (1981) described 61 cases of transient neurologic dysfunction in men seen during a 15-year period at the United States (US) Air Force School of Aerospace Medicine. These cases were derived from a selected group of highly trained young men whose profession required outstanding visual abilities. Age of onset was 12–44 years. Family history was present in 15 (24.6%), and a personal history of migraine was present only in 2 (3.3%). Eighteen subjects (29.5%) had nonvisual neurologic deficits during the episodes. Permanent neurologic deficiency occurred in one patient.

Cohen et al. (1984) reported 31 cases of TVD attributed to migraine. Headache was present in 20 patients (64.5%). A family history of migraine was found in 61%; and 57% had a personal history of migraine. After approximately 2 years, one patient died of cardiac disease, none had a stroke, one developed amaurosis fugax, and one developed transient global amnesia.

Mattsson and Lundberg (1999) estimated the prevalence and characteristics of TVD of possible migraine origin in both the clinical and general population. One hundred consecutive women migraine patients (17–69 years) and 245 women (40–75 years) from the general population were interviewed. Lifetime prevalence was 37% in migraine patients and 13% in the general population. There were no differences in the TVD characteristics between the groups. Slightly less than half of each group had a gradual onset of 5 or more minutes (45% and 46% of the groups, respectively). Headache following TVDs had more migrainous features in patients than in controls. The TVDs that did not fulfill the IHS criteria for migraine with aura probably represented abortive migraine phenomena.

Visual migrainous phenomena are not rare,—they occur in 1.33% of women and in 1.08% of men in a general population sample—and are usually benign. Transient migrainous accompaniments (scintillating scotomata, numbness, aphasia, dysarthria, and motor weakness) may occur for the first time after the age of 45 and be easily confused with TIAs of cerebrovascular origin. Diagnosis in all but the most classical cases is still by exclusion (Table 10–7).

TABLE 10–7 Familial Hemiplegic Migraine.

Description

Migraine with aura including hemiparesis and where at least one first-degree relative has identical attacks

Diagnostic criteria

A. Fulfills criteria for 1.2
B. The aura includes some degree of hemiparesis and may be prolonged
C. At least one first-degree relative has identical attacks

Migraine with Aura

In 2004, the criteria for *Migraine with aura* (1.2) were substantially altered (Table 10–8). The typical aura of migraine is characterized by focal neurologic features that usually precede migrainous headache but may accompany it or occur in the absence of the headache (Olesen et al., 1990). Typical aura symptoms develop over ⩾5 minutes and last no more than 60 minutes, and visual aura is overwhelmingly the most common (Jensen et al., 1986). Typical visual auras have a hemianopic distribution. Scotomas (graying out of vision), photopsia or phosphenes, and other visual manifestations may occur. This mixing of positive and negative features is the hallmark of migraine aura. Visual distortions such as metamorphopsia, micropsia, and macropsia are more common in children (Lippman 1952; Silberstein and Young, 1995; Klee and Willanger 1966; Kelman 2004b).

Auras are not always visual. Sensory symptoms occur in up to one-third of patients who have migraine with aura (Manzoni et al., 1985). Sensory auras include numbness (negative symptom) *and* tingling or paresthesia (positive symptoms). The distribution may be cheiro-oral (face and hand). Word-finding difficulty or dysphasia may be part

TABLE 10–8 ICHD-2 Criteria for 1.2.1 *Typical Aura with Migraine Headache.*

A. At least two attacks fulfilling criteria B–D
B. Aura consisting of at least one of the following, but no motor weakness:
   1. Fully reversible visual symptoms including positive features (e.g., flickering lights, spots or lines) and/or negative features (i.e., loss of vision)
   2. Fully reversible sensory symptoms including positive features (i.e., pins and needles) and/or negative features (i.e., numbness)
   3. Fully reversible dysphasic speech disturbance
C. At least two of the following:
   1. Homonymous visual symptoms and/or unilateral sensory symptoms
   2. At least one aura symptom develops gradually over ⩾5 minutes and/or different aura symptoms occur in succession over ⩾5 minutes
   3. Each symptom lasts ⩾5 and ⩽60 minutes
D. Headache fulfilling criteria B–D for 1.1 *Migraine without aura* begins during the aura or follows aura within 60 minutes
E. Not attributed to another disorder

of typical aura. Motor weakness, symptoms of brain stem dysfunction, and changes in level of consciousness all occur (Russel and Olesen, 1996) usually signaling particular subtypes of migraine with aura (hemiplegic, and basilar-type).

Typical migraine aura sometimes occurs with headache types other than migraine (i.e., headache not fulfilling the criteria of 1.1). *Typical aura with nonmigraine headache* (1.2.2) is the correct diagnosis. Typical aura occurs with cluster headache, chronic paroxysmal hemicrania, and hemicrania continua (Silberstein et al., 2000; Matharu and Goadsby, 2001; Peres et al., 2002). These cases are classified based on the aura and the headache (*Typical aura with nonmigraine headache*).

When typical aura occurs in the absence of headache (Whitty, 1967; Willey, 1979; Ziegler and Hanassein, 1990), it is coded *Typical aura without headache* (1.2.3), a disorder most often reported by middle-aged men (Staehelin-Jensen et al., 1981). Differentiating this benign disorder from TIA, a medical emergency, may require investigation, especially when it first occurs after age 40, when negative features (i.e., hemianopia) are predominant or when the aura is of atypical duration (Fisher, 1980).

Familial hemiplegic migraine (1.2.4, FHM) is the first migraine syndrome to be linked to a specific set of genetic polymorphisms (Haan et al., 1997; Carrera et al., 2001; Ducros, 2001; De Fusco et al., 2003). The criteria for this disorder (Klee and Willanger, 1966) include those of *Migraine with aura* (1.2) except that aura includes some degree of motor weakness (hemiparesis) and may be more prolonged than 60 minutes (up to 24 hours); additionally, at least one first-degree relative has had similar attacks (also meeting these criteria) (Table 10–7). Cerebellar ataxia may occur in 20% of FHM sufferers. The onset of weakness may be abrupt, but usually lasts less than 1 hour (Staehelin-Jensen et al., 1981). A person with FHM may develop migraine with aura in adulthood and migraine without aura later in life (Staehelin-Jensen et al., 1981).

The three known loci for FHM are on chromosome 1, 2, and 19, but some families do not link to any of these, indicating that there is at least one additional locus (Ophoff et al., 1996, 1997; Thomsen et al., 2007).

Patients otherwise meeting these criteria but who have no family history of this disorder are classified as having *sporadic hemiplegic migraine* (SHM, 1.2.5), a disorder new to the revised classification (Thomsen et al., 2003).

Basilar-type migraine (1.2.6) is a new term, replacing "basilar migraine." The change is intended to remove the implication that the basilar artery (or, necessarily, its territory) is involved. The distinguishing feature of basilar-type migraine is a symptom profile that suggests posterior fossa involvement (Kuhn et al., 1997). Diagnosis requires at least two of the following aura symptoms, all fully reversible: dysarthria, vertigo, tinnitus, decreased hearing, double vision, visual symptoms simultaneously in both temporal and nasal fields of both eyes, ataxia, decreased level of consciousness, simultaneous bilateral paresthesias. Because 60% of patients with FHM have basilar-type symptoms, basilar-type migraine should be diagnosed only when weakness is absent. The headache meets criteria for 1.1 *Migraine without aura* (Table 10–5).

Childhood Periodic Syndromes That Are Commonly Precursors of Migraine

A number of more or less well-described disorders are classified under this heading (Hosking, 1988) including *Cyclical vomiting* (1.3.1), *Abdominal migraine* (1.3.2), and *Benign paroxysmal vertigo* (1.3.3). These disorders are discussed in Chapter 27.

Retinal Migraine

Retinal migraine is a rare disorder defined by recurrent (at least two) attacks of monocular visual disturbances associated with migraine headache. Visual disturbances may include scintillations, scotomata, or blindness, affecting one eye only, accompanied or followed within 1 hour by migraine headache (fulfilling criteria for 1.1). Other causes of monocular visual loss, including TIA, optic neuropathy and retinal detachment must be ruled out by appropriate investigation (Troost and Zagami, 2000). Though the ICHD-2 criteria require that the visual features be fully reversible, a recent review suggests patients with monocular "aura" experience retinal infarction of migrainous origin (Grosberg et al., 2006). These patients should be coded as *Migrainous infarction* (1.5.4) in the current version of ICHD-2.

Complications of Migraine

The ICHD-2 criteria include a number of complications of migraine starting with *Chronic migraine* (1.5.1), as discussed in Chapter 10.

Status migrainosus (1.5.2) refers to an attack of migraine with a headache phase lasting more than 72 hours (Bento and Esperanca, 2000). The pain is severe (a diagnostic criterion) and debilitating. Non-debilitating attacks lasting more than 72 hours are coded as *Probable migraine without aura* (1.6.1).

Persistent aura without infarction (1.5.13) is diagnosed when aura symptoms, otherwise typical of past attacks, persist for more than 1 week. Investigation shows no evidence of infarction. It is an unusual but well-documented complication of migraine that is now being introduced into the IHS classification (Bento and Esperanca, 2000). If aura symptoms last more than 1 hour (typical aura), but less than 1 week (persistent aura without infarction), a code of 1.6.2 (probable migraine with aura), specifying the atypical feature (prolonged aura), should be assigned.

Migrainous infarction (1.5.4) is an uncommon occurrence. One or more otherwise typical aura symptoms persist beyond 1 hour and neuroimaging confirms ischemic infarction. Strictly applied, these criteria distinguish this disorder from other causes of stroke, which must be excluded (Rothrock et al., 1988). The neurologic deficit develops during the course of an apparently typical attack of migraine with aura, and exactly mimics the aura of previous attacks.

Migraine and epilepsy are comorbid disorders (below). Headaches are common in the postictal period, but epilepsy can be triggered by migraine (migralepsy). The criteria for *Migraine-triggered seizure* (1.5.5) require that a seizure fulfilling diagnostic criteria for one type of epileptic attack occurs during or within 1 hour after a migraine aura (Table 10–9).

Probable Migraine

A significant proportion (between 10% and 45%) of patients with features of migraine fail to meet all criteria for migraine (or any of its subtypes) (Rains et al., 2001). If a single criterion is missing (and the full set of criteria for another disorder are not met), the applicable code is *Probable migraine* (1.6). Epidemiologic studies demonstrate that probable migraine is common and associated

TABLE 10–9 Migraine-triggered seizure

Description:
A seizure triggered by a migraine aura.
Diagnostic criteria:
A. Migraine fulfilling criteria for 1.2 Migraine with aura
B. A seizure fulfilling diagnostic criteria for one type of epileptic attack occurs during or within 1 hour after a migraine aura

Source: Headache Classification committee of the International Headache Society (2004)

with temporary disability and reduction in the health-related quality of life (Patel et al., 2003; Bigal Kolodner, et al., 2006). In a recent large epidemiological study conducted in the US, where 162,576 individuals aged 12 years or more were interviewed, the 1-year period prevalence of probable migraine was 4.5% (3.9% in men and 5.1% in women). In both women and men, prevalence was higher in middle life, between the ages of 30 and 59 years. The prevalence was significantly higher in African–Americans than in Caucasians (female 7.4% versus 4.8%; male 4.8% versus 3.7%) and inversely related to household income. During their headaches, most sufferers (48.2%) had at least some impairment, while 22.1% were severely disabled (Silberstein et al., 2007).

Comorbidities of Migraine

The term "comorbidity," coined by Feinstein, is now widely used to refer to the greater than coincidental association of two conditions in the same individual (Feinstein, 1970). Population-based and clinical studies have provided evidence that migraine sufferers are more likely than others of the same age and gender to have a number of comorbid conditions (Table 10–10), with the strongest data for depression, anxiety disorders, epilepsy, and ischemic cardiovascular disease (CVD). Understanding the comorbidity of migraine is potentially important from a number of different perspectives. True comorbidity implies that having diagnosed one disorder, the comorbid disorder is more likely, not less likely, to be present. This principle of concomitant diagnosis is the opposite of diagnostic parsimony. In addition, comorbidity may impose limitations on treatment opportunities as well as treatment itself.

Table 10–10 Comorbidities of Migraine.

Neurologic
Epilepsy
Stroke
Psychiatric
Depression
Bipolar disease
Anxiety disorders
Panic disorder
Cardiac
Myocardial infarction
Angina
Patent foramen ovale
Other
Raynaud's syndrome
Irritable bowel syndrome
Asthma
Other pain disorders

Methodological Issues

Studies of migraine comorbidity require the consistent application of reliable and valid case definitions, for both migraine and the other disorders being studied, to representative samples. Studies must be adequately powered and bias must be limited. It is ideal to conduct population-based, bi-directional incidence studies. Using this approach persons with migraine, free of the comorbidity, are recruited from the population and followed to estimate rates of onset of the comorbid condition of interest. Similarly, individuals with the comorbidity but free of migraine are followed to estimate the rate of migraine onset. These bi-directional or reciprocal incidence studies have been conducted for depression and anxiety disorders, for nonheadache pain disorders (e.g., back pain), and, to some degree, for epilepsy.

Apparent comorbidity may arise as a diagnostic artifact. For example, TIA may be confused with migraine aura and vice versa. As a consequence, migraine with aura may appear to be comorbid with vascular disease because it is confused with TIA. Migraine and epilepsy both can cause transient alterations of consciousness and headache. Thus, diagnostic uncertainty may lead to a spurious association between disorders.

Migraine and Vascular Disease

The association between migraine and ischemic stroke is well known and has been demonstrated in case–control and cohort studies. Recent studies are summarized in Table 10–4. Until recently, the evidence has been strongest for stroke in young women, particularly for migraine with aura and even more so for women who smoke or use oral contraceptives. (Welch et al., 2003). A recent prospective analysis by Kurth et al. (2005) from the Women's Health Study extended findings to women over age 45. Almost 40,000 female health professionals aged 45 and older were followed for an average of 10 years (Kurth et al., 2005). Classification of migraine and aura were based on self-report. Aura was considered positive if respondents reported they had an "aura or any indication a migraine is coming." Thus defined, migraine with aura was associated with incident ischemic stroke [HR=1.71(1.1–2.7)], with no increased risk for hemorrhagic stroke. The risk of ischemic stroke was most evident for those less than 55 years of age at baseline [HR=2.25 (1.3–3.39)]. Migraine with aura was also a risk factor for other forms of ischemic vascular disease (below). It should be noted that the migraine with aura case group may have been contaminated both with false positives [e.g., TIA misclassified as aura, hypothetically leading to a spurious increased odds ratio (OR)] and with false negatives (e.g., nonspecific prodromal features classified as aura, hypothetically attenuating the OR).

More recently, these results have been extended to male physicians over 40 (Kurth et al., 2007). In this analysis from the Physicians' Health Study, 20,084 men aged 40–84 were followed for a mean of 15.7 years. Migraine diagnosis was based on self-report and there was no information on aura. Results failed to show an increased risk of ischemic stroke [HR=1.12(0.8–1.5)], although there was an interaction by age, with increased risk for the younger men (age 40–54 years at baseline) relative to the older men (age 55–84 at baseline).

Migraine has also been associated with white matter abnormalities (WMAs), although there have been some inconsistencies in results. A meta-analysis by Swartz et al. summarized results from seven case-control studies that considered this question (Swartz and Kern, 2004). The pooled risk of WMA associated with migraine was increased four-fold [3.9 (2.3(6.7)], with the OR similar for studies that included [OR = 3.6 (1.5(8.4)] or excluded [OR=4.1 (2.1–8.4)] individuals with cerebrovascular disease risk factors.

An important population-based study by Kruit et al. demonstrated that some migraineurs are at increased risk for sub-clinical stroke apparent on magnetic resonance imaging (MRI) (Kruit et al., 2004). A cohort of migraineurs with and without aura and a gender- and age-matched comparison group received an MRI and standard neurologic examination. No participants reported a history of stroke, TIA, or had an abnormal neurologic examination. This study had a number of methodological strengths: migraine sufferers and controls were recruited from the general population, headache diagnosis was supervised by expert headache diagnosticians, participants with aura drew their visual symptoms, and evaluation of MRI was done by a neuro-radiologist blind to migraine case status. There was no difference overall in the prevalence of clinically relevant infarcts between the migraineurs and controls. However the migraineurs, particularly those with aura, had an increased likelihood of sub-clinical infarcts in the cerebellar region of the posterior circulation. The highest risk for these lesions was seen in those with migraine with aura and with more than one attack per month [OR = 15.8 (1.8(140)]. In addition, women with migraine (both with and without aura) were roughly twice as likely to have deep white matter lesions as the nonmigraineurs [OR=2.1(1.0–4.1)].Consistent with the earlier studies on clinical stroke and WMAs, these findings were independent of the presence of measured cardiovascular risk factors.

Coronary Heart Disease

Data on the association of migraine and coronary heart disease (CHD) have been inconsistent. Most studies have been positive for an association between migraine and angina and negative for an association with myocardial infarction (MI). Early negative findings emerged from the Physicians Health Study (Cook et al., 2002), the Women's Health Study (Cook et al., 2002), the ARIC study (Rose et al., 2004), a study based on a managed care cohort (Sternfeld et al., 1995)and an earlier study by Waters (Waters et al., 1983). All of these studies were either based on middle-aged or older adults or did not present risk separately for migraine with and without aura. Notably, female migraineurs in the Cook study had a negative CHD risk profile compared to the nonheadache controls based on traditional coronary risk factors (Cook et al., 2002).

Two recent re-analyses (Kurth et al., 2006, 2007) of initially negative results (Cook et al., 2002) from the Women's Health and Physicians' Health Studies suggest that longer follow-up (in this case, an additional 4 years) was necessary to detect a statistically evident increased risk of CHD outcomes in these cohorts. The re-analysis of the Women's Health Study found that migraine with aura was a risk factor for all cause, CVDs including MI [OR=2.08(1.3–3.3)], coronary revascularization [OR=1.74 (1.2(2.5)], and angina [OR = 1.71 [1.2(2.5)] and ischemic CVD death [OR=2.33 (1.2–4.5)] (Kurth et al., 2006). Results were substantially similar after adjustment for many baseline risk factors for coronary artery disease. Migraine without aura was not associated with increased risk of any CVD outcome. The re-analysis of the Physician's Health Study data showed that self-reported migraine was associated with an increased risk of major CVD, [HR=1.24(1.1–1.5)], driven largely by MI [HR=1.4(1.2–1.8)]. No increased risk was seen for ischemic stroke overall (however, note age interaction above), coronary revascularization, angina, or ischemic cardiovascular death.

Finally, in a recent study from an Australian population-based cohort of older men and women (age 49–97) using standardized diagnostic criteria, women with migraine with aura had a (nonsignificantly) increased risk of CHD death [relative risk (RR) = 2.2 (0.8(5.8)] over a 6-year follow-up. No increased risk was seen for male migraineurs (Liew et al., 2007).

A population study by Scher et al. based on a cohort of adults aged 20–65 from the Netherlands, considered whether migraineurs had an elevated risk profile for CHD based on classic risk factors (Scher Bigal, et al., 2005). Results suggested that the migraineurs—particularly those with aura—had an increased likelihood for some CHD risk factors, including an unfavorable cholesterol profile, high blood pressure (for the nondiagnosed migraineurs with aura), and parental history of early MI. Some risk factors (body mass index, waist hip ratio) were not elevated in the migraineurs. It is unclear what, if any, clinical significance these findings mean on an individual basis. However, physicians should be aware that migraineurs—particularly those with aura—may be more likely than expected to have an elevated risk profile for CVD. As this study (as well as the Kurth et al., 2007 study) found an increased likelihood of parental history of early MI in migraineurs with aura, inquiring about family history of early MI or of stroke should also be considered.

Congenital Heart Defects

Patent foramen ovale (PFO) and atrial septal aneurysm (ASA) have been reported to be present more often than expected in persons with migraine with aura. All studies to date have been based on patients in specialty care. As PFO may play a role in cryptogenic stroke—particularly in younger adults—via presumed paradoxical embolism through a right-to-left shunt, might some of the migraine with aura/stroke association be mediated by co-existing PFO? A number of studies have been conducted—all in specialty care patients—measuring the association between migraine and PFO and ASA (Table 10–11). Some trials evaluated the effect on migraine after percutaneous closure of PFO (Table 10–11). Results generally support the notion that migraineurs with aura—at least in specialty care—are more likely than others to have a clinically significant PFO. Further, some early trials or observational studies suggest improvement of migraine after PFO closure.

For example, a study by Schwerzmann et al. 2004 was based on 72 patients with presumed PFO-mediated paradoxical embolism and pre-existing headache (37 with aura, 11 without aura, and 28 with nonmigraine headaches). At follow-up, monthly headache frequency reduced in the MA group (1.2–0.6 attacks/month) and the MO group (1.2–0.4 attacks/month), but not the nonmigraine headache group (1.4–1.0 attacks per month). A similar second study examined 66 patients, of whom 26 had pre-existing migraine (Post et al., 2004). Six months after PFO closure, there was a decrease in the prevalence of MA (from 12/66 to 3/47, $p < 0.05$) but not of MO (from 14/66 to 6/57, $p = 0.11$). Most patients were also treated with low-dose aspirin. Results from these and other (Morandi et al., 2003; Reisman et al., 2003; Kimmelstiel et al., 2007) studies may be limited by the effects of regression towards the mean, as well as

TABLE 10–11 Selected Recent Comorbidity Studies.

	Country	*Year*	*Comorbid condition*	*Source of participants*
Stroke				
Kurth et al., 2006	US	2006	Stroke-female	Female health professionals
Swartz and Kern, 2004	Various	2004	White matter abnormalities	Meta-analysis
Kruit et al., 2004	Netherlands	2004	Sub-clinical stroke, WML	Population
CHD				
Rose et al., 2004	US	2004	Rose angina	Population
Scher Terwindt, et al., 2005	US	2005	CHD risk factors	Population
Kurth et al., 2006	US	2007	CHD	Female health professionals
Kurth et al., 2007	US	2007	CHD	Male physicians
Congenital Heart Defects				
Carerj et al., 2003	Italy	2003	Atrial septal aneurysm	Patients
Lamy et al., 2002	Multicenter	2002	PFO, stroke	Patients
Marcovitz et al., 2003	US	2003	PFO	Patients
Schwerzmann et al., 2005	Switzerland	2005	PFO	Patients
Wilmshurst et al., 2004	UK	2004	PFO, ASD	Patients
Morandi et al., 2003	Italy	2003	PFO closure	Patients (trial)
Post et al., 2004	Belgium	2004	PFO closure	Patients (trial)
Reisman et al., 2005	US	2005	PFO closure	Patients (trial)
Schwerzmann et al., 2004	Switzerland	2004	PFO closure	Patients (trial)

(continued)

TABLE 10–11 (continued)

	Country	*Year*	*Comorbid condition*	*Source of participants*
Kimmelstiel et al., 2007	US	2007	PFO closure	Patients (trial)
Psychiatric				
Breslau et al., 2003	US	2003	Depression	Population
McWilliams et al., 2004	US	2004	Depression, anxiety	Population
Patel et al., 2004	US	2004	Depression	HMO Participants
Smoller et al., 2003	US	2003	Panic attacks	Population
Zwart et al., 2003	Norway	2003	Depression, anxiety	Population
Pain				
El Metwally et al., 2004	Finland	2004	Musculoskeletal pain	3rd, 5th grade children
Hestbaek et al., 2004	Denmark	2004	Low back pain	Population
Von Korff et al., 2005	US	2005	Chronic spinal pain	Population

Abbreviations: ASD, artrial septal defect; CHD, coronary heart disease; HMO, health maintenance organization; PFO, patent foramen ovale; WMLs, white matter lesions.

the influence of natural history, or concomitant treatment.

The MIST trial is the only prospective placebo (sham procedure) controlled randomized trial of PFO closure on migraine. Initial results have been presented in abstract form (Dowson, 2006). Results confirmed a high prevalence (38%) of moderate to large PFOs in this population of migraineurs with aura with frequent (5+ days per month) but not daily (7+ headache-free days per month) headaches who were somewhat refractory to preventive medications. Complete resolution of headache, the primary endpoint, was not different between treatment groups. A secondary endpoint, 50% or more reduction in migraine days, was reached in 42% in the treatment versus 23% of sham patients ($p < 0.038$). The efficacy of PFO closure as a treatment for migraine with aura will presumably become clearer after publication of peer-reviewed results from the initial trial and completion of ongoing studies in the US and the UK (Tepper et al., 2007).

Epilepsy

The association between migraine and epilepsy has been assessed in controlled clinic and voluntary organization-based studies, but not in population-based studies. In the Family Study of Columbia University, 1948 adult probands with epilepsy and 1411 of their parents and siblings were examined to assess the comorbidity of migraine and epilepsy (Lipton et al., 1994; Ottman and Lipton, 1994; Ottman and Lipton, 1996). They reported a two-fold increased risk of migraine in probands with epilepsy. The risk was independent of type of epilepsy, age, and sex. The association was shown to be bi-directional; from migraine to epilepsy and from epilepsy to migraine. In other studies, findings have been inconsistent.

Psychiatric Comorbidity

Cross-sectional associations and bi-directional associations between migraine and a variety of psychiatric and somatic conditions have been reported in numerous studies (Merikangas et al., 1997; Low and Merikangas, 2003;). Herein, we highlight studies which examine the relationship between migraine, depression and anxiety.

Depression is the most extensively studied psychiatric comorbidity of migraine. The odds of depression given migraine in cross-sectional studies range from 2.0 to 4.0 (Crisp et al., 1977; Paulin et al., 1985; Devlen, 1994; Wang et al., 1999; Lipton et al., 2000; Kececi et al., 2003; Zwart et al., 2003; Oedegaard et al., 2006). Breslau et al. measured the bi-directional associations of migraine, severe nonmigraine headache, and depression in a 2-year longitudinal population-based cohort from the Detroit metropolitan area (Breslau et al., 2003). The study examined the relationship between migraine and incident depression as well as depression and incident migraine. The study also assessed the specificity of this association for migraine versus other severe headaches. Results showed that over a 2-year period, having baseline depression increased the risk of incident migraine [RR=3.4(1.4–8.7)], but did not increase the risk of other severe headaches. In addition, the risk of incident depression was higher in those with baseline migraine [RR=5.8(2.7–12.3)], and (marginally higher) in those with severe headache [RR=2.7(0.9–8.1)].

A cross-sectional study of over 50,000 adults aged 20 and older by Zwart et al. (the Nord-Trøndelag Health Study) measured the co-occurrence of headache and depression or anxiety disorders. Measurements included headache diagnosis, a medical examination, and administration of the Hospital Anxiety and Depression scale (Zwart et al., 2003) Overall, the individuals with migraine headache were more likely to have depression [OR=2.7(2.3–3.2)] or anxiety disorders [OR=3.2(2.8–3.6)] than the nonheadache controls. Similar associations were seen for nonmigraine headache and depression [OR=2.2(2.0–2.5)] or anxiety disorders [OR=2.7(2.4–3.0)]. There was a linear trend associated with headache frequency. Thus, for migraine headache of more than 7 days/month, 7–14 days/month, 15+ days/month respectively, the association with depression was OR = 2.0 (1.6(2.5), OR = 4.2 (3.2(5.6), and OR = 6.4 (4.4(9.3). A similar trend was seen for anxiety disorders and for nonmigraine headache with depression or anxiety disorders.

Other studies have linked anxiety disorders to migraine in both clinic- and community-based studies (Harper and Roth, 1962; Garvey et al., 1984; Merikangas et al., 1990; Breslau et al.,

1991; Breslau and Davis, 1993; Stewart et al., 1994; Merikangas, 1996; Breslau, 1998; Smoller et al., 2003; Hung et al., 2005). In general, anxiety tends to precede the onset of depression (Merikangas et al., 1990; Breslau et al., 1991).

It is of interest whether other chronic pain conditions are associated with depression and anxiety to a similar extent as migraine. McWilliams et al. measured the cross-sectional associations between three pain conditions (migraine, arthritis, back pain) and three psychiatric disorders (depression, generalized anxiety disorder, panic attacks) using data from a large adult US population (McWilliams et al., 2004). The associations between the three psychiatric disorders were roughly similar for the three pain conditions (i.e., the association between migraine and depression was roughly similar to the association between back pain and depression). However, the authors noted that the association between pain and anxiety was generally stronger than the association between pain and depression.

Studies assessing migraine and bipolar disease are less convincing than the studies of unipolar depression and anxiety. In clinic-based studies, the prevalence of migraine is elevated in persons with bipolar disease relative to the general population (Cassidy and Flanagan, 1957; Younes et al., 1986; Blehar et al., 1998; Mahmood, 1999; Low et al., 2003). In community studies, bipolar spectrum disorders (Merikangas et al., 1990) bipolar 1 and bipolar 2 are associated with migraine (Breslau).

Comorbid Pain

Migraine is comorbid with other chronic pain conditions in childhood, adolescence, and adulthood (Scher et al., 2006). El-Metwally et al. evaluated 1756 3rd and 5th grade schoolchildren in Finland for the presence of nontraumatic musculoskeletal pain symptoms (El Metwally et al., 2004). They were re-evaluated after 1 and 4-years to determine factors related to the prognosis of musculoskeletal pain. The children with comorbid headache were more likely to have persistent musculoskeletal pain at follow-up compared to the children without comorbid headache.

In a study of over 9000 adolescents and young adults, Hestbaek et al. described conditions comorbid with low back pain (Hestbaek et al., 2004). Headache (not characterized by type) was associated with both moderate low back pain [$\leq$30 days/year; OR=2.1(1.8–2.5)] and with high frequency low back pain [>30 days/year; OR=3.4 (2.3–5.0)].

In the Nord-Trøndelag Health Study the co-occurrence of headache and musculoskeletal symptoms, defined as musculoskeletal pain and/or stiffness in muscles and joints lasting continuously for at least 3 months was studied (Hagen et al., 2002). According to this study, individuals with headache were roughly twice as likely to report musculoskeletal symptoms as those without headache. The elevated risk was similar in those with nonmigrainous [OR=1.8(1.8–1.9)] and migrainous [OR=1.9(1.8–2.0)] headaches. Notably, headache frequency was a stronger predictor of comorbid musculoskeletal symptoms than headache type.

A population-based study by Von Korff et al. studied the comorbidity of chronic back and neck pain with other physical and mental disorders (Von Korff et al., 2005). Data are from the National Comorbidity Survey Replication (NCS-R), a nationally representative face-to-face household survey of adults 18 years of age or older. Chronic spinal pain was defined as self-reported "chronic back or neck problems." Comorbid mental disorders were based on DSM-IV criteria, and included mood disorders, anxiety disorders, and substance use disorders.

Results showed that chronic spinal pain was associated with mood disorders [OR=2.5 (1.9–3.2)], anxiety disorders [OR=2.3(1.9–2.7)], and substance use disorders (primarily alcohol abuse or dependence) [1.6 (1.2–2.2)]. In addition, chronic spinal pain was associated with other chronic pain [OR=4.8(3.9–5.8)], which included arthritis [OR=3.9(3.2–4.7)], migraine [5.2 (4.1–6.4)], other headache [OR=4.0(2.9–5.3)], and any other chronic pain [OR=3.7(2.9–4.7)].

The presence of these disorders can impose therapeutic challenges and limit treatment options. A restricted therapeutic armamentarium can severely compromise treatment. Additionally, patients with major comorbid psychiatric disorders may require ongoing care from a mental health professional appropriate to the disorder.

References

Amery, WK, Waelkens, J, and Caers, I (1986). Dopaminergic mechanisms in premonitory phenomena. In *The Prelude to the Migraine Attack* (WK Amery and A Wauquier, eds.), pp. 64–77. Bailliere Tindall, London.

Amery, WK, Waelkens, J, and Van den Bergh, V (1986). Migraine warnings. *Headache*, 26:60–66.

Anthony, M, Rasmussen, B.K. (1993). Migraine without aura. In *The headaches* (J Olesen, P Tfelt-Hansen, and MA Welch, eds.), pp. 255–261. Raven Press, New York.

Bento, MS and Esperanca, P (2000). Migraine with prolonged aura. *Headache*, 40:52–53.

Bigal, ME, Kolodner, KB, Lafata, JE, et al. (2006). Patterns of medical diagnosis and treatment of migraine and probable migraine in a health plan. *Cephalalgia*, 26(1):43–49.

Bigal, ME, Liberman, JN, and Lipton, RB (2006). Age-dependent prevalence and clinical features of migraine. *Neurology*, 67(2):246–251.

Bigal, ME, Sheftell, FD, Rapoport, AM, et al. (2002). Chronic daily headache in a tertiary care population: correlation between the International Headache Society diagnostic criteria and proposed revisions of criteria for chronic daily headache. *Cephalalgia*, 22(6):432–438.

Blau, JN (1980). Migraine prodromes separated from the aura: complete migraine. *Br Med J*, 281:658–660.

Blau JN (1982). Resolution of migraine attacks: sleep and the recovery phase. *J Neurol Neurosurg Psychiatry*, 45:223–226.

Blehar, MC, DePaulo, JR, Gershon, ES, et al. (1998). Women with bipolar disorder: findings from the NIMH Genetics Initiative sample. *Psychopharmacol Bull*, 34(3):239–243.

Boyle R, Behan PO, Sutton JA (1990). A correlation between severity of migraine and delayed gastric emptying measured by an epigastric impedance method. *Br J Clin Pharmacol*, 30:405–409.

Breslau, N, Davis, GC, and Andreski, P (1991). Migraine, psychiatric disorders and suicide attempts: an epidemiologic study of young adults. *Psychiatr Res*, 37 (1):11–23.

Breslau, N, Lipton, RB, Stewart, WF, et al. (2003). Comorbidity of migraine and depression: investigating potential etiology and prognosis. *Neurology*, 60 (8):1308–1312.

Breslau N, Davis GC (1993). Migraine, physical health and psychiatric disorder: a prospective epidemiologic study in young adults. *J Psychiatr Res*, 27:211–221.

Breslau N, Kessler RC, Chilcoat HD et al (1998). Trauma and posttraumatic stress disorder in the community: the 1996 Detroit Area Survey of Trauma. *Arch Gen Psychiatry*, 55:626–632.

Burstein, R, Yarnitsky, D, Goor-Aryeh, I, et al. (2000). An association between migraine and cutaneous allodynia. *Ann Neurol*, 47:614–624.

Cady, RK, Gutterman, D, Saiers, JA, et al. (1997). Responsiveness of nonIHS migraine and tension-type headache to sumatriptan. *Cephalalgia*, 17:588–590.

Cady RK, Wendt JK, Kirchner JR et al (1991). Treatment of acute migraine with subcutaneous sumatriptan. *JAMA*, 265:2831–2835.

Carrera, P, Stenirri, S, Ferrari, M, et al. (2001). Familial hemiplegic migraine: a ion channel disorder. *Brain Res Bull*, 56:239–241.

Carerj, S, Narbone, MC, Zito, C, et al. (2003). Prevalence of atrial septal aneurysm in patients with migraine: an echocardiographic study. *Headache*, 43(7):725–728.

Cassidy, WL and Flanagan, NB (1957). Clinical observations in manic-depressive disease. *J Am Med Assoc*, 164:1535–1546.

Celentano, DD, Stewart, WF, and Linet, MS (1990). The relationship of headache symptoms with severity and duration of attacks. *J Clin Epidemiol*, 43:983–994.

Cohen GR, Harbison JW, Blair CJ et al (1984). Clinical significance of transient visual phenomena in the elderly. *Ophthalmology*, 91:436–442.

Cook, NR, Bensenor, IM, Lotufo, PA, et al. (2002). Migraine and coronary heart disease in women and men. *Headache*, 42(8):715–727.

Crisp, AH, Kalucy, RS, McGuinness, B, et al. (1977). Some clinical, social and psychological characteristics of migraine subjects in the general population. *Postgrad Med J*, 53(625):691–697.

Dalessio, DJ (1980). Migraine. In *Wolff's headache and other head pain*. (Dalessio, DJ, ed.) pp. 56–130. Oxford University Press, New York.

Davies PT, Peatfield RC, Steiner TJ et al (1991). Some clinical comparisons between common and classical migraine: a questionnaire-based study. *Cephalalgia*, 11:223–227.

De Fusco, M, Marconi, R, Silvestri, L, et al. (2003). Haploinsufficiency of ATP1A2 encoding the Na/K pump a2 subunit associated with familial hemiplegic migraine type 2. *Nat Genet*, 33(2):192–196.

Devlen, J (1994). Anxiety and depression in migraine. *J Roy Soc Med*, 87:338–341.

Diamond, S, Bigal, ME, Silberstein, S, et al. (2007). Patterns of diagnosis and acute and preventive treatment for migraine in the United States: results from the American Migraine Prevalence and Prevention study. *Headache*, 47(3):355–363.

Diamond, S, Freitag, FG, Prager, J, et al. (1985). Olfactory aura in migraine. *N Eng J Med*, 312:1390–1391.

Dodick, D, Kaniecki, R, Mathew, N, et al. (2007). Traditional and non-traditional migraine-associated symptoms: incidence and consistent responsiveness across 4 migraine attacks with sumatriptan 85 RT Technology and naproxen sodium 500 mg (SumaRT/Nap). *Neurology*, 68(Suppl. 1):A195.

Dowson, A. Platform presentation at American Academy of Neurology Annual Meeting, 2006.

Drummond, PD (1987). Scalp tenderness and sensitivity to pain in migraine and tension headache. *Headache*, 27:45–50.

Drummond PD, Lance JW. Clinical diagnosis and computer analysis of headache symptoms. J Neurol Neurosurg Psychiatry 1984 Feb;47:128–133.

Drummond PD (1986). A quantitative assessment of photophobia in migraine and tension headache. *Headache*, 26:465–469.

Ducros, A, Denier, C, Joutel, A, et al. (2001). The clinical spectrum of familial hemiplegic migraine associated with mutations in a neuronal calcium channel. *N Engl J Med*, 345:17–24.

El Metwally, A, Salminen, JJ, Auvinen, A, et al. (2004). Prognosis of non-specific musculoskeletal pain in preadolescents: a prospective 4-year follow-up study till adolescence. *Pain*, 110(3):550–559.

Feinstein, AR (1970). The pretherapeutic classification of comorbidity in chronic disease. *J Chron Dis*, 23:455–468.

Ferrari, MD, Roon, KI, Lipton, RB, et al. (2001). Oral triptans (serotonin 5-HT(1B/1D) agonists) in acute migraine treatment: a meta-analysis of 53 trials. *Lancet*, 358(9294):1668–1675.

Fisher, CM (1980). Late life migraine accompaniments as a cause of unexplained transient ischemic attacks. *Can J Neurol Sci*, 7:9–17.

Friedman, AP, Diserio, FJ, and Hwang, DS (1989). Symptomatic relief of migraine: multicenter comparison of cafergot pb, cafergot, and placebo. *Clin Therap*, 11:170–182.

Garvey, MJ, Tollefson, GD, and Schaffer, CB (1984). Migraine headaches and depression. *Am J Psychiatr*, 141(8):986–988.

Giffin, NJ, Ruggiero, L, Lipton, RB, et al. (2003). Premonitory symptoms in migraine: an electronic diary study. *Neurology*, 60(6):935–940.

Goadsby, P, Lipton, RB, and Ferrari, MF (2002). Migraine—current understanding and treatment. *N Engl J Med*, 346(4):257–270.

Grosberg BM, Solomon S, Friedman DI, et al (2006). Retinal migraine reappraised. *Cephalalgia*, 26:1275–1286.

Haan, J, Terwindt, GM, and Ferrari, MD (1997). Genetics of migraine. *Neurol Clin*, 15:43–60.

Hachinski, VC, Porchawka, J, and Steele, JC (1973). Visual symptoms in the migraine syndrome. *Neurology*, 23:570–579.

Hagen, K, Einarsen, C, Zwart, JA, et al. (2002). The co-occurrence of headache and musculoskeletal symptoms amongst 51 050 adults in Norway. *Eur J Neurol*, 9(5):527–533.

Headache Classification Committee of The International Headache Society (1988). Classification and diagnostic criteria for headache disorders, cranial neuralgias and facial pain. *Cephalalgia*, 8(Suppl. 7):1–96.

Headache Classification Committee of The International Headache Society (2004). International classification of headache disorders (Second Edition). *Cephalalgia*, 24(Suppl. 1):1–160.

Hestbaek, L, Leboeuf-Yde, C, Kyvik, KO, et al. (2004). Comorbidity with low back pain: a cross-sectional population-based survey of 12- to 22-year-olds. *Spine*, 29(13):1483–1491.

Hosking, G (1988). Special forms: variants of migraine in childhood. In *Migraine in Childhood* (JM Hockaday, ed.), pp. 35–53. Butterworths, Boston.

Hung, C, Wang, SJ, Hsu, KH, et al. (2005). Risk factors associated with migraine or chronic daily headache in out-patients with major depressive disorder. *Acta Psychiatr Scand*, 111:310–315.

Hupp, SL, Kline, LB, and Corbett, JJ (1989). Visual disturbances of migraine. *Surv Ophthalmol*, 33:221–236.

Isler, H (1986). Frequency and time course of premonitory phenomena. In *The prelude to the migraine attack* (WK Amery, A Wauquier, eds) pp. 44–53. Bailliere Tindall, London.

Iversen HK, Langemark M, Andersson PG et al. (1990). Clinical characteristics of migraine and episodic tension-type headache in relation to old and new diagnostic criteria. *Headache*, 30:514–519.

Jensen, K, Tfelt-Hansen, P, Lauritzen, M, et al. (1986). Classic migraine, a prospective recording of symptoms. *Acta Neurol Scand*, 73:359–362.

Kececi, H, Dener, S, and Analan, E (2003). Co-morbidity of migraine and major depression in the Turkish population. *Cephalalgia*, 23(4):271–275.

Kelman, L (2004a). The aura: a tertiary care study of 952 migraine patients. *Cephalalgia*, 24(9):728–734.

Kelman, L (2004b). The premonitory symptoms (prodrome): a tertiary care study of 893 migraineurs. *Headache*, 44(9):865–872.

Kimmelstiel, C, Gange, C, and Thaler, D (2007). Is patent foramen ovale closure effective in reducing migraine symptoms? A controlled study. *Catheter Cardiovasc Interv*, 69:740–746.

Klee, A and Willanger, R (1966). Disturbances of visual perception in migraine. *Acta Neurol Scand*, 42:400–414.

Kruit, MC, van Buchem, MA, Hofman, PA, et al. (2004). Migraine as a risk factor for subclinical brain lesions. *JAMA*, 291(4):427–434.

Kuhn, WF, Kuhn, SC, and Daylida, L (1997). Basilar migraine. *Eur J Emerg Med*, 4:33–38.

Kuritzky, A, Ziegler, KE, and Hassanein, R (1981). Vertigo, motion sickness and migraine. *Headache*, 21:227–231.

Kurth, T, Slomke, MA, Kase, CS, et al. (2005). Migraine, headache, and the risk of stroke in women: a prospective study. *Neurology*, 64:1020–1026.

Kurth, T, Gaziano, JM, Cook, NR, et al. (2007). Migraine and risk of cardiovascular disease in men. *Arch Intern Med*, 167:795–801.

Kurth, T, Gaziano, JM, Cook, NR, et al. (2006). Migraine and risk of cardiovascular disease in women. *JAMA*, 296:283–291.

Lamy, C, Giannesini, C, Zuber, M, et al. (2002). Clinical and imaging findings in cryptogenic stroke patients with and without patent foramen ovale: the PFO-ASA Study. Atrial Septal Aneurysm. *Stroke*, 33 (3):706–711.

Lance, JW and Anthony M (1966). Some clinical aspects of migraine. *Arch Neurol*, 15:356–361.

Levy, DE (1988). Transient CNS deficits: a common, benign syndrome in young adults. *Neurology*, 38:831–836.

Liew, G, Wang, JJ, and Mitchell, P (2007). Migraine and coronary heart disease mortality: a prospective cohort study. *Cephalalgia*, 27(4):368–371.

Lippman, CV (1952). Certain hallucinations peculiar to migraine. *J Nerv Ment Dis*, 116:346.

Lipton, RB, Ottman, R, Ehrenberg, BL, et al. (1994). Comorbidity of migraine: the connection between migraine and epilepsy. *Neurology*, 44:S28–S32.

Lipton, RB and Silberstein, SD (1994). Why study the comorbidity of migraine? *Neurology*, 44(10 Suppl. 7): S4–S5.

Lipton, RB, Stewart, WF, Cady, R, et al. (2000). Sumatriptan for the range of headaches in migraine sufferers: results of the Spectrum Study. *Headache*, 40:783–791.

Lipton RB, Hamelsky, SW, Kolodner, KB, et al. (2000). Migraine, quality of life and depression: a population-based case-control study. *Neurology*, 55(5):629–635.

Lipton, RB, Diamond, S, Reed, M, et al. (2001). Migraine diagnosis and treatment: results from the American Migraine Study II. *Headache*, 41:638–645.

Lipton, RB, Stewart, WF, Diamond, S, et al. (2001). Prevalence and burden of migraine in the United States: data from the American Migraine Study II. *Headache*, 41:646–657.

Lipton, RB, Bigal, ME, Diamond, M, et al. (2007). Migraine prevalence, disease burden, and the need for preventive therapy. *Neurology*, 68(5):343–349.

Low, NC, DuFort, GG, and Cervantes, P (2003). Prevalence, clinical correlates, and treatment of migraine in bipolar disorder. *Headache*, 43(9):940–949.

Low, NC and Merikangas, KR (2003). The comorbidity of migraine. *CNS Spectr*, 8(6):433–434, 437–444.

Mahmood, T, Romans, S, and Silverstone, T (1999). Prevalence of migraine in bipolar disorder. *J Affect Disord*, 52(1–3):239–241.

Manzoni, G, Farina, S, Lanfranchi, M, et al. (1985). Classic migraine: clinical findings in 164 patients. *Eur Neurol*, 24:163–169.

Marcovitz, PA, Tobin, KJ, and Cronin, L (2003). Patent Foramen ovalle is more common in migraine headache sufferers than in controls. *J Am Coll Cardiol*, 41(6):466A.

Matharu, MJ and Goadsby, PJ (2001). Post-traumatic chronic paroxysmal hemicrania (CPH) with aura. *Neurology*, 56:273–275.

Mattsson P, Lundberg PO (1999). Characteristics and prevalence of transient visual disturbances indicative of migraine visual aura. *Cephalalgia*, 19:479–484.

McWilliams, LA, Goodwin, RD, and Cox, BJ (2004). Depression and anxiety associated with three pain conditions: results from a nationally representative sample. *Pain*, 111(1–2):77–83.

Merikangas, KR, Angst, J, and Isler, H (1990). Migraine and psychopathology. *Arch Gen Psychiatr*, 47:849–853.

Merikangas, KR, Fenton, BT, Cheng, SH, et al. (1997). Association between migraine and stroke in a large-scale epidemiological study of the United States. *Arch Neurol*, 54(4):362–368.

Merikangas KR, Angst J, Isler H (1981). (Archives of General Psychiatry). Migraine and psychopathology. Results of the Zurich cohort study of young adults. *Arch Gen Psychiatry*, 47:849–853.

Morandi, E, Anzola, GP, Angeli, S, et al. (2003). Transcatheter closure of patent foramen ovale: a new migraine treatment? *J IntervCardiol*, 16(1):39–42.

O'Connor PS, Tredici TJ (1981). Acephalgic migraine. Fifteen years experience. *Ophthalmology*, 88:999–1003.

Oedegaard, K, Neckelmann, D, Mykletun, A, et al. (2006). Migraine with and without aura: association with depression and anxiety disorder in a population-based study. The HUNT Study. *Cephalalgia*, 26(1):1–6.

Olesen, J (1978). Some clinical features of the acute migraine attack. An analysis of 750 patients. *Headache*, 18:268–271.

Olesen, J, Friberg, L, Olsen, TS, et al. (1990). Timing and topography of cerebral blood flow, aura, and headache during migraine attacks. *Ann Neurol*, 28:791–798.

Olesen, J and Lipton, RB (1994). Migraine classification and diagnosis. International Headache Society criteria. *Neurology*, 44(6 Suppl. 4):S6–S10. Review.

Olesen, J, Tfelt-Hansen, P, and Welch, KMA (2000). *The Headaches* (2nd edn). Lippincott, Williams & Wilkins, Philadelphia.

Ophoff, RA, Terwindt, GM, Vergouwe, MN, et al. (1996). Familial hemiplegic migraine and episodic ataxia type-2 are caused by mutations in the Ca^{2+} channel gene CACNL1A4. *Cell*, 87:543–552.

Ophoff, RA, Terwindt, GM, Vergouwe, MN, et al. (1997). Wolff Award 1997. Involvement of a Ca2+ channel gene in familial hemiplegic migraine and migraine with and without aura. Dutch Migraine Genetics Research Group. *Headache*, 37:479–485.

Ottman, R and Lipton, RB (1994). Comorbidity of migraine and epilepsy. *Neurology*, 44:2105–2110.

Ottman, R and Lipton, RB (1996). Is the comorbidity of epilepsy and migraine due to a shared genetic susceptibility? *Neurology*, 47:918–924.

Patel, N, Bigal, ME, Kolodner, K, et al. (2003). Disability and health-related quality of life in strict migraine vs probable migraine (migrainous headache) and control subjects within a health plan. *Cephalalgia*:593. Presented at the XI Congress of the International Headache Society, September 13–16, 2003.

Patel, NV, Bigal, ME, Kolodner, KB, et al. (2004). Prevalence and impact of migraine and probable migraine in a health plan. *Neurology*, 63(8):1432–1438.

Paulin, JM, Waal-Manning, HJ, Simpson, FO, et al. (1985). The prevalence of headache in a small New Zealand town. *Headache*, 25(3):147–151.

Peres, MF, Siow, HC, and Rozen, TD (2002). Hemicrania continua with aura. *Cephalalgia*, 22:246–248.

Post, MC, Thijs, V, Herroelen, L, et al. (2004). Closure of a patent foramen ovale is associated with a decrease in prevalence of migraine. *Neurology*, 62(8):1439–1440.

Rains, JC, Penzien, DB, Lipchik, GL, et al. (2001). Diagnosis of migraine: empirical analysis of a large clinical sample of atypical migraine (IHS 1.7) patients and proposed revision of the IHS criteria. *Cephalalgia*, 21:584–595.

Raskin, NH and Schwartz, RK (1980). Icepick-like pain. *Neurology*, 30:203–205.

Rasmussen, BK and Olesen, J (1992a). Migraine with aura and migraine without aura: an epidemiological study. *Cephalalgia*, 12:221–228.

Rasmussen, BK and Olesen, J (1992b). Symptomatic and nonsymptomatic headaches in a general population. *Neurology*, 42:1225–1231.

Rasmussen BK, Jensen R, Schroll M, et al. (1991). Epidemiology of headache in a general population–a prevalence study. *J Clin Epidemiol*, 44:1147–1157.

Reisman, M, Gray, WA, and Olsen, JV (2003). Relief of migraine headaches associated with closure of patent foramen ovale. *J Am Coll Cardiol*, 41(6):474A.

Reisman M, Christofferson RD, Jesurum J, et al. (2005). Migraine headache relief after transcatheter closure of patent foramen ovale. *J American College of Cardiology*, 15;45:493–495.

Rose, KM, Carson, AP, Sanford, CP, et al. (2004). Migraine and other headaches: associations with Rose angina and coronary heart disease. *Neurology*, 63(12):2233–2239.

Rothrock, JF, Walicke P, Swenson MR, et al. Migrainous stroke. Arch Neurol 1988,45:63–67.

Russel MB and Olesen, J (1996). A nosographic analysis of the migraine aura in a general population. *Brain*, 119:355–361.

Russell MB, Rasmussen BK, Brennum J et al. (1992). Presentation of a new instrument: the diagnostic headache diary. *Cephalalgia*, 12:369–374.

Sacks, O (1985). Migraine: understanding a common disorder. University of California Press, Berkeley.

Saper, JR (1983). Headache disorders: current concepts in treatment strategies. Wright-PSG, Littleton.

Scher, AI, Stewart, WF, Liberman, J, et al. (1998). Prevalence of frequent headache in a population sample. *Headache*, 38:497–506.

Scher, AI, Bigal, ME, and Lipton, RB (2005). Comorbidity of migraine. *Curr Opin Neurol*, 18:305–310.

Scher, AI, Terwindt, GM, Picavet, HSJ, et al. (2005). Cardiovascular risk factors and migraine: the GEM population-based study. *Neurology*, 64:614–620.

Scher AI, Stewart WF, Lipton RB (2006). The comorbidity of headache with other pain syndromes. *Headache*, 46:1416–1423.

Schoonman, GG, Evers, DJ, Terwindt, GM, et al. (2006). The prevalence of premonitory symptoms in migraine: a questionnaire study in 461 patients. *Cephalalgia*, 26(10):1209–1213.

Schwerzmann, M, Nedeltchev, K, Lagger, F, et al. (2005). Prevalence and size of directly detected patent foramen ovale in migraine with aura. *Neurology*, 65:1415–1418.

Schwerzmann, M, Wiher, S, Nedeltchev, K, et al. (2004). Percutaneous closure of patent foramen ovale reduces the frequency of migraine attacks. *Neurology*, 62:1399–1401.

Selby, G and Lance, JW (1960). Observation on 500 cases of migraine and allied vascular headaches. *J Neurol Neurosurg Psychiatr*, 23:23–32.

Silberstein S, Loder E, Diamond S et al. (2007). Probable migraine in the United States: results of the American Migraine Prevalence and Prevention (AMPP) study. *Cephalalgia*, 27:220–234.

Silberstein, SD and Lipton, RB (1994). Overview of diagnosis and treatment of migraine. *Neurology*, 44:6–16.

Silberstein, SD and Young, WB (1995). Migraine aura and prodrome. *Seminars Neurol*, 45:175–182.

Silberstein, SD,(1995). Migrane symptoms: results of a survey of self-reported migraineurs. *Headache*, 35:387–396.

Silberstein, SD and Rosenberg, J (2000). Multispecialty consensus on diagnosis and treatment of headache. *Neurology*, 54:1553.

Silberstein, SD and Lipton, RB (2001). Chronic daily headache, including transformed migraine, chronic tension-type headache, and medication overuse. In *Wolff's Headache and Other Facial Pain* (SD Silberstein, RB Lipton, and DJ Dalessio, eds.), pp. 247–282. Oxford University Press, New York London.

Silberstein, SD (2005). Preventive treatment of headaches. *Curr Opin Neurol*, 18(3):289–292.

Smoller, JW, Pollack, MH, Wassertheil-Smoller, S, et al. (2003). Prevalence and correlates of panic attacks in postmenopausal women: results from an ancillary study to the women's health initiative. *Arch Intern Med*, 163:2041–2050.

Staehelin-Jensen, T, Olivarius, B, Kraft, M, et al. (1981). Familial hemiplegic migraine. A reappraisal and long-term follow-up study. *Cephalalgia*, 1:33–39.

Sternfeld, B, Stang, P, and Sidney, S (1995). Relationship of migraine headaches to experience of chest pain and subsequent risk for myocardial infarction. *Neurology*, 45(12):2135–2142.

Stewart WF, Shechter A, Lipton RB (1994). Migraine heterogeneity. Disability, pain intensity, and attack frequency and duration. *Neurology*, 44:S24–S39.

Swartz, RH and Kern, RZ (2004). Migraine is associated with magnetic resonance imaging white matter abnormalities: a meta-analysis. *Arch Neurol*, 61 (9):1366–1368.

Tepper, SJ, Sheftell, FD, and Bigal, ME (2007). The patent foramen ovale-migraine question. *Neurol Sci*, 28 (Suppl. 2):S118–S123.

Thomsen, LL, Ostergaard, E, Olesen, J, et al. (2003). Evidence for a separate type of migraine with aura: sporadic hemiplegic migraine. *Neurology*, 60:595–601.

Thomsen, LL, Kirchmann, M, Bjornsson, A, et al. (2007). The genetic spectrum of a population-based sample of familial hemiplegic migraine. *Brain*, 130(Pt 2):346–356.

Troost, T and Zagami, AS (2000). Ophthalmoplegic migraine and retinal migraine. In *The Headaches* (J Olesen, P Tfelt-Hansen, and KMA Welch, eds), pp. 511–516. Lippincott Willians & Wilkins, Philadelphia.

Younes, RP, DeLong, GR, Neiman, G, et al. (1986). Manic-depressive illness in children: treatment with lithium carbonate. *J Child Neurol*, 1(4):364–368.

Volans GN (1978). Migraine and drug absorption. *Clin Pharmacokinet*, 3:313–318.

Von Korff, M, Crane, P, Lane, M, et al. (2005). Chronic spinal pain and physical-mental comorbidity in the United States: results from the national comorbidity survey replication. *Pain*, 113:331–339.

Wang, SJ, Liu, HC, Fuh, JL, et al. (1999). Comorbidity of headaches and depression in the elderly. *Pain*, 82 (3):239–243.

Waters, WE, Campbell, MJ, and Elwood, PC (1983). Migraine, headache, and survival in women. *Br Med J (Clin Res Ed)*, 287(6403):1442–1443.

Welch KM (2003). Stroke and migraine—the spectrum of cause and effect. *Funct Neurol*, 18:121–126.

Whitty, CVM (1967). Migraine without headache. *Lancet*, ii:283–285.

Wijman CA, Wolf PA, Kase CS, Kelly-Hayes M et al. (1998). Migrainous Visual Accompaniments Are Not Rare in Late Life : The Framingham Study. *Stroke*, 29:1539–1543.

Wilkinson, M (1986). Clinical features of migraine. In *Handbook of Clinical Neurology* (FC Rose, ed.), pp. 117–133. Elsevier, New York.

Willey, RG (1979). The scintillating scotoma without headache. *Ann Ophthalmol*, 11:581–585.

Wilmshurst, PT, Pearson, MJ, Nightingale, S, et al. (2004). Inheritance of persistent foramen ovale and atrial septal defects and the relation to familial migraine with aura. *Heart*, 90(11):1315–1320.

Ziegler, DK and Hanassein, RS (1990). Specific headache phenomena: their frequency and coincidence. *Headache*, 30:152–160.

Zwart, JA, Dyb, G, Hagen, K, et al. (2003). Depression and anxiety disorders associated with headache frequency. The Nord-Trondelag Health Study. *Eur J Neurol*, 10 (2):147–152.

11 Migraine Treatment

Stephen D Silberstein, Frederick G Freitag, and Marcelo E Bigal

INTRODUCTION

Migraine is a chronic neurologic disease characterized by episodic attacks of headache and associated symptoms (Headache Classification Committee, 2004). In U.S. population studies, migraine prevalence is approximately 18% in women and 6% in men (Lipton and Silberstein, 2001; Lipton et al., 2001, 2007). Approximately 90% of migraine sufferers have moderate or severe pain. Three-quarters of migraineurs have a reduced ability to function and one-third require bed rest during their attacks (Lipton et al., 2001; Lipton et al., 2007). Therefore, effective treatments and treatment strategies play a critical role in reducing the disability, burden, and cost of care for these patients (Matchar et al., 2000). This chapter relied on the triptan meta-analysis (Ferrari et al., 2001), the Technical Reports of the Agency for Healthcare Policy and Research (Goslin et al., 1999; Gray, Goslin, et al., 1999; Gray et al., 1999b, 1999c), U.S. Headache Consortium Guidelines (Ramadan et al., 1999; Matchar et al., 2000), and the recent update of the headache guidelines (SDS in future press).

Effective migraine treatment begins with making an accurate diagnosis, ruling out alternate causes, ordering appropriate studies, and addressing the headache's effect on the patient. An accurate diagnosis should be established before instituting treatment, because a medication that is specific for migraine may be without value or even harmful if used to treat a condition that looks like, but is not, migraine. For example, a patient's acute symptomatic headache due to a stroke or subarachnoid hemorrhage (SAH) may respond to a triptan but the neurologic deficit may be adversely influenced (Rosenberg and Silberstein, 2005).

Once a diagnosis has been made, patients benefit from a full explanation. Patients with recurrent headaches often believe that their complaints have not been taken seriously. They worry that they have a life-threatening condition, such as a brain tumor or an aneurysm. Just as they want headache relief, patients want to know what is wrong with them (Packard, 1979) and to be assured that their physician is committed to relieving their distress. Patients are relieved to find out that their headache is neither secondary to an organic disorder nor psychogenic.

Migraine varies widely in its frequency, severity, and impact on the patient's quality of life. A treatment plan should consider not only the patient's diagnosis, symptoms, and any coexistent or comorbid conditions, but also his or her expectations, needs, and goals. The pharmacologic treatment of migraine may be acute (abortive) or preventive (prophylactic), and patients with frequent, severe headaches often require both approaches. Acute treatment attempts to relieve or stop the progression of an attack or the pain and impairment once an attack has begun. Preventive therapy is given, even in the absence of a headache, to reduce the frequency and severity of anticipated attacks. Additional benefits of preventive therapy include improved responsiveness to acute attack treatment, improved function, and reduced disability. Acute treatment is appropriate for most attacks and should be used a maximum of 2–3 days a week. Preventive therapy is used more selectively.

The patient's most disturbing symptoms must be dealt with in the most appropriate way (Lipton and Silberstein, 1994). Patients have the expectation and the right to participate in their treatment.

Patient commitment improves compliance and fosters the patient–physician relationship. Patients need to be informed of the goals of treatment, the purpose of the various components of their treatment plan, the need for follow-up care, and their medications' adverse effects (AEs). Meeting treatment needs and patient preferences may not always be possible. It is often not possible to fulfill the goals of both complete relief and maintenance of normal function. Patients may prefer one to the other depending on the situation, that is, they would accept sedation from a rescue medication but not from a first-line therapy.

Comorbidity is the presence of two or more disorders, the association of which is more likely than chance. Conditions that occur in migraineurs with a higher prevalence than coincidence include stroke, epilepsy, mitral valve prolapse, Raynaud's syndrome, and certain psychologic disorders, which include depression, mania, anxiety, and panic (Table 11–1). Co-occurring (any other disorder present) and comorbid disease and the presence of nonheadache symptoms present both therapeutic opportunities and limitations. For example, if nausea and vomiting (both migraine-associated symptoms) are prominent, a nonoral route of drug administration is needed.

Table 11–1 Migraine Comorbid Disease.

Cardiovascular
Hyper-/hypotension
Raynaud's
Mitral valve prolapse
Angina/myocardial infarction
PFO (aura) Stroke
Psychiatric
Depression
Mania
Panic disorder
Anxiety disorder
Neurologic
Epilepsy
Essential tremor
Positional vertigo
Restless legs syndrome
GI
Irritable bowel syndrome
Other
Asthma
Allergies

Migraineurs should be educated about their condition and its treatment and encouraged to participate in its management. A headache calendar will help to establish the frequency, intensity, and duration of headache and the presence of associated symptoms, such as aura or nausea and vomiting. Provoking factors, such as menses, missed meals, or too little sleep, can be identified. Once a treatment program has been prescribed, the calendar can be used to show the effectiveness of both acute and preventive treatment (Dalessio, 1987).

A comprehensive headache treatment plan includes (1) education and reassurance; (2) avoiding triggers to prevent attacks; (3) nonpharmacologic treatments, such as relaxation and biofeedback, and life style regulation, such as maintaining a regular schedule, getting adequate sleep and exercise, and stopping smoking; (4) treating the acute attack to stop its progression and relieve pain and impairment; (5) long-term preventive therapy to reduce attack frequency, severity, and duration; (6) physical and alternative medicine when appropriate; and (7) periodic reassessment of the treatment plan.

PROVOKING/ACTIVATING FACTORS (TRIGGERS)

Migraineurs are physiologically and perhaps psychologically hyperresponsive to a variety of internal and external stimuli, including hormonal changes, dietary factors, environmental changes, sensory stimuli, and stress (Saper, 1983; Silberstein and Silberstein, 1990) (Table 11–2). Too much or too little sleep, missed or delayed meals, menstruation, alcohol, food and food additives, chemical and drug ingestion and withdrawal, light glare, and odors have all been reported to provoke or activate migraine in susceptible individuals. Their association is based on anecdotal data and reports of adverse drug reactions. The fact that these stimuli are associated with headache does not prove causality or eliminate the need to consider other etiologies. Since headache is a complaint often attributed to placebo, substance-related headache may arise as a result

TABLE 11–2 Migraine Triggers.

Diet
Hunger
Alcohol
Additives
Certain foods
Chronobiologic
Sleep (too much or too little)
Schedule change
Hormonal changes
Menstruation
Environmental factors
Light glare
Odors
Altitude
Weather Change
Head or neck pain
Of another cause
Physical exertion
Exercise
Sex
Stress and anxiety
Letdown
Head trauma

of expectation. Premonitory symptoms of migraine (chocolate craving, anxiety, exhilaration, or depression) can be mistaken for migraine triggers. Putative migraine triggers may not consistently incite a migraine attack because the migraine threshold may vary with time, depending on intrinsic or extrinsic factors not yet fully understood. This variability may make a migraineur more sensitive to trigger factors at certain times than at others. Several trigger factors occurring within close proximity may be more likely to elicit a migraine than a single trigger factor.

The association between a headache and an exposure may be coincidental (occurring just on the basis of chance) or due to a concomitant illness or a direct or indirect effect of a drug, and may depend on the condition being treated. Headache can be a symptom of a systemic disease, and drugs given to treat such a condition will be associated with headache. Some disorders may predispose to substance-related headache. Alone, neither the drug nor the condition would produce headache. A nonsteroidal anti-inflammatory drug (NSAID) may produce headache by inducing aseptic meningitis in susceptible individuals. The possible relationships between drugs and headache are outlined in Table 11–3 (Silberstein, 1998).

Van den Bergh et al. (1987) collected information on provoking factors in 217 migraineurs. Most patients (85%) were aware of the presence of one or more factors. The most prevalent activating factors were specific foods (44.7%), menstruation (49%), alcoholic beverages (51.0%), and stress (48.8%).

Chabriat et al. did a prospective study of precipitating factors in migraine as part of a national control-matched survey conducted in France. Three hundred eighty-five migraineurs (group 1) and 313 nonmigraineurs (group 2) kept a diary for a 3-month period (a total of 35,805 days in group 1 and 29,109 days in group 2). The most frequent precipitating factors [reported at least once by more than 10% of subjects (range 18%–80% in both groups)] were fatigue and/or sleep, stress, food and/or drinks, menstruation, heat/cold/weather, and infections in both groups. All these factors except infections were reported to cause headache more frequently in migraineurs than in nonmigraineurs (Chabriat et al., 1999).

Zivadinov et al. studied precipitating factors in subjects with migraine and tension-type headache (TTH) in the adult population of Bakar, Croatia. They performed a population-based survey using a "face-to-face door-to-door" interview of 5173 residents aged between 15 and 65 years. A total of 720 lifetime migraine sufferers and 1319 TTH sufferers were identified. The most common precipitants for both migraine and TTH were stress and frequent traveling. Stress [odds ratio (OR) 1.4, 95% confidence interval (CI) 1.17, 1.69] was

TABLE 11–3 Drug and Substance Related Headache.

A. Coincidental
B. Reverse causality
C. Interaction headache
D. Causal
    I. Acute
        a. Primary effect
        b. Secondary effect

associated with migraine, whereas physical activity (OR 0.72, 95% CI 0.59, 0.87) was related to TTH. Frequent traveling (OR 2.2, 95% CI 1.59, 2.99), food items (OR 2.2, 95% CI 1.35, 3.51) and changes in weather conditions and temperature (OR 1.75, 95% CI 1.27, 2.41) exhibited a significant positive association with migraine with aura. Lifetime migraineurs experienced headache attacks preceded by triggering factors more frequently than TTH sufferers. Migraine with aura was more frequently associated with precipitating factors than migraine without aura (Zivadinov et al., 2003).

Karli et al. investigated trigger factors of migraine and TTH in 96 patients. Only five individual trigger factors were significantly different between groups. Hunger and odor were significantly more common in migraine patients. Foods were a significant precipitating factor for headache for migraine with aura patients. Head and neck movements were important trigger factors in episodic TTH (Karli et al., 2005).

Wöber et al. examined potential trigger factors of migraine and TTH in both clinic patients and subjects from the population. One hundred and twenty subjects (66 patients with migraine and 22 with TTH) from a headache outpatient clinic and 32 persons with headache (migraine or TTH) from the population were included. The most common trigger factors were weather (82.5%), stress (66.7%), menstruation (51.4%), and relaxation after stress (50%). Most triggers occurred occasionally and not consistently. The number of triggers experienced was smallest in the population group ($p = 0.002$), whereas the number of triggers known did not differ in the three study groups (Wober et al., 2006). Because common events happen commonly, the association between a headache and an exposure to a substance may be mere coincidence. The possible relationships between drugs and headache are outlined in Table 11–3.

Coincidental. The association between a headache and an exposure may be coincidental (occurring just on the basis of chance). In a population-based study, 1-day point prevalence for any headache was 11% in men and 22% in women (Rasmussen et al., 1991). Headache can be a symptom of a systemic disease, and drugs given to treat such a condition will be associated with headache. For example, drugs used to treat the common cold may have headache identified incorrectly as an adverse drug reaction, since headache can be a symptom of a cold. In acute migraine drug trials, headache, as well as other associated symptoms, are listed as adverse drug reactions despite the fact that they are symptoms of the disorder and not the result of treatment (Silberstein, 1998).

Reverse causality. Premonitory symptoms of migraine (chocolate craving, anxiety, exhilaration, or depression) can mistakenly be believed to be migraine triggers. Thus, the desire for and the consumption of the food may be part of the migraine complex rather than a migraine trigger (Saper, 1983; Silberstein, 1998).

Interaction headache. Some disorders may predispose to substance-related headache or other adverse drug reaction. Alone, neither the drug nor the condition would produce headache. A NSAID may produce headache by inducing aseptic meningitis in susceptible individuals; a lactose intolerant individual might develop a headache after drinking milk (Silberstein, 1998).

Causal. Acute or chronic drug, food, or chemical exposure may be causally related to the headache.

Diet

The role that food allergy plays in migraine is controversial. The most common cause of what patients commonly call "food allergy" is food aversion—a psychological response to the food itself (Bix et al., 1984). Most food reactions are chemically mediated, for example, lactose intolerance (Bayless et al., 1975), nitrites ("hot dog headache") (Raskin, 1981), monosodium glutamate (MSG), which is believed to be responsible for the "Chinese restaurant syndrome" (Schaumberg et al., 1969), red wine (Littlewood et al., 1988), alcohol (Raskin, 1981), and perhaps aspartame (Schiffman et al., 1987; Koehler and Glaros, 1988;) and sucralose (Bigal and Krymchantowski, 2006). Chocolate is probably not a migraine-provoking factor (Moffett et al., 1974) and in a recent double-blind study was not found to be more likely to provoke a migraine headache than carob (Marcus et al., 1997).

Chocolate, alcohol, citrus fruits, and cheese and dairy products are the foods that patients most commonly believe trigger their migraine, but the evidence is not persuasive.

Amino acids. MSG (Schamburg et al., 1969) and aspartame, the active ingredient of "Nutrasweet," may cause headache in susceptible individuals (Schiffmann et al., 1987). Phenylethylamine, tyramine, and aspartame have been incriminated, but their headache-inducing potential is not sufficiently validated.

MSG can induce headache and the Chinese restaurant syndrome in susceptible individuals. The headache is typically dull or burning and nonpulsating, but may be pulsating in migraine sufferers. It is commonly associated with other symptoms, including pressure in the chest, pressure and/or tightness in the face, burning sensations in the chest, neck or shoulders, flushing of the face, dizziness, and abdominal discomfort (Schamburg et al., 1969).

Aspartame, a sugar substitute, is an *o*-methyl ester of the dipeptide L-α-aspartyl-L-phenylalanine that blocks the increase in brain tryptophan, 5-hydroxytryptamine (5-HT), and 5-hydroxyindoleacetic acid normally seen after carbohydrate consumption (Schiffmann et al., 1987). It produced headache in two controlled studies but not in the third (Silberstein, 1998).

Tyramine. Tyramine is a biogenic amine that is present in mature cheeses. It is probably not a migraine trigger (Silberstein, 1998).

Phenylethylamine. Chocolate contains large amounts of β-phenylethylamine, a vasoactive amine that is, in part, metabolized by monoamine oxidase. The evidence to support it as a trigger is weak (Silberstein, 1998).

Ethanol. Ethanol, alone or in combination with congeners (as in wine or liquor), can induce headache in susceptible individuals, often within hours of ingestion (Olesen, 1984). In the United Kingdom, red wine is more likely to trigger migraine than white is, while in France and Italy white wine is more likely to produce headache than red is. Headaches are more likely to develop in response to white wine if red coloring matter has been added (Masyczek and Pugh, 1983). Migraineurs who believed that red wine (but not plain alcohol) provoked their headaches were challenged either with red wine or a vodka mixture of equivalent alcoholic content. The red wine provoked migraine in 9/11 subjects, the vodka in 0/11. Neither provoked headache in other migraine subjects or controls (Littlewood et al., 1988). It is not known which component of red wine triggers headache. Some have suggested that the specific phenolic flavonoids may be the trigger (Littlewood et al., 1987). The headache related to red wine may be blocked by prostaglandin synthesis inhibitors (Kaufman and Starr, 1991).

The susceptibility to hangover headache has not been determined. Migraineurs can suffer a migraine the next day after only modest alcoholic intake, while nonmigraineurs usually need a high intake of alcoholic beverages to develop hangover headache. A few subjects develop headache due to a direct effect of alcohol or alcoholic beverages (cocktail headache). This is much rarer than delayed alcohol-induced headache (hangover headache).

Lactose intolerance is a common genetic disorder that occurs in more than two-thirds of African–Americans, native Americans, and Ashkenazic Jews, and in 10% of individuals of Scandinavian ancestry. The most common symptoms are abdominal cramps and flatulence. How lactose intolerance triggers migraine is uncertain (Silberstein, 1998).

Chocolate. Chocolate is the food most frequently believed to trigger headache, but the evidence supporting this belief is inconsistent (Scharff and Marcus, 1999). Chocolate is probably not a migraine trigger, despite the fact that many migraineurs believe that it triggers their headache. It is the most commonly craved food in the United States. Women are more likely than men to have migraine, and they crave chocolate more than men. Sweet craving is a premonitory symptom of migraine and menses is often associated with an increase in carbohydrate and chocolate craving.

Sucralose. Bigal and Krymchantowski reported a patient with attacks of migraine consistently triggered by sucralose. Withdrawal was associated with complete resolution of the attacks. Single-blind exposure (versus sugar) triggered the attacks, after an attack-free period (Bigal and Krymchantowski, 2006).

Rajendrakumar et al. found a potential causal relationship between sucralose and migraines; it may be important for physicians to remember this can be a possible trigger during dietary history taking (Patel et al., 2006).

The use of elimination diets and clinical ecology is controversial (Egger et al., 1983; MacDonald et al., 1989; Ferguson, 1990; Jewett et al., 1990). Most diet-restriction studies have lacked adequate control groups. Rather than having a "placebo" diet to control for expectation, they have used the patient's usual diet as a baseline control (Salfield et al., 1987). These studies frequently show that headaches are decreased on the restrictive diet compared with baseline (Applebaum, 1984; Bentley et al., 1984; Podell, 1984; Scharff and Marcus, 1999). Carter et al. (1985) have recommended protein-tryptophan and carbohydrate rich diets (Hasselmark et al., 1987).

Medina and Diamond (1978) found no differences in headache indices in 41 migraineurs who were given either a free diet, tyramine-free diet, or tyramine-containing diet.

Dietary manipulation can result in headache improvement, regardless of the type of diet used. Controlled draconian studies have identified differences between restricted and control diets. Ninety-five migraineurs from a neurology clinic were placed on a strict elimination diet (McQueen et al., 1989). Thirty-six (37.9%) dropped out and 37 became headache-free for at least 2 weeks. Nineteen of these 37 individuals then participated in double-blind challenges and went on to the test diet. Response rates to the dietary challenges varied from 21% to 58%. The response to the two placebos was 20% (sucrose) and 32% (starch), respectively. An appropriate diet based on the challenge was then administered to the 19 subjects, this time with a control diet consisting of trigger foods to which the individuals had responded during the challenges. Subjects were randomly assigned either to the approved diet or to the trigger diet, and crossed-over to the other diet after 4 weeks. A 50% reduction in headache occurred in nine subjects in the trigger-elimination diet and in three subjects in the trigger-inclusion diet. Thus, only a small subset of migraineurs could benefit from a strict diet.

Egger (1983) studied 99 children with severe, frequent migraine who had been referred to a tertiary care center. Eighty-eight were able to complete an oligoantigenic diet; of these, 48 were atopic, 41 were hyperactive, and 14 had seizures. Only 40 of 74 completed a double-blind trial. Twenty-six of 40 responded to a previously identified food. However, the challenges were not carried out under medical supervision, and not all of the 40 subjects developed headaches.

MacDonald (1989) used an elimination diet for 60 children with migraine. He concluded that the diet was expensive, difficult to administer, nutritionally inadequate, and not of major benefit in treating migraine.

Practitioners have diagnosed food intolerance by unusual bizarre techniques of laboratory and clinical investigation, such as hair analysis, cytotoxic blood tests, iridology, and sublingual and injection provocation tests (Ferguson, 1990). Jewett et al. (1990), in a double-blind manner, attempted to reproduce allergic symptoms, including headache, by intradermally injecting extracts of suspected allergens. He found that the diagnostic and neutralization procedure, which had been assumed to be fully effective in unblinded use, was due to the placebo response.

It had been believed that vasoactive amines, such as tyramine and phenylethylamines, were responsible for triggering migraine in certain patients. It was suggested that some migraine patients have a tyramine metabolism-conjugating defect (Youdim et al., 1971; Glover et al., 1983). A clinical trial was devised to determine whether dietary triggers in migraine and other headaches could be related to patient suggestibility or allergic mechanisms. While a subset of migraine with aura patients did have headaches related to specific foods, this did not correlate with apparent allergy mediation (Nattero, Savi, et al., 1991).

Previous studies suggested a correlation between foods that reportedly triggered attacks in migraineurs and the levels of the vasoactive amines present. However, recent work using current technology suggests that there is no link between foods that trigger migraine and their vasoactive amine content. Any effect is probably coincidental or purely idiosyncratic (Mosniam et al., 1996; Shulman and Walker, 1999).

Thus, based on current data, most migraineurs do not require severely restricted diets, but they should avoid foods or additives that they feel might provoke their headaches. Migraineurs should consume alcohol, particularly red wine, with caution. They should avoid large amounts of MSG, aspartamine, and perhaps cured meats (nitrites). They should not skip meals. The value of avoiding strong cheeses, pickled herring, chicken liver, and chocolate is unproven and should be restricted only when patients demonstrate a reliable pattern of migraine in conjunction with eating these foods. Patients with a lactase deficiency should use supplemental lactase (Lactaid). Elimination diets are rarely necessary.

Sleep

Alterations in chronobiology, such as too much or too little sleep, can provoke migraine, as can shift work or jet lag. Patients with migraine need to maintain proper sleep practices; that is, keep a regular bedtime and avoid sleeping in on weekends. It has been theorized that migraineurs have a defect in chronobiologic synchronizing systems (Saper et al., 1993).

Hormonal Factors and Migraine

Menstrual Migraine

Menstrual migraine is defined as an attack that occurs up to 1 day before and up to 3 days after the onset of menses. Premenstrual migraine occurs 7 days to 1 day before the onset of menses. Migraine attacks occur around the menses in 60% of women, and exclusively during this period (true menstrual migraine) in 14% (Epstein et al., 1975). Premenstrually it may be accompanied by other features of premenstrual dysphoric disorders, including mood changes, backache, nausea, and breast tenderness and swelling (American Psychiatric Association, 1994). During menstruation, migraine is often associated with dysmenorrhea. Menstrual migraine is most likely due to estrogen withdrawal, which may trigger migraine attacks in susceptible women (Somerville, 1971; Silberstein and Merriam, 1997; Silberstein, 2007b).

Migraine and Pregnancy

Migraine may worsen in the first trimester of pregnancy but significantly improve during the later half of the pregnancy. Twenty-five percent of women have no change. Women with a history of menstrual migraine typically have an improvement of all their migraine types with pregnancy, perhaps because of sustained high estrogen levels (Lance and Anthony, 1966; Somerville, 1972; Bousser et al., 1990; Ratinahirana et al., 1990; Silberstein and Lipton, 1996; Silberstein, 2007b).

Migraine and Menopause

Migraine prevalence decreases with advancing age (Goldstein and Chen, 1982). Menopause may bring regression, worsening, or no change in migraine. Estrogen replacement therapy can exacerbate migraine or prevent natural improvement (Silberstein, 2007b). Women with natural menopause often show an improvement in their migraines while women with surgical menopause often worsen (Neri et al., 1993).

Migraine and Hormonal Contraception

The oral contraceptives (OCs) that are most commonly used in the United States contain combinations of estrogen and progestin and are taken 21 days each month. The older high-estrogen OCs had an increased risk of stroke, but this risk has been significantly reduced with the new, low-estrogen formulations. Progestin-only OCs are also available, as are implantable and injection progestins. New formulations are packaged with an 84-day dosing regimen that results in only four menstrual periods per year (Silberstein, 2007b). Combination OCs can induce, change, or alleviate headache. OCs can provoke the first migraine attack, most often in women with a family history of migraine. Existing migraine may exacerbate, and headaches may predictably occur on the days when women are off the OC. The headache pattern may become more severe and/or frequent and may be associated with neurologic symptoms. The headaches may become refractory to standard treatment. Generally, data from neurologic or migraine clinics show an increased incidence, severity, and refractoriness of migraine in OC users; however, studies from contraceptive clinics and general practitioners are more favorable (Silberstein and Merriam, 1997).

Women with cardiovascular or cerebrovascular risk factors or moderate-to-severe neurologic events in migraine, especially those who smoke, should avoid OCs. Progestin-only hormonal contraception may be safer but probably aggravates headache (Silberstein and Merriam, 1997; Silberstein, 2007b).

OTHER PROVOKING PHENOMENA

Environmental factors, including weather or temperature change, light glare, pungent odors, and high altitude can provoke migraine headache in susceptible individuals (Van den Bergh et al., 1987). Head and neck pain of another cause may also provoke migraine. Physical exertion from exercise or sexual activity can incite headache (Blau, 1987). Stress and anxiety, particularly the post-stress letdown phase, can precipitate a migraine headache, as can head trauma (Diamond, 1964; Lance, 1982; Saper, 1983; Blau, 1987; Van den Bergh et al., 1987; Speed, 1989). Some headache experts believe that most migraine attacks occur from intrinsic provocation or timing not related to external events.

Nonpharmacologic Treatment

Behavioral interventions that are believed to benefit migraineurs include regular exercise, good health practices, regular mealtimes, adequate sleep, and maintenance of accustomed patterns of activity (Saper, 1983). Chronobiologic phenomena may play an important role in provoking migraine. Migraineurs are less capable of adjusting to changes in expected external stimuli, such as mealtimes, stress, or awakening and retiring times. They should maintain a regular pattern of activities of daily living. Mealtimes should be approximately the same time every day, as should retiring and awakening times. The weekends should approximate the rest of the week, including breakfast time and the amount of food eaten early in the morning.

The nonpharmacologic techniques of relaxation training, biofeedback, and formal psychotherapy are useful for selected patients (see Chapter 10). Biofeedback and relaxation therapy also serve to engage patients in cognitive behavioral therapy. These techniques are especially useful for children, pregnant women, and those individuals for whom stress is a trigger. During an acute attack, the patient should avoid uncomfortable sensory stimuli and if possible, retire to a dark, quiet room. Ice packs or heat may be useful adjuncts.

Some migraineurs may find biofeedback using training in electromyography (EMG) and thermal and hand-warming techniques helpful. Those patients who are not depressed, do not have chronic daily headache or medication overuse headache, and are well motivated will probably benefit from these techniques, which can be taught to them by trained technicians (Diamond et al., 1979; Diamond and Montrose, 1984; Duke University and Center for Clinical Health Policy Research, 1999).

Since migraine is a recurrent episodic disorder, periodic follow-up medical management is required. At each visit, the benefits and detrimental effects of treatments should be reviewed and the headache calendar examined. Routine blood work, blood levels of medications, and drug screens can be obtained if necessary (Dalessio, 1987).

NEUROPHARMACOLOGY OF MIGRAINE TREATMENT

Serotonin

Serotonin, or 5-HT, is widely distributed throughout the body, with major concentrations in the gastrointestinal tract (90%), the platelets (8%), and the brain (Table 11–4). The principal cell bodies of 5-HT neurons are located in the raphe nuclei of the brainstem and project throughout the brain and spinal cord. 5-HT, in addition to being released at synapses, may also be released at sites of axonal swelling, termed *varicosities*. When 5-HT is released at nonsynaptic varicosities, it acts by diffusing to its targets. 5-HT is synthesized from L-tryptophan and rapidly accumulated in synaptic vesicles. The 5-HT released by nerve-impulse flow is reaccumulated into the presynaptic terminal by an Na^+-dependent carrier, the 5-HT transporter (Sanders-Bush and Mayer, 2001).

5-HT "recognizes" at least three distinct types of molecular structures: seven guanine nucleotide binding G-protein-coupled receptors, one ligand-gated ion channel, and one transporter (Table 11–4) (Mamounas et al., 1992; Miguel and Hamon, 1992; Waeber and Palacios, 1991; Palacios et al., 1991; Weinshank et al., 1992; Silberstein, 1994; Hoyer et al., 1994b).

TABLE 11–4 5-HT Receptors.

Subtypes	*Gene structure*	*Signal transduction*
G protein-coupled receptors		
5-HT₁ $_{(1A,1B,1C,1E,1F)}$	Intronless	Inhibition of AC
5-HT₂ $_{(2A,2B,2C)}$	Introns	Activation of PLC
$5\text{-}HT_4$	Introns	Activation of AC
$5\text{-}HT_5$ $_{(5A,\ 5B)}$	Introns	Activation of AC for $_{5A}$
$5\text{-}HT_6$	Introns	Activation of AC
$5\text{-}HT_7$	Introns	Activation of AC
Ligand gated ion channels		
$5\text{-}HT_3$	Introns	Ligand-operated ion channel
Transporters		
5-HT uptake site		

AC = adenylyl cyclase;
PLC = phospholipase C

The $5\text{-}HT_1$ family of inhibitory G-protein-linked receptors has five heterogeneous subtypes: A, B, D, E, and F. The $5\text{-}HT_2$ G-protein-linked receptors stimulate phosphoinositol hydrolysis. Other G-protein-coupled receptors are the $5\text{-}HT_4$, $5\text{-}HT_5$, $5\text{-}HT_6$, and $5\text{-}HT_7$ receptors. The $5\text{-}HT_3$ receptor is coupled to an ion channel (Branchek et al., 1991; Monsma et al., 1992; Humphrey et al., 1993; Ruat et al., 1993; Silberstein, 1994; Hoyer et al., 1994b).

The five $5\text{-}HT_1$ family member subtypes can be grouped together on the basis of the absence of introns in the cloned genes, common G-protein transduction systems [including inhibition of adenylate cyclase (AC), with a reduction in cyclic adenosine monophosphate (cAMP) production], and elevation of intracellular calcium concentrations and stimulation of phospholipase-C in transfected cells.

The $5\text{-}HT_{1A}$ receptor has a high selective affinity for 8-OH-DPAT. Drugs such as buspirone act as agonists in cell lines that have a large number of receptors and as antagonists in cell lines that have few receptors, suggesting that this property of a ligand is dependent on receptor density (Humphrey et al., 1993; Peroutka, 1993). The $5\text{-}HT_{1A}$ receptor also activates a receptor-operated K^+ channel and inhibits a voltage-gated Ca^{2+} channel, a common property of receptors coupled to the pertussis toxin-sensitive G_i/G_o family of G proteins. It is found in the raphe nuclei of the brainstem, where it functions as an inhibitory, somatodendritic autoreceptor on cell bodies of serotonergic neurons (Sanders-Bush and Mayer, 2001).

The $5\text{-}HT_{1D}$ receptor subfamily has of two closely related subtypes, $5\text{-}HT_{1D}$ and $5\text{-}HT_{1B}$. Both the human and rodent B and D receptors have been cloned. The rodent $5\text{-}HT_{1B}$ receptor is 97% homologous to the $5\text{-}HT_{1B}$ human receptor, which had been called the $5\text{-}HT_{1D\beta}$ receptor, with the original $5\text{-}HT_{1D}$ receptor being called $5\text{-}HT_{1D\alpha}$.

Both $5\text{-}HT_{1D}$ and $5\text{-}HT_{1B}$ messenger RNA (mRNA) is expressed in human trigeminal ganglia. However, immunoreactivity to $5\text{-}HT_{1D}$ receptors is present on trigeminal nerve endings, while $5\text{-}HT_{1B}$ immunoreactivity is present on cranial blood vessels (Beer et al., 1993; Longmore et al., 1997). The triptans and ergot alkaloids have high affinity for both the human $5\text{-}HT_{1B}$ and $5\text{-}HT_{1D}$ receptors (Waeber and Palacios, 1991; Russell and Olesen, 1995). The $5\text{-}HT_{1D}$ receptor functions as an autoreceptor on axon terminals, inhibiting 5-HT release, as does its rat homolog, $5\text{-}HT_{1B}$. $5\text{-}HT_{1D}$ receptors, abundantly expressed in the substantia nigra and basal ganglia, may regulate the firing rate of dopamine-containing cells and the release of dopamine (DA) at axonal terminals (Sanders-Bush and Mayer, 2001).

The cloned human $5\text{-}HT_{1E}$ receptor has low affinity for 5-carboxamidotriptamine (5-CT) and sumatriptan, unlike other 5-HT_1 receptors (McAllister et al., 1992; Zgombick et al., 1992). The cloned human 5-HT_{1F} receptor, like its closest genetic relative, the 5-HT_{1E} receptor, has low affinity for 5-CT, but differs in its high affinity for sumatriptan (Adham et al., 1993). 5-HT_{1F} receptors do not mediate vasoconstriction. Using autoradiography, 5-HT_{1F} receptors have been localized to areas of the human brain associated with pain transmission (trigeminal nucleus caudalis, substantia gelatinosa of the spinal cord). The density of 5-HT_{1F} receptors in these areas is greater than that of 5-HT_{1D} receptors (Connor and Beattie, 1999).

A selective 5-HT_{1F} receptor agonist, LY334370, that shows approximately 100-fold selectivity for 5-HT_{1F} over other 5-HT_{1B} and 5-HT_{1D} receptors has now been identified (Johnson et al., 1997). This compound inhibits dural plasma protein extravasation (PPE) in guinea pigs at very low doses.

Alniditan has high affinity for 5-HT_{1B} and 5-HT_{1D} receptors but, in contrast to sumatriptan, has relatively low 5-HT_{1F} receptor affinity. Alniditan is more potent than sumatriptan in blocking neurogenic PPE in the dura of anesthetized rats (Limmroth et al., 1997). Thus, 5-HT_{1F} receptor activity is not necessary but could be sufficient for antimigraine activity (Connor and Beattie, 1999).

The 5-HT_2 receptor has three subtypes (5-HT_{2A}, 5-HT_{2B}, 5-HT_{2C}) with close sequence homology, similar intron/exon gene products, the same G-protein-linked transduction system [stimulation of phospholipase-C with the generation of two second messengers, diacylglycerol (DAG) [a cofactor in the activation of protein kinase C (PKC)] and inositol trisphosphate (which mobilizes intracellular stores of Ca^{2+})], and similar operational profiles. The 5-HT_{2A}, 5-HT_{2B}, and 5-HT_{2C} human receptors are all found in the human central nervous system (CNS). The 5-HT_2 classic receptor is now called 5-HT_{2A}. High densities of 5-HT_{2A} receptors are found in the prefrontal, parietal, and somatosensory cortex, the claustrum, and in platelets. The 5-HT_{2B} receptors were originally described in the stomach fundus (hence their original name "5-HT_{2F} fundus receptor"). The expression of 5-HT_{2B} receptor mRNA is highly restricted in the CNS. The 5-HT_{1C} receptor, originally named a "1" receptor on the basis of its high affinity for serotonin, has been renamed the 5-HT_{2C} receptor because of its second messenger and operational properties. The 5-HT_{2C} receptor is regulated by RNA editing, a posttranscriptional event that alters expression of the genetic code at the level of RNA. Multiple receptor isoforms exist within the second intracellular loop; these edited isoforms have modified G protein-coupling efficiencies (Sanders-Bush et al., 2003). 5-HT_{2C} receptors have a very high density in the choroid plexus, an epithelial tissue that is the primary site of cerebrospinal fluid production.

The 5-HT_3 receptors are distinct; they are the only monoamine neurotransmitter receptors that function as ligand-operated ion channels. Evidence suggests the existence of splice variants of the 5-HT_3 receptor. Their activation elicits a rapidly desensitizing depolarization. 5-HT_3 receptors are located on parasympathetic terminals in the gastrointestinal (GI) tract. In the CNS, a high density of 5-HT_3 receptors is found in the solitary tract nucleus and in the area postrema. 5-HT_3 receptors in both the gastrointestinal tract and the CNS participate in the emetic response. Selective 5-HT_3 receptor antagonists are antiemetics and may be useful for irritable bowel syndrome (Fozard, 1992; Humphrey et al., 1993; Peroutka, 1993).

5-HT_4 receptors are G-protein-coupled receptors positively linked to AC (Silberstein, 1994) and were first characterized in the CNS. 5-HT_4 receptors couple to G_s to activate adenylyl cyclase, leading to a rise in intracellular levels of cAMP. In the CNS, they are found on neurons of the superior and inferior colliculi and in the hippocampus. In the GI tract, 5-HT_4 receptors are located on neurons of the myenteric plexus and on smooth muscle and secretory cells. The 5-HT_4 receptor is thought to evoke secretion in the alimentary tract and to facilitate the peristaltic reflex (Sanders-Bush and Mayer, 2001). 5-HT_4 receptor activation may have a role in learning and memory, anxiolysis and analgesia, with proconceptive as well as antinociceptive effects. It has yet to be determined whether there is any role for 5-HT_4 receptors in migraine pathogenesis, or for selective ligands in migraine treatment (Connor and Beattie, 1999).

The 5-HT_5 receptor is subdivided into 5-HT_{5A} and 5-HT_{5B} subtypes. The 5-HT_{5A} receptor inhibits adenylyl cyclase. The signal transduction pathway(s) and physiologic role of the 5-HT_{5B}

receptor are unclear. The cloned 5-HT_6 receptor is positively coupled to AC and expressed within the CNS (Hoyer et al., 1994a; Hoyer and Martin, 1997). It is abundant in extrapyramidal and limbic areas, consistent with a role in the serotonergic control of motor function and mood, respectively. The antipsychotic activity of some neuroleptic agents (e.g., clozapine) may be due to an interaction with 5-HT_6 receptors (Roth et al., 1994).

The 5-HT_7 receptor has now been cloned and sequenced, and its functional properties characterized. It is positively coupled to AC in both neuronal and nonneuronal tissue. The 5-HT_7 receptor is the previously described "5-HT_1-like" receptor that mediates smooth muscle relaxation. 5-HT_7 receptor activation may be involved in cranial vasodilation and nociceptive processing (Watson and Girdlestone, 1996; Eglen et al., 1997; Connor and Beattie, 1999). Multiple splice variants of the 5-HT_7 receptor exist.

Catecholamines (5-HT, NE), Neuropeptides, Triptans, and Migraine

The evidence linking 5-HT to migraine is circumstantial. During a migraine attack, platelet 5-HT decreases, urinary 5-HT increases in some patients, and 5-hydroxyindole acetic acid (5-HIAA), a major metabolite of 5-HT, may increase (Ferrari et al., 1989). These changes in 5-HT are most likely epiphenomena, since changes in the plasma 5-HT levels are probably not of clinical significance in regulating cerebral arterial tone. Other supporting evidence is the observation that headache can be precipitated by reserpine, a 5-HT releaser, relieved by 5-HT or 5-HT_1 agonists, and blocked by pretreatment with methysergide, a 5-HT_2 antagonist (Kimball et al., 1960; Anthony et al., 1967; Somerville, 1976; Fozard, 1982; Ferrari et al., 1989; Lance, 1992; Ferrari and Saxena, 1993b; Silberstein, 1994).

Headaches similar to migraine can be triggered by 5-HT-releasing agents, such as fenfluramine or reserpine, and exacerbated by selective inhibition of 5-HT reuptake (Fozard, 1982). Metachlorophenylpiperazine (mCPP), a metabolite of trazadone, can trigger migraine, conceivably by activating the 5-HT_{2B} or 5-HT_{2C} receptors (Fozard and Gray, 1989). 5-HT infusion has been said to abort a migraine attack, but this could not be replicated by Somerville (1976). 5-HT_1 agonists such as ergotamine, dihydroergotamine (DHE), and the triptans can abort an acute migraine attack. This is not evidence for 5-HT deficiency, as their effectiveness is because, in part, of (1) agonism of 5-HT_1 inhibitory heteroreceptors on the trigeminal nerve blocking neurogenic inflammation and pain transmission (Moskowitz, 1990), and (2) their direct inhibitory effects on pain transmission in the trigeminal nucleus caudalis (Goadsby and Hoskin, 1996; Cumberbatch et al., 1997). DHE and the centrally penetrant triptans have been shown to bind to and inhibit the activity of the nucleus caudalis of the trigeminal complex in the brainstem (Goadsby and Gundlach, 1991). (3) the drugs also being vasoconstrictors and close arteriovenous anastomoses (AVAs). The relevance of this to their mechanism of action is unclear.

Ergotamine, DHE, and the triptans have affinity for the 5-HT_{1B} and 5-HT_{1D} receptors. They have variable affinity for the 5-HT_{1E} and 5-H_{1F} receptors. Ergotamine and DHE also bind to the 5-HT_2, α_1 and α_2 noradrenergic and DA receptors. The acute antimigraine action of both classes of drugs is probably related to their high affinity and agonism for the 5-HT_1 receptor. Some believe that a selective 1D neuronal mechanism is all that is needed and others suggest that 1B agonism is required.

PNU 142633 is a highly selective $5HT_{1D}$ agonist that has the expected pharmacologic effects on biochemical processes. However the drug was comparable to the placebo in a placebo-controlled double-blind trial (McCall, 1999).The 5-HT_{1F} receptor agonists, which are devoid of vasoconstriction activity, have antimigraine activity (Johnson et al., 1997).

Trigeminal sensory neurons contain substance P (SP), calcitonin gene-related peptide (CGRP), and neurokinin A (Uddman et al., 1985). Stimulation results in SP and CGRP release from sensory C-fiber terminals (Buzzi et al., 1991) and neurogenic inflammation (Markowitz et al., 1988). The neuropeptides interact with the blood vessel wall, producing dilation, PPE, and platelet activation (Dimitriadou et al., 1992). One study suggests that neurogenic inflammation occurs in humans (Pappagalo et al., 2002). Neurogenic inflammation sensitizes nerve fibers (peripheral sensitization) that now respond to previously innocuous stimuli, such as blood vessel pulsations (Strassman et al., 1996), causing, in part, the pain of migraine (Moskowitz and Cutrer, 1993). Central sensitization (CS) can also occur. After meningeal irritation, c-fos expression (a marker for neuronal activation) occurs in the trigeminal nucleus caudalis (Nozaki et al., 1992) and in the dorsal horn at the C_1 and C_2 levels (Kaube et al., 1993; Goadsby and Hoskin, 1997).

Superior sagittal sinus stimulation results in CGRP, but not SP, release (Zagami et al., 1990). This is important: CGRP, not SP, is elevated in external jugular venous blood during migraine (Goadsby et al., 1990). Sumatriptan reduced elevated CGRP levels in a migraine attack and in experimental animals during trigeminal ganglion stimulation (Goadsby and Edvinsson, 1993; Edvinsson and Goadsby, 1998). CGRP may play a role in migraine headache (O'Connor and van der Kooy, 1986; O'Connor and Van der Kooy, 1988). A potent specific CGRP antagonist (Doods et al., 2000) has been reported to be effective in acute migraine treatment (Olesen et al., 2003).

Applying an inflammatory soup to the dura sensitizes second-order trigeminovascular neurons (increased spontaneous activity and response to mechanical and thermal skin stimulation) (Strassman et al., 1996). Triptans administered early prevented CS: dural and facial receptive fields did not expand; spontaneous activity and mechanical and thermal sensitivity did not increase. Late triptan intervention did not reverse CS but shrank the expanded dural receptive fields and normalized intracranial mechanosensitivity. CS may play a key role in maintaining the headache (Burstein et al., 2001; Burstein et al., 2002).

Patients often develop cutaneous allodynia (CA) during migraine attacks due to trigeminal sensitization (Burstein et al., 2002). Triptans can prevent, but not reverse, CA (Burstein et al., 2001). CA can be used to predict the effectiveness of triptans (Burstein et al., 2002). When allodynia was not present, triptans completely relieved the headache and blocked the development of allodynia. In 90% of attacks with established allodynia, triptans provided little or no headache relief and did not suppress allodynia. However, late triptan therapy eliminated peripheral sensitization (throbbing pain aggravated by movement) even when pain relief was incomplete and allodynia was not suppressed (Burstein et al., 2002). Early intervention may work by preventing CA and CS. Specific migraine drugs (ergotamine, DHE, and the triptans) that are agonists at presynaptic 5-HT_{1D} and/or 5-HT_{1F} receptors inhibit the release of these neuropeptides, blocking neurogenic inflammation (Saito et al., 1988a; Connor and Beattie, 1999). Methysergide works in this model only after chronic administration; this is consistent with its clinical usefulness as a prophylactic antimigraine drug (Moskowitz, 1990). The NSAIDs block neurogenic inflammation by a direct effect on dural blood vessels (see Chapters 6 and 7 by Goadsby and Karl messlinger, Andrew M Strassman and Rami Burstein).

DHE (Goadsby and Gundlach, 1991) and the brain-penetrant triptans pass through the blood–brain barrier and label nuclei in the brain stem and spinal cord that are intimately involved in pain transmission and modulation. The trigeminal caudalis nucleus, the major relay nucleus for head and face pain, is activated by stimulation of the sagittal sinus, and this activity is transmitted to the thalamus. Both ergots and the brain-penetrant triptans (and sumatriptan, after disruption of the blood–brain barrier), in clinically relevant doses, suppress this activation. These data strongly suggest that the specific migraine drugs exert their antimigraine effect, in part, by a receptor-mediated neural pathway in the CNS with inhibition of pain transmission (Lance, 1986). (Sumatriptan may access the CNS through a more porous blood–brain barrier during a migraine attack.) (see Chapter 7 by Goadsby).

Levy et al. have shown that sumatriptan effectively terminates sensitization in central trigeminovascular neurons (recorded in the dorsal horn), but not in peripheral trigeminovascular neurons (recorded in the trigeminal ganglion). After sensitization was established in both types of neuron, sumatriptan effectively normalized intracranial mechanical sensitivity of central neurons, but failed to reverse hypersensitivity in peripheral neurons. In both the peripheral and central neurons, the drug failed to attenuate the increased spontaneous activity established during sensitization. This suggests that neither peripheral nor central trigeminovascular neurons are directly inhibited by sumatriptan. Rather, triptans act at presynaptic 5HT1B/1D receptors in the dorsal horn to block synaptic transmission between axon terminals of the peripheral trigeminovascular neurons and cell bodies of their central counterparts. This suggests that the analgesic action of triptans can be attained specifically in the absence, but not in the presence, of CS (Levy et al., 2004).

Migraine-specific drugs also constrict meningeal, dural, cerebral, and pial vessels by stimulating vascular 5-HT_{1B} receptors (Humphrey and Feniuk, 1991; Ferrari and Saxena, 1993a; Longmore et al., 1997). They do not have an effect on cerebral hemisphere blood flow (Hachinski et al., 1978; Andersen et al., 1987), which suggests that their effect in migraine is independent of any cerebrovascular vasoconstrictor properties in the arterioles. The ergots and triptans close cerebral AVAs in cats and dogs. Heyck has proposed that migraine is due to the opening of these shunts in humans, but there is no strong supporting data for this theory (Spierings, 1984). The efficacy of the selective 5HT_{1F} receptor agonists suggests that vasoconstriction is not necessary for migraine efficacy.

Before the characterization of 5-HT_2 subtypes, it was believed that 5-HT_2 (now 5-HT_{2A}) receptor antagonism was required for preventive drugs to be effective. The efficacy of the classic serotonin antagonist prophylactic drugs, pizotifen, cyproheptadine, and methysergide, had been ascribed to their 5-HT_2 receptor antagonism. However, there is no correlation between their 5-HT_{2A} receptor affinity and their clinical effectiveness. This suggests that 5-HT_{2A} receptor binding is not relevant. Supporting evidence comes from the observation that some 5-HT_{2A} receptor antagonists, such as mianserin, sergolexole, ketanserin, and ICI 169,369, are not effective migraine preventives (Fozard, 1982, 1990; Silberstein, 1994).

The antiserotonin migraine-preventive drugs are potent 5-HT_{2B} and 5-HT_{2C} receptor antagonists, while mCPP, a 5-HT_{2B} and 5-HT_{2C} receptor agonist, induces migraine in susceptible individuals (Brewerton et al., 1988; Silberstein et al., 1992; Gordon et al., 1993; Baxter et al., 1995). Methysergide, cyproheptadine, and pizotifen, effective migraine prophylactic drugs, are 5-HT_{2B} and 5-HT_{2C} receptor antagonists, while ketanserin, a selective 5-HT_{2A} and a poor 5-HT_{2B} and 5-HT_{2C} receptor antagonist, is not (Fozard and Kalkman, 1994; Fozard, 1995; Kalkman, 1999). Methysergide, pizotifen, cyproheptadine, amitriptyline, propranolol, ketanserin, ritanserin, and mianserin do not discriminate between 5-HT_{2B} and 5-HT_{2C} sites (Kalkman, 1999). The average daily prophylactic human doses of the drugs correlate with their affinity for both 5-HT_{2B} and 5-HT_{2C} receptors (Fozard and Kalkman, 1994; Kalkman, 1999). Ketanserin (Winther, 1995), which lacks affinity for both the 5-HT_{2B} and the 5-HT_{2C} receptor, is not an effective preventive drug.

Brewerton et al. (1988) studied subjects with a prior personal or family history of migraine and found that mCPP, a major metabolite of the antidepressants trazadone and nefazodone, induces migraine hours after the immediate pharmacologic response to the drug (monitored by elevation of plasma cortisol and prolactin) is over. Gordon et al. (1993) used a lower dose of oral mCPP (0.25 mg/kg) than did Brewerton et al. (1988) and found a similar delay in headache onset. Gordon et al. (1993) found that mCPP induced headache in both migraineurs (5 of 8) and nonmigraine controls (4 of 10). No significant differences were found between the migraineurs and normal subjects in terms of their neuroendocrine or headache responses to mCPP, but highly significant associations between the cortisol responses and headache severity and duration existed. The increases in cortisol and body temperature induced by mCPP in humans can be abolished by 5-$HT_{2B/2C}$ receptor antagonists such as ritanserin (Seibyl et al., 1991), metergoline (Mueller et al., 1986; Kahn et al., 1990; Pigott et al., 1991) or methysergide (Kahn et al., 1990).

Pizotifen and methylergometrine are potent rabbit jugular vein endothelial cell 5-HT_2 receptor antagonists. RNA for 5-HT_{2B} receptors is expressed in the endothelial cells of human cerebral vessels (Bouchelet et al., 1996). Fozard (1990, 1995) has speculated that 5-HT_{2B} or 5-HT_{2C} receptor activation by mCPP or endogenously released 5-HT could dilate cerebral vessels. Vasodilation, however, is neither necessary nor sufficient to cause headache (Moskowitz, 1992a, 1992b), but endothelium-derived nitric oxide (NO) can activate sensory trigeminovascular fibers resulting in CGRP release, which mediates pial artery vasodilation (Wei et al., 1992) and neurogenic inflammation (Fozard, 1990, 1995; Moskowitz, 1992b). mCPP itself can produce extravasation in the dural membrane, which can be blocked by selective 5-HT_{2B} antagonists (Nelson, 1996).

Fozard's (1995) speculations cannot explain the delay of head pain in humans following mCPP ingestion. Subjects experience the premonitory symptoms of migraine during the delay time: feelings of exhilaration, exhaustion, anxiety, depression, or cognitive difficulties. mCPP may induce not the headache but incite the prodrome of migraine, which may be of hypothalamic origin.

Methysergide is also a 5-HT_1 receptor agonist that contracts canine, bovine, and human cerebral arteries [the latter is a model for the human 5-HT_{1B} receptor (Muller, 1986, 1992)]. Methysergide has lower affinity for the 5-HT_1 than for the 5-HT_2 binding site (Peroutka and Snyder, 1979). Methysergide-induced contraction of dog isolated saphenous vein is also mediated by 5-HT_{1B} receptors (Saxena and DeVlaam, 1974). Mianserin, cyproheptadine, and, to a large extent, methysergide do not antagonize the serotonin-induced vasoconstriction in the canine carotid vascular bed (Saxena et al., 1971; Saxena, 1972; Saxena and DeVlaam, 1974; Saxena et al., 1986). Methysergide selectively decreases carotid blood flow (Saxena et al., 1971; Saxena, 1974; Humphrey et al., 1990;) by closing AVAs via 5-$HT_{ID/B}$ receptors (Saxena and Verdouw, 1984). This effect, in part due to its metabolite, methylergometrine, is less marked than that of sumatriptan or ergotamine (Bom et al., 1989; DenBoer et al., 1991a; DenBoer et al., 1991b; MacLennan and Martin, 1990).

Chronic, but not acute, treatment with methysergide attenuates dural plasma extravasation following electric stimulation of the rat trigeminal ganglion in the Moskowitz model (Saito et al., 1988b). The difference between acute and chronic drug administration could be due to the accumulation of the active metabolite, methylergometrine. Moskowitz has postulated that methysergide (or methylergometrine) presynaptically inhibits the release of CGRP from perivascular sensory nerves. However, functional antagonism (via vasoconstriction) of the vasodilator effects of CGRP also occurs (Krootila et al., 1992). In addition, there is an interaction with neuropeptide Y (NPY).

Saxena (1974) believes that methysergide's efficacy is due to its vasoconstrictor action within the carotid vascular bed closing AVAs (Saxena and Verdouw, 1984). However, its carotid vasoconstrictor effect is less than that of ergotamine (Saxena, 1972; Bom et al., 1989; DenBoer et al., 1991a; DenBoer et al., 1991b) or sumatriptan (DenBoer et al., 1991b), while its therapeutic effect may be due to its more potent vasoconstricting metabolite, methylergometrine (MacLennan and Martin, 1990; Muller, 1992).

NPY, a 36-amino acid peptide, is co-localized with norepinephrine (NE) in some sympathetic nerves. Both act as vasoconstrictors. In addition, it is one of the most abundant brain peptides found in high concentration in the hypothalamus. NPY is involved in control of body weight. It is a potent appetite stimulant that also reduces energy expenditure by inhibiting the sympathetic nerves that stimulate brown adipose tissue. 5-HT is an anorectic agent when acting via 5-$HT_{2B/2C}$ receptors; when stimulated they inhibit the production and release of NPY. mCPP acting through the 5-$HT_{2B/2C}$ receptor induces anorexia and reduces NPY levels in the paraventricular nucleus (Dryden et al., 1994). Methysergide blocks 5-$HT_{2B/2C}$ receptors and acutely increases NPY secretion and chronically increases NPY mRNA levels. This may account, in part, for the weight gain seen with 5-HT_2 antagonists. NPY also blocks neurogenic inflammation. Could an increase in NPY, in the vicinity of trigeminal nerve endings, account in part for the preventive effect of 5-HT_2 antagonists (Dryden et al., 1995)?

Opioid Receptors

Opioid receptors belong to the large superfamily of seven transmembrane-spanning G protein-coupled receptors (Table 11–5). As a class, G protein-coupled receptors are of fundamental physiologic importance, mediating the actions of the majority of known neurotransmitters and hormones (Waldhoer et al., 2004; Holden et al., 2005).

Four distinct opioid receptor types exist. These are: μ, δ, κ and the N/OFQ receptor (Piros et al., 1996; Bovill, 1997; Darland et al., 1998). Four opioid receptors have been cloned: the MOP1 (μ =_ mu for morphine), the KOP (κ = kappa for ketocyclazocine), the DOP (δ = delta for deferens because it was first identified in the vas deferens of mice), and the NOP-R [initially called LC132 (8), ORL-1 (9), or nociceptin/orphanin FQ receptor]

TABLE 11–5 Opioids.

Receptor	*Cloned receptor*	*Endogenous ligand*	*Agonist*	*Antagonist*
Mu (μ_1, μ_2, μ_3,)	MOP-R	β-Endorphin	Morphine	Naloxone
Delta (δ_1, δ_2,)	DOP-R	Enkephalin		Naloxone
Kappa (κ_1, κ_2, κ_3)	KOP-R	Dynorphin (κ_1)	Butorphanol	Naloxone (κ_3)
Nociceptin/ orphanin FQ receptor Orphan	NOP-R	OFQ/N		

(Waldhoer et al., 2004). There is a disparity between the existence of only four opioids receptor genes and the substantial pharmacologic evidence for additional opioid receptor phenotypes. Post-translational modifications, alternative mRNA splicing, tissue distribution of more than one receptor gene and/or scaffolding with additional proteins, or homo- or heterodimerization of the existing DOP, MOP, KOP, and NOP receptor proteins could result in these various additional pharmacologic phenotypes.

The μ receptor, important in sensory processing, including the modulation of nociceptive stimuli, extrapyramidal functioning, and limbic and neuroendocrine regulation, has three pharmacologic subtypes: a high-affinity μ_1, a low-affinity μ_2, and a μ_3 subtype (Bovill, 1997). MOP receptor (MOP-R) genes have been cloned from rat, mouse, human, and many other species. A number of alternative mRNA splice variants have also been cloned, but their pharmacology does not appear to differ in ligand binding assays. Thus, it is unlikely that these splice variants explain the observation of pharmacologically distinct MOP-R subtypes (Waldhoer et al., 2004). Opioids produce analgesia because of their ability to inhibit the ascending transmission of nociceptive information from the spinal cord dorsal horn and to activate pain control circuits that descend from the midbrain via the rostral ventromedial medulla (RVM) to the spinal cord dorsal horn. Opioids produce analgesia primarily through μ-receptor activation, which also produces respiratory depression, miosis, reduced gastrointestinal motility, and feelings of well-being (euphoria) (Pasternak, 1993). μ-Opioid receptor mRNA and/or ligand binding is seen throughout the periaqueductal gray (PAG), pontine reticular formation, median raphe, nucleus raphe magnus, and adjacent gigantocellular reticular nucleus in the RVM and spinal cord. Most of these spinal μ-receptor ligand-binding sites are located presynaptically on the terminals of primary afferent nociceptors. μ-Opioid receptor mRNA is present in medium- and large-diameter dorsal root ganglion (DRG) cells (Gutstein and Akil, 2006). The supraspinal mechanisms of analgesia produced by μ-opioid agonist drugs are thought to involve the μ_1 receptor, whereas spinal analgesia, respiratory depression, and the effects of opioids on gastrointestinal function are associated with the μ_2 receptor (Reisine and Pasternak, 1996). The μ_3 receptor binds opioid alkaloids, such as morphine, but has exceedingly low or no affinity for the naturally occurring endogenous opioid peptides. The μ_3 receptor occurs in macrophages, astrocytes, and endothelial cells and may be involved in immune processes. The endogenous ligand for this receptor may be morphine or codeine (Bovill, 1997).

Three pharmacologic κ receptor subtypes exist (Table 11–5). Dynorphin A is the natural ligand for the κ_1 receptor, which elicits spinal analgesia. κ_2 sites bind (Arg6, Phe7) Met-enkephalin and DADLE, and the so-called κ_3 site is sensitive to naloxone benzoylhydrazone (Waldhoer et al., 2004). κ-Opioid receptor mRNA and ligand binding are widespread throughout the PAG, pontine reticular formation, median raphe, nucleus raphe magnus, and adjacent gigantocellular reticular nucleus. κ-receptor ligand binding but minimal mRNA have been found in the dorsal horn, κ-opioid receptor mRNA in small- and medium-diameter cells (Gutstein and Akil, 2006). Selective κ-receptor agonists continue to produce analgesia in animals that have been made tolerant to μ agonists. κ_1-receptor agonists act primarily in the spinal cord and cause less intense miosis and respiratory depression than do μ agonists. κ_3 receptor analgesia is mediated supraspinally. Instead of euphoria, κ agonists produce dysphoric psychotomimetic effects (disoriented and/or depersonalized feelings) (Pfeiffer et al., 1986; Reisine and Pasternak, 1996). Cloned KOP-R has high affinity for the endogenous peptide dynorphin A (1–17), similar to the κ_1 receptor (Waldhoer et al., 2004).

Two subtypes of the δ receptor, whose natural ligand is the enkephalins, have been identified (Bovill, 1997). The first opioid receptor to be cloned was the mouse DOP receptor (DOP-R), followed by the discovery of the rat DOP-R, and the human DOP-R in 1994. The cloned DOP-R resembles the δ_1-subtype when expressed in heterologous systems. Whether there is a specific gene or a splice variant encoding for a DOP-R of the δ_2-type remains to be seen (Waldhoer et al., 2004). δ-Opioid receptor mRNA and ligand binding have been demonstrated in the ventral and ventrolateral quadrants of the PAG, the pontine reticular formation, and the gigantocellular reticular nucleus, but only low levels are seen in the median raphe and nucleus raphe magnus. Significant numbers of δ-opioid receptor-binding sites are present in the dorsal horn but there is no detectable mRNA expression, suggesting an important role for presynaptic actions of the δ-opioid receptor in spinal analgesia. (Gutstein and Akil, 2006).

The NOP receptor (NOP-R) was first identified in 1994 because of its extensive nucleotide sequence homology with the δ receptor (Darland et al., 1998). It has been found in human, rat, mouse, pig, and guinea pig. It has greater than 90% sequence identity and approximately 60% homology with the three classical opioid receptors, DOP-R, KOP-R, and MOP-R. Because early ligand-binding studies on the cloned NOP-R found very low levels of binding to all known opioid ligands, this receptor was considered to be an orphan receptor and termed "orphanin FQ," "nociceptin," or "ORL-1" (for opioid receptor-like 1) receptor. The natural ligand for this receptor, an endogenous peptide [nociception/orphanin FQ (N/ORQ)] is part of a larger protein (preoORQ/N), whose gene maps to human chromosome 8p21 (Darland et al., 1998). N/OFQ mRNA and peptides are present throughout descending pain control circuits. N/OFQ-containing neurons are present in the PAG, the median raphe, throughout the RVM, and in the superficial dorsal horn. N/OFQ-receptor ligand binding and mRNA are seen in the PAG, median raphe, and RVM. The effects of N/OFQ on pain responses appear to depend on the preexisting state of pain in the animal and the specific neural circuitry inhibited by N/OFQ (Waldhoer et al., 2004).

The sigma receptor was initially classified as an opioid receptor. However, since the time it was cloned, it has become evident that the sigma receptor is a single transmembrane-spanning protein targeted by other drugs of abuse, for example phencyclidine and its analogs, and it is no longer regarded as a member of the opioid receptor family (Waldhoer et al., 2004).

The opioids have been divided into three groups: morphine and related opioid agonists; opioids with mixed actions, such as nalorphine, butorphanol, and pentazocine, which are agonists at some receptors and antagonists or very weak partial agonists at others; and opioid antagonists, such as naloxone. Mixed agonist/antagonists, such as pentazocine and nalorphine, can produce disturbing psychotomimetic effects that are not effectively blocked by naloxone (Pasternak, 1993; Reisine and Pasternak, 1996).

Most clinically used opioid agonists exert their effects through μ-opioid receptors. δ-Opioid receptor agonists also are potent analgesics in animals, and in some cases they have proved useful in humans. Agonists selective for κ-receptors produce analgesia that is mediated primarily at spinal sites in animals. Instead of euphoria, κ-receptor agonists produce dysphoric and psychotomimetic effects. In neural circuitry mediating reward and analgesia, μ- and κ-agonists have been shown to have antagonistic effects (Waldhoer et al., 2004).

Although many compounds have pharmacologic properties that are similar to morphine, none is clinically superior in relieving pain. Morphine-like drugs produce analgesia without loss of consciousness, and often without drowsiness, changes in mood, or mental clouding. Mixed agonist/antagonists and partial agonists differ from morphine in that they are not full agonists at all opioid receptor subtypes. Nalorphine, cyclazocine, and nalbuphine are competitive μ antagonists but κ receptor agonists. Pentazocine and butorphanol are weaker μ antagonists or partial μ agonist and κ receptor agonists. The combination of μ antagonism and κ agonism is responsible for the designation of these drugs as mixed agonist/antagonist agents (Reisine and Pasternak, 1996).

Second Messengers

The receptor is located on and in the plasma membrane. To transfer information, it is coupled to effectors located in the plasma membrane that include ion channels and multiple G-proteins. The G-proteins that function in transmembrane signaling are heteromers consisting of alpha and beta (subunits in increasing order of molecular weight (Berridge, 1989; Gilman, 1989; Krebs, 1989; Nishizuka, 1989; Simon et al., 1991; Mikoshiba, 1993). G-proteins can be either stimulatory or inhibitory.

After an agonist binds to a G-protein-coupled receptor, a complex rearrangement occurs. In the resting state, guanosine diphosphate (GDP) is bound to the α-subunit. When an agonist binds to the receptor, signaling begins by activating the G-protein. This results in the exchange of GDP for guanosine triphosphate (GTP) on the α subunit of the G-protein and the dissociation of the α-GTP subunit from the beta-(dimer. A single receptor can activate multiple G-protein molecules. The α-GTP and β- subunits may then interact with ion channels or enzymes to generate or prevent generation of regulatory molecules or second messengers. The beta- dimer functions as an anchor for the beta- subunit to the plasma membrane (Gilman, 1989; Simon et al., 1991).

Termination of the signal occurs when the GTP that is bound to the α-subunit is hydrolyzed to GDP. The α-subunit then reassociates with the beta- dimer. Multiple distinct G-proteins have been identified. Pertussis toxin uncouples the receptor from some G-proteins by interacting with the α-subunit, which blocks signal transduction. Some α-subunits are activated by cholera toxin. Intestinal epithelial G-α is the natural target for the toxin: activation results in enhanced fluid secretion into the gut. Inhibitory α-subunits (part of inhibitory G-proteins) also exist that, when activated, result in the inhibition of second message production (Gilman, 1989; Simon et al., 1991).

The cell membrane is like a switchboard, with multiple receptors and different effectors. Ligands can both activate and inhibit receptors that are linked to excitatory and inhibitory G-proteins. The G-protein α-subunit cycles between an inactive GDP-bound state to an active GTP-bound state. The G-protein subunits modulate the activity of membrane and cytoplasmic enzymes. A single α-subunit can interact with more than one effector. (1) G-proteins can stimulate AC activity, leading to cAMP formation and enhanced activity of protein kinase A (PKA). (2) Other pertussis toxin–sensitive G-proteins inhibit AC activity. (3) Some G-proteins can activate the enzyme phospholipase, which hydrolyzes phosphatidylinositol 4,5-biphosphate (PIP_2) into two active messengers, DAG and inositol 1,4,5-triphosphate (IP_3). IP_3 is water soluble, diffuses into the cytosol, and results in the release of calcium. DAG, which is membrane bound, activates PKC. (4) Some G-proteins are directly linked to ion channels, including calcium channels (Gilman, 1989; Nishizuka, 1989).

Phospholipase C beta (PLCβ) is activated through G_q-mediated transduction of signals. Activation leads to cleavage of phosphoinositol 4,5-bisphosphate in the plasma membrane to generate IP_3 and DAG. IP_3 interacts with a specific receptor that is present on the endoplasmic reticulum membrane to promote release of Ca^{2+} into the cytoplasmic compartment. The increased calcium may activate protein kinases, promote secretion, or foster contractile activity. Depletion of intracellular calcium pools by IP_3 results in enhanced uptake of calcium across the plasma membrane. Other phospholipases may also be important in hormone-dependent signaling. Phospholipase D employs phosphatidylcholine as a substrate to generate choline and phosphatidic acid. As with PLC_{PC} above, no IP_3 is generated as a consequence of this reaction. Phospholipase A_2 triggers release of arachidonic acid, a precursor of prostaglandins, leukotrienes, endoperoxides, and thromboxanes, all signaling molecules in their own right (Gardner and Nissenson, 2004).

Protein kinases (PKs) are a large family of proteins (e.g., α, β, γ) with important roles in the regulation of cell function. Some are receptors for tumor promoters. One, PKA, is the effector for cAMP. Another, PKC, is a calcium (Ca^{2+}) and phospholipid (DAG) dependent serine/threonine PK. Activation of PKC through signal transduction is mediated by DAG. However, not all PKC activity derives from the breakdown of PIP_2 substrate. Metabolism of phosphatidylcholine by PLC_{PC} leads to the generation of phosphocholine and DAG. This latter pathway is believed to be responsible for the more protracted elevations in PKC activity seen following exposure to agonists. Other phospholipases may also be important in hormone-dependent signaling (Gardner and Nissenson, 2004). PKC plays an important role in many physiologic functions, including adhesion, secretion, exocytosis, modulation of ion conduction, downregulation of receptors, and gene expression. PKC activates the Ca^{2+} transport ATPase and Na^+/Ca^{2+} exchange protein, both of which remove Ca^{2+} from the cytosol. PKC is also involved in gene expression and C-fos activation, which may be responsible for its role in learning and long-term potentiation (Nishizuka, 1989; Simon et al., 1991; Mikoshiba, 1993).

Inositol triphosphate (IP_3), another second messenger, releases calcium stores and results in intracellular calcium oscillations. IP_3, produced by the G-protein activation of phosphoinositidase, is one part of a bifurcating signaling system, the other limb of which is controlled by DAG. Both are produced by the hydrolysis of PIP_2. IP_3 diffuses into the cytoplasm to release calcium. Its action is terminated by hydrolysis. Ultimately, free inositol, the precursor of PIP_2, is formed. Lithium lowers brain inositol levels by blocking the hydrolysis of inositol monophosphate, resulting in a depletion of the PIP_2 precursor producing receptor desensitization. IP_3 releases calcium from an IP_3-sensitive localized nonmitochondrial pool through one of at least two different high-affinity receptors linked to calcium channels (Mikoshiba, 1993). The IP_3 calcium signal often initiates within a discrete region of the cell and is followed at times by a wave of increased cellular calcium. In some tissues, the Ca^{2+} oscillation frequency is dependent on the external 5-HT concentration. The Ca^{2+} channel activity of the IP_3 receptor is modulated by PKA and PKC. The frequency, as opposed to the amplitude of intracellular calcium oscillations, induced by pulse secretions of IP_3, may be the intracellular signal (Nishizuka, 1989; Simon et al., 1991; Mikoshiba, 1993).

NO is a highly diffusible free-radical gas initially identified in macrophages and endothelial cells, where it is the vascular relaxing factor released in response to acetylcholine. NO is synthesized from the guanidonitrogen of L-arginine by the enzyme NO synthase (NOS). It activates soluble guanyl cyclase, resulting in increased intracellular cyclic GMP (cGMP). In the CNS, NOS is localized in neurons scattered throughout the brain and spinal cord. NO is formed in the postsynaptic neuron following activation of the N-methyl-D-aspartate (NMDA) receptor. Once formed, it can diffuse into the presynaptic neuron, acting as an intercellular messenger. It may induce changes in the synaptic contact between the pre- and postsynaptic neurons, creating synaptic memory. NO may also be involved in the genesis of the headache caused by nitroglycerine. Nitroglycerine is metabolized to NO, which releases CGRP from certain neurons, potentially producing vasodilation and headache. NO may also be the link between activity and cerebral blood flow (Ferrari et al., 1989; Dawson et al., 1992; Ladecola, 1993).

MIGRAINE TREATMENT

Treatment of the Prodrome

Some premonitory symptoms, such as elation, hunger, thirst, and drowsiness, which precede the headache by as much as 24 hours, suggest a hypothalamic disturbance, perhaps mediated by DA and serotonin (Pasternak, 1993). The periodicity of migraine attacks experienced by some migraineurs and the flow of symptoms from prodrome to aura to headache may be regulated by the hypothalamic arcuate nucleus. (see Goadsby, this volume.)

Two studies examined the effect of administering domperidone (an antidopaminergic drug that does not cross the blood–brain barrier) during the migraine prodrome. The first, conducted among patients with migraine with aura found that domperidone, taken at the onset of premonitory symptoms, was significantly more effective than placebo in preventing the headache phase (Amery and Waelkens, 1983). A subsequent study found evidence of a dose–response relationship, with a 40-mg dose significantly more effective than a 20-mg dose (Waelkens, 1984). Domperidone, 30 mg, taken at the earliest appearance of the premonitory symptoms, prevented 66% of headache attacks. No AEs were reported when domperidone was administered during the prodrome.

For maximum efficacy, the drug must be taken at the first appearance of the nonevolutive premonitory symptoms (those that do not merge into the headache and that occur at least 6 hours before the attack). Taking the medication for evolutive prodromal symptoms (occurring within 6 hours of the attack) was not as effective. Spierings (1989) suggested that metoclopramide may be as effective as domperidone.

A single small trial of DHE nasal spray (NS) during the migraine prodrome also demonstrated statistically significant superiority over placebo in preventing the anticipated migraine attack (Massiou, 1987).

Finally, a single open-label trial of naratriptan, 2.5 mg taken at the time subjects knew their headache was inevitable, was positive. Patients with three prodromes separated by at least 48 hours were treated. Twenty patients completed both phases. During the baseline phase, 59 prodromes were reported and all were followed by headache. During the treatment phase, 63 prodromes were reported. Of these, 38 (60%) were not followed by headache. If headaches did occur, most occurred within 2 hours of naratriptan administration (Luciani et al., 2000). The evidence of triptans given during the premonitory phase of migraine is not compelling, however. Preemptive treatment of the migraine attack (except for menstrual migraine) may be of benefit but is still unproven.

Treatment of the Aura

It was previously believed that the migraine aura was caused by cerebral vasoconstriction and the headache by reactive vasodilation (Wolff, 1963). It is now believed that the migraine aura is due to neuronal dysfunction, not ischemia (ischemia rarely, if ever, occurs) (Olesen et al., 1990; Cutrer et al., 1998; Sanchez-del Rio et al., 1999), and the headache is secondary to neurogenic inflammation, not to simple reflex vasodilation (Hadjikhani et al., 2001).

The migrainous aura corresponds to an event moving across the cortex at 2–3 mm/minute (Lashley, 1941). Noxious stimulation of the rodent cerebral cortex produced a spreading decrease in electrical activity that moved at 2–3 mm/minute [cortical spreading depression (CSD)] (Leao, 1944). CSD is characterized by shifts in cortical steady state potential, transient increases in potassium, NO, and glutamate, and transient increases in cerebral blood flow (CBF), followed by sustained decreases (Olesen et al., 1990).

The aura is associated with an initial hyperemic phase followed by reduced CBF, which moves across the cortex (spreading oligemia) (Olesen et al., 1981). Olesen and Lauritzen (Olesen et al., 1981; Olesen, 1991) found 17%–35% reductions in posterior CBF, which spread anteriorly at 2–3 mm/minute. It crossed brain areas supplied by separate vessels and is, thus, not due to segmental vasoconstriction (Olesen, 1991). The absence of diffusion abnormalities at neuroimaging suggests that ischemia does not occur during the aura (Cutrer and O'Donnell, 1999).

Using transcranial magnetic stimulation, which applies magnetic fields of increasing intensity to evaluate occipital cortex excitability, Aurora et al. (1999) and Young et al. (2001) but not Afra et al. (1998) found that phosphenes were generated at lower thresholds in migraineurs than in controls, and that it was easier to visually trigger headaches in those with lower thresholds. Other evidence of increased CNS excitability comes from studies of visual and brainstem auditory evoked potentials (Schoenen and Thomsen, 2000). Migraine with aura may be due to neuronal hyperexcitability, perhaps due to cortical disinhibition.

Treatments for migraine aura are limited and most are based on clinical experience or empiricism. Wolff found that inhaling 10% CO_2 in air for 5 minutes was temporarily effective in decreasing the visual aura of migraine (Dalessio, 1980). Inhaling 10% CO_2 with 90% O_2 was always effective in abolishing the aura of migraine and preventing the development of the expected headache. When headache was present, the effect of 10% CO_2 with 90% O_2 was unpredictable. Alvarez (1934) found that inhaling 100% O_2 for 15–120 minutes produced relief in 42% of his patients. The earlier the treatment, the better the result. Alvarez's patients had a more unpredictable result and required longer treatment than Wolff's patients.

Wolff concluded that the migraine aura was caused by a primary vasoconstriction that could be overridden by the administration of the potent vasodilator arterial carbon dioxide (Dalessio, 1980). However, experimental studies on CSD offer another explanation. Hypercapnic hyperoxia inhibits the propagation of CSD. Thus, the effects of hypercapnia on the migraine aura may be mediated by CSD inhibition (Lauritzen, 1986).

Wolff found that inhaling small amounts of amyl nitrite could temporarily reverse the preheadache scotoma in some subjects (Dalessio, 1980). Inhaling larger amounts of amyl nitrite produced generalized vasodilation, hypotension, and an enlargement of the scotoma.

Kupersmith et al. (1987) found that inhaling isoproterenol (using a Medihaler) at the onset of the aura could abort the neurologic or visual deficit of migraine with aura and basilar migraine. In some cases, the resulting headache was unaffected; in others it became more severe with the use of isoproterenol. Kunkel demonstrated the utility of vasodilators in a small number of patients who had migraine with aura. Administering the vasodilators nitroglycerin or amyl nitrate early in the aura phase of the attacks resulted in resolution of the neurologic symptoms in about half the cases. There was minimal impact on the headache phase or severity (Kunkel, 1982).

Sublingual nifedipine 10 mg was effective in reversing the focal neurologic symptoms of migraine with prolonged aura (including aphasia and a mild right hemianopia) (Miller and Santoro, 1985; Goldner and Levitt, 1987). Scholtz and Hoffer (1987) found that nifedipine was not effective in treating the headache when it was given during the aura of migraine. Subcutaneous (SC) sumatriptan is not effective in treating the headache of migraine when given during the aura (Ensink, 1991).

We have anecdotally found that corticosteroids, neuroleptics, intravenous (IV) magnesium, and IV lasix were effective to treat prolonged or continuous auras with the addition of concomitant preventive medication. Rozen reported two patients with spells of prolonged aura that were treated and apparently aborted with IV furosemide. Furosemide was chosen because IV furosemide has inhibited the generation of CSD in animals (Rozen, 2000). Two patients with prolonged auras were treated with intravenous prochlorperazine combined with intravenous magnesium sulfate. One of the patients was pregnant. This combination was successful at aborting the aura and the headache (Rozen, 2003). In a study of patients seen in emergency departments, patients with migraine with aura who received magnesium sulfate, 1000 mg IV, had reduced aura duration and improvement in their other migraine symptoms (Bigal et al., 2001).

In experimental animals, CSD is mediated through excitatory amino acids and can be blocked by glutamate NMDA receptor antagonists. Kaube et al. studied the effect of the NMDA antagonist ketamine (25 mg intranasally) on the disabling aura symptoms of 11 patients with familial hemiplegic migraine. In five of eleven patients, ketamine reproducibly reduced the severity and duration of the neurologic deficits. Ketamine may offer a possible treatment option for severe and prolonged aura (Kaube et al., 2000).

Calcium channel antagonists (verapamil and flunarizine), anticonvulsants (divalproex, lamotrigine, and gabapentin), and carbonic anhydrase inhibitors may prevent the occurrence of the aura even in the absence of a headache (Lampl et al., 1999). Forteza et al. reported a new North American family with genetically proven cerebral autosomal-dominant arteriopathy with subcortical infarcts and leukoencephalopathy (CADASIL). Their proband experienced resolution of frequent migraines with aura following treatment with acetazolamide. Its transient discontinuation resulted in rapid recurrence of the symptoms and its reinstitution was again successful (Forteza et al., 2001).

Treatment of the Acute Migraine Headache

Migraine treatment is determined by the subtype, severity, and frequency of attacks the patient experiences. Acute medication is indicated even if patients are using preventive medication. It is important to treat the headache as early as possible both to prevent its escalation and to increase the drug's effectiveness, although overuse of acute medication should always be avoided. Often migraine begins with mild to moderate pain and is described as similar to a TTH. As the headache increases in severity, it takes on more migraine-like features. Mild and severe migraine forms respond, in migraineurs, to triptans (Silberstein, 1984; Lipton et al., 1999).

Medication for an acute attack can be specific or nonspecific. Nonspecific medications are used to control the pain and associated symptoms of migraine as well as other pain disorders, while specific medications control the migraine attack but are not useful for nonheadache pain disorders. Nonspecific acute headache medications include analgesics (NSAIDs and combination analgesics), antiemetics, opioids, corticosteroids, and DA antagonists. Specific acute headache medications include ergotamine, DHE, and the selective 5-HT_1 agonists (triptans). It is advisable to develop a treatment strategy for headaches of different severity, using one or more of these drug classes (Silberstein, 1991) that includes initial treatment, a backup treatment, and a rescue treatment, taking into consideration the patient's age and any coexistent illnesses, the migraine type, and the severity, frequency, disability, and associated features (including nausea and vomiting) of the attack.

The following treatment tips are recommended. Tailor the treatment to the attack and to the individual in whom it occurs. Determine the previous response, if any, to previous treatment and the potential for drug overuse. Be aware of all the drugs that the patient is using, both prescription and over-the-counter (OTC). Acute headache medication overuse often causes treatment failure. Headaches are stratified primarily by severity and disability and treated with the medications that are the most likely to be effective for that attack, taking into account the drug's efficacy, safety, and AEs. Maximize the chance that treatment will be effective by using the correct dose and appropriate formulation and treating the attack early.

Strategies for the Acute Treatment of Migraine—Step Care and Stratified Care

Individualize treatment. Patients with mild to moderate attacks can use NSAIDs or combinations such as aspirin plus acetaminophen plus caffeine, or acetaminophen, plus isometheptene, plus dichloralphenazone for initial therapy. Patients with more severe migraine and those whose headaches are known to respond poorly to simple NSAIDs and combination analgesics should be treated with specific agents (triptans, or DHE, and ergotamine in special situations). It is important to get the treatment "right" as soon as possible to reduce pain, disability, and dropouts. Patients who had moderate or nonsevere headache and were stratified to a triptan based on a migraine disability assessment (MIDAS) score that showed moderate or severe disability did better than patients who were given aspirin and metoclopramide. There was less escalation of medication and higher efficacy (Lipton, Stewart, et al., 2000). Failure to use a more effective treatment early may increase the pain, impairment, and impact of the headache. A backup medication is needed in case initial treatment fails. Triptans or DHE can be used if analgesics fail; neuroleptics or parenteral ketorolac or combination analgesics (with opioids or butalbital) can be used if triptans or ergots fail.

The two basic strategies for the acute treatment of migraine are step care and stratified care (Lipton and Silberstein, 2001; Silberstein, Stark, et al., 2006). When step care is used, treatment is escalated across or within attacks. In step care across attacks, patients with migraine progress through a sequence of medications, usually ordered by a combination of perceived safety, cost, and efficacy. This process can last from weeks to months, and many patients lapse from care before effective treatment is found. Simple analgesics are often given as first-line acute treatment. If the treatment is ineffective, an analgesic plus an antiemetic or another therapeutic combination may be prescribed. Only when these simple, often low-cost treatments have failed are specific migraine therapies (e.g., triptans or DHE) considered. Step care within attacks can also consist of initial, nonspecific therapy. However, in contrast to step care across attacks, if the relief is unsatisfactory within a period of time (e.g., 2 hours), the patient may escalate treatment (e.g., from analgesics to migraine-specific therapy) within the attack until relief is achieved or symptoms resolve over time.

The risk of this approach is that the patient may take several different medications to treat a single attack, and there may be a significant delay in taking the necessary migraine-specific medication.

In contrast, stratified care bases treatment selection on an initial assessment of illness severity, much in the way that diabetes, hypertension, asthma, or any other illness that requires ongoing treatment is managed. Patients with minimal or no migraine disability may be well controlled using nonspecific therapies or OTC medications (Lipton and Silberstein, 2001). Patients with significant migraine-related disability may be better controlled with medications that have been proven effective for acute treatment of migraine (e.g., evidence-based recommendations reviewed herein), and effective migraine preventive treatments (evidence-based recommendations reviewed elsewhere) (Silberstein, Stark, et al., 2006). One large, randomized, double-blind, controlled trial (Class I) compared stratified care with step care treatment strategy for migraine and showed that stratified care is associated with better acute treatment efficacy (Lipton, Baggish, et al., 2000). Two additional studies demonstrated that, relative to step care, stratified care is more cost effective for patients and payers (Williams et al., 2001; Sculpher et al., 2002). Therefore, Class I evidence supports the use of stratified care over step care in the acute management of migraine.

In accordance with the recommendations from the U.S. Headache Consortium Guidelines (Matchar et al., 2000; Silberstein, 2000b; Silberstein et al., 2007 guidelines submitted), we endorse the principle of matching treatment with illness severity or disease burden. Migraine care is likely to be effective when treatment is based on attack frequency, severity, the presence and level of disability, and associated nonheadache symptoms (e.g., nausea and vomiting). A stratified-care approach to migraine management may lead to an initial increase in relatively expensive migraine-specific medication, which may in turn produce an initial rise in the direct costs associated with the acute care of migraine. However, studies show that migraine-specific drugs lead to a significant decrease in the number of migraine-related physician office visits, emergency department visits, and medical procedures for patients with migraine-related disability (Williams et al., 2001; Sculpher et al., 2002). Additional studies show that health-related quality of life significantly improved in subjects with higher disability who used migraine-specific therapies compared with those who used nonspecific therapies (Dahlof et al., 1997; Santanello et al., 1997).

Choosing the Right Formulation and Rescue Drug

The formulation and route of administration are based on the attack severity, how rapidly the attack escalates, the patient's preference, the presence or absence of severe nausea or vomiting, and the need for rapid relief. Use a nonoral route and consider an antiemetic when significant early nausea or vomiting is present. Do not restrict antiemetics just to patients who are vomiting or likely to vomit. Nausea itself is one of the most disabling symptoms of migraine and should be treated appropriately (Silberstein, 1997b). Antiemetics, in combination with analgesics, are commonly used in European centers (Olesen et al., 1979; Wilkinson, 1988). In general, for the same chemical entity, injections are faster and more effective than suppositories and NS, which in turn are generally faster acting and more effective than tablets.

For severe migraine, a self-administered rescue medication is needed when other treatments fail. Rescue medications may not completely eliminate pain and return patients to normal activities, but they provide relief without the discomfort and expense of a visit to the physician's office or emergency department. Rescue medications include potent opioids, neuroleptics, and corticosteroids.

Preventing Medication Overuse

Acute headache medication is the best approach when attacks are infrequent or compliance is a problem. Do not give a preventive medication for infrequent headaches that are generally well controlled by acute headache treatment. Treat at least two different attacks before deciding that a drug is ineffective. If there is no benefit from the drug, be sure that the dose is adequate and no other factors interfere with its effect. It may be necessary to change formulation or route of administration or add an adjuvant. Consider changing the drug when the response is incomplete or too slow, the headache recurs, the results are inconsistent after an adequate trial at an adequate dose, or the AEs are bothersome. Guard against medication-overuse headache. In general, limit treatment with acute headache treatment to 2–3 days per week. Medication-overuse headache results from the too frequent use of acute headache medications, often resulting in more frequent headaches that are refractory to treatment (see Chapter 13).

Patients with frequent disabling headaches often overuse analgesics, opioids, ergotamine, and triptans. Overuse is now defined in terms of treatment days per month (ICHD-2) (Headache Classification Committee, 2004). It is crucial that treatment occur both frequently and regularly, that is, several days each week. For example, the diagnostic criterion of use on 10 or more days a month (15 for simple analgesics) translates into 2–3 treatment days every week. The amount of use that constitutes overuse depends on the drug. Ergotamine-overuse headache requires intake on 10 or more days a month on a regular basis for 3 or more months. The headache is often daily and constant. Triptan-overuse headache is usually frequent, intermittent, and migrainous. Triptan intake (any formulation) on 10 or more days a month may increase migraine frequency to that of chronic migraine. Evidence suggests that this occurs sooner with triptan overuse than with ergotamine overuse. The actual limit of symptomatic drug use and duration beyond which rebound occurs are unknown (Headache Classification Committee, 2004; Headache Classification Committee, 2006).

Medication overuse by headache-prone patients can incite chronic daily headache, with growing dependence and habituation to symptomatic medication (Saper, 1983, 1986) (see Chapter 10—CDH). Following discontinuation of acute medication, withdrawal symptoms (including increased headache) and refractoriness to preventive medications are characteristic (Kudrow, 1982; Saper, 1983, 1986; Mathew, 1990). Stopping the acute medication will usually result in headache improvement after a period of increased headache (analgesic washout period) (Saper, 1986; Rapoport and Weeks, 1988; Baumgartner et al., 1989; Silberstein et al., 1996). In addition to the induction of chronic refractory headache, each class of medication has unique AEs: ergotism, analgesic nephropathy, gastrointestinal problems (including dyspepsia and ulcers), and anemia.

Nonpharmacologic treatment can be helpful. At the first sign of the attack, patients should remove themselves from situations of sensory overstimulation; if possible, they should rest in a dark, quiet room, apply an ice pack, and use acute medication. Pressure over the superficial temporal artery on the affected side is often temporarily effective.

For practical purposes, we have provided general and arbitrary guidelines. To maintain a drug-free interval between the days of drug use, it is important to limit the number of treatment days the drug is used per week (events) as well as the maximum amount of drug used per month. Another empiric strategy to limit overuse is to use alternate classes of medications. For example, alternate an NSAID with a triptan or DHE with a neuroleptic. However, no evidence exists to prove this strategy works.

Early Versus Late Treatments—The State of the Evidence

Since stratified care is the recommended approach for the acute management of migraine, and because migraineurs who seek care have attack-related disability, most migraineurs who seek care should receive a triptan (or DHE), unless contraindicated. When is the proper time to treat the attack? Assessing early intervention studies with triptans is complicated and potentially misleading for a number of reasons, most of them related to trial design (Moschiano et al., 2005; Dowson et al., 2006). Regardless of the trial design, results consistently support that early intervention strategies are associated with an increase in pain-free rates at 2 hours, compared with late intervention. This has been demonstrated in trials with sumatriptan (Scholpp et al., 2004), zolmitriptan (Klapper et al., 2004), rizatriptan (Mathew et al., 2004), almotriptan (Mathew, 2003), eletriptan (Brandes et al., 2005), and frovatriptan (Cady et al., 2004).

We endorse the recommendations of the U.S. Headache Consortium (Silberstein et al, 2007):

- Acute treatment choice should be based on attack-related disability, which encompasses the severity, duration, and frequency of migraine attacks and the presence of associated symptoms. Stratified care specifically matches illness severity to treatment need, including acute treatment and/or preventive treatments (Level B).
- Patients should be instructed to treat a migraine early in the course of the pain phase of an attack. Treatment of migraine when pain is mild and when CS is not established confers therapeutic benefits to triptans (Level A).

In the following sections, we review the classes of medications that are useful for the acute treatment of migraine. The evidence and recommendations are in accordance with the recently U.S. Headache Consortium Guidelines (Silberstein et al., submitted).

Analgesics Including NSAIDs

Using the stratified care approach, migraine attacks with no more than mild attack-related disability may be treated with nonspecific medications. In such cases, where there is no substantial disability, most people obtain headache relief with a simple analgesic, such as aspirin (Murray, 1964) or acetaminophen, either alone or in combination with caffeine or other adjuvants. Combination analgesics have some advantages over analgesics alone: (1) Combining two analgesics that have different mechanisms of action can enhance analgesia (Beaver, 1984; McQuay et al., 1999). (2) Caffeine not only substantially enhances the analgesia of aspirin and acetaminophen (Beaver, 1984) and ibuprofen (Forbes et al., 1991), but is itself analgesic (Ward et al., 1991). (3) Lower doses of different drugs reduce AEs. (4) Analgesic combination drugs also offer product convenience (Beaver, 1984). The use of barbiturates or benzodiazepam is controversial. Any value of the barbiturate may be via a central effect: sedation or pain modulation (Saper, 1990). Some physicians believe that these combinations are more likely to lead to overuse and dependence and may not offer enough additional pain control to justify their use.

Acetaminophen's efficacy in acute migraine treatment has been established, and the danger of Reye syndrome makes acetaminophen preferable to aspirin for children who have nonspecific headache and are younger than 15 years of age (Silberstein, 1990). Two placebo-controlled studies to assess acetaminophen's efficacy as monotherapy for the acute treatment of migraine have been performed: the earlier one failed to demonstrate a significant effect over placebo (Larsen et al., 1990), and the second, later, trial excluded patients who were severely disabled (requiring bed rest or vomiting >20% of the time) (Lipton, Baggish, et al., 2000). In the second trial, acetaminophen was more effective than placebo at primary and secondary end points in the treatment of migraine pain. Acetaminophen was not effective in treating migraine-associated nausea. A third study tested a combination containing acetaminophen, aspirin, and caffeine versus the single constituents (including acetaminophen alone) versus placebo, and acetaminophen as monotherapy was significantly better than placebo in primary and other end points (Diener, Pfaffenrath, Pageler, et al., 2005). Acetaminophen is an option for patients for whom aspirin or the other NSAIDs are contraindicated because of gastritis or bleeding disorder.

The combination of aspirin, acetaminophen, and caffeine (AAC) is discussed below.

Nonsteroidal Anti-inflammatory Drugs

At least five different chemical classes of NSAIDs (Pradalier et al., 1988) have been used for headache treatment (Table 11–6). These include the salicylates, arylpropionic acids, aryl and heterocyclic acids, fenamic acids, and enolic acids. The major mechanism of action of NSAIDs is the differential inhibition of one of the two subtypes of the enzyme cyclooxygenase (COX1 and COX2), preventing prostaglandin synthesis (Campbell, 1990). NSAIDs can now be distinguished on the basis of their relative inhibitory activity on COX1 and COX2. In addition, some NSAIDs (ketoprofen, indomethacin, diclofenac) decrease the synthesis of leukotrienes by inhibiting 5-lipooxygenase (Campbell, 1990; Brooks and Day, 1991). One NSAID (meclofenamate) may be a direct prostaglandin receptor antagonist. In

TABLE 11–6 NSAIDs: Chemical Classification.

Salicylic acids
Aspirin
Choline magnesium salicylate
Salsalate
Sodium salicylate
Arylpropionic acids
Ibuprofen
Naproxen
Fenoprofen
Ketoprofen
Flurbiprofen
Oxaprozin
Indole/heteroaryl acetic acids
Tolectin
Indomethacin
Diclofenac
Sulindac
Ketorolac
Fenamic acids
Mefenamic acid
Meclofenamate
Enolic acids
Phenylbutazone
Piroxicam

addition, NSAIDs interfere with a variety of membrane-associated processes, including the activity of nicotinamide adenosine dinucleotide phosphate (NADPH) oxidase in neutrophils and phospholipase C in macrophages (Brooks and Day, 1991). NSAIDs may also interfere with cell adhesion molecules and have direct antinociceptive effects on neurons (McCormack, 1994).

VonEuler (1937) coined the term prostaglandin to describe the semen extract that contracts uterine smooth muscle. The 20-carbon polyunsaturated essential fatty acid, arachidonic acid, is the major source of prostaglandins in mammalian tissues (Cashman and McAnulty, 1995).

Prostaglandin synthesis requires the release of arachidonic acid from cell membrane phospholipids by phospholipase. Arachidonic acid is the substrate for the COX enzymes, which are membrane-bound glycoproteins (Hemler et al., 1976). COX catalyzes the oxidation of arachidonic acid to a cyclic [doperoxide (PGG2)] and in a peroxidase step reduces the C15 hydroperoxide to a hydroxy (PGH2) (Frölich, 1997). Most prostanoids do not directly activate nociceptors, but rather sensitize them. Prostaglandins of the E series are involved in the hyperalgesia seen in acute inflammation. PGE2 is the predominant eicosanoid in such inflammatory conditions, acting synergistically with other mediators to produce inflammatory pain. PGE2 sensitizes receptors on afferent nerve endings to bradykinin and histamine.

There are two different COX enzymes encoded by two genes: COX1, the constitutive, and COX2, the induced form. COX1 is produced in normal quiescent conditions and is important when prostaglandins have a protective function, such as gastric mucus production and renal blood flow maintenance (Cashman and McAnulty, 1995). COX1 is found in platelets, where it is essential for thromboxane A2 synthesis. Inhibition of thromboxane synthesis leads to loss of normal platelet aggregation. COX1 activation leads to prostacyclin production, which is antithrombogenic in the endothelium and cytoprotective in the stomach. In the kidney, prostaglandins are synthesized in the renal medulla, the ascending loop of Henle, and the cortex (Frölich, 1997).

The COX2 isoenzyme is found in endothelial cells, macrophages, and synovial fibroblasts (Frölich, 1997). It is found in small amounts in normal human lung, rat kidney, and fetal membranes, but most is the result of induction. It can be induced by interleukin 1 (IL1) and endotoxin, and its expression is unregulated at sites of inflammation, increasing more than 20-fold during inflammation (Frölich, 1997).

NSAIDs are among the most commonly prescribed drugs in the world, but their use as antinflammatory, antipyretic, antithrombotic, and analgesic is often limited by their gastric toxicity secondary to the suppression of prostaglandin synthesis (mainly through inhibition of COX1 activity), although several NSAIDs also have topical irritant properties (Wallace and Cirino, 1994). The ratio of inhibition of COX1 to COX2 by NSAIDs determines the likelihood of specific AEs. NSAIDs such as aspirin and indomethacin with a high ratio have more AEs than ibuprofen, which has a low ratio. Dexamethasone, at anti-nflammatory concentrations, inhibits COX2 (Wallace and Cirino, 1994).

Aspirin at very low doses is a selective COX1 platelet inhibitor. At intermediate doses the COX1 inhibition is generalized, and the active metabolite of aspirin, salicylate, adds to its overall anti-nflammatory effect. Salicylate is a fairly selective COX2 inhibitor. It does not block platelet aggregation in humans in anti-inflammatory dosage and it does not produce gastrointestinal blood loss (Wallace and Cirino, 1994).

Nonselective COX inhibitors inhibit both COX1 and COX2 and include aspirin, indomethacin, piroxicam, diclofenac and ibuprofen. Selective COX2 inhibitors include salicylate and nimesulide (Wallace and Cirino, 1994). Salicylates (sodium salicylate, salicylamide, and magnesium trisalicylate) can be used safely by patients with aspirin-induced asthma (Wallace and Cirino, 1994).

Highly selective COX2 inhibitors show COX2: COX1 ratios of <0.001 in intact cells and include celecoxib (Monsanto/Seale), rofecoxib (Merck-Frosst), CGP28238 (Ciba–Geigy), DuP697 (Dupont), and NS398 (Taiso) (Frölich, 1997).

If COX2 is primarily responsible for the production of prostanoids that mediate inflammation, pain, and fever, it is unlikely that highly selective COX2 inhibitors will be more therapeutically effective than existing NSAIDs, since many of the existing NSAIDs are very effective COX2 inhibitors and since it is possible that prostanoids produced via COX1 contribute to the inflammation, pain, and fever (Wallace and Cirino, 1994).

Some of the AEs of NSAIDs may be related to their ability to suppress COX2 activity. It is possible that COX2 is constitutively expressed in some tissues, and that the prostanoids produced via this enzyme are physiologically important (Wallace and Cirino, 1994). Unlike the damage NSAIDs produce in the stomach, NSAID-induced small intestinal injury may not be related to suppression of prostaglandin synthesis. Thus the sparing of intestinal prostaglandin synthesis by a selective COX2 inhibitor would not necessarily result in reduced intestinal toxicity (Wallace and Cirino, 1994).

Gastrointestinal toxicity can be reduced by linking the NSAID to a NO-releasing moiety. NO maintains gastric mucosal blood flow, prevents leukocyte adherence within the gastric microcirculation, and counteracts the detrimental effects of COX suppression. They produce markedly less gastric injury than the native NSAIDs after both acute and chronic administration and do not cause detectable small intestinal injury (Wallace and Cirino, 1994). Recently cardiac AEs have led to the withdrawal of two selective COX2 inhibitors and have raised a safety issue.

Since the potential risk of cardiac AE is of major interest, Hernández-Díaz et al. conducted a systematic review of cohort and case-control studies on NSAIDs and selective inhibitors of cyclooxygenase-2 (Coxibs), and myocardial infarction published between 2000 and 2005. Ibuprofen was associated with neither an increased risk nor with protection; diclofenac was associated with an increased risk. Naproxen was associated with a 17% reduced risk among people who do not use aspirin, a population with a relatively low risk of coronary heart disease. For Coxibs, there appeared to be a dose–response relationship between rofecoxib and the risk of myocardial infarction, but no significantly elevated risk for celecoxib, irrespective of dose, in clinical practice (Hernandez-Diaz et al., 2006).

The *Acute Section of the Headache Guidelines* (Bigal et al., in Silberstein et al., submitted) analyzed 33 controlled trials of NSAIDs and other nonopiate analgesics and found them to be consistently effective for acute migraine headache pain relief compared with placebo. *Aspirin* (Hakkarainen et al., 1979; Tfelt-Hansen and Olesen, 1984; Boureau et al., 1994), *ibuprofen* (doses >400 mg) (Havanka-Kanniainen, 1989; Kloster et al., 1992), *tolfenamic acid* (Hakkarainen et al., 1979; Tokola et al., 1984), and *naproxen sodium* (Sargent et al., 1988; Johnson, Ratcliffe, et al., 1985) were superior to placebo. One new trial reported that *naproxen sodium* was as effective as *lysine clonixinate* in achieving a headache response and there were no differences between treatments (Krymchantowski et al., 2005). Two studies show that *naproxen sodium added to sumatriptan 85 mg* in a fixed-dose formulation offers more clinical benefits than the constituent therapies given alone (Silberstein, Stark, et al., 2006).

In the first edition of the U.S. Headache Consortium Guideline, three studies supported the superiority of *conventional aspirin* over placebo. Two recent studies compared 1000 mg *effervescent aspirin*, 50 mg encapsulated sumatriptan, 400 mg ibuprofen and placebo (Diener, Bussone, et al.,

2004; Diener, Eikermann, et al., 2004). With Regard to headache relief, aspirin was as effective as 50 mg sumatriptan and 400 mg ibuprofen in the treatment of migraine attacks (Diener, Bussone, et al., 2004). Regarding the patient being pain-free at 2 hours, sumatriptan was the most effective of the treatments tested. One additional second study reports that effervescent aspirin was effective in the management of the associated symptoms of migraine as well (Diener, Eikermann, et al., 2004). Dispersible aspirin, at the dose of 900 mg, was also tested against placebo and found to be effective in reducing migraine pain as early as 30 minutes (MacGregor et al., 2002). The *combination of aspirin 900 mg with metoclopramide 10 mg* was tested against zolmitriptan 2.5 mg (Geraud et al., 2002). The percentage of patients with a 2-hour headache response after the first dose for all three attacks was similar among active treatment groups. Another study comparing aspirin plus metoclopramide and lysine acetylsalicylate plus metoclopramide with oral sumatriptan showed no significant differences between the analgesic compounds and sumatriptan for headache relief (Oral Sumatriptan and Aspirin-plus-Metoclpramide Comparative Study Group, 1992). Collectively, these studies show that aspirin (conventional tablet, effervescent, or dispersible formulations) is effective for the acute treatment of migraine, and in some patients may be as effective as selected triptan therapy (e.g., zolmitriptan or sumatriptan).

Clinical trials reviewed for the first edition of the U.S. Headache Consortium Guidelines demonstrated that *ibuprofen* was more effective than placebo in the acute treatment of migraine (Matchar et al., 2000). In a trial that excluded subjects with migraine-related disability, doses of ibuprofen 200 and 400 mg were more effective than placebo for 2-hour pain relief of mild or moderate headache; but only 400 mg was effective for relief of severe migraine attacks (Codispoti et al., 2001). In four additional studies, ibuprofen was used as an active comparator to rofecoxib (Misra et al., 2004; Saper et al., 2006), aspirin (Diener, Bussone, et al., 2004), and AAC (Goldstein et al., 2006) and was found comparable to aspirin and refexoxib (Diener, Bussone, et al., 2004; Misra et al., 2004; Saper et al., 2006) but less effective than AAC (Goldstein et al., 2006). Ibuprofen is effective for the acute treatment of migraine. The relative efficacy suggests that ibuprofen is as effective as other selected simple analgesics, but may not be as effective as combination therapies, such as AAC.

Individual positive placebo-controlled studies of *diclofenac-K* (Dahlof and Bjorkman, 1993), *flurbiprofen* (Awidi, 1982), *naproxen* (Andersson et al., 1989), *piroxicam SL* (Nappi et al., 1993), *pirprofen* (Kinnunen et al., 1988), and *proquazone* (Diserio et al., 1989) exist. *Diclofenac sodium* intramuscular (IM) was superior to placebo (Delbene et al., 1987) and low doses of acetaminophen IM (Karachalios et al., 1992). Another more recent study compared *diclofenac sodium softgel* 100 mg versus diclofenac sodium softgel 100 mg plus caffeine 100 mg versus placebo plus caffeine 100 mg (but not diclofenac alone). This study found diclofenac sodium softgel formulations to be significantly more effective than placebo in achieving a 1-hour headache reduction (Peroutka et al., 2004). In comparative trials, *tolfenamic acid* was superior to acetaminophen (Larsen et al., 1990) but no different from aspirin (Hakkarainen et al., 1979) or ibuprofen (Pearce et al., 1983). In some trials, adding an antiemetic or caffeine had no additional effect (Hakkarainen et al., 1982; Tfelt-Hansen and Olesen, 1984; Tokola et al., 1984). *Ketoprofen,* at the doses of 75 and 150 mg, was compared with zolmitriptan 2.5 mg and placebo in a double-blind, placebo-controlled, cross-over trial (Dib et al., 2002). No differences between treatments were reported for headache relief among the two doses of ketoprofen and zolmitriptan 2.5 mg, and all treatments reported a greater than 60% headache relief.

As reviewed in the first edition of the U.S. Headache Consortium Guidelines, three trials tested the efficacy of *AAC* versus placebo for migraine patients. All three studies excluded patients with severe disability (vomiting in a significant proportion of attacks or requiring bed rest in a significant proportion of attacks). All three trials were positive versus placebo (Lipton et al., 1998). Since the first edition report, AAC has also been compared to other antimigraine therapies, including triptans and other analgesics. In one trial, the combination of AAC was more effective than 50 mg sumatriptan for mild to moderate migraine (Goldstein et al., 2005). In this trial, sumatriptan (previously proven effective for the acute treatment of migraine) was equivalent to placebo, and this raises important concerns about the sample size and potential randomization bias in this study. In another randomized, controlled trial that included patients who usually used OTC medications to treat their headaches (migraine or TTHs), the fixed combination of AAC was statistically significantly superior to the combination without caffeine, or the individual components, or placebo (Diener, Pfaffenrath, Pageler, et al., 2005). Aspirin and acetaminophen both differed significantly in achieving pain relief versus placebo, but caffeine as monotherapy was equivalent to placebo. This study further tested the efficacy of AAC (acetaminophen 250 mg, aspirin 250 mg, and caffeine 65 mg) versus ibuprofen (200 mg) in migraine patients of any severity (no exclusion for migraine disability) and found that both treatments were more effective than placebo in achieving pain relief, but AAC also was significantly more effective than ibuprofen (Goldstein et al., 2006). Collectively, these studies show that the AAC combination is more effective than placebo for the acute treatment of migraine in patients with mild or no disability. This study also suggests that the AAC combination may be more effective than simple analgesics given as monotherapy.

Comparative trials showed that *opiate-containing aspirin compounds* were more efficacious than aspirin alone (Hakkarainen et al., 1978, 1980). *Ergotamine* was superior to aspirin in two trials (Hakkarainen et al., 1978, 1980). No significant differences were observed between ergotamine ((caffeine) and ketoprofen PR (Kangasniemi and Kaaja, 1992), naproxen sodium (Pradalier et al., 1985; Sargent et al., 1988; Treves et al., 1992), or tolfenamic acid (Hakkarainen et al., 1979). Oral sumatriptan was not significantly different than either aspirin plus metoclopramide (Oral Sumatriptan and Aspirin-plus-Metoclpramide Comparative Study Group, 1992) or lysine acetylsalicylate plus metoclopramide (Tfelt-Hansen et al., 1995). The clinical efficacy of ketorolac IM in comparative trials was inconclusive (Duarte et al., 1992; Larkin and Prescott, 1992; Davis et al., 1995; Shrestha et al., 1996).

AEs with all the NSAIDs include GI upset, peptic ulcers and bleeding, abdominal pain, constipation, diarrhea, nausea, occasional paradoxical headache, lightheadedness, dizziness, somnolence, tinnitus, and fluid retention. In the short-term trials reviewed in the AHCPR Technical Report (Gray et al., 1999c), aspirin was generally well tolerated. Other NSAIDs were associated with higher rates of gastric irritation/discomfort, nausea, and vomiting. NSAIDs were consistently associated with lower overall AE rates when compared with ergotamine; in particular, lower rates of nausea and vomiting were noted. Antiemetics did not reduce the adverse gastrointestinal events typically associated with NSAIDs (Gray et al., 1999, 1999c). The more lipid-soluble NSAIDs penetrate the CNS more effectively and may have greater central effects (Brooks and Day, 1991). All NSAIDs, which are both COX1 + COX2 inhibitors, are associated with an increased risk of peptic ulcer disease, the risk increasing with the dosage of the NSAID (Griffin et al., 1991) and aggravation of existing gastrointestinal inflammatory disease. Selective COX2 inhibitors may not have this risk. Contraindications to NSAIDs include active ulcer disease, gastritis, kidney disease, and bleeding disorders. The prolonged use of NSAIDs, especially those with more potent COX-2 inhibition, should be cautiously monitored, owing to cardiovascular concerns (McGettigan and Henry, 2006).

NSAIDs can be used symptomatically or, in special situations, preventively, and should be considered a first-line choice for the treatment of chronic paroxysmal hemicrania, menstrual migraine, exertional migraine, benign orgasmic cephalgia, hemicrania continua, and ice-pick headache. To be effective, NSAIDs must be given in adequate doses. If one NSAID is ineffective, another should be tried.

The most consistent evidence for efficacy exists for aspirin, ibuprofen, naproxen sodium, tolfenamic acid, and AAC. Their low cost and favorable tolerability make them a first-line treatment choice for mild-to-moderate migraine attacks or severe attacks that have been responsive in the past to similar NSAIDs or nonopiate analgesics. The NSAIDs most commonly used for headache relief are listed in Table 11–6. The dose should not exceed the maximum for each drug. In some cases it can be repeated in 1–2 hours (naproxen, ibuprofen) as long as the maximal dose is not exceeded.

Indomethacin (Indocin) is available as a 50 mg rectal suppository, which is useful for patients with severe nausea and vomiting.

Ketorolac (Toradol) can be given by injection (available as 15, 30, and 60 mg Cartrix for IM injection). No placebo-controlled trials testing the efficacy of ketorolac IM for treatment of acute migraine attack have been performed. Small comparative trials suggest possible equivalence to some agents, and a single comparison trial with meperidine demonstrated inferiority. Ketorolac IM is an option that may be used in a physician-supervised setting, although conclusions regarding clinical efficacy cannot be made at this time.

Injectable lysine ASA (iLAS) has been used in the acute treatment of migraine. In a double-blind, multicenter trial that included 278 patients, iLAS was compared to SC sumatriptan and placebo. Both drugs were superior to placebo. Two hours following the administration of sumatriptan, iLAS, and placebo, 76.3%, 43.7%, and 14.3% of the patients, respectively, were pain-free. iLAS was significantly better tolerated than sumatriptan: AEs were 7.6% for iLAS and 37.8% for sumatriptan (Diener, 1999).

Scientific evidence now exists regarding the efficacy of the selective COX2 inhibitors in migraine and other types of headache; in addition they have been shown to be analgesic in dental pain models (Morrison et al., 1999). Because of cardiovascular safety concerns with long-term use, two (rofecoxib and valdecoxib) have been withdrawn from the market.

Celecoxib is a 1,5-diaryl pyrazole-based compound that inhibits recombinant COX2 with an IC50 of 4×10^{-8} mol/L compared with 1.5×10^{-5} mol/L for COX1. Single doses of celecoxib 100 or 400 mg were superior to placebo and as effective as aspirin for pain relief following dental extraction. Phase 2 studies have established dose ranges of 100–400 mg per day for osteoarthritis and 200–800 mg per day for rheumatoid arthritis. An acute endoscopic study showed that levels of gastric mucosal injury with celecoxib 100 or 200 mg twice daily for 7 days were similar to those with placebo and reduced compared with naproxen 500 mg twice a day.

Patients using NSAIDs other than acetaminophen and selective COX2 inhibitors should be monitored for GI blood loss, renal dysfunction, worsening of hypertension, and aggravation of colitis. Perimenstrual use should be limited to 1 week at a time or three times a week when used regularly. It is not known whether NSAIDs can produce rebound headache, but some authors have implicated these drugs (Henry et al., 1985).

Isometheptene and Isometheptene Combination Agents

The combination of acetaminophen, isometheptene (a sympathomimetic), and dichloralphenazone (a chloral hydrate derivative) is used in the treatment of migraine and TTH (Yuill et al., 1972; Ryan, 1974). In two placebo-controlled trials, isometheptene attained borderline statistical significance in relieving headache pain (Ogden, 1963; Ryan, 1974; Diamond and Medina, 1975). Isometheptene mucate plus acetaminophen plus dichloralphenazone was significantly more effective than placebo in two of three trials, although the magnitude of the effect was relatively modest (Ryan, 1974; Diamond and Medina, 1975; Diamond, 1976).

The combination was compared with its constituents (acetaminophen and isometheptene, respectively) and no significant advantages were found (Ryan, 1974; Diamond, 1976). The combination was significantly more effective at reducing headache intensity (Yuill et al., 1972) and was associated with significantly less nausea and vomiting than was ergotamine plus caffeine. A recent multicenter, double-blind, randomized, parallel trial found no statistically significant difference in efficacy between the isometheptene-containing combination and sumatriptan for mild-to-moderate migraine with or without aura (Freitag, Cady, et al., 1999). Headache recurrence was not significantly different over the 24-hour evaluation period for patients who respond in the first 4 hours. AEs associated with isometheptene combinations were not significantly more frequent than with placebo or with the comparator medications described above. Recently, a comparative study tested five capsules of the isometheptene combination given over 3 hours versus sumatriptan 25 mg repeated in 2 hours in the early treatment of nondisabling mild, moderate, or severe migraine. This study showed that both regimens were equally effective in reducing migraine pain, and other secondary end points may have favored the isometheptene combination (Freitag, Cady, et al., 2001). Collectively, these studies show that isometheptene combination therapy is effective for the acute treatment of migraine, and the magnitude of effect is modest. On the basis of clinical evidence and favorable tolerability, they may be a reasonable choice for patients with mild-to-moderate headache. The initial dose is two capsules, with a maximum of five capsules per attack. Contraindications include glaucoma, renal failure, significant hypertension, heart or liver disease, and use of MAO inhibitors. Adverse reactions include transient dizziness and skin rash.

U.S. Headache Consortium Conclusions and Recommendations for NSAIDS and Analgesics That Do Not Contain Opioids or Barbiturates

Conclusions

- Aspirin (conventional tablet, effervescent, or dispersible formulations) with or without the addition of metoclopramide is established as effective for the acute treatment of migraine.
- Acetaminophen is probably effective for the acute treatment of nondisabling migraine.
- AAC combination therapy is effective for *nondisabling* migraine.
- AAC combination therapy is *more effective* than acetaminophen, aspirin, or ibuprofen monotherapy for the treatment of nondisabling migraine.
- Isometheptene mucate, dichloralphenazone, acetaminophen combination is effective for the treatment of *nondisabling* migraine. Ibuprofen, naproxen sodium, ketoprofen are established as effective for the acute treatment of migraine.
- Diclofenac-K is established as effective for acute treatment of migraine, with one of these studies showing similar efficacy to sumatriptan.
- Diclofenac sodium softgel (100 mg plus caffeine 100 mg) is probably effective for the acute treatment of migraine.
- Ketorolac IV or IM for treatment of acute migraine attack is probably effective for the acute treatment of migraine.

Recommendations

- Aspirin, naproxen sodium, ibuprofen, and diclofenac-K should be used for the acute treatment of nondisabling migraine (Level A).
- Ketorolac IV or IM should be considered for the acute treatment of migraine for patients requiring parenteral therapy (Level B).
- Acetaminophen should be considered for the acute treatment of nondisabling migraine (Level B).
- AAC should be use for the acute treatment of migraine (Level A).
- Isometheptene mucate, dichloralphenazone, acetaminophen combination should be used for the treatment of migraine (Level A).

BARBITURATE HYPNOTICS

The AHCPR Technical Report (Silberstein and McCrory, 2001) identified ten separate controlled trials of butalbital-containing agents for headache treatment. Only one was conducted among migraineurs, and it did not include a placebo arm. This trial compared butalbital plus aspirin plus caffeine plus codeine (Fiorinal with codeine) with butorphanol NS (Stadol NS) (Goldstein et al., 1988). Butorphanol was superior in efficacy to the butalbital combination with codeine at 2 hours, but differences between the two treatments were not significant at 4 hours. Butalbital combined with codeine (Fiorinal with codeine) was associated with significantly fewer AEs than butorphanol NS (Goldstein et al., 1988; Silberstein and McCrory, 2001).

No randomized, placebo-controlled studies have established the efficacy of butalbital-containing agents in the treatment of acute migraine headaches. Because of concerns about overuse, medication-overuse headache, and withdrawal, the use of butalbital-containing analgesics should be limited and carefully monitored. Their use should be limited to situations wherein a more specific or less potentially problematic agent cannot be used or is ineffective. They may be very effective as back-up medications when other migraine medications have failed. For an individual attack, patients should take one or two tablets or capsules, with a maximum of six per attack. The most frequent adverse reactions are drowsiness and dizziness. Drug use should be limited to no more than two to three treatment days per week.

U.S. Headache Consortium Conclusions and Recommendations

Conclusions

- No Class-I studies exist that show that butalbital compounds are effective in the acute treatment of migraine. Therefore, the data are inadequate to support their use in the acute treatment of migraine. Level-B evidence supports the efficacy of butalbital-containing analgesics in the treatment of *nonspecified headache*.
- Limit and carefully monitor patients' use of butalbital-containing analgesics because of the high risk of dependency, medication-overuse headache, and withdrawal concerns (Level B).

Recommendations

- None (Level U). Butalbital-containing analgesics are *not recommended as a first-line therapy* for the acute treatment of migraine.
- Limit and carefully monitor patient's use of butalbital-containing analgesics because of the risk of dependency, medication-overuse headache, and withdrawal concerns (Level U).

OPIOIDS

Opium is the Greek term for the juice of the poppy plant. Opiates are drugs derived from opium (Ferrante, 1996). Opioid is a more inclusive term that applies to all agonists or antagonists that have morphine-like activity, such as opiates or endogenous or synthetic opioid peptides (Reisine and Pasternak, 1996). The term narcotic is derived from the Greek word for stupor but, because of its legal meaning, it is no longer used pharmacologically. Three families of endogenous opioid peptides, each derived from a different polypeptide precursor, have been identified: the enkephalins (from proenkephalin), the endorphins (from pro-opiomelanocortin), and the dynorphins (from prodynorphin). In addition, good evidence for the presence of endogenous morphine and codeine exists. Morphine- and codeine-like substances have been isolated from the brain of several species, and biosynthetic pathways for morphine production, similar to that used by the opium poppy, have been demonstrated in mammals (Silberstein and McCrory, 1999).

Saper and colleagues (Saper et al., 2000) reported the results of a 5-year prospective study using sustained, long-acting opioids in the treatment of more than 300 patients with intractable daily or almost-daily headache. Of 160 patients treated for 3–5 years, only 23% demonstrated evidence of significant improvement, although a slightly larger group reported feeling better, but without corroborative evidence, such as reduction in previous medication usage or an increase in daily activity. Up to 40% of patients showed some evidence of noncompliance (self-adjustment of doses, etc.) in the first year, despite the highly structured program that required monthly or bimonthly visits during the entire course of the study. The authors recommended that only patients who have failed all reasonable methods of treatment, including intense, advanced care interventions, including full detoxification and hospitalization, should be placed on sustained opioid therapy. Exceptions might include pregnant women and patients with profound medical illnesses or medication requirements that would make the use of standard medications inappropriate. On the basis of clinical observations during the period of the study, the authors also suggest that patients with severe Axis I psychiatric illness and those with cluster B personality disorders (borderline, histrionic, antisocial, and narcissistic) not be given sustained opioids.

Clinical Studies in Migraine and TTH

The AHCPR Technical Report supports the effectiveness of several opioids for episodic treatment of acute migraine and TTH (Table 11–7). However, opioid drugs are often used as rescue medications after other treatments have failed, and the available trials do not address this situation. Clinical trials of opioid drugs are all conducted over short time-frames. Because they focus on relieving the pain of acute headache attacks, these studies do not address clinically important issues about frequent or prolonged use of opioid analgesics, such as rebound headache, tolerance, and dependence (Silberstein and McCrory, 1999). In a recent study published after the first edition of the Guideline, meperidine IV (1.5 mg/Kg) was compared with droperidol IM 2.5 mg, and both treatments were equally effective (Richman et al., 2002).

Opioids may be considered for patients who have infrequent disabling migraines that do not respond to standard medication. Opioids are

TABLE 11–7 Clinical Trials of Opioids.

Drug	*Population*	*Findings*
APAP/Codeine	Migraine	Better HA relief than placebo (2 of 3 trials) No better than aspirin (1 trial)
	Tension-type	No better complete relief than Fioricet @ 2 hours (1 trial) Less complete relief than Fioricet @ 4 hours (1 trial)
APAP/codeine/ doxylamine	Migraine	No better (HA complete relief, SPID) than placebo (2 of 2 trials) No better SPID than APAP/codeine (1 trial)
APAP/codeine/ buclizine	Migraine	Better HA relief than placebo (1 of 3 trials) No better HA severity than ergotamine/cyclizine/caffeine (Migril®)
Butorphanol (IM)	Migraine	No better HA relief than meperidine/hydroxyzine (IM) (1 trial) No better HA relief than dihydroergotamine/ metoclopramide (IV) (1 trial)
Butorphanol (IN)	Migraine	Better HA severity than placebo (2 of 2 trials)
Doleron	Migraine	Better HA relief than aspirin (1 of 1 trial) No better HA relief than ergotamine tartrate
Doleron novum	Migraine	Better HA relief than aspirin (1 of 1 trial) No better HA relief than ergotamine tartrate
Fiorinal with codeine	Tension-type	Better PID than placebo (3 of 3 trials) Better PID than Fiorinal (1 of 3 trials) Less HA relief than butorphanol (1 trial)
Meperidine (IV)	Migraine	No better than ketorolac (IM) (1 trial)
Meperidine/ promethazine (IV)	Migraine	No better than placebo (1 trial) No better than ketorolac (IM) (2 of 2 trials) No better HA relief than dihydroergotamine/metoclopramide (IV) (1 trial)
Meperidine/ dimenhydrinate (IV)	Migraine	Less reduction in HA severity than chlorpromazine (IV) (1 trial) No better HA severity than methotrimeprazine (IV) (1 trial)
Meperidine/ hydroxyzine IM	Migraine	No better HA relief than butorphanol (IM) Less HA relief than dihydroergotamine/metoclopramide (IV) (2 trials) No better HA relief than ketorolac (IM) (1 trial)

Abbreviations: IM, intramuscular; IV, intravenous.

particularly useful for patients who cannot use specific headache medications because of coexisting disease or the lack of a diagnosis (such as a patient who presents to the emergency department with a new headache). They are a *safe treatment* for pregnant women when given in limited amounts. They are useful for severe, middle-of-the-night headache and as a rescue medication. (A self-administered rescue medication should be prescribed for severe migraine since most treatments do not always work. In fact, the triptans may not work at all in as many as 20% to 30% of attacks.) Although rescue medications often do not maintain normal function, they permit the patient to achieve relief of pain and suffering without the discomfort and expense of a visit to the physician's office or emergency department. Rescue medications include opioids and neuroleptics (Silberstein and McCrory, 1999).

Opioids can be used for patients who have not overused or abused medication or violated treatment recommendations. They should be avoided or used cautiously and restrictively in patients who have demonstrated severe addictive tendencies and perhaps have a family history of addictive disease. Strict limits (no more than two treatment days per week) should be set and small amounts of medication prescribed to avoid the risk of excessive use in treatment-resistant patients (Portenoy et al., 1990; Saper et al., 1999a). In addition, use the lowest dose and least potent agent available when possible; carefully review other concurrently used medications to avoid enhanced sedation, respiratory suppression, or other untoward reactions; calculate and prescribe the appropriate number of pills to be used between visits, on the basis of frequency of attacks and attack requirements (refills are discouraged, as are call-in requests for additional medication); carefully delineate the guidelines for usage, including for which type of headache, how many times per day, and how frequently per week the drug can be used; and establish a visit pattern that is consistent with the headache frequency and the amount and type of medications prescribed (Saper et al., 1999b). The limits can be relaxed for pregnant women and migraineurs with menstrual headache. Opioids are often useful for the pregnant patient, and their occasional use by patients who cannot tolerate or do not respond to ergots, triptans, or other symptomatic medications is appropriate.

Opioids should be administered by the most appropriate route for the clinical circumstance. The dosages should be adjusted to account for differences in bioavailability between the oral, parenteral, and rectal routes of administration (Table 11–8). The selection of a specific drug should be based on its route of administration, AE profile, time to peak drug levels, and bioavailability. A nonoral route should be considered when there is severe nausea or vomiting. The agonist–antagonist opioids, such as butorphanol and nalbuphine, seem to have lower abuse potential than the pure agonists. Parenteral butorphanol (2–3 mg) produces analgesia and respiratory depression equal to that of 10 mg of morphine (with similar onset, peak, and duration of action) or 80 mg of meperidine. Butorphanol's plasma half-life is approximately 3 hours; higher values

TABLE 11–8 Doses of Opioids Equivalent to 10 mg Parenteral Morphine.

Drug	*Oral dose (mg)*	*Oral-to-parenteral dose ratio*	*Parenteral dose (mg)*
Butorphanol	NA	NA	2
Codeine	200	1.5:1	130
Hydromorphone	7.5	5:1	1.5
Meperidine	300	4:1	75
Methadone	20	2:1	10
Morphine	60	6:1	10
Single dose	30	3:1	10
Repeated dose			
Oxycodone	15	2:1	30

are observed in the elderly. Like other κ receptor agonists, there is much less of an increase in respiratory depression with higher doses compared with morphine and other μ receptor agonists. Excessive administration, improper selection, and use for frequent headaches have led to numerous cases of physical and psychologic dependence. Usage patterns exceeding a bottle of butorphanol a day are not uncommon. Recent work suggests that withdrawal from butorphanol results in focal increases in extracellular glutamate levels within the locus ceruleus that may act through the NMDA glutamate receptor (Hoshi et al., 1996; Saper et al., 1999b).

Butorphanol NS (1 mg followed by an additional 1 mg spray 1 hour later) was compared with IM administered methadone 10 mg, in a placebo-controlled, double-blind, double-dummy study of 96 patients. Both active agents provided statistically significant pain relief over placebo during the entire course of the study. Butorphanol was statistically superior at the $p < 0.05$ level in the first 2 hours of the study. Global satisfaction and time to remedication both favored butorphanol NS (transnasal butorphanol) in the acute treatment of migraine (Diamond et al., 1991).

The major AEs of butorphanol are drowsiness, weakness, sweating, feelings of floating, and nausea. The incidence of psychotomimetic AEs is lower than that with equianalgesic doses of pentazocine, but qualitatively similar.

Oral opioid combinations (e.g., aspirin or acetaminophen plus codeine) may be considered for acute migraine when sedation AEs will not put the patient at risk and the risk for abuse has been addressed. Commonly used combinations include aspirin or acetaminophen plus butalbital, a short-acting barbiturate effective in reducing anxiety (Silberstein, 1984). These combinations, available with or without caffeine, may be prescribed.

Parenteral opioids may be considered as a choice for rescue therapy in a supervised setting for acute migraine when sedation AEs will not put the patient at risk and the risk for abuse has been addressed.

In general, we recommend no more than two usage-days per week, with strict monthly limits of these agents to prevent overuse. Monthly limits should be established below maximal allowable usage, although individual consideration on a patient-by-patient basis is appropriate. Nonetheless we recognize that some patients use and have benefits using higher amount of opioids. These patients should be the exception.

U.S. Headache Consortium Conclusions and Recommendations

Conclusions

- Oral opioids, including agents containing codeine, are effective for the acute treatment of migraine but are associated with a risk of dependency and overuse (Level A).
- Butorphanol NS is an effective treatment for some patients with migraine and is associated with dependency (Level A).
- Other oral opioids are effective in the treatment of some patients with migraine but should be used cautiously owing to the risk of dependency (Level B).
- The injectable form of methadone (IM) is effective in reducing migraine headache pain (Level C).
- No clear differences in analgesic efficacy were demonstrated when parenteral opioid analgesic treatments were compared (butorphanol IM versus meperidine IM plus hydroxyzine IM; methadone IM versus butorphanol IN) (Level C).
- Butorphanol IM failed to show superiority compared with DHE plus metoclopramide IV, as measured by pain outcomes 30 minutes following treatment (Level C).
- Meperidine is not superior to other effective medications (chlorpromazine IV, droperidol IM, ketorolac IM, DHE plus metoclopramide IV). However, large, randomized placebo-controlled trials with meperidine are lacking (Level C).
- The evidence supporting meperidine IV is inadequate to support its use as acute treatment in migraine.

Recommendations

- Oral opiate and butorphanol NS are effective for use in the acute treatment of migraine (Level A); however their use should be limited and reserved for back-up or rescue therapy, or when other medications, such as triptans or NSAIDs cannot be used (e.g., pregnancy, lactation, contraindications to triptans or NSAIDs) (Level U).

- Parenteral opoids should be used as a back-up for acute migraine when sedation side effects will not put the patient at risk and when the risk of abuse has been addressed (Level B).
- No recommendations can be made for the acute treatment of migraine with meperidine IV for patients requiring parenteral therapy (Level U).

SPECIFIC MIGRAINE MEDICATIONS

Ergotamine and DHE

Ergotamine is a choice for moderate-to-severe migraine if analgesics produce significant AEs or do not provide headache relief (Ziegler, 1987) and cost is a factor, therefore, precluding treatment with triptans. Some patients still respond preferentially to rectal ergotamine. Ergotamine tartrate, originally derived from a rye fungus (Claviceps Purpurea), is an ergopeptide, which consists of a natural D-lysergic acid linked to a tricyclic peptide moiety by a peptide bond.

Ergotamine has α-adrenergic and serotonergic agonist activity and vasoconstricting actions, stimulating arterial smooth muscle through serotonin receptors. It also constricts venous capacitance vessels. Both ergotamine and DHE are agonists at the serotonin 5-HT_{1A}, 5-HT_{1B}, 5-HT_{1D}, 5-HT_{1E}, and 5-HT_{1F} receptors (Peroutka, 1990a, 1990b). DHE is a derivative of ergotamine that has been reduced at the nine to ten double bond on the D-lysergic acid moiety. Ergotamine and DHE bind avidly to their receptor sites, producing a long k_{off}. This produces a multiphasic metabolism and excretion pattern of drug elimination that may require up to 72 hours for a single dose of ergotamine.

DHE differs from ergotamine (Berde and Stuermer, 1978). While both DHE and ergotamine inhibit the reuptake of noradrenaline at sympathetic nerve endings, DHE is a weaker arterial vasoconstrictor but almost as potent a venoconstrictor as ergotamine, constricting venous capacitance vessels while having a negligible effect on resistance vessels. DHE is a more potent α-adrenergic blocker than ergotamine and inhibits the baroreceptor circulatory reflex. In both animals and humans, DHE is much less emetic and has less effect on the uterus than ergotamine. It is very difficult to induce experimental gangrene in the rat's tail with high doses of DHE.

Dosage Forms and Bioavailability

Ergotamine tartrate is available as a sublingual preparation and, in combination with caffeine, as an oral tablet and a suppository. Caffeine may enhance ergotamine oral absorption (Schmidt and Fanchamps, 1974) and is an analgesic itself (Ward et al., 1991). The oral absorption of ergotamine is erratic. Ergotamine's bioavailability is highly dependent on the route of administration. Ergotamine given by suppository to normal volunteers produced blood levels 20- to 30-fold higher than the same dose given orally (Sanders et al., 1986).

Efficacy and Safety

The AHCPR reviewed 23 controlled trials of ergotamine tartrate, ergotamine-containing compounds, and ergostine-containing compounds. The results were not consistent and were difficult to interpret owing to the fact that many of these trials are older and used outdated dosing strategies and outcome measures Gray, RN, McCrory, DC, Eberlein, K, Westman, EC, and Hasselblad, V (199b) (1999c). (More recent studies testing the efficacy of ergot alkaloids, specifically DHE, used current headache outcome measures and reported improved efficacy results.)

Five placebo-controlled trials of ergotamine had findings that ranged from no effect to finding large differences favoring ergotamine (Ostfeld, 1961; Waters, 1970; Behan, 1978; Hakkarainen et al., 1982; Kangasniemi and Kaaja, 1992). Three trials comparing ergotamine plus caffeine with placebo also reported mixed results (Ryan, 1970; Sargent et al., 1988; Friedman et al., 1989). One placebo-controlled trial supported the efficacy of ergostine plus caffeine (Ryan, 1970). A proprietary combination of ergotamine, caffeine, pentobarbital, and Bellafolline was shown, in one trial each, to be superior to placebo and ergotamine plus caffeine (Friedman et al., 1989). Otherwise, no significant differences were shown among ergotamine tartrate, ergotamine plus caffeine, ergotamine plus caffeine plus butalbital plus belladonna alkaloids (Kinnunen et al., 1988), and ergostine (Ryan, 1970; Kinnunen et al., 1988).

Ergotamine was significantly more effective than was aspirin in two of three studies (Hakkarainen et al., 1978, 1979). Ergotamine was not significantly different from ketoprofen PR (Kangasniemi and Kaaja, 1992), naproxen sodium (Treves et al., 1992), tolfenamic acid (Hakkarainen et al., 1979), aspirin plus dextropropoxyphene chloride plus phenazone plus (2-diaminoethyl) phentiazin carboxyl chloride plus caffeine (Hakkarainen et al., 1978), aspirin plus dextropropoxyphene napsylate plus phenazone (Hakkarainen et al., 1980), metoclopramide (Hakkarainen and Allonen, 1982), or an isometheptene combination (Behan, 1978). Ergotamine plus caffeine was less effective than oral sumatriptan (Multinational Oral Sumatriptan and Cafergot Comparative Study Group, 1991) or the combination of isometheptene, dichloralphenazone, and acetaminophen (Yuill et al., 1972), and not significantly different from DHE NS (Hirt et al., 1989) or naproxen sodium (Sargent et al., 1988).

Since the first edition of the Guideline, another crossover comparison of efficacy and preference for rizatriptan 10 mg versus ergotamine plus caffeine found rizatriptan superior to ergotamine plus caffeine in all end points (Christie et al., 2003). These studies suggest, but with some mixed results, that ergotamine (with or without caffeine) is more effective than placebo in the acute treatment of migraine. Superiority or equivalency of ergotamine to analgesics, NSAIDs, combination products, or triptans has not been clearly established.

Ergot alkaloids were consistently associated with higher rates of AEs—especially nausea and vomiting—than were placebo, sumatriptan, isometheptene, NSAIDs, and dextropropoxyphene compounds. Most ergotamine combinations (ergotamine plus caffeine, ergotamine plus caffeine plus pentobarbital plus Bellafoline, and ergotamine plus metoclopramide) had lower rates of nausea and vomiting than ergotamine alone (Gray et al., 1999b).

Ergotamine Usage

The evidence to support the efficacy of ergotamine for the treatment of migraine is inconsistent. Ergots had more AEs than placebo, sumatriptan, isometheptene, NSAIDs, or dextropropoxyphene compounds. Ergotamine is consistently inferior to triptans (Lipton, Bigal, et al., 2004). Selected patients with moderate-to-severe migraine will definitively respond to ergot derivatives. For individual attacks, patients can take up to six 1 mg tablets or two suppositories over 24 hours. Use should not exceed two dosage days per week (Saper, 1986). In certain circumstances (e.g., cluster headache) or over shorter periods of time (e.g., menstrual migraine) these limits may be liberalized. Determine the subnauseating dose of ergotamine before its initial use, at a time when the patient is headache free. This will avoid overdosing and increased headache and nausea, and underdosing and lack of efficacy (Silberstein, 1991). Since the rectal route of administration produces higher blood levels than the oral route, the patient should start with the predetermined subnauseating dose (one-third to one-half of a suppository) at the time of the acute headache attack (Silberstein, 1991).

Patients who cannot tolerate ergotamine because of nausea can be pretreated with metoclopramide (Volans, 1978), prochlorperazine (Kanto et al., 1981), phenergan (Silberstein, 1991), or a mixture of a barbiturate and a belladonna alkaloid. Oral metoclopramide might also enhance oral absorption of ergotamine. Patients who cannot tolerate ergotamine or obtain no relief from it and still need an ergot should use DHE. Overuse of ergotamine and most acute migraine medications can lead to CDH and their use must be limited (see Chapter 20).

U.S. Headache Consortium Conclusions and Recommendations

Conclusions

- Class-I studies repeated establish ergot alkaloids as effective for the acute treatment of migraine, although the magnitude of effect and relative efficacy compared with other acute migraine medications appears to vary across studies and treatments.

Recommendations

- Ergotamine tablets (with or without caffeine) may be considered for the treatment of selected patients with migraine, although the magnitude of effect may be modest (Level B).

DIHYDROERGOTAMINE

DHE is available in 1 mg/ml ampules, which can be administered IM, SC, or IV, and it is also available as an NS. Bioavailability and blood levels are highest with IV injection (Kanto et al., 1981), and most erratic with SC injection (Schran and Tse, 1985). Patients can be taught to self-administer DHE IM. Bioavailability of the NS is approximately 40%.

Nine placebo-controlled trials reported on the efficacy and safety of DHE NS (Bousser and Loria, 1985; Krause and Bleicher, 1985; Paiva et al., 1985; Rohr and Dufresne, 1985; Massiou, 1987; Tulunay et al., 1987; Ziegler et al., 1994; Dihydroergotamine Nasal Spray Multicenter Investigators, 1995; Gallagher, 1996). These trials demonstrated the superiority of DHE NS, although the magnitude of the benefit was small to moderate. Three comparisons of different doses of DHE NS were inconclusive (Krause and Bleicher, 1985; Paiva et al., 1985; Gallagher, 1996). Two placebo-controlled trials did not clearly establish whether DHE IV (with an added antiemetic) is effective or ineffective for the treatment of acute migraine (Callaham and Raskin, 1986; Klapper and Stanton, 1991b).

Two trials compared DHE NS to other treatments. One found no significant difference between DHE and ergotamine plus caffeine (Hirt et al., 1989). The other trial found that 6 mg of SC sumatriptan was significantly better than 1 mg with the option for a second 1-mg dose of DHE NS 1 hour later (Touchon et al., 1996). One milligram of DHE SC was less effective than 6 mg of sumatriptan SC for headache relief at 1 and 2 hours, but this difference was not seen at 3, 4, and 24 hours following treatment (Winner et al., 1996). DHE SC had a significantly lower incidence of headache recurrence than did SC sumatriptan. DHE (plus metoclopramide IV) afforded better headache pain relief at 30 and 60 minutes than did meperidine IM plus hydroxyzine IM (Belgrade et al., 1989; Klapper and Stanton, 1993). A single trial compared a 50% lower dose of DHE (0.5 mg) plus metoclopramide (1 mg) IV to meperidine (75 mg) plus promethazine (25 mg) IM and found no differences between treatments (Scherl and Wilson, 1995). In a more recent trial (not included in the AHCPR Technical Report) (Gray et al., 1999b) DHE IM plus hydroxyzine was as effective as meperidine plus hydroxyzine IM (Carleton et al., 1998). In a recent large multicenter trial, DHE 1 mg IM was equally effective compared with meperidine 1.5 mg/kg IM (Leniger et al., 2005). Collectively, these studies support a therapeutic role for DHE IV or IM in the acute treatment of migraine in the emergency department setting.

The most common AE associated with DHE NS was mild-to-moderate rhinitis, which was clearly related to the route of administration. Compared with ergotamine plus caffeine, DHE NS had a similar incidence of adverse events. Compared with SC sumatriptan, it had a significantly lower rate of adverse events. Nausea and vomiting are the most common adverse events associated with IV DHE treatment (Gray et al., 1999c).

DHE NS is rapidly absorbed, with peak plasma concentrations occurring within 45 minutes. The bioavailability is 40% of the same dose given IM. The AEs of nasal DHE are mild and transient and include nasal stuffiness, nausea, and (rarely) vomiting (Lataste, 1989).

DHE NS is safe and effective for the treatment of acute migraine attacks. It is an appropriate treatment choice and should be considered a first-line drug for selected patients with moderate-to-severe migraine. Because of their inability to tolerate or take oral medications, patients with nausea and vomiting may be given DHE NS. Initial treatment with DHE NS is a reasonable choice when the headache is moderate-to-severe or an adequate trial of NSAIDs or other nonopoid analgesics (including combination NSAIDs, such as AAC) has failed to provide adequate relief in the past. After priming the device, the patient delivers one spray (approximately 0.5 mg) into each nostril. This is repeated in 10–15 minutes. An additional set of sprays may be used in 2 hours, for a total dose of 3 mg.

Contraindications to the use of ergotamine tartrate or DHE include renal or hepatic failure, pregnancy, hypertension, sepsis, and coronary, cerebral, and peripheral vascular disease.

No placebo-controlled trials in migraine patients have demonstrated the efficacy and safety of DHE SC, IM, or IV as monotherapy. Clinical opinion suggests that DHE SC is relatively safe and effective when compared with other migraine therapies, and DHE SC has fewer AEs than DHE. Because of their inability to tolerate or take oral medication, patients with nausea and vomiting may be given DHE SC, IV, and IM. Initial treatment with DHE SC is a reasonable choice when the headache is moderate to severe or an adequate trial of NSAIDs or other nonopoid analgesics (including combination NSAIDs such as acetaminophen plus aspirin plus caffeine) has failed to provide adequate relief in the past. DHE IM may be considered for patients with moderate-to-severe migraine. A trial to determine the subnauseating dose of DHE may be undertaken when the patient is headache-free. The patient should take up 1 mg of DHE in a 3 ml syringe with a 1″ 22 gauge needle. Start by instructing the patient to inject DHE 0.25 mg (0.25 cc) IM and then inject additional 0.25 mg increments every 15 minutes, until a maximum of 1.0 mg has been injected or nausea has developed. The incidence of nausea is much lower with IM than with IV injection and lower still than is seen with oral or rectal ergotamine tartrate (Tillgren, 1947). Dosage for individual attacks should be limited to 1 mg IM or IV (maximum of 3 mg per day). Monthly limits are 18 ampules or 12 events. DHE, unlike ergotamine, may not produce rebound headache, but this remains uncertain. We recommend limiting its use to prevent overuse of IM injections and the development of refractoriness. Exceptions include cluster headache, menstrual migraine, and use during detoxification.

DHE IV plus antiemetics has been shown to be effective and moderately safe in the treatment of moderate-to-severe migraine compared with parenteral opioids. DHE IV plus antiemetics is an appropriate treatment choice for patients with severe migraine. DHE may produce nausea in some patients. Pretreatment with metoclopramide, promethazine, or a combination of atropine and a barbiturate, or perhaps ondansetron, might counter this side effect and treat the nausea associated with the migraine as well.

The combination of prochlorperazine IV 5 mg followed by DHE IV is a safe and effective means of terminating a migraine attack (Callaham and Raskin, 1986). The combination of metoclopramide IV and DHE IV was more effective in treating an acute migraine attack than is meperidine IM (Belgrade et al., 1989). One can mix 10 mg (2 ml) of prochlorperazine and 1 mg (1 ml) of DHE in a syringe and inject 2 cc of the mixture IV. If the headache is not relieved in 15–30 minutes, the remainder of the dose can be injected (Raskin, 1990).

Repetitive IV DHE. IV DHE has become the mainstay of acute symptomatic treatment for intractable headache (Raskin, 1986; Edmeads, 1988; Silberstein et al., 1990). Repetitive IV DHE was effective in eliminating intractable headache in 89% of patients within 48 hours (Raskin, 1986). IV diazepam was only partially effective in eliminating such headaches (13% within 3–6 days). Silberstein et al. (1990) also found that repetitive IV DHE was effective in eliminating prolonged migraine, cluster headache, and chronic daily headaches with or without rebound.

IV DHE has a sustained therapeutic effect, but it is uncertain whether this is directly related to the effects of the DHE itself (Silberstein et al., 1990), the active metabolite 8-OH-DHE (Aellig, 1984; Muller-Schweinitzer, 1984), the termination of drug "rebound" (Saper, 1986; Diener et al., 1988), or removing the patient from a stressful environment (Silberstein et al., 1990).

Patients treated with DHE should have a heparin lock inserted for medication administration. The patients may be pretreated with an antinauseant, such as metoclopramide 10 mg IV or ondansetron 8 mg IV, which is continued as needed before each infusion of DHE. DHE is initially administered at a test dose of 0.5 mg (0.25 in children) given via IV push over 3–5 minutes. If the headache persists, another 0.5 mg of DHE is given and 1.0 mg of DHE is administered every 8 hours (Fig. 11–1). If the patient is controlled on 0.5 mg of DHE, the dose is continued every 8 hours. If nausea persists, the next dose of DHE can be reduced to 0.25 mg. DHE is tapered and discontinued (after 3–5 days) if the patient is headache-free or fails to respond to the medication. Alternative delivery methods include an IV drip of DHE diluted in normal saline. There are two methods of doing this. In the first method, DHE is diluted in 50 cc of normal saline and administered over 30–60 minutes. In the second method, DHE is infused continuously for up to 3 days (Ford and Ford, 1997). These alternative delivery methods may reduce local venous reactions as well as other AEs, such as nausea and chest pain.

U.S. Headache Consortium Conclusions and Recommendations Conclusions

- DHE NS is effective for the acute treatment of migraine and may be considered for treatment of selected patients with migraine.
- There is limited evidence to support the use of DHE IM, SC, IV with or without an anti-emetic (Level B).

Recommendations

- DHE NS should be used for the acute treatment of migraine in adults (Level A).
- DHE IM, SC, IV may be used in the treatment of migraine (Level B).

SELECTIVE SEROTONIN (5-HT$_1$) AGONISTS (TRIPTANS)

The first selective 5-HT$_{1B/1D}$ agonist to be developed and tested was sumatriptan, followed by zolmitriptan, naratriptan, rizatriptan, almotriptan, eletriptan, and frovatriptan (Tables 11–9 and 11–10). Sumatriptan was first available as a SC injection, then as an oral tablet, a NS and, more recently, as a dispersible tablet, which replaced the conventional tablet. In the sections that follow, we discuss sumatriptan first, since it was the first triptan to be available. We then discuss the other triptans (usually termed the second generation triptans) in alphabetic order. We close by briefly discussing the combination of sumatriptan and naproxen, expected to be launched in the United States in 2007.

Sumatriptan is extensively metabolized in the liver by MAO-A and therefore its use as an oral or NS formulation is contraindicated in patients who are on MAO inhibitors. The injectable form, however, has been shown to be safe and well tolerated (Freitag et al., 1998). Substantial drug–drug interaction with other traditional migraine preventive medications, including β-blockers, calcium channel antagonists, selective serotonin reuptake inhibitors (SSRIs), and tricyclic antidepressants (TCAs), were not found. No difference was found in the likelihood of improved response with preventive therapies or between preventive therapies. Headache recurrence and AEs were also similar in the various treatment groups.

SC sumatriptanatriptan. Fourteen placebo-controlled trials consistently showed that SC sumatriptan (6 mg) was superior to placebo for headache relief and complete relief at 1 and 2 hours (Jackson, 1996; Mushet et al., 1996; Scott et al., 1996; Visser et al., 1996; Carpay et al., 1997; Cull et al., 1997; Gruffydd-Jones et al., 1997; Kelly et al., 1997; Ryan et al., 1997; Cady et al., 1998; Diamond et al., 1998; Myllyla et al., 1998; Pfaffenrath et al., 1998; Tepper et al., 1998; Matchar et al., 2000). A second dose of sumatriptan SC, administered 1 hour after the first, provided no

TABLE 11–9 Selective 5-HT$_1$ Receptor Agonists (Saxena and Tfelt-Hansen, 2006).

Drug	*Company*	T_{max} (hours)	*Half-life (hours)*
Almotriptan	Almirall/OthoMcNeil	2.1	3.1
Eletriptan	Pfizer	1.8	5
Frovatriptan	Vanguard/Endo	~2.5	~26
Naratriptan	GlaxoSmithKlein	3–5	6
Rizatriptan	Merck	2–3	5
Sumatriptan	Glaxo Smith Klein	2	2
Zolmitriptan	AstraZeneca	2.5	3

TABLE 11–10 Headache Response and Therapeutic Gain for Triptans at 2 Hours (Saxena and Tfelt-Hansen, 2006).

	Headache response (2 hours)	*Therapeutic gain* for response (2 hours)*
Almotriptan (25 mg)	61%	27%
Eletriptan (40 mg)	60%	36%
Eletriptan (80 mg)	64%	45%
Frovatriptan (2.5 mg)	44%	20%
Naratriptan (2.5 mg)	48%	21%
Rizatriptan (10 mg)	69%	36%
Sumatriptan (20 mg NS)	61%	31%
Sumatriptan (50 mg)	59%	29%
Sumatriptan (100 mg)	61%	33%
Sumatriptan (6 mg SC)	80%–85%	51%
Zolmitriptan (2.5 mg)	63%	34%
Zolmitriptan (5 mg NS)	70%	39%

Abbreviations: NS, nasal spray; SC, subcutaneous.

* Therapeutic gain is the difference between the response to active drug and the response to placebo. It can be used to compare drugs tested in different clinical trials and is presented here with 95% confidence intervals based on published and abstracted studies.

added benefit (Cady et al., 1991; SC Sumatriptan International Study Group, 1991). One additional large, randomized, controlled, double-blind study demonstrated the efficacy of *sumatriptan SC 4 mg in* the acute treatment of migraine (Wendt et al., 2006). The primary end point was pain relief at 2 hours, and this was reached by 70% of the patients receiving sumatriptan 4 mg SC versus 22% of those receiving placebo. Adverse events included injection-site reactions (43%), tingling (12%), and other known triptan side effects. All 15 of these Class-I trials demonstrate that the 4- and 6-mg dose of sumatriptan SC is superior to placebo in achieving headache relief.

Two trials directly compared SC and oral formulations of sumatriptan. Methodological differences between the trials complicated their comparison and interpretation, but both studies found SC sumatriptan to be significantly more effective than oral sumatriptan at 2 and 4 hours (Carpay et al., 1997; Gruffydd-Jones et al., 1997).

One trial each compared SC sumatriptan with SC DHE (Winner et al., 1996) and DHE NS (Touchon et al., 1996). In both trials, 1- and 2-hour data on headache relief and complete relief favored sumatriptan, while 2- to 24-hour recurrence rates favored DHE.

Sumatriptan SC was effective for treatment of recurrent headache after initially successful treatment with sumatriptan (Henry and D'allens, 1993), but sumatriptan administered during the migraine aura, before the onset of headache pain, was no more effective than placebo at preventing the development of a moderate-to-severe headache (Ensink, 1991).

Significantly more patients reported AEs with SC sumatriptan than with placebo or DHE NS, but less than with SC DHE. The most commonly reported AEs with sumatriptan SC were injection site reactions, flushing, dizziness/vertigo, and paresthesia/tingling. Some patients reported transient chest symptoms in many of the trials included in the analysis (Gray, Goslin, et al., 1999).

Oral sumatriptan—conventional tablets. Eleven placebo-controlled trials provided consistent evidence that oral sumatriptan, in a dose of 100 mg, is significantly more effective than is placebo for headache relief and complete relief at 2 and 4 hours (Oral Sumatriptan Dose-Defining Study Group, 1991; Oral Sumatriptan International Multiple-Dose Study Group, 1991; Nappi et al., 1994; Cutler et al., 1995; Pini et al., 1995; Sargent et al., 1995; Tfelt-Hansen et al., 1995; Cutler et al., 1996; Jackson, 1996; Myllyla et al., 1998). In the

United States, sumatriptan is currently available in 25- and 50-mg doses. Three trials supported the efficacy of these lower doses (25 and 50 mg) (Cutler et al., 1995; Sargent et al., 1995; Pfaffenrath et al., 1998; Matchar et al., 2000). In the only multidose study reporting 4-hour outcomes, headache relief and complete relief rates with the 50-mg dose were comparable to those reported with the 100-mg dose and superior to the 25-mg dose (Pfaffenrath et al., 1998). In general, the proportions of patients who reported relief with oral sumatriptan were lower than with SC sumatriptan. Two trials directly comparing SC and oral sumatriptan suggested that the SC formulation provides superior relief (Carpay et al., 1997; Gruffydd-Jones et al., 1997).

Oral sumatriptan—dispersible tablets. Two newer studies with the new formulation of sumatriptan rapidly dispersible tablets have been reported. Both randomized, double-blind, placebo-controlled trials demonstrated that sumatriptan dispersible tablet is significantly more effective than is placebo in achieving pain relief at 2 hours following treatment (Sheftell et al., 2005; Carpay and Dowson, 2006). One study enrolled 2996 patients with moderate or severe pain and after 2 hours, 72% of the patients receiving the 100-mg dose versus 67% of those receiving the 50-mg dose achieved pain relief (42% with placebo). The two doses were not statistically different, although the time to achieve pain relief was faster in the 100-mg group. In the second study, 481 patients were enrolled, and both doses were significantly better than placebo in achieving a pain-free response at 1 and 2 hours. No studies have been reported comparing sumatriptan dispersible tablet with either the conventional tablet or other triptans. Collectively these studies show that sumatriptan as a regular tablet or in the newer rapidly dispersible tablet are effective in achieving pain relief versus placebo.

One trial each compared sumatriptan 100 mg with aspirin plus metoclopramide (Oral Sumatriptan and Aspirin-plus-Metoclpramide Comparative Study Group, 1992), lysine acetylsalicylate plus metoclopramide (Tfelt-Hansen et al., 1995), and a rapid-release formulation of tolfenamic acid (Myllyla et al., 1998). They demonstrated no significant differences between the analgesic compounds and sumatriptan for headache relief at 2 hours, and only one of the three trials found sumatriptan to be significantly better for complete relief (Oral Sumatriptan and Aspirin-plus-Metoclpramide Comparative Study Group, 1992). Sumatriptan was significantly more effective than ergotamine plus caffeine for both headache relief and complete relief at 2 hours (Multinational Oral Sumatriptan and Cafergot Comparative Study Group, 1991).

A second dose of oral sumatriptan, 2–4 hours after the first dose, did not provide any additional relief of the initial headache (Ferrari et al., 1994; Scott et al., 1996) and did not prevent headache recurrence (Ferrari et al., 1994; Scott et al., 1996; Rapoport et al., 1995). Four trials of sumatriptan showed it to be significantly better than placebo in relieving recurrent headache pain (Pini et al., 1995; Ferrari et al., 1994; Cady et al., 1994; Teall et al., 1998).

Sumatriptan NS. Six placebo-controlled trials support the efficacy of sumatriptan NS for headache relief at one and two hours (Finnish Sumatriptan Group and the Cardiovascular Clinical Research Group, 1991; Salonen et al., 1994; Ryan et al., 1997; Diamond et al., 1998). A dose–response relationship was demonstrated, with superiority to placebo at the 10-, 20-, and 40-mg doses. Results with the 5-mg dose were mixed, and the 1-mg dose was shown to be ineffective. Significantly more patients reported AEs with sumatriptan NS than with placebo, the most common symptom being "taste disturbance."

Other delivery methods of sumatriptan. One trial each tested the efficacy of sumatriptan IM (Kelly et al., 1997) and sumatriptan PR (Tepper et al., 1998). Sumatriptan IM 6 mg was as effective as chlorpromazine IV at 1 and 2 hours posttreatment. Sumatriptan PR (12.5 or 25 mg) was significantly more effective than placebo at 2 hours, with a stronger clinical benefit observed with the higher dose.

Sumatriptan relieves headache pain, nausea, photophobia, and phonophobia, and restores the patient's ability to function normally. Sumatriptan (or another triptan) is often prescribed at the initial consultation as a first-line drug for severe attacks and as backup medication for less severe attacks that do not adequately respond to simple or combination analgesics. We prefer the SC injection or the NS for patients who need rapid relief or have severe nausea or vomiting. Oral sumatriptan is used for gradual-onset headache when rapid pain relief is not required. Although 80% of patients get pain relief from an initial SC dose of sumatriptan, headache recurs in about one-third of patients within a day. Recurrences respond well to a second dose of sumatriptan and sometimes to simple and combination analgesics.

Almotriptan. Almotriptan was compared with placebo in three double-blind trials (Cabarrocas and Zayas, 1998; Pascual et al., 2000). Doses ranged from 2 to 25 mg across the three trials, and the 12.5-mg dose was used in all three studies. Headache relief was achieved in each of these trials and supported the utility of 6.25–25 mg. Sumatriptan 100 mg was used as an active comparator in one trial, and no differences were seen between drugs regarding efficacy, although almotriptan was better tolerated. These studies show that almotriptan 6.25 and 12.5 mg are more effective than placebo in achieving headache relief and are similar in efficacy to sumatriptan 100-mg oral tablet; some patients may tolerate almotriptan better than sumatriptan 100 mg.

Eletriptan. Oral eletriptan is rapidly absorbed, with high bioavailability (50%) and a long half-life (5 hours). There is some concern, however, regarding eletriptan's possible interaction with other compounds that are metabolized at the cytochrome p450 site.

Eletriptan, 20, 40, and 80 mg, was tested in three double-blind, placebo-controlled trials (80-mg dose not available in the United States) (Farkkila, 1996; Stark et al., 2002; Sheftell et al., 2003). Headache response at 2 hours was the primary end point for all three studies, and all three doses were effective versus placebo. Eletriptan 40-mg was more effective than 20-mg and had fewer side effects than the 80-mg dose. These studies show that eletriptan is more effective than placebo in achieving pain relief within 2 hours following treatment.

Pryse-Phillips (1999) compared oral eletriptan (40–80 mg) and oral sumatriptan (50–100 mg) for the treatment of acute migraine in a randomized, placebo-controlled trial in sumatriptan-naive patients. Eletriptan was also more effective than sumatriptan at providing relief of functional disability, nausea, photophobia, and phonophobia. Headache recurrence rates were low in the eletriptan groups (19% and 16% for 40 mg and 80 mg). In general, treatment-related AEs were transient and mild or moderate in intensity. These findings were supported by two other studies; where sumatriptan was encapsulated but demonstrated to be bioequivalent to nonencapsulated sumatriptan also suggested the superiority of eletriptan 40 mg over sumatriptan 50 mg (Goadsby et al., 2000; Diener, Ryan, et al., 2004).

Frovatriptan. Frovatriptan is a $5HT_{1B/1D}$ receptor agonist with a high affinity for the $5HT_{1B/1D}$ receptors, potent agonism in isolated human cerebral arteries, functional selectivity for isolated cerebral arteries compared with coronary arteries, and limited coronary constrictor activity relative to sumatriptan.

Two randomized, placebo-controlled efficacy studies have been reported for frovatriptan, with dose ranges between 0.5 and 5 mg (Rapoport et al., 2002; Goldstein and Keywood, 2002). These studies found that frovatriptan 2.5 mg was significantly better than placebo in achieving headache relief at 2 hours. All doses were significantly superior to placebo at 4 hours, but the 2.5-mg dose was selected for clinical use.

Frovatriptan 2.5 mg was tested in patients with substantial coronary artery disease risk factors, including an active diagnosis of coronary artery disease. No substantial changes in blood pressure, pulse rate, or electrocardiogram were found over a 24-hour continuously monitored patient study. No chest pain was reported by frovatriptan-treated patients, and there was a statistically significant greater incidence of 12-lead electrocardiogram changes among placebo patients as compared with the frovatriptan patients at 4 hours (Rosenorn et al., 1988). However, the risk of an adverse cardiovascular AE with any triptan is very rare and perhaps idiosyncratic.

Naratriptan. Oral naratriptan differs from sumatriptan primarily in its longer half-life, longer T-max, higher oral bioavailability (70%), and lipophilicity. Studies of more than 4000 patients indicate that the drug has a well-defined dose–response relationship for headache relief, with a mean response of 48% at 2 hours after administration, but therapeutic gains are comparatively modest (21%). Two trials tested the efficacy of naratriptan and found a significant clinical benefit over placebo for the 1 and 2.5-mg doses at 4 hours posttreatment (Klassen et al., 1997; Mathew et al., 1997). Relief rates with naratriptan were lower than with the other oral 5-$HT_{1B/1D}$ agonists. A direct comparative crossover study of patients prone to headache recurrence showed that about one-third fewer experienced recurrence when they used naratriptan compared with sumatriptan. However, 24-hour comparisons of naratriptan and sumatriptan found relief rates to be similar. The studies showed excellent tolerability for the 2.5-mg dose of naratriptan, with an adverse event rate close to that of placebo.These data support the efficacy of naratriptan in the acute treatment of migraine 4 hours after treatment, but efficacy at early time points (within two hours following treatment) is not established.

Rizatriptan. Rizatriptan has rapid oral absorption and high oral bioavailability at 45% for the 10-mg dose. Four double-blind trials found that rizatriptan was significantly better than placebo for headache relief and complete relief at 2 hours; doses tested ranged from 5 to 40 mg, with higher rates of relief reported with the higher doses (doses currently available in United States: rizatriptan 5 and 10 mg) (Cutler et al., 1996; Visser et al., 1996; Gijsman et al., 1997; Teall et al., 1998). One published study directly compared oral sumatriptan (100 mg) and rizatriptan (10, 20, 40 mg), and found that a high dose of rizatriptan (40 mg) produced significantly better results at 2 hours (Visser et al., 1996). No significant differences were found between sumatriptan and the lower doses of rizatriptan at 2 hours. When directly compared with sumatriptan 100 mg, rizatriptan 10 mg had a cumulative benefit of approximately 20% in terms of patients who achieved headache response in the first 2 hours and a cumulative advantage of approximately 15% when compared with sumatriptan 50 mg. Rizatriptan has high consistency from attack to attack in formal blinded consistency studies and a useful wafer (Melt) formulation that many patients, particularly those with nausea as a prominent feature, find convenient, as it dissolves on the tongue and requires no water, although absorption is gastrointestinal and transbuccal. Rizatriptan has a significant interaction with propranolol, which requires that the dose be halved to 5 mg and is contraindicated with monoamine oxidase inhibitors (MAOIs), because of its route of metabolism. Rizatriptan was significantly better than placebo at relieving recurrent headache pain (Teall et al., 1998). The efficacy of rizatriptan orally dissolving tablet also has been established in two double-blind, placebo controlled trials (Ahrens et al., 1999; Klapper and O'Connor, 2000). These Class-I studies show that both the 5-mg and the 10-mg tablets and orally disintegrating wafers are superior to placebo within 2 hours following treatment.

Zolmitriptan. Zolmitriptan has high oral bioavailability (40%), a T-max of approximately 2.5 hours, and is metabolized by the cytochrome P450 system to an active metabolite that is degraded by MAO-A. Therefore, patients taking MAOIs are limited to a total zolmitriptan dose of 5 mg/day. In four randomized, controlled trials, zolmitriptan 2.5-mg or 5-mg tablets were significantly more effective than placebo for headache relief and complete relief at 2 and 4 hours (Rapoport et al., 1997; Solomon et al., 1997; Dahlof et al., 1998) (Visser et al., 1998) The only trial that directly compared the 2.5- and 5-mg doses of zolmitriptan found no significant difference between them (Rapoport et al., 1997). Zolmitriptan demonstrated a headache response of 64% with a therapeutic gain of 34% for the 2.5-mg dose and a headache response of 65% and a 37% therapeutic gain for the 5-mg dose. The recommended starting dose of 2.5 mg provides the best balance of benefit and AEs, although some patients may benefit from the higher 5-mg dose. In all studies, zolmitriptan reduced the incidence of photophobia, phonophobia, and nausea compared with placebo. In formal comparisons with sumatriptan 100 mg, zolmitriptan 5 mg was no different, and in a recent comparison with zolmitriptan 2.5 mg, no clinically relevant differences were seen. The most frequently reported AEs include asthenia, nausea, somnolence, dizziness, and paresthesias. A randomized, controlled, parallel trial that compared sumatriptan 25 and 50 mg with zolmitriptan 2.5 and 5 mg over the course of a series of headaches showed that both doses of zolmitriptan were either comparable or statistically superior to both doses of sumatriptan for headache relief, consistency of response, and 24-hour headache relief rates (Rapoport et al., 1997). Zolmitriptan (Solomon et al., 1997) was significantly better than placebo at relieving recurrent headache pain. One small study did not support the use of zolmitriptan during the aura phase for the short-term prevention of migraine (Dowson, 1996). Three new trials compared zolmitriptan orally disintegrating tablet and placebo (Dowson and Charlesworth, 2002; Spierings et al., 2004; Loder et al., 2005). Two studies tested the efficacy of the 2.5-mg dose (Dowson and Charlesworth, 2002; Loder et al., 2005), and one tested the 5-mg dose. Both doses were positive in achieving pain relief at 2 hours (pain free in 2 hours and headache relief in 2 hours). One trial reported zolmitriptan 5 mg was more effective than placebo in achieving headache response at 30 minutes (primary end point) (Spierings et al., 2004). These studies confirm that zolmitriptan 2.5- and 5-mg doses are effective in achieving pain relief within 2 hours following treatment.

Zolmitriptan NS was compared with placebo in three recent double-blind trials. In one trial, the doses ranged from 0.5 to 5 mg and the zolmitriptan 2.5-mg tablet was used as an active control (Charlesworth et al., 2003). Response rates at 2 hours for the 0.5-, 1.0-, 2.5-, and 5-mg doses were 41%, 55%, 59% ,and 70%, respectively, compared with 30% for placebo (all $p < 0.001$) and 61% for zolmitriptan 2.5-mg tablet. In a second trial, zolmitriptan 5-mg NS confirmed the efficacy of the 5-mg dose and also repeated the finding that this formulation provides pain relief in some patients as early as 15 minutes onward (Dodick et al., 2005). The third study reported that zolmitriptan 5 mg was superior to placebo in achieving complete symptom relief (no pain and no migraine symptoms) at 30 minutes and thereafter (Gawel et al., 2005).

AEs—most commonly malaise/fatigue, dizziness/vertigo, asthenia, and nausea—were generally more frequent (and in some cases significantly more frequent) with the oral triptans than with placebo. The incidence of AEs was dose-dependent with rizatriptan and zolmitriptan. Significantly more patients reported adverse events with sumatriptan than with aspirin/lysine acetylsalicylate plus metoclopramide. For all treatments in this drug class, small numbers of patients reported transient chest symptoms (Gray et al., 1999b). Warnings are now included in the product information for all triptans regarding the risk of serotonin syndrome in patients taking other serotonin agonists.

None of the triptans should be used by patients who have or are at high risk for clinical ischemic heart disease, Prinzmetal's angina, uncontrolled hypertension, or strictly vertebrobasilar migraine. Sumatriptan's common AEs include pain at the injection site, tingling, flushing, burning, and warm or hot sensations. Dizziness, heaviness, neck pain, and dysphoria can also occur. These AEs generally abate within 45 minutes. Sumatriptan causes noncardiac chest pressure in approximately 4% of patients. We get an electrocardiogram on patients over the age of 40 and those who have risk factors for heart disease before using any of the triptans. We often give the first triptan dose in the office at a time when the patient does not have a headache.

The triptans are effective and relatively safe for the acute treatment of migraine headaches. To date, no evidence supports their use during the aura phase of a migraine attack. They are appropriate first-line treatment choices and may be considered for patients with moderate-to-severe migraine who have no contraindications to these agents. Because of their inability to take oral medications, patients with nausea and vomiting may be given intranasal or SC sumatriptan. Initial treatment with any triptan is a reasonable choice when the headache is moderate to severe or an adequate trial of NSAIDs or other nonopioid analgesics (including combination of NSAIDs such as acetaminophen plus aspirin plus caffeine) has failed to provide adequate relief in the past.

Sumatriptan plus naproxen sodium. The literature contains several studies that suggest that the efficacy of triptans is improved when naproxen sodium is given concomitantly (Krymchantowski, 2000; Smith et al., 2005). Therefore, a new single-tablet, fixed-dose, combination agent that combines sumatriptan 85 mg with naproxen sodium 500 mg in a patented RT Technology formulation has been developed. Two studies report that this new fixed-dose combination is more effective than placebo or either agent (sumatriptan 85 mg or naproxen 500 mg) given as monotherapy in achieving headache relief at 2 hours (Silberstein, Stark, et al., 2006). This combination of therapies appears to also offer improvement in 24-hour outcome measures, such as higher 24-hour headache response rates and lower recurrence rates. This combination is expected to be available in the U.S. market in 2007.

U.S. Headache Consortium Conclusions and Recommendations

Conclusions

- The triptans have several advantages when compared with other specific migraine therapies in that they have selective pharmacology, simple and consistent pharmacokinetics, evidence-based dose recommendations, and established efficacy based on large, well-designed, controlled trials (Lipton, Bigal, et al., 2004). The limitations for triptans is that they are more expensive than ergotamine compounds and, like ergot derivatives, they are contraindicated in the presence of cardiovascular disease (Dodick et al., 2004).
- On the basis of a review of the multiple Class-I studies, all seven triptans in all formulations are effective for the acute treatment of migraine in adults.
- A combination of sumatriptan 85 mg plus 500 mg naproxen is effective in the treatment of migraine and offers improved clinical response over sumatriptan or naproxen given as monotherapy (Level A).

Recommendations

- All seven triptans in all formulations (oral tablets, orally disintegrating tablets, NSs, and injectable formulations) should be used for the acute treatment of mild, moderate or severe migraine (Level A).
- For patients who experience migraine-related disability, triptans should be used by adults for the acute treatment of migraine unless contraindicated (Level A).
- Combination of triptans plus naproxen sodium should be used in the acute treatment of migraine and offers improved clinical response over either treatment given as monotherapy (Level A).

NEUROLEPTICS AND ANTIEMETICS

The associated symptoms of migraine, such as nausea and vomiting, can be as disabling as the headache pain itself (Table 11–1). The gastric stasis and delayed gastric emptying that are associated with migraine can decrease the effectiveness of oral medication (Volans, 1978; Tfelt-Hansen et al., 1980; Boyle et al., 1990). The medications used to treat migraine can produce nausea, as can migraine itself. In addition, many antiemetics are themselves effective in migraine headache treatment.

Neuroleptics may be used as an adjunct treatment for nausea or as primary therapy. Neuroleptics can be administered orally, rectally, IM, or IV. Monitor for hypotension and sedation. Avoid orthostatic hypotension by maintaining the patient supine for several hours following IV neuroleptics and using supplementary IV fluids if necessary.

Sixteen trials (AHCPR Technical Report) compared the efficacy of rectally and parenterally administered medications that are commonly recognized as antiemetics (Amery and Waelkens, 1983; Waelkens, 1984; McEwen et al., 1987; Lane et al., 1989; Bell et al., 1990; Tek et al., 1990; Rowat et al., 1991; Stiell et al., 1991; Ellis et al., 1993; Chappell et al., 1994; Jones et al., 1994; Cameron et al., 1995; Coppola et al., 1995; Jones et al., 1996; Shrestha et al., 1996).

Intravenous Antidopaminergic Medications

Metoclopramide. The first edition of the Guideline showed that metoclopramide IV was superior to placebo (in three of five trials) and ibuprofen (one trial) for the acute treatment of migraine (Matchar et al., 2000; Silberstein, 2000b). Since this report, one additional trial used repeated doses of metoclopramide plus dimenhydrinate IM and found it as effective as SC sumatriptan in the treatment of migraine in the emergency department (Friedman et al., 2005). These studies confirm the role of metoclopramide IV or IM as an emergency department treatment for the acute care of migraine.

Prochlorperazine. Studies have shown that prochlorperazine IV or IM significantly relieved headache pain compared with placebo (Matchar et al., 2000; Silberstein, 2000b). In one more recent trial, IV prochlorperazine was superior to IV divalproex in relieving pain and nausea of migraine (no placebo group) (Tanen et al., 2003).

Chlorpromazine. Prior small studies show chlorpromazine IV to be superior to meperidine IV and lidocaine IV for the acute treatment of migraine; however, large prospective, controlled, randomized trials are lacking (Matchar et al., 2000; Silberstein, 2000b). In a single study, chlorpromazine IM was not more effective than placebo (McEwen et al., 1987). In a double-blind emergency room study, chlorpromazine IV 0.1 mg/Kg was effective in achieving significant pain-free response at 30 minutes versus placebo (Bigal, Bordini, and Speciali, 2002). Relative to placebo, fewer patients in the chlorpromazine group reported nausea. The study also randomized separately attacks with or without aura, and chlorpromazine separated from placebo in both groups. These few studies suggest a therapeutic role for chlorpromazine IV in the acute treatment of migraine in the emergency department setting.

Metoclopramide, prochlorperazine, and chlorpromazine all had the common AE of drowsiness or sedation. Acute dystonic reactions and akathisia were rare (Gray et al., 1999b, 1999c).

Oral Antidopaminergic Medications

Studies of specific oral agents, such as domperidone and prochlorperazine, suggest some clinical benefit, but studies were limited. No studies were identified for other oral antiemetics as monotherapy to manage acute migraine attacks for headache relief. Oral antiemetics may be used as an adjunct in the treatment of nausea associated with migraine.

Metoclopramide. Oral metoclopramide given as monotherapy for the acute treatment of migraine is not well studied and the results are difficult to interpret (Matchar et al., 2000). However, in a number of clinical trials, oral metoclopramide administered as adjuvant medication for the treatment of migraine pain has been proven effective, although these trials did not include assessment of metoclopramide as monotherapy (Matchar et al., 2000). The first edition of the guideline showed that metoclopramide IV was superior to placebo (in three out of five trials) and ibuprofen (one trial) for the acute treatment of migraine (Matchar et al., 2000; Silberstein, 2000b). Pretreatment with metoclopramide IV seems to reduce nausea in patients with migraine (Cete et al., 2005). IM metoclopramide was not effective as monotherapy for treatment of acute migraine headache. Since this report, one additional trial used repeated doses of metoclopramide plus dimenhydrinate IM and found it as effective as SC sumatriptan in the emergency department treatment of migraine (Friedman et al., 2005). These studies confirm the role of metoclopramide IV or IM as an emergency room treatment for the acute care of migraine.

Metoclopramide IV may be an appropriate choice as adjunct therapy for the treatment of headache pain or nausea in the appropriate setting. Metoclopramide IV may be considered as monotherapy for migraine pain relief. Metoclopramide (Reglan) is available as tablets, syrup, and injectable form (dose 10–20 mg), and is useful in the treatment of migraine. It decreases gastric atony and enhances the absorption of coadministered medications (Albibi and McCallum, 1983).

In the previous guideline, prochlorperazine IM, IV, or PR was proven to be relatively safe and effective for the treatment of migraine headache and associated nausea and vomiting (Matchar et al., 2000; Silberstein, 2000b). In one newer small trial, buccal prochlorperazine at the dose of 3 mg was superior to 1 mg ergotamine plus caffeine 100 mg and placebo for relief of headache pain and migraine symptoms (Sharma et al., 2002). In another trial, IV prochlorperazine was superior to IV divalproex in relieving pain and nausea of migraine (no placebo group) (Tanen et al., 2003).

Prochlorperazine IV, IM, and PR may be a therapeutic choice for migraine in the appropriate setting. Prochlorperazine PR may be considered an adjunct in the treatment of acute migraine with nausea and vomiting. Prochlorperazine (Compazine) can be administered IV 7.5–15 mg over 5–10 minutes via a saline drip or "slow push" (Callaham and Raskin, 1986; Jones et al., 1989).

Promethazine, available in tablet, liquid, suppository, and injectable forms (dose 25–50 mg) is also useful for the control of nausea and vomiting but, unlike metoclopramide, does not enhance gastric emptying. Some patients find promethazine more tolerable than metoclopramide because it has fewer extrapyramidal AEs.

Hydroxyzine (dose 50–100 mg orally, 75 mg IM) may be useful in controlling both nausea and headache. Perphenazine (dose 2–4 mg orally,

5 mg IM), chlorpromazine (dose 25–50 mg orally, 25–100 mg PR), and prochlorperazine (dose 10 mg IM or PR) may be similarly useful, and are discussed in more detail later.

Chlorpromazine (Thorazine) can be administered IV (10–25 mg three–four times per day) diluted in 20–30 ml of saline by rapid drip or "slow push" over several minutes. Chlorpromazine can also be administered IM or PR.

Perphenazine (Trilafon 5 mg IM), haloperidol (Haldol 5 mg IM), and thiothixene (Navane 5 mg IM) can also be used as primary or adjunct treatment for intractable migraine. Haloperidol was shown to be effective in acute migraine treatment in an open case series (Fisher, 1995).

Droperidol is a parenteral neuroleptic. A pilot study of IV droperidol in 35 patients (32 women and 3 men; mean age 43) with status migrainosus (N = 25) or refractory migraine (N = 10) was conducted in an ambulatory infusion center. Headache was graded as severe in 21 patients and moderate in 14. Droperidol (2.5 mg) was given IV every 30 minutes until either three doses were given or the patient was completely or almost headache-free (Wang et al., 1997).

The success rate (headache-free or mild headache) was 88% (22/25) in patients with status migrainosus and 100% (10/10) in patients with refractory migraine. Sedation was common (34/35), akathisia unusual (5/35), and dystonia rare (1/35). At follow-up 24 hours after discharge, the recurrence rate (headache intensity from none or mild to moderate or severe) was 23% in status migrainosus patients and 10% in refractory migraine patients. Krusz et al. (Krusz et al., 1999) treated 45 patients, taken from a population of migraineurs in a headache clinic, with IV droperidol. The average dose per treatment was 3.2 mg, using increments of 0.625 mg per dose. The average reduction in headache severity was 86.1%, using a 0–10 visual analog scale rated by each patient. The average time to maximum reduction of headache was approximately 40 minutes. Droperidol is useful in aborting ongoing migraine headache, acts rapidly, and was devoid of AEs when used in the dosage range employed in this study.

In a newer randomized, double-blind, controlled trial, droperidol 0.1, 2.75, 5.5, and 8.25 mg was tested for the acute treatment of moderate-to-severe migraine versus placebo (Silberstein, Young, et al., 2003). Headache relief at 2 hours was significantly different among treatment groups; droperidol doses 2.75 mg (87%), 5.5 mg (81%), and 8.25 mg (85%) were superior to placebo (57%). There was significant difference among the doses tested. Droperidol 2.75 mg was significantly better in reducing nausea at 1, 1.5, 3, and 4 hours after treatment assessments. Droperidol appears to be safe and effective in treating status migrainosus and refractory migraine. Hypotension was uncommon. Patients should be warned of sedation and akathisia (Wang et al., 1997), which can be treated with diphenhydramine or benzotropine.

Serotonin receptor (5-HT$_3$) antagonists. Studies testing the efficacy of granisetron (Rowat et al., 1991) and zatosetron (Chappell et al., 1994) did not demonstrate a statistically significant clinical benefit for headache relief. Sufficient studies to demonstrate the clinical efficacy of this class of drug have not been done. Evidence is insufficient at this time to establish, or refute, a role for 5-HT$_3$ antagonists as monotherapy in the management of acute attacks. 5-HT$_3$ antagonists may be considered as adjunct therapy to control nausea in selected patients with migraine attacks. Ondansetron, a selective 5-HT$_3$ receptor antagonist that has no antidopaminergic activity and no effect on gastrointestinal motility, is available as an IV for the nausea associated with migraine (dose 0.15 mg/kg diluted in 50 ml of D5W or NSS).

U.S. Headache Consortium Conclusions and Recommendations

Conclusions

- Metoclopramide as oral monotherapy is ineffective for the acute treatment of migraine. However, when given as adjunct therapy with NSAIDs or triptans, the combination therapy is probably effective.
- Metoclopramide IV is probably effective for the acute treatment of migraine.
- Metoclopramide IM is probably ineffective for the acute treatment of migraine.
- One study suggests that buccal prochlorperazine 3 mg and another study suggests that

IV droperidol 2.75 mg is probably effective for the acute treatment of migraine.

- Prochlorperazine PR may be a therapeutic choice for selected cases of moderate or severe migraine (Level B).
- Chlorpromazine IV and prochlorperazine IV are effective for the acute treatment of migraine in the emergency room setting.
- Serotonin receptor (5-HT_3) antagonists (i.e., ondansetron and granisetron) are probably ineffective for the acute treatment of migraine.

Recommendations

- Oral metoclopramide as monotherapy should not be used for the acute treatment of migraine (Level A). However, oral metoclopramide probably should be considered as adjunct therapy to NSAIDs or triptans for acute treatment of migraine (Level B).
- Metoclopramide IM should probably not be used as monotherapy for the acute treatment of migraine for patients requiring parenteral therapy.
- Metoclopramide IV should be considered for the acute treatment of migraine for patients requiring parenteral therapy (Level B).
- Chlorpromazine IV and prochlorperazine IV should be used for the acute treatment of migraine for patients requiring parenteral therapy (Level A).
- Prochlorperazine buccal and droperidol should be considered for the acute treatment of selected cases of moderate or severe migraine (Level B).
- Ondansetron and granisetron should not be considered for the acute treatment of migraine (Level B).

OTHER ACUTE TREATMENT

Preventive Medications Used in the Acute Treatment of Migraine

β adrenergic blockers. Featherstone (1983) and Tokola and Hokkanan (1978) have suggested that propranolol (40–80 mg) can abort an acute attack of migraine with or without aura. However, Fuller and Guiloff (1990) could not demonstrate propranolol's effectiveness in a placebo-controlled, double-blind study. This could be a result of a large placebo effect in the open studies or failure to study a subset of migraineurs who might respond to propranolol (Table 11–11).

Calcium antagonists. IV verapamil (10 mg) and sublingual nimodipine (40 mg) have not been effective in treating acute attacks of migraine (Andersson and Vinge, 1990). Nifedipine may be useful for treating the aura of migraine but is ineffective in treating the headache (Scholz and Hoffert, 1987). Some recent studies suggest that IV (Soyka et al., 1989; Pfaffenrath et al., 1990) or sublingual (Takeshima et al., 1988) flunarizine is effective in the acute treatment of migraine, perhaps in part due to its dopaminergic blocking effect.

Divalproex. In the first edition of the Guideline, small open studies suggested that IV divalproex is effective in acute migraine treatment (Matchar et al., 2000). Fourteen consecutive patients with moderate-to-severe headaches of 24–72 hours' duration were given 500 mg of valproate IV over 15–30 minutes or 10 mg metoclopramide with 1

TABLE 11–11 Preventive Prescription Drugs.

ACE inhibitors/angiotensins/receptor antagonists
Anticonvulsants
Valproate, gabapentin, topiramate
Antidepressants
TCAs, SSRIs, SNRIs
β-Adrenergic blockers
Propranolol/nadolol/metoprolol/atenolol
Calcium channel antagonists
Verapamil/flunarizine
Neurotoxins
Serotonin antagonists
Methysergide/methergine
Others
NSAIDs, riboflavin, magnesium, feverfew, butteroot, neuroleptics?

Abbreviations: ACE, angiotensin-converting enzyme; NSAID, nonsteroidal anti-nflammatory drug; SNRIs, selective serotonin norepinephrine reuptake inhibitors; SSRIs, selective serotonin reuptake inhibitors; TCA, tricyclic antidepressant.

mg DHE IM. In the IV valproate group, 71.4% of patients improved to a state of mild or no headache at 1 hour, 85.7% at 2 hours, and 71.4% at 4 hours. Migraine-associated symptoms of nausea, photophobia, and phonophobia showed similar improvement. In the DHE group, 42.8% of patients improved to a state of mild or no headache at 1 and 2 hours and 57.1% at 4 hours (Edwards et al., 1999).

Czapinski and Motyl (1999) studied 25 patients (18 women and 7 men) with an acute migraine attack, with or without aura, within 6 hours of onset. They were given either valproate over 5 minutes IV at the dosage of 15 mg/kg of body weight, or 0.9% NaCl according to the same protocol. Ten of thirteen patients treated with valproate showed a decrease or subsidence of pain, in contrast to four of twelve patients in the placebo group. Complete pain relief occurred as soon as 10 minutes, with a range of 10–25 minutes (Mathew, Kailasam, et al., 1999).

Three additional trials have been reported on the use of parenteral antiepileptic agents for the acute treatment of migraine. In an open-label study, patients received either 500 mg valproate IV or 10 mg metoclopramide IM plus 1 mg DHE (Edwards et al., 2001). Response to both regimens was similar, showing comparable efficacy. In another study, valproate 500 mg IV was inferior to prochlorperazine 10 mg IV in reducing pain and nausea associated with migraine (Tanen et al., 2003). A third study compared valproate 800 mg IV with lysine-acetylsalicylic acid (1000 mg) IV in acute migraine attacks using a cross over design (Leniger et al., 2005). Both drugs were equally effective in acute migraine attacks, with a nonsignificant trend in favor of lysine. Collectively these studies provide little additional support for the efficacy of divalproex or sodium valproate for the acute treatment of migraine in the emergency room setting.

U.S. Headache Consortium Conclusions and Recommendations

Conclusions

- The evidence is inadequate for the use of sodium valproate in the acute treatment in migraine.

Recommendations

- No recommendations can be made for the acute treatment of migraine with sodium valproate for patients requiring parenteral therapy.

OTHER ACUTE TREATMENT

Lidocaine IV demonstrated limited benefit over placebo in one small study that failed to demonstrate clinically significant benefit or harm (Reutens et al., 1991). In a second trial, lidocaine was significantly less effective than chlorpromazine IV and not more effective than DHE IV (Bell et al., 1990). Recent evidence suggests that continuous IV lidocaine given over days may be effective (Rosen et al., 2006). Three double-blind studies assessed the efficacy of intranasal lidocaine for the acute treatment of migraine, and these studies showed mixed results for its efficacy in the acute treatment of migraine (Maizels et al., 1996; Maizels, 1998; Blanda et al., 2001). Collectively, there is little consistent evidence to support the use of lidocaine IM or intranasal for the acute treatment of migraine.

Corticosteroids. Studies have suggested that corticosteroids are effective in the treatment of headache (Gallagher, 1986). The mechanism by which the corticosteroids exert their effect in migraine is uncertain. They may control neurogenic inflammation or have an effect on the hypothalamic-pituitary axis. One study suggests that the addition of dexamethasone to an opioid regimen provides added relief (Gallagher, 1986). Two small studies have been done that provide insufficient data from which to draw conclusions about the efficacy or safety of either dexamethasone IV or hydrocortisone IV for acute treatment of migraine (Klapper and Stanton, 1991b; Kozubski, 1992). In one study, dexamethasone given IV at a dose of 6 mg following pretreatment with IV-administered metoclopramide was said to be effective in the treatment of acute migraine headache (Klapper and Stanton, 1991a). No good quality studies support or refute the effectiveness of steroids for acute migraine. Corticosteroids may be considered as a treatment choice for rescue therapy for patients with status migrainosus. Clinical experience also supports the view that oral steroids can assist in terminating an otherwise refractory migraine (Saper, 1989). We believe that high-dose IV steroids, alone or in conjunction with neuroleptics or DHE, can terminate a refractory headache cycle (Saper, 1990; Silberstein et al., 1990).

Hydrocortisone or Solu-Medrol (methyl prednisolone sodium succinate) can be given IV in the following manner: 100 mg via a saline drip over 10 minutes every 6 hours for 24 hours; every 8 hours for 24 hours; every 12 hours for 24 hours; and then a final dose. Dexamethasone (Decadron) can be administered IV or IM, starting at a dose of 8–20 mg per day in divided doses, rapidly tapering over 2–3 days. Oral dexamethasone 1.5 mg twice daily for 2 days with a taper over 3 more days has also proven useful for less disabled migraineurs with prolonged migraine headache.

U.S. Headache Consortium Conclusions and Recommendations

Conclusions

- The evidence is inadequate for the use of corticosteroids IV in the acute treatment in migraine.

Recommendations

- No recommendations can be made for the acute treatment of migraine with corticosteroids IV for patients requiring parenteral therapy.

Magnesium. The efficacy of IV magnesium sulfate ($MgSO_4$) 1 g was evaluated and the clinical response was correlated to the basal serum ionized magnesium (IMg^{2+}) level. In an outpatient headache clinic, a consecutive sample of patients with a moderate or severe headache of any type (migraine without aura, cluster headaches, chronic TTHs, and chronic migrainous headaches) were studied. Total serum magnesium was measured with atomic absorption spectroscopy and IMg^{2+} was measured with ion selective electrodes. Complete pain relief was observed in 80% of the patients within 15 minutes of $MgSO_4$ infusion. No recurrence or worsening of pain was observed within 24 hours in 56% of patients. Patients treated with $MgSO_4$ also had complete elimination of migraine-associated symptoms such as nausea, photophobia, and phonophobia. Of the 18 patients who did well, 16 (89%) had a low serum IMg^{2+} level. Of the eight patients with no relief, only 37.5% had a low IMg^{2+} level. IV infusion of 1 g of $MgSO_4$ may relieve headache pain in patients with low serum IMg^{2+} levels (Gray et al., 1999a). One new double-blind study tested magnesium sulfate IV, at the dose of 1000 mg, in the treatment of migraine (Bigal, Bordini, Tepper, et al., 2002). Patients with migraine with aura and migraine without aura were treated separately. In migraine without aura, magnesium sulfate was not better than placebo in treating pain, but improved photo- and phonophobia. In migraine with aura, statistically significant improvement of pain, nausea, photophobia, and phonophobia were seen with magnesium sulfate treatment. In a separate trial, Cete and colleagues (Cete et al., 2005) evaluated the relative efficacy of intravenous magnesium 2 g IV versus metoclopramide 10 mg IV versus placebo. They found no difference among treatments for the reduction of pain using a visual analog scale, although use of rescue medication was higher in the placebo group. These studies provide conflicting evidence on the usefulness of $MgSO_4$ for the acute treatment of migraine in the emergency department setting.

U.S. Headache Consortium Conclusions and Recommendations

Conclusion

- Magnesium IV is probably effective for the acute treatment of migraine with aura. The evidence is conflicting to support the use of magnesium IV in the acute treatment of migraine without aura.

Recommendations

- Magnesium IV should be considered for the acute treatment of migraine with aura for patients requiring parenteral therapy (Level B).

Neuroactive steroids alter the excitability of membrane-bound receptors in the nervous system and thus differ from steroid hormones, which regulate gene transcription through interactions with intracellular receptors. Neuroactive steroids modulate neurotransmission through specific, positive allosteric interaction with a steroid recognition site on the γ-aminobutyric acid ($GABA_A$) receptor ion-channel complex and inhibit voltage-gated Ca^{2+} currents and NMDA receptor function (Gasior et al., 1999).

Ganaxolone is a member of a novel class of neurosteroids called epalons, which modulate $GABA_A$ receptors in the CNS by interacting with the epalon receptor. The epalons, chemically related to progesterone, have no hormonal activity, but have potent antiepileptic, anxiolytic, sedative, and hypnotic activity. Chemically ganaxolone is 3-hydroxy-3-methyl-5-pregnan-20-one. It is being developed for the treatment of epilepsy and migraine. In a Phase II migraine trial, 252 premenopausal women between the ages of 18 and 55 were given a liquid suspension of one of four doses of ganaxolone or placebo. There was a substantial increase in response as a function of the plasma during level 2 and 4 hours postdose. Patients with a plasma drug level of 80 mg/ml or more were more likely to experience pain relief. A tablet formulation, designed to increase the predictability of absorption, will be used for further relevant trials (Kapicioglu et al., 1997).

Octreotide, a long acting somatostatin analogue, inhibits 5-HT, bradykinin, prostaglandin, SP, and vasoactive intestinal peptide (VIP) release. In a double-blind, placebo-controlled trial, Octreotide 100 μg SC was more effective than placebo in reducing headache at 2 hours.

NOS Inhibitors: Nitric oxide (NO) is formed from the amino acid L-arginine, catalyzed by a family of enzymes known as etNOS. Some of these enzymes are constitutive (cNOS) and calcium/calmodulin-dependent, and result in the release of NO from endothelium and neurons in response to receptor stimulation. Other NOSs are inducible (iNOS) and cause the release of NO from macrophages, astrocytes, and microglia (Thomsen et al., 1994).

NO exerts many of its actions by stimulating soluble guanylate cyclase. NO is a powerful vasodilator. It is the most important of the so-called endothelium-derived relaxing factors. NO is a noxious molecule (Hibbs et al., 1988), and pain, by definition, is a sensation elicited by noxious stimulation. NO plays a role in the central processing of pain by interacting with CNS NMDA receptors resulting in hyperalgesia (Kolesnikov et al., 1992). NO donors cause the release of CGRP from perivascular nerve endings in animals.

NO may play a pivotal role in migraine pain. Migraineurs are hypersensitive to nitroglycerin, and the NO donor nitroglycerin (glyceryl trinitrate) triggers genuine migraine attacks.

In a double-blind study, 15 patients were randomized to receive the NOS inhibitor L-N^a methylarginine hydrochloride (546C88) and 3 patients to receive placebo. The placebo-treated patients were used in the statistical evaluation, together with 11 historical controls who had received IV placebo in recent double-blind studies. Patients were treated in hospital with 6 mg/kg 546C88 or placebo (5% dextrose) given IV over 15 minutes for a single spontaneous migraine attack. Of those treated in the trial, 10 of 15 had headache relief at 2 hours compared with 2 of 14 in the control group. Most of these patients were historic (i.e., came from prior trials). It is thus possible that the relief could be due to a placebo effect (Lassen et al., 1997).

Krusz and Belanger (1999) reported on the effectiveness of propofol (2,6, diidopropylphenol), an IV anesthetic agent, in treating acute migraine and other headaches in the outpatient headache clinic. Forty-two patients were treated for intractable headaches that were refractory to the usual therapy. Headaches were rated as 7 or higher (out of 10) on visual analog scale. Propofol was administered IV, 20–30 mg every 3–5 minutes. In no case was the patient asleep during any phase of treatment. The average reduction in headache severity was 94.7%. Time to maximal reduction was 15–30 minutes. The average dose of propofol was 95 mg. Propofol has numerous mechanisms of action, which includes at GABA-A receptors, with reduction in sympathetic neuronal activity, stimulation of NO release, depression of spinal nociceptive neurotransmission, and depression of NMDA receptor excitation.

Civamide, chemically related to capsaicin, a vanniloid receptor agonist that blocks the release of CGRP and SP, was studied in a multicenter blinded trial. Both doses (20 and 150 (g) were effective in at least 50% of patients; however, nasal burning also occurred in 88% of the subjects (Diamond, Phillips, et al., 1999).

Failed Drugs

Neurokinin. Lanepitant, a high affinity selective neurokinin-1 (NK-1) receptor antagonist effective in the dural inflammation model, was not effective in acute migraine treatment. Lanepitant 30, 80, and 240 mg given orally was no more effective than placebo in a controlled, double-blind, crossover trial. However, absorption of the drug during a migraine attack is less than 10% of that of fasted volunteers. This suggests the negative result is due to inadequate plasma concentration of the drug and says nothing about drug efficacy or the predictive value of the Moskowitz model (Goldstein et al., 1997). RPR100893-201, another NK-1 antagonist, was also not effective in acute migraine treatment at a 20 mg oral dose. Again sufficient plasma concentration may not have been achieved (Diener, 1996).

Endothelial antagonists. The endothelin family of peptides are potent endogenous vasoconstrictor and pressor agents. Two receptor subtypes, ET_A and ET_B, have been cloned and are both found on smooth muscle cells. ET_B is also found on endothelial cells and mediates endothelin-dependent vasodilation by the release of NO and prostacyclin (Ferro and Webb, 1996). Bosantan, a mixed ($ET_{A/B}$) endothelin receptor antagonist, was ineffective in the treatment of migraine even when administered IV. In this case, the pharmacokinetics of oral absorption was circumvented (Clozel et al., 1994; Brandli et al., 1996).

PREVENTIVE TREATMENT

The goal of preventive therapy is to reduce the frequency, duration, or severity of attacks. In addition, reduced disability and improved function and responsiveness to acute attack treatment may result. Preventive treatment may also prevent episodic migraine's progression to chronic migraine and result in health care cost reductions (Silberstein, Winner, et al., 2003). The changes in healthcare utilization occur at a variety of levels, beginning with a decrease in triptan use (Etemad et al., 2005).

Silberstein et al. (Silberstein, Winner, et al., 2003) retrospectively analyzed resource utilization information in a large claims database. The addition of migraine preventive drug therapy to therapy that consisted of only an acute medication was effective in reducing resource consumption. Compared with the 6 months preceding preventive therapy, migraine diagnosis-related office and other outpatient visits decreased by 51.1%, emergency department visits with a migraine diagnosis decreased 81.8%, computed tomography (CT) scans decreased 75.0%, magnetic resonance imagings (MRIs) decreased 88.2%, and other migraine medication dispensements decreased 14.1% during the second 6 months after the initial preventive medication (Silberstein, Winner, et al., 2003).

In another study, Silberstein et al. evaluated the medical resource utilization and overall cost of care among patients treated with topiramate for migraine prevention in a commercially insured population that included 2645 plan members. These patients were drawn from a diverse set of health plans and were receiving topiramate for migraine prevention. Significant decreases in resource use were observed within 6 months of topiramate initiation (follow-up period 1), and this trend continued in follow-up period 2 (6–12 months after initiation). Although an initial increase in total headache-related costs resulted when topiramate was introduced (follow-up period 1), the cost in follow-up period 2 was similar to that in the preindex period, suggesting that benefits of long-term treatment with topiramate can be achieved without increasing total cost. Topiramate utilization was associated with significantly less triptan utilization: in postindex period 1, there was a 46% decrease in emergency department visits, a 39% decrease in diagnostic procedures (e.g., CT scans and MRIs), and a 33% decrease in hospital admissions; physician office visits were unchanged. In postindex period 2, there was a 46% decrease in emergency department visits, a 72% decrease in diagnostic procedures, a 61% decrease in hospital admissions, and a 35% decrease in physician office visits (Silberstein et al., 2007).

While controlling healthcare costs is of significant importance to insurers and patients, so, too, are the employment-related costs to businesses. A British study examined the impact of topiramate treatment for migraine and found that not only was treatment associated with a decrease in the number of migraine attacks per month, but also with improved quality of life and a significant reduction in lost work time that would more than compensate for the cost of treatment (Brown et al., 2006). Using educational programs in addition to optimizing medical management of migraine with acute and preventive therapies not only reduced loss of productivity and time lost from work, but also resulted in a significant reduction in total medical costs related to migraine (Vicente-Herrero et al., 2004).

Several studies have examined the impact of preventive therapy on quality of life. These have included specific therapies, such as topiramate, as well a more far reaching assessment. Using the SF36 to examine quality of life, several studies (Bordini et al., 2005) (D'Amico et al., 2006) have demonstrated highly statistically significant changes across the range of scores with as little as 6 months of treatment. With a migraine-specific quality of life assessment, Diamond and colleagues (Diamond et al., 2005) found broad improvement across the domains of at least moderate size and an effect that was persistent over a prolonged period of observation.

Preventive treatment can be either preemptive, short-term (miniprophylaxis), or chronic. Preemptive treatment is used when there is a known headache trigger, such as exercise or sexual activity. Patients can be instructed to pretreat before the exposure or activity. For example, single doses of indomethacin can be used to prevent exercise-induced migraine. Short-term prevention is used when patients are undergoing a time-limited exposure to a provoking factor, such as ascent to a high altitude or menstruation. These patients can be treated with daily medication just before and during the exposure (Silberstein et al., 1998). The Revised U.S. Evidence-Based Guidelines for Migraine (Silberstein, 2004a; Silberstein on behalf of the Quality Standards Improvement Committee, 2007) and the European Guidelines (Evers et al., 2006) have established the circumstances that might warrant preventive treatment. These include:

- Recurring migraine attacks that, in the patient's opinion, significantly interfere with his or her daily routines, despite appropriate acute treatment.
- Frequent headaches (>4 attacks/month)
- Contraindication to, failure with, overuse of, or intolerance to acute therapies
- Patient preference
- Frequent, very long, or uncomfortable auras
- Presence of uncommon migraine conditions, including hemiplegic migraine, basilar migraine, migraine with prolonged aura, or migrainous infarction (to possibly reduce neurologic damage)

The use of preventive medication during pregnancy is the exception to the rule. Most medications with proven benefit in migraine prevention are given a C classification for drugs in pregnancy, with divalproex sodium being rated Class D. The severity of the migraine episodes, their frequency, their response to acute medications, and the views of the mother and her significant other regarding medication during pregnancy must be considered. The progress of the pregnancy will also bear on this decision-making process, since the potential greatest effects of the preventive medication on the developing fetus occurs in the first trimester. (Silberstein, 1997a; Silberstein, 2007a)

Prevention is not being used to the extent it should be; only 13% of all migraineurs currently use medication that can be used as preventive therapy to control their attacks (Lipton et al., 2005). According to the American Migraine Prevalence and Prevention (AMPP) Study, 38.8% of patients with migraine should be considered for (13.1%) or offered (25.7%) migraine preventive therapy on the basis of migraine frequency and disability associated with the headaches (Silberstein et al., 2005).

The major medication groups (Table 11–1) for preventive migraine treatment include β-adrenergic blockers, antidepressants, calcium channel antagonists, serotonin antagonists, anticonvulsants, NSAIDs, and others (including riboflavin, minerals, and herbs). If preventive medication is indicated, the agent should be preferentially chosen from one of the first-line categories, on the basis of the drug's side effect profile and the patient's coexistent and comorbid conditions (Tfelt-Hansen and Lipton, 1993). The following principles will help increase the chance of success:

- Start the chosen drug at a low dose and increase it slowly until therapeutic effects develop, the ceiling dose for the chosen drug is reached, or side effects become intolerable. (Migraineurs often require a lower dose of a preventive medication than is needed for other indications. While some patients may respond to lower doses of preventive medications, it may be necessary to increase the dose to tolerance before assuming that the agent is ineffective.)
- Give each treatment an adequate trial. A full therapeutic trial may take 2–6 months. In controlled clinical trials, efficacy is often first noted at 4 weeks and continues to increase for 3 months. In practice, a common mistake is to treat a patient with a new preventive medication for 1 or 2 weeks without effect and discontinue treatment after a breakthrough headache.
- Avoid interfering, overused, and contraindicated drugs. To obtain maximal benefit from preventive medication, the patient should not overuse analgesics, opioids, triptans, or ergot derivatives.
- Reevaluate therapy. Migraine headaches may improve independent of treatment; if the headaches are well controlled, slowly taper and, if possible, discontinue the drug. Many patients experience continued relief with a lower dose of the medication and others may not require it at all.
- A woman of child bearing potential should be on adequate contraception before starting migraine medication. However, some women who are pregnant or attempting to become pregnant may still require preventive medications. If this is absolutely necessary, inform the patient and her partner of any potential risks and pick the medication that will have the least AE on the fetus (Silberstein, 1997a).
- To maximize compliance, involve patients in their care. Take patient preferences into account when deciding between drugs of relatively equivalent efficacy. Discuss the rationale for a particular treatment, when and how to use it, and what side effects are likely. Address patient expectations. Discuss with the patient the expected benefits of therapy and how long it will take to achieve them. Set realistic goals. Success is defined as a 50% reduction in attack frequency. Other measures that may be important include a significant decrease in attack duration, an improved response to acute medication, improved quality of life, and less time lost from work and family activities.
- Set realistic expectations regarding AEs. The risk and extent of AEs vary greatly from patient to patient and we have no way of predicting the presence or severity of AEs in an individual patient. Most AEs are self-limited and dose-dependent, and patients should be encouraged to tolerate the early AEs that may develop when a new medication is started.
- Consider comorbidity, which is the presence of two or more disorders whose association is more likely than chance. Conditions that are comorbid with migraine include stroke, epilepsy, mitral valve prolapse, Raynaud's syndrome, irritable bowel syndrome, and certain psychologic disorders, including depression, mania, anxiety, and panic (Table 11–2) (Ryan and Sudilovsky, 1983; Ryan, 1984; Olerud et al., 1986; Sudilovsky et al., 1986; Cole et al., 2006).

Mechanism of Action of Preventive Medications

The migraine aura is probably due to CSD. CSD is characterized by a slowly spreading wave (at a rate of 2–3 mm/minute) of neuronal and glial depolarization that lasts approximately 1 minute (Gold et al., 1998; Bradley et al., 2001). CSD develops within brain areas, such as the cerebral cortex, cerebellum, or hippocampus, after electrical or chemical stimulation. CSD is associated with a marked decrease in neuronal membrane resistance, a massive increase in extracellular K^+ and neurotransmitters, and an increase in intracellular Na^+ and Ca^{++}. The threshold for CSD is believed to be reduced in patients with migraine; this has been shown to be true for familial hemiplegic migraine-1. How CSD is triggered in the human cortex during a migraine attack is uncertain (Dichgans et al., 2005).

Headache probably results from activation of meningeal and blood vessel nociceptors combined with a change in central pain modulation. Headache and its associated neurovascular changes are subserved by the trigeminal system. Trigeminal sensory neurons contain SP, CGRP, and neurokinin A. Stimulation results in the release of SP and CGRP from sensory C-fiber terminals and neurogenic inflammation. The neuropeptides interact with the blood vessel wall, producing dilation, PPE, and platelet activation (Dimitriadou et al., 1992). Neurogenic inflammation sensitizes nerve fibers (peripheral sensitization), which now respond to previously innocuous stimuli, such as blood vessel pulsations, causing, in part, the pain of migraine. CS of trigeminal nucleus caudalis neurons can also occur. CS may play a key role in maintaining the headache. Brainstem activation also occurs in migraine without aura, in part owing to increased activity of the endogenous antinociceptive system. The migraine aura can trigger headache: CSD activates trigeminovascular afferents. How does a headache begin in the absence of aura? CSD may occur in silent areas of the cortex or the cerebellum. In addition, direct activation of the trigeminal nerve can occur. Stress can also activate meningeal plasma cells via a parasympathetic mechanism, leading to nociceptor activation (Kandere-Grzybowska et al., 2003).

Migraine may be a result of a change in pain and sensory input processing. The aura is triggered in the hypersensitive cortex (CSD). Headache is generated by central pain facilitation and neurogenic inflammation. CS can occur, in part mediated by supraspinal facilitation. Decreased antinociceptive system activity and increased peripheral input may be present.

Most migraine preventive drugs were designed to treat other disorders. Serotonin antagonists were developed on the basis of the pathophysiologic concept that migraine is due to excess 5-HT. Antidepressants downregulate 5-HT2 and B-adrenergic receptors. Anticonvulsant medications decrease glutamate and enhance $GABA_A$. Potential mechanisms of migraine preventive medications include raising the threshold to migraine activation by stabilizing a more reactive nervous system; enhancing antinociception; inhibiting CSD; inhibiting peripheral and CS; blocking neurogenic inflammation; and modulating sympathetic, parasympathetic, or serotonergic tone. Oshinsky has shown that descending control from the upper brainstem, through serotonergic and noradrenergic systems, modulates the trigeminal nucleus caudalis and prevents CS (Oshinsky and Luo, 2006). Moskowitz has shown that preventive medications given chronically, but not acutely, block CSD (Silberstein, 2004b). Chronic daily administration of migraine prophylactic drugs (topiramate, valproate, propranolol, amitriptyline, and methysergide) dose-dependently suppressed CSD frequency by 40%–80% and increased the cathodal stimulation threshold, whereas acute treatment was ineffective. Longer treatment durations produced stronger CSD suppression. Chronic D-propranolol (the inactive enantiomer of propranolol) treatment did not differ from saline control. Assessing CSD threshold may prove useful for developing new prophylactic drugs and improving upon existing ones (Ayata et al., 2006).

New targets are being evaluated. Gap junctions, intercellular channels that allow diffusion of small molecules up to 1 KDa, play a central role in mechanisms that underlie initiation and propagation of spreading depression (SD). Vertebrate gap junction channels are composed of 12 protein subunits, called connexins. Gap-junction inhibitors abolish both astrocytic Ca^{2+} waves in culture and SD (Theis et al., 2005). Tonabersat (SB-220453), a gap-junction inhibitor, has entered clinical trials for migraine. Tonabersat inhibits CSD, CSD-induced NO release, and cerebral vasodilation. It does not constrict isolated human blood vessels, but it does inhibit trigeminally induced craniovascular effects (Goadsby, 2005).

Antidepressants

Antidepressants consist of a number of different classes of drugs with different mechanisms of action: (1) MAOIs: (a) selective and reversible and (b) nonselective and irreversible; (2) monoamine reuptake inhibitors; (a) nonselective TCAs; (b) SSRIs; and (c) selective serotonin and NE reuptake inhibitors (SNRIs): (3) monoamine receptor targeted drugs: (a) serotonin (trazadone); (b) norepinephrine α_2 NE antagonist (mirtazepine); and (c) DA (bupropion). Future drugs may be based on SP antagonism.

TCAs, SSRIs, and SNRIs increase synaptic NE or serotonin (5-HT) by inhibiting high-affinity reuptake. Some are more potent inhibitors of NE, others of 5-HT reuptake. Bupropion is both a DA and NE reuptake inhibitor.

MAOIs block the degradation of catecholamines. The therapeutic action of antidepressant treatment was initially believed to be a consequence of increased synaptic NE and 5-HT. However, this does not account for the temporal discrepancy between the rapid drug-induced effects on amine uptake, which occur within hours, the antidepressant effects, which take 2–3 weeks, and prophylactic headache response, which takes 3–10 days or longer (Heninger and Charney, 1987).

The most consistent neurochemical finding with antidepressant treatment (including TCAs, SSRIs, MAOIs, and electroconvulsive therapy) is a decrease in β adrenergic receptor density and NE-stimulated cAMP response. Increased α1 receptor system sensitivity is not seen as consistently with antidepressant treatment. Long-term antidepressant treatment decreases 5-HT_2 receptor-binding and imipramine-binding sites (related to the 5-HT uptake system) but does not change 5-HT_1 receptor binding. A strong interaction exists between the NE and 5-HT systems. Antidepressant treatment β-receptor downregulation is dependent on an intact 5-HT system, while lesions of the NE system block the decrease in 5-HT_2 receptor binding (Heninger and Charney, 1987).

The decrease in 5-HT_2 receptor binding sites does not correlate with a decrease in function; in fact, there may be enhanced physiologic responsiveness. Long-term antidepressant treatment actually enhances the efficacy of 5-HT synaptic transmission. The mechanisms underlying this enhanced synaptic transmission differ according to the type of treatment administered. TCAs and electroconvulsive shocks enhance 5-HT synaptic transmission by increasing the sensitivity of postsynaptic 5-HT1A receptors, whereas selective 5-HT reuptake blockers reduce the function of terminal 5-HT autoreceptors, thereby increasing the amount of 5-HT released per stimulation-triggered action potential (Heninger and Charney, 1987).

TCAs up-regulate the GABA-B receptor, down-regulate the histamine receptor, and enhance the neuronal sensitivity to SP. Some TCAs are 5-HT_2 receptor antagonists. TCAs also interact with endogenous adenosine systems. They inhibit adenosine and augment its electrophysiologic actions that contribute to antinociception. Adenosine A_1 receptor activation results in antinociception mediated by inhibition of AC, while adenosine A_2 receptor activation is pronociceptive owing to stimulation of AC within the sensory nerve terminal (Taiwo and Levine, 1991). Adenosine A_3 receptors facilitate pain due to release of histamine and 5-HT from mast cells (Sawynok et al., 1998, 1999).

Neurotrophic factors may also mediate the long-term effects of antidepressants. The neurotrophins [a protein class comprising nerve growth factor (NGF), brain-derived neurotrophic factor (BDNF), neurotrophin-3 (NT-3), NT-4/5, and NT-6] positively modulate monoaminergic neurotransmission (Siuciak et al., 1996) and CNS neuron survival, outgrowth, and neuroprotection (Lindsay et al., 1994). BDNF binds to and phosphorylates its high-affinity tyrosine kinase receptor (TrkB) and activates intracellular signaling pathways, including microtubule-associated protein (MAP) kinase and cAMP (Skolnick et al., 2001). BDNF promotes serotonin neuron development, augments serotonin synthesis and turnover, and increases serotonergic axon fiber density. Serotonergic axon densities are decreased in the prefrontal cortex of suicide patients with major depressive disorder (Austin et al., 2002). In the neocortex and hippocampus, BDNF mRNA and protein are highly expressed (Altar, 1999), and these regions are widely implicated in the pathophysiology of depressive disorders. Environmental stressors, such as immobilization, that produce learned helplessness in animals and precipitate depression in humans decrease BDNF mRNA (Smith et al., 1995). Intraventricular, dorsal raphe, or hippocampal infusions of BDNF in rats reduce learned helplessness behavior and reduce immobility in the forced swim and inescapable shock models, indicating an antidepressant-like effect. BDNF mRNA increases in animals treated with antidepressant drugs and following seizures (Altar et al., 2003). Antidepressants increase BDNF mRNA in the brain via 5-HT2A and β-adrenoceptor subtypes and prevent the stress-induced decreases in BDNF mRNA.

In the hippocampus of depressed patients treated with unspecified antidepressants, BDNF protein immunoreactivity was elevated compared with subjects who were not so treated at the time of death (Altar et al., 2003). Clinical trials are currently evaluating the antidepressant activity of small molecules that increase BDNF mRNA and protein release from cultured cells (Skolnick et al., 2001). BDNF protein levels were measured with a two-site enzyme-linked immunosorbent assay (ELISA) in six brain regions of adult male rats that received daily Electro convulsive seizures (ECS) or daily injections of antidepressant drugs. BDNF increased gradually in the hippocampus and frontal cortex, with a peak response by the 4th day of ECS. Increases peaked at 15 hours after the last ECS and lasted at least 3 days thereafter. Two weeks of daily injections with the MAO-A and MAO-B inhibitor tranylcypromine (8–10 mg/kg, IP) increased BDNF by 15% in the frontal cortex, and 3 weeks of treatment increased it by 18% in the frontal cortex and 29% in the neostriatum. Tranylcypromine, fluoxetine, and desmethylimipramine did not elevate BDNF in the hippocampus. Elevations in BDNF protein in brain are consistent with the greater treatment efficacy of ECS and MAO inhibitors in drug-resistant major depressive disorder and may be predictive for the antidepressant action of the more highly efficacious interventions (Altar et al., 2003).

The mechanism by which antidepressants work to prevent headache is uncertain, but it does not result from treating masked depression. Antidepressants are useful in treating many chronic pain states, including headache, independent of the presence of depression, and the response occurs sooner than the expected antidepressant effect (Couch et al., 1976; Kishore-Kumar et al., 1990; Panerai et al., 1990). In animal pain models, antidepressants potentiate the effects of coadministered opioids (Feinmann, 1985). The clinically effective antidepressants in headache prophylaxis either inhibit 5-HT reuptake or are antagonists at the 5-HT_2 receptors (Richelson, 1990).

A total of 17 controlled trials investigated the efficacy of the TCAs amitriptyline and clomipramine, and the SSRIs fluoxetine and fluvoxamine (Jacobs, 1972; Gomersall and Stuart, 1973; Couch and Hassanein, 1976; Couch and Hassanein, 1979; Noone, 1980; Andersson and Petersen, 1981; Mathew, 1981; Zeeberg et al., 1981; Bonuso et al., 1983; Kangasniemi et al., 1983; Langohr et al., 1985; Monro et al., 1985; Orholm et al., 1986; Ziegler et al., 1987; Adly et al., 1992; Bank, 1994; Saper et al., 1994). Amitriptyline has been more frequently studied than the other agents, and is the only antidepressant with fairly consistent support for efficacy in migraine prevention. Three placebo-controlled trials found amitriptyline significantly better than placebo at reducing headache index or frequency (Gomersall and Stuart, 1973; Couch and Hassanein, 1976, 1979; Ziegler et al., 1987). One trial conducted in patients with frequent severe or disabling headaches found no significant difference between amitriptyline and propranolol (Ziegler et al., 1987). In another trial, amitriptyline was significantly more efficacious than propranolol for patients with mixed migraine and TTH, while propranolol was significantly better for patients with migraine alone (Mathew, 1981). Amitriptyline was significantly better than timed-released DHE (TR-DHE) at reducing headache index in a group of patients with mixed migraine and TTH (Ahuja and Verma, 1985). However, an analysis of the data on headache duration, stratified by severity, showed that amitriptyline was significantly better than TR-DHE at reducing the number of hours of moderate and mild TTH-like pain. In contrast, TR-DHE was significantly better than amitriptyline at reducing the number of hours of extremely severe and severe migraine-like pain. More recently, Dodick and colleagues compared the relative efficacy and tolerability profiles of topiramate (100 mg/day) and amitriptyline (100 mg/day) as preventive treatment for migraine. This was a large, randomized, double-blind, parallel-treatment group, comparative study powered to examine a noninferiority hypothesis in patients with episodic migraine ($N = 347$; ≥ 18 years). Both treatments were associated with a lower mean monthly attack frequency, although treatment with topiramate was associated with a significant improvement of daily activities in all three domains of the migrane specific questionnaire (MSQ) compared with amitriptyline (Dodick et al., 2007). These studies showed that amitriptyline is effective for migraine prevention (efficacious doses in clinical trials: 30–150 mg/day) (Ramadan et al., 2000). Additional new studies further suggest a possible role of amitriptyline for migraine prevention in children (Hershey et al., 2002), in combination with nonpharmacologic therapies or in combination with other therapies (Krymchantowski et al., 2002; Rampello et al., 2004). Collectively, these studies confirm that amitriptyline is effective for migraine prevention.

The evidence was insufficient to support the efficacy of clomipramine (Noone, 1980; Langohr et al., 1985) and fluvoxamine (Bank, 1994) for migraine prevention. Fluoxetine was significantly better than placebo in one (Adly et al., 1992) but not a second (Saper et al., 1994) migraine prevention trial. In a small retrospective study, Adelman reported that mean reduction in migraine fell from 16.1 to 11.1 headaches per month with venlafaxine treatment (Adelman et al., 2000). Bulut and colleagues also assessed the relative efficacy of venlafaxine versus amitriptyline and found that the two agents were equally effective in reducing pain outcomes for migraine, but venlafaxine may be better tolerated, on the basis of study drop-out rates (Bulut et al., 2004).

Anticholinergic symptoms were frequently reported with the TCAs studied, including amitriptyline. Adverse events were less common with SSRIs, with nausea and sexual dysfunction the most frequently observed symptoms (Gray, Goslin, et al., 1999).

The TCAs most commonly used for migraine (and tension-type) headache prophylaxis include amitriptyline, nortriptyline, doxepin, and protriptyline. Imipramine and desipramine have been used at times. Most have not been vigorously evaluated; their use is based on anecdotal or uncontrolled reports.

Pharmacology of the TCAs. There is wide individual variation in the absorption, distribution, and excretion of the TCAs, with a 10- to 30-fold variation in individuals' drug metabolism. A therapeutic window above or below which the TCAs are ineffective may exist, but this has been evaluated only for amitriptyline, nortriptyline, and imipramine for treatment of depression. No therapeutic window was found, however, for amitriptyline in the treatment of chronic pain (Brenne et al., 1997). Therapeutic windows may also exist for the SSRI and SNRI antidepressants. The presence of a therapeutic window and the wide variation in TCA metabolism necessitates individualized dosing and may prompt monitoring of TCA plasma levels if there are issues of toxicity or compliance. TCAs are lipid soluble, have a high volume of distribution, and avidly bind to plasma proteins. The antihitamine and antimuscarinic activity of the TCAs account for many of their AEs (Richardson and Richelson, 1984). A useful rule of thumb is to start low and aim for a dose of 1–1.5 mg/kg body weight.

Principles of antidepressant use

- The TCA dose range is wide and must be individualized.
- With the exception of protriptyline, TCAs are prone to causing sedation. Start with a low dose of the chosen TCA at bedtime, except when using protriptyline, which should be administered in the morning.
- If the TCA is too sedating, switch from a tertiary TCA (amitriptyline, doxepin) to a secondary TCA (nortriptyline, protriptyline). If a patient develops insomnia or nightmares, give the TCA in the morning.
- SSRIs can be given as a single dose in the morning or evening. They are less sedating than the TCAs and some patients may require a hypnotic for sleep induction or use during the daytime.
- SNRIs have an AE profile similar to SSRIs, although they may cause nausea and be more activating.
- Bipolar patients in a depressed state can become manic on antidepressants.

AEs are common with TCA use. Their AEs are due to their interaction with multiple neurotransmitters and their receptors. The antimuscarinic AEs are most common; they include dry mouth, a metallic taste, epigastric distress, constipation, dizziness, mental confusion, tachycardia, palpitations, blurred vision, and urinary retention. Antihistaminic activity may be responsible for carbohydrate cravings, which contribute to weight gain. Adrenergic activity is responsible for the orthostatic hypotension, reflex tachycardia, and palpitations that patients may experience. Paradoxically, excess sweating can also occur. Rarely amitriptyline and others will cause inappropriate secretion of ADH. Any antidepressant treatment may change depression to hypomania or frank mania (particularly in bipolar patients). Ten percent of patients may develop tremors, and confusion or delirium may occur, particularly in older patients who are more vulnerable to the muscarinic AEs. Antidepressant treatments may also reduce the seizure threshold, although this is not generally a problem in antimigraine treatment (Baldessarini, 1990). Differences exist among the TCAs and they have properties that may be useful in selecting an agent and modifying drug regimens to reduce AEs.

Clinical Use

Tertiary Amines

Amitriptyline (Elavil, Endep) is a tertiary amine tricyclic that is sedating (Table 11–12). Patients with depression are more tolerant and require higher doses of amitriptyline than patients with migraine. Start at a dose of 10–25 mg at bedtime. The dose ranges from 10 to 400 mg a day.

Doxepin (Sinequan, Adapin) is a sedating tertiary amine TCA. Start at a dose of 10 mg at bedtime. The dose ranges from 10 to 300 mg a day.

Secondary Amines

Nortriptyline (Pamelor, Aventyl) is a secondary amine that is less sedating than amitriptyline. Nortriptyline is a major metabolite of amitriptyline. If insomnia develops, give the drug earlier in the day or in divided doses. Start at a dose of 10–25 mg at bedtime. The dose ranges from 10 to 150 mg a day.

Protriptyline (Vivactil) is a secondary amine that is similar to nortriptyline. Start at a dose of 5 mg a day taken in the morning. The dose ranges from 5 to 60 mg a day.

Table 11–12 Antidepressants in the Preventive Treatment of Migraine.

Agent	*Daily dose*	*Comment*
Tertiary Amines		
Amitriptyline	10–400 mg	• Start at 10 mg at bedtime
Doxepin	10–300 mg	• Start at 10 mg at bedtime
Secondary Amines		
Nortriptyline	10–150 mg	• Start at 10–25 mg at bedtime • If insomnia, give early in the morning
Protriptyline	5–60 mg	• Start at 10–25 mg in the morning
Selective Serotonin Reuptake Inhibitors (SSRI)		
Citalopram	10–80 mg	• Evidence in the treatment of migraine is controversial. • Some may worsen the migraine pattern • May be used as an adjuvant in the treatment of migraine and severe depression
Escitalopram	10–20 mg	
Fluoxetine tablets	10–80 mg	
Sertraline tablets	25–100 mg	
Paroxetine tablets	10–30 mg	
Selective Serotonin Norepinephrine Reuptake Inhibitors (SNRI)		
Venlafaxine tablets	37.5–300 mg 20–60 mg	• Some evidence in the treatment of migraine
Duloxetine		
Other		
Mirtazapine tablets	15–45 mg	
Monoamine Oxidase Inhibitors		
Phenelzine	30–90 mg	• Strict diet considerations

MONOAMINE REUPTAKE INHIBITORS

Selective Serotonin Reuptake Inhibitors

Evidence for the use of SSRIs is poor. They are helpful for patients with comorbid depression because their tolerability profile is superior to tricyclics. Fluoxetine, fluvoxamine, paroxetine, sertraline, and citalopram are specific SSRIs that have minimal antihistaminic and antimuscarinic activity. These drugs may produce weight gain, unlike the original impression, but have fewer cardiovascular side effects than the TCAs (Abramowicz, 1990). The most common AEs include anxiety, nervousness, insomnia, drowsiness, fatigue, tremor, sweating, anorexia, nausea, vomiting, and dizziness or lightheadedness. Headache was noted in 20.3% of patients on fluoxetine; however, it was also noted in 19.9% of patients on placebo (Barnhart, 1991). A discontinuation syndrome that resembles serotonin syndrome may occur with the shorter half-life drugs. The combination of an SSRI and a TCA can be beneficial in treating refractory depression (Weilburg et al., 1989) and, in our experience, resistant cases of migraine. The combination may require dose adjustment of the TCA because levels may significantly increase.

The efficacy analysis summarized in the AHCPR Evidence Report did not indicate a clear benefit of the racemic mixture of fluoxetine over placebo. In contrast, a recent randomized controlled trial of S-fluoxetine indicated a possible clinical benefit in migraine prevention, as measured by a reduction in migraine frequency, as early as 1 month after initiation of therapy (Steiner et al., 1998). Anecdotal reports (Markley et al., 1991) and our experience seem to indicate its benefit in migraine prophylaxis where coexistent depression is a prominent issue. Some researchers have reported that fluoxetine does not improve or may worsen headache (Solomon and Kunkel, 1990). One new study provides additional evidence showing fluoxetine 20 mg/day was more effective than placebo in reducing total pain index scores at 6 months (d'Amato et al., 1999). Fluoxetine should be started at a dose of 10 mg in the morning. The dose ranges from 10 to 80 mg a day.

No evidence exists that the other SSRIs are effective in migraine (Moja et al., 2005).

Selective Serotonin and NE Reuptake Inhibitors

Venlafaxine is available in a variety of doses (25, 37.5, 50, 75, or 100 mg) and a twice- daily and extended-release formulation (37.5, 75, or 150 mg). It has been shown to be effective in a double-blind, placebo-controlled trial and a separate placebo and amitriptyline controlled trial (Bulut et al., 2004). The effective dose is 150 mg/day. Start with the extended release tablet of 37.5 mg for 1 week, then 75 mg for 1 week, and then 150 mg extended release 150 mg in the morning. Side effects included insomnia and nervousness, mydriasis and seizures. As with the TCAs and SSRIs, weight gain may occur.

Duloxetine is available as 20, 30, or 60 mg capsules. The dose ranges from 20 to 60 mg/day. A 20 mg daily starting dose is begun and slowly titrated upward.

Monoamine Oxidase Inhibitors

MAO exists in two subtypes: MAO-A, which preferentially deaminates NE and 5-HT, and MAO-B, which preferentially deaminates DA. Phenelzine is a nonspecific inhibitor of MAO-A and -B. L-Deprenyl is a selective MAO-B inhibitor that may be effective in the treatment of Parkinson's disease.

The MAOI phenelzine (Nardil), at a dose of 15 mg TID, was effective in an open study in 80% of 25 patients who were resistant to other forms of treatment (including cyproheptadine and methysergide) (Anthony and Lance, 1969). However, no placebo-controlled, double-blind trials exist. Many authorities find that phenelzine can be extremely effective in migraine prophylaxis when simpler treatments fail (Lance, 1986; Raskin, 1988a; Saper et al., 1993).

The dose of phenylzine ranges from 30 to 90 mg a day in divided doses. All patients on MAOI-A must be on a restricted diet and avoid the use of certain medications to prevent hypertensive crisis. Meperidine, sympathomimetics (including Midrin), alcohol, and foods with a high tyramine or DA content (cheddar cheese, fava beans, banana peel, tap beers, Marmite and Veggie-Mite concentrated, yeast extract, sauerkraut, soy sauce, and other soybean condiments) must be avoided

(Tollefson, 1983; Raskin, 1988a; Mosniam et al., 1996; Shulman and Walker, 1999).

The most common AEs of MAOIs include insomnia, orthostatic hypotension, constipation, increased perspiration, weight gain, peripheral edema, and, less commonly, inhibition of ejaculation or reduced libido. Insomnia can be reduced by giving most of the medication early in the day. The risk of hypertensive crisis may be reduced by having the patient take the MAOI 3–4 hours before or after eating or taking the entire dose at bedtime, as MAO activity in the liver rapidly returns to normal (Raskin, 1988b). Sublingual nifedipine has been used to treat hypertensive crisis when it occurs in MAOI users (Clary and Schweitzer, 1987). Labetalol and Thorazine have also been used.

The MAOI and amitriptyline combination has been reported to be relatively safe and effective in the treatment of refractory depression when the two drugs are started concurrently (Lader, 1983; Saper, 1989). Some headache experts have used this combination to treat refractory migraine (Freitag et al., 1987; Raskin, 1988b; Saper, 1989). Combination therapy may decrease the risk of hypertensive crisis. A clinical trial demonstrated that administering amitriptyline to patients who were on an MAOI could prevent the occurrence of hypertensive crisis from the ingestion of cheeses or other high tyramine foods (Pare et al., 1982). However, severe reactions, including hyperthermia, delirium, and seizures, have been reported (White and Simpson, 1984). The newer atypical antidepressants, such as fluoxetine, must not be combined with an MAOI, since fatal outcomes have been reported. One must wait 5 weeks after stopping fluoxetine before starting an MAOI and 2–3 weeks after stopping an MAOI before starting fluoxetine.

Other Antidepressants

Mirtazepine is an antagonist at central a_2 presynaptic NE receptor resulting in increased NE and 5-HT action. In addition it is a potent 5-HT_2 and 5-HT_3 receptor antagonist. The dose ranges from 15 to 45 mg at bedtime.

Pies (1983) found trazodone, an atypical nontricyclic antidepressant that is a highly selective 5-HT reuptake inhibitor, to be effective in a patient with features of both migraine and TTH; most investigators, including ourselves, rarely find it effective. Trazodone is metabolized to m-chlorophenylpiperazone (m-CPP), a known migraine precipitant, perhaps by being a 5-HT1C receptor agonist (Brewerton et al., 1988). Plasma levels of m-CPP in patients on trazodone are 40% that of the parent drug (Curzon et al., 1990). An open-label study of its related compound found it to be effective in chronic daily headache (Saper et al., 2001).

Other antidepressants can be tried in resistant cases, particularly those complicated by depression. Bupropion is useful for smoking cessation and neuropsychiatric comorbidity.

Antiepileptic Drugs

Antiepileptic drugs are increasingly recommended for migraine prevention because of placebo-controlled, double-blind trials that prove them effective (Table 11–13). Despite earlier researchers' belief that anticonvulsants are more effective in children who have paroxysmal electroencephalograms (Rapoport et al., 1989), they are effective regardless of the electroencephalogram (Prensky, 1987). With the exception of valproic acid and phenobarbital, many anticonvulsants interfere with the efficacy of the OCs (Coulam and Annagers, 1979; Hanston and Horn, 1985).

Nine controlled trials of five different anticonvulsants were included in the AHCPR Technical Report (Rompel and Bauermeister, 1970; Anthony et al., 1972; Stensrud and Sjaastad, 1979; Jensen et al., 1994b; Klapper, 1995; Mathew et al., 1995a; Klapper, 1997).

Carbamazepine. The only placebo-controlled trial of carbamazepine suggested a significant benefit, but this trial was inadequately described in several important respects (Rompel and Bauermeister, 1970). Another trial, comparing carbamazepine with clonidine and pindolol, suggested that carbamazepine had a weaker effect on headache frequency than either comparator treatment, although differences from clonidine were not statistically significant (Anthony et al., 1972). A significantly higher percentage of patients reported adverse events with carbamazepine than

TABLE 11–13 Selected Antiepileptic Drugs in the Preventive Treatment of Migraine.

Agent	*Daily dose*	*Comment*
Carbamazepine	600–1200 mg	• TID
Gabapentin	600–2400 mg	• Dose can be increased to 3000 mg
Lamotrigine	100–200 mg	• Start 25 mg very slow titration • May be effective in migraine with aura • DC if rash
Topiramate	100–600 mg	• Start 15 to 25 bedtime • Increase 15–25 mg per week • Attempt to reach 50–100 mg • Increase further if necessary • Associated with weight loss
Valproate/Divalproex	500–1500 mg/day	• Start 250–500 mg day. • Monitor levels if compliance is an issue • Max dose is 60 mg/Kg day

with placebo or pindolol; there was no significant difference in this respect between carbamazepine and clonidine. Since this original Guideline report, no new trials have been reported. There is insufficient evidence to clearly demonstrate carbamazepine as an effective migraine preventive treatment.

In our experience, carbamazepine (Tegretol), 600–1200 mg a day (beginning at 100 mg twice a day), may be effective in the preventive treatment of migraine, particularly for patients who have coexisting mania or hypomania, especially if there is rapid cycling; however, monitoring of plasma levels and white blood count is essential.

Gabapentin (600–1800 mg) was effective in episodic migraine and chronic migraine in a 12-week open-label study (Mathew, 1996). Gabapentin was not effective in one placebo-controlled, double-blind study (Wessely et al., 1987), but a more recent trial (not included in the AHCPR Technical Report and reported in abstract form with limited information on AEs) reported clinical efficacy for gabapentin in migraine prevention (Mathew et al., 1998). This randomized, placebo-controlled, double-blind trial showed that gabapentin 1800–2400 mg was superior to placebo in reducing the frequency of migraine attacks. The study involved 145 subjects (81% women) who experienced.

3–8 migraine episodes a month and who had failed no more than two prophylactic antimigraine regimes. The responder rate was 36% for gabapentin and 14% for placebo ($p = 0.02$). The two treatment groups were comparable with respect to treatment-limiting AEs.

Limited data were reported on AEs. The most common were dizziness or giddiness and drowsiness. Relatively high patient withdrawal rates due to AEs were reported in some trials (Gray, Goslin, et al., 1999).

Lamotrigine. Lamotrigine blocks voltage-sensitive sodium channels, leading to inhibition of neuronal glutamate release of glutamate, which is essential in the propagation of CSD. Lamotrigine was studied as combination therapy for headache prevention in one relatively large, prospective, open-label trial of 65 patients, most of whom had chronic migraine (Wheeler, 2001). Only 35 patients were compliant with treatment to warrant inclusion in the analysis, with 12 dropping out because of AEs. There were 17 (48.6%) responders, at a mean dose of 55 mg/day. Those who had migraine with aura had a better response rate (12/18 or 67%). Another open label study assessed the impact of lamotrigine on aura itself, and found that the drug significantly reduced both the frequency and duration of aura (Wheeler, 2001). Chen et al. (Chen et al., 2001) reported two patients with migraine with persistent aura-like visual phenomena for months to years. After 2 weeks of lamotrigine treatment, both had resolution of the visual symptoms.

Steiner et al. (Steiner et al., 1997) compared the safety and efficacy of lamotrigine (200 mg/day) and placebo in migraine prophylaxis in a double-blind, randomized, parallel-groups trial. Improvements were greater on placebo, and these changes, not statistically significant, indicate that lamotrigine was ineffective for migraine prophylaxis. There were more AEs on lamotrigine than on placebo, the most common being rash. With slow dose-escalation, their frequency was reduced and the rate of withdrawal for AEs was similar in both treatment groups.

Despite lamotrigine's overall lack of efficacy in migraine headache prevention, it may have a special role in the treatment of migraine with aura.

Oxcarbazepine. Silberstein and colleagues evaluated the efficacy, safety, and tolerability of oxcarbazepine (1200 mg/day) versus placebo as prophylactic therapy for patients suffering from migraine headaches. Oxcarbazepine did not show efficacy in the prophylactic treatment of migraine headaches (Silberstein on behalf of the Quality Standards Improvement Committee, 2007).

Topiramate is a structurally unique anticonvulsant that was discovered by serendipity. It was originally synthesized as part of a research project to discover structural analogs of fructose-1, 6-diphosphate capable of inhibiting the enzyme fructose 1,6-bisphosphatase, thereby blocking gluconeogenesis, but has not to date demonstrated clinical evidence of hypoglycemic activity. Topiramate is a derivative of the naturally occurring monosaccharide D-fructose and contains a sulfamate moiety. The structural resemblance of its O-sulfamate moiety to the sulfonamide moiety in acetazolamide prompted an evaluation of possible anticonvulsant effects. Topiramate was originally marketed for the treatment of epilepsy (Shank et al., 1994); it is now Food and Drug Administration (FDA)-approved for migraine.

Topiramate is rapidly and almost completely absorbed. The blood plasma concentration increases linearly as a function of dose in humans over the pharmacologically relevant range (Easterling et al., 1988; Streeter et al., 1994). It is not extensively metabolized in humans and is eliminated predominantly unchanged in the urine. The average elimination half-life is approximately 21 hours (Easterling et al., 1988). Topiramate readily enters the CNS parenchyma; in rats, the concentration in whole brain was approximately one-third that in blood plasma 1 hour after oral dosing.

In a pharmacokinetic interaction study with a concomitantly administered combination OC product containing 1 mg norethindrone plus 35 mcg ethinyl estradiol, topiramate at doses of 50–200 mg/day was not associated with statistically significant changes in mean exposure (area under the curve) to either component of the OC (Doose et al., 2003). Topiramate is therefore not associated with significant reductions in estrogen exposure at doses below 200 mg per day. At doses above 200 mg per day, there may be a dose-related reduction in exposure to the estrogen component of OCs.

The anticonvulsant activity of most antiepileptic drugs is thought to be due to a state-dependent blockade of voltage-dependent Na^+ or Ca^{2+} channels or an ability to enhance the activity of γ-aminobutyrate (GABA) at $GABA_A$ receptors (MacDonald and McLean, 1986; Rogawski and Porter, 1990). Topiramate can influence the activity of some types of voltage-activated Na^+ and Ca^{2+} channels, $GABA_A$ receptors, and the α-amino-3-hydroxy-5-methylisoxazole-4-proprionic acid (AMPA)/kainate subtype of glutamate receptors. Topiramate also inhibits some isozymes of carbonic anhydrase (CA) and exhibits selectivity for CA II and CA IV (Shank et al., 1994; Dodgson et al., 2000). Topiramate blocks Na^+ channels in a voltage-sensitive, use-dependent manner (DeLorenzo et al., 2000). Topiramate can reduce the amplitude of tetrodotoxin-sensitive voltage-gated Na^+ currents in rat cerebellar granule cells as measured by whole-cell current-clamp recordings (Zona et al., 1997).

Topiramate selectively, but not specifically, inhibits two of six isozymes of CA (CA II and CA IV). In humans the K_i is between 1 and 10 μM. At high therapeutic doses (200 mg twice daily) the concentration of topiramate in the blood plasma of humans can be approximately 25 μM (Sachdeo et al., 1996), and based on the brain-to-plasma concentration ratio in rats, the concentration in the CNS parenchyma may be 10 μM. Therefore, CA II and CA IV are likely to be inhibited appreciably in various tissues, including the CNS, in patients receiving high doses of topiramate. The relevance of the carbonic anhydrase inhibitory activity to the anticonvulsant activity of topiramate is not known (Anderson et al., 1989).

The effects of topiramate on voltage-activated NA^+ channels, voltage-activated calcium channels, $GABA_A$ receptors, and AMPA/kainate receptors are regulated by protein phosphorylation (Krebs, 1994; Sigel, 1995; Wang and Kelly, 1995; Roche et al., 1996). One or more subunits of each complex is phosphorylated by PKA, PKC, and possibly CA^{2+}/CaM-activated kinases. The consensus peptide sequence at the PKA-mediated phosphorylation site exhibits homology; that is, the GluR6 subunit of the AMPA/kainate receptor contains an RRQS, the subunit of the $GABA_A$ receptor contains RRAS, and some subtypes of the primary subunit of Na^+ and Ca^{2+} channels contain RRNS and RRPT, respectively (R = arginine, Q = glutamine, S = serine, T = threonine, A = alanine, N = asparagine). Immediately upon binding to the site, topiramate could exert either a positive or negative allosteric modulatory effect; secondarily, topiramate would prevent PKA from accessing the serine hydroxyl site, thereby preventing phosphorylation, which, over time, would shift a population of channels toward the dephosphorylated state (Shank et al., 2000). Thus topiramate may bind to the membrane channel complexes at phosphorylation sites in the inner loop and thereby allosterically modulate ionic conductance through the channels (Shank et al., 2000).

Storer and Goadsby (Storer and Goadsby, 2003) studied topiramate's effect on trigeminocervical activation in the anesthetized cat. Activation of neurons within the trigeminocervical complex is likely to be the biological substrate for pain in migraine and cluster headache. The superior sagittal sinus was isolated and electrically stimulated. Units linked to superior sagittal sinus stimulation were recorded in the most caudal part of the trigeminal nucleus. Topiramate reduced superior sagittal sinus-evoked neuron firing in the trigeminocervical complex in a dose-dependent fashion. Its inhibition is a plausible mechanism of the action of migraine or cluster headache preventive medicines.

Clinical Profile

Topiramate has been shown to be effective in a number of open label and pilot studies (Shuaib et al., 1999; Edwards et al., 2000; Potter et al., 2000). In addition, its chronic use has been associated with weight loss, not weight gain (a common reason to discontinue preventive medication).

In a preliminary safety and efficacy study (Silberstein, Hulihan, et al., 2006), 213 patients were randomized (2:1) to topiramate or placebo and were titrated to either 200 mg/day or maximum tolerated dose over an 8-week period, followed by a 12-week maintenance period. More topiramate patients dropped out during the first 4 weeks of the study. Analysis of covariance was insensitive for detecting drug-placebo differences in the intention-to-treat (ITT) population, but was sensitive enough to demonstrate superiority of topiramate versus placebo for patients completing the trial ($n = 155$, $p = 0.03$). However, a repeated measures analysis using the ITT population demonstrated statistically significant reductions in monthly migraine rate ($p = 0.04$), migraine days ($p = 0.04$), and percent reduction in migraine episodes ($p = 0.02$) for patients on topiramate versus those on placebo. A weighted regression analysis also demonstrated a statistically significant reduction in migraine rate for topiramate patients versus placebo patients ($p = 0.05$). Analyses of the migraine-with-aura population demonstrated a significant reduction not only in occurrence of aura, but also in migraine frequency, migraine days, and migraine duration compared with the placebo treatment (Freitag, 2003).

Two large, pivotal, multicenter, randomized, double-blind, placebo-controlled clinical trials assessed the efficacy and safety of topiramate (50, 100, and 200 mg/day) in migraine prevention. In the first pivotal placebo-controlled clinical trial of 487 patients, Silberstein et al. (Silberstein et al., 2004) assessed the efficacy and safety of topiramate (50, 100, and 200 mg/day) in migraine prevention in a 26-week, multicenter, randomized, double-blind, placebo-controlled study (MIGR-001). The responder rate (patients with >50% reduction in monthly migraine frequency) was 52% with topiramate 200 mg/day ($p < 0.001$); 54% with topiramate 100 mg ($p < 0.001$); 36% with topiramate 50 mg/day ($p = 0.039$); compared with 23% with placebo.

Topiramate treatment was also associated with reduced consumption of acute-treatment medications. The onset of efficacy was observed within the first week of treatment using the combined data from the primary efficacy trials (Freitag et al., 2007). The 200 mg dose was not significantly more effective than the 100 mg dose. However AEs, including AEs resulting in patients discontinuing the study, were more common at the 200-mg dose. The most common AEs were paresthesias, fatigue, nausea, anorexia, and abnormal taste. Body weight was reduced an average of 3.8% in the 100 mg and 200 mg groups (Silberstein et al., 2004).

In the second (MIGR-002) pivotal trial (Brandes, Saper, et al., 2004), significantly more patients exhibited at least a 50% reduction in mean monthly migraines in the groups treated with 50 mg/day of topiramate (39%, $p = 0.009$), 100 mg/day of topiramate (49%, $p = 0.001$), and 200 mg/day of topiramate (47%, $p = 0.001$).

A third (MIGR-003) randomized, double-blind, parallel-group, multicenter trial (Diener, Tfelt-Hansen, et al., 2004) compared two doses of topiramate (100 mg/day or 200 mg/day) to placebo or propranolol (160 mg/day) in 575 subjects in 13 countries. Topiramate 100 mg/day was superior to placebo as measured by reduction in monthly migraine frequency, overall 50% responder rate (37%), reduction in monthly migraine days, and reduction in the rate of daily rescue medication use. Propranolol 160 mg/day and topiramate 100 mg/day were similar with respect to reductions in migraine frequency, responder rate (43%), migraine days, and daily rescue medication usage. Topiramate 100 mg and propranol 160 mg had similar AE rates and both were better tolerated than topiramate 200 mg.

Safety and Tolerability

Topiramate's most common AE is paresthesia, which occurred in 51% of patients in the topiramate 100 group and 49% of patients in the topiramate 200 group, compared with 6% in the placebo group. Most patients rated paresthesias as mild to moderate, and they were treatment-limiting in only 8% of these subjects; when they are bothersome, they can be controlled with potassium supplementation (Silberstein, 2002). The other common AEs were fatigue, decreased appetite, nausea, diarrhea, weight decrease, taste perversion, hypoesthesia, and abdominal pain. In the migraine trials, body weight was reduced an average of 2.3% in the 50 mg group, 3.2% in the 100 mg group, and 3.8% in the 200 mg group. Patients on propranolol gained 2.3% of their baseline body weight.

The most common CNS AEs were somnolence, insomnia, difficulty with memory, language problems, difficulty with concentration, mood problems, and anxiety. Renal calculi can occur with topiramate use. The reported incidence is approximately 1.5%, representing a two- to fourfold increase over the estimated occurrence in the general population (Sachedo et al., 1997).

Patients receiving topiramate infrequently develop a syndrome that consists of acute myopia associated with secondary angle closure glaucoma. No cases of this condition were reported in the clinical studies. Symptoms include the acute onset of decreased visual acuity and/or ocular pain. The primary treatment to reverse symptoms is to discontinue topiramate as rapidly as possible, according to the judgment of the treating physician. Other measures, in conjunction with discontinuation, may be helpful (Thomson Healthcare, 2003).

Oligohidrosis (decreased sweating), infrequently resulting in hospitalization, has been reported in association with an elevation in body temperature. Some of the cases were reported after exposure to elevated environmental temperatures. Most of the reports have involved children.

The occurrence of AEs related to treatment with topiramate, while more common in the 200 mg/day treatment group compared with the 100 mg/day treatment group, were found to be most common during the dose titration period and to dissipate to a low frequency of events by the time the maintenance phase of treatment had begun (Freitag et al., 2005).

The MIGR-001, MIGR-002, and MIGR-003 trials represent the largest controlled clinical trials of topiramate in migraine prevention to date, and together represent the largest controlled trials of a migraine preventive. Treatment with topiramate 100 or 200 mg/day was associated with significant reductions in migraine frequency, migraine days, and number of migraine attacks per month. Treatment with topiramate was also associated with reduced use of acute medications (Limmroth et al., 2002). The 100-mg dose seems to have the best efficacy/tolerability ratio. Cognitive side effects are of less concern with doses of 100 mg or less.

Clinical Usage

Topiramate is available as a 15-mg spansule and as 25-, 50-, 100-, and 200-mg tablets. Start at a dose of 15–25 mg at bedtime. Increase by a dose of 15–25 mg/week. Do not increase the dose if bothersome AEs develop; wait until they resolve (they usually do). If they do not resolve, decrease the drug to the last tolerable dose, then increase by a lower dose more slowly. Attempt to reach a dose of 50 mg/day given twice a day. It is our experience that patients who tolerate the lower doses with only partial improvement often have increased benefit with higher doses. The dose can be increased to 600 mg/day or higher.

Tiagabine was studied by Freitag, Diamond, et al. (1999) in an open-label clinical trial of 41 patients. All patients had been previously treated with divalproex sodium and discontinued therapy owing to AEs or relative lack of efficacy. Tiagabine was initiated at a dose of 4 mg at bedtime for 1 week and then increased to 4 mg twice a day. Patients were reevaluated at 1 month intervals and further dosage adjustments made. Five patients experienced a remission, and thirty-three of forty-one patients had at least a 50% reduction in their attacks. The mean duration of treatment at final assessment was 3.9 months. The mean dose of tiagabine was 10 mg/day. There were no apparent differences between men and women, age-related responses, nor type of migraine. Fourteen AEs were reported by twelve patients.

Valproic Acid

Valproic acid possesses anticonvulsant activity in a wide variety of experimental epilepsy models. Valproate at high concentrations increases GABA levels in synaptosomes, perhaps by inhibiting its degradation; it enhances the postsynaptic response to GABA, and, at lower concentrations, it increases potassium conductance, producing neuronal hyperpolarization. Valproate turns off the firing of the 5-HT neurons of the dorsal raphe, which are implicated in controlling head pain.

Five studies provided strong and consistent support for the efficacy of divalproex sodium (Behan, 1985; Klapper, 1995; Klapper, 1997) and sodium valproate (Hering and Kuritzky, 1992; Jensen et al., 1994a). Two placebo-controlled trials of each of these agents showed them to be significantly better than placebo at reducing headache frequency (Jensen et al., 1994a; Mathew et al., 1995a; Klapper, 1997). A single study, reported in abstract form only, compared divalproex sodium with propranolol and found differences favoring divalproex sodium; however, the statistical significance of these results could not be determined (open-label study with high dropout rates) (Klapper, 1995). A more recent study (published after December 1996 and therefore not included in the AHCPR Technical Report) found divalproex sodium more effective compared with placebo, but not significantly different compared with propranolol, for prevention of migraine in patients without aura (Kaniecki, 1997). One new double-blind, randomized, controlled trial showed that extended-release divalproex sodium 500–100 mg (once a day) significantly reduced the mean 4-week migraine headache rate versus placebo. No significant differences were detected between treatment groups in either the overall incidence or in the incidence of any specific treatment-emergent AE. This study suggests that extended-release divalproex sodium is also efficacious for migraine prophylaxis (Freitag et al., 2002).

Valproic acid is a simple 8 carbon, 2 chain fatty acid with 80% bioavailability after oral administration. It is highly protein bound, with an elimination half-life between 8 and 17 hours.

Nausea, vomiting, and gastrointestinal distress are the most common AEs of valproate therapy. These are generally self-limited and are slightly less common with divalproex sodium than with sodium valproate. When the therapy is continued, the incidence of gastrointestinal symptoms decreases, particularly after 6 months. Later, tremor and alopecia can occur. Valproate has little effect on cognitive functions and it rarely causes sedation. On rare occasions, valproate administration is associated with severe adverse reactions, such as hepatitis or pancreatitis. The frequency varies with the number of concomitant medications used, the patient's age, the presence of genetic and metabolic disorders, and the patient's general state of health. These idiosyncratic reactions are unpredictable (Pellock and Willmore, 1991).

The risk of valproate hepatotoxicity is highest in children under the age of 2 years, especially those treated with multiple antiepileptic drugs, those with metabolic disorders, and those with severe epilepsy accompanied by mental retardation and organic brain disease (Driefuss et al., 1987). The relative risk of hepatotoxicity from valproate is low in migraineurs. Hepatic failure, however, cannot be predicted by laboratory monitoring, since hepatic function tests can be normal until the clinical symptoms are advanced. Some patients progress to fatal hepatotoxicity without ever developing any specific hepatic function abnormalities. Vomiting was the most frequently reported initial symptom in fatal cases of hepatotoxicity. Combined symptoms of nausea and vomiting and anorexia occurred in 82% of valproate-associated hepatotoxicity cases, whereas lethargy, drowsiness, and coma were described in 40%.

Valproate is potentially teratogenic and should not be used by pregnant women or women considering pregnancy (Silberstein, 1996). Hyperandrogenism, resulting from elevated testosterone levels, ovarian cysts, and obesity, is of particular concern in young women with epilepsy who use valproate (Vainionpaa et al., 1999). It is uncertain if valproate can cause these symptoms in young women with migraine or mania.

Because of valproate's potential idiosyncratic interactions with barbiturates (severe sedation, coma), migraine patients who are on valproate should not be given barbiturate-containing combination analgesics for symptomatic headache relief. If these drugs are used, they should be given with caution and at a low dose. Absolute contraindications to valproate are pregnancy and a history of pancreatitis or a hepatic disorder such as chronic hepatitis or cirrhosis of the liver. Hematologic disorders, including thrombocytopenia, pancytopenia, and bleeding disorders, are also important contraindications.

Valproic acid is available as 250-mg capsules and as a syrup (250 mg/5 ml) (Table 11–13). Divalproex sodium is a stable coordination complex comprised of sodium valproate and valproic acid in a 1:1 molar ratio. An enteric-coated form of divalproex sodium is available as 125-, 250-, and 500-mg capsules and a sprinkle formulation. Start with 250–500 mg a day in divided doses and slowly increase the dose. Monitor serum levels if there is a question of toxicity or compliance. (The usual therapeutic level is from 50 to 100 mg/ml.) The maximum recommended dose is 60 mg/kg/day. An extended release form of divalproex sodium demonstrated comparable efficacy to the tablet formulation. The AE profile in the clinical trial, however, showed almost identical AE rates for the placebo and active treatment arms (Freitag, Diamond, et al., 2001).

Silberstein (1996) published practical recommendations and clinical guidelines for using valproate in headache prophylaxis. These include the following: (1) before initiating divalproex sodium, perform a physical examination and take a thorough medical history, with special attention to hepatic, hematologic, and bleeding abnormalities. Obtain screening baseline laboratory studies to help identify risk factors that could influence drug selection. (2) to minimize gastrointestinal AEs, use the enteric coated divalproex sodium formulation if available. Begin with a dose of 250 mg at bedtime. If nausea still occurs, use the sprinkle formulation (125 mg) and very slowly increase the dose. Slowly increase the dose to 500–750 mg a day. (3) obtain follow-up divalproex levels to test for compliance, toxicity, and drug reactions as needed. (4) see the patient on a regular basis (every 1–2 months) during the first 6–9 months of therapy. (5) it is not necessary to monitor blood and urine in otherwise healthy and asymptomatic patients on monotherapy. (6) if mild hepatic transaminase elevation occurs, continue divalproex sodium at the same dose or a lower dose until the enzymes normalize. (7) 10% of treated patients may develop tremor. If this occurs and is bothersome, decrease the dose of divalproex sodium or use propranolol to reduce the occurrence and severity of the tremor.

Vigabatrin, an anticonvulsant similar pharmacologically to sodium valproate, was compared with placebo in a double-blind study in drug-resistant migraineurs. Seventeen women and six men who had migraine with or without aura and were between 25 and 60 years of age, randomly received either vigabatrin or matched placebo tablets for 12 weeks. After a 4-week washout period, alternative treatment was given. The dose was increased slowly to 1000–2000 mg daily, according to the patients' tolerance and response, during the first 6 weeks of each phase; after that no further dosage adjustment was made. Serum drug levels were monitored at 4 weekly intervals. Four patients dropped out of the study and three patients were withdrawn for poor compliance. The treated patients had a 40%–90% reduction in their migraine attack frequency. Analysis of variance indicated a significant reduction in migraine attack frequency in women but not in men. Vigabatrin possibly decreased migraine attack frequency in women who previously derived no benefit from any other medication (Ghose et al., 1996).

Zonisamide. Two retrospective, open-label studies of zonisamide in the preventive treatment of episodic migraine have been performed (Drake et al., 2001; Krusz, 2001). In the study conducted by Drake et al. (Drake et al., 2001), 34 patients with refractory migraine with or without aura were treated adjunctively with zonisamide at doses as high as 400 mg/day (Drake et al., 2001). Headache data were obtained from patient headache diaries and telephone reports. A 40% reduction in headache severity, a 50% reduction in headache duration, and a 25% decrease in headache frequency were found at 3 months compared with baseline values. Four patients (12%) discontinued the drug because of AEs and nine stopped the medicine because they believed it was not working. Krusz reported improvement in 14/33 (42%) patients, with 4 dropouts due to AEs (Krusz, 2001). Zonisamide was also examined as monotherapy in a small, prospective, open-label study of nine patients with episodic migraine with or without aura (Cochran, 2002). The drug was titrated to a mean dose of 244 mg/day, and investigator efficacy ratings were made for all patients who remained on a stable dose of drug for 6 weeks. It was effective or very effective in 6/9 (67%) patients.

Beta (β)-adrenergic Blockers

β-Blockers, the most widely used class of drugs in prophylactic migraine treatment, are 60%–80% effective in producing a greater than 50% reduction in attack frequency (Table 11–14). Rabkin et al. (1966) serendipitously discovered propranolol's effectiveness in headache treatment in patients who were being treated for angina (Weber and Reinmuth, 1972; Diamond and Medina, 1976).

The AHCPR Technical Report analyzed 74 controlled trials of β-blockers for migraine prevention, including 46 trials of propranolol, 14 trials of metoprolol, and trials of acebutolol, alprenolol, atenolol, bisoprolol, nadolol, oxprenolol, pindolol, practolol, and timolol (Gray, Goslin, et al., 1999).

Evidence consistently showed propranolol's efficacy in a daily dose of 120–240 mg for migraine prevention. Twelve of twenty-one placebo-controlled trials of propranolol allowed estimation of effect sizes for headache frequency or headache index (Borgesen et al., 1974; Wideroe and Vigander, 1974; Forssman et al., 1976; Stensrud and Sjaastad, 1976a; Pita et al., 1977; Mikkelsen and

Table 11–14 β-Blockers in the Preventive Treatment of Migraine.

Agent	*Daily dose*	*Comment*
β-Blockers		
Atenolol	50–200 mg	• Use it QID • Fewer side effects than propranolol
Metoprolol	100–200 mg	• Use the short-acting form BID • Use the long acting form QID
Nadolol	20–160 mg	• Use it QID • Fewer side effects than propranolol
Propranolol	40–400 mg	• Use the short-acting form BID or TID • Use the long acting form QID or BID • 1–2 mg/kg in children
Timolol	20–60 mg	• Divide the dose • Short half life

Falk, 1982; Tfelt-Hansen et al., 1984; Ahuja and Verma, 1985; Sargent et al., 1985; Johnson et al., 1986; Dahlof, 1987; Pradalier et al., 1989). The 12-effect size estimates were statistically homogeneous and, when combined, indicated a high degree of certainty that propranolol provides a moderate reduction in headache frequency or index.

The relative efficacy of the different β-blockers has not been clearly established, and most studies show no significant difference between drugs. Direct comparisons demonstrated few significant differences in efficacy between propranolol and flunarizine (Lucking et al., 1988; Ludin, 1989; Shimell et al., 1990; Gawel et al., 1992), amitriptyline (Mathew, 1981; Ziegler et al., 1987), naproxen sodium (Sargent et al., 1985), mefenamic acid (Johnson et al., 1986), tolfenamic acid (Mikkelsen et al., 1986; Kjaersgaard-Rasmussen et al., 1994), divalproex sodium (Kaniecki, 1997), and methysergide (Behan and Reid, 1980; Steardo et al., 1982). These treatments were all effective for migraine prevention. One trial comparing propranolol and amitriptyline suggested that propranolol is more efficacious in patients with migraine alone and amitriptyline is superior for patients with mixed migraine and TTH (Mathew, 1981).

Results from four trials comparing metoprolol with placebo reported mixed results (Andersson et al., 1983; Langohr et al., 1985; Kangasniemi et al., 1987; Steiner et al., 1988). Direct comparisons of metoprolol with propranolol (Steardo et al., 1982; Andersson et al., 1983; Olsson et al., 1984; Gerber et al., 1991) flunarizine (Grotemeyer et al., 1990; Sorensen et al., 1991), and pizotifen (Vilming et al., 1985) demonstrated few significant differences, suggesting that metoprolol is efficacious for the prevention of migraine. Timolol (Stensrud and Sjaastad, 1976b; Briggs and Millac, 1979; Stellar et al., 1984), atenolol (Stensrud and Sjaastad, 1974; Forssman et al., 1983; Johannsson et al., 1987), and nadolol (Ryan and Sudilovsky, 1983; Freitag and Diamond, 1984; Ryan, 1984; Olerud et al., 1986; Sudilovsky et al., 1986; Tobita et al., 1987) are also likely to be beneficial on the basis of comparisons with placebo or with propranolol.

β-blockers with intrinsic sympathomimetic activity (acebutolol, alprenolol, oxprenolol, pindolol) have not been found to be effective for the prevention of migraine (Ekbom and Lundberg, 1972; Sjaastad and Stensrud, 1972; Ekbom and Zetterman, 1977; Nanda et al., 1978; Ekbom, 1994). These drugs, which are partial agonists, exert intrinsic sympathomimetic activity, and this property may make them ineffective (Fanchamps, 1985). A review of the pharmacologic characteristics of the various β-blockers suggested that the only factor that correlates with their efficacy is the absence of partial agonist activity (Shanks, 1987). Since all of the negative studies are small and of low power, the possibility that beneficial effects have escaped detection cannot be excluded. In fact, pindolol (Anthony et al., 1972) and practolol (Sales and Bada, 1975) were found to be effective in open-label studies.

A few trials used long-acting or extended-release preparations of propranolol or metoprolol, but evidence was insufficient to determine whether these preparations were more efficacious and/or better tolerated than regular formulations of these agents (Wideroe and Vigander, 1974; Pita et al., 1977; Steardo et al., 1982; Andersson et al., 1983; Solomon, 1986; Kuritzky and hering, 1987).

Since the first edition of this Guideline, three new randomized, double-blind trails (Level-I) tested the efficacy of β-blockers in migraine prevention (Rao et al., 2000; Diener et al., 2001, 2002). Diener and colleagues (Diener et al., 2001) found that metoprolol (200 mg/day) was more effective than aspirin (300 mg/day) in achieving a 50% reduction in migraine frequency. Diener et al. (Diener et al., 2002) reported that propranolol LA 120 mg/day was similar in efficacy to flunarizine 5 or 10 mg/day as measured by attack frequency and responder rates (reduction of >50% attack frequency from baseline). Rao and colleagues (Rao et al., 2000) reported that propranolol (80 mg/day) was as effective as cyproheptadine (4 mg/day) in reducing migraine frequency and severity. The combination of cyproheptadine and propranolol was more effective than monotherapy.

These studies further support previous recommendations that propranolol is effective for migraine prevention. Additionally, combination therapy (e.g., propranolol with cyproheptadine) may offer additional clinical benefit; however, this is among the first studies investigating combination therapy for migraine prevention. Additional Level-1 evidence using standard primary end points is needed before conclusions can be made regarding the therapeutic benefit of combination therapies in migraine prevention.

No absolute correlation has been found between propranolol's dose and its clinical efficacy (Andersson and Vinge, 1990). One meta-analysis of 53 studies (2403 treated patients) revealed that, on average, propranolol yielded a 44% reduction in migraine activity compared with a 14% reduction in migraine activity with placebo. Variations in propranolol dose levels across studies were unrelated to the magnitude of the propranolol treatment effect. Overall, one out of six patients discontinued propranolol treatment (Holroyd et al., 1991).

The choice of β-blocker should be based on specific properties, such as β_1 selectivity, convenience of drug formulation, and idiosyncratic drug effectiveness. Before giving up on β-blockers as a group, it may be worthwhile to use combined or alternate trials. There may be continued improvement after the drug is discontinued. In a 6-month clinical trial of propranolol, approximately 46% of patients who experienced a reduction in migraine frequency maintained their improvement for up to 6 additional months after discontinuation (Diamond et al., 1982).

The mechanism of action of β-blockers is not certain, but it appears that their antimigraine effect is due to inhibition of β_1-mediated mechanisms (Ablad and Dahlof, 1986).

β blockade results in inhibition of NE release by blocking prejunctional β receptors. In addition, it results in a delayed reduction in tyrosine hydroxylase activity (the rate-limiting step in NE synthesis) in the superior cervical ganglia. In the rat brainstem, a delayed reduction of the locus ceruleus neuron firing rate has been demonstrated after propranolol administration (Ablad and Dahlof, 1986). This could explain the delay in the prophylactic effect of the β-blocker. The potential for a peripheral effect of β-blockers is suggested by the finding that pindolol is ineffective in migraine prevention yet shares the central effects on neurons, similar to propranolol (Lejeune and Millan, 2000).

The action of β-blockers most likely is central and could be mediated by: (1) inhibiting central β receptors interfering with the vigilance-enhancing adrenergic pathway, (2) interaction with 5-HT receptors (but not all β-blockers bind to the 5-HT receptors), and (3) cross modulation of the serotonin system (Koella, 1985; Silberstein and Silberstein, 1990). Propranolol inhibits NO production by blocking inducible NOS. Propranolol also inhibits kainate-induced currents and is synergistic with NMDA blockers, which reduce neuronal activity, and has membrane-stabilizing properties.(Ramadan, 2004)

Schoenen et al. (1986) have shown that contingent negative variation (CNV), an event-related slow negative scalp potential, is significantly increased and its habituation reduced in patients with untreated common migraine. CNV normalizes after treatment with β-blockers, consistent with central adrenergic hyperactivity in migraine. Migraineurs with elevated CNV scores have a much better response to β-blocker therapy (80% effective) than migraineurs with a low or normal score (22% effective), suggesting that the CNV may predict the response to β-blocker treatment (Schoenen et al., 1986). Migraineurs exhibit an enhanced centrally mediated secretion of epinephrine after exposure to light (Stoica and Enulescu, 1990); this returns to normal after treatment with propranolol.

β-blockers that are clinically useful in the treatment of migraine consist of both the nonselective blocking agents (propranolol, nadolol, and timolol) and the selective β_1-blockers (metoprolol and atenolol).

All β-blockers can produce behavioral AEs, such as drowsiness, fatigue, lethargy, sleep disorders, nightmares, depression, memory disturbance, and hallucinations, indicating that they all affect the CNS. AEs most commonly reported in clinical trials of β-blockers were fatigue, depression, nausea, dizziness, and insomnia. These symptoms appear to be fairly well tolerated and were seldom the cause of premature withdrawal from trials (Gray, Goslin, et al., 1999). In animals, β-blockers reduce spontaneous motor activity, counteract amphetamine-induced hyperactivity, and produce slow-wave and paradoxical sleep disturbances. The central effect of β-blockers is used to treat anxiety (Koella, 1985). Common AEs include gastrointestinal complaints and decreased exercise tolerance. Less common are orthostatic hypotension, significant bradycardia, impotence, and aggravation of intrinsic muscle disease. Propranolol has been reported to have an AE on the fetus (Featherstone, 1983). Severe congestive heart failure, asthma, and insulin-dependent diabetes are contraindications to the use of nonselective β-blockers.

Case reports (Prendes, 1980; Gilbert, 1982; Bardwell and Trott, 1987; Kumar and Cooney, 1990) have suggested that propranolol might be implicated in the development of migrainous infarction or the increase in visual symptoms experienced by patients with migraine with aura. However, Kangasniemi et al. (1987), in a double-blind placebo-controlled study, found that metoprolol was effective in the prevention of migraine with aura. Hedman et al. (1988) looked at the modification of aura symptoms by metoprolol. They found that patients had fewer migraine attacks during metoprolol treatment and those that occurred were less severe. There was no change in the total visual and nonvisual aura symptoms, but scintillations and paresthesias were more common, while speech disturbances were less frequent.

At this time, it appears that β-blockers are not absolutely contraindicated in migraine with aura unless a clear stroke risk is present; the reported adverse reactions to propranolol may be either coincidental or idiosyncratic, but the actual risk is uncertain.

Treatment with β-blockers must be individualized following the principles of prophylactic therapy. If the first β-blocker is ineffective or has significant AEs, it may be worthwhile to try a second β-blocker. Some authors have commented on continued improvement (Rosen, 1983) and lack of rebound (Diamond et al., 1982) after discontinuing propranolol. However, it seems more reasonable to slowly taper β-blockers, since stopping them abruptly can cause increased headache (Kangasniemi et al., 1987) and the withdrawal symptoms of tachycardia and tremulousness (Frishman, 1987).

Clinical Use

Propranolol (Inderal; approved by the FDA for migraine) is a nonselective β-blocker with a half-life of 4–6 hours, also available in an effective long-acting formulation (Inderal LA) (Diamond et al., 1987; Pradalier et al., 1989) (Table 11–14). The therapeutically effective dose of propranolol ranges from 40 to 400 mg a day, with no correlation between propranolol and 4-hydroxypropranolol plasma levels and headache relief (Cortelli et al., 1985). The short-acting form can be given three to four times a day, the long-acting form once or twice a day (we recommend twice a day). Start with 40 mg a day in divided doses of propranolol (Inderal 60 LA) and slowly increase to tolerance. An advantage of the regular propranolol is its greater dosing flexibility. The dose for children is 1–2 mg/kg a day.

Nadolol (Corgard) is a nonselective β-blocker with a long half-life. It is less lipid-soluble than propranolol and has fewer CNS side effects. The dose ranges from 20 to 160 mg a day given once daily or in split doses. Some authorities prefer it to propranolol since it has fewer side effects (Sudilovsky et al., 1987).

Timolol (Blocadren; approved by the FDA for migraine) is a nonselective β-blocker with a short half-life. The dose ranges from 20 to 60 mg a day in divided doses.

Atenolol (Tenormin) is a selective β_1-blocker with fewer side effects than propranolol. The dose ranges from 50 to 200 mg a day once daily.

Metoprolol (Lopressor) is a selective β_1-blocker with a short half-life. The dose ranges from 100 to 200 mg a day in divided doses. The long acting preparation may be given once a day.

Calcium Channel Antagonists

Calcium, in combination with a calcium-binding protein such as calmodulin or troponin, regulates many functions, including muscle contraction, neurotransmitter and hormone release, and enzyme activity (Table 11–15). Its extracellular

TABLE 11–15 Selected Calcium Channel Blockers in the Preventive Treatment of Migraine.

Agent	*Daily dose*	*Comment*
Verapamil	120–640 mg	• Start 80 mg BID or TID • Sustained release can be given QID or BID
Flunarizine	5–10 mg	• Give at bedtime • Weight gain is the most common side effect

concentration is high; its intracellular free concentration is 10,000-fold smaller. The concentration gradient is established by membrane pumps and the intracellular sequestering of free calcium. When stimulated, the cell can open calcium channels in the plasma membrane or release intracellular stores of calcium (Snyder and Reynolds, 1985).

Two types of calcium channels exist: calcium entry channels, which allow extracellular calcium to enter the cell, and calcium release channels, which allow intracellular calcium (in storage sites in organelles) to enter the cytoplasm. They include ryanodine and inositol 1,4,5-triphosphate receptors (Greenberg, 1997). Calcium entry channel subtypes include voltage-gated, opened by depolarization; ligand-gated, opened by chemical messengers, such as glutamate; and capacitative, activated by depletion of intracellular calcium stores.

Voltage-gated calcium channels mediate calcium influx in response to membrane depolarization and regulate intracellular processes, such as contraction, secretion, neurotransmission, and gene expression. They are members of a gene superfamily of transmembrane ion channel proteins that includes voltage-gated potassium and sodium channels. There are six functional subclasses of voltage gated calcium (Ca^{2+}) channels that are named T, L, N, P, Q, and R. They fall into two major categories: high-voltage activated channels and the unique low-voltage activated T-type, which is activated at negative potentials (Varadi et al., 1995).

Voltage-gated calcium channels are heteromers composed of four or five distinct subunits, which are encoded by multiple genes. The α_1 subunit of 190–250 KDa is the largest; it incorporates the conduction pore, the voltage sensor and gating apparatus, and the known sites of channel regulation by second messengers, drugs, and toxins.

Mammalian α_1 subunits are encoded by at least 10 distinct genes. It is associated with auxiliary subunits, including a membrane-spanning α_2-δ complex that increases the amplitude of calcium currents and binds the anticonvulsant gabapentin, and a cytoplasmic β subunit that modifies the channel's current amplitude, voltage dependence, and activation and inactivation properties (Greenberg, 1997). The α_1 subunit of voltage-gated calcium channels is organized in four homologous domains (I–IV) with six transmembrane segments (S1–S6) in each. The S4 segment serves as the voltage sensor. The pore loop between transmembrane segments S5 and S6 in each domain determines ion conductance and selectivity, and changes of only three amino acids in the pore loops in domains I, III, and IV will convert a sodium channel to calcium selectivity. An intracellular β subunit and a transmembrane, disulfide-linked $\alpha_2\delta$ subunit complex are components of most types of calcium channels. A γ subunit has also been found in skeletal muscle calcium channels, and related subunits are expressed in heart and brain. Although these auxiliary subunits modulate the properties of the channel complex, the pharmacologic and electrophysiologic diversity of calcium channels arises primarily from the existence of multiple α_1 subunits (Catterall et al., 2003).

Calcium currents have diverse physiologic and pharmacologic properties. L-type (long-lasting) calcium currents require a strong depolarization for activation and are long-lasting (Varadi et al., 1995). L-type calcium channels are expressed in a variety of cardiovascular, endocrine, and neural tissues and are involved in muscle contraction and hormone release. N-type, P/Q-type, and R-type calcium currents also require strong depolarization for activation. They are expressed primarily in neurons, where they initiate neurotransmission at most fast synapses and also mediate calcium entry into cell bodies and dendrites. T-type (transient) calcium channels, in contrast to most other channel subtypes, are activated by weak depolarization and are transient. They are expressed in a wide variety of cell types, where they are involved in shaping the action potential and controlling patterns of repetitive firing (Catterall et al., 2003). The novel calcium channel antagonist mibefradil blocks T-type channels preferentially.

Calcium channels are named using the chemical symbol of the principal permeating ion (Ca) with the principal physiologic regulator (voltage) indicated as a subscript (Ca_V). The numerical identifier corresponds to the Ca_V channel α_1 subunit gene subfamily (1–3 at present) and the order of discovery of the α_1 subunit within that subfamily (1 through m). According to this nomenclature, the Ca_V1 subfamily ($Ca_V1.1$ to $Ca_V1.4$) includes channels containing α_{1S}, α_{1C}, α_{1D}, and α_{1F}, which mediate L-type Ca^{2+} currents. The Ca_V2 subfamily ($Ca_V2.1$ to $Ca_V2.3$) includes channels containing α_{1A}, α_{1B}, and α_{1E}, which mediate P/Q-, N-, and R-type Ca^{2+} currents, respectively. The Ca_V3 subfamily ($Ca_V3.1$ to $Ca_V3.3$) includes channels containing α_{1G}, α_{1H}, and α_{1I}, which mediate T-type Ca^{2+} currents (Catterall et al., 2003).

The pharmacology of the three families of calcium channels is distinct. The Ca_V1 channels are the molecular targets of the organic calcium channel blockers used widely in treatment of cardiovascular diseases. The three major classes of L-type Ca^{2+} channel blockers are the dihydropyridines (e.g., nifedipine), benzothiazepines (e.g., diltiazem), and phenylalkylamines (e.g., verapamil). Regions of the α_1 subunit contain the binding sites for all of these drugs (Varadi et al., 1995). Phenylalkylamines are intracellular pore blockers. Dihydropyridines can be channel activators or inhibitors and therefore are thought to act allosterically to shift the channel toward the open or closed state, rather than by occluding the pore. Diltiazem and related benzothiazepines are thought to bind to a third receptor site (Catterall et al., 2003).

The Ca_V2 family of calcium channels is relatively insensitive to dihydropyridine calcium channel blockers, but these calcium channels are specifically blocked with high affinity by peptide toxins from spiders and marine snails (Miljanich and Ramachandran, 1995).

The $Ca_V2.1$ channels are blocked specifically by ω-agatoxin IVA from funnel web spider venom. The $Ca_V2.2$ channels are blocked specifically by ω-conotoxin GVIA and related cone snail toxins. The $Ca_V2.3$ channels are blocked specifically by the synthetic peptide toxin SNX-482 derived from tarantula venom. These peptide toxins are potent blockers of synaptic transmission because of their specific effects on the Ca_V2 family of calcium channels (Miljanich and Ramachandran, 1995; Catterall et al., 2003).

The Ca_V3 family of calcium channels is insensitive to both the dihydropyridines that block Ca_V1 channels and the spider and cone snail toxins that block the Ca_V2 channels. There are no widely useful pharmacologic agents that block T-type calcium currents (Miljanich and Ramachandran, 1995; Catterall et al., 2003).

Mechanism of Action in Migraine

The mechanism of action of the calcium channel antagonists in migraine prevention is uncertain. They were introduced into the treatment of migraine on the assumption that they prevent hypoxia of cerebral neurons, contraction of vascular smooth muscles, and inhibition of CA^{2+} dependent enzymes involved in prostaglandin formation. Perhaps it is their ability to block 5-HT release, interfere with neurovascular inflammation, or interfere with the initiation and propagation of spreading depression that is critical (Wauquier et al., 1985). The discovery that an abnormality in an α_{1A} subunit (P/Q channel) can produce familial hemiplegic migraine (Ophoff et al., 1996) has led to a search for more fundamental associations. (see Chapter 10).

The AHCPR Technical Report identified 45 controlled trials of calcium antagonists, including flunarizine (25 trials), nimodipine (11 trials), nifedipine (5 trials), verapamil (3 trials), cyclandelate (3 trials), and nicardipine (1 trial) (Gray, Goslin, et al., 1999). Flunarizine was compared with placebo in eight migraine prevention trials and effect sizes could be calculated for seven studies (Louis, 1981; Mendenopoulos et al., 1985; Pini et al., 1985; Sorensen et al., 1986; Thomas et al., 1991; Aldeeb et al., 1992; Aldeeb et al., 1992; Diamond and Freitag, 1993), but not the eighth study (Frenken and Nuijten, 1984). A meta-analysis of these seven heterogeneous trials was statistically significant in favor of flunarizine. Flunarizine was not significantly different than propranolol (Lucking et al., 1988; Ludin, 1989; Shimell et al., 1990; Gawel et al., 1992), metoprolol (Grotemeyer et al., 1987; Sorensen et al., 1991, pizotifen (Cerbo et al., 1986; Rascol et al., 1986; Gabai and Spierings, 1989), or methysergide (Steardo et al., 1986). Two new studies meet Level-I criteria (Diener et al., 2002) reported that flunarizine (5–10 mg/day; not available in the United States) was as effective as propranolol 160 mg/day in reducing attack frequency. Bussone and colleagues found that flunarizine and α dihydroergocryptine titrated up to 20 mg/day) were both effective in reducing frequency of migraine and days with migraine.

Nimodipine had mixed results in placebo-controlled trials. Three placebo-controlled studies suggested no significant differences [Ansell et al.,

1988; Migraine-Nimodipine European Study Group (MINES), 1989], while two reported relatively large and statistically significant differences in favor of nimodipine (Gelmers, 1983; Ansell et al., 1988). Nimodipine was not different than flunarizine (Bussone et al., 1987), pizotifen (Louis and Spierings, 1982; Cerbo et al., 1986; Rascol et al., 1986), or propranolol (Formisano et al., 1991).

The evidence for nifedipine was difficult to interpret. Two comparisons with placebo yielded similar effect sizes that were statistically insignificant, but the 95% CI associated with these estimates were large and did not exclude either a clinically important benefit or harm associated with nifedipine (McArthur et al., 1989; Shukla et al., 1995). Similarly ambiguous results were reported in one comparison with flunarizine (Lamsudin and Sadjimin, 1993) and in two comparisons with propranolol (Albers et al., 1989; Gerber et al., 1991). One trial found that metoprolol was significantly better than nifedipine at reducing headache frequency (Gerber et al., 1991).

Verapamil was more effective than placebo in two of three trials, but both positive trials had high dropout rates, rendering the findings uncertain (Markley et al., 1984; Solomon, 1986). The single negative placebo-controlled trial included a propranolol treatment arm. This trial reported no significant difference between verapamil, propranolol, and placebo (Solomon, 1986). The efficacy of nicardipine is supported by a single comparison with placebo in 30 patients with migraine with aura (Leandri et al., 1990). Recently, dotarzine at 50 and 100 mg has been shown to have statistically significant efficacy in a multicenter, placebo-controlled, parallel trial. However, long-term studies beyond 3 months of active treatment may be required to attain maximal benefit (Diamond, Ryan et al., 1999; Diamond et al., 1999b).

Diltiazem (60–90 mg QID) was effective in two small open studies (Riopelle and McCans, 1982; Smith and Schwartz, 1984).

AEs of the Ca^{2+} antagonists are dependent on the drug, and include dizziness and headache (particularly with nifedipine), depression, vasomotor changes, tremor, gastrointestinal complaints (including constipation), peripheral edema, orthostatic hypotension, and bradycardia. Patients frequently report an initial increase in headache. Headache improvement frequently requires weeks of treatment. The AHCPR Technical Report provided little useful information on the risk of AEs with these agents. AEs most commonly associated with flunarizine were sedation, weight gain, and abdominal pain. Symptoms reported with other calcium channel antagonists included dizziness, edema, flushing, and constipation. Two trials of verapamil and one of nifedipine reported high dropout rates due to AEs (Gray, Goslin, et al., 1999). AEs with nifedipine were frequent (54%) and included dizziness, edema, flushing, headache, and mental symptoms (McArthur et al., 1989).

Clinical Use

Verapamil (Calan, Isoptin) is available as a 40-, 80-, or 120-mg tablet or as a 120-, 180-, or 240-mg sustained-release preparation (Table 11–15). Start at a dose of 80 mg two to three times a day, with a maximum of 640 mg a day in divided doses. The sustained-release preparation of verapamil can be given once or twice a day, but unreliable absorption reduces reliability. The most common AE is constipation; dizziness, nausea, hypotension, headache, and edema are less common. Bioavailability is 20%. The absorbed drug is tightly protein bound. Peak plasma levels occur in 5 hours; the half-life ranges from 2.5 to 7.5 hours.

Diltiazem (Cardizem) is available in 30, 60, 90, and 120 mg tablets. Start at a dose of 30 mg two to three times a day, with a maximal dose of 360 mg a day in divided doses. AEs are infrequent: hypotension, A–V block, and headaches are occasionally seen. Bioavailability is 50%; the drug is tightly protein bound.

Nifedipine (Procardia) is available in 10- or 20-mg capsules. Start at a dose of 10 mg a day. This can be increased to a maximum of 120 mg a day in divided doses. AEs are common and include hypotension, headache, nausea, and vomiting. Bioavailability is 50%; almost all the drug is protein bound.

Nimodipine (Nimotop) is available in 30-mg capsules. The dose is 30–60 mg four times a day. AEs are infrequent. However, the cost of the drug may be prohibitive in the United States.

Flunarizine (Sibellium) is not available in the United States. The dose is 5–10 mg a day.

The most prominent AEs include weight gain, somnolence, dry mouth, dizziness, hypotension, and occasional extrapyramidal reactions. The elimination half-life of flunarizine is 19 days.

Serotonin Antagonists

Methysergide (Sansert)

Methysergide is a semisynthetic ergot alkaloid that is structurally related to methylergonovine (Table 11–16). It is a 5-HT_2 receptor antagonist and 5-$HT_{1B/D}$ agonist. It was one of the first drugs developed for migraine prevention, but its usefulness is limited by reports of retroperitoneal and retropleural fibrosis associated with long-term, mostly uninterrupted, administration. The AHCPR Technical Report identified 17 controlled trials of methysergide for migraine prevention (Lance et al., 1963; Shekelle and Ostfeld, 1964; Pedersen and Moller, 1966; Hudgson et al., 1967; Barrie et al., 1968; Ryan, 1968; Presthus, 1971; Forssman et al., 1972; Andersson, 1973; Sicuteri, 1973; Behan and Reid, 1980; Steardo et al., 1982; Steardo et al., 1986; Cangi et al., 1989). Four placebo-controlled trials suggested that methysergide was significantly better than placebo at reducing headache frequency (Lance et al., 1963; Shekelle and Ostfeld, 1964; Pedersen and Moller, 1966; Ryan, 1968).

Four comparison trials showed no statistically significant differences between methysergide and pizotifen (Ryan, 1968; Presthus, 1971; Forssman et al., 1972; Andersson, 1973). Two trials that directly compared methysergide and propranolol failed to demonstrate any statistically significant differences between these treatments (Behan and Reid, 1980; Steardo et al., 1982). The only trial that

TABLE 11–16 Miscellaneous Medication in the Preventive Treatment of Migraine.

Agent	*Daily dose*	*Comment*
Serotonin Antagonists		
Methysergide	2–8 mg	• Higher doses given BID or TID • Start 1 mg and increase 1 mg every 3 days • Should not be taken continuously for long periods
Cyproheptadine	12–36 mg	• BID or TID • Useful in children • Weight gain in most patients
Pizotifen	1.5–3 mg	• TID • Weight gain and drowsiness are common side effects
α_2-agonists		
Clonidine	0.05–0.3 mg/day	• Limited evidence in migraine
Guanfacine	1 mg	• Limited evidence in migraine.
Miscellaneous		
Lisinopril	10–40 mg	• Positive small controlled trial
Candesartan	8–32 mg	• Positive small controlled trial
Feverfew	50–82 mg	• Controversial evidence
Petasites	50–100 mg	• 75 and 100 mg better than placebo in independent trials
Riboflavin	400 mg	• Positive small controlled trial
Coenzyme Q	150–300 mg	• Two positive controlled trials
Magnesium	400–600 mg	• Controversial evidence

compared methysergide with metoprolol reported an unusually low response to metoprolol (6%) and thus a misleading relative increase in methysergide efficacy (Behan and Reid, 1980).

Methysergide was associated with a higher incidence of AEs than was placebo. AEs noted in trials and clinical practice included transient muscle aching, claudication, gastrointestinal complaints (nausea, vomiting, abdominal pain, and diarrhea), leg cramps, hair loss, weight gain, dizziness, giddiness, drowsiness, lassitude, paresthesia, and hallucinations. Frightening hallucinatory experiences after the first dose are not uncommon (Curran et al., 1967). Curran and Lance (1964) have treated leg claudication with vasodilators with some enhancement of methysergide's effectiveness, suggesting that its action on headache is not a result of vasoconstriction. The major complication of methysergide is the rare (1/5000) development of retroperitoneal, pulmonary, or endocardial fibrosis (Graham, 1967; Elkind et al., 1968).

Methysergide is indicated for the treatment of migraine and cluster headache. The dose ranges from 2 to 8 mg a day, with the higher doses being given two or three times a day. Some clinicians find they can use higher doses, up to 14 mg a day, without AEs and with higher efficacy (Raskin, 1988a). To minimize early AEs, patients can start with a dose of 1 mg a day and increase the dose gradually by 1 mg every 2–3 days. (This can be accomplished by breaking the 2 mg tablets.) Methysergide, in general, should not be taken continuously for long periods, since doing so may produce retroperitoneal fibrosis (Graham et al., 1966; Graham, 1967; Bana et al., 1974). Instead, the drug should be given for 6 months, stopped for 1 month, and then restarted. To avoid an increase in headache when methysergide is stopped, the patient should be weaned off the drug over a 1-week period. Some authorities use methysergide on a continuous basis with careful monitoring (Raskin, 1988a), which includes auscultation of the heart and yearly echocardiography, chest X-ray, and abdominal MRI. The drug should be discontinued immediately if pulmonary or cardiac retroperitoneal fibrosis is suspected (Raskin, 1988a).

Contraindications to methysergide use include pregnancy, peripheral vascular disorders, severe arteriosclerosis, coronary artery disease, severe hypertension, thrombophlebitis or cellulitis of the legs, peptic ulcer disease, fibrotic disorders, lung diseases, collagen disease, liver or renal function impairment, valvular heart disease, debilitation, or serious infection. Patients who receive methysergide should remain under the treating physician's supervision and be examined regularly for development of pulmonary/cardiac or peritoneal fibrosis or vascular complications.

Methysergide is an effective migraine preventive medication that is an appropriate consideration in resistant headaches with a high attack frequency. All of the open and controlled studies attest to its efficacy. In addition to being effective in reducing attack frequency, it often acts synergistically with ergotamine for breakthrough attacks. Owing to its side effect profile, it should be reserved for severe cases in which other migraine preventive drugs are not effective. It is no longer readily available in the United States.

Ergonovine is an ergot alkaloid 5-HT antagonist which is anecdotally said to be an effective migraine preventive drug (Raskin, 1988b). Gallagher (1989) found it useful in the treatment of menstrual migraine in an open trial. AEs are uncommon and include nausea, abdominal pain, and aching legs. The dose is 0.2–0.4 mg three to four times a day. Contraindications include Prinzmetal's angina, peripheral vascular disease, asthma, and pregnancy.

Ergonovine is no longer commercially available. We have used methylergonovine maleate, a principal metabolite of methysergide and a 5-HT antagonist, in place of ergonovine. The dose is 0.2–0.4 mg three to four times a day. AEs and contraindications are the same as for methysergide.

Cyproheptadine (Periactin), an antagonist at the 5-HT_2, histamine H_1, L-calcium channels and muscarinic cholinergic receptors, is widely used in the prophylactic treatment of migraine in children (Barlow, 1984; Forsythe and Hockaday, 1988; Raskin, 1988b). Curran and Lance (1964) found cyproheptadine more effective than placebo but less effective than methysergide. Cyproheptadine (Periactin) is available as 4-mg tablets. The total dose ranges from 12 to 36 mg a day (given two to three times a day or at bedtime). Common AEs are sedation and weight gain; dry mouth, nausea, lightheadedness, ankle edema, aching legs, and diarrhea are less common. Cyproheptadine may inhibit growth in children (Smyth and Lazarus, 1974) and reverse the effects of SSRIs. Rao and colleagues reported that cyproheptadine (4 mg/day) was as effective as propranolol (80 mg/day) in reducing migraine frequency and severity (Rao et al., 2000). The combination of cyproheptadine and propranolol was more effective than monotherapy. These four studies suggest a possible role of histamine, but not leukotriene, therapy in migraine prevention, but because only single studies that include 60–300 patients for each of these drugs have been performed, additional studies are needed to confirm these results. Additional studies are needed on the potential role of histamine and cyproheptadine in migraine prevention, but preliminary studies suggest a possible therapeutic benefit in migraine prevention.

*Pizotifen*a, 5-HT_2 receptor antagonist structurally similar to cyproheptadine, is not available in the United States. The U.S. Headache Consortium guidelines (Silberstein, 2000b) found that evidence was inconsistent for its efficacy from 11 placebo-controlled trials (Lance and Anthony, 1968; Ryan, 1968; Sjaastad and Stensrud, 1969; Arthur and Hornabrook, 1971; Hughes and Foster, 1971; Ryan, 1971; Krakowski and Engisch, 1973; Carroll and Maclay, 1975; Lawrence et al., 1977; Osterman, 1977; Bellavance and Meloche, 1990) and 19 comparisons with other agents (Ryan, 1968; Presthus, 1971; Forssman et al., 1972; Andersson, 1973; Hubbe, 1973; Osterman, 1977; Kangasniemi, 1979; Bono et al., 1982; Louis and Spierings, 1982; Behan, 1985; Micieli et al., 1985; Vilming et al., 1985; Cerbo et al., 1986; Rascol et al., 1986; Gawel, 1987; Havanka-Kanniainen et al., 1987; Nappi et al., 1987; Bellavance and Meloche, 1990; Nattero, Biale, et al., 1991). Analysis of the placebo-controlled trials suggested a large clinical effect that was statistically significant. In direct comparisons with other agents known to be efficacious for migraine prevention, no significant differences between pizotifen and flunarizine were demonstrated (Louis and Spierings, 1982; Cerbo et al., 1986; Rascol et al., 1986), methysergide (Ryan, 1968; Presthus, 1971; Forssman et al., 1972; Andersson, 1973), naproxen sodium (Bellavance and Meloche, 1990), or metoprolol (Vilming et al., 1985). However, in the 26 trials reviewed, pizotifen was generally poorly tolerated (Gray, Goslin, et al., 1999). Substantial weight gain, tiredness, and drowsiness were frequently reported. Pizotifen was associated with a high withdrawal rate due to AEs. Controlled and uncontrolled studies in Europe (Peatfield, 1986) have shown this drug to be of benefit in 40%–79% of patients. The dose recommendation is 0.5–1 mg, one three times daily by titration. Side effects include drowsiness and weight gain (Capildeo and Rose, 1982).

Miscellaneous Prophylactic Drugs

Clonidine (Catapres) is an imidazoline that activates (2 adrenergic receptors (Table 11–16). Clonidine inhibits the firing of locus ceruleus neurons (the major source of noradrenergic neurons) induced by opoid withdrawal by activating presynaptic inhibitory $\alpha 2$ receptors. This is the basis of clonidine's clinical effectiveness in treating opioid (Bakris et al., 1982; Aghajanian, 1978), alcohol, and cigarette withdrawal (Baumgartner and Rowen, 1987) and in controlling menopausal hot flashes (Nagamani et al., 1987).

The AHCPR Technical Report included 16 controlled trials of clonidine (Wilkinson, 1970; Sjaastad and Stensrud, 1971; Anthony et al., 1972; Shafar et al., 1972; Ryan and Diamond, 1975; Stensrud and Sjaastad, 1976a; Kallanranta et al., 1977; Mondrup and Moller, 1977; Adam et al., 1978; Boisen et al., 1978; Das et al., 1979; Kass and Nestvold, 1980; Behan, 1985; Louis et al., 1985; Bredfeldt et al., 1989; Elkind et al., 1989). The evidence from these trials suggests that $\alpha 2$ agonists are minimally, and not conclusively, efficacious. Three of 11 placebo-controlled trials of clonidine found a significant difference in favor of the active agent, but the magnitude of the effect was small (Sjaastad and Stensrud, 1971; Stensrud and Sjaastad, 1976a; Kallanranta et al., 1977).

Two comparative trials comparing clonidine with the β-blockers metoprolol (Louis et al., 1985) and propranolol yielded mixed results (Kass and Nestvold, 1980). Two additional comparative trials showed no significant differences among clonidine, practolol (Kallanranta et al., 1977), and pindolol (Anthony et al., 1972). (The latter two agents are β-blockers with intrinsic sympathomimetic activity.) One trial each found no significant differences between clonidine and pizotifen (Behan, 1985) or between clonidine and carbamazepine (Anthony et al., 1972).

The most common AEs reported with clonidine in clinical trials were drowsiness and tiredness, but these were usually neither serious nor cause for withdrawal from the trials. In studies comparing clonidine with β-blockers, AEs occurred at similar rates for both interventions.

Clonidine (Catapres) is available as 0.1-, 0.2-, and 0.3-mg tablets and as a patch delivering 0.1 mg (TTS #1), 0.2 mg (TTS #2), and 0.3 mg (TTS #3) a day. The dose ranges from 0.1 to 2 mg a day.

Calcitonin is a single chain polypeptide hypocalcemic hormone secreted by the thyroid gland. Salmon calcitonin (100 IU a day) is effective in treating pain, perhaps by increasing the circulating levels of β endorphin, adrenocorticotropic hormone (ACTH), and cortisol (Ustdal et al., 1989). Salmon calcitonin given IM (Gennari et al., 1986) or by NS (Micieli et al., 1988) and an analog of eel calcitonin given IM (Patti et al., 1987) are proposed as effective in migraine prophylaxis.

Angiotensin Converting Enzyme Inhibitors and Angiotensin II Receptor Antagonists

Lisinopril. Schrader et al. (Schrader et al., 2001) conducted a double-blind, placebo-controlled, crossover study of lisinopril, an angiotensin converting enzyme inhibitor, in migraine prophylaxis. The treatment period was 12 weeks, with one 10 mg lisinopril tablet once daily for 1 week then two 10 mg lisinopril tablets once daily for 11 weeks, followed by a 2-week wash-out period. The second treatment period consisted of one placebo tablet once daily for 1 week and then two placebo tablets for 11 weeks. Hours with headache, days with headache, days with migraine, and headache severity index were significantly reduced by 20% (95% CI 5%–36%), 17% (5%–30%), 21% (9%–34%), and 20% (3%–37%), respectively, with lisinopril compared with placebo. Days with migraine were reduced by at least 50% in 14 participants for active treatment versus placebo and 17 patients for active treatment versus run-in period. Fourteen participants had at least 50% fewer days with migraine with active treatment versus placebo. Intention to treat analysis of data from 55 patients supported the differences in favor of lisinopril for the primary end points.

Candesartan. Tronvik et al. (Tronvik et al., 2003) performed a randomized, double-blind, placebo-controlled, crossover study of candesartan, an angiotensin II receptor blocker, in migraine prevention. Sixty patients aged 18–65 years with two to six migraine attacks per month were recruited. A placebo run-in period of 4 weeks was followed by two 12-week treatment periods separated by 4 weeks of placebo washout. Thirty patients were randomly assigned to receive one 16-mg candesartan cilexetil tablet daily in the first treatment period, followed by one placebo tablet daily in the second period. The remaining 30 patients received placebo followed by candesartan. In a period of 12 weeks, the mean number of days with headache was 18.5 with placebo versus 13.6 with candesartan ($p = .001$) in the ITT analysis ($n = 57$). The number of candesartan responders (reduction of 50% compared with placebo) was 18 of 57 (31.6%) for days with headache and 23 of 57 (40.4%) for days with migraine. AEs were similar in the two periods. In this study, the angiotensin II receptor blocker candesartan was effective, with a tolerability profile comparable with that of placebo.

Lanepitant is a potent inhibitor of neurogenic dural inflammation. Patients with three to eight migraine headaches during a 1 month placebo lead-in period were randomized to a double-blind, parallel comparison of 200-mg QD lanepitant ($n = 42$) and placebo ($n = 42$). Lanepitant was ineffective in preventing or reducing severity of migraine. The fact that absorption was not impaired by gastric stasis associated with the migraine attack suggests that lack of effect in the acute migraine study was due to ineffectiveness of the NK-1 blockade rather than insufficient plasma concentration (Goldstein et al., 1999).

Leukotriene Receptor Antagonist (Montelukast)

Montelukast. A previous small, open-label study of migraine patients suggested prophylactic efficacy for montelukast, an antagonist of the cysteinyl leukotriene receptor that is used to treat asthma. Brandes et al. (Brandes, Visser, et al., 2004) evaluated the efficacy and tolerability of montelukast 20 mg in the prophylactic treatment of migraine in a multicenter, randomized, double-blind, placebo-controlled, parallel-groups study. Over 3 months of treatment, there was no significant difference between the two groups in the percentage of patients who reported at least a 50% decrease in migraine attack frequency per month: 15.4% for montelukast versus 10.3% for placebo ($p = 0.304$). Montelukast 20 mg was not an effective drug for prevention of migraine.

Histamine and N-α Methyl Histamine

The use of histamine in headache dates to the work of Horton (Horton et al., 1939) in the 1930s as a treatement for cluster headache. Since then, its use has ebbed and flowed, lacking well designed clinical trials to verify its efficacy. Histamine 1 ng infusion twice weekly was more effective than placebo in reducing headache frequency at 4 and 8 weeks (Millan-Guerrero et al., 2003). In a separate study, Millan-Guerrero et al. (Millan-Guerrero et al., 2006) reported that N-α methyl histamine (1–3 ng BIW) was effective in reducing migraine frequency, severity and duration as measured at 12 weeks.

These studies suggest a possible role of histamine, but not leukotriene, therapy in migraine prevention; however, because only single studies that include 60–300 patients for each of these drugs have been conducted, additional studies are needed to confirm these results. Additional studies on the potential role of histamine and cyproheptadine in migraine prevention are also needed, but preliminary studies suggest a possible therapeutic benefit in migraine prevention.

Medicinal Herbs, Vitamins, and Minerals

According to a national survey (Eisenberg et al., 1998), the use of herbal medicinal products by the general U.S. population increased by a staggering 480% between 1990 and 1997. (Table 11–16)

Feverfew (Tanacetum parthenium) is a medicinal herb used in self-treatment of migraine. Four trials were conducted, two in the AHCPR and two after the report. The AHCPR Technical Report listed two trials, distinctly different in design, that compared feverfew with placebo and no treatment. One trial was conducted in a self-selected group of feverfew users and showed that withdrawing feverfew led to a statistically significant increase in headache frequency (Johnson, Kadam, et al., 1985). A pilot study of 17 migraineurs who ate fresh feverfew leaves daily was undertaken at the City of London Migraine Clinic. Patients were given capsules of freeze–dried feverfew or placebo. Those receiving placebo had a tripling in the frequency of migraine attacks. Patients on placebo reported increased nervousness, tension headaches, insomnia, or joint stiffness constituting a "post feverfew syndrome" (perhaps another example of rebound).

The other, more conventional, trial was conducted in a larger group of migraineurs, most of whom (71%) had never used feverfew (Murphy et al., 1988). This trial reported a smaller difference between feverfew and the control treatment than did the other trial, but still found the difference to be statistically significant in favor of feverfew. Two trials were not included in the AHCPR report. One was a double-blind, randomized, crossover trial that tested the efficacy of feverfew compared with placebo, and reported that treatment with feverfew was associated with a significant reduction in pain intensity and nonheadache symptoms (nausea, vomiting, photophobia, and phonophobia) (Palevitch et al., 1997). The other trial reported no significant differences between feverfew given as an alcoholic extract and placebo for reducing migraine frequency (Deweerdt et al., 1996). One new Level-II study compared the efficacy of placebo versus the combination of magnesium (300 mg) + riboflavin (400 mg) + feverfew (100 mg). Both treatment groups showed improvement over baseline, but no between-group differences were noted (Maizels et al., 2004).

Limited information indicates that AEs were no more common with feverfew than with the control treatment (Gray, Goslin, et al., 1999). Feverfew's AEs include mouth ulceration and a more widespread oral inflammation associated with loss of taste. Feverfew's mechanism of action is uncertain. It is rich in sesquiterpene lactones, especially parthenolide, which may be a nonspecific NE, 5-HT, bradykinin, prostaglandin, and acetylcholine antagonist. The biologic variation in the sesquiterpene lactone content and the long-term safety and effectiveness of feverfew are of concern (Johnson, Kadam, et al., 1985).

Until recently, it was generally assumed that parthenolides represent the active principle of feverfew. This hypothesis was supported by in vitro experiments that emphasized its biological activity. These studies have demonstrated that the plant has inhibitory effects on platelet aggregation and release of serotonin from blood platelets and leukocytes (Heptinstall et al., 1985, 1987). One trial that used feverfew extract with a standardized and constant concentration of parthenolides to treat migraine did not show any beneficial effect (Deweerdt et al., 1996). Thus, the clinical effectiveness of feverfew for migraine prevention has not been established beyond reasonable doubt. More clinical trials are needed, both on a larger scale and with various feverfew extracts, including parthenolide-free sesquiterpene lactone chemotypes (Vogler et al., 1998).

MIG-99. MIG-99 is a relatively new stable extract of *Tanacetum parthenium* (feverfew), which is reproducibly manufactured with supercritical CO_2 from feverfew (*T. parthenium*). Since the first part of the Guidelines, three new studies on MIG 99 for migraine prophylaxis have been published, two of which meet Level-I criteria for review herein. One dose-finding trial of MIG-99 (2.08 mg, 6.25 mg, 18.75 mg TID) reported the highest reduction in attack frequency with the 6.25-mg dose (Pfaffenrath et al., 2002). A second study confirmed that MIG-99 (6.25-mg TID) is effective in reducing mean number of migraine attacks versus placebo (Diener, Pfaffenrath, Schnitker, et al., 2005).

Riboflavin. A mitochondrial dysfunction resulting in impaired oxygen metabolism may play a role in migraine pathogenesis (Welch et al., 1989; Montagna et al., 1994; Sangiorgi et al., 1994; Watanabe et al., 1996). Riboflavin (vitamin B_2) is the precursor of flavin mononucleotide and flavin adenine dinucleotide, which are required for the activity of flavoenzymes involved in the electron transport chain. Given to patients with MELAS or mitochondrial myopathies on the assumption that at large doses it might augment activity of mitochondrial complexes I and II, riboflavin improved clinical as well as biochemical parameters (Arts et al., 1983; Penn et al., 1992; Antozzi et al., 1994; Scholte et al., 1995).

On the basis of the results of an open trial in migraine, a placebo-controlled, double-blind trial of high dose of vitamin B_2 (400 mg) was performed and showed significant benefit (Schoenen et al., 1998). Schoenen et al. (1998) compared riboflavin (400 mg) with placebo in migraineurs in a randomized trial of 3 months' duration. Riboflavin was significantly superior to placebo in reducing the attack frequency ($p = 0.005$), headache days ($p = 0.012$), and migraine index (0.012). The proportion of patients who improved by at least 50% in headache days, that is, "responders," was 15% for placebo, 59% for riboflavin ($p = 0.002$) and the number-needed-to-treat for effectiveness was 2.3. Only three AEs occurred: two in the riboflavin group (diarrhea and polyuria) and one in the placebo group (abdominal cramps). None was serious. Because of its high efficiency, excellent tolerability, and low cost, riboflavin is an interesting option for prophylaxis and a candidate for a comparative trial with an established prophylactic drug.

Coenzyme Q10. Rozen et al. (Rozen et al., 2002) assessed the efficacy of coenzyme Q10 as a preventive treatment for migraine headaches in an open label trial. Thirty-two patients with a history of episodic migraine with or without aura were treated with coenzyme Q10 at a dose of 150 mg per day. Thirty-one of thirty-two patients completed the study; 61.3% of patients had a greater than 50% reduction in number of days with migraine headache. There were no AEs noted with coenzyme Q10. From this open label investigation, coenzyme Q10 appears to be a good migraine preventive. Sandor et al. (Sandor et al., 2003) performed a double-blind, placebo-controlled trial of coenzyme Q10 (100-mg TID)in 42 patients for 3 months. The 50% responder rate was 47.6% for coenzyme Q10 and 14.3% for placebo.

Petasites hybridus root (butterbur) is a perennial shrub whose extracts have been used for therapeutic purposes in traditional medicine for centuries. Lipton et al. (Lipton, Gobel, et al., 2004) conducted a randomized, double-blind, placebo-controlled trial of Petasites' efficacy in migraine prophylaxis. Two-hundred and forty-five eligible IHS migraine patients were randomized to one of three arms: Petasites extract 50-mg BID, Petasites extract 75-mg BID, or placebo BID. Over 4 months of treatment, migraine attack frequency was reduced by 26% for placebo, 48% for Petasites extract 75-mg

BID ($p = 0.0012$ versus placebo), and 36% for Petasites extract 50-mg BID ($p = 0.127$ versus placebo). The most frequently reported AE was mild gastrointestinal events, predominantly burping. This study demonstrates that a standardized Petasites extract, 75-mg BID, is more effective than placebo and is well tolerated as a preventive therapy for migraine.

Diener et al. (Diener, Rahlfs, et al., 2004) performed an independent reanalysis of a randomized, placebo-controlled, parallel-group study on the efficacy and tolerability of a special butterbur root extract (Petadolex) for the prophylaxis of migraine. In order to follow regulatory requirements, an independent reanalysis of the original data was performed. Following a 4-week baseline phase, 33 patients were randomized to treatment with two 25-mg capsules of butterbur twice a day and 27 to placebo. The mean monthly attack frequency decreased from 3.4 at baseline to 1.8 after 3 months ($p = 0.0024$) in the active group and from 2.9 to 2.6 in the placebo group (n.s.). The responder rate (improvement of migraine frequency >50%) was 45% in the active group and 15% in the placebo group. Butterbur was well tolerated and may be effective in the prophylaxis of migraine.

Mineral Salts

Lithium is effective in the treatment of cluster headache. On the basis of the analogy to cluster, Medina (1982) found lithium carbonate effective in treating cyclic migraine, a disorder in which patients have bouts of migrainous headaches separated by headache-free periods. Lithium may be a particularly useful adjunctive medication for bipolar or manic patients. AEs include hand tremor, polyuria, thirst, and ankle edema. Long-term complications include hypothyroidism, oliguric renal failure, and diabetes insipidus. The dose of lithium is 900–1800 mg a day, titrated to give a serum level between 0.6 and 1.2 mEq/l. Combining lithium with verapamil can cause adverse responses (lithium toxicity) at standard doses. The lithium dose must be substantially reduced when it is given with verapamil, even when the blood level is in the therapeutic range (Price and Giannini, 1986; Price and Shalley, 1987).

Magnesium supplementation has been shown to be effective in one of two trials. One study enrolled 81 patients who had IHS migraine. Their mean attack frequency was 3.6 per month. After a prospective baseline period of 4 weeks, these patients received 600 mg (24 mmol) of oral magnesium (trimagnesium dicitrate) or placebo daily for 12 weeks. In weeks 9–12 the attack frequency was reduced by 41.6% in the magnesium group and by 15.8% in the placebo group compared to the baseline ($p < 0.05$). The number of days with migraine and symptomatic drug consumption also decreased significantly in the magnesium group. AEs were diarrhea (18.6%) and gastric irritation (4.7%) (Peikert et al., 1996).

In another multicenter, prospective, randomized, double-blind, placebo-controlled study, the migraine prophylactic effect of 20mmol magnesium-L-aspartate-hydrochloride trihydrate given in divided doses was evaluated. Included in this study were patients with a 2-year history of two to six attacks a month of migraine without aura. The efficacy end-point was a reduction of at least 50% in intensity or duration of migraine attacks at the end of the 12th week of treatment compared to baseline. With a calculated total sample size of 150 patients, an interim analysis was planned after treatment of at least 60 patients was completed; this analysis, in fact, was performed with 69 patients (64 women, 5 men). Of these, 35 had received magnesium and 34 placebo. There were 10 responders in each group (28.6% magnesium and 29.4% placebo). The trial was discontinued for this reason as determined by the study protocol. There was no benefit from magnesium compared with placebo in the number of migraine days or migraine attacks (Pfaffenrath et al., 1996).

The studies differed in the amount of magnesium (24 mmol versus 20 mmol) and in the salt (dicitrate versus aspartate). Those differences may produce differences in bioavailability and efficacy and account for the reported difference.

In one recent study, magnesium oxide (9 mg/kg/PO) was given to children (age 3–17 years) and was shown to be more effective than placebo in reducing headache days and headache severity (Wang et al., 2003). Two previous studies (Peikert et al., 1996; Pfaffenrath et al., 1996) report conflicting results regarding the efficacy of magnesium in migraine prevention in adults (doses tested: 400–600). One Level-II study compared the efficacy of placebo versus the combination of magnesium (300 mg) + riboflavin (400 mg) + feverfew (100 mg). Both treatment groups showed improvement over baseline, but no between-group differences were noted and no comparisons were reported for monotherapy (Maizels et al., 2004).

Use of Abortive Agents for Migraine Prophylaxis

Aspirin. O'Neill and Mann (O'Neill and Mann, 1979) and Masel et al. (1980) found that aspirin (650 mg a day) decreased headache frequency. Two major multicenter trials, however, clearly proved the efficacy of aspirin in the prophylaxis of migraine: in 1988 "The British Physician Trial" showed that a daily dose of 500 mg aspirin reduced the frequency of migraine by an average of 30% (Peto et al., 1988). In a double-blind trial of low-dose aspirin (325 mg every other day) in 22,071 U.S. male physicians (Physician Health Study), Buring et al. (1990) found a 20% reduction in headache frequency. Although this is statistically significant, it may not be clinically significant. In a small open trial, Baldratti et al. (1983) compared the efficacy of aspirin (13.5 mg/kg) with propranolol (1.8 mg/kg). In this trial, both drugs were equally effective and reduced the frequency, duration, and intensity of the attacks to the same extent. In a double-blind crossover trial, aspirin (500 mg daily) was statistically less effective than 200 mg of propranolol daily (Grotemeyer et al., 1990). A trial comparing 300 mg of aspirin to 200 mg of metoprolol in a parallel design found that while metoprolol was more effective than aspirin in preventing migraine, it was associated with a higher AE rate (Diener et al., 2001). High-dose aspirin use may lead to overuse and the development of rebound headaches. Aspirin in low doses clearly is indicated for the prophylaxis of myocardial infarction and transient ischemic attacks. We would use aspirin only for patients with prolonged or nonvisual aura.

NSAIDs

Some NSAIDs may be effective in migraine prophylaxis. These include sodium naproxen, naproxen, fenoprofen, ketoprofen, and tolfenamic acid (Pradalier et al., 1988). Some headache disorders (chronic paroxysmal hemicrania, hemicrania continua) are defined by their responsiveness to indomethacin (Sjaastad and Dale, 1976; Sjaastad and Spierings, 1984; Bordini et al., 1991). Although NSAIDs are effective, they must be used with caution because of their AEs on gastrointestinal and renal function (Solomon, 1989).

Ergotamine

The prophylactic use of ergotamine is discouraged. The exception is women with primarily menstrual migraine, who can use ergotamine only at the time of headache vulnerability without the danger of developing rebound headache.

Dihydroergotamine

Some studies have shown that an oral programmed release form of DHE (DHE methanesulfonate, DHE retard) at a dose of 5 mg three times a day is effective in the prophylactic treatment of migraine (Centonze et al., 1983; Fontanari et al., 1983; Martucci et al., 1983; Mastrosimone and Iaccarino, 1987). DHE retard is not available in the United States.

Newer Treatments

Botulinum toxin type A (Botox). Mathew, Saper, et al. (1999) evaluated the safety and efficacy of pericranial botulinum toxin type A injections as prophylactic treatment of chronic moderate-to-severe migraine. One hundred twenty three patients who had chronic IHS-defined migraine and a history of two to eight moderate-to-severe migraine attacks during a 1-month baseline were randomized to treatment with either 0, 25, or 75 U of botulinum toxin type A injected symmetrically into glabellar, frontalis, and temporalis muscles. Diaries were kept for 3 months postinjection. At 12 centers, 41, 42, and 40 patients were randomized to 0, 25, and 75 U Botulinum toxin type A treatment groups and had baseline frequencies of migraine of 4.41, 4.45, and 3.95 attacks per month, respectively. The 25 U Botulinum toxin type A treatment group fared significantly better than the placebo group by the following measures: reduction in mean frequency of moderate-to-severe migraines during days 31–60; incidence of 50% reduction and incidence of two headache decrease in mild to severe migraines at days 61–90; reduction in mild to severe migraine during days 61–90; reduction of days with phonophobia during days 31–90; and improvement by patient global assessment for days 31–60 postinjection. The 75 U botulinum toxin type A treatment group was significantly better than the placebo group on patient global assessment for days 31–60, but not other parameters. Botulinum toxin type A treatment was well tolerated, but high-dose botulinum toxin type A showed significantly more treatment-related AEs than placebo. No serious treatment-related AEs were reported. Pericranial injection of botulinum toxin type A (25 U) showed significant differences compared to vehicle in reducing migraine frequency and associated symptoms during 90 days following injection.

Some studies support the efficacy of botulinum toxin type A in migraine treatment. A double-blind, vehicle-controlled trial of 123 patients with moderate-to-severe migraine found that subjects treated with a single injection of 25 U botulinum toxin type A (but not those treated with 75 U) showed significantly fewer migraine attacks per month, as well as reductions in severity, number of days requiring acute medication, and incidence of migraine-induced vomiting (Silberstein et al., 2000). The lack of significant effect in the higher-dose group may be related to baseline group differences, for example, fewer migraines or a longer time since onset. Another double-blind, placebo-controlled, region-specific study found a significant reduction in migraine pain among patients who received simultaneous injections of botulinum toxin type A in the frontal and temporal regions, as well as an overall trend toward botulinum toxin type A superiority to placebo in reducing migraine frequency (Brin et al., 2000). A randomized, double-blind, placebo-controlled study compared the efficacy of placebo, botulinum toxin type A 16 U, and botulinum toxin type A 100 U as migraine prophylaxis when injected into the frontal and neck muscles (Evers et al., 2004). While there were no statistically significant differences in reduction of migraine frequency among the groups, the accompanying symptoms of migraine were reduced in the botulinum toxin type A 16 U group.

However, new studies have failed to demonstrate significant improvements over placebo. A recent study (Saper et al., 2007) of patients (N = 232) with moderate-to-severe episodic (4–8 episodes/month) migraine compared placebo to regional (frontal, temporal or glabellar) or combined treatment with botulinum toxin type A. Reductions from baseline in migraine frequency, maximum severity, and duration occurred with botulinum toxin type As and placebo, but there were no significant between-group differences. Elkind et al. (Elkind et al., 2006) conducted a series of three sequential studies of 418 patients with a history of four to eight moderate-to-severe migraines per month with re-randomization at each stage and doses ranging from 7.5 to 50 U. Botulinum toxin type A and placebo produced comparable decreases from baseline in migraine frequency at each time-point examined, with no consistent, statistically significant, between-group differences observed.

RECOMMENDATIONS

The goals of preventive treatment are to reduce the frequency, duration, or severity of attacks, improve responsiveness to acute attack treatment, improve function, and reduce disability (Table 11–17). It may also prevent episodic migraine's progression to chronic migraine and result in health care cost reductions. The medications used to treat migraine can be divided into five major categories: (1) drugs that have been proven effective (some β-blockers, amitriptyline, topiramate, and divalproex); (2) drugs that are probably effective; (3) drugs that are possibly effective; (4) drugs for which evidence is inadequate or conflicting; and (5) drugs that are probably ineffective.

Group 1. The following medications are established as effective for migraine prevention on the basis of multiple Class-I randomized controlled trials:

- AEDs: topiramate and divalproex sodium (Grade A).
- Antidepressants: amitriptyline (Grade A).
- β-Blockers: metoprolol, propranolol and timolol (Grade A).
- Serotonin agonists: frovatriptan for short-term prevention of menstrually related migraine (Grade A).
- Petasites or MIG-99 (Grade A).
- Serotonin antagonists: methysergide (severe AEs) (Grade A).

TABLE 11–17 Preventive Therapies for Migraine.

Group 1	*Group 2*	*Group 3*	*Group 4*	*Group 5*
Antiepileptic drugs	ACE-inhibitors	α-Agonists	Anticoagulants	Antiepileptic drugs
Divalproex sodium	Lisinopril	Clonidine	Acenocoumarol	Clonazepam
Sodium valproate	Candasartan		Coumadin	Oxycarbamazepine
Topiramate		Anticonvulsants	Picotamide	
	Antiepileptic drugs	Carbamazepine		Acetazolamide
Antidepressants	Gabapentin		Antiepileptic drugs	Lanepitant
Amitriptyline		Ca++ blockers	Lamotrigine	Montelukast
	Antidepressants/SSRI/	Diltiazem	Tiagabine	ω-3
β-blockers	SNRI	Nicardipine		Vitamine E
Metoprolol	Fluoxetine	Nifedipine	Antidepressants TCAs	
Propranolol	Venlafaxine	Nimodipine	Doxepin	
Timolol	Antihistamines/	Verapamil	Imipramine	
	leukotriene antagonists		Nortriptyline	
Other	Cyproheptadine		Protriptyline	
Petasites	Histamine			
			SSRI/SNRI	
Serotonin agonists (MRM)	Beta-blockers		Fluvoxamine	
Frovatriptan	Atenolol		Paroxetine	
	Nadolol		Sertraline	
Serotonin antagonists				
Methysergide	NSAIDs		Other	
	Aspirin		Mirtazepine	
	Fenoprofen		Phenylzine	
	Flurbiprofen			
	Ibuprofen			

(continued)

Table 11–17 (continued)

Group 1	*Group 2*	*Group 3*	*Group 4*	*Group 5*
	Ketoprofen		Beta-Blockers	
	Mefenamic acid		Acebutolol	
	Naproxen		Bisoprolol	
	Naproxen sodium		Pindolol	
	Other		Serotonin antagonists	
	Coenzyme Q10		Methylergonovine	
	MIG-99 (feverfew)			
	Vitamin B2			
	Serotonin agonists (MRM)			
	Naratriptan[a]			
	Zolmitriptan[a]			

Abbreviations: ACE, angiotensin-converting enzyme; SNRIs, selective serotonin norepinephrine reuptake inhibitors, SSRIs, selective serotonin reuptake inhibitors; TCA, tricyclic antidepressant.

[a] For short-term prophylaxis menstrually related migraine (MRM)

Group 1: Medications with proven high efficacy based on two Class-I trials a

Group 2: Medications are probably effective based on one Class-I or two Class II studies

Group 3: Medications use are possibly effective based one Class-II studies or two Class III studies or conflicting studies

Group 4: Medication use cannot be recommended based on inadequate or conflicting data with no Class I-III trials (Class IV studies or no studies).

Group 5: Medications probably ineffective (based on one Class-I or two Class II studies)

Group 2. The following medications are probably effective migraine prevention (on the basis of at least one Class I or two Class II studies).

- ACE inhibitors/antagonists: candesartan and lisinopril
- AEDs: gabapentin
- Antidepressants: fluoxetine and venlafaxine
- β-Blockers: atenolol, nadolol
- Histamine and cyproheptadine
- Other: MIG-99 (feverfew)
- NSAIDS: aspirin, fenoprofen, flurbiprofen, ibuprofen, ketoprofen, mefenamic acid, naproxen, naproxen sodium
- Serotonin agonists: naratriptan and zolmitriptan for short-term prevention of menstrually related migraine .
- Vitamins: Riboflavin (vitamin B2), CO-Q10, magnesium

Group 3. The following agents are possibly effective (one Class-II or two Class III studies) for migraine prevention

- α-Agonists: guanfacine, clonidine
- AEDs: carbamezapine
- Calcium-channel blockers: verapamil, nicardipine, nifedipine, nimodipine

Group 4. Evidence is inadequate or conflicting to support their use for migraine prevention:

- Anticoagulants: picotamide, acenocoumarol, coumadin
- AEDs: lamotrigine, and tiagabine
- Antidepressants
- SSRIs: clomipramine, fluvoxamine, s-fluoxetine
- TCAs: doxepin, imipramine, nortriptyline, protriptyline
- β-Blockers: acebutolol, bisoprolol, pindolol,
- MAOIs: phenylzine (see special considerations)
- Serotonin agonists: DHE

Group 5. The following medications are probably ineffective (on the basis of one Class-I or two Class II studies) for migraine prevention:

- AEDs: clonazapem, oxycarbamazepine
- Acetazolamide
- Montelukast
- Lanepitant
- Vitamins: vitamin E, Omega-3

RECOMMENDATIONS

All drugs in Group 1 should be used for the preventive treatment of migraine (Level A).

All drugs in Group 2 should be considered for the preventive treatment of migraine (Level B).

All groups in Group 3 may be considered for the preventive treatment of migraine (Level C).

All drugs in Group 4 have no recommendation (Level U).

All drugs in Group 5 should not be considered for migraine prevention (Level B).

Choice of a preventive medication should be made on the basis of a drug's proven efficacy, the patient's preferences and headache profile, the drug's AEs, and the presence or absence of coexisting or comorbid disease (Table 11–1). The drug used should be the one that has the best risk-to-benefit ratio for the individual patient and takes advantage of the drug's AE profile. An underweight patient would be a candidate for one of the medications that commonly produce weight gain, such as a TCA; in contrast, one would try to avoid these drugs in the overweight patient and consider using topiramate. Tertiary TCAs that have a sedating effect would be useful at bedtime for patients with insomnia. Older patients with cardiac disease or patients with significant hypotension may not be able to use TCAs or calcium channel or β-blockers, but could use divalproex or topiramate. Caution should be used when prescribing β-blockers for the athletic patient. Medication that can impair cognitive functioning should be avoided when patients are dependent on their wits (Silberstein et al., 1998; Silberstein and Goadsby, 2002).

Comorbid and coexistent diseases have important implications for treatment. The presence of a second illness provides therapeutic opportunities but also imposes certain therapeutic limitations. In some instances, two or more conditions may be treated with a single drug. However, there are limitations to using a single medication to treat two illnesses. Giving a single medication may not treat two different conditions optimally: although one of the two conditions may be adequately treated, the second illness may require a higher or lower dose, and therefore the patient is at risk of the second illness not being adequately treated. In an effort to use a single medication to treat two conditions, the physician may choose a second- or third-tier drug for treating either or both conditions, and this may not provide adequate efficacy for either illness. The risk is that one condition is managed appropriately, but the second condition requires a higher dose or additional therapy. Therapeutic independence may be needed should monotherapy fail. For example, a higher or lower dose of medication may be needed for migraine prophylaxis than the dose commonly used for other indications. Usually, medicine is started with a minimally effective dose and then titrated over weeks or months. Avoiding drug interactions or increased AEs is a primary concern when using polypharmacy. For example, when a patient is undergoing treatment for depression, adding a β-blocker for migraine management may exacerbate the depression and put the patient at unnecessary risk.

For some patients, a single medication may adequately manage comorbid conditions. When migraine and hypertension and/or angina occur together, β-blockers or calcium channel blockers may be effective for all conditions (Solomon, 1989). However, this is likely to be the exception rather than the rule. A β-blocker may be poorly tolerated (or even contraindicated) in the presence of other conditions, such as depression or coexisting asthma. Co-pharmacy may enable therapeutic adjustments based on the status of each illness. TCAs are often recommended for patients with migraine and depression (Silberstein et al., 1995). However, appropriate management of depression often requires higher doses of TCAs, which may be associated with more AEs. A better approach might be to treat the depression with an SSRI or SNRI and the migraine with a cortical excitability stabilizer (antiepileptic drug, e.g., topiramate). For the patient with migraine and epilepsy (Mathew et al., 1995b), one may achieve control of both conditions with AEDs, such as topiramate or divalproex sodium. Divalproex and topiramate are the drugs of choice for the patient with migraine and bipolar illness (Bowden et al., 1994; Silberstein, 1996). The pregnant migraineur who has a comorbid condition that needs treatment should be given a medication that is effective for both conditions and has the lowest potential for fetal AEs. When individuals have more than one disease, certain categories of treatment may be relatively contraindicated. For example, β-blockers should be used with caution in the depressed migraineur, while TCAs or neuroleptics may lower the seizure threshold and should be used with caution for the epileptic migraineur.

Although monotherapy is preferred, it is often not the best choice and it may sometimes be necessary to combine preventive medications. Antidepressants are often used with β-blockers or calcium channel blockers and topiramate or divalproex sodium may be used in combination with any of these medications (Table 11–18).

TABLE 11–18 Drug Combinations.

Suggested
- Antidepressant
  - β-Blocker
  - Calcium channel blocker
  - Divalproex
- Methysergide
  - Calcium channel blocker
- SSRIs
  - TCAs

Cautious use
- β-Blocker
  - Calcium channel blocker
  - Methysergide
- MAOIs
  - Amitriptyline or nortriptyline
- Methysergide
  - Dihydroergotamine

Contraindications
- MAOIs
  - SSRIs
  - Most TCAs (except amitriptyline or nortriptyline)
  - Doxepin and trazadone
  - Carbamazepine
- Midrin
  - Most triptans (cautions with zolmitriptan and SC sumatriptan, safe with naratriptan)
- NSAIDs
  - Lithium
- Methysergide
  - Ergotamine, triptans (cautions with dihydroergotamine)

Abbreviations: SSRIs, selective serotonin reuptake inhibitors; TCA, tricyclic antidepressant;MAOIs, monoamine oxidase inhibitors; NSAID, nonsteroidal anti-inflammatory drug.

Use of Acute Medication for Patients on Preventive Treatment

Preventive medication is considered to be effective if it decreases the frequency of attacks by more than 50%. Thus, patients treated with preventive medication may continue to have attacks of episodic migraine and TTH. Menstrual migraine attacks often persist to a greater extent than nonmenstrual attacks. Preventive medication may also decrease the intensity and duration of the attacks, and may make acute medications more effective. Using preventive and acute medication together presents a new set of complexities.

The amount of acute medication taken must be limited to prevent the development of drug-induced daily rebound headache and loss of efficacy of the preventive medication. This is one of the causes of secondary failure of preventive medication.

Certain acute medications should be used with caution in the presence of certain preventive medications (Table 11–19). Ergotamine, DHE, and sumatriptan could potentially have enhanced vasospastic properties in the presence of methysergide. However, many authorities have found that the ergots are more effective for patients being treated with methysergide (Curran et al., 1967). MAOIs decrease first-pass metabolism of the triptans, other than naratriptan, frovatriptan, and almotriptan. This increases the half-life and the area under the curve of these agents. Therefore, the dose of oral zolmitriptan should be reduced and it should be used cautiously, if at all, and all but SC sumatriptan and oral naratriptan should not be used in patients taking MAOIs. Meperidine, tramadol, and sympathomimetics are a potentially lethal addition to MAOIs and may result in serotonin syndrome or hypertensive crisis.

Summary

Most patients require acute headache treatment. Some require preventive treatment. Patients on preventive medication still require acute treatment for breakthrough attacks. Many patients find that their acute attacks are more manageable if they are on a preventive medication. The choice of preventive treatment depends on the individual drug's efficacy and AEs, the patient's clinical features, frequency, and response to prior treatment, and the presence of any comorbid or coexistent disease.

Special Situations

Status Migrainosus

The IHS defines status migrainosus as an attack of migraine, the headache phase of which lasts more than 72 hours whether it is treated or not (Headache Classification Committee, 2004) (Table 11–20). The headache is continuous throughout the attack or is interrupted by headache-free intervals that last less than 4 hours. Relief during periods of sleep is disregarded. No clear distinction is made between transformed migraine and prolonged status migrainosus because no upper time limit is given to status migrainosus.

TABLE 11–19 Cautions in Acute Medication Use.

	Caution	*Contraindicated*
Methysergide	Ergotamine, DHE, 5-HT_1 agonists	
Monoamine oxidase Inhibitors	Sumatriptan SC, naratriptan, zolmitriptan, eletriptan, and frovatriptan	Meperidine, sympatho-mimetics (Midrin), dextromethorphan, rizatriptan, sumatriptan (po, IN)
NSAIDs	Other NSAIDs or aspirin-containing compounds	
Divalproex	Overuse of short-acting barbiturates, or benzodiazepines	
SSRI/SNRI	Triptans??	

Abbreviations: DHE, dihydroergotamine; NSAID, nonsteroidal anti-inflammatory drug; SC, subcutaneous; SNRIs, selective serotonin norepinephrine reuptake inhibitors, SSRIs, selective serotonin reuptake inhibitors.

Table 11–20 Treatment of Status Migrainosus.

Start an IV
Pretreat with: prochlorperazine (5–10 mg IV) or metoclopramide (10 mg IV)
Treat with: dihydroergotamine (0.6–1.0 mg IV)
If headache persists: in 1 hour give additional dihydroergotamine (0.5 mg IV)
Additions: dexamethasone (4 mg IV); diazepam (5–10 mg IV)
Alternatives: ketorolac (30–60 mg IM); opioids; chlorpromazine (0.1 mg/kg); sumatriptan (6 mg SC)
Consider IV fluids

Abbreviations: IM, intramuscular; IV, intravenous; SC, subcutaneous.

Factors responsible for triggering status migrainosus include emotional stress, depression, abuse of medications, anxiety, diet, hormonal factors, and multiple nonspecific factors (Couch and Diamond, 1983). Status migrainosus may be secondary to an acute neurologic disorder. However, acute CNS events can trigger an otherwise typical migraine.

There are no large series or double-blind treatment trials in status migrainosus, although reports of the treatment of isolated migraine attacks may include many patients whose attacks approximate the 72 hour criterion mentioned above (Callaham and Raskin, 1986; Jones et al., 1989; Saadah, 1992; Lane and Ross, 1995). Patients with status migrainosus need aggressive treatment. They usually present in the emergency department, but can be treated in outpatient infusion centers. The principles of treatment for status migrainosus include: (1) fluid and electrolyte replacement (if indicated); (2) drug detoxification; (3) intravenous pharmacotherapy to control pain; (4) treatment of associated symptoms of nausea and vomiting; and (5) concurrent implementation of migraine prophylaxis (if indicated).

For details of aggressive treatment see Chapter 10 on chronic daily headache. Oral, rectal, IM, or intravenous neuroleptics may be used as primary therapy or as adjunct treatment for nausea. Patients who receive neuroleptics must be monitored carefully for hypotension, sedation, and dystonic reactions. Orthostatic hypotension can be avoided by maintaining the patient supine for several hours following neuroleptic administration.

Five milligrams of prochlorperazine intravenously followed by intravenous DHE is a safe and effective means of terminating a migraine attack (Callaham and Raskin, 1986). The combination of intravenous metoclopramide and intravenous DHE is more effective for an acute migraine attack than is IM meperidine (Belgrade et al., 1989). One can mix 10 mg (2 ml) of prochlorperazine and 1 mg (1 ml) of DHE in a syringe and inject 2 cc of the mixture intravenously. If the headache is not relieved in 15–30 minutes, the remainder of the dose can be injected. At times, the addition of 5–10 mg of intravenous diazepam will help terminate the headache attack (Raskin, 1990). Other choices include haloperidol and droperidol (Wang et al., 1997).

Patients who have truly intractable headaches should be admitted to the hospital.

After acute treatment is completed, many patients with status migrainosus require continuing care. This should include a preventive treatment program using standard migraine preventive drugs.

References

Ablad, B, Dahlof, C (1986). Migraine and β-blockade: modulation of sympathetic neurotransmission. *Cephalalgia*, 6:7–13.

Abramowicz, M (1990). Fluoxetine (Prozac) revisited. *Medical Letter Drugs Ther*, 32(826):83–85.

Adam, EI, Gore, SM, and Price, WH (1978). Double-blind trial of clonidine in the treatment of migraine in a general practice. *J R Coll Gen Pract*, 28:587–590.

Adelman, LC, Adelman, JU, Von Seggern, R, et al. (2000). Venlafaxine extended release (XR) for the prophylaxis of migraine and tension-type headache: a retrospective sutdy in a clinical setting. *Headache*, 40:572–580.

Adham, N, Kao, HT, and Schechter, LE (1993). Cloning of another human serotonin receptor (5-HT_{1F}): a fifth 5-HT_1 receptor subtype coupled to the inhibition of adenylate cyclase. *Neurobiol*, 90:408–412.

Adly, C, Straumanis, J, and Chesson, A (1992). Fluoxetine prophylaxis of migraine. *Headache*, 32:101–104.

Aellig, WH (1984). Investigation of the venoconstrictor effect of 8'hydroxydihydroergotamine, the main metabolite of dihydroergotamine, in man. *Eur J Clin Pharmacol*, 26:239–242.

Afra, J, Mascia, A, Gerard, P, et al. (1998). Interictal cortical excitability in migraine: a study using transcranial magnetic stimulation of motor and visual cortices. *Ann Neurol*, 44:209–215.

Aghajanian, GK (1978). Tolerance of locus coeruleus neurones to morphine and suppression of withdrawal response by clonidine. *Nature*, 276:186–188.

Ahrens, SP, Farmer, MV, Williams, DL, et al. (1999). Efficacy and safety of rizatriptan wafer for the acute treatment of migraine. Rizatriptan Wafer Protocol 049 Study Group. *Cephalalgia*, 19:525–530.

Ahuja, GK and Verma, AK (1985). Propranolol in prophylaxis of migraine. *Indian J Med Res*, 82:263–265.

Albers, GW, Simon, LT, Hamik, A, et al. (1989). Nifedipine versus propranolol for the initial prophylaxis of migraine. *Headache*, 29:215–218.

Albibi, R and McCallum, RW (1983). Metoclopramide: pharmacology and clinical application. *Ann Intern Med*, 98:86–95.

Aldeeb, SM, Biary, N, Bahou, Y, et al. (1992). Flunarizine in migraine: a double-blind placebo-controlled study (in a Saudi population). *Headache*, 32:461–462.

Altar, CA (1999). Neurotrophins and depression. *TiPS*, 20:59–61.

Altar, CA, Whitehead, RE, Chen, R, et al. (2003). Effects of electroconvulsive seizures and antidepressant drugs on brain-derived neurotrophic facor protein in rat brain. *Biol Psychiatry*, 54:703–709.

Alvarez, WC (1934). The present day treatment of migraine. *Mayo Clin Proc*, 9:22.

American Psychiatric Association (1994). *Diagnostic and Statistical Manual Of Mental Disorders*, Washington.

Amery, WK and Waelkens, J (1983). Prevention of the last chance: an alternative pharmacologic treatment of migraine. *Headache*, 23:37–38.

Andersen, AR, Tfelt-Hansen, P, and Lassen, NA (1987). The effect of ergotamine and dihydroergotamine on cerebral blood flow in man. *Stroke*, 18:120–123.

Anderson, RE, Chiu, P, and Woodbury, DM (1989). Mechanisms of tolerance to the anticonvulsant effects of acetazolamide in mice: relation to the activity and amount of carbonic anhydrase in brain. *Epilepsia*, 30:208–216.

Andersson, K and Vinge, E (1990). Beta-adrenoceptor blockers and calcium antagonists in the prophylaxis and treatment of migraine. *Drugs*, 39:355–373.

Andersson, PG (1973). BC105 and deseril in migraine prophylaxis: a double-blind study. *Headache*, 13:68–73.

Andersson, PG, Dahl, S, Hansen, JH, et al. (1983). Prophylactic treatment of classical and nonclassical migraine with metoprolol: a comparison with placebo. *Cephalalgia*, 3:207–212.

Andersson, PG, Hinge, HH, Johansen, O, et al. (1989). Double-blind study of naproxen vs placebo in the treatment of acute migraine attacks. *Cephalalgia*, 9:29–32.

Andersson, PG and Petersen, EN (1981). Propranolol and femoxetine, a 5HT-uptake inhibitor, in migraine prophylaxis: a double-blind crossover study. *Acta Neurol Scand*, 64:280–288.

Ansell, E, Fazzone, T, Festenstein, R, et al. (1988). Nimodipine in migraine prophylaxis. *Cephalalgia*, 8:269–272.

Anthony, M, Hinterberger, H, and Lance, JW (1967). Plasma serotonin in migraine and stress. *Arch Neurol*, 16:544–592.

Anthony, M and Lance, JW (1969). Monoamine oxidase inhibition in the treatment of migraine. *Arch Neurol*, 21:263–268.

Anthony, M, Lance, JW, and Somerville, B (1972). A comparative trial of prindolol, clonidine and carbamazepine in the interval therapy of migraine. *Med J Aust*, 6:1343–1346.

Antozzi, C, Garavaglia, B, Mora, M, et al. (1994). Late-onset riboflavin-responsive myopathy with combined multiple acyl coenzyme. A dehydrogenase and respiratory chain deficiency. *Neurology*, 44:2153–2158.

Applebaum, RS (1984). Diet and migraine. *J Am Diet Assoc*, 84:942.

Arthur, GP and Hornabrook, RW (1971). The treatment of migraine with BC105 (pizotifen): a double-blind trial. *N Z Med J*, 73:5–9.

Arts, WF, Scholte, HR, Boggard, JM, et al. (1983). NADH-CoQ reductase deficient myopathy: successful treatment with riboflavin. *Lancet*, 2:581–582.

Aurora, SK, Cao, Y, Bowyer, SM, et al. (1999). The occipital cortex is hyperexcitable in migraine: experimental evidence. *Headache*, 39:469–476.

Austin, MC, Whitehead, RE, Edgar, CL, et al. (2002). Localized decrease in serotonin transporter-immunoreactive axons in the prefrontal cortex of depressed subjects committing suicide. *Neuroscience*, 114:807–815.

Awidi, AS (1982). Efficacy of flurbiprofen in the treatment of acute migraine attacks: a double-blind cross-over study. *Curr Ther Res*, 32:492–497.

Ayata, C, Jin, H, Kudo, C, et al. (2006). Suppression of cortical spreading depression in migraine prophylaxis. *Ann Neurol*, 59:652–661.

Bakris, GL, Cross, PD, and Hammarstein, JE (1982). The use of clonidine for the management of opiate abstinence in a chronic pain patient. *Mayo Clin Proc*, 57:657–660.

Baldessarini, RJ (1990). Drugs and the treatment of psychiatric disorders. In The Pharmacological Basis of Therapeutics (AG Gilman, TW Rall, AS Nies, et al., eds.), pp. 383–435. Pergamon, New York.

Baldratti, A, Cortelli, P, Proccaccianti, G, et al. (1983). Propranolol and acetylsalicylic acid in migraine prophylaxis. Double-blind crossover study. *Acta Neurol Scand*, 67:181–186.

Bana, DS, MacNeal, PS, LeCompte, PM, et al. (1974). Cardiac murmurs and endocardial fibrosis associated with methysergide therapy. *Amer Heart J*, 88:640–655.

Bank, J (1994). A comparative study of amitriptyline and fluvoxamine in migraine prophylaxis. *Headache*, 34:476–478.

Bardwell, A and Trott, J (1987). Stroke in migraine as a consequence of propranolol. *Headache*, 27:381–383.

Barlow, CF (1984). JB Lippincott Co. *Headaches and Migraine in Children*. Philadelphia.

Barnhart, ER (1991). *Physicians' Desk Reference*. Medical Economics Inc., Oradell.

Barrie, MA, Fox, WR, Weatherall, M, et al. (1968). Analysis of symptoms of patients with headaches and their response to treatment with ergot derivatives. *Q J Med*, 146:319–336.

Baumgartner, C, Wessly, P, Bingol, C, et al. (1989). Long-term prognosis of analgesic withdrawal in patients with drug-induced headaches. *Headache*, 29:510–514.

Baumgartner, GR and Rowen, RC (1987). Clonidine vs chlordiazepoxide in the management of acute alcohol withdrawal syndrome. *Arch Intern Med*, 147:1223–1226.

Baxter, G, Kennett, G, Blaney, F, et al. (1995). 5-HT_2 receptor subtypes: a family reunited. *TiPS*, 16:105–110.

Bayless, TM, Rothfeld, B, Massa, L, et al. (1975). Lactose and milk intolerance: clinical implications. *N Engl J Med*, 292:1156–1159.

Beaver, WT (1984). Combination analgesics. *Am J Med*, 77:38–53.

Beer, MS, Middlemiss, DN, and McAllister, G (1993). 5-HT_1-like receptors: six down and still counting. *TiPS*, 14:228–231.

Behan, PO (1978). Isometheptene compound in the treatment of vascular headache. *Practitioner*, 221:937–939.

Behan, PO (1985). Prophylactic treatment for migraine: a comparison of pizotifen and clonidine. *Cephalalgia*, 5:524–525.

Behan, PO and Reid, M (1980). Propranolol in the treatment of migraine. *Practitioner*, 224:201–204.

Belgrade, MJ, Ling, LJ, Schleevogt, MB, et al. (1989). Comparison of single-dose meperidine, butorphanol, and dihydroergotamine in the treatment of vascular headache. *Neurology*, 39:590–592.

Bell, R, Montoya, D, Shuaib, A, et al. (1990). A comparative trial of three agents in the treatment of acute migraine headache. *Ann Emerg Med*, 19:1079–1082.

Bellavance, AJ and Meloche, JP (1990). A comparative study of naproxen sodium, pizotyline, and palcebo in migraine prophylaxis. *Headache*, 30:710–715.

Bentley, D, Katchbuvian, A, and Brostoff, J (1984). abdominal migraine and food insensitivity in children. *Am Int Med*, 5:713–728.

Berde, B and Stuermer, E (1978). Introduction to the pharmacology of ergot alkaloids and related compounds as a basis of their therapeutic application. In *Ergot Alkaloids and Related Compounds* (B Berde and HO Schild, eds.), pp. 1–28. Springer-Verlag, Berlin.

Berridge, MJ (1989). Inositol triphosphate, calcium, lithium, and cell signaling. *JAMA*, 262:1834–1841.

Bigal, ME, Bigal, JO, Bordini, CA, et al. (2001). [Evaluation of placebo use in migraine without aura, migraine with aura and episodic tension-type headache acute attacks]. *Arq Neuropsiquiatr*, 59:552–558.

Bigal, ME, Bordini, CA, and Speciali, JG (2002). Intravenous chlorpromazine in the emergency department treatment of migraines: a randomized controlled trial. *J Emerg Med*, 23:141–148.

Bigal, ME, Bordini, CA, Tepper, SJ, et al. (2002). Intravenous magnesium sulphate in the acute treatment of migraine without aura and migraine with aura. A randomized, double-blind, placebo-controlled study. *Cephalalgia*, 22:345–353.

Bigal, ME and Krymchantowski, AV (2006). Migraine triggered by sucralose—a case report. *Headache*, 46:515–517.

Bix, KJ, Pearson, DJ, and Bentley, SJ (1984). A psychiatric study of patients with supposed food allergy. *Br J Psychiatry*, 145:121–126.

Blanda, M, Rench, T, Gerson, LW, et al. (2001). Intranasal lidocaine for the treatment of migraine headache: a randomized, controlled trial. *Acad Emerg Med*, 8:337–342.

Blau, JN (1987). Adult migraine: the patient observed. In Clinical and Research Aspects (JN Blau, ed.), pp. 3–30. Johns Hopkins University Press, Baltimore.

Boisen, E, Deth, S, Hubbe, P, et al. (1978). Clonidine in the prophylaxis of migraine. *Acta Neurol Scand*, 58:288–295.

Bom, AH, Heiligers, JP, Saxena, PR, et al. (1989). Reduction of cephalic arteriovenous shunting by ergotamine is not mediated by 5-HT_1-like or 5-HT_2 receptors. *Br J Pharmacol*, 97:383–390.

Bono, G, Criscuoli, M, Martignoni, E, et al. (1982). Serotonin precursors in migraine prophylaxis. *Adv Neurol*, 33:357–363.

Bonuso, S, DiStasio, E, Barone, P, et al. (1983). Timed-release dihydroergotamine in the prophylaxis of mixed headache: a study versus amitriptyline. *Cephalalgia*, 3:175–178.

Bordini, C, Antonaci, F, Stovner, LJ, et al. (1991). "Hemicrania Continua"—a clinical review. *Headache*, 31:20–26.

Bordini, CA, Mariano da Silva, H, Garbelini, RP, et al. (2005). Effect of preventive treatment on health-related quality of life in episodic migraine. *J Headache Pain*, 6:387–391.

Borgesen, SE, Nielsen, JL, and Moller, CE (1974). Prophylactic treatment of migraine with propranolol: a clinical trial. *Acta Neurol Scand*, 50:651–656.

Bouchelet, I, Z.Cohen, W, Yong, D, et al. (1996). Molecular basis for a possible role of 5-hydroxytryptamine (T-HT) 2B receptors in the aetiology of migraine headache. Proceedings of the International Business Communications Conference on serotonin receptors in the central nervous system. Philadelphia, January 25–26.

Boureau, F, Joubert, JM, Lasserre, V, et al. (1994). Double-blind comparison of an acetaminophen 400 mg-codeine 25 mg combination versus aspirin 1000mg and placebo in acute migraine attack. *Cephalalgia*, 14:156–161.

Bousser, MG and Loria, Y (1985). Efficacy of dihydroergotamine nasal spray in the acute treatment of migraine attacks. *Cephalalgia*, 5:554–555.

Bousser, MG, Ratinahirana, H, and Darbois, X (1990). Migraine and pregnancy: a prospective study in 703 women after delivery. *Neurology*, 40:437 (Abstract).

Bovill, JG (1997). Mechanisms of actions of opioids and nonsteroidal antiinflammatory drugs. *Eur J Anesthesiol*, 14:9–15.

Bowden, CL, Brugger, AM, and Swann, AC (1994). Efficacy of divalproex vs lithium and placebo in the treatment of mania. *JAMA*, 271:918–924.

Boyle, R, Behan, PO, and Sutton, JA (1990). A correlation between severity of migraine and delayed emptying measured by an epigastric impedance method. *Br J Clin Pharmacol*, 30:405–409.

Bradley, DP, Smith, MI, Netsiri, C, et al. (2001). Diffusion-weighted MRI used to detect in vivo modulation of cortical spreading depression: comparison of sumatriptan and tonabersat. *Exp Neurol*, 172:342–353.

Branchek, T, Zgombick, J, Macchi, M, et al. (1991). Cloning and expression of a human 5-HT_{1D} receptor. In *Serotonin-molecular Biology, Receptors and Functional Effects* (JR Fozard and PR Saxena, eds.), pp. 21–32. Birkhauser, Switzerland.

Brandes, JL, Kudrow, D, Cady, R, et al. (2005). Eletriptan in the early treatment of acute migraine: influence of pain intensity and time of dosing. *Cephalalgia*, 25:735–742.

Brandes, JL, Saper, JR, Diamond, M, et al. (2004). Topiramate for migraine prevention: a randomized controlled trial. *JAMA*, 291:965–973.

Brandes, JL, Visser, H, Farmer, MV, et al. (2004). Montelukast for migraine prophylaxis: a randomized, double-blind, placebo-controlled study. On behalf of the protocol 125 study group. *Headache*, 44:581–586.

Brandli, P, Loffler, BM, Breu, V, et al. (1996). Role of endothelin in mediating neurogenic plasma extravasation in rat aura mater. *Pain*, 64:315–322.

Bredfeldt, RC, Sutherland, JE, and Kruse, JE (1989). Efficacy of transdermal clonidine for headache prophylaxis and reduction of narcotic use in migraine patients. A randomized crossover trial. *J Fam Pract*, 29:153–156.

Brenne, E, van der Hagen, K, Maehlum, E, et al. (1997). Treatment of chronic pain with amitriptyline. A double-blind dosage study with determination of serum levels. *Tidsskr Nor Laegeforen*, 117:3491–3494.

Brewerton, TD, Murphy, DL, Mueller, EA, et al. (1988). Induction of migraine like headaches by the serotonin agonist m-chlorophenylpiperazine. *Clin Pharmacol Ther*, 43:605–609.

Briggs, RS and Millac, PA (1979). Timolol in migraine prophylaxis. *Headache*, 19:379–381.

Brin, MF, Swope, DM, O'Brien, C, et al. (2000). Botox for migraine: double-blind, placebo-controlled, region-specific evaluation. *Cephalalgia*, 20:421–422 (Abstract).

Brooks, PM and Day, RO (1991). Nonsteroidal antiinflammatory drugs: differences and similarities. *N Engl J Med*, 324:1716–1725.

Brown, JS, Papadopoulos, G, Neumann, PJ, et al. (2006). Cost-effectiveness of migraine prevention: the case of topiramate in the UK. *Cephalalgia*, 26:1473–1482.

Bulut, S, Berilgen, MS, Baran, A, et al. (2004). Venlafaxine versus amitriptyline in the prophylactic treatment of migraine: randomized, double-blind, crossover study. *Clin Neurol Neurosurg*, 107:44–48.

Buring, JE, Peto, R, and Hennekens, CH (1990). Low-dose aspirin for migraine prophylaxis. *JAMA*, 264:1711–1713.

Burstein, R, Collins, B, Bajwa, Z, et al. (2002). Triptan therapy can abort migraine attacks if given before the establishment or in the absence of cutaneous allodynia and central sensitization: clinical and preclinical evidence. *Headache*, 42:390–391 (Abstract).

Burstein, R, Cutrer, and MF, Yarnitsky, D (2001). The development of cutaneous allodynia during a migraine attack: clinical evidence for the sequential recruitment of spinal and supraspinal nociceptive neurons in migraine. *Brain*, 123:1703–1709.

Bussone, G, Baldini, S, D'Andrea, G, et al. (1987). Nimodipine versus flunarizine in common migraine: a controlled pilot trial. *Headache*, 27:76–79.

Buzzi, MG, Moskowitz, MA, Shimizu, T, et al. (1991). Dihydroergotamine and sumatriptan attenuate levels of CGRP in plasma in rat superior sagittal sinus during electrical stimulation of the trigeminal ganglion. *Neuropharmacol*, 30:1193–1200.

Cabarrocas, X and Zayas, JM (1998). Efficacy data on oral almotriptan, a novel 5HT1B/1D agonist. *Headache*, 38:377.

Cady, R, Elkind, A, Goldstein, J, et al. (2004). Randomized, placebo-controlled comparison of early use of frovatriptan in a migraine attack versus dosing after the headache has become moderate or severe. *Curr Med Res Opin*, 20:1465–1472.

Cady, RC, Ryan, R, Jhingran, P, et al. (1998). Sumatriptan injection reduces productivity loss during a migraine attack: results of a double-blind, placebo-controlled trial. *Arch Intern Med*, 158:1013–1018.

Cady, RK, Rubino, J, Crummett, D, et al. (1994). Oral sumatriptan in the treatment of recurrent headache. *Arch Fam Med*, 3:766–772.

Cady, RK, Wendt, JK, Kirchner, JR, et al. (1991). Treatment of acute migraine with subcutaneous sumatriptan. *JAMA*, 265:2831–2835.

Callaham, M and Raskin, N (1986). A controlled study of dihydroergotamine in the treatment of acute migraine headache. *Headache*, 26:168–171.

Cameron, JD, Lane, PL, and Speechley, M (1995). Intravenous chlorpromazine vs intravenous metoclopramide in acute migraine headache. *Acad Emerg Med*, 2:597–602.

Campbell, WB (1990). Lipid-derived autocoids: eicosanoids and platelet-activating factor. In *The Pharmacological Basis of Therapeutics* (AG Gilman, TW Rall, P Taylor, eds), pp. 600–617. Pergamon Press, New York.

Cangi, F, Boccuni, M, Zanotti, A, et al. (1989). Dihydroergokryptine (DEK) in migraine prophylaxis in a double-blind study vs methysergide. *Cephalalgia*, 9:448–449.

Capildeo, R and Rose, FC (1982). Single-dose pizotifen, 1.5mg nocte: a new approach in the prophylaxis of migraine. *Headache*, 22:272–275.

Carleton, SC, Shesser, RF, Pietrzak, MP, et al. (1998). Double-blind, multicenter trial to compare the efficacy of intramuscular dihydroergotamine plus hydroxyzine versus intramuscular meperidine plus hydroxyzine for the emergency department treatment of acute migraine headache. *Ann Emerg Med*, 32:129–138.

Carpay, HA and Dowson, AJ (2006). Sumatriptan fast-disintegrating/rapid-release tablets: viewpoints. *Drugs*, 66:891–892.

Carpay,7 HA, Matthijsse, P, Steinbuch, M, et al. (1997). Oral and subcutaneous sumatriptan in the acute treatment of migraine: an open randomized cross-over study. *Cephalalgia*, 17:591–595.

Carroll, JD and Maclay, WP (1975). Pizotifen (BC105) in migraine prophylaxis. *Curr Med Res Opin*, 3:68–71.

Carter, CM, Egger, J, and Soothill, JF (1985). A dietary management of severe childhood migraine. *Hum Nutr Appl Nutr*, 39:294–303.

Cashman, J and McAnulty, G (1995). Nonsteroidal antiinflammatory drugs in perisurgical pain management: mechanisms of action and rationale for optimum use. *Drugs*, 49:51–70.

Catterall, WA, Striessnig, J, Snutch, TP, et al. (2003). Compendium of voltage-gated ion channels: calcium channels. *Pharmacol Rev*, 55:579–581.

Centonze, V, Attolini, E, Santoiemma, L, et al. (1983). DHE retard for prophylactic therapy of migraine: efficacy and tolerability. *Cephalalgia*, 3:179–184.

Cerbo, R, Casacchia, M, Formisano, R, et al. (1986). Flunarizine-pizotifen single-dose double-blind cross-over trial in migraine prophylaxis. *Cephalalgia*, 6:15–18.

Cete, Y, Dora, B, Ertan, C, et al. (2005). A randomized prospective placebo-controlled study of intravenous magnesium sulphate vs. metoclopramide in the management of acute migraine attacks in the Emergency Department. *Cephalalgia*, 25:199–204.

Chabriat, H, Danchot, J, Michel, P, et al. (1999). Precipitating factors of headache. A prospective study in a national control-matched survey in migraineurs and nonmigraineurs. *Headache*, 39:335–338.

Chappell, AS, Bay, JJ, Botzum, GD, et al. (1994). Zatosetron, a 5HT3 receptor antagonist in a multicenter trial for acute migraine. *Neuropharmacology*, 33:509–513.

Charlesworth, BR, Dowson, AJ, Purdy, A, et al. (2003). Speed of onset and efficacy of zolmitriptan nasal spray in the acute treatment of migraine: a randomised, double-blind, placebo-controlled, dose-ranging study versus zolmitriptan tablet. *CNS Drugs*, 17:653–667.

Chen, WT, Fuh, JL, Lu, SR, et al. (2001). Persistent migrainous visual phenomena might be responsive to lamotrigine. *Headache*, 41:823–825.

Christie, S, Gobel, H, Mateos, V, et al. (2003). Crossover comparison of efficacy and preference for rizatriptan 10 mg versus ergotamine/caffeine in migraine. *Eur Neurol*, 49:20–29.

Clary, C and Schweitzer, E (1987). The treatment of MAOI hypertensive crisis with sublingual nifedipine. *Clin Psychiatry*, 48:249–250.

Clozel, M, Breu, V, Gray, AG, et al. (1994). Pharmacologic characterization of bosentan, a new potent orally active nonpeptide endothelin receptor antagonist. *J Pharmacol Exp Ther*, 270:228–235.

Cochran, JW (2002). Efficacy of zonisamide in prophylactic treatment of migraine headaches with or without aura: open-label experience in 7 patients. *J Pain*, 3:39 (Abstract).

Codispoti, JR, Prior, MJ, Fu, M, et al. (2001). Efficacy of nonprescription doses of ibuprofen for treating migraine headache. a randomized controlled trial. Headache 41:665–679.

Cole, JA, Rothman, KJ, Cabral, HJ, et al. (2006). Migraine, fibromyalgia and depression among people with IBS; a prevalence study. *BMC Gastroenterol*, 26 (Abstract).

Connor, HE and Beattie, DT (1999). 5-Hydroxytryptamine receptor subtypes: relation to migraine. In *Migraine and Headache Pathophysiology* (L Edvinsson, ed.), pp. 43–52. Martin Dunitz Limited, London.

Coppola, M, yealy, DM, and Leibold, RA (1995). Randomized, placebo-controlled evaluation of prochlorperazine versus metoclopramide for emergency department treatment of migraine headache. *Ann Emerg Med*, 26:541–546.

Cortelli, P, Sacquegna, T, Albani, F, et al. (1985). Propranolol plasma levels and relief of migraine. *Arch Neurol*, 42:46–48.

Couch, JR and Diamond, S (1983). Status migrainosus: causative and therapeutic aspects. *Headache*, 23:94–101.

Couch, JR and Hassanein, RS (1976). Migraine and depression: effect of amitriptyline prophylaxis. *Trans Am Neurol Assoc*, 101:234–237.

Couch, JR and Hassanein, RS (1979). Amitriptyline in migraine prophylaxis. *Arch Neurol*, 36:695–699.

Couch, JR, Ziegler, D, and Hassanein, R (1976). Amitriptyline in the prophylaxis of migraine: effectiveness and relationship of antimigraine and antidepressant effects. *Neurology*, 26:121–127.

Coulam, CB and Annagers, JR (1979). New anticonvulsants reduce the efficacy of oral contraception. *Epilepsia*, 20:519–525.

Cull, RE, Price, WH, and Dunbar, A (1997). The efficacy of subcutaneous sumatriptan in the treatment of recurrence of migraine headache. *J Neurol Neurosurg Psychiatry*, 62:490–495.

Cumberbatch, MJ, Hill, RG, and Hargreaves, RJ (1997). rizatriptan has central antinociceptive effects against durally evoked responses. *Eur J Pharmacol*, 328:37–40.

Curran, DA, Hinterberger, H, and Lance, JW (1967). Methysergide. *Res Clin Stud Headache*, 1:74–122.

Curran, DA and Lance, JW (1964). Clinical trial of methysergide and other preparations in the management of migraine. *J Neurol Neurosurg Psychiatry*, 27:463–469.

Curzon, G, Kennett, GA, Shah, K, et al. (1990). Behavioral effects of m-chlorophenylpiperazine (m-CPP), a reported migraine precipitant. In *Migraine, A Spectrum of Ideas*, (M Sandler and G Collins, eds) pp. 173–181. Oxford Medical Publishers, Oxford.

Cutler, N, Mushet, GR, Davis, R, et al. (1995). Oral sumatriptan for the acute treatment of migraine: evaluation of three dosage strengths. *Neurology*, 45:S5–S9.

Cutler, NR, Claghorn, J, Sramek, JJ, et al. (1996). Pilot study of MK462 in migraine. *Cephalalgia*, 16:113–116.

Cutrer, FM and O'Donnell, A (1999). Recent advances in functional neuroimaging. *Cur Opin Neurol*, 12:255–259.

Cutrer, FM, Sorenson, AG, Weisskoff, RM, et al. (1998). Perfusion-weighted imaging defects during spontaneous migrainous aura. *Ann Neurol*, 43:25–31.

Czapinski, P and Motyl, R (1999). Randomized comparative placebo-controlled assessment of intravenous valproic acid effectiveness and safety in patients with acute migraine. *Cephalalgia*, 19:372–373 (Abstract).

d'Amato, CC, Pizza, V, marmolo, T, et al. (1999). Fluoxetine for migraine prophylaxis: a double-blind trial. *Headache*, 39:716–719.

D'Amico, D, Solari, A, Usai, S, et al. (2006). Improvement in quality of life and activity limitations in migraine patients after prophylaxis. A prospective longitudinal multicentre study. *Cephalalgia*, 26:691–696.

Dahlof, C (1987). No clear-cut long-term prophylactic effect of one month of treatment with propranolol in migraineurs. *Cephalalgia*, 7:459–460.

Dahlof, C and Bjorkman, R (1993). Diclofenac-K (50 and 100mg) and placebo in the acute treatment of migraine. *Cephalalgia*, 13:117–123.

Dahlof, C, Bouchard, J, Cortelli, P, et al. (1997). A multinational investigation of the impact of subcutaneous sumatriptan. II: Health-related quality of life. *Pharmacoeconomics*, 11(Suppl. 1):24–34.

Dahlof, C, Diener, HC, Goadsby, PJ, et al. (1998). Zolmitriptan, a 5-HT1B/1D receptor agonist for the acute oral treatment of migraine: a multicentre, dose-range finding study. *Eur J Neurol*, 5:535–543.

Dalessio, DJ (1980). *Wolff's Headache and Other Head Pain*. Oxford University Press, Oxford.

Dalessio, DJ (1987). *Wolff's Headache and Other Head Pain*. Oxford University Press, Oxford.

Darland, T, Heinricher, MM, and Grandy, DK (1998). Orphanin FQ/nociceptin: a role in pain and analgesia, but so much more. *TINS*, 21:215–221.

Das, SM, Ahuja, GK, and Narainaswamy, AS (1979). Clonidine in prophylaxis of migraine. *Acta Neurol Scand*, 60:214–217.

Davis, CP, Torre, PR, Williams, C, et al. (1995). Ketorolac versus meperidine-plus-promethazine treatment of migraine headache: evaluations by patients. *Am J Emerg Med*, 13:146–150.

Dawson, TM, Dawson, VL, and Snyder, SH (1992). A novel neuronal mesenger mlecule in brain: the free radical, nitric oxide. *Ann Neurol*, 32:297–311.

Delbene, E, Poggioni, M, Garagiola, U, et al. (1987). Intramuscular treatment of migraine attacks using diclofenac sodium: a crossover clinical trial. *J Int Med Res*, 15:44–48.

DeLorenzo, RJ, Sombati, S, and Coulter, DA (2000). Effects of topiramate on sustained repetitive firing and spontaneous recurrent seizure discharges in cultured hippocampal neurons. *Epilepsia*, 41:S40–S44.

DenBoer, MO, Villain, CM, Heiligers, JP, et al. (1991a). The role of 5-HT_1-like receptors in the reduction of porcine cranial arteriovenous anastomotic shunting by sumatriptan. *Br J Pharmacol*, 102:323–330.

DenBoer, MO, Villalon, CM, Heiligers, JP, et al. (1991b). The role of 5-HT_1-like receptors. *Br J Pharmacol*, 104:183–189.

Deweerdt, CJ, Bootsma, HP, and Hendriks, H (1996). Herbal medicines in migraine prevention: randomized double-blind placebo-controlled crossover trial of feverfew preparation. *Phytomedicine*, 3:225–230.

Diamond, M, Dahlof, C, Papadopoulos, G, et al. (2005). Topiramate improves health-related quality of life when used to prevent migraine. *Headache*, 45:1023–1030.

Diamond, S (1964). Depressive headaches. *Headache*, 4:255–259.

Diamond, S (1976). Treatment of migraine with isometheptene, acetaminophen, and dichloralphenazone combination: a double-blind, crossover trial. *Headache*, 15:282–287.

Diamond, S, Elkind, A, Jackson, RT, et al. (1998). Multiple-attack efficacy and tolerability of sumatriptan nasal spray in the treatment of migraine. *Arch Fam Med*, 7:234–240.

Diamond, S and Freitag, FG (1993). A double-blind trial of flunarizine in migraine prophylaxis. *Headache Q*, 4:169–172.

Diamond, S, Freitag, FG, Chu, G, et al. (1991). A placebo-controlled comparative study versus intramuscular methadone. In *New Advances in Headache Research* (C Rose, ed.), pp. 319–324. Smith Gordon, London.

Diamond, S, Kudrow, L, Stevens, J, et al. (1982). Long-term study of propranolol in the treatment of migraine. *Headache*, 22:268–271.

Diamond, S, Medina, J, Diamond-Falk, J, et al. (1979). The value of biofeedback in the treatment of chronic headache: a five-year retrospective study. *Headache*, 19:90–96.

Diamond, S and Medina, JL (1975). Isometheptene—a nonergot drug in the treatment of migraine. *Headache*, 15:211–213.

Diamond, S and Medina, JL (1976). Double-blind study of propranolol for migraine prophylaxis. *Headache*, 16:24–27.

Diamond, S and Montrose, D (1984). The value of biofeedback in the treatment of chronic headache: a four-year retrospective study. *Headache*, 24:5–18.

Diamond, S, Phillips, SB, and Bernstein, JE (1999). Intranasal Civamide for the acute treatment of migraine headache. *Headache*, 39:350.

Diamond, S, Ryan, RE, Klapper, JA, et al. (1999). Dotarizine in the prophylaxis of migraine headaches. *Headache*, 39:350.

Diamond, S, Solomon, GD, Freitag, FG, et al. (1987). Long-acting propranolol in the prophylaxis of migraine. *Headache*, 27:70–72.

Dib, M, Massiou, H, Weber, M, et al. (2002). Efficacy of oral ketoprofen in acute migraine: a double-blind randomized clinical trial. *Neurology*, 58:1660–1665.

Dichgans, M, Freilinger, T, Eckstein, G, et al. (2005). Mutation in the neuronal voltage-gated sodium channel SCN1A in familial hemiplegic migraine. *Lancet*, 366:371–377.

Diener, HC (1996). Substance-P antagonist RPR100893-201 is not effective in human migraine attacks. Proceedings of the VIth International Headache Seminar (J Olesen and P Tfelt-Hansen, eds.) Lippincott-Raven, New York.

Diener, HC (1999). The efficacy and safety of acetylsalicylic acid lysinate compared to subcutaneous sumatriptan and parenteral placebo in the acute treatment of migraine. A double-blind, double-dummy, randomized multicenter, parallel group study. The ASASUMAMIG Study Group. *Cephalalgia*, 19 (6):581–588.

Diener, HC, Bussone, G, de, LH, et al. (2004a). Placebo-controlled comparison of effervescent acetylsalicylic acid, sumatriptan and ibuprofen in the treatment of migraine attacks. *Cephalalgia*, 24:947–954.

Diener, HC, Eikermann, A, Gessner, U, et al. (2004). Efficacy of 1,000 mg effervescent acetylsalicylic acid and sumatriptan in treating associated migraine symptoms. *Eur Neurol*, 52:50–56.

Diener, HC, Gerber, WD, and Geiselhart, S (1988). Short and long-term effects of withdrawal therapy in drug-induced headache. In *Drug-induced Headache* (HC Diener and M Wilkinson, eds), pp. 133–142. Springer-Verlag, Berlin.

Diener, HC, Hartung, E, Chrubasik, J, et al. (2001). A comparative study of oral acetylsalicyclic acid and metoprolol for the prophylactic treatment of migraine. A randomized, controlled, double-blind, parallel group phase III study. *Cephalalgia*, 21:120–128.

Diener, HC, Matias-Guiu, J, Hartung, E, et al. (2002). Efficacy and tolerability in migraine prophylaxis of flunarizine in reduced doses: a comparison with propranolol 160 mg daily. *Cephalalgia*, 22:209–221.

Diener, HC, Pfaffenrath, V, Pageler, L, et al. (2005). The fixed combination of acetylsalicylic acid, paracetamol and caffeine is more effective than single substances and dual combination for the treatment of headache: a multicentre, randomized, double-blind, single-dose, placebo-controlled parallel group study. *Cephalalgia*, 25:776–787.

Diener, HC, Pfaffenrath, V, Schnitker, J, et al. (2005). Efficacy and safety of 6.25 mg t.i.d. feverfew CO2-extract (MIG-99) in migraine prevention—a randomized, double-blind, multicentre, placebo-controlled study. *Cephalalgia*, 25:1031–1041.

Diener, HC, Rahlfs, VW, and Danesch, U (2004). The first placebo-controlled trial of a special butterbur root extract for the prevention of migraine: reanalysis of efficacy criteria. *Eur Neurol*, 51:89–97.

Diener, HC, Ryan, R, Sun, W, et al. (2004). The 40-mg dose of eletriptan: comparative efficacy and tolerability versus sumatriptan 100 mg. *Eur J Neurol*, 11:125–134.

Diener, HC, Tfelt-Hansen, P, Dahlof, C, et al. (2004). Topiramate in migraine prophylaxis—results from a placebo-controlled trial with propranolol as an active control. *J Neurol*, 251:943–950.

Dihydroergotamine Nasal Spray Multicenter Investigators (1995). Efficacy, safety, and tolerability of dihydroergotamine nasal spray as monotherapy in the treatment of acute migraine. *Headache*, 35:177–184.

Dimitriadou, V, Buzzi, MG, Theoharides, TC, et al. (1992). Ultrastructural evidence for neurogenically mediated changes in blood vessels of the rat aura mater and tongue following antidromic trigeminal stimulation. *Neuroscience*, 48:187–203.

Diserio, F, Patin, J, and Friedman, A (1989). USA trials of dihydroergotamine nasal spray in the acute treatment of migraine headache. *Cephalalgia*, 9:344–345.

Dodgson, SJ, Shank, RP, and Maryanoff, BE (2000). Topiramate as an inhibitor of carbonic anhydrase isoenzymes. *Epilepsia*, 41:35–39.

Dodick, D, Brandes, J, Elkind, A, et al. (2005). Speed of onset, efficacy and tolerability of zolmitriptan nasal spray in the acute treatment of migraine: a randomised, double-blind, placebo-controlled study. *CNS Drugs*, 19:125–136.

Dodick, DW, Martin, VT, Smith, T, et al. (2004). Cardiovascular tolerability and safety of triptans: a review of clinical data. *Headache*, 44(Suppl. 1):S20–S30.

Dodick, DW, Silberstein, SD, and Frietag, F (2007). Topiramate versus amitriptyline for migraine prophylaxis: a multicenter randomized, double-blind, parallel treatment group trial. *Cephalalgia*, 26:1373 (Abstract).

Doods, H, Hallermayer, G, Wu, D, et al. (2000). Pharmacological profile of BIBN-4096BS, the first selective small molecule CGRP antagonist. *Br J Pharmacol*, 129:420–423.

Doose, DR, Wang, S-S, Padmanabhan, M, et al. (2003). Effect of topiramate or carbamazepine on the pharmacokinetics of an oral contraceptive containing norethindrone and ethinyl estradiol in healthy obese and nonobese female subjects. *Epilepsia*, 44:540–549.

Dowson, A (1996). Can oral 311C90, a novel 5HT1D agonist, prevent migraine headache when taken during an aura? *Eur Neurol*, 36:28–31.

Dowson, AJ and Charlesworth, B (2002). Review of zolmitriptan and its clinical applications in migraine. *Expert Opin Pharmacother*, 3:993–1005.

Dowson, AJ, Mathew, NT, and Pascual, J (2006). Review of clinical trials using early acute intervention with oral triptans for migraine management. *Int J Clin Pract*, 60:698–706.

Drake, ME, Greathouse, NI, Armenthright, AD, et al. (2001). Zonisamide in the prophylaxis of migraine headache. *Cephalalgia*, 21:374 (Abstract).

Driefuss, FE, Santilli, N, Langer, DH, et al. (1987). Valproic acid hepatic fatalities: a retrospective review. *Neurology*, 37:379–385.

Dryden, S, Frankish, HM, Kilpatrick, A, et al. (1994). The serotonin agonist mCPP reduces neuropeptide Y concentrations in the paraventricular nucleus of the rat: could this explain its hypophagic action? *Clin Sci*, 86:43.

Dryden, S, Wang, Q, Frankish, HM, et al. (1995). The serotonin (5-HT) antagonist methysergide increases neuropeptide Y (NPY) synthesis and secretion in the hypothalamus of the rat. *Brain Res*, 699:12–18.

Duarte, C, Dunaway, F, Turner, L, et al. (1992). Ketorolac versus meperidine and hydroxyzine in the treatment of acute migraine headache: a randomized, prospective, double-blind trial. *Ann Emerg Med*, 21:1116–1121.

Duke University and Center for Clinical Health Policy Research (1999). Behavioral and physical treatments for migraine headache.*Technical Review 2.2*:1–116.

Easterling, DE, Zakszewski, T, and Moyer, MD (1988). Plasma pharmacokinetics of topiramate, a new anticonvulsant, in humans. *Epilepsia*, 29:662.

Edmeads, J (1988). Emergency management of headache. *Headache*, 28:675–679.

Edvinsson, L and Goadsby, PJ (1998). Neuropeptides in headache. *Eur J Neurol*, 5:329–341.

Edwards, K, Santarcangelo, V, Shea, P, et al. (1999). Intravenous valproate for acute treatment of migraine headaches. *Cephalalgia*, 19:356 (Abstract).

Edwards, KR, Glantz, MJ, Shea, P, et al. (2000). A double-blind, randomized trial of topiramate versus placebo in the prophylactic treatment of migraine headache with and without aura. *Cephalalgia*, 20:316 (Abstract).

Edwards, KR, Norton, J, and Behnke, M (2001). Comparison of intravenous valproate versus intramuscular dihydroergotamine and metoclopramide for acute treatment of migraine headache. *Headache*, 41:976–980.

Egger, J, Wilson, J, Carter, CM, et al. (1983). Is migraine food allergy? *Lancet ii*,:865–869.

Eglen, RM, Hasper, JR, Chang, DJ, et al. (1997). The 5-HT7 receptor: orphan found. *Trends Pharmacol Sci*, 18:104–107.

Eisenberg, DM, Davis, RB, Ettner, SL, et al. (1998). Trends in alternative medicine use in the United States, 1990-1997: results of a follow-up national survey. *JAMA*, 280:1569–1575.

Ekbom, K (1994). Alprenolol for migraine prophylaxis. *Headache*, 34:476–478.

Ekbom, K and Lundberg, PO (1972). Clinical trial of LB-56 (d, 1-4-(2-hydroxy-3-isopropylaminopropoxy)indol): an adrenergic beta-receptor blocking agent in migraine prophylaxis. *Headache*, 12:15–17.

Ekbom, K and Zetterman, M (1977). Oxprenolol in the treatment of migraine. *Acta Neurol Scand*, 56:181–184.

Elkind, AH, Friedman, AP, Bachman, A, et al. (1968). Silent retroperitoneal fibrosis associated with methysergide therapy. *JAMA*, 206:1041–1044.

Elkind, AH, O'Carroll, P, Blumenfeld, A, et al. (2006). A series of three sequential, randomized, controlled studies of repeated treatments with botulinum toxin type A for migraine prophylaxis. *J Pain*, 7:688–696.

Elkind, AH, Webster, C, and Herbertson, RK (1989). Efficacy of guanfacine in a double-blind parallel study for migraine prophylaxis. *Cephalalgia*, 9:369–370.

Ellis, GL, Delaney, J, Dehart, DA, et al. (1993). The efficacy of metoclopramide in the treatment of migraine headache. *Ann Emerg Med*, 22:191–195.

Ensink, F (1991). Subcutaneous sumatriptan in the acute treatment of migraine. *J Neurol*, 238:S66–S69.

Epstein, MT, Hockaday, JM, and Hockaday, TDR (1975). Migraine and reproductive hormones throughout the menstrual cycle. *Lancet*, 1:543–548.

Etemad, LR, Wang, W, Globe, D, et al. (2005). Costs and utilization of triptan users who receive drug prophylaxis for migraine versus triptan users who do not receive drug prophylaxis. *J Manag Care Pharm*, 11:137–144.

Evers, S, Afra, J, Frese, A, et al. (2006). EFNS guideline on the drug treatment of migraine—report of an EFNS task force. *Eur J Neurol*, 13:560–572.

Evers, S, Vollmer-Haase, J, Schwaag, S, et al. (2004). Botulinum toxin A in the prophylactic treatment of migraine—a randomized, double-blind, placebo-controlled study. *Cephalalgia*, 24:838–843.

Fanchamps, A (1985). Why do not all beta-blockers prevent migraine? *Headache*, 25:61–62.

Farkkila, M (1996). A dose-finding study of eletriptan (UK-116,044) (5-30 mg) for the acute treatment of migraine. *Cephalalgia*, 16:387–388.

Featherstone, HJ (1983). Low dose propranolol therapy for aborting acute migraine. *West J Med*, 138:416–417.

Feinmann, C (1985). Pain relief by antidepressants: possible modes of action. *Pain*, 23:1–8.

Ferguson, A (1990). Food sensitivity or self-deception? *N Engl J Med*, 323:476.

Ferrante, FM (1996). Principles of opioid pharmacotherapy: practical implications of basic mechanisms. *J Pain Symptom Mgt*, 11:265–273.

Ferrari, MD, James, MH, Bates, D, et al. (1994). Oral sumatriptan: effect of a second dose, and incidence and treatment of headache recurrences. *Cephalalgia*, 14:330–338.

Ferrari, MD, Odink, J, Tapparelli, C, et al. (1989). Serotonin metabolism in migraine. *Neurology*, 39:1239–1242.

Ferrari, MD, Roon, KI, Lipton, RB, et al. (2001). Oral triptans (serotonin $5\text{-HT}_{1B/1D}$ agonists) in acute migraine treatment: a metaanalysis of 53 trials. *Lancet*, 358:1668–1675.

Ferrari, MD and Saxena, PR (1993a). Clinical and experimental effects of sumatriptan in humans. *TiPS*, 14:129–133.

Ferrari, MD and Saxena, PR (1993b). On serotonin and migraine: a clinical and pharmacological review. *Cephalalgia*, 13:151–165.

Ferro, CJ and Webb, DJ (1996). The clinical potential of endothelin receptor antagonists in cardiovascular medicine. *Drugs*, 51:12–27.

Finnish Sumatriptan Group and the Cardiovascular Clinical Research Group (1991). A placebo-controlled study of intranasal sumatriptan for the acute treatment of migraine. *Eur Neurol*, 31:332–338.

Fisher, H (1995). A new approach to emergency department therapy of migraine headache. *J Emerg Med*, 136:119–122.

Fontanari, D, Perulli, L, Conte, F, et al. (1983). Planned release dihydroergotamine in common migraine and "tension-vascular headache" multicenter clinical trial. *Cephalalgia*, 3:189–191.

Forbes, JA, Beaver, WT, Jones, KF, et al. (1991). Effect of caffeine on ibuprofen analgesia in postoperative surgery pain. *Clin Pharmacol Ther*, 49:674–684.

Ford, RG and Ford, KT (1997). Continuous intravenous dihydroergotamine in the treatment of intractable headache. *Headache*, 37:129–136.

Formisano, R, Falaschi, P, Cerbo, R, et al. (1991). Nimodipine in migraine: clinical efficacy and endocrinological effects. *Eur J Clin Pharmacol*, 41:69–71.

Forssman, B, Henriksson, KG, Johannsson, V, et al. (1976). Propranolol for migraine prophylaxis. *Headache*, 16:238–245.

Forssman, B, Henriksson, KG, and Kihlstrand, S (1972). A comparison between BC105 and methysergide in the prophylaxis of migraine. *Acta Neurol Scand*, 48:204–212.

Forssman, B, Lindblad, CJ, and Zbornikova, V (1983). Atenolol for migraine prophylaxis. *Headache*, 23:188–190.

Forsythe, I and Hockaday, JM (1988). Management of childhood migraine. In *Migraine in Childhood* (JM Hockaday, ed.), pp. 63–74. Butterworths, London.

Forteza, AM, Brozman, B, Rabinstein, AA, et al. (2001). Acetazolamide for the treatment of migraine with aura in CADASIL. *Neurology*, 57:2144–2145.

Fozard, JR (1982). Serotonin, migraine and platelets. *Progressive Pharmacol*, 414:135–146.

Fozard, JR (1990). 5-HT in migraine: evidence from 5-Ht receptor antagonists for a neuronal etiology. In *Migraine: A Spectrum of Ideas* (M Sandler and GM Collins, eds.), pp. 128–146. Oxford University Press, New York.

Fozard, JR (1992). Pharmacological relevance of 5-HT_3 receptors. In *Serotonin Receptor Subtypes: Pharmacological Significance and Clinical Implications* (SZ Langer, N Brunello, G Racagni, et al., eds), pp. 44–55. Karger, Basel.

Fozard, JR (1995). The 5-hydroxytryptamine-nitric oxide connection: the key link in the initialization of migraine? *Arch Int Pharmacodyn*, 329:111–119.

Fozard, JR and Gray, JA (1989). 5-HT_{1C} receptor activation: a key step in the initiation of migraine? *Trends Pharmacol Sci*, 10:307–309.

Fozard, JR and Kalkman, HO (1994). 5-Hydroxytryptamine (5-HT) and the initiation of migraine: new perspectives. *Arch Pharmacol*, 350:225–229.

Freitag, F, Diamond, S, Diamond, M, et al. (1998). Subcutaneous sumatriptan in patients treated with monoamine oxidase inhibitors and other prophylactic agents. *Headache Q*, 9:165–171.

Freitag, FG (2003). Topiramate prophylaxis in patients suffering from migraine with aura: results from a randomized, double-blind, placebo-controlled trial. *Advanced Studies in Med*, 3:S562–S564.

Freitag, FG, Cady, R, Diserio, F, et al. (2001). Comparative study of a combination of isometheptene mucate, dichloralphenazone with acetaminophen and sumatriptan succinate in the treatment of migraine. *Headache*, 41:391–398.

Freitag, FG, Cady, R, Elkind, A, et al. (1999). Comparative study of Midrin® and sumatriptan succinate in the treatment of migraine headache. *Headache*, 19:355 (Abstract).

Freitag, FG, Collins, SD, Carlson, HA, et al. (2002). A randomized trial of divalproex sodium extended-release tablets in migraine prophylaxis. *Neurology*, 58:1652–1659.

Freitag, FG and Diamond, S (1984). Nadolol and placebo comparison study in the prophylactic treatment of migraine. *J Am Osteopath Assoc*, 84:343–347.

Freitag, FG, Diamond, S, Diamond, M, et al. (2001). Divalproex in the long-term treatment of chronic daily headache. *Headache*, 41:271–278.

Freitag, FG, Diamond, S, Diamond, ML, et al. (1999). The prophylaxis of migraine with the GABA-agonist, tiagabine: a clinical report. *Headache*, 19:(Abstract).

Freitag, FG, Diamond, S, and Solomon, GD (1987). Antidepressants in the treatment of mixed headache: MAO inhibitors and combined use of MAO inhibitors and tricyclic antidepressants in the recidivist headache patient. In *Advances in Headache Research* (FC Rose, ed.), pp. 271–275. John Libbey and Co. Ltd, London.

Freitag, FG, Forde, G, Neto, W, et al. (2007). Topiramate effectively prevents migraine: analyzing pooled data from pivotal controlled trials. *JAOA* (in press).

Freitag, FG, Lainez, MJ, Neto, W, et al. (2005). Comparing the incidence of adverse events in the titration and maintenance phases of placebo-controlled trials of topiramate for migraine prevention. *Headache*, 55:821 (Abstract).

Frenken, CW and Nuijten, ST (1984). Flunarizine, a new preventive approach to migraine: a double-blind comparison with placebo. *Clin Neurol Neurosurg*, 86:17–20.

Friedman, AP, Diserio, FJ, and Hwang, DS (1989). Symptomatic relief of migraine: multicenter comparison of cafergot pb, cafergot, and placebo. *Clin Ther*, 11:170–182.

Friedman, BW, Corbo, J, Lipton, RB, et al. (2005). A trial of metoclopramide vs sumatriptan for the emergency department treatment of migraines. *Neurology*, 64:463–468.

Frishman, WH (1987). Beta adrenergic blocker withdrawal. *Am J Cardiol*, 59:32F.

Frölich, JC (1997). A classification of NSAIDs according to the relative inhibition of cyclooxygenase isoenzymes. *Trends Pharmacol Sci*, 18:30–34.

Fuller, GN and Guiloff, RJ (1990). Propranolol in acute migraine: a controlled study. *Cephalalgia*, 10:229–233.

Gabai, IJ and Spierings, ELH (1989). Prophylactic treatment of cluster headache with verapamil. *Headache*, 29:167–168.

Gallagher, RM (1986). Emergency treatment of intractable migraine. *Headache*, 26:74–75.

Gallagher, RM (1989). Menstrual migraine and intermittent ergonovine therapy. *Headache*, 29:366–367.

Gallagher, RM (1996). Acute treatment of migraine with dihydroergotamine nasal spray. Dihydroergotamine Working Group. *Arch Neurol*, 53:1285–1291.

Gardner, DG and Nissenson, RA (2004). Mechanisms of hormone action. In *Basic and Clinical Endocrinology* (FS Greenspan and DG Gardner, eds.), pp. 61–84. McGraw-Hill, New York.

Gasior, M, Carter, RB, and Witkin, JM (1999). Neuroactive steroids: potential therapeutic use in neurological and psychiatric disorders. *TiPS*, 20:107–112.

Gawel, M (1987). A double blind, cross over study of nimodipine versus pizotyline in common and classical migraine. *Cephalalgia*, 7:453–454.

Gawel, M, Aschoff, J, May, A, et al. (2005). Zolmitriptan 5 mg nasal spray: efficacy and onset of action in the acute treatment of migraine—results from phase 1 of the REALIZE study. *Headache*, 45:7–16.

Gawel, MJ, Kreeft, J, Nelson, RF, et al. (1992). Comparison of the efficacy and safety of flunarizine to propranolol in the prophylaxis of migraine. *Can J Neurol Sci*, 19:340–345.

Gelmers, HJ (1983). Nimodipine, a new calcium antagonist, in the prophylactic treatment of migraine. *Headache*, 23:106–109.

Gennari, C, Chierichetti, MS, Gonnelli, S, et al. (1986). Migraine prophylaxis with salmon calcitonin: a crossover, double-blind, placebo-controlled study. *Headache*, 26:13–16.

Geraud, G, Compagnon, A, and Rossi, A (2002). Zolmitriptan versus a combination of acetylsalicylic acid and metoclopramide in the acute oral treatment of migraine: a double-blind, randomised, three-attack study. *Eur Neurol*, 47:88–98.

Gerber, WG, Diener, H, Scholz, E, et al. (1991). Responders and nonresponders to metoprolol, propranolol and nifedipine treatment in migraine prophylaxis: a dose-range study based on time-series analysis. *Cephalalgia*, 11:37–45.

Ghose, K, Niven, B, McLeod, A, et al. (1996). Vigabatrin in the prophylaxis of drug resistant migraine: a double-blind crossover comparison with placebo. *Cephalalgia*, 16:367.

Gijsman, H, Kramer, MS, Sargent, J, et al. (1997). Double-blind, placebo-controlled, dose-finding study of rizatriptan (MK-462) in the acute treatment of migraine. *Cephalalgia*, 17:647–651.

Gilbert, GJ (1982). An occurrence of complicated migraine during propranolol therapy. *Headache*, 22:81–83.

Gilman, AG (1989). G proteins and regulation of adenylyl cyclase. *JAMA*, 262:1819–1825.

Glover, V, Littlewood, J, Sandler, M, et al. (1983). Biochemical predisposition to dietary migraine: the role of phenolsulfotransferase. *Headache*, 23:53–58.

Goadsby, PJ (2005). Can we develop neurally acting drugs for the treatment of migraine? *Nat Rev Drug Discov*, 4:741–750.

Goadsby, PJ and Edvinsson, L (1993). The trigeminovascular system in migraine: studies characterizing cerebrovascular and neuropeptide changes seen in humans and cats. *Ann Neurol*, 33:48–56.

Goadsby, PJ, Edvinsson, L, and Ekman, R (1990). Vasoactive peptide release in the extracerebral circulation of humans during migraine headache. *Ann Neurol*, 28:183–187.

Goadsby, PJ, Ferrari, MD, Olesen, J, et al. (2000). Eletriptan in acute migraine: a double-blind, placebo-controlled comparison to sumatriptan. Eletriptan Steering Committee. *Neurology*, 54:156–163.

Goadsby, PJ and Gundlach, AL (1991). Localization of [3H]-dihydroergotamine binding sites in the cat central nervous system: relevance to migraine. *Ann Neurol*, 29:91–94.

Goadsby, PJ and Hoskin, KL (1996). Inhibition of trigeminal neurons by intravenous administration of the serotonin (5HT)-1-D receptor agonist zolmitriptan (311C90): are brainstem sites a therapeutic target in migraine? *Pain*, 67:355–359.

Goadsby, PJ and Hoskin, KL (1997). The distribution of trigeminovascular afferents in the non-human primate brain. *J Anatomy*, 190:367–375.

Gold, L, Black, T, Arnold, G, et al. (1998). Cortical spreading depression-associated hyperemia in rats: involvement of serotonin. *Brain Res*, 783:1983.

Goldner, JA and Levitt, LP (1987). Treatment of complicated migraine with sublingual nifedipine. *Headache*, 27:484–486.

Goldstein, DJ, Offen, WW, Klein, EG, et al. (1999). Lanepitant, an NK-1 antagonist, in migraine prophylaxis. *Cephalalgia*, 19:377 (Abstract).

Goldstein, DJ, Wang, O, Saper, JR, et al. (1997). Ineffectiveness of neurokinin-1 antagonist in acute migraine: a crossover study. *Cephalalgia*, 17:785–790.

Goldstein, J, Gawel, MJ, Winner, P, et al. (1988). Comparison of butorphanol nasal spray and fiorinal with codeine in the treatment of migraine. *Headache*, 38:516–522.

Goldstein, J and Keywood, C (2002). Frovatriptan for the acute treatment of migraine: a dose-finding study. *Headache*, 42:41–48.

Goldstein, J, Silberstein, SD, Saper, JR, et al. (2005). Acetaminophen, aspirin, and caffeine versus sumatriptan succinate in the early treatment of migraine: results from the ASSET trial. *Headache*, 45:973–982.

Goldstein, J, Silberstein, SD, Saper, JR, et al. (2006). Acetaminophen, aspirin, and caffeine in combination versus ibuprofen for acute migraine: results from a multicenter, double-blind, randomized, parallel-group, single-dose, placebo-controlled study. *Headache*, 46:444–453.

Goldstein, M and Chen, TC (1982). The epidemiology of disabling headache. In *Advances in Neurology*, Vol. 33. (M Critchley, ed.), pp. 377–390. Raven Press, New York.

Gomersall, JD and Stuart, A (1973). Amitriptyline in migraine prophylaxis. Changes in pattern of attacks during a controlled clinical trial. *J Neurol Neurosurg Psychiatry*, 36:684–690.

Gordon, ML, Lipton, RB, Brown, SL, et al. (1993). Headache and cortical responses to m-chlorophenylpiperazine are highly correlated. *Cephalalgia*, 13:400–405.

Goslin, RE, Gray, RN, McCrory, DC, et al. (1999). Behavioral and physical treatments for migraine headache.

Prepared for the Agency for Health Care Policy and Research, Contract No. 290-94-2025. Available from the National Technical Information Service. Accession No 127946. February (Technical Review 2.2).

Graham, J (1967). Cardiac and pulmonary fibrosis during methysergide therapy for headache. *Am J Med Sci*, 254:1–12.

Graham, JR, Suby, HI, LeCompte, PR, et al. (1966). Fibrotic disorders associated with methysergide therapy for headache. *N Engl J Med*, 274:360–368.

Gray, RN, Goslin, RE, McCrory, DC, et al. (1999). Drug treatments for the prevention of migraine headache. Prepared for the Agency for Health Care Policy and Research, Contract No. 290-94-2025. Available from the National Technical Information Service Accession No. 127953.

Gray, RN, McCrory, DC, Eberlein, K, et al. (1999a). Drug treatments for acute migraine headache. Prepared for the Agency for Health Care Policy and Research, Contract No. 290-94-2025. Available from the National Technical Information Service, Accession No. 127854.

Gray, RN, McCrory, DC, Eberlein, K, et al. (1999b). Parenteral drug treatments for acute migraine headache. Prepared for the Agency for Health Care Policy and Research, Contract No. 290-94-2025. Available from the National Technical Information Service, Accession No. 127862. February (Technical Review 2.5).

Gray, RN, McCrory, DC, Eberlein, K, et al. (1999c). Self-administered drug treatments for acute migraine headache. Prepared for the Agency for Health Care Policy and Research, Contract No. 290-94-2025. Available from the National Technical Information Service, Accession No. 127854. February (Technical Review 2 4).

Greenberg, DA (1997). Calcium channels in neurological disease. *Ann Neurol*, 42:275–282.

Griffin, MR, Piper, JM, Daugherty, JR, et al. (1991). Nonsteroidal antiinflammatory drug use and increased risk for peptic ulcer disease in elderly persons. *Ann Intern Med*, 114:257–263.

Grotemeyer, KH, Scharafinski, HW, Schlake, HP, et al. (1990). Acetylsalicylic acid vs metoprolol in migraine prophylaxis: a double-blind crossover study. *Headache*, 30:639–641.

Grotemeyer, KH, Schlake, HP, Husstedt, IW, et al. (1987). Metoprolol versus flunarizine: a double blind crossover study. *Cephalalgia*, 7:465–466.

Gruffydd-Jones, K, Hood, CA, and Price, DB (1997). A within-patient comparison of subcutaneous and oral sumatriptan in the acute treatment of migraine in general practice. *Cephalalgia*, 17:31–36.

Gutstein, HB and Akil, H (2006). Opioid analgesics. In *Goodman & Gilman's The Pharmacological Basis of Therapeutics* (LL Brunton, JS Lazo, and KL Parker, eds), pp. 547–590. McGraw-Hill, New York.

Hachinski, V, Norris, JW, Edmeads, J, et al. (1978). Ergotamine and cerebral blood flow. *Stroke*, 9:594–596.

Hadjikhani, N, Sanchez delRio, M, Wu, O, et al. (2001). Mechanisms of migraine aura revealed by functional MRI in human visual cortex. *Proc Nat Acad Sci USA*, 98:4687–4692.

Hakkarainen, H and Allonen, H (1982). Ergotamine vs metoclopramide vs their combination in acute migraine attacks. *Headache*, 22:10–12.

Hakkarainen, H, Gustafsson, B, and Stockman, O (1978). A comparative trial of ergotamine tartrate acetyl salicylic acid and dextropropoxyphene compound in acute migraine attacks. *Headache*, 18:35–39.

Hakkarainen, H, Parantainen, J, Gothoni, G, et al. (1982). Tolfenamic acid and caffeine: a useful combination in migraine. *Cephalalgia*, 2:173–177.

Hakkarainen, H, Quiding, H, and Stockman, O (1980). Mild analgesics as an alternative to ergotamine in migraine. A comparative trail with acetylsalicylic acid, ergotamine tartrate, and dextropropoxyphene compound. *J Clin Pharmacol*, 20:590–595.

Hakkarainen, H, Vapaatalo, H, Gothoni, G, et al. (1979). Tolfenamic acid is an effective as ergotamine during migraine attacks. *Lancet*, 2:326–328.

Hanston, PP and Horn, JR (1985). Drug interaction. *Newsletter*, 5:7–10.

Hasselmark, L, Malingren, R, and Hanneiz, J (1987). Effect of carbohydrate-rich low in protein tryptophan in classic and common migraine. *Cephalalgia*, 7:87–92.

Havanka-Kanniainen, H (1989). Treatment of acute migraine attack: ibuprofen and placebo compared. *Headache*, 29:507–509.

Havanka-Kanniainen, H, Hokkanen, E, and Myllyla, VV (1987). Efficacy of nimodipine in comparison with pizotifen in the prophylaxis of migraine. *Cephalalgia*, 7:7–13.

Headache Classification Committee (2004). *The International Classification of Headache Disorders* (2nd Edn). *Cephalalgia*, 24:1–160.

Headache Classification Committee (2006). New appendix criteria open for a broader concept of chronic migraine. *Cephalalgia*, 26:742–746.

Hedman, C, Andersen, AR, Andersson, PG, et al. (1988). Symptoms of classic migraine attacks: modifications brought about my metoprolol. *Cephalalgia*, 8:279–284.

Hemler, M, Lands, WE, and Smith, WL (1976). Purification of the cyclooxygenase that forms prostaglandins. Demonstration of two forms of iron in the holoenzyme. *J Biol Chem*, 251:2629–2636.

Heninger, GR and Charney, DS (1987). Mechanism of action of antidepressant treatments: implications for the etiology and treatment of depressive disorders. In *Psychopharmacology: The Third Generation of Progress* (HY Meltzer, ed.). pp. 535–544. Raven Press, New York.

Henry, P and D'allens, H (1993). Subcutaneous sumatriptan in the acute treatment of migraine in patients using dihydroergotamine as prophylaxis. *Headache*, 33:432–435.

Henry, P, Dartigues, JF, and Benetier, MP, et al. (1985). Ergotamine- and analgesic-induced headaches. In *Migraine* (C Rose, ed.), pp. 197–205. Proceedings of the 5th International Migraine Symposium, London.

Heptinstall, S, Groenewegen, WA, Spangenberg, P, et al. (1987). Extracts of feverfew may inhibit platelet behavior via neutralization of sulphydryl groups. *J Pharm Pharmacol*, 39:459–465.

Heptinstall, S, White, A, Williamson, L, et al. (1985). Extracts of feverfew inhibit granule secretion in blood platelets and polymorphonuclear leukocytes. *Lancet*, i:1071–1074.

Hering, R and Kuritzky, A (1992). Sodium valproate in the prophylactic treatment of migraine: a double-blind study versus placebo. *Cephalalgia*, 12:81–84.

Hernandez-Diaz, S, Varas-Lorenzo, C, and Garcia Rodriguez, LA (2006). Non-steroidal antiinflammatory drugs and the risk of acute myocardial infarction. *Basic Clin Pharmacol Toxicol*, 98:266–274.

Hershey, AD, Powers, SW, Vockell, AL, et al. (2002). Effectiveness of topiramate in the prevention of childhood headaches. *Headache*, 42:810–818.

Hibbs, JB, Taintor, RR, Vavrin, Z, et al. (1988). Nitric oxide: a cytotoxic activated macrophage effector molecule. *Biochem Biophys Res Commun*, 157:87–94.

Hirt, D, Lataste, X, and Taylor, P (1989). A comparison of DHE nasal spray and cafergot in acute migraine. *Cephalalgia*, 9:410–411.

Holden, JE, Jeong, Y, and Forrest, JM (2005). The endogenous opioid system and clinical pain management. *AACN Clin Issues*, 16:291–301.

Holroyd, KA, Penzien, DB, and Coordingley, GE (1991). Propranolol in the management of recurrent migraine: a meta-analytic review. *Headache*, 31:333–340.

Horton, BT, MacLean, AR, and Craig, WM (1939). A new syndrome of vascular headache: results of treatment with histamine: preliminary report. *Mayo Clin Proc*, 14:257–260.

Hoshi, K, Ma, T, and Ho, IK (1996). Precipitated kappa-opioid receptor agonist withdrawal increases glutamate in rat locus coeruleus. *Eur J Pharmacol*, 314:301–306.

Hoyer, D, Clarke, DE, and Fozard, JR, et al (1994a). The IUPHAR classification of receptors for 5-hydroxytryptamine (serotonin). *Pharmacol Rev*, 46:157–204.

Hoyer, D, Clarke, DE, Fozard, JR, et al. (1994b). VII International union of pharmacology classification of receptors for 5-hydroxytryptamine (serotonin). *Pharmacol Rev*, 46:157–203.

Hoyer, D and Martin, GR (1997). 5-HT receptor classification and nomenclature: towards a harmonization with the human genome. *Neuropharmacology*, 36:419–428.

Hubbe, P (1973). The prophylactic treatment of migraine with an antiserotonin pizotifen. *Acta Neurol Scand*, 49:108–114.

Hudgson, P, Foster, JB, and Newell, DJ (1967). Controlled trial of demigran in the prophylaxis of migraine. *Br Med J*, 2:91–93.

Hughes, RC and Foster, JB (1971). BC 105 in the prophylaxis of migraine. *Curr Ther Res Clin Exp*, 13:63–68.

Humphrey, PP, Apperley, E, Feniuk, W, et al. (1990). A rational approach to identifying a fundamentally new drug for the treatment of migraine. In *Cardiovascular Pharmacology of 5-hydroxytryptamine: Prospective Therapeutic Applications* (PR Saxena, DI Wallis, W Wouters, et al., eds), pp. 416–431. Kluwer Academic Publishers, Dodrecht.

Humphrey, PP and Feniuk, W (1991). Mode of action of the antimigraine drug sumatriptan. *Trends Pharmacol Sci*, 12:444–446.

Humphrey, PP, Hartig, P, and Hoyer, D (1993). A proposed new nomenclature for 5-HT receptors. *Trends Pharmacol Sci*, 14:233–238.

Jackson, NC (1996). A comparison of oral eletriptan (UK-116,044) (20-80mg) and oral sumatriptan (100mg) in the acute treatment of migraine, for the Eletriptan Steering Committee. *Cephalalgia*, 16:368–369 (Abstract).

Jacobs, H (1972). A trial of opipramol in the treatment of migraine. *J Neurol Neurosurg Psychiatr*, 35:500–504.

Jensen, R, Brinck, T, and Olesen, J (1994a). Sodium valproate has a prophylactic effect in migraine without aura. *Neurology*, 44:647–651.

Jensen, R, Brinck, T, and Olesen, J (1994b). Sodium valproate has prophylactic effect in migraine without aura: a triple-blind, placebo-controlled crossover study. *Neurology*, 44:241–244.

Jewett, DL, Fein, G, and Greenberg, MH (1990). A double-blind study of symptom provocation to determine food sensitivity. *N Engl J Med*, 323:429–433.

Johannsson, V, Nilsson, LR, Widelius, T, et al. (1987). Atenolol in migraine prophylaxis: a double-blind crossover multicenter study. *Headache*, 27:372–374.

Johnson, ES, Kadam, NP, Hylands, DM, et al. (1985). Efficacy of feverfew as prophylactic treatment of migraine. *Br Med J*, 291:569–573.

Johnson, ES, Ratcliffe, DM, and Wilkinson, M (1985). Naproxen sodium in the treatment of migraine. *Cephalalgia*, 5:5–10.

Johnson, KW, Schaus, JM, and Durkin, MM, et al (1997). 5HT1F receptor agonists inhibit neurogenic dural inflammation in guinea pigs. *Neuroreport*, 8:2237–2240.

Johnson, RH, Hornabrook, RW, and Lambie, DG (1986). Comparison of mefenamic acid and propranolol with placebo in migraine prophylaxis. *Acta Neurol Scand*, 73:490–492.

Jones, EB, Gonzales, ER, Boggs, JG, et al. (1994). Safety and efficacy of rectal prochlorperazine for the treatment of migraine in the emergency department. *Ann Emerg Med*, 24:237–241.

Jones, J, Pack, S, and Chun, E (1996). Intramuscular prochlorperazine versus metoclopramide as single-agent therapy for the treatment of acute migraine headache. *Am J Emerg Med*, 14:262–264.

Jones, J, Sklar, D, Dougherty, J, et al. (1989). Randomized double-blind trial of intravenous prochlorperazine for the treatment of acute headache. *JAMA*, 261:1174–1176.

Kahn, RS, Kalus, O, Wetzler, S, et al. (1990). Effects of serotonin antagonists on m-chlorophenylpiperazine-mediated responses in normal subjects. *Psychiatry Res*, 33:189–198.

Kalkman, HO (1999). Minireview: is migraine prophylactic activity caused by 5-HT_{2B} or 5-HT_{2C} receptor blockade? *Life Sci*, 54:641–644.

Kallanranta, T, Hakkarainen, H, Hokkanen, E, et al. (1977). Clonidine in migraine prophylaxis. *Headache*, 17:169–172.

Kandere-Grzybowska, K, Gheorghe, D, Priller, J, et al. (2003). Stress-induced dura vascular permeability does not develop in mast cell-deficient and neurokinin-1 receptor knockout mice. *Brain Res*, 980:213–220.

Kangasniemi, P (1979). 1-isopropylnoradrenochrome-5-monosemicarbazono, and pizotifen in migraine prophylaxis. *Headache*, 19:219–222.

Kangasniemi, P, Andersen, AR, Andersson, PG, et al. (1987). Classic migraine: effective prophylaxis with metoprolol. *Cephalalgia*, 7:231–238.

Kangasniemi, P and Kaaja, R (1992). Ketoprofen and ergotamine in acute migraine. *J Intern Med*, 231:551–554.

Kangasniemi, PJ, Nyrke, T, Lang, AH, et al. (1983). Femoxetine—a new 5HT uptake inhibitor–and propranolol in the prophylactic treatment of migraine. *Acta Neurol Scand*, 68:262–267.

Kaniecki, RG (1997). A comparison of divalproex with propranolol and placebo for the prophylaxis of migraine without aura. *Arch Neurol*, 54:1141–1145.

Kanto, J, Allonen, H, and Koski, K (1981). Pharmacokinetics of dihydroergotamine in healthy volunteers and in neurological patients after a single intravenous injection. *Int J Clin Pharmacol Ther Toxicol*, 19:127–130.

Kapicioglu, S, Gokce, E, Kapicioglu, Z, et al. (1997). Treatment of migraine attacks with a long-acting somatostatin analogue (octreotide, SMS 201-995). *Cephalalgia*, 17:27–30.

Karachalios, GN, Fotiadou, A, Chrisikos, N, et al. (1992). Treatment of acute migraine attack with diclofenan sodium: a double-blind study. *Headache*, 32:98–100.

Karli, N, Zarifoglu, M, Calisir, N, et al. (2005). Comparison of pre-headache phases and trigger factors of migraine and episodic tension-type headache: do they share similar clinical pathophysiology? *Cephalalgia*, 25:444–451.

Kass, B and Nestvold, K (1980). Propranolol (Inderal) and clonidine (Catapressan) in the prophylactic treatment of migraine: a comparative trial. *Acta Neurol Scand*, 61:351–356.

Kaube, H, Herzog, J, Kaufer, T, et al. (2000). Aura in some patients with familial hemiplegic migraine can be stopped by intranasal ketamine. *Neurology*, 55:139–141.

Kaube, H, Keay, K, Hoskin, KL, et al. (1993). Expression of c-fos like immunoreactivity in the trigeminal nucleus caudalis and high cervical cord following stimulation of the sagittal sinus in the cat. *Brain Res*, 629:95–102.

Kaufman, HS and Starr, D (1991). Prevention of red wine headache (RWH): a blind controlled study. In *Advances in Headache Research* (FC Rose, ed.), pp. 369–373. Smith Gordon, London.

Kelly, AM, Ardagh, M, Curry, C, et al. (1997). Intravenous chlorpromazine versus intramuscular sumatriptan for acute migraine. *J Accid Emerg Med*, 14:209–211.

Kimball, RW, Friedman, AP, and Vallejo, E (1960). Effect of serotonin in migraine patients. *Neurology*, 10:107–111.

Kinnunen, E, Erkinjuntti, T, and Färkkilä, M (1988). Placebo controlled double-blind trail of pirprofen and an ergotamine tartrate compound in migraine attacks. *Cephalalgia*, 8:175–179.

Kishore-Kumar, R, Max, MB, Schafer, SC, et al. (1990). Desipramine relieves post-herpetic neuralgia. *Clin Pharmacol Ther*, 47:305–312.

Kjaersgaard-Rasmussen, MJ, Holt-Larsen, B, Borg, L, et al. (1994). Tolfenamic acid versus propranolol in the prophylactic treatment of migraine. *Acta Neurol Scand*, 89:446–450.

Klapper, J, Lucas, C, Rosjo, O, et al. (2004). Benefits of treating highly disabled migraine patients with zolmitriptan while pain is mild. *Cephalalgia*, 24:918–924.

Klapper, JA (1995). An open label crossover comparison of divalproex sodium and propranolol HCl in the prevention of migraine headaches. *Headache Q*, 5:50–53.

Klapper, JA (1997). Divalproex sodium in migraine prophylaxis: a dose-controlled study. *Cephalalgia*, 17:103–108.

Klapper, JA and O'Connor, S (2000). Rizatriptan wafer—sublingual vs. placebo at the onset of acute migraine. *Cephalalgia*, 20:585–587.

Klapper, JA and Stanton, J (1993). Current emergency treatment of severe migraine headaches. *Headache*, 33:560–562.

Klapper, JA and Stanton, JS (1991a). Ketorolac versus DHE and metoclopramide in the treatment of migraine headaches. *Headache*, 31:523–524.

Klapper, JA and Stanton, JS (1991b). The emergency treatment of acute migraine headache; a comparison of intravenous dihydroergotamine, dexamethasone, and placebo. *Cephalalgia*, 11:159–160.

Klassen, A, Elkind, A, Asgharnjad, M, et al. (1997). Naratriptan tablets are effective and well-tolerated in the acute treatment of migraine: results of a double-blind, placebo-controlled, parallel group trial. *Headache*, 37:640–645.

Kloster, R, Nestvold, K, and Vilming, ST (1992). A double-blind study of ibuprofen versus placebo in the treatment of acute migraine attacks. *Cephalalgia*, 12:169–171.

Koehler, SM and Glaros, A (1988). The effect of aspartame on migraine headache. *Headache*, 28:10–13.

Koella, WP (1985). CNS-related (side-)effects of β-blockers with special reference to mechanisms of action. *Eur J Clin Pharmacol*, 28:55–63.

Kolesnikov, Y, Pick, CG, and Pasternack, GW (1992). N^G-nitro-1-arginine prevents morphine tolerance. *Eur J Pharmacol*, 221:399–400.

Kozubski, W (1992). Metamizole and hydrocortisone for the interruption of a migraine attack—preliminary study. *Headache Q*, 3:326–228.

Krakowski, AJ and Engisch, R (1973). A new agent for chemotherapy of migraine headaches: a controlled study. *Psychosomatics*, 14:302–308.

Krause, KH and Bleicher, MA (1985). Dihydroergotamine nasal spray in the treatment of migraine attacks. *Cephalalgia*, 5:138–139.

Krebs, EG (1989). Role of the cyclic AMP-dependent protein kinase in signal transduction. *JAMA*, 262:1815–1818.

Krebs, EG (1994). The growth of research on protein phosphorylation. *Trends Biochem Sci*, 19:439.

Krootila, K, Oksala, O, Zschauer, A, et al. (1992). Inhibitory effect of methysergide on calcium gene-related peptide-induced vasodilatation and ocular irritative changes in the rabbit. *Br J Pharmacol*, 106:404–408.

Krusz, JC (2001). Zonisamide in the treatment of headache disorders. *Cephalalgia*, 21:374–375 (Abstract).

Krusz, JC and Belanger, J (1999). Propofol—a highly effective treatment for acute headaches. *Cephalalgia*, 19:358 (Abstract).

Krusz, JC, Scott, V, and Belanger, J (1999). IV droperidol as a treatment for acute migraine headaches. *Cephalalgia*, 19:356 (Abstract).

Krymchantowski, AV (2000). Naproxen sodium decreases migraine recurrence when administered with sumatriptan. *Arq Neuropsiquiatr*, 58:428–430.

Krymchantowski, AV, Peixoto, P, Higashi, R, et al. (2005). Lysine clonixinate vs naproxen sodium for the acute treatment of migraine: a double-blind, randomized, crossover study. *Med Gen Med*, 7:69.

Krymchantowski, AV, Silva, MT, Barbosa, JS, et al. (2002). Amitriptyline versus amitriptyline combined with fluoxetine in the preventative treatment of transformed migraine: a double-blind study. *Headache*, 42:510–514.

Kudrow, L (1982). Paradoxical effects of frequent analgesic use. *Adv Neurol*, 33:335–341.

Kumar, KL and Cooney, TG (1990). Visual symptoms after atenolol therapy for migraine. *Ann Intern Med*, 112:712–713.

Kunkel, RS (1982). Vasodilator therapy for classical migraine headaches. In *Advances in Migraine Research and Therapy* (FC Rose, ed.), pp. 205–209. Raven Press, New York.

Kupersmith, MJ, Hass, WK, and Chase, NE (1987). Isoproterenol treatment of visual symptoms in migraine. *Stroke*, 27:484–486.

Kuritzky, A and Hering, R (1987). Prophylactic treatment of migraine with long acting propranolol: a comparison with placebo. *Cephalalgia*, 7:457–458.

Ladecola, C (1993). Regulation of the cerebral microcirculation during neural activity: is nitric oxide the missing link? *TiPS*, 16:206–214.

Lader, M (1983). Combined use of tricyclic antidepressants and monoamine oxidase inhibitors. *J Clin Psychiatry*, 44:20–24.

Lampl, C, Buzath, A, Klinger, D, et al. (1999). Lamotrigine in the prophylactic treatment of migraine aura—a pilot study. *Cephalalgia*, 19:58–63.

Lamsudin, R and Sadjimin, T (1993). Comparison of the efficacy between flunarizine and nifedipine in the prophylaxis of migraine. *Headache*, 33:335–338.

Lance, JW (1982). *Mechanisms and Management of Headache*. Butterworth Scientific, London.

Lance, JW (1986). The pharmacotherapy of migraine. *Med J Aust*, 144:85–88.

Lance, JW (1992). History of involvement of 5-HT in primary headaches. In *5-Hydroxytryptamine Mechanisms in Primary Headaches* (J Olesen and PR Saxena, eds), pp. 19–28. Raven Press, New York.

Lance, JW and Anthony, M (1966). Some clinical aspects of migraine. *Arch Neurol*, 15:356–361.

Lance, JW and Anthony, M (1968). Clinical trial of a new serotonin antagonist, BC105, in the prevention of migraine. *Med J Aust*, 1:54–55.

Lance, JW, Fine, RD, and Curran, DA (1963). An evaluation of methysergide in the prevention of migraine and other vascular headaches. *Med J Aust*, 1:814–818.

Lane, PL, McLellan, BA, and Boggoley, CJ (1989). Comparative efficacy of chlorpromazine and meperidine with dimenhydrinate in migraine headache. *Ann Emerg Med*, 18:360–365.

Lane, PL and Ross, R (1995). Intravenous chlorpromazine—preliminary results in acute migraine. *Headache*, 25:302–304.

Langohr, HD, Gerber, WD, Koletzki, E, et al. (1985). Clomipramine and metoprolol in migraine prophylaxis: a double-blind crossover study. *Headache*, 25:107–113.

Larkin, GL and Prescott, JE (1992). A randomized, double-blind, comparative study of the efficacy of ketorolac tromethamine versus meperidine in the treatment of severe migraine. *Ann Emerg Med*, 21:919–924.

Larsen, BH, Christiansen, LV, Andersen, B, et al. (1990). Randomized double-blind comparison of tolfenamic acid and paracetamol in migraine. *Acta Neurol Scand*, 81:464–467.

Lashley, KS (1941). Patterns of cerebral integration indicated by the scotomas of migraine. *Arch Neurol*, 46:331–339.

Lassen, LH, Ashina, M, Christiansen, I, et al. (1997). Nitric oxide synthase inhibition in migraine. *Lancet*, 349:401–402.

Lataste, X (1989). Dihydroergotamine nasal spray. In *Migraine and Other Headaches* (MD Ferrari and X Lataste, eds), pp. 249–260. Parthenon, Park Ridge, New Jersey.

Lauritzen, M (1986). Spreading cortical depression as a mechanism of the aura in classic migraine. In *The prelude to the Migraine Attack* (WK Amery and A Wauquier, eds), pp. 134–141. Bailliere Tindall, London.

Lawrence, ER, Hossain, M, and Littlestone, W (1977). Sanomigran for migraine prophylaxis: controlled multicenter trial in general practice. *Headache*, 17:109–112.

Leandri, M, Rigardo, S, Schizzi, R, et al. (1990). Migraine treatment with nicardipine. *Cephalalgia*, 10:111–116.

Leao, AAP (1944). Spreading depression of activity in cerebral cortex. *J Neurophysiol*, 7:359–390.

Lejeune, F and Millan, MJ (2000). Pindolol excites dopaminergic and adrenergic neurons, and inhibits serotonergic neurons, by activation of 5-HT1A receptors. *Eur J Neurosci*, 12:3265–3275.

Leniger, T, Pageler, L, Stude, P, et al. (2005). Comparison of intravenous valproate with intravenous lysine-acetylsalicylic acid in acute migraine attacks. *Headache*, 45:42–46.

Levy, D, Jakubowski, M, and Burstein, R (2004). Disruption of communication between peripheral and central trigeminovascular neurons mediates the antimigraine action of 5HT1B-1D receptor agonists. *PNAS*, 101:4274–4279.

Limmroth, V, Katsarava, Z, Fritsche, G, et al. (2002). Features of medication overuse headache following overuse of different acute headache drugs. *Neurology*, 59:1011–1014.

Limmroth, V, Wermelskirchen, D, Tegtmeier, F, et al (1997). Alniditan blocks neurogenic edema by activation of 5HT1B/1D receptors in anesthetized rats more effectively than sumatriptan. *Cephalalgia*, 17:402.

Lindsay, RM, Wiegand, SJ, Altar, CA, et al. (1994). Neurotrophic factors: from molecule to man. *Trends Neurosci*, 17:182–190.

Lipton, RB, Baggish, JS, Stewart, WF, et al. (2000a). Efficacy and safety of acetaminophen in the treatment of migraine: results of a randomized, double-blind, placebo-controlled, population-based study. *Arch Intern Med*, 160:3486–3492.

Lipton, RB, Bigal, M, and Diamond, M (2007). Migraine prevalence, disease burden and the need for preventive therapy. *Neurology*, 68(5):343–349.

Lipton, RB, Bigal, ME, and Goadsby, PJ (2004). Double-blind clinical trials of oral triptans vs other classes of acute migraine medication—a review. *Cephalalgia*, 24:321–332.

Lipton, RB, Cady, RK, O'Quinn, S, et al. (1999). Sumatriptan treats the full spectrum of headache in individuals with disabling IHS migraine. *Headache*, 40:783–791.

Lipton, RB, Diamond, M, Freitag, F, et al. (2005). Migraine prevention patterns in a community sample: results from the American migraine prevalence and prevention (AMPP) study. *Headache*, 45:792–793 (Abstract).

Lipton, RB, Gobel, H, Einhaupl, KM, et al. (2004). Petasites hybridus root (butterbur) is an effective preventive treatment for migraine. *Neurology*, 63:2240–2244.

Lipton, RB and Silberstein, SD (1994). Why study the comorbidity of migraine? *Neurology*, 44:4–5.

Lipton, RB and Silberstein, SD (2001). The role of headache-related disability in migraine management: implications for headache treatment guidelines. *Neurology*, 56:S35–S42.

Lipton, RB, Stewart, WF, Diamond, S, et al. (2001). Prevalence and burden of migraine in the United States: data from the American Migraine Study II. *Headache*, 41:646–657.

Lipton, RB, Stewart, WF, Ryan, RE, et al. (1998). Efficacy and safety of the nonprescription combination of acetaminophen, aspirin, and caffeine in alleviating headache pain of an acute migraine attack: three double-blind, randomized, placebo-controlled trials. *Arch Neurol*, 55:210–217.

Lipton, RB, Stewart, WF, Stone, AM, et al. (2000). Stratified care vs step care strategies for migraine. The disability in strategies of care (DISC) study: a randomized trial. *JAMA*, 284:2599–2505.

Littlewood, JT, Gibb, C, Glover, V, et al. (1987). Red wine as a migraine trigger. In *Advances in Headache Research*, (FC Rose, ed.), pp. 123–127. John Libbey, London.

Littlewood, JT, Glover, V, Davies, PT, et al. (1988). Red wine as a cause of migraine. *Lancet*, 1 (8585):558–559.

Loder, E, Freitag, FG, Adelman, J, et al. (2005). Pain-free rates with zolmitriptan 2.5 mg ODT in the acute treatment of migraine: results of a large double-blind placebo- controlled trial. *Curr Med Res Opin*, 21:381–389.

Longmore, J, Shaw, D, Smith, D, et al. (1997). Differential distribution of 5HT(1D)- and 5HT(1B)-immunoreactivity within the human trigeminocerebrovascular system: implications for the discovery of new antimigraine drugs. *Cephalalgia*, 17:833–842.

Louis, P (1981). A double-blind placebo-controlled prophylactic study of flunarizine (Sibelium) in migraine. *Headache*, 21:235–239.

Louis, P, Schoenen, J, and Hedman, C (1985). Metoprolol vs clonidine in the prophylactic treatment of migraine. *Cephalalgia*, 5:159–165.

Louis, P and Spierings, EL (1982). Comparison of flunarizine (Sibelium) and pizotifen (Sandomigran) in migraine treatment: a double-blind study. *Cephalalgia*, 2:197–203.

Luciani, R, Carter, D, Mannix, L, et al. (2000). Prevention of migraine during prodrome with naratriptan. *Cephalalgia*, 20:122–126.

Lucking, CH, Oestreich, W, Schmidt, R, et al. (1988). Flunarizine vs propranolol in the prophylaxis of migraine: two double-blind comparative studies in more than 400 patients. *Cephalalgia*, 8:21–26.

Ludin, HP (1989). Flunarizine and propranolol in the treatment of migraine. *Headache*, 29:219–224.

MacDonald, A, Forsythe, I, and Wall, C (1989). Dietary treatment of migraine. In *Headache in Children and Adolescents*, (G Lanzi, U Balottin, and A Cernibori, eds), pp. 333–338. Elsevier, New York.

MacDonald, RL and McLean, MJ (1986). Anticonvulsant drugs: mechanisms of action. In *Advances in Neurology*, (AD Escueta, AA Ward, DM Woodbury, et al., eds), pp. 713–736. Raven Press, New York.

MacGregor, EA, Dowson, A, and Davies, PT (2002). Mouth-dispersible aspirin in the treatment of migraine: a placebo-controlled study. *Headache*, 42:249–255.

MacLennan, SJ and Martin, GR (1990). Comparison of the effects of methysergide and methylergometrine with GR 43175 on feline carotid blood flow distribution. *Br J Pharmacol*, 99:221.

Maizels, M (1998). Intranasal lidocaine for migraine in an outpatient population. *Headache*, 38:391.

Maizels, M, Blumenfeld, A, and Burchette, R (2004). A combination of riboflavin, magnesium, and feverfew for migraine prophylaxis: a randomized trial. *Headache*, 44:885–890.

Maizels, M, Scott, B, Cohen, W, et al. (1996). Intranasal lidocaine for treatment of migraine: a randomized, double-blind, controlled trial. *JAMA*, 276:319–321.

Mamounas, LA, Wilson, MA, Axt, KJ, et al. (1992). Morphological aspects of serotonergic innervation. In *Serotonin, CNS Receptors and Brain Function* (PB Bradley, SL Handley, SJ Cooper, et al., eds), pp. 97–118. Pergamon Press, New York.

Marcus, DA, Scharff, L, Turk, D, et al. (1997). A double-blind provocative study of chocolate as a trigger of headache. *Cephalalgia*, 17:855–862.

Markley, HG, Cleronis, JCD, and Piepko, RW (1984). Verapamil prophylactic therapy of migraine. *Neurology*, 34:973–976.

Markley, HG, Gasser, PA, Markley, ME, et al. (1991). Fluoxetine in prophylaxis of migraine: clinical experience. *Cephalalgia*, 11:164–165.

Markowitz, S, Saito, K, and Moskowitz, MA (1988). Neurogenically mediated plasma extravasation in dura mater: effect of ergot alkaloids. A possible mechanism of action in vascular headache. *Cephalalgia*, 8:83–91.

Martucci, N, Manna, V, Mattesi, P, et al. (1983). Ergot derivatives in the prophylaxis of migraine: a multicentric study with a timed-release dihydroergotamine formulation. *Cephalalgia*, 3:151–155.

Masel, BE, Chesson, AL, Peters, BH, et al. (1980). Platelet antagonists in migraine prophylaxis: a clinical trial using aspirin and dipyridamole. *Headache*, 20:13–18.

Massiou, H (1987). Dihydroergotamine nasal spray in prevention and treatment of migraine attacks: two controlled trials versus placebo. *Cephalalgia*, 7:440–441.

Mastrosimone, F and Iaccarino, C (1987). Progress in migraine: treatment with dihydroergotamine-retard. *Cephalalgia*, 7:168–170.

Masyczek, R and Pugh, CS (1983). The 'red wine' reaction. *Ann J Enol Vitic*, 34:260–264.

Matchar, DB, Young, WB, Rosenberg, JA, et al. (2000). Evidence-based guidelines for migraine headache in the primary care setting: pharmacological management of acute attacks. *Neurology* available from http://www.aan.com.

Mathew, N, Saper, J, and Magnus-Miller, L (1998). Efficacy and safety of gabapentin (Neurontin®) in migraine prophylaxis. 17th Annual Meeting of the American Pain Society. San Diego, California (Abstract).

Mathew, NT (1981). Prophylaxis of migraine and mixed headache. A randomized controlled study. *Headache*, 21:105–109.

Mathew, NT (1990). Drug induced headache. *Neurol Clin*, 8:903–912.

Mathew, NT (1996). Gabapentin in migraine prophylaxis. *Cephalalgia*, 16:367.

Mathew, NT (2003). Early intervention with almotriptan improves sustained pain-free response in acute migraine. *Headache*, 43:1075–1079.

Mathew, NT, Kailasam, J, Meadors, L, et al. (1999). Intravenous valproate sodium (Depacon®) aborts migraine rapidly: a preliminary report. *Cephalalgia*, 19:373 (Abstract).

Mathew, NT, Kailasam, J, and Seifert, T (2004). Early treatment of migraine with rizatriptan: a placebo-controlled study. *Neurology*, 62:A183 (Abstract).

Mathew, NT, Peykamian, M, Laurenza, A, et al. (1997). Efficacy and tolerability of naratriptan tablets in the treatment of migraine: results of a double-blind, placebo-controlled, crossover trial. Neurology (Abstract).

Mathew, NT, Saper, JR, Silberstein, SD, et al. (1999). A multicenter, double-blind, placebo-controlled trial of two dosages of botulinum toxin type A (BOTOX[R]) in the prophylactic treatment of migraine. Submitted for publication (Abstract).

Mathew, NT, Saper, JR, Silberstein, SD, et al. (1995a). Migraine prophylaxis with divalproex. *Arch Neurol*, 52:281–286.

Mathew, NT, Saper, JR, Silberstein, SD, et al. (1995b). Prophylaxis of migraine headaches with divalproex sodium. *Arch Neurol*, 52:281–286.

McAllister, G, Charlesworth, A, Snodin, C, et al. (1992). Molecular cloning of a serotonin receptor from human brain (5HT1E): a fifth 5HT1-like subtype. *Proc Natl Acad Sci USA*, 89:5517–5521.

McArthur, JC, Marek, K, Pestronk, A, et al. (1989). Nifedipine in the prophylaxis of classic migraine: a crossover, double-masked, placebo-controlled study of headache frequency and side effects. *Neurology*, 39:284–286.

McCall, RB (1999). Preclinical and clinical studies in migraine using the selective $5HT_{1D}$ receptor agonist PNU-142633. IBC Third Annual Conference on Migraine: Novel Drug and Therapeutic Development. Philadelphia, May 20.

McCormack, K (1994). Nonsteroidal antiinflammatory drugs and spinal nociceptive processing. *Pain*, 59:9–43.

McEwen, JI, O'Connor, HM, and Dinsdale, HB (1987). Treatment of migraine with intramuscular chlorpromazine. *Ann Emerg Med*, 16:758–763.

McGettigan, P and Henry, D (2006). Cardiovascular risk and inhibition of cyclooxygenase: a systematic review of the observational studies of selective and nonselective inhibitors of cyclooxygenase 2. *JAMA*, 296:1633–1644.

McQuay, HJ, Carroll, D, Watts, PG, et al. (1999). Codeine 20 mg increases relief from ibuprofen 400 mg after third molar surgery. Repeat dose comparison in an ibuprofen-codeine combination. *Pain*, 37:7–13.

McQueen, J, Loblay, RH, Savain, AR, et al. (1989). A controlled trial of dietary modification in migraine. In *New Advances in Headache Research* (FC Rose, ed.), pp. 235–242. Smith Gordon, London.

Medina, JC and Diamond, S (1978). The role of diet in migraine. *Headache*, 18:31–34.

Medina, JL (1982). Cyclic migraine: a disorder responsive to lithium carbonate. *Psychosomatics*, 23:625–637.

Mendenopoulos, G, Manafi, T, Logothetis, I, et al. (1985). Flunarizine in the prevention of classical migraine: a placebo-controlled evaluation. *Cephalalgia*, 5:31–37.

Micieli, G, Cavallini, A, Martignoni, E, et al. (1988). Effectiveness of salmon calcitonin nasal spray preparation in migraine treatment. *Headache*, 28:196–200.

Micieli, G, Trucco, M, Agostinis, C, et al. (1985). Nimodipine vs pizotifen in common migraine: results of a double-blind crossover trial. *Cephalalgia*, 5:532–533.

Migraine-Nimodipine European Study Group (MINES) (1989). European multicenter trial of nimodipine in the prophylaxis of common migraine (migraine without aura). *Headache*, 29:633–638.

Miguel, MD and Hamon, M (1992). 5-HT_1 receptor subtypes: pharmacological heterogeneity. In *Serotonin Receptor Subtypes: Pharmacological Significance and Clinical Implications* (SZ Langer, N Brunello, G Racagni, et al., eds), pp. 13–30. Karger, Basel.

Mikkelsen, B, Pedersen, KK, and Christiansen, LV (1986). Prophylactic treatment of migraine with tolfenamic acid, propranolol, and placebo. *Acta Neurol Scand*, 73:423–427.

Mikkelsen, BM and Falk, JV (1982). Prophylactic treatment of migraine with tolfenamic acid: a comparative double-blind crossover study between tolfenamic acid and placebo. *Acta Neurol Scand*, 66:105–111.

Mikoshiba, K (1993). Inositol 1,4,5-triphosphate receptor. *TiPS*, 14:86–89.

Miljanich, GP and Ramachandran, J (1995). Antagonists of neuronal calcium channels: structure, function, and therapeutic implications. *Annu Rev Pharmacol Toxicol*, 35:707–734.

Millan-Guerrero, RO, Isais-Millan, R, Benjamin, TH, et al. (2006). Nalpha-methyl histamine safety and efficacy in migraine prophylaxis: phase III study. *Can J Neurol Sci*, 33:195–199.

Millan-Guerrero, RO, Pineda-Lucatero, AG, Hernandez-Benjamin, T, et al. (2003). Nalpha-methylhistamine safety and efficacy in migraine prophylaxis: phase I and phase II studies. *Headache*, 43:389–394.

Miller, FW and Santoro, TJ (1985). Nifedipine in the treatment of migraine headache and amaurosis fugax in patients with systemic lupus erythematosus. *N Eng J Med*, 311:921.

Misra, UK, Jose, M, and Kalita, J (2004). Rofecoxib versus ibuprofen for acute treatment of migraine: a randomised placebo controlled trial. *Postgrad Med J*, 80:720–723.

Moffett, AM, Swash, M, and Scott, DF (1974). Effect of chocolate: a double-blind study. *J Neurol Neurosurg Psychiatry*, 37:445–448.

Moja, PL, Cusi, C, Sterzi, RR, et al. (2005). Selective serotonin reuptake inhibitors (SSRIs) for preventing migraine and tension-type headaches. *Cochrane Database Syst Rev* 3.

Mondrup, K and Moller, CE (1977). Prophylactic treatment of migraine with clonidine: a controlled clinical trial. *Acta Neurol Scand*, 56:405–412.

Monro, P, Swade, C, and Coppen, A (1985). Mianserin in the prophylaxis of migraine: a double-blind study. *Acta Psychiatr Scand*, 72:98–103.

Monsma, FJ, Shen, Y, Ward, RP, et al. (1992). Cloning and expression of a novel serotonin receptor with high affinity for tricyclic psychotropic drugs. *Molecular Pharmacol*, 43:320–327.

Montagna, P, Cortelli, P, Monari, L, et al. (1994). ^{31}P-Magnetic resonance spectroscopy in migraine without aura. *Neurology*, 44:666–669.

Morrison, BW, Christensen, S, Yuan, W, et al. (1999). Analgesic efficacy of the cyclooxygenase-2-specific inhibitor rofecoxib in postdental surgery pain: a randomized, controlled trial. *Clin Ther*, 21:943–953.

Moschiano, F, D'Amico, D, Allais, G, et al. (2005). Early triptan intervention in migraine: an overview. *Neurol Sci*, 26(Suppl. 2):s108–s110.

Moskowitz, MA (1990). Basic mechanisms in vascular headache. *Neurol Clin*, 8:801–815.

Moskowitz, MA (1992a). Interpreting vessel diameter changes in vascular headaches. *Cephalalgia*, 12:5–7.

Moskowitz, MA (1992b). Neurogenic versus vascular mechanisms of sumatriptan and ergot alkaloids in migraine. *TiPS*, 13:307–311.

Moskowitz, MA and Cutrer, FM (1993). Sumatriptan: a receptor-targeted treatment for migraine. *Ann Rev Med*, 44:145–154.

Mosniam, A, Freitag, FG, Ignacio, R, et al. (1996). Apparent lack of correlation between tyramine and phenylethylamines content and the occurrence of food precipitated migraine. *Headache Q*, 7:239–249.

Mueller, EA, Murphy, DL, and Sunderland, T (1986). Further studies of the putative serotonin agonist, m-chlorophenylpiperazine: evidence for a serotonin receptor mediated mechanism of action in humans. *Psychopharmacology*, 89:388–391.

Muller, SE (1986). Serotonergic receptors in brain vessels. In *Neural Regulation of Brain Circulation* (C Owman and JE Hardebo, eds), pp. 219–234. Elsevier, Amsterdam.

Muller, SE (1992). Ergot alkaloids in migraine: is the effect via 5-HT receptors. In *5-Hydroxytryptamine Mechanisms in Primary Headaches* (J Olesen and PR Saxena, eds), pp. 297–304. Raven Press, New York.

Muller-Schweinitzer, E (1984). Pharmacological actions of the main metabolites of dihydroergotamine. *Eur J Clin Pharmacol*, 26:699–705.

Multinational Oral Sumatriptan and Cafergot Comparative Study Group (1991). A randomized, double-blind comparison of sumatriptan and cafergot in the acute treatment of migraine. *Eur Neurol*, 31:314–322.

Murphy, JJ, Heptinstall, S, and Mitchell, JR (1988). Randomized double-blind placebo controlled trial of feverfew in migraine prevention. *Lancet*, 2:189–192.

Murray, WJ (1964). Evaluation of aspirin in treatment of headache. *Clin Pharmacol Ther*, 5:21–25.

Mushet, GR, Miller, D, Clements, B, et al. (1996). Impact of sumatriptan on workplace productivity, nonwork activities, and health-related quality of life among hospital employees with migraine. *Headache*, 36:137–143.

Myllyla, VV, Havanka, H, Herrala, L, et al. (1998). Tolfenamic acid rapid release versus sumatriptan in the acute treatment of migraine: comparable effect in a double-blind, randomized, controlled, parallel-group study. *Headache*, 38:201–207.

Nagamani, M, Kelver, ME, and Smith, ER (1987). Treatment of menopausal hot flashes with transdermal administration of clonidine. *Am J Obstet Gynecol*, 156:561–565.

Nanda, RN, Johnson, RH, Gray, J, et al. (1978). A double-blind trial of acebutolol for migraine prophylaxis. *Headache*, 18:379–381.

Nappi, G, Micieli, G, Tassorelli, C, et al. (1993). Effectiveness of a piroxicam fast dissolving formulation sublingually administered in the symptomatic treatment of migraine without aura. *Headache*, 33:296–300.

Nappi, G, Sandrini, G, Savoini, G, et al. (1987). Comparative efficacy of cyclandelate versus flunarizine in the prophylactic treatment of migraine. *Drugs*, 33:103–198.

Nappi, G, Sicuteri, F, Byrne, M, et al. (1994). Oral sumatriptan compared with placebo in the acute treatment of migraine. *J Neurol*, 241:138–144.

Nattero, G, Biale, L, and Savi, L (1991). Lisuride and pizotifen in the treatment of migraine without aura. *Cephalalgia*, 11:218–219.

Nattero, G, Savi, I, Cadario, G, et al. (1991). Food and headache: adverse reaction or psychic suggestion? In *New Advances in Headache Research* (FC Rose, ed.), pp. 199–203. Smith Gordon, London.

Nelson, DL (1996). Proceedings of the International Business Communications conference on serotonin receptors in the central nervous system. Philadelphia, January:25–26.

Neri, I, Granella, F, Nappi, RMGC, et al. (1993). Characteristics of headache at menopause: a clinico-epidemiologic study. *Maturitas*, 17:31–37.

Nishizuka, Y (1989). The family of protein kinase C for signal transduction. *JAMA*, 262:1833.

Noone, JF (1980). Clomipramine in the prevention of migraine. *J Int Med Res*, 8:49–52.

Nozaki, K, Boccalini, P, and Moskowitz, MA (1992). Expression of c-fos-like immunoreactivity in brainstem after meningeal irritation by blood in the subarachnoid space. *Neuroscience*, 49:669–680.

O'Connor, TP and Van der Kooy, D (1988). Enrichment of vasoactive neuropeptide (calcitonin gene related peptide) in trigeminal sensory projection to the intracranial arteries. *J Neurosci*, 8:2468–2476.

O'Connor, TP and vanderKooy, D (1986). Pattern of intracranial and extracranial projections of trigeminal ganglion cells. *J Neurosci*, 6:2200–2207.

O'Neill, BP and Mann, JD (1979). Aspirin prophylaxis in migraine. *Lancet*, 2:1179–1181.

Ogden, HD (1963). Controlled studies of a new agent in vascular headache. *Headache*, 3:29–31.

Olerud, B, Gustavsson, CL, and Furberg, B (1986). Nadolol and propranolol in migraine management. *Headache*, 26:490–493.

Olesen et al. (2003). Note—Will have full reference at time of proofs. Cephalalgia.

Olesen, J (1984). The significance of trigger factors in migraine. In *Progress in Migraine Research* (FC Rose, ed.), pp. 21–22. Pitman, London.

Olesen, J (1991). Cerebral and extracranial circulatory disturbances in migraine: pathophysiological implications. *Cerebrovasc Brain Metab Rev*, 3:1–28.

Olesen, J, Aebelholt, A, and Veilis, B (1979). The Copenhagen acute headache clinic: organization, patient material and treatment results. *Headache*, 19:223–227.

Olesen, J, Friberg, L, and Skyhoj-Olsen, T (1990). Timing and topography of cerebral blood flow, aura and headache during migraine attacks. *Ann Neurol*, 28:791–798.

Olesen, J, Larsen, B, and Lauritzen, M (1981). Focal hyperemia followed by spreading oligemia and impaired activation of RCBF in classic migraine. *Ann Neurol*, 9:344–352.

Olsson, JE, Behring, HC, Forssman, B, et al. (1984). Metoprolol and propranolol in migraine prophylaxis: a double-blind multicenter study. *Acta Neurol Scand*, 70:160–180.

Ophoff, RA, Terwindt, GM, and Vergouwe, MN (1996). Familial hemiplegic migraine and episodic ataxia type-2 are caused by mutations in the Ca^{2+} channel gene CACNLA4. *Cell Tiss Res*, 87:543–552.

Oral Sumatriptan and Aspirin-plus-Metoclpramide Comparative Study Group (1992). A study to compare oral sumatriptan with oral aspirin plus oral metoclopramide in the acute treatment of migraine. *Eur Neurol*, 32:177–184.

Oral Sumatriptan Dose-Defining Study Group (1991). Sumatriptan—an oral dose-defining study. *Eur Neurol*, 31:300–305.

Oral Sumatriptan International Multiple-Dose Study Group (1991). Evaluation of a multiple-dose regimen of oral sumatriptan for the acute treatment of migraine. *Eur Neurol*, 31:306–313.

Orholm, M, Honor, PF, and Zeeberg, I (1986). A randomized general practice group-comparative study of femoxetine and placebo in the prophylaxis of migraine. *Acta Neurol Scand*, 74:235–239.

Oshinsky, M and Luo, J (2006). Neurochemistry of a rat migraine model USE REF 7335. *Headache*, 46(Suppl. 1):S39–S44.

Osterman, PO (1977). A comparison between placebo, pizotifen, and 1-isopropyl-3-hydroxy-5-semicarbazono-6-oxo-2.3.5.6-tetrahydroindol (Divascan) in migraine prophylaxis. *Acta Neurol Scand*, 56:17–28.

Ostfeld, AM (1961). A study of migraine pharmacotherapy. *Am J Med Sci*, 241:192–198.

Packard, RC (1979). What does the headache patient want? *Headache*, 19:370–374.

Paiva, T, Esperanca, P, Marcelino, L, et al. (1985). A double-blind trial with dihydroergotamine nasal spray in migraine crisis. *Cephalalgia*, 5:140–141.

Palacios, JM, Waeber, C, Mengod, G, et al. (1991). Molecular neuroanatomy of 5-HT receptors. In *Serotonin-molecular Biology, Receptors and Functional Effects.* (JR Fozard and PR Saxena, eds), pp. 5–20. Birkhauser, Switzerland.

Palevitch, D, Earon, G, and Carusso, R (1997). Feverfew (Tanacetum parthenium) as a prophylactic treatment for migraine: a double-blind placebo-controlled study. *Phytother Res,* 11:508–511.

Panerai, AE, Monza, G, Movilia, P, et al. (1990). A randomized, within-patient, cross-over, placebo-controlled trial on the efficacy and tolerability of the tricyclic antidepressants chlorimipramine and nortriptyline in central pain. *Acta Neurol Scand,* 82:34–38.

Pappagalo, M, Szabo, Z, Esposito, G, et al. (2002). Imaging neurogenic inflammation inpatients with migraine headaches. *Neurology,* 52:274–275.

Pare, CM, Kline, N, Hallstrom, C, et al. (1982). Will amitriptyline prevent the "cheese" reaction of monoamine-oxidase inhibitors? *Lancet,* 9:183–186.

Pascual, J, Falk, RM, Piessens, F, et al. (2000). Consistent efficacy and tolerability of almotriptan in the acute treatment of multiple migraine attacks: results of a large, randomized, double-blind, placebo-controlled study. *Cephalalgia,* 20:488–496.

Pasternak, GW (1993). Review: pharmacological mechanisms of opioid analgesics. *Clin Neuropharmacol,* 16:1–18.

Patel, RM, Sarma, R, and Grimsley, E (2006). Popular sweetner sucralose as a migraine trigger. *Headache,* 46:1303–1304.

Patti, F, Scapagnini, U, Nicoletti, F, et al. (1987). A short-term trial of an analogue of eel-calcitonin in headache. *Headache,* 27:334–339.

Pearce, I, Frank, GJ, and Pearce, JM (1983). Ibuprofen compared with paracetamol in migraine. *Practitioner,* 227:465–467.

Peatfield, R (1986). Drugs acting by modification of serotonin function. *Headache,* 26:129–131.

Pedersen, E and Moller, CE (1966). Methysergide in migraine prophylaxis. *Pharmacol Ther,* 7:520–526.

Peikert, A, Wilimzig, C, and Kohne-Volland, R (1996). Prophylaxis of migraine with oral magnesium: results from a prospective, multicenter, placebo-controlled and double-blind randomized study. *Cephalalgia,* 16:257–263.

Pellock, JM and Willmore, LJ (1991). A rational guide to routine blood monitoring in patients receiving antiepileptic drugs. *Neurology,* 41:961–964.

Penn, AM, Lee, JW, Thuillier, P, et al. (1992). MELAS syndrome with mitochondrial $tRNA^{LEU(UUR)}$ mutation: correlation of clinical state, nerve conduction, and muscle ^{31P} magnetic resonance spectroscopy during treatment with nicotinamide and riboflavin. *Neurology,* 42:2147–2152.

Peroutka, SJ (1990a). Developments in 5-hydroxytryptamine receptor pharmacology in migraine. *Neurol Clin,* 8:829–838.

Peroutka, SJ (1990b). The pharmacology of current antimigraine drugs. *Headache,* 30:5–11.

Peroutka, SJ (1993). 5-hydroxytryptamine receptors. International Society for Neurochemistry. Short review. *J Neurochem,* 60:408–416.

Peroutka, SJ, Lyon, JA, Swarbrick, J, et al. (2004). Efficacy of diclofenac sodium softgel 100 mg with or without caffeine 100 mg in migraine without aura: a randomized, double-blind, crossover study. *Headache,* 44:136–141.

Peroutka, SJ and Snyder, SH (1979). Multiple serotonin receptors: differential binding of 3H-5-hydroxytryptamine, 3H-lysergic acid diethylamide and 3H-spiroperidol. *Mol Pharmacol,* 16:687–689.

Peto, R, Gray, R, Collins, R, et al. (1988). Randomized trial of prophylactic daily aspirin in British male doctors. *Br Med J,* 296:313–316.

Pfaffenrath, V, Cunin, G, Sjonell, G, et al. (1998). Efficacy and safety of sumatriptan tablets (25mg, 50mg, and 100mg) in the acute treatment of migraine: defining the optimum doses of oral sumatriptan. *Headache,* 38:184–190.

Pfaffenrath, V, Diener, HC, Fischer, M, et al. (2002). The efficacy and safety of Tanacetum parthenium (Feverfew) in migraine prophylaxis: a double-blind, multicenter, randomized, placebo-controlled, dose-response study. *Cephalalgia,* 22:523–532.

Pfaffenrath, V, Oestreich, W, and Haase, W (1990). Flunarizine (10 and 20mg) i.v. versus placebo in the treatment of acute migraine attacks: a multicenter double-blind study. *Cephalalgia,* 10:77–81.

Pfaffenrath, V, Wessely, P, Meyer, C, et al. (1996). Magnesium in the prophylaxis of migraine—a double-blind, placebo-controlled study. *Cephalalgia,* 16:436–440.

Pfeiffer, A, Brantl, V, Herz, A, et al. (1986). Psychotomimesis mediated by κ opiate receptors. *Science,* 233:774–776.

Pies, R (1983). Trazodone and intractable headaches. *J Clin Psychiatry,* 44:317.

Pigott, TA, Zohar, J, Hill, JL, et al. (1991). Metergoline blocks the behavioral and neuroendocrine effects of orally administered m-chlorophenylpiperazine in patients with obsessive-compulsive disorder. *Biol Psychiatry,* 29:418–426.

Pini, LA, Ferrari, A, Guidetti, G, et al. (1985). Influence of flunarizine on the altered electronystagmographic (ENG) recordings in migraine. *Cephalalgia,* 5:173–175.

Pini, LA, Sternieri, E, Fabbri, L, et al. (1995). High efficacy and low frequency of headache recurrence after oral sumatriptan. The Oral sumatriptan Italian Study Group. *J Int Med Res,* 23:96–105.

Piros, ET, Hales, TG, and Evans, CJ (1996). Functional analysis of cloned opioid receptors in transfected cell lines. *Neurochemical Res,* 21:1277–1285.

Pita, E, Higueras, A, Bolanos, J (1977). Propranolol and migraine: a clinical trial. *Arch Farmacol Toxicol,* 3:273–278.

Podell, RN (1984). Is migraine a manifestation of food allergy? *Postgrad Med*, 75:221–224.

Portenoy, RK, Foley, KM, and Inturrisi, CE (1990). The nature of opioid responsiveness and its implications for neuropathic pain: new hypotheses derived from studies of opioid infusions. *Pain*, 43:273–286.

Potter, DL, Hart, DE, Calder, CS, et al. (2000). A double-blind, randomized, placebo-controlled, parallel study to determine the efficacy of topiramate in the prophylactic treatment of migraine. *Neurology*, 54:A15 (Abstract).

Pradalier, A, Clapin, A, and Dry, J (1988). Treatment review: nonsteroid antiinflammatory drugs in the treatment and long-term prevention of migraine attacks. *Headache*, 28:550–557.

Pradalier, A, Rancurel, G, Dordain, G, et al. (1985). Acute migraine attack therapy: comparison of naproxen sodium and an ergotamine tartrate compound. *Cephalalgia*, 5:107–113.

Pradalier, A, Serratrice, G, Colard, M, et al. (1989). Long-acting propranolol on migraine prophylaxis: results of a double-blind, placebo-controlled study. *Cephalalgia*, 9:247–253.

Prendes, JL (1980). Consideration on use of propranolol in complicated migraine. *Headache*, 20:93–95.

Prensky, AL (1987). Migraine in children. In *Migraine: Clinical and Research Aspects* (JN Blau, ed.), pp. 31–53. Johns Hopkins University Press, Baltimore.

Presthus, J (1971). BC105 and methysergide (deseril) in migraine prophylaxis. *Acta Neurol Scand*, 47:514–518.

Price, WA and Giannini, AJ (1986). Neurotoxicity caused by lithium-verapamil synergism. *J Clin Pharmacol*, 26:717–719.

Price, WA and Shalley, JE (1987). Lithium-verapamil toxicity in the elderly. *JAGS*, 35:177–179.

Pryse-Phillips, W (1999). Comparison of oral eletriptan (40–80 mg) and oral sumatriptan (50–100 mg) for the treatment of acute migraine: a randomized, placebo-controlled trial in sumatriptan-naive patients. *Cephalalgia*, 19:355 (Abstract).

Rabkin, R, Stables, DP, Levin, NW, et al. (1966). The prophylactic value of propranolol in angina pectoris. *Am J Cardiol*, 18:370–383.

Ramadan, NM (2004). Prophylactic migraine therapy: mechanisms and evidence. *Curr Pain Headache Rep*, 8:91–95.

Ramadan, NM, Silberstein, SD, Freitag, FG, et al. (1999). Evidence-based guidelines of the pharmacological management for prevention of migraine for the primary care provider. *Neurology*. Available: http://www.neurology.org

Ramadan, NM, Silberstein, SD, Freitag, FG, et al. (2000). Evidence-based guidelines for migraine headache in the primary care setting: pharmacological management for prevention of migraine. *Neurology*. Available: http://www.neurology.org.

Rampello, L, Alvano, A, Chiechio, S, et al. (2004). Evaluation of the prophylactic efficacy of amitriptyline and citalopram, alone or in combination, in patients with comorbidity of depression, migraine, and tension-type headache. *Neuropsychobiology*, 50:322–328.

Rao, BS, Das, DG, Taraknath, VR, et al. (2000). A double blind controlled study of propranolol and cyproheptadine in migraine prophylaxis. *Neurol India*, 48:223–226.

Rapoport, A, Ryan, R, Goldstein, J, et al. (2002). Dose range-finding studies with frovatriptan in the acute treatment of migraine. *Headache*, 42(Suppl. 2): S74–S83.

Rapoport, AM, Ramadan, NM, Adelman, JU, et al. (1997). Optimizing the dose of zolmitriptan (Zomig, 311C90) for the acute treatment of migraine: a multicenter, double-blind, placebo-controlled, dose range-finding study. 017 Clinical Trial Study Group. *Neurology*, 49:1210–1218.

Rapoport, AM, Sheftell, FD, and Gordon, B (1989). The successful treatment of migraine with anticonvulsant medication in patients with abnormal EEGs. *Headache*, 29:309.

Rapoport, AM, Visser, WH, Cutler, NR, et al. (1995). Oral sumatriptan in preventing headache recurrence after treatment of migraine attacks with subcutaneous sumatriptan. *Neurology*, 45:1505–1509.

Rapoport, AM and Weeks, RE (1988). Characteristics and treatment of analgesic rebound headache. In *Drug-induced Headache* (HC Diener and M Wilkinson, eds), pp. 162–167. Springer-Verlag, Berlin.

Rascol, A, Montastruc, JL, and Rascol, O (1986). Flunarizine versus pizotifen: a double-blind study in the prophylaxis of migraine. *Headache*, 26:83–85.

Raskin, NH (1981). Chemical headaches. *Ann Rev Med*, 32:63–71.

Raskin, NH (1986). Repetitive intravenous dihydroergotamine as therapy for intractable migraine. *Neurology*, 36:995–997.

Raskin, NH (1988a). *Headache*. Churchill-Livingstone, New York.

Raskin, NH (1988b). Migraine treatment. In *Headache* (NH Raskin, ed.), Churchill-Livingstone, New York.

Raskin, NH (1990). Modern pharmacotherapy of migraine. *Neurol Clin*, 8:857–865.

Rasmussen, BK, Jensen, R, Schroll, M, et al. (1991). Epidemiology of headache in a general population-a prevalence study. *J Clin Epidemiol*, 44:1147–1157.

Ratinahirana, H, Darbois, Y, and Bousser, MG (1990). Migraine and pregnancy: a prospective study in 703 women after delivery. *Neurology*, 40:437.

Reisine T, Pasternak G (1996). Opioid analgesics and antagonists. In *Goodman & Gilman's The Pharmacological Basis of Therapeutics* (JG Hardman, LE Limbird, PB Molinoff, et al., eds), pp. 521–556. McGraw-Hill, New York.

Reutens, DC, Fatovich, DM, Stewart-Wynne, EG, et al. (1991). Is intravenous lidocaine clinically effective in acute migraine? *Cephalalgia*, 11:245–247.

Richardson, JW and Richelson, E (1984). Antidepressants: a clinical update for medical practitioners. *Mayo Clin Proc*, 59:330–337.

Richelson, E (1990). Antidepressants and brain neurochemistry. *Mayo Clin Proc*, 65:1227–1236.

Richman, PB, Allegra, J, Eskin, B, et al. (2002). A randomized clinical trial to assess the efficacy of intramuscular droperidol for the treatment of acute migraine headache. *Am J Emerg Med*, 20:39–42.

Riopelle, R and McCans, JL (1982). A pilot study of the calcium channel antagonist diltiazem in migraine syndrome prophylaxis. *Can J Neurol Sci*, 9:269.

Roche, KW, O'Brien, RJ, Mammen, AL, et al. (1996). Characterization of multiple phosphorylation sites on the AMP receptor GluR1 subunit. *Neuron*, 16:1179–1188.

Rogawski, MA and Porter, RJ (1990). Antiepileptic drugs: pharmacological mechanisms and clinical efficacy with consideration of promising development stage compounds. *Pharmacol Rev*, 42:223–286.

Rohr, J and Dufresne, JJ (1985). Dihydroergotamine nasal spray for the treatment of migraine attacks: a comparative double-blind crossover study with placebo. *Cephalalgia*, 5:142–143.

Rompel, H and Bauermeister, PW (1970). Aetiology of migraine and prevention with carbamazepine (Tegretol). *S Afr Med J*, 44:75–80.

Rosen, JA (1983). Observations on the efficacy of propranolol for the prophylaxis of migraine. *Ann Neurol*, 13:92–93.

Rosen, N, Silberstein, S, and Abbas, MA (2006). Effect of lidocaine infusion in the treatment of refractory chronic daily headache—a retrospective study. *Neurology*, 66: A224 (Abstract).

Rosenberg, JH and Silberstein, SD (2005). The headache of SAH responds to sumatriptan. *Headache*, 45:597–598.

Rosenorn, J, Eskesen, V, and Schmidt, K (1988). Unruptured intracranial aneurysms: an assessment of the annual risk of rupture based on epidemiological and clinical data. *J Neurosurg*, 2:369–377.

Roth, BL, Craigo, SC, Choudhary, MS, et al. (1994). Binding of typical and atypical antipsychotic agents to 5-hydroxytryptamine-6 and 5-hydroxytryptamine-7 receptors. *J Pharmacol Exp Ther*, 268:1403–1410.

Rowat, BM, Merrill, CF, Davis, A, et al. (1991). A double-blind comparison of granisetron and placebo for the treatment of acute migraine in the emergency department. *Cephalalgia*, 11:207–213.

Rozen, TD (2000). Treatment of a prolonged migrainous aura with intravenous furosemide. *Neurology*, 55:732–733.

Rozen, TD (2003). Aborting a prolonged migrainous aura with intravenous prochlorperazine and magnesium sulfate. *Headache*, 43:901–903.

Rozen, TD, Oshinsky, ML, Gebeline, CA, et al. (2002). Open label trial of coenzyme Q10 as a migraine preventive. *Cephalalgia*, 22:137–141.

Ruat, M, Traiffort, E, Arrang, JM, et al. (1993). A novel rat serotonin (5-HT6) receptor: molecular cloning, localization, and stimulation of cAMP accumulation. *Biochem Biophys Res Commun*, 193:268–276.

Russell, MB and Olesen, J (1995). Increased familial risk and evidence of genetic factor in migraine. *Br Med J*, 311:541–544.

Ryan, R, Elkind, A, Baker, CC, et al. (1997). Sumatriptan nasal spray for the acute treatment of migraine: results of two clinical studies. *Neurology*, 49:1225–1230.

Ryan, RE (1968). Double-blind crossover comparison of BC105, methysergide, and placebo in the prophylaxis of migraine headache. *Headache*, 8:118–126.

Ryan, RE (1970). Double-blind clinical evaluation of the efficacy and safety of ergostine–caffeine and placebo in migraine headache. *Headache*, 9:212–220.

Ryan, RE (1971). BC105, a new preparation for the interval treatment of migraine: a double blind evaluation compared with placebo. *Headache*, 11:6–18.

Ryan, RE (1974). A study of Midrin[R] in the symptomatic relief of migraine headache. Headache 14:33–42.

Ryan, RE (1984). Comparative study of nadolol and propranolol in prophylactic treatment of migraine. *Am Heart J*, 108:1156–1159.

Ryan, RE and Diamond, S (1975). Double-blind study of clonidine and placebo for the prophylactic treatment of migraine. *Headache*, 15:202–210.

Ryan, RE and Sudilovsky, A (1983). Nadolol: its use in the prophylactic treatment of migraine. *Headache*, 23:26–31.

Saadah, HA (1992). Abortive headache therapy in the office with interavenous dihydroergotamine plus prochlorperazine. *Headache*, 32:143–146.

Sachdeo, RC, Sachdeo, SK, Walker, SA, et al. (1996). Steady-state pharmacokinetics of topiramate and carbamazepine in patients with epilepsy during monotherapy and concomitant therapy. *Epilepsia*, 37:774–780.

Sachedo, RC, Reife, RA, Lim, P, et al. (1997). Topiramate monotherapy for partial onset seizures. *Epilepsia*, 38:294–300.

Saito, K, Markowtiz, S, and Moskowitz, MA (1988a). Ergot alkaloids block neurogenic extravasation in dura mater: proposed action in vascular headaches. *Ann Neurol*, 24:732–737.

Saito, K, Markowtiz, S, and Moskowitz, MA (1988b). Ergot alkaloids specifically block the development of neurogenic inflammation within the dura mater induced by chemical or electrical stimulation. *Ann Neurol*, 24:732–737.

Sales, F and Bada, JL (1975). Practolol and migraine. *Lancet*, 1:742.

Salfield, SA, Waywardly, BL, and Houlsby, WT (1987). Controlled study of exclusion of dietary vasoactive amines in migraine. *Arch Dis Childhood*, 62:458–460.

Salonen, R, Ashford, E, Dahlof, C, et al. (1994). Intranasal sumatriptan for the acute treatment of migraine.

International Intranasal Sumatriptan Study Group. *J Neurol*, 241:463–469 (Abstract).

Sanchez-del Rio, M, Bakker, D, Wu, O, et al. (1999). Perfusion weighted imaging during migraine: spontaneous visual aura and headache. *Cephalalgia*, 19:701–707.

Sanders, SW, Haering, N, Mosberg, H, et al. (1986). Pharmacokinetics of ergotamine in healthy volunteers following oral and rectal dosing. *Eur J Clin Pharmacol*, 30:331–334.

Sanders-Bush, E, Fentress, H, and Hazelwood, L (2003). Serotonin 5-ht2 receptors: molecular and genomic diversity. *Mol Interv*, 3:319–330.

Sanders-Bush, E and Mayer, SE (2001). 5-Hydroxytryptamine (serotonin): receptor agonists and antagonists. In *Goodman & Gilman's The Pharmacological Basis Of Therapeutics* (JG Hardman, LE Limbird, and A Goodman-Gilman, eds), pp. 269–290. McGraw-Hill, New York.

Sandor, PS, diClemente, L, Coppola, G, et al. (2003). Coenzyme Q10 for migraine prophylaxis: a randomized controlled trial. *Cephalalgia*, 23:577 (Abstract).

Sangiorgi, S, Mochi, M, Riva, R, et al. (1994). Abnormal platelet mitochondrial function in patients affected by migraine with and without aura. *Cephalalgia*, 14:21–23.

Santanello, NC, Polis, AB, Hartmaier, SL, et al. (1997). Improvement in migraine-specific quality of life in a clinical trial of rizatriptan. *Cephalalgia*, 17:867–872.

Saper, J, Dahlof, C, So, Y, et al. (2006). Rofecoxib in the acute treatment of migraine: a randomized controlled clinical trial. *Headache*, 46:264–275.

Saper, JR (1983). *Headache Disorders: Current Concepts in Treatment Strategies*. Wright-PSG, Littleton.

Saper, JR (1986). Changing perspectives of chronic headache. *Clin J Pain*, 2:19–28.

Saper, JR (1989). Chronic headache syndromes. *Neurol Clin*, 7:387–412.

Saper, JR (1990). Chronic headache syndromes. *Neurol Clin*, 8:891–901.

Saper, JR, Lake, AE, Hamel, RH, et al. (2000). Sustained, scheduled opioid therapy for patients with intractable headache: a 5-year prospective study. Presented to the American Headache Society, ACHE Award Lecture, Montreal, Quebec, June.

Saper, JR, Lake, AE, and Tepper, SJ (2001). Nefazodone for chronic daily headache prophylaxis: an open-label study. *Headache*, 41:465–474.

Saper, JR, Mathew, NT, Loder, EW, et al. (2007). A double-blind, randmoized, placebo-controlled comparison of botulinum toxin type A injection sites and doses in the prevention of episodic migraine. *Pain Med*, published articles online: 1-Feb-2007.

Saper, JR, Silberstein, SD, Gordon, CD, et al. (1993). *Handbook of Headache Management*. Williams & Wilkins, Baltimore.

Saper, JR, Silberstein, SD, Gordon, CD, et al. (1999a). *Handbook of Headache Management: A Practical Guide to Diagnosis and Treatment of Head, Neck, and Facial Pain*. Lippincott Williams & Wilkins, Inc., Baltimore.

Saper, JR, Silberstein, SD, Gordon, CD, et al. (1999b). Medications used in the pharmacotherapy of headache. In *Handbook of Headache Management: A Practical Guide to Diagnosis and Treatment of Head, Neck, and Facial Pain*. (JR Saper, SD Silberstein, CD Gordon, et al., eds), pp. 61–145. Lippincott Williams & Wilkins, Inc., Baltimore.

Saper, JR, Silberstein, SD, Lake, AE, et al. (1994). Double-blind trial of fluoxetine: chronic daily headache and migraine. *Headache*, 34:497–502.

Sargent, J, Kirchner, JR, Davis, R, et al. (1995). Oral sumatriptan is effective and well tolerated for the acute treatment of migraine: results of a multicenter study. *Neurology*, 45:S10–S14.

Sargent, J, Solbach, P, Damasio, H, et al. (1985). A comparison of naproxen sodium to propranolol hydrochloride and a placebo control for the prophylaxis of migraine headache. *Headache*, 25:320–324.

Sargent, JD, Baumel, B, Peters, K, et al. (1988). Aborting a migraine attack: naproxen sodium versus ergotamine plus caffeine. *Headache*, 28:263–266.

Sawynok, J, Reid, A, and Poon, A (1998). Peripheral antinociceptive effect of an adenosine kinase inhibitor, with augmentation by an adenosine deaminase inhibitor, in the rat formalin test. *Pain*, 74:75–81.

Sawynok, J, Reid, AR, and Esser, MJ (1999). Peripheral antinociceptive action of amitriptyline in the rat formalin test: involvement of adenosine. *Pain*, 80:45–55.

Saxena, PR (1972). The effects of antimigraine drugs on the vascular responses evoked by 5-hydroxytryptamine and related biogenic substances on the external carotid bed of dogs: possible pharmacologic implications to their antimigraine action. *Headache*, 12:44–54.

Saxena, PR (1974). Selective vasoconstriction in carotid vascular bed by methysergide: possible relevance to its antimigraine effect. *Eur J Pharmacol*, 27:99–105.

Saxena, PR and DeVlaam, SG (1974). Role of some biogenic substances in migraine and relevant mechanism in antimigraine action of ergotamine. Studies in an animal experimental model for migraine. *Headache*, 13:142–163.

Saxena, PR, Duncker, DJ, Bom, AH, et al. (1986). Effects of MDL72222 and methiothepin on carotid vascular responses to 5-hydroxytryptamine in the pig: evidence for the presence of vascular 5-hydroxytryptamine1-like receptors. *Arch Pharmacol*, 333:198–204.

Saxena, PR and Tfelt-Hansen, P (2006). Triptans, 5-HT1B/1D receptor agonists in the acute treatment of migraines. In *The Headaches*, (J Olesen, PJ Goadsby, NM Ramadan, et al., eds), pp. 459–468. Lippincott Williams &Wilkins, Philadelphia.

Saxena, PR, VanHouwelingen, P, and Bonta, IL (1971). The effect of mianserin hydrochloride on the vascular responses to 5-hydroxytryptamine and related substances. *Eur J Pharmacol*, 13:295–305.

Saxena, PR and Verdouw, PD (1984). Effects of methysergide and 5-hydroxytryptamine on carotid blood flow distribution in pigs: further evidence for the presence of atypical 5-HT receptors. *Br J Pharmacol*, 82:817–826.

Schamburg, HH, Byck, R, Gerstl, R, et al. (1969). Monosodium L-glutamate: its pharmacology and role in the Chinese restaurant syndrome. *Science*, 163:826–828.

Scharff, L and Marcus, DA (1999). The association between chocolate and migraine: a review. *Headache Q*, 10:199–205.

Scherl, ER and Wilson, JF (1995). Comparison of dihydroergotamine with metoclopramide versus meperidine with promethazine in the treatment of acute migraine. *Headache*, 35:256–259.

Schiffman, SS, Buckley, CE III, Sampson, HA, et al. (1987). Aspartame and susceptibility to headache. *N Eng J Med*, 317:1181.

Schiffmann, SS, Buckley, CE, Sampson, HA, et al. (1987). Aspartame and susceptibility to headache. *N Engl J Med*, 317:1181–1185.

Schmidt, R and Fanchamps, A (1974). Effect of caffeine on intestinal absorption of ergotamine in man. *Eur J Clin Pharmacol*, 7:213–216.

Schoenen, J, Jacquy, J, and Lenaerts, M (1998). Effectiveness of high-dose riboflavin in migraine prophylaxis. A randomized controlled trial. *Neurology*, 50:466–470.

Schoenen, J, Maertens de Noordout, A, Timsit-Bertheir, M, et al. (1986). Contingent negative variation and efficacy of β-blocking agents in migraine. *Cephalalgia*, 6:231–233.

Schoenen, J and Thomsen, LL (2000). Neurophysiology and autonomic dysfunction in migraine. In *The Headaches* (J Olesen, P Tfelt-Hansen, KMA Welch, eds), pp. 301–312. Lippincott Williams & Wilkins, Philadelphia.

Scholpp, J, Schellenberg, R, Moeckesch, B, et al. (2004). Early treatment of a migraine attack while pain is still mild increases the efficacy of sumatriptan. *Cephalalgia*, 24:925–933.

Scholte, HR, Busch, HF, Bakker, HD, et al. (1995). Riboflavin-responsive complex I deficiency. *Biochimica et Biophysica Acta*, 1271:75–83.

Scholz, M and Hoffert, M (1987). Low dose nifedipine is no better than vehicle in abortive treatment of classic migraine headache. 5th World Congress on Pain IASP.

Schrader, H, Stovner, LJ, Helde, G (2001). Prophylactic treatment of migraine with angiotensin converting enzyme inhibitor (lisinopril): randomized, placebo-controlled, crossover study. *Br Med J*, 322:19–22.

Schran, HF and Tse, FLS (1985). Pharmacokinetics of dihydroergotamine following subcutaneous administration in humans. *Int J Clin Pharmacol Ther Toxicol*, 23:1–4.

Scott, RJ, Aitchison, WR, Barker, PR, et al. (1996). Oral sumatriptan in the acute treatment of migraine and migraine recurrence in general practice. *QJM*, 89:613–622.

Sculpher, M, Millson, D, Meddis, D, et al. (2002). Cost-effectiveness analysis of stratified versus stepped care strategies for acute treatment of migraine: the Disability in Strategies for Care (DISC) Study. *Pharmacoeconomics*, 20:91–100.

Seibyl, JP, Krystal, JH, Price, LH, et al. (1991). Effects of ritanserin on the behavioral, neuroendocrine, and cardiovascular responses to metachlorophenylpiperazine in healthy human subjects. *Psychiatry Res*, 38:227–236.

Shafar, J, Tallett, ER, and Knowlson, PA (1972). Evaluation of clonidine in prophylaxis of migraine. Double-blind trial and followup. *Lancet*, 1:403–407.

Shank, RP, Gardocki, JF, Streeter, AJ, et al. (2000). An overview of the preclinical aspects of topiramate: pharmacology, pharmacokinetics, and mechanism of action. *Epilepsia*, 41:S3–S9.

Shank, RP, Gardocki, JF, Vaught, JL, et al. (1994). Topiramate: preclinical evaluation of structurally novel anticonvulsant. *Epilepsia*, 35:450–460.

Shanks, RG (1987). A review of the relationship between beta-adrenoreceptor antagonists and their action in migraine. In *Advances in Headache Research* (FC Rose, ed.), pp. 161–166. John Libbey, London.

Sharma, S, Prasad, A, Nehru, R, et al. (2002). Efficacy and tolerability of prochlorperazine buccal tablets in treatment of acute migraine. *Headache*, 42:896–902.

Sheftell, F, Ryan, R, and Pitman, V (2003). Efficacy, safety, and tolerability of oral eletriptan for treatment of acute migraine: a multicenter, double-blind, placebo-controlled study conducted in the United States. *Headache*, 43:202–213.

Sheftell, FD, Dahlof, CG, Brandes, JL, et al. (2005). Two replicate randomized, double-blind, placebo-controlled trials of the time to onset of pain relief in the acute treatment of migraine with a fast-disintegrating/rapid-release formulation of sumatriptan tablets. *Clin Ther*, 27:407–417.

Shekelle, RB and Ostfeld, AM (1964). Methysergide in the migraine syndrome. *Clin Pharmacol Ther*, 5:201–204.

Shimell, CJ, Fritz, VU, and Levien, SL (1990). A comparative trial of flunarizine and propranolol in the prevention of migraine. *S Afr Med J*, 77:75–77.

Shrestha, M, Singh, R, Moreden, J, et al. (1996). Ketorolac vs chlorpromazine in the treatment of acute migraine without aura. A prospective, randomized, double-blind trial. *Arch Intern Med*, 156:1725–1728.

Shuaib, A, Ahmed, F, Muratoglu, M, et al. (1999). Topiramate in migraine prophylaxis: a pilot study. *Cephalalgia*, 19:379–380 (Abstract).

Shukla, R, Garg, RK, Nag, D, et al. (1995). Nifedipine in migraine and tension headache: a randomized double-blind crossover study. *J Assoc Physicians India*, 43:770–772.

Shulman, KI and Walker, SE (1999). Refining the MAOI diet. Tyramine content of pizzas and soy products. *J Clin Psychiatr*, 60:191–193.

Sicuteri, F (1973). The ingestion of serotonin precursors (L-5-hydroxytryptophan and L-tryptophan) improves migraine headache. *Headache*, 13:19–22.

Sigel, E (1995). Functional modulation of ligand-gated $GABA_A$ and NMDA receptor channels by phosphorylation. *J Receptor Signal Transduction Res*, 15:325–332.

Silberstein, S, Diamond, S, Loder, E, et al. (2005). Prevalence of migraine sufferers who are candidates for preventive therapy: results from the American migraine study (AMPP) study. *Headache*, 45:770–771 (Abstract).

Silberstein, SD (1984). Treatment of headache in primary care practice. *Am J Med*, 77:65–72.

Silberstein, SD (1990). Twenty questions about headaches in children and adolescents. *Headache*, 30:716–727.

Silberstein, SD (1991). Appropriate use of abortive medication in headache treatment. *Pain Mgt*, 4:22–28.

Silberstein, SD (1994). Review: serotonin (5-HT) and migraine. *Headache*, 34:408–417.

Silberstein, SD (1996). Divalproex sodium in headache—literature review and clinical guidelines. *Headache*, 36:547–555.

Silberstein, SD (1997a). Migraine and pregnancy. *Neurologic Clin*, 15:209–231.

Silberstein, SD (1997b). Preventive treatment of migraine: an overview. *Cephalalgia*, 17:67–72.

Silberstein, SD (1998). Drug-induced headache. *Neurol Clin N Amer*, 16:107–123.

Silberstein, SD (2000a). Drug, food, and chemical related headaches. In (Cooney TG, Kumar K, eds) (in press).

Silberstein, SD (2000b). Practice parameter—evidence-based guidelines for migraine headache (an evidence-based review): Report of the Quality Standards Subcommittee of the American Academy of Neurology for the United States Headache Consortium. *Neurology*, 55:754–762.

Silberstein, SD (2002). Control of topiramate-induced paresthesias with supplemental potassium (Letter). *Headache*, 42:85.

Silberstein, SD (2004a). Headaches in pregnancy. *Neurol Clin*, 22:727–756.

Silberstein, SD (2004b). Migraine pathophysiology and its clinical implications. *Cephalalgia*, 24(Suppl. 2):2–7.

Silberstein, SD (2007a). Migraine, pregnancy and lactation. In *Sex Hormones and Headache* (S Silberstein, ed.), pp. 109–131. Current Medicine Group LLC, Philadelphia.

Silberstein, SD (2007b). *Sex Hormones and Headache*, Current Medicine Group, Philadelphia.

Silberstein, SD, Feliu, AL, Rupow, MFT, et al. (2007). Topiramate in migraine prophylaxis: long-term impact on resource utilization and cost. *Headache*, 47:500–510.

Silberstein, SD, Fozard, JR, and Murphy, L (1992). Letter to the editor. *Headache*, 32:242–243.

Silberstein, SD and Goadsby, PJ (2002). Migraine: preventive treatment. *Cephalalgia*, 22:491–512.

Silberstein, SD, Hulihan, J, Karim, MR, et al. (2006). Efficacy and tolerability of topiramate 200 mg/d in the prevention of migraine with/without aura in adults: a randomized, placebo-controlled, double-blind, 12-week pilot study. *Clin Ther*, 28:1002–1011.

Silberstein, SD and Lipton, RB (1996). Migraine epidemiology. *Neurol Clin*, 14:421–434.

Silberstein, SD, Lipton, RB, and Breslau, N (1995). Migraine: association with personality characteristics and psychopathology. *Cephalalgia*, 15:337–369.

Silberstein, SD, Lipton, RB, and Goadsby, PJ (1998). Migraine: diagnosis and treatment. In *Headache in Clinical Practice* (SD Silberstein, RB Lipton, and PJ Goadsby, eds), pp. 61–90. Isis Medical Media Ltd., Oxford.

Silberstein, SD, Lipton, RB, and Sliwinski, M (1996). Classification of daily and near-daily headaches: field trial of revised IHS criteria. *Neurology*, 47:871–875.

Silberstein, SD, Mathew, N, Saper, J, et al. (2000). Botulinum toxin type A as a migraine preventive treatment: for the Botox® Migraine Clinical Research Group. *Headache*, 40:445–450.

Silberstein, SD and McCrory, DC (1999). Opioids. In (HC Diener, ed.) Karger, Switzerland.

Silberstein, SD and McCrory, DC (2001). Butalbital-containing compounds for the treatment of tension-type and migraine headache. *Headache*, 41:953–967.

Silberstein, SD and Merriam, GR (1997). Sex hormones and headache. In *Headache* (PJ Goadsby and SD Silberstein, eds), pp. 143–173. Butterworth-Heinemann, Newton.

Silberstein, SD, Neto, W, Schmitt, J, et al. (2004). Topiramate in migraine prevention: results of a large controlled trial. *Arch Neurol*, 61:490–495.

Silberstein, SD and on behalf of the Quality Standards Improvement Committee (2007). Practice parameter: evidence-based guidelines for treatment of migraine headache. *Neurology* (in press).

Silberstein, SD, Schulman, EA, and Hopkins, MM (1990). Repetitive intravenous DHE in the treatment of refractory headache. *Headache*, 30:334–339.

Silberstein, SD and Silberstein, MM (1990). New concepts in the pathogenesis of headache. Part II. *Pain Mgt*, 3:334–342.

Silberstein, SD, Stark, S, DeRossett, SE, et al. (2006). Superior clinical benefits of a new single-tablet formulation of sumatriptan formulated with RT technology and naproxen sodium. *Neurology*, 66(Suppl. 2):A254 (Abstract).

Silberstein, SD, Young, WB, Mendizabal, JE, et al. (2003). Acute migraine treatment with droperidol: a randomized, double-blind, placebo-controlled trial. *Neurology*, 60:315–321.

Silberstein, SD, Winner, PK, and Chmiel, JJ (2003). Migraine preventive medication reduces resource utilization. *Headache*, 43:171–178.

Simon, MI, Strathmann, MP, and Gautam, N (1991). Diversity of G proteins in signal transduction. *Science*, 252:802–909.

Siuciak, JA, Boylan, C, Fritsche, M, et al. (1996). BDNF increases monoaminergic activity in rat brain following intracerebroventricular or intraparenchymal administration. *Brain Res*, 710:11–20.

Sjaastad, O and Dale, I (1976). A new (?) clinical headache entity: chronic paroxysmal hemicrania. 2. *Acta Neurol Scand*, 54:140–159.

Sjaastad, O and Spierings, EL (1984). Hemicrania continua: another headache absolutely responsive to indomethacin. *Cephalalgia*, 4:65–70.

Sjaastad, O and Stensrud, P (1969). Appraisal of BC105 in migraine prophylaxis. *Acta Neurol Scand*, 45:594–600.

Sjaastad, O and Stensrud, P (1971). 2-(2.6-dichlorophenylamino)-2-imidazoline hydrochloride (ST 155 or Catapresan) as a prophylactic remedy against migraine. *Acta Neurol Scand*, 47:120–122.

Sjaastad, O and Stensrud, P (1972). Clinical trial of a beta-receptor blocking agent (LB46) in migraine prophylaxis. *Acta Neurol Scand*, 48:124–128.

Skolnick, P, Legutko, B, Li, X, et al. (2001). Current perspectives on the development of non-biogenic amine-based antidepressants. *Pharmacol Res*, 43:411–423.

Smith, MA, Makino, S, Kvetnansky, R, et al. (1995). Stress and glucocorticoids affect the expression of brain-derived neurotrophic factor and neurotrophin-3 mRNAs in the hippocampus. *J Neurosci*, 15:1768–1777.

Smith, R and Schwartz, A (1984). Diltiazem prophylaxis in refractory migraine. *N Engl J Med*, 310:1327–1328.

Smith, TR, Sunshine, A, Stark, SR, et al. (2005). Sumatriptan and naproxen sodium for the acute treatment of migraine. *Headache*, 45:983–991.

Smyth, GA and Lazarus, L (1974). Suppression of growth hormone secretion by melatonin and cyproheptadine. *J Clin Invest*, 54:116–121.

Snyder, SH and Reynolds, IJ (1985). Calcium-antagonist drugs: receptor interactions that clarify therapeutic effects. *N Eng J Med*, 313:995–1002.

Solomon, G and Kunkel, R (1990). Effects of fluoxetine on premenstrual syndrome in chronic headache sufferers. *Headache*, 30:301.

Solomon, GD (1986). Verapamil and propranolol in migraine prophylaxis: a double-blind crossover study. *Headache*, 26:325.

Solomon, GD (1989). Management of the headache patient with medical illness. *Clin J Pain*, 5:95–99.

Solomon, GD, Cady, RK, Klapper, JA, et al. (1997). Clinical efficacy and tolerability of 2.5mg zolmitriptan for the acute treatment of migraine. *Neurology*, 49:1219–1225.

Somerville, BW (1971). The role of progesterone in menstrual migraine. *Neurology*, 21:853–859.

Somerville, BW (1972). A study of migraine in pregnancy. *Neurology*, 22:824–828.

Somerville, BW (1976). Platelet-bound and free serotonin levels in jugular and forearm venous blood during migraine. *Neurology*, 26:41–45.

Sorensen, PS, Hansen, K, and Olesen, J (1986). A placebo-controlled, double-blind, cross-over trial of flunarizine in common migraine. *Cephalalgia*, 6:7–14.

Sorensen, PS, Larsen, BH, Rasmussen, MJ, et al. (1991). Flunarizine versus metoprolol in migraine prophylaxis: a double-blind, randomized parallel group study of efficacy and tolerability. *Headache*, 31(10):657.

Soyka, D, Taneri, Z, Oestreich, W, et al. (1989). Flunarizine IV in the acute treatment of common or classical migraine attacks—a placebo-controlled double-blind trial. *Headache*, 29:21–27.

Speed, WG (1989). Closed head injury sequelae: changing concepts. *Headache*, 29:643–647.

Spierings, EL (1984). The role of arteriovenous shunting in migraine. In *The Pharmacological Basis of Migraine Therapy* (WK Amery, JV VanNueten, and A Wauquier, eds), pp. 36–49. Pitman, London.

Spierings, EL (1989). Treatment of the migraine attack. In *Migraine and Other Headaches* (MD Ferrari and X Lataste, eds), pp. 241–248. Parthenon, Park Ridge, New Jersey.

Spierings, EL, Rapoport, AM, Dodick, DW, et al. (2004). Acute treatment of migraine with zolmitriptan 5 mg orally disintegrating tablet. *CNS Drugs*, 18:1133–1141.

Stark, R, Dahlof, C, Haughie, S, et al. (2002). Efficacy, safety and tolerability of oral eletriptan in the acute treatment of migraine: results of a phase III, multicentre, placebo-controlled study across three attacks. *Cephalalgia*, 22:23–32.

Steardo, L, Bonuso, S, DiStasio, E, et al. (1982). Selective and nonselective beta-blockers: are both effective in prophylaxis of migraine? A clinical trial versus methysergide. *Acta Neurol*, 4:196–204.

Steardo, L, Marano, E, Barone, P, et al. (1986). Prophylaxis of migraine attacks with a calcium-channel blocker; flunarizine versus methysergide. *J Clin Pharmacol*, 26:524–528.

Steiner, TJ, Ahmed, F, Findley, LJ, et al. (1998). S-fluoxetine in the prophylaxis of migraine: a phase II double-blind randomized placebo-controlled study. *Cephalalgia*, 18:283–286.

Steiner, TJ, Findley, LJ, and Yuen, AW (1997). Lamotrigine versus placebo in the prophylaxis of migraine with and without aura. *Cephalalgia*, 17:109–112.

Steiner, TJ, Joseph, R, Hedman, C, et al. (1988). Metoprolol in the prophylaxis of migraine: parallel-groups comparison with placebo and dose-ranging followup. *Headache*, 28:15–23.

Stellar, S, Ahrens, SP, Meibohm, AR, et al. (1984). Migraine prevention with timolol: a double-blind crossover study. *JAMA*, 252:2576–2580.

Stensrud, P and Sjaastad, O (1974). Clinical trial of a new antibradykinin, antiinflammatory drug, ketoprofen (19.583 r.p.) in migraine prophylaxis. *Headache*, 14:96–100.

Stensrud, P and Sjaastad, O (1976a). Clonidine (Catapresan)-double-blind study after long-term treatment with the drug in migraine. *Acta Neurol Scand*, 53:233–236.

Stensrud, P and Sjaastad, O (1976b). Short-term trial of propranolol in racemic form (Inderal), d-propranolol and placebo in migraine. *Acta Neurol Scand,* 53:229–232.

Stensrud, P and Sjaastad, O (1979). Clonazepam (rivotril) in migraine prophylaxis. *Headache,* 19:333–334.

Stiell, IG, Dufour, DG, Moher, D, et al. (1991). Methotrimeprazine versus meperidine and dimenhydrinate in the treatment of severe migraine: a randomized, controlled trial. *Ann Emerg Med,* 20:1201–1205.

Stoica, E and Enulescu, O (1990). Propranolol corrects the abnormal catecholamine response to light during migraine. *Eur Neurol,* 30:19–22.

Storer, RJ and Goadsby, PJ (2003). Topiramate inhibits trigeminovascular traffic in the cat: a possible locus of action in the prevention of migraine. *Neurology,* 60: A238 (Abstract).

Strassman, AM, Raymond, SA, and Burstein, R (1996). Sensitization of meningeal sensory neurons and the origin of headaches. *Nature,* 384:560–564.

Streeter, AJ, Stahle, PL, Hills, JF, et al. (1994). Pharmacokinetics of topiramate in the rat. *Pharm Res,* 11:372.

Subcutaneous Sumatriptan International Study Group (1991). Treatment of migraine attacks with sumatriptan. *N Engl J Med,* 325:316–321.

Sudilovsky, A, Elkind, AH, Ryan, RE, et al. (1987). Comparative efficacy of nadolol and propranolol in the management of migraine. *Headache,* 27:421–426.

Sudilovsky, A, Stern, MA, and Meyer, JH (1986). Nadolol: the benefits of an adequate trial duration in the prophylaxis of migraine. *Headache,* 26:325.

Taiwo, YO and Levine, JD (1991). Further confirmation of the role of adenyl cyclase and of cAMP-dependent protein kinase in primary afferent hyperalgesia. *Neurosci,* 44:131–135.

Takeshima, T, Nishikawa, S, and Takashashi, K (1988). Sublingual administration of flunarizine for acute migraine: will flunarizine take the place of ergotamine? *Headache,* 28:602–606.

Tanen, DA, Miller, S, French, T, et al. (2003). Intravenous sodium valproate versus prochlorperazine for the emergency department treatment of acute migraine headaches: a prospective, randomized, double-blind trial. *Ann Emerg Med,* 41:847–853.

Teall, J, Tuchman, M, Cutler, N, et al. (1998). Rizatriptan (MAXALT) for the acute treatment of migraine and migraine recurrence. A placebo-controlled, outpatient study (Rizatriptan 022 Study Group). *Headache,* 38:281–287.

Tek, DS, McClellan, DS, Olshaker, JS, et al. (1990). A prospective, double-blind study of metoclopramide hydrochloride for the control of migraine in the emergency department. *Ann Emerg Med,* 19:1083–1087.

Tepper, SJ, Cochran, A, Hobbs, S, et al. (1998). Sumatriptan suppositories for the acute treatment of migraine. S2B351 Study Group. *Int J Clin Pract,* 52:31–35.

Tfelt-Hansen, P, Henry, P, Mulder, LJ, et al. (1995). The effectiveness of combined oral lysine acetylsalicylate and metoclopramide compared with oral sumatriptan for migraine. *Lancet,* 346:923–926.

Tfelt-Hansen, P and Lipton, RB (1993). Prioritizing treatment. In *The Headaches* (J Olesen, P Tfelt-Hansen, and KMA Welch, eds), pp. 359–362. Raven Press, New York.

Tfelt-Hansen, P and Olesen, J (1984). Effervescent metoclopramide and aspirin (Migravess) versus effervescent aspirin or placebo for migraine attacks: a double-blind study. *Cephalalgia,* 4:107–111.

Tfelt-Hansen, P, Olesen, J, Aebelholt-Krabbe, A, et al. (1980). A double blind study of metoclopramide in the treatment of migraine attacks. *J Neurol Neurosurg Psychiatry,* 43:369–371.

Tfelt-Hansen, P, Standnes, B, Kangasniemi, P, et al. (1984). Timolol vs propranolol vs placebo in common migraine prophylaxis: a double-blind multicenter trial. *Acta Neurol Scand,* 69:1–8.

Tfelt-Hansen P, Teall J, Rodriguez F, Giacovazzo M, Paz J, Malbecq W, Block GA, Reines SA, Visser WH. <http://www.ncbi.nlm.nih.gov.proxy1.lib.tju.edu:2048/sites/entrez?Db=pubmed&Cmd=ShowDetailView&TermToSearch=11284463&ordinalpos=12&itool=EntrezSystem2. PEntrez.Pubmed.Pubmed_ResultsPanel.Pubmed_RVDocSum>Oral rizatriptan versus oral sumatriptan: a direct comparative study in the acute treatment of migraine. Rizatriptan 030 Study Group.Headache. 1998 Nov-Dec;38(10):748–755.

Theis, M, Sohl, G, Eiberger, J, et al. (2005). Emerging complexities in identity and function of glial connexins. *Trends Neurosci,* 28:188–195.

Thomas, M, Behari, M, and Ahuja, GK (1991). Flunarizine in migraine prophylaxis: an Indian trial. *Headache,* 31:613–615.

Thomsen, LL, Iversen, HK, Lassen, LH, et al. (1994). The role of nitric oxide in migraine pain: therapeutic implications. *CNS Drugs,* 2:417–422.

Thomson Healthcare (2003). *Physicians' Desk Reference.* Thomson PDR, Montvale.

Tillgren, N (1947). Treatment of headache with dihydroergotamine tartrate. *Acta Med Scand,* 196:222–228.

Tobita, M, Hino, M, Ichikawa, N, et al. (1987). A case of hemiplegic migraine treated with flunarizine. *Headache,* 487–488.

Tokola, R and Hokkanan, E (1978). Propranolol for acute migraine. *Br Med J,* 2:1089.

Tokola, RA, Kangasniemi, P, Neuvonen, PJ, et al. (1984). Tolfenamic acid, metoclopramide, caffeine and their combinations in the treatment of migraine attacks. *Cephalalgia,* 4:253–263.

Tollefson, GD (1983). Monoamine oxidase inhibitors: a review. *J Clin Psychiatry,* 44:280–288.

Touchon, J, Bertin, L, Pilgrim, AJ, et al. (1996). A comparison of subcutaneous sumatriptan and dihydroergotamine nasal spray in the acute treatment of migraine. *Neurology,* 47:361–365.

Treves, TA, Streiffler, M, and Korczyn, AD (1992). Naproxen sodium versus ergotamine tartrate in the treatment of acute migraine attacks. *Headache*, 32:280–282.

Tronvik, E, Stovner, LJ, Helde, G, et al. (2003). Prophylactic treatment of migraine with an angiotensin II receptor blocker: a randomized controlled trial. *JAMA*, 289:65–69.

Tulunay, FC, Karan, O, Aydin, N, et al. (1987). Dihydroergotamine nasal spray during migraine attacks. A double-blind crossover study with placebo. *Cephalalgia*, 7:131–133.

Uddman, R, Edvinsson, L, Ekman, R, et al. (1985). Innervation of the feline cerebral vasculature by nerve fibers containing calcitonin gene-related peptide: trigeminal origin an co-existence with substance P. *Neurosci Lett*, 62:131–136.

Ustdal, M, Dogan, P, Soyeur, A, et al. (1989). Treatment of migraine with salmon calcitonin: effects on plasma beta-endorphin, ACTH, and cortisol levels. *Biomed Pharmacother*, 43:687–691.

Vainionpaa, LK, Rattya, J, Knip, M, et al. (1999). Valproate-induced hyperandrogenism during pubertal maturation in girls with epilepsy. *Ann Neurol*, 45:444–450.

Van den Bergh, V, Amery, WK, and Waelkens, J (1987). Trigger factors in migraine: a study conducted by the Belgian migraine society. *Headache*, 27:191–196.

Varadi, G, Mori, Y, Mikala, G, et al. (1995). Molecular determinants of Ca^{2+} channel function and drug action. *TiPS*, 2:43–49.

Vicente-Herrero, T, Burke, TA, and Lainez, MJ (2004). The impact of a worksite migraine intervention program on work productivity, productivity costs, and non-workplace impairment among Spanish postal service employees from an ermployer perspective. *Curr Med Red Opin*, 20:1805–1814.

Vilming, S, Standnes, B, and Hedman, C (1985). Metoprolol and pizotifen in the prophylactic treatment of classical and common migraine: a double-blind investigation. *Cephalalgia*, 5:17–23.

Visser, WH, Teall, JH, Malbecq, W, et al. (1998). Early onset of action of rizatriptan versus sumatriptan in the acute treatment of migraine, on behalf of the Rizatriptan Sumatriptan Comparison Group. *Lancet* (in press).

Visser, WH, Terwindt, GM, Reines, SA, et al. (1996). Rizatriptan vs sumatriptan in the acute treatment of migraine. A placebo-controlled, dose-ranging study. Dutch/United States Rizatriptan Study Group. *Arch Neurol*, 53:1132–1137.

Vogler, BK, Pittler, MH, and Ernst, E (1998). Feverfew as a preventive treatment for migraine: a systematic review. *Cephalalgia*, 18:704–708.

Volans, GN (1978). Research review: migraine and drug absorption. *Pharmacokinetics*, 3:313–318.

VonEuler, US (1937). On the specific vasodilating and plain muscle stimulating substance from accessory genital glands in man and certain animals (prostaglandin and vesiglandin). *J Physiol*, 88:213–234.

Waeber, C and Palacios, JM (1991). 5-HT1C, 5-HT1D and 5-HT2 receptors in mammalian brain: multiple affinity states with a different regional distribution. In *Serotonin-molecular Biology, Receptors and Functional Effects* (JR Fozard and PR Saxena, eds), pp. 107–131. Birkhauser, Switzerland.

Waelkens, J (1984). Dopamine blockade with domperidone: bridge between prophylactic and abortive treatment of migraine? A dose-finding study. *Cephalalgia*, 4:85–90.

Waldhoer, M, Bartlett, SE, and Whistler, JL (2004). Opioid receptors. *Annu Rev Biochem*, 73:953–990.

Wallace, JL and Cirino, G (1994). The development of gastrointestinal-sparing nonsteroidal antiinflammatory drugs. *Trends Pharmacol Sci*, 15:405–406.

Wang, F, Van Den Eeden, SK, Ackerson, LM, et al. (2003). Oral magnesium oxide prophylaxis of frequent migrainous headache in children: a randomized, double-blind, placebo-controlled trial. *Headache*, 43:601–610.

Wang, JH and Kelly, PT (1995). Postsynaptic injection of CA^{2+}/CaM induces synaptic potentiation requiring CaMKII and PKC activity. *Neuron*, 15:443–452.

Wang, SJ, Silberstein, SD, and Young, WB (1997). Droperidol treatment of status migrainosus and refractory migraine. *Headache*, 37:377–382.

Ward, N, Whitney, C, Avery, D, et al. (1991). The analgesic effects of caffeine in headache. *Pain*, 44:141–155.

Watanabe, H, Kuwabara, T, Ohkubo, M, et al. (1996). Elevation of cerebral lactate detected by localized ^{1}H-magnetic resonance spectroscopy in migraine during the interictal period. *Neurology*, 47:1093–1095.

Waters, WE (1970). A randomized controlled trial of ergotamine tartrate. *Br J Prev Soc Med*, 24:65.

Watson, S and Girdlestone, D (1996). 1996 receptor & ion channel nomenclature supplement. *Trends Pharmacol Sci*, (Suppl.):1–81.

Wauquier, A, Ashton, D, and Marranes, R (1985). The effects of flunarizine in experimental models related to the pathogenesis of migraine. *Cephalalgia*, 5:119–120.

Weber, RB and Reinmuth, OM (1972). The treatment of migraine with propranolol. *Neurology*, 22:366–369.

Wei, EP, Moskowitz, MA, Boccalini, P, et al. (1992). Calcitonin gene-related peptide mediqates nitroglycerine and sodium nitroprusside-induced vasodilation in feline cerebral arterioles. *Circ Res*, 70:1313–1319.

Weilburg, JB, Rosenbaum, JF, Biederman, J, et al. (1989). Fluoxetine added to nonMAOI antidepressants converts nonresponders to responders: a preliminary report. *J Clin Psychiatry*, 50:447–449.

Weinshank, RL, Adham, N, Zgombick, J, et al. (1992). Molecular analysis of serotonin receptor subtypes. In *Serotonin Receptor Subtypes: Pharmacological Significance and Clinical Implications* (SZ Langer, N Brunello, G Racagni, et al., eds), pp. 1–12. Karger, Basel.

Welch, KMA, Levine, SRDG, Schultz, L, et al. (1989). Preliminary observations on brain energy metabolism in migraine studied by in vivo ^{31}phosphorus NMR spectroscopy. *Neurology*, 39:538–541.

Wendt, J, Cady, R, Singer, R, et al. (2006). A randomized, double-blind, placebo-controlled trial of the efficacy and tolerability of a 4-mg dose of subcutaneous sumatriptan for the treatment of acute migraine attacks in adults. *Clin Ther*, 28:517–526.

Wessely, P, Baumgartner, C, Klinger, D, et al. (1987). Preliminary results of a double-blind study with the new migraine prophylactic drug Gabapentin. *Cephalalgia*, 7:477–478.

Wheeler, SD (2001). Lamotrigine efficacy in migraine prevention. *Cephalalgia*, 21:374 (Abstract).

White, K and Simpson, G (1984). The combined use of MAOIs and tricyclics. *J Clin Psychiatry*, 45:67–69.

Wideroe, TE and Vigander, T (1974). Propranolol in the treatment of migraine. *Br Med J*, 2:699–701.

Wilkinson, M (1970). Preliminary report on the use of clonidine (Boehringer Ingelheim) in the treatment of migraine. *Res Clin Stud Headache*, 3:315–320.

Wilkinson, M (1988). Introduction. In *Drug Induced Headache* (HC Diener and M Wilkinson, eds), pp. 1–2. Springer-Verlag, Berlin.

Williams, P, Dowson, AJ, Rapoport, AM, et al. (2001). The cost effectiveness of stratified care in the management of migraine. *Pharmacoeconomics*, 19:819–829.

Winther, K (1995). Ketanserin: a selective serotonin antagonist in relation to platelet aggregation and migraine attack rate. *Cephalalgia*, 5:402–403.

Winner, P, Ricalde, O, Leforce, B, et al. (1996). A double-blind study of subcutaneous dihydroergotamine vs subcutaneous sumatriptan in the treatment of acute migraine. *Arch Neurol*, 53:180–184.

Wober, C, Holzhammer, J, Zeitlhofer, J, et al. (2006). Trigger factors of migraine and tension-type headache: experience and knowledge of the patients. *J Headache Pain*, 7:188–195.

Wolff, HG (1963). *Headache and Other Head Pain*. Oxford University, New York.

Youdim, MBH, Bonham-Carter, SM, Sandler, M, et al. (1971). Conjugation defect in tyramine sensitive migraine. *Nature*, 230:127–128.

Young, WB, Oshinsky, ML, Shechter, AL, et al. (2001). Consecutive transcranial magnetic stimulation induced phosphene thresholds in migraineurs and controls. *Neurology*, 56:A142 (Abstract).

Yuill, GM, Swinburn, WR, and Liversedge, LA (1972). A double-blind crossover trial of isometheptene mucate compound and ergotamine in migraine. *Br J Clin Prac*, 26:76–79.

Zagami, AS, Goadsby, PJ, and Edvinsson, L (1990). Stimulation of the superior sagittal sinus in the cat causes release of vasoactive peptides. *Neuropeptides*, 16:69–75.

Zeeberg, I, Orholm, M, Nielsen, JD, et al. (1981). Femoxetine in the prophylaxis of migraine: a randomized comparison with placebo. *Acta Neurol Scand*, 64:452–459.

Zgombick, JM, Schechter, LE, Macchi, M, et al. (1992). Human gene S31 encodes the pharmacologically defined serotonin 5-hydroxytryptamine1E receptor. *Mol Pharmacol*, 42:180–185.

Ziegler, D, Ford, R, Kriegler, J, et al. (1994). Dihydroergotamine nasal spray for the acute treatment of migraine. *Neurology*, 44:447–453.

Ziegler, DK (1987). The treatment of migraine. In Wolff's headache and other head pain, (Dalessio DJ, ed.) pp. 87–111. Oxford University Press, New York.

Ziegler, DK, Hurwitz, A, Hassanein, RS, et al. (1987). Migraine prophylaxis. A comparison of propranolol and amitriptyline. *Arch Neurol*, 44:486–489.

Zivadinov, R, Willheim, K, Sepic-Grahovac, D, et al. (2003). Migraine and tension-type headache in Croatia: a population-based survey of precipitating factors. *Cephalalgia*, 23:336–343.

Zona, C, Ciotti, MT, and Avoli, M (1997). Topiramate attenuates voltage-gated sodium currents in rat cerebellar granule cells. *Neurosci Lett*, 231:123–126.

12 Tension-type Headache

Marc E. Lenaerts and Lawrence C. Newman

INTRODUCTION

Tension-type headache (TTH) is a highly prevalent disorder. Overall, and especially compared to migraine, symptoms remain mild or moderate. Therefore episodic TTH (ETTH) is rarely seen in headache clinics or even primary care settings. In contrast, even if only slightly more severe, chronic TTH (CTTH) is, because of its frequency at least, a reason to seek medical attention and is more commonly seen in clinical practice. The clinical picture is vague mainly because its symptomatology is based on the absence of symptoms. Environmental factors appear to predominate genetic influence. Comorbidity affects a large proportion of patients and must be recognized and appropriately managed. With the exception of outstanding contributions from Scandinavian research teams, the condition has been largely neglected by investigators compared to migraine, in part due to the lack of funding because of low interest by health authorities and the pharmaceutical industry alike. A surprisingly dubious attitude by many physicians, even neurologists, regarding the nature of this headache itself, adds to its reputation of "parent pauvre" of headaches. Many patients may experience at different times symptoms of TTH and symptoms of migraine, but the concept of a migraine spectrum remains a subject of debate.

The pathophysiology of TTH remains largely unknown, but recent investigations have begun to clarify the role and contribution of peripheral nociception and central sensitization. Patient education and lifestyle modification need to be an integral part of management, and comorbidities need to be recognized and addressed for therapeutic success, especially in patients with CTTH. Acute treatment of ETTH and CTTH are similar, though preventive treatment is appropriate in the management of CTTH. There is a paucity of evidence to support alternative and complementary treatments, though they may be considered in selected patients. Education of young physicians is integral to improve the care of TTH in the future. With better understanding of central sensitization as well as new therapeutic options against it, increased interest in TTH is expected.

EPIDEMIOLOGY AND IMPACT

TTH is the most common primary headache disorder in the general population (Rasmussen et al., 1991b; Rasmussen, 1995; Schwartz et al., 1998, Lyngberg et al., 2005a), yet the heterogeneity of this disorder makes prevalence estimates difficult. Further complicating the issue is that nearly all of the epidemiological studies published were conducted before the introduction of the International Classification of Headache Disorders (ICHD)-II criteria. Two Danish population studies conducted 12 years apart estimated the lifetime prevalence of TTH increased from 78% to 87% (Rasmussen et al., 1991b; Lyngberg et al., 2005a). The majority (51%–59%) had TTH 1 day or less per month. In other studies, several attacks per month of TTH were reported by 18%–37% whereas 10%–25% reported weekly attacks (Rasmussen et al., 1991b; Pryse-Phillips et al., 1992; Göbel, Petersen-Braun et al., 1994; Lavados and Tenhamm, 1998; Schwartz *et al.*, 1998; Castillo et al., 1999; Rasmussen, 1999; Cheung, 2000). In the United States, the 1-year prevalence of ETTH is approximately 38% (Schwartz et al., 1998); similar estimates have been reported in other countries (Bigal et al., 2001; Da Costa et al., 2002; Pop et al., 2002). A recent population-based study using ICHD-II criteria noted that 1-year prevalence of infrequent

ETTH was 63.5%, frequent ETTH was 21.6%, and CTTH was 0.9% (Russell, Levi et al., 2006). Another study employing ICHD-II criteria in those over the age of 40 reported a 1-year prevalence for infrequent ETTH of 48%, frequent ETTH 34%, and CTTH 2% (Russell, 2005). In Chile, however, the prevalence of TTH was reported to be 72% (Lavados and Tenhamm, 1998).

TTH affects women slightly more often than men. The age of onset is usually between 20 and 30 years (Rasmussen et al, 1991b; Göbel, Petersen-Braun et al., 1994; Schwartz et al., 1998; Lyngberg et al., 2005a), and peak prevalence is between the ages of 30–39 for both sexes (Schwartz et al., 1998a). The decline in later years may be indicative of a strong environmental effect. In schoolchildren, TTH has an equal prevalence in boys and girls, and like migraine a female predominance begins in adolescence (Laurell et al., 2003; Milovanovic et al., 2007). In the United States, ETTH was reported to be more prevalent with higher levels of education (Schwartz et al., 1998). A population-based study of twins found a higher concordance rate in monozygotic versus same-gender dizygotic twins for frequent ETTH. No differences were noted for infrequent ETTH, and not enough data was available for CTTH (Russell, Saltyte-Benth et al., 2006).

CTTH affects 2%–3% of the population (Rasmussen et al., 1991b; Pryse-Phillips et al., 1992; Göbel, Petersen-Braun et al., 1994; Schwartz et al., 1998; Castillo et al., 1999; Wang et al., 2000). The prevalence of CTTH is higher in women, and unlike ETTH, declines with increasing levels of education (Schwartz et al., 1998).

The natural history of TTH is variable. In a Danish study of 62 patients followed over a 10-year period, 75% with ETTH remained episodic while 25% evolved into CTTH. Of those patients with CTTH, one-third continued to have chronic headaches, nearly half improved to an episodic form, and approximately 20% developed medication overuse headaches (Moerk and Jensen, 2000). Most sufferers of CTTH initially began with the episodic subtype (Langemark et al., 1988; Moerk and Jensen, 2000). In a long-term follow-up study of children and adolescents with migraine and TTH, approximately 30% were headache free, and 20%–25% shifted from TTH to migraine or vice versa when reevaluated 5–8 years later (Kienbacher et al., 2006).

Despite the fact that most sufferers do not seek medical care, TTH has a significant socioeconomic impact (Rasmussen et al., 1992; Schwartz et al., 1998; Bigal et al., 2001; Silva et al., 2004). TTH is responsible for 820 days of lost work days yearly per 1000 employees (Rasmussen et al., 1992). In the United States, 8% of ETTH subjects miss work and 44% report diminished effectiveness at home, work, or school. Subjects with CTTH lose more days from work and have more days of reduced effectiveness than do ETTH sufferers (Schwartz *et al.*, 1997). Similar findings were reported in other countries as well (Rasmussen et al., 1992; Bigal et al., 2001).

The burden of TTH is significant. One-third of patients experience more than 14 days of headache per year (Schwartz et al., 1998). The overall personal, professional, and societal impact of TTH, especially the chronic form, should be a cause of concern for physicians and health care policymakers alike (Lenaerts, 2006). The prevalence of TTH, like that of migraine, is greatest at the height of professionally active years. The disability imparted by TTH is therefore more significant. The rate of consultation for TTH varies from 31% to 44 % (Edmeads et al., 1993; Lavados and Tenhamm 2001; Wang SJ et al., 2001; Lyngberg et al., 2005b).

A Dutch study highlighted the individual work productivity loss for TTH (ETTH and CTTH): it amounted to $22 per month which, at the level of society, is considerable (Pop et al., 2002). In a survey including 40 TTH patients, the monthly average number of missed days of work was 2.3 for ETTH and 8.9 for CTTH, whereas the average numbers of missed days of house activity were 1.6 and 10.3, respectively (Cassidy et al., 2003).

The personal and societal impact of TTH also accounts for comorbidities, especially depression, which is more common in TTH patients as opposed to headache-free individuals (Breslau et al., 2000). Similarly fibromyalgia is comorbid with TTH (Lenaerts and Gill, 2006).

A tendency to delay consultation for TTH increases therapeutic failure rates and consequently tends to prompt more ancillary investigations thereby driving up medical care cost (Lenaerts, 2006). Finally whereas ETTH is usually less severe and easier to treat than CTTH, it nonetheless causes most of the impact on society's productivity by its sheer prevalence.

CLASSIFICATION AND CLINICAL FEATURES

The ICHD-I classified TTH as episodic and chronic subtypes (Headache Classification Committee of the International Headache Society, 1988). The second edition of the ICHD classification has divided TTH into three separate categories based upon attack frequency; an infrequent episodic form in which headaches occur 1 day or less per month on average, a frequent episodic form in which headaches occur an average of 1–14 days per month, and a chronic form with 15 or more headache days per month. All three subtypes may be further subcategorized based on the presence or absence of associated pericranial tenderness. The diagnostic criteria for TTH are listed in Tables 12–1 to 12–3. All three subtypes have identical headache characteristics; however, minor differences in the associated features are listed for the chronic form. These criteria were established primarily to distinguish TTH from migraine.

In clinical practice, patients with TTH usually describe their headaches as a dull, nonthrobbing ache, or as a tightness, heaviness, or pressure sensation (Rasmussen et al., 1991a). Many report a feeling as if their head is in a "vice" or like a "belt" or "band" encircling their head (Friedman, 1979). Greater than 80% of patients report that they "seldom" or "never" experience pulsating pain (Rasmussen et al., 1991b; Rasmussen, 1995). Most patients have bilateral pain although the pain often changes locations during an individual attack (Pfaffenrath and Isler, 1993). The pain may also involve the posterior neck and shoulders.

According to the ICHD-II criteria, the pain of TTH is mild or moderately intense. A population-based study found that 87%–99% of subjects with ETTH do in fact experience mild or moderate pain (Rasmussen et al., 1991a). As attack frequency increases however, the severity of pain may increase to moderate or severe levels (Rasmussen *et al.*,

Table 12–1 Infrequent ETTH.

A. At least 10 episodes occurring on <1 days/month (<12 days/year) and fulfilling criteria B–D
B. Headache lasting from 30 minutes to 7 days
C. Headache has two or more of the following characteristics:
   1. Bilateral location
   2. Pressing/tightening (nonpulsating) quality
   3. Mild or moderate intensity
   4. Not aggravated by routine physical activity
D. Both of the following:
   1. No nausea or vomiting (anorexia may occur)
   2. No more than one of photophobia or phonophobia
E. Not attributed to another disorder

Table 12–2 Frequent ETTH.

A. At least 10 episodes occurring on more than 1 but <15 days/month for 3 months or more (12 or more and <180 days/year) and fulfilling criteria B–D
B. Headache lasting from 30 minutes to 7 days
C. Headache has two or more of the following characteristics:
   1. Bilateral location
   2. Pressing/tightening (nonpulsating) quality
   3. Mild or moderate intensity
   4. Not aggravated by routine physical activity
D. Both of the following:
   1. No nausea or vomiting (anorexia may occur)
   2. No more than one of photophobia or phonophobia
E. Not attributed to another disorder

Table 12–3 CTTH.

A. Headache occurring on 15 or more days/month (180 days/year or more) for >3 months and fulfilling criteria B–D
B. Headache lasts hours or may be continuous
C. Headache has 2 or more of the following characteristics:
   1. Bilateral location
   2. Pressing/tightening (nonpulsating) quality
   3. Mild or moderate intensity
   4. Not aggravated by routine physical activity
D. Both of the following:
   1. Not >1 of photophobia, phonophobia, mild nausea
   2. Neither moderate or severe nausea nor vomiting
E. Not attributed to another disorder

1991a; Ulrich et al., 1996; Scher et al., 2003). A hallmark of TTH, and a major distinguishing factor from migraine, is the absence of worsening head pain with movement or activity. Indeed, 72%–84% of ETTH sufferers report no worsening of their headache with activity (Rasmussen et al., 1992; Jensen et al., 1993; Göbel, Petersen-Braun et al., 1994).

Many clinicians view TTH as a featureless headache, because when compared to other headache disorders, most patients with TTH have no associated symptoms. The ICHD-II criteria for both of the episodic subtypes of TTH (infrequent and frequent) mandate that the headaches cannot be associated with nausea or vomiting, and no more than one of photophobia or phonophobia (Tables 12–1 and 12–2). Both subtypes may be associated with anorexia (ICHD-II). In epidemiologic studies of patients with ETTH, 10% of subjects reported mild photophobia, 7% reported mild phonophobia, but these symptoms accompanied the headaches only occasionally (Rasmussen et al., 1991a, 1992).

The duration of TTH varies from 30 minutes to 7 days for the episodic forms, and may last hours or be continuous with the chronic subtype (ICHD-II). TTH may coexist with migraine, and when it does, the features of TTH differs in that the it is more frequent and longer lasting in migraine sufferers than in nonmigraineurs (Ulrich et al., 1996).

As with all primary headache disorders, proper diagnosis of TTH is predicated on the exclusion of secondary mimics, and as such, patients with TTH should have normal medical and neurological examinations. An exception to this is the presence of pericranial muscle tenderness that may be experienced by some patients with TTH; these findings, when present, worsen with increasing frequency and severity of the headache (Jensen et al., 1993; Jensen, 2001). The increased prevalence of TTH over a 12-year period noted in the Danish study mentioned earlier (Lyngberg et al., 2005a) is associated with an increase in pain sensitivity (Buchgreitz et al., 2007). Manual palpation of the frontal, temporal, masseter, pterygoid, sternocleidomastoid, splenius, and trapezius muscles should be performed on all patients with TTH according to the new criteria, and if present, the diagnosis of TTH *associated with pericranial tenderness* should be assigned (ICHD-II). The use of pressure algometers and electromyography (EMG) recordings to measure muscle sensitivity is no longer required in the new guidelines.

Despite misconceptions to the contrary, TTH is not caused by psychological stress and emotional tension, but these may be triggers. In fact, these factors, as well as lack of sleep, fatigue, and missing meals are reported by sufferers of both migraine and ETTH (Ulrich et al., 1996; Spierings et al., 2001). The personality of TTH patients is comparable to that of migraine patients (Pffafenrath *et al.*, 1991). Depression and anxiety levels in TTH patients in general appear higher than those of controls, but comparable for young adults (Hatch et al., 1991; Merikangas et al., 1994). Daily stress correlates with frequency of headache in TTH (De Benedittis et al., 1992). Triggers typically thought of as specific for migraine, such as menstruation, weather changes, relaxation after stress, exposure to bright lights, strong odors and loud noises, and ingestion of alcoholic beverages, may also precipitate TTH in some patients (Ulrich et al., 1996; Spierings et al., 2001; Wober et al., 2006).

DIAGNOSTIC PITFALLS

Although the ICHD-II lists criteria for the various forms of TTH, it is important to realize that none of the criteria are mandatory for establishing the diagnosis. In fact, the criteria for TTH are based on negative features; the clinician makes a diagnosis of TTH by noting what is not present. The diagnosis is made, therefore, by excluding other primary and secondary headache syndromes. Clearly most sufferers will meet the criteria as delineated in the ICHD-II. Since TTH is a heterogeneous disorder, sharing symptomatology with other primary and secondary headache disorders, diagnostic difficulties may arise. Primary headache disorders for which ETTH may be mistaken include migraine without aura, cervicogenic headache, and probable migraine. TTH may be mistaken for migraine without aura when the headache is bilateral, has a nonthrobbing character, and is not associated with photophobia and phonophobia or nausea. When patients endorse triggers typically thought of as specific for migraine, TTH may also be misdiagnosed. Cervicogenic headache is characterized by unilateral headaches and trigger points in the neck that when palpated elicit pain. Clinicians may confuse the trigger points of cervicogenic headache for the *tender points* occasionally seen with TTH. Probable migraine is the ICHD-II designation given for migraine headaches that fulfill all but one of the necessary criteria needed for diagnosis. A patient with probable migraine might complain of a bilateral nonthrobbing headache of moderate severity that is associated with photophobia, but not nausea, vomiting, or phonophobia. This description meets the criteria for both probable migraine and TTH, but in fact, the ICHD-II criteria states that a definitive diagnosis is always given over a probable diagnosis. Nonetheless, these disorders while similar, are distinct, and respond to different therapeutic options. In these situations, the clinician needs to take a more thorough history, inquiring about family history, trigger factors, and other features in an attempt to render an accurate diagnosis.

CTTH has a more extensive differential diagnosis and is more easily mistaken for other disorders. The primary headache disorders for which CTTH may be mistaken include chronic migraine (Mathew et al., 1982; Mathew, 1987), new daily persistent headache (Rozen, 2003), and hemicrania continua (Sjaastad and Spierings, 1984) (Table 12–4). These disorders fall under the clinical classification of chronic daily headaches (CDHs) of long duration; disorders that occur more than 15 days per month with individual headache episodes lasting longer than 4 hours (Silberstein et al., 1996). CDH is not recognized by the ICHD-II classification and is discussed in more detail in other chapters. The relationship between temporomandibular joint dysfunction and TTH is debatable. Large surveys in the general population reveal a consistent 13% prevalence of temporomandibular joint dysfunction but no statistically significant association with headache, tension-type or other, is found (Locker et al., 1988; Jensen et al., 1993). The criteria for headache attributed to temporal mandibular joint (TMJ) disorder include pain precipitated by jaw movements, reduced range of or irregular jaw opening, and tenderness of the joint capsule(s) of one or both TMJs. Pain from the temporomandibular joint or related tissues is common and may be associated with myofascial pain and headache. The ICHD-II criteria for TTH also specify that TTH should *not* be attributed to an underlying condition, de facto closing the debate for classification. A mere co-occurrence between the two disorders is likely (Pilley et al., 1997). Nonetheless, in-depth evaluation of patients is necessary for accurate diagnosis of these often comorbid conditions (Graff-Radford, 2007).

Of greater clinical concern is that CTTH may be mimicked by some secondary headache disorders—misdiagnosis or diagnostic delay in these situations may have potentially dire consequences. Intracranial lesions such as primary or metastatic tumors often present with headaches that resemble CTTH—77% of patients with brain tumors were reported to have headaches resembling CTTH; the headaches were often bifrontal and pressure-like (Forsyth and Posner, 1993). Unlike CTTH, however, brain tumor headaches sometimes worsen with activity and changes in position. High and low cerebral spinal fluid pressure syndromes may also produce headaches with features of CTTH; here too, a change in headache severity with positional changes would be expected. Neurological findings such as papilledema, sixth nerve palsy, or altered levels of alertness or consciousness are usually evident with intracranial hypertension. Giant cell arteritis must be considered as a cause of new persistent headache in a patient older than age 60; failure to rapidly diagnose this condition may lead to blindness.

TTH IN CHILDREN

Studying headache in children poses several challenges. Gathering detailed symptoms is limited by their verbal and recall abilities and their lack of prior comparative experience. Complex notions such as sensoriphobia may rely on observation (Anttila, 2006). It is also likely that, in children as in adults TTH is underreported compared to migraine because it is milder (Hershey et al., 2006). Furthermore, the ICHD-II criteria for TTH and migraine in children tend to be too restrictive (Anttila, 2006).

The overall population prevalence of TTH in young patients varies significantly according to studies, from 9%–72 % (Barea et al., 1996; Laurell et al., 2004).

While girls and boys are initially equally affected, later in adolescence the prevalence in girls surpasses that in boys. (Laurell et al., 2004). Commonly TTH starts around the age of seven

TABLE 12–4 Pharmacologic agents with dosages, adverse events, levels of efficacy and of evidence.

Name	*Dosage*	*Adverse events and contraindications*	*Efficacy*	*Evidence*
Analgesics and NSAIDs				
Acetaminophen	1000 mg PRN, max thrice daily	Hepatotoxicity		I
ASA	1000 mg PRN, max twice daily	Gastric irritation/bleeding; nephrotoxicity long-term		I
Ibuprofen	200–400 mg PRN, max thrice daily	Same		I
Ketoprofen	25 mg PRN, max thrice daily	Same		I
Ketorolac	60 mg IV	Same		I
Tri- or tetracyclic				
Amitriptyline	10–200 mg total daily; QD or BID regimen	Xerostomia, constipation, lightheadedness, sedation, confusion; avoid in prostate hypertrophy, glaucoma, old age	High	I
Protriptyline	Same	Same	Moderate	IV
Clomipramine	25–75 mg; QD regimen	Same	Moderate	II
Other antidepressants				
Venlafaxine	75 mg daily, QD regimen	Sedation or insomnia, agitation, nausea, anorexia, diaphoresis, anorgasmia	Moderate	IV
Fluvoxamine	50–100 mg daily; BID regimen	Same	Low	IV
Mirtazapine		Xerostomia, constipation, sedation, confusion	Moderate	II

(continued)

Table 12–4 (continued)

Name	*Dosage*	*Adverse events and contraindications*	*Efficacy*	*Evidence*
	15–30 mg daily, QD regimen; ± ibuprofen			
Other drugs				
Topiramate	50–100 mg daily; BID regimen	Acroparesthesias, nephrolithiasis, anorexia, cognitive slowing	Low	IV
Tizanidine	12–24 mg daily; BID or TID regimen	Sedation, lightheadedness	Low	II
Buspirone	15 mg daily; QD regimen	Sedation	Low	IV
Other treatments				
Physiotherapy			Low	III
Stress management + tricyclic			Low	III
Acupuncture + other treatments			Low	IV
Relaxation, BFB, CBT			Moderate	IV
Occlusal adjustment			Moderate	II
Hypnotherapy			Moderate	III

Abbreviations: ASA, acetylsalicylic acid; BFB, biofeedback; BID, twice per day; CBT, cognitive-behavioral therapy; NSAIDS, nonsteroidal anti-inflammatory drugs; QD, once per day; PRN, as needed (pro rata necessitas); TID, thrice per day.

and the average frequency of headaches is two per month and the duration 2 hours. Headache intensity, duration, frequency, and medication use are lower in TTH than in migraine (Anttila *et al.*, 2002).

The prevalence of CTTH in children is expectedly much higher in headache clinics, as high as 7%, than in the general population, as low as 0.9% (Abu-Arafeh and Russell, 1994; Wöber-Bingöl et al., 1995). In a headache specialty pediatric clinic, of 115 consecutive patients, CTTH was the most prevalent diagnosis (81%). Stressful life events, major illnesses, and psychopathology represented significant risk factors. (Abu-Arafeh, 2001).

Because migraine in children tends to last less than that in adults, even less than 2 hours as accepted by the IHS criteria, and is more often bilateral, it can be misclassified as TTH. Hence TTH is probably overrepresented in epidemiological studies (Maytal et al., 1997).

An interesting long-term study (6 years) of children and adolescents in a headache clinic shows that 30% become headache-free, 20%–25% shift from migraine to TTH or the reverse, and poor prognosis is indicated by an initial diagnosis of migraine, changing headache location, time delay to consultation, and female gender (Kienbacher et al., 2006).

Diagnosis requires the use of calendars completed by patients and often facilitated by parents (Anttila, 2006). Electronic diaries are attractive too and are more accurate with young patients (Palermo et al., 2004).

Proper management includes long-term follow-up because of a common waxing and waning headache course. Besides pharmacotherapy, hygienic measures are essential, and more effective than in adults, and education is essential, including on issues such as pregnancy must be addressed (Lenaerts, 2005).

TTH IN THE ELDERLY

Although TTH peaks in the fifth decade of life and the prognosis is relatively favorable, it is still observed at the approximate prevalence of 25% in older people (Schwartz et al., 1998; Wang et al., 2000; Couch, 2005).

In the older patients the mere prevalence of underlying diseases necessitates great caution to establish the diagnosis of a primary headache such as TTH (Kaniecki, 2006). Therefore the most important aspect of geriatric headache care will be the screening of headache causes such as cancer, giant cell arteritis, or intracranial space-occupying lesions. Proper ancillary investigations must be considered at least in the following conditions: first, worst, or progressive headache, focal neurological symptoms or signs, fever, weight loss, or a history of prior malignancy. Pharmacologic recommendations are similar in the elderly adult, but particular caution should be applied to monitoring adverse effects such as those of tricyclic antidepressants and polytherapy since creatinine clearance decreases with age (Kaniecki, 2006).

PATHOPHYSIOLOGY

While the pathophysiology of TTH is not known, it has been observed that cephalic and generalized pain sensitivity (perception of pain from a suprathreshold stimulus) is consistently abnormal in CTTH, whereas studies on pain thresholds have yielded conflicting results (Schoenen, Bottin, et al.,1991; Bendtsen, 2000; Ashina et al., 2006). In CTTH as in fibromyalgia syndrome, the stimulus-response curve is abnormal: a left shift and linear pressure-pain ratio correlates with abnormal pain processing involved in central sensitization (Bendtsen et al., 1996c). TTH patients are more likely to develop shoulder and neck pain in response to static exercise than healthy controls (Christensen et al., 2005) It appears that trapezius muscle, a frequent site of pain in patients with CTTH, shows higher muscle pain sensitivity when compared to anterior tibialis (Ashina et al., 2003). Sensitization of muscle A-delta and C-fiber nociceptors contributes to not only abnormal thresholds but the propagation of pain to a more diffuse area (Mense, 1993).

Excessive pericranial myofascial tenderness is the most crucial physical finding in CTTH patients (Langemark and Olesen, 1987; Jensen *et al.*, 1993; Bendtsen et al., 1995; Lipchick et al., 1997). Pericranial as well as distal muscle pain sensitivity is increased and pain thresholds decreased in frequent episodic as well as chronic TTH, and this is observed regardless of whether headache is ongoing at the time of testing or not

(Schmidt-Hansen et al., 2007.) However, electromyographic activity overall is not abnormal or useful in the evaluation of TTH (Wittrock, 1997; Jensen et al., 1998). In contrast, pressure-pain thresholds have been found normal, decreased specifically in the frontalis, or decreased diffusely (Sandrini et al., 1994; Jensen et al., 1996, 1998). Pain thresholds and tolerance to mechanical stimuli are abnormally low in CTTH (Schoenen, Bottin, et al., 1991; Jensen, 1995; Bendtsen et al., 1996b). More important than absolute thresholds, the pressure-pain relationship becomes linear, which indicates abnormal central processing (Bendtsen et al., 1996c). Moreover these abnormalities are not dependant on the very presence of the headache (Bove and Nilsson, 1999). On these premises it is likely that chronic headache develops through central sensitization of the trigeminal nucleus caudalis after prolonged nociceptive inputs (Bendtsen and Ashina, 2000). It appears from comparable populations of TTH sufferers that pericranial tenderness and pressure-pain sensitivity have increased over the 1990s in women with frequent TTH. This observation accredits the hypothesis of increased central sensitization in the genesis of CTTH, and the effect of long-term peripheral nociception in the development of central sensitization itself (Buchgreitz et al., 2007).

The underlying mechanism of sensitization and myofascial tenderness is unclear. Magnesium levels are abnormal not only in migraine but also in TTH and may contribute to central sensitization by facilitation of N-methyl D-aspartate (NMDA) receptor function (Schoenen, Sianard-Gainko, et al.,1991; Mauskop et al., 1993). There also appears to be a deficit in diffuse noxious inhibitory control mechanisms for electrical detection and pain thresholds in CTTH (Pielsticker et al., 2005). On the other hand, there might be possibly compensatory increased brainstem opioid receptor hyperactivity (Schoenen et al., 1993).

The role of nitric oxide (NO) in the pathogenesis of TTH has recently emerged. NO contributes to central sensitization at various levels: medullary dorsal horn, trigeminal nucleus caudalis, and even periacqueductal gray matter (Hamalainen and Lovick, 1997; Wu et al., 1998). Glyceryl trinitrate, a NO donor, induces a typical headache in TTH patients (Ashina et al., 2000). Trials on CTTH patients showed a reduction in headache as well as in muscle hardness with L-N^G methyl arginine hydrochloride (L-NMMA), an inhibitor of NO synthase (NOS), likely through decreased central sensitization although the ultimate mechanism remains uncertain (Ashina, Bendtsen, et al., 1999; Ashina, Lassen, et al., 1999). This pharmacological approach is promising not only for CTTH but also for chronic migraine and other chronic pain syndromes (Ashina, 2002; Ashina, 2004).

While blood flow in pericranial muscles in CTTH patients is normal at rest, it is impaired in temporal muscle postexercise and in tender points of trapezius muscle in response to static exercise, possibly because of abnormal sympathetic function in this chronic pain syndrome, although changes appear conflicting (Langemark et al., 1990; Wallash, 1993; Ashina et al., 2002).

The recent finding of decreased gray matter in the brain of CTTH patients, especially in areas pertinent to pain such as the periaqueductal gray matter and the anterior cingulate cortex, suggests a structural basis for the condition, whether cause or consequence (Schmidt-Wilcke et al., 2005).

The impact of genetic factors in TTH is far lower than in migraine. There is no known single chromosome or gene for TTH and twin studies remain nonrevealing. In CTTH there is a higher concordance in first- and second-degree relatives, indicative of a genetic factor (Østergaard et al., 1997) The relative effect of environmental factors is even higher for ETTH than for CTTH (Ulrich et al., 2004). Twin studies in ETTH show no significant differences in symptom expression between mono- and dizygotic pairs, pointing to a low potential for genetic influence. Prevalence of ETTH varies geographically, further indicating a predominantly environmental effect. This is not true for CTTH (Rasmussen et al., 1992; Schwartz et al., 1998; Ho and Ong, 2003; Wang, 2003) In twin pair studies the relative role of nonshared environmental factors was found to be much higher in ETTH (81%) (the value for CTTH could not be separately calculated) than for migraine without (39%) and with (35%) aura (Gervil et al., 1999; Ulrich et al., 1999, 2004).

TTH AND MIGRAINE; DISTINCT SYNDROMES OR TWO POINTS ON A CONTINUUM

Scientific study of TTH is hampered by its frequent co-occurrence with migraine. Analyzing subjects with pure TTH or pure migraine eliminates the problem yet becomes less representative of reality in clinical practice. TTH is clinically nonspecific and milder than other headaches; its pathophysiology remains difficult to comprehend; it is commonly comorbid with other headaches, primary or secondary, and can mimic the latter. These are some of the reasons why a relative lack of attention is paid to this headache category. Accordingly the amount of research and publications, funding from governments and pharmaceutical industries and, at an individual level, the attention received by physicians are insufficient, particularly in view of its extreme prevalence (Jensen and Bendtsen, 2006).

Among controversies in TTH, a common argument is that many patients may actually suffer from a mild phenotype of migraine. However, the two disorders are likely separate, rather than two points on a continuum. The reasons for this position are several; first, the sex ratio is different. Second, while triptans appear to benefit all headaches in patients suffering from comorbid migraine and TTH (Lipton et al., 2000), they are ineffective in pure TTH sufferers (Brennum et al., 1996). Third, prevalence in the population is clearly different, with the yearly prevalence of ETTH and CTTH at 38% and CTTH at 3% respectively (Schwartz et al., 1998), compared to a 13% prevalence of migraine (Lipton et al., 2002).

COMORBIDITY

Comorbidity between two conditions can result from a causal relationship between the two, in either or both directions, from a common environmental effect or genetic predisposition, or a combination thereof. In the case of diseases associated with TTH, the relations are often complex and incompletely elucidated.

Although the association between epilepsy and headache often points to migraine, the prevalence of TTH in that setting is not negligible (Guidetti et al., 1987; Ottmann and Lipton, 1994; Lenaerts, 1999).

Overall TTH is associated with an increased risk of psychiatric disease, namely depression and anxiety. Greater headache frequency in TTH correlates with higher psychiatric comorbidity: the prevalence in CTTH subjects is significantly more than that in ETTH subjects (Mitsikostas and Thomas, 1999; Puca et al., 1999). Besides, the rate of mood disorders in CTTH is comparable to that in migraine (Siniatchkin et al., 1999; Cassidy et al., 2003). Since this is also observed in migraine the effect may be attributable in part to headache frequency per se. Clinic studies, probably in part due to a selection bias, depict a higher prevalence of psychiatric comorbidity than do general population studies with, for instance, in ETTH subjects, mean rates of depression and anxiety at 13% and 30% in clinics, respectively, compared to 9.5% and 13% in population studies (Guidetti et al., 1998; Mitsikostas and Thomas, 1999; Puca et al., 1999; Holroyd et al., 2000; Juang et al., 2000; Mongini et al., 2004).

Among psychiatric conditions associated with TTH, anxiety, especially generalized anxiety disorder, is the most prevalent (Puca et al., 1999).

Some personality profiles are more common in TTH but remained thus far understudied and this is of little value in clinical practice (Heckman and Holroyd, 2006).

On the other hand, maladaptative coping mechanisms such as avoidance and catastrophizing affect TTH patients and correlate with mood disorders (Wittrock and Myers, 1998; Materazzo et al., 2000). However even if these mechanisms may have an impact in therapeutic implementation and success, the response to treatment and overall prognosis of TTH seems unaffected by a given psychiatric disease, albeit different in the presence of multiple mental conditions (Jacob et al., 1983; Guidetti et al., 1998).

Expectedly with tricyclic antidepressants and behavioral therapies, associated psychopathology tends to improve with the treatment of TTH although both responses can be observed independently (Blanchard et al., 1991).

Age influences the rate of psychiatric comorbidity: in a 1-year prevalence observation, young adults with ETTH did not appear to be at greater risk for mood disorders (Merikanagas et al., 1993). In another study older adults with CTTH were observed to have a twice-greater chance to suffer from depression (Wang et al., 1999).

In a large, multicentric study in Italy, TTH was found comorbid with psychiatric disorders overall in 84.8%, 52.5% anxiety and 36.4% depression (Puca et al., 1999).

Fibromyalgia syndrome is a chronic condition with recurrent or fluctuating musculoskeletal pain, multifocal or diffuse, and muscular tenderness. It affects approximately 2% of the general population (Lawrence et al.,1998). More that half of patients with fibromyalgia syndrome complain of headache (Yunus, 2005b). In a systematic controlled study, 23% patients with fibromyalgia syndrome had a prior diagnosis of CTTH, and 5% fit the ICHD-II criteria at the time of the study (Aaron et al., 2000). Common exacerbators or triggers include head trauma, obesity, anxiety, depression, psychological stressors, and sleep deprivation (Gerster and Hadj-Djilani, 1984; Yunus *et al.*, 1989; Affleck et al., 1996; Dionne, 1999; Inanici et al., 1999; Benjamin et al., 2000; Al Allaf et al., 2002; White et al., 2002; Yunus et al., 2002; Lenaerts et al., 2004). It is conceivable that central sensitization is their common pathogenic mechanism, focal in one, more diffuse in the other (Schoenen, 2004; Yunus 2005a). Myorelaxants, however, are useful in fibromyalgia syndrome but not in TTH (Lenaerts, 2005). Pharmacologic neuro-modulation and nonpharmacologic approaches are beneficial to both conditions (Lenaerts and Gill, 2006). As in TTH, medical care and lost productivity contribute to the high personal and societal cost of fibromyalgia syndrome (Robinson et al., 2003).

THERAPY

The overall evidence of efficacy of TTH therapies remains scarce (Zhao and Stillman, 2003) The scientific literature must be interpreted critically, especially therapeutic trials that are uncontrolled or nonrandomized. Guidelines for therapeutic trials, both prophylactic and abortive, have been established by the International Headache Society.

Treatment must be individualized. Indeed the intensity, time course, and disabling characteristics of symptoms vary significantly. Likewise comorbidities and general physical condition may impact the therapeutic choice. Finally, patient's informed preference must be considered when selecting from among the therapeutic choices.

While acute therapy remains the cornerstone, prophylaxis must always be considered for chronic and frequent episodic TTH.

Prophylactic treatments should be evaluated for their ability to reduce headache indices (frequency, duration, intensity), to decrease the need for abortive therapy, and to improve quality of life. It should be considered for a headache frequency even below 15 days a month. Although the long-term prognosis of TTH is better than that of migraine, the functional impairment it can impart deserves adequate prevention (Couch, 2005)

Treatment must be holistic.

Lifestyle modification, especially trigger recognition and avoidance for ETTH and exacerbating factors for CTTH, must be emphasized. For instance sleep deprivation is a trigger for TTH in 39% patients (Blau, 1990).

Patient education is paramount. Explanation of the mechanism of action, side effect profile, and treatment expectations (measures of success) facilitates compliance.

Multimodal therapeutic approaches are useful: pharmacotherapy, alternative methods, and psychological therapies are mutually beneficial and synergistic.

Although tricyclic antidepressants prevent headaches regardless of their effect on mood, they may be beneficial on potential comorbid depression, anxiety, and/or insomnia.

Pharmacologic

Table 12–4 lists main phramacologic agents with dosages, adverse events, level of efficacy, and of evidence.

Analgesics

Acute treatments for TTH should be limited to an average of 2 days per week. Daily use of abortive therapy is highly discouraged because of the medical complications and the risk of medication overuse headache.

Nonsteroidal anti-inflammatory drugs are more potent than acetaminophen and more effective for the acute treatment of TTH. Ketoprofen, even at the low dose of 25 mg, and the solubilized ibuprofen relieve TTH more effectively than acetaminophen (Steiner and Lange, 1998; Packman et al., 2000). In another comparative trial, ketoprofen 25 mg was more effective than 12.5 mg, 1000 mg acetaminophen, and placebo (Mehlisch et al., 1998). Ketorolac is also very effective for the acute treatment of TTH (Harden et al., 1998).

Acetylsalicylic acid (1000mg) has been shown to be effective for the acute treatment of ETTH (Martinez-Martin et al., 2001).

Tricyclic Antidepressants

Tricyclic antidepressants, especially amitriptyline, but also nortriptyline, clomipramine, mianserin (actually a *tetra*cyclic), have been evaluated for the prophylactic treatment of TTH (Lance and Curran, 1964; Mathew, 1981; Langemark et al., 1990; Pfaffenrath et al., 1994; Bendtsen et al., 1996a; Cohen, 1997; Cerbo et al., 1998; Bendtsen and Jensen, 2000; Tomkins et al., 2001; Bendtsen and Jensen, 2002; Boz, 2002). Amitriptyline is effective in chronic yet not episodic TTH (Cerbo et al., 1998). To compensate for the lag in efficacy of tricyclics, an interesting approach consists of administering an initial boosting 3-week course of tizanidine 4 mg per day to amitriptyline 20 mg per day. An open-label, randomized trial on 18 CTTH patients pointed to a beneficial effect with 52 versus 40% headache frequency improvement at 3 months (Bettucci *et al.*, 2006).

A minimum duration of therapeutic trial of 6 weeks is necessary before considering the drug inefficient (Göbel, Hamouz, et al., 1994). Effective treatments should be maintained for at least 3 months. Thereafter, a slow taper should be considered (Lenaerts, 2005).

While the mechanism of action of tricyclics in TTH is unclear, the benefits for headache do not appear to be mediated by mood alteration. (Couch et al., 1976; Cerbo et al., 1998) The improvement appears to correlate more with pericranial tenderness. Because serotonin-specific re-uptake inhibitors (SSRIs) are ineffective for TTH, it is likely that the inhibition of norepinephrin re-uptake and/or NMDA antagonism associated with amitriptyline are more important than the inhibition of serotonin re-uptake. (Bendtsen and Jensen, 2000; Ashina et al., 2004).

Side effects of tricyclic antidepressants include *anticholinergic muscarinic* effects such as xerostomia, urinary retention, decreased sweating, mydriasis, and constipation; *antihistaminic* effects such as sedation, confusion and bulimia; *serotonergic* effects such as nausea; α_1-*adrenergic* effects such as tachycardia and postural hypotension; and *dopaminergic* effects such as tremor. Slow titration is recommended for better tolerance. Toxicity can include seizures, syncope, and even death by arrhythmia. These drugs should be used with caution or avoided in the elderly, hypotensive, epileptic, and closed-angle glaucoma patients.

SSRIs and Serotonin-Norepinephrin Re-uptake Inhibitors

Clinical trials evaluating the efficacy of SSRIs for the prophylactic treatment of TTH have been underwhelming. In a double-blind, placebo-controlled comparative trial in CTTH patients, amitriptyline 75 mg daily improved the headache index by 30, headaches were shorter and needed fewer analgesics while citalopram 20 mg daily proved nonbeneficial (Bendtsen et al., 1996a). In an open-label trial, CTTH patients who failed amitriptyline did not respond to paroxetine (Holroyd et al., 2003). In a prospective, randomized, placebo-controlled trial, sertraline reduced analgesic consumption but remained ineffective on headache index in 50 CTTH patients (Singh and Misra, 2002). In another study it compared negatively to amitriptyline (Boz et al., 2002).

However mirtazapine, 15–30 mg daily, significantly improved headache intensity, duration and frequency in 24 previously intractable but nondepressed CTTH patients in a double-blind, randomized, cross-over design (Bendtsen and Jensen, 2004). Unfortunately however, an investigation into the efficacy of a combination of mirtazapine (a serotonin-norepinephrin re-uptake inhibitor) and ibuprofen failed to benefit a group of CTTH patients (Bendtsen et al., 2007).

Muscle Relaxants

Tizanidine was modestly beneficial for TTH in two controlled studies, one on women only, and negative in another (Fogelholm and Murros, 1992; Murros et al., 2000; Saper et al., 2002). One can therefore not draw definite conclusions as to the role of this α-$_2$ adrenergic drug in TTH.

Other and Potential Future Pharmacological Treatments

Interestingly, a survey assessing response to sumatriptan injection for headache sufferers in the emergency department showed no difference between migraine and TTH (Miner et al., 2007). Sumatriptan is ineffective in pure TTH sufferers (Brennum et al., 1996).

Sodium valproate failed to benefit patients with mixed migraine and TTH (Lenaerts et al., 1996).

In an open-label prospective trial in 46 patients, topiramate demonstrated approximately 50% improvement in headache frequency and severity. The responder rate (percentage of patients with at least 50% improvement) was 73% (Lampl et al., 2006).

Based on the central sensitization theory involving NO, an experimental NOS inhibitor L-NMMA decreased pain significantly in 16 CTTH patients (Ashina, Lassen, et al. 1999). NOS inhibition may represent a promising therapeutic modality for the treatment of CTTH and other chronic pain syndromes (Ashina, 2002; Ashina and Ashina, 2003).

A recent report indicates long-term benefit of botulinum toxin type A in chronic headache, yet the study is limited by the lack of therapeutic control (Farinelli et al., 2006). A large multicentric placebo-controlled randomized trial of botulinum toxin for 6 months did not reach its primary end point of significantly reducing the frequency of headache-free days (Silberstein et al., 2005).

Although the overall evidence remains controversial, a recent trial reported a significant benefit from the addition of osteopathic therapy to relaxation (Anderson and Seniscal, 2006).

Physiotherapy appears to decrease headache frequency in TTH, with better results for CTTH and in women (Torelli et al., 2004).

Added to regular physical therapy specific cranio-cervical training proved beneficial (van Ettekoven and Lucas,2006).

Greater occipital nerve steroid injection appears ineffective in preventing CTTH (Leinisch-Dahlke et al., 2005).

Complementary and Alternative Therapy

The rationale for the use of complementary and alternative therapies is multifold: conventional treatments may be contra-indicated, have limited efficacy, or become associated with sometimes intolerable side effects. They also enhance the patient's ability to develop an internal locus of control.

The use of complementary and alternative therapies for headaches is on the rise. In one survey, up to 34% of headache sufferers consulted non-physicians and only 24% had a prescription-type treatment (Edmeads et al., 1993). Among 110 patients with CTTH in an Italian headache clinic, 40% had used those therapies even though 41% perceived them as inefficacious. In 41%, the treatment was suggested by a friend, and 60% did not tell their physician (Rossi et al., 2006). The efficacy of some alternative therapies such as acupuncture is inherently difficult to evaluate but improved trial methods and outcome measures afford the ability to assess the efficacy of these therapies (Vernon et al., 1999). For instance large-scale investigations assess the effect of acupuncture in various pain syndromes with strict sham placebos (Endres et al., 2004). Furthermore, personal factors such as patient's expectation can play a significant role in efficacy assessment, and this is not universally screened for (Linde et al., 2007).

Compared to migraineurs, CTTH patients appear less confident to gain control over their condition, which cognitive-behavior therapy can improve (Holroyd et al., 2005; Romanek et al., 2005).

Most often the mechanism of action of alternative therapies is unknown but presumably the activation of natural endogenous analgesic processes may be involved.

Age can have a determining effect: complementary and alternative therapies are most successful in young patients, especially children. They often require significant personal participation; hence, subjects must be chosen carefully. Combining this treatment approach with conventional, for example, pharmacologic, measures appears synergistic. A meta-analysis of psychological interventions clearly assert their overall efficacy (success rate of 70%) in children and adolescents although most included trials on TTH involved migraine as well (Trautmann et al., 2006). However this should not be confused with a known increased placebo response in younger individuals. Patients most likely to benefit from physical therapy, including massage, relaxation, biofeedback, and thermal therapy are younger patients with pericranial tenderness and absence of psychological stressors.

Despite the term alternative, these therapies are best used in *conjunction with* conventional therapy—as well as with each other—in the broader spectrum of a holistic therapeutic approach. Indeed the mechanisms of action differ between these modalities and a synergistic effect can benefit the patient (Detar and Chessman, 2007). In a randomized, controlled trial of CTTH patients (N = 203) comparing placebo, tricyclic antidepressants (amitriptyline up to 100 mg or nortriptyline up to 75 mg), stress management therapy or a combination thereof, headache indices, need for analgesics and headache-related disability decreased modestly from those with either therapy alone (respectively by 38 and 35% versus 29% for placebo,) but the benefit was significantly increased with combination treatment (64%) (Holroyd et al., 2001).

There appears to be some benefit of physical therapy, increasingly with headache frequency. Physiotherapy for 8 weeks benefited TTH patients, especially women, and CTTH where more than 50 patients experienced at least 50% reduction in headache frequency (Torelli et al., 2004). Chiropraxy appears effective but the evidence is low (Biondi, 2005). Overall the level of scientific proof for manual and physical therapies in TTH remains insufficient (Lenssinck et al., 2004; Fernandez-de-Las-Penas et al., 2006).

The overall evidence for Botulinum Toxin shows no benefit in TTH (Padberg et al., 2004; Evers, 2006).

The relative lack of scientific evidence for the efficacy of such therapies does not specifically spell a lack of biological effect but the overall methodological quality—lack of placebo, small samples, etc.—precludes definite conclusions. Future rigorous studies are likely to answer this clinical question in the future (Fernandez-de-las-Penas et al., 2006).

In an evidence-based review, the efficacy of relaxation on TTH in children is unclear, whereas biofeedback and cognitive therapy appear inefficient (Verhagen et al., 2005). Relaxation therapy seems to be accepted by younger patients than pharmacotherapy (Bussone et al., 1998; Grazzi et al., 2004).

Relaxation techniques are meant to be integrated in patients' daily life to be most effective. The therapeutic impact of this is decreased if the patient is either unwilling or unable to actively participate in the treatment program (Nash, 2003).

Techniques such as biofeedback or cognitive-behavioral therapy enhance relaxation but also modify central sensitization that is believed to be exacerbated by depression and anxiety. A review of evidence of efficacy of different techniques found that at least 40% patients with TTH benefit from relaxation training, EMG biofeedback with or without relaxation, and cognitive-behavioral therapy with or without relaxation (McCrory et al., 2001).

Acupuncture represents another alternative therapeutic avenue. Despite the high number of trials for acupuncture in primary headaches, the limitations imposed by methodology limit their reliability and significance (Manias et al., 2000).

A retrospective analysis of acupuncture in Germany on headache sufferers, 2 022 patients receiving an average of eight treatments, revealed that at least 50% of 791 patients with TTH (440 Chronic) had at least 50% reduction in headache frequency at 6 months. While this is a study of uncontrolled and coadministered therapies and a placebo effect in it may confound results, it shows a probable benefit of acupuncture that warrants further prospective controlled trials (Melchart et al., 2006). A randomized controlled trial showed acupuncture to be better than no treatment but not significantly different from minimal acupuncture, that is, sham (Melchart et al., 2005). In 25 CTTH patients, laser acupuncture, 10 sessions over 3 weeks, decreased headache intensity, duration, and frequency. The responses were significant at each of the following 3 months, and expectedly decremental. (Ebneshahidi et al., 2005).

There now exists new methods to apply a placebo to acupuncture studies but their use is still limited (Fink et al., 2001). In a large review of 14 trials comparing true with sham acupuncture in patients with migraine and TTH, treatment efficacy was statistically significant in eight studies, showed a trend in four and was absent in the remaining two (Melchart et al., 2001). However, this technique failed to help 39 CTTH patients when compared to placebo/sham (Cummings, 2001). Electro-acupuncture improved headache frequency, duration, pain intensity and disability for up to 3 months in 37 TTH patients in a single-blind, 4-week treatment (Xue et al., 2004). Therapies aiming at reducing pericranial and neck muscle activity have therefore been studied for long, and a number of trials or observations indicate several efficacious methods. Massage mobilizes deep interstitial fluid, thereby decreasing edema, freeing connective adherences, and relaxing muscles. It can be associated with thermotherapy but no controlled study exists to this date. Often patients are unaware of excessive pericranial muscle contraction. Biofeedback is a technique by which a device recording a biological function indicates the result to the patient. Applied to muscle contraction, an electromyographic machine delivers a visual or an auditory signal to the patient; combined with relaxation therapy it can benefit TTH.

In an open label, yet controlled and randomized trial, young CTTH sufferers failed to respond significantly to relaxation therapy (Fichtel and Larsson, 2004).

Eight weeks of physical therapy in TTH modestly improved headache days but not severity, duration or analgesic use (Torelli et al., 2004).

In a large literature review less than 50% of studies on physical therapies in headaches met sufficient quality. As far as TTH was concerned, spinal manipulation, electrotherapy, transcutaneous electrical nerve stimulation with or without stretching were considered effective, although weaker than amitriptyline (Bronfort et al., 2004).

Treatment of oromandibular dysfunction consists of modification of the occlusion with the aid of a splint or orthodontics or even complex surgeries. The latter must be considered only rarely and in the wake of a specific dental need as opposed to just pain as a symptom (Graff-Radford and Forssell, 2000). Although recent literature is scant, an older placebo-controlled occlusal adjustment indicated long-term benefit in headaches frequency in CTTH patients with oromandibular dysfunction (Forssell et al., 1987).

Homeopathy is of no benefit. Besides, its putative mechanism of action are difficult to integrate to TTH pathophysiology. The initial negative report of 98 chronic headache sufferers was thought to be due to too short an observation period not allowing dissipating the uncertainty effect, but a long-term follow-up did not demonstrate any difference (Walach et al., 2001).

An older trial of hypnotherapy in CTTH compared favorably to a waiting list group (control) in headaches frequency, duration and intensity (Melis et al., 1991).

Much, obviously, remains to be done to establish several of them in the therapeutic armamentarium of TTH. It must be emphasized that a relative lack of evidence for the efficacy of alternative treatments justifies caution when applying treatments that could be costly. The reader must not be discouraged, however, to try these therapies and obviously a continuous follow-up of the literature is advised in this ever evolving field. Ideally these treatments must be part of a *holistic* approach including pharmaco- and, whenever applicable, psycho-therapy, and, always, patient education. Finally, it must be reminded that the very nature of the placebo effect remains unknown but is believed to be in part linked to the attitude of the caregiver, leaving an obvious window of opportunity (Lenaerts, 2004).

Psychological and Behavioral Therapy

Psychological and behavioral therapies are often used in combination with pharmacotherapy, but in certain circumstances, these nonmedical approaches may be the mainstay of treatment. Situations in which these treatments are used without pharmacotherapy include; when medications are poorly tolerated, cause adverse effects, or are contraindicated; in childhood, during pregnancy or nursing; or when the patient preference is to avoid medication therapy. The goals of these therapeutic modalities are to decrease headache frequency and its attendant disability, as well as to teach coping skills that lessen stress and thereby enable patients to care better for themselves. In general, these treatments are used as a preventive strategy, but may reduce the impact of individual headache attacks as well.

Behavioral therapies that are useful in the treatment of TTH include relaxation training, EMG biofeedback, cognitive behavioral therapy, and identification and management of headache precipitants (Nash, 2003). Meta-analyses of these modalities, both as solo therapy, or in combination with pharmacotherapy, have supported their efficacy (McCrory et al., 2001; Raines, et al., 2005). A randomized study of patients with CTTH, most of whom also experienced episodic migraine, found that treatment combining tricyclic antidepressants with relaxation and cognitive behavioral skills resulted in a 64% decrease in headache at 8 months; whereas a 38% decrease was seen in those using tricyclics alone, 35% decrease using only stress management, and 29%

decrease with placebo anti-depressants (Holroyd et al., 2001).

PROGNOSIS

A 2-year follow-up of adolescents with chronic headache revealed that TTH has a better prognosis than migraine. Its prevalence regressed from 86 to 46%. Poor outcome was predicted by psychopathology and female gender (Wang et al., 2007). Psychopathology in chronic headache creates a negative impact on prognosis; therefore the clinician must assess, address, and arrange for therapy of comorbid psychiatric conditions to increase therapeutic success (Baskin et al., 2006).

In an 8-year long follow-up study of adolescents, the presence of 2 or more psychiatric comorbidities had a negative prognostic value, with persistence or aggravation of the headache. In children somatic symptoms and family problems appear moderately more frequent headache patients than in nonheadache patients but, contrary to migraine, depression is not very frequent (Anttila et al., 2004). Because of significant psychiatric comorbidity, proper assessment of the TTH patient requires evaluation of psychological profile and status. Depression assessment tools such as Hamilton's scale and Beck's inventory, anxiety scales such as State-Trait Anxiety Inventory, are commonly used in trials on TTH. Minnesota Multiple Personality Inventory has also served extensively to characterize these patients.

References

Aaron, L, Burke, M, and Buchwald, D (2000). Overlapping conditions among patients with chronic fatigue syndrome, fibromyalgia and temporomandibular disorder. *Arch Intern Med*, 160:221–227.

Abu-Arafeh, I (2001). Chronic tension-type headache in children and adolescents. *Cephalalgia*, 21:360–366.

Abu-Arafeh, I and Russell, G (1994) Prevalence of headache and migraine in schoolchildren. *BMJ*, 309:765–769.

Affleck, G, Urrows, S, Tennen, H, et al (1996). Sequential daily relations of sleep, pain intensity and attention to pain among women with fibromyalgia. *Pain*, 8:363–368.

Al Allaf, AW, Dunbar, KL, Hallum, NS, et al. (2002). A case-control study examining the role of physical trauma in the onset of fibromyalgia syndrome. *Rheumatology*, 41:450–453.

Anderson, RE and Seniscal, C (2006). A comparison of selected osteopathic treatment with relaxation for tension-type headache. *Headache*, 46:1273–1280.

Anttila, P (2006). Tension-type headache in childhood and adolescence. *Lancet Neurol*, 5:268–274.

Anttila, P, Metashonkala, L, Aromaa, M, et al (2002). Determinants of tension–type headache in children. *Cephalalgia*, 22:401–408.

Anttila, P, Sourander, A, Metsahonkala, L, et al (2004). Psychiatric symptoms in children with primary headache. *J Am Acad Child Adolesc Psychiatry*, 43:412–419.

Ashina, M (2002). Nitric oxide synthase inhibitors for the treatment of tension–type headache. *Expert Opin Pharmacother*, 3:395–399.

Ashina, M (2004). Neurobiology of chronic tension–type headache. *Cephalalgia*, 24:161–172.

Ashina, M, Bendtsen, L, Jensen, R, et al (1999). Possible mechanisms of action of nitric oxide synthase inhibitors in chronic tension–type headache. *Brain*, 122:1629–1635.

Ashina, M, Bendtsen, L, Jensen, R, et al (2000). Nitric Oxide–induced headache in patients with chronic tension–type headache. *Brain*, 123:1830–1837.

Ashina, M, Stallknecht, B, Bendtsen, L, et al (2002). In vivo evidence of altered skeletal muscle blood flow in chronic tension–type headache. *Brain*, 125:320–326.

Ashina, M, Lassen, LH, Bendtsen, L, et al (1999). Effect of inhibition of nitric oxide synthase on chronic tension–type headache: a randomized crossover trial. *Lancet*, 353:287–289.

Ashina, S and Ashina, M (2003). Current and potential future drug therapies for tension–type headache. *Curr Headache Pain Rep*, 7:466–474.

Ashina, S, Bendtsen, L, Ashina, M, et al (2006). Generalized hyperalgesia in patients with chronic tension–type headache. *Cephalalgia*, 26:940–948.

Ashina, S, Bendtsen, L, and Jensen, R (2004). Analgesic effect of amitriptyline in chronic tension–type headache is not directly related to serotonin reuptake inhibition. *Pain*, 108:108–114.

Ashina, S, Jensen, R, and Bendtsen, L (2003). Pain sensitivity in pericranial and extracranial regions. *Cephalalgia*, 23:456–462.

Barea, LM, Tannhauser, M, and Rotta, NT (1996). An epidemiologic study of headache among children and adolescents in southern Brazil. *Cephalalgia*, 16:545–549.

Baskin, SM, Lipchik, GL, and Smitherman, TA (2006). Mood and anxiety disorders in chronic headache. *Headache*, 46 : S76–S87.

Bendtsen, L (2000). Central sensitization in tension–type headache—possible pathophysiological mechanisms. *Cephalalgia*, 20:486–508.

Bendtsen, L and Ashina, M (2000). Sensitization of myofascial pain pathways in tension–type headache. In *The Headaches* (2nd edn) (J Olesen, P Tfelt-Hansen, KMA Welch, eds), pp. 573–577. Philadelphia: Lippincott Williams & Wilkins.

Bendtsen, L, Buchgreitz, L, Ashina, S, et al (2007). Combination of low–dose mirtazapine and ibuprofen for prophylaxis of chronic tension–type headache. *Eur J Neurol*, 14:187–193.

Bendtsen, L and Jensen, R (2000). Amitriptyline reduces myofascial tenderness in patients with chronic tension–type headache. *Cephlalagia*, 20:603–610.
Bendtsen, L and Jensen, R (2000). Amitriptyline reduces myofascial tenderness in patients with chronic tension–type headache. *Headache*, 20:603–610.
Bendtsen, L and Jensen, R (2000). Mirtazapine is effective in the prophylactic treatment of chronic tension–type headache. *Neurology*, 62:1706–1711.
Bendtsen, L, Jensen, R, Jensen, NK, et al (1995). Pressure–controlled palpation: a new technique which increases the reliability of manual palpation. *Cephalalgia*, 15:205–210.
Bendtsen, L, Jensen, R, and, Olesen J (1996a). A non–selective (amitriptyline) but not a selective (citalopram) serotonin reuptake inhibitor is effective in the prophylactic treatment of chronic tension–type headache. *J Neurol Neurosurg Psychiatry*, 61:285–290.
Bendtsen, L, Jensen, R, and Olesen, J (1996b). Decreased pain detection and tolerance thresholds in chronic tension–type headache. *Arch Neurol*, 53:373–376.
Bendtsen, L, Jensen, R, and Olesen, J (1996c). Qualitatively altered nociception in chronic myofascial pain. *Pain*, 65:259–264.
Benjamin, S, Morris, S, McBeth, J, et al (2000). The association between chronic widespread pain and mental disorder: a population–based study. *Arthritis Rheum*, 43:561–567.
Bettucci, D, Testa, L, Calzoni, S, et al (2006). Combination of tizanidine and amitriptyline in the prophylaxis of chronic tension–type headache: evaluation of efficacy and impact on quality of life. *J Headache Pain*, 7:34–36.
Bigal, ME, Bigal, JM, Betti, M, et al (2001). Evaluation of the impact of migraine and episodic tension–type headache on the quality of life and performance of a university student population. *Headache*, 41:710–719.
Biondi, DM (2005) Physical treatments for headache: a structured review. *Headache*, 45:738–746.
Blanchard, EB, Steffek, BD, Jaccard, J, et al (1991). Psychological changes accompanying non--pharmacological treatment of chronic headache: the effects of outcome. *Headache*, 31:249–253.
Blau, JN (1990). Sleep-deprivation headache. *Cephalalgia*, 10:157–160.
Bove, GM and Nilsson, N (1999) Pressure–pain threshold and pain tolerance in episodic tension–type headache do not depend on the presence of headache. *Cephalalgia*, 19:174–178.
Boz, C, Altunayoglu, V, Velioglu, S, et al (2002). Sertraline versus amitriptyline in the prophylactic therapy of non–depressed chronic tension–type headache patients. *Headache*, 4:72–78.
Brennum, J, Brinck, T, Schriver, L, et al (1996). Sumatriptan has no clinically relevant effect in the treatment of episodic tension–type headache. *Eur J Neurol*, 3:23– 28.
Breslau, N, Schultz, LR, Stewart, WF, et al (2000). Headache and major depression. Is the association specific to migraine? *Neurology*, 54:308–313.
Bronfort, G, Nilsson, N, Haas, M, et al (2004). Non–invasive physical treatments for chronic/recurrent headache. *Cochrane Database Syst Rev*, 3: CD001878.
Buchgreitz, L, Lyngberg, A, Bendtsen, L, et al (2007). Increased prevalence of tension–type headache over a 12–year period is related to increased pain sensitivity. A population study. *Cephalalgia*, 27: 145–152.
Bussone, G, Grazzi, L, D'Amico, D, et al (1998). Biofeedback–assisted relaxation training for young adolescents with tension–type headache: a controlled study. *Cephalalgia*, 18:463–467.
Cassidy, EM, Tomkins, E, Hardiman, O, et al (2003). Factors associated with burden of primary headache in a specialty clinic. *Headache*, 43:638–644.
Castillo, J, Munoz, P, Guitera, V, et al (1999). Epidemiology of chronic daily headache in the general population. *Headache*, 38:497–506.
Cerbo, R, Barbanti, P, Fabbrini, G, et al (1998). Amitriptyline is effective in chronic but not in episodic tension–type headache: pathogenetic implications. *Headache*, 38:453–457.
Cheung, RT (2000). Prevalence of migraine, tension–type headache, and other headaches in Hong Kong. *Headache*, 40:473–479.
Christensen, M, Bendtsen, L, Ashina, M, et al (2005). Experimental induction of muscle tenderness and headache in tension–type headache patients. *Cephalalgia*, 25:1061–1067.
Cohen, GL (1997). Protriptyline, tension–type headaches and weight loss in women. *Headache*, 37:433–436.
Couch, JR (2005). The long–term prognosis of tension–type headache. *Curr Pain Headache Rep*, 9:436–441.
Couch, JR, Ziegler, DK and Hassanein, R (1976). Amitriptyline in the prophylaxis of migraine. Effectiveness and relationship of antimigraine and antidepressant effects. *Neurology*, 26:121–127.
Cummings, M (2001). No difference between acupuncture and sham in chronic tension–type headache (n = 39). *Acupunct Med*, 19:51–53.
Da Costa, MZ, Soares, CB and Heinisch, RH (2002). Frequency of headache in the medical students of Santa Catarina's Federal University. *Headache*, 40:740–744.
De Benedittis, G, Lorenzetti, A (1992). The role of stressful life events in the persistance of primary headache: major events vs. daily hassles. *Pain*, 51:35–42.
Detar, DT and Chessman, AW (2007). Physiotherapy plus a craniocervical training programme was better than physiotherapy alone in tension type headache. *Evid Based Med*, 12:14.
Dionne, CE (1999). Low back pain. In *Epidemiology of Pain: A Report of the Task Force on Epidemiology of the International Association for the Study of Pain* (IK Crombie, PR Croft, SJ Linton, et al., eds) pp. 283–297. IASP Press: Seattle, WA.
Ebneshahidi, NS, Heshmatipour, M, Moghaddami, A, et al. (2005). The effects of laser acupuncture on chronic tension headache—a randomized controlled trial. *Acupunct Med*, 23:13–18.
Edmeads, J, Findlay, H, Tugwell, P, et al (1993). Impact of migraine and tension–type headache on life–style, consulting behaviour, and medication use: a Canadian population survey. *Can J Neurol Sci*, 20:131–137.

Endres, HG, Zenz, M, Schaub, C, et al (2004). Haake M, Streitberger K, Skipka G, Maier C. German Acupuncture Trials (gerac) address problems of methodology associated with acupuncture studies. *Cochrane Database Syst Rev*, 3:CD001878.

Evers, S (2006). Investigating prophylactic botulinum toxin type A for chronic headache disorders. *Expert Opin Investig Drugs*, 15:1161–1166.

Farinelli, I, Coloprisco, G, De Filippis, S, et al (2006). Long–term benefits of botulinum toxin type A (BOTOX) in chronic daily headache: a five–year long experience. *J Headache Pain*, 7:407–412.

Fernandez-de-Las-Penas, C, Alonso-Blanco, C, Cuadrado, ML, et al (2006). Are manual therapies effective in reducing pain from tension–type headache?: a systematic review. *Clin J Pain*, 22:278–275.

Fernandez-de-las-Penas, C, Alonso-Blanco, C, San-Roman, J, et al (2006). Methodological quality of randomized controlled trials of spinal manipulation and mobilization in tension–type headache, migraine, and cervicogenic headache. *J Orthop Sports Phys Ther*, 36:160–169.

Fichtel, A and Larsson, B (2004). Relaxation treatment administered by school nurses to adolescents with recurrent headaches. *Headache*, 44:545–554.

Fink, M, Gutenbrunner, C, Rollnik, J, et al (2001). Credibility of a newly designed placebo needle for clinical trials in acupuncture research. *Forsch Komplementarmed Klass Naturheilkd*, 8:368–372.

Fogelholm, R and Murros, K (1992). Tizanidine in chronic tension–type headache: a placebo–controlled, double–-blind, cross–over study. *Headache*, 32:509–513.

Forssell, H, Kirveskari, P and Kangasniemi, P (1987). Response to occlusal treatment in headache patients previously treated with mock occlusal treatment. *Acta Odontol Scand*, 45:77–80.

Forsyth, PA and Posner, JB (1993). Headaches in patients with brain tumors: a study of 111 patients. *Neurology*, 43:1678–1683.

Friedman, AP (1979). Characteristics of tension headache: a profile of 1420 cases. *Psychosomatics*, 20:451–461.

Gerster, JC and Hadj-Djilani, A (1984). Hearing and vestibular abnormalities in primary fibrositis syndrome. *J Rheumatol*, 11:678–680.

Gervil, M, Ulrich, V, Kaprio, J, et al (1999). The relative role of genetic and environmental factors in migraine without aura. *Neurology*, 53:995–999.

Göbel, H, Hamouz, V, Hansen, C, et al (1994). Chronic tension–type headache: amitriptyline reduces clinical headache–duration and experimental pain sensitivity but does not alter pericranial muscle activity readings. *Pain*, 59:241–249.

Göbel, H, Petersen-Braun, M, Soyka, D (1994). The epidemiology of headache in Germany: a nationwide survey of a representative sample on the basis of the headache classification of the International Headache Society. *Cephalalgia*, 14:97–106.

Grazzi, L, Andrasik, F, Usai, S, et al (2004). Pharmacological behavioural treatment for children and adolescents with tension–type headache: preliminary data. *Neurol Sci*, 25:S270–S271.

Graff-Radford, SB and Forssell, H (2000). Oro–mandibular treatment of tension–type headache. In *The Headaches* (2nd edn) (J Olesen, P Tfelt-hansen, KMA Welch, eds.), pp. 657–660. Lippincott, Williams & Wilkins, Philadelphia.

Graff-Radford, SB (2007). Temporomandibular disorders and other causes of facial pain. *Curr Pain Headache Rep*, 11:75–81.

Guidetti, V, Fornara, R, Marchini, R, et al (1987). Headache and epilepsy in childhood: analysis of a series of 620 children. *Funct Neurol*, 2:323–341.

Guidetti, V, Galli, F, Fabrizi, P, et al (1998). Headache and psychiatric comorbidity: clinical aspects and outcome in an 8–year followup study. *Cephalalgia*, 18:455–462.

Hamalainen, MM and Lovick, TA (1997). Involvement of NO and and serotonin in modulation of antinociception and pressor responses evoked by stimulation in the dorsolateral region of the periacqueductal gray matter in the rat. *Neuroscience*, 80:821–827.

Harden, RN, Rogers, D, Kink, K, et al (1998). Controlled trial of ketorolac in tension–type headache. *Neurology*, 50:507–509.

Hatch, JP, Schoenfeld, LS, Boutros, NN, et al (1991). Anger and hostility in tension-type headache. *Headache*, 31:302–304.

Headache Classification Committee of the International Headache Society. (1998). Classification and diagnostic criteria for headache disorders, cranial neuralgias, and facial pain. *Cephalalgia*, 8 (Suppl. 7):1–96.

Headache Classification Committee of the International Headache Society. (2004). The international classification of headache disorders, 2nd edition. *Cephalalgia*, 24 (Suppl. 1):1–160.

Heckman, BD and Holroyd, KA (2006). Tension–type headache and psychiatric comorbidity. *Cur Pain Headache Rep*, 10:439–447.

Hershey, AD, Kabbouche, MA, and Powers, SW (2006). Tension–type headache in the young. *Curr Pain Headache Rep*, 10:467–470.

Ho, KH and Ong, BK (2003). A community–based study of headache diagnosis and prevalence in Singapore. *Cephalalgia*, 23:6–13.

Holroyd, KA, Labus, JS, O'Donnell, FJ, et al (2003). Treating chronic tension–type headache not responding to amitriptyline hydrochloride with paroxetine hydrochloride: a pilot evaluation. *Headache*, 43:999–1004.

Holroyd, KA, O'Donnell, FJ, Stensland, M, et al (2001). Management of chronic tension–type headache with tricyclic antidepressant medication, stress management therapy, and their combination: a randomized, controlled trial. *JAMA*, 285:2208–2215.

Holroyd, KA, Stensland, M, and Hill, K (2005). Separate and combined effects of cognitive–behavior therapy and antidepressant medication in the treatment of chronic tension–type headache: psychological outcomes. *Headache*, 45:776–790.

Holroyd, K, Stensland, M, Lipchik, G, et al (2000). Psychosocial correlates and impact of chronic tension–type headaches. *Headache*, 40:3–16.

Inanici, F, Yunus, MB, and Aldag, JC (1999). Clinical features and psychological factors in regional soft tissue pain: comparison with fibromyalgia syndrome. *J Musculoskelet Pain*, 7:293–301.

Jacob, RG, Turner, SN, Szekely, BC, et al (1983). Predicting outcome of relaxation therapy in headaches: the role of "depression." *Behav Ther*, 14:457–465.

Jensen, R (1995). Mechanisms of spontaneous tension–type headaches: An analysis of tenderness, pain thresholds and EMG. *Pain*, 64:251–256.

Jensen, R (2001). Chronic tension–type headache. *Adv Studies Med*, 1:449–450.

Jensen, R and Bendtsen, L (2006). Tension–type headache: Why does this condition have to fight for its recognition? *Curr Pain Headache Rep*, 10:454–458.

Jensen, R, Bendtsen, R, and Olesen, J (1998). Muscular factors are of importance in tension–type headache. *Headache*, 38:10–17.

Jensen, R and Rasmussen, BK (1996). Muscular disorders in tension–type headache. *Cephalalgia*, 16:97–103.

Jensen, R, Rasmussen, BK, Pedersen, B, et al (1993). Muscle tenderness and pressure pain thresholds in headache. A population study. *Pain*, 52:193–199.

Juang, K, Wang, S, Fuh, J, et al (2000). Comorbidity of depressive and anxiety disorders in chronic daily headache and its subtypes. *Headache*, 40:818–823.

Kaniecki, RG (2006). Tension–type headache in the elderly. *Curr Pain Headache Rep*, 10:448–453.

Kienbacher, C, Wober, C, Zesch, HE, et al (2006). Clinical features, classification and prognosis of migraine and tension–type headache in children and adolescents: a long–term follow–up study. *Cephalalgia*, 26:820–830.

Lampl, C, Marecek, S, May, A, et al (2006). A prospective, open–label, long–term study of the efficacy and tolerability of topiramate in the prophylaxis of chronic tension–type headache. *Cephalalgia*, 26:1203–1208.

Lance, JW and Curran, DA (1964). Treatment of tension–type headache. *Lancet*, 1:1236–1239.

Langemark, M, Jensen, K, and Olesen, J (1990). Temporal muscle blood flow in chronic tension–type headache. *Arch Neurol*, 47:654–658.

Langemark, M, Loldrup, D, Bech, P, et al (1990). Clomipramine and mianserin in the treatment of chronic tension–type headache: a double–blind, controlled study. *Headache*, 30:118–121.

Langemark, M and Olesen, J (1987). Pericranial tenderness in tension headache. A blind, controlled study. *Cephalalgia*, 7:249–255.

Langemark, M, Olesen, J, Poulsen, DL, et al (1988). Clinical characteristics of patients with tension–type headache. *Headache*, 28:590–596.

Laurell, K, Larsson, B, and Eeg-Olofsson, O (2003). Headache in schoolchildren: agreement between different sources of information. *Cephalalgia*, 23:420–428.

Laurell, K, Larsson, B, and Eeg-Olofsson, O (2004). Prevalence of headache in Swedish schoolchildren, with a focus on tension–type headache. *Cephalalgia*, 24:380–388.

Lavados, PM and Tenhamm, E (2001). Consulting behaviour in migraine and tension–type headache sufferers: a population–based survey in Santiago, Chile. *Cephalalgia*, 21:733–737.

Lavados, PM, Tenhamm, E (1998). Epidemiology of tension-type headache in Santiago, chile: a prevalance study. *Cephalalgia*, 18:552–558.

Lawrence, RC, Helmick, CG, Arnett, FC, et al (1998). Estimates of the prevalence of arthritis and selected musculoskeletal disorders in the United States. *Arthritis Rheum* 41:778–799.

Leinisch-Dahlke, E, Jurgens, T, Bogdahn, U, et al (2005). Greater occipital nerve block is ineffective in chronic tension type headache. *Cephalalgia*, 25:704–708.

Lenaerts, M (1999). *Migraine and epilepsy: comorbidity and temporal relationship*. 9th Congress of the International Headache Society, Barcelona, Spain, June 1999.

Lenaerts, M (2005). Pharmacoprophylaxis of tension–type headache. *Curr Pain Headache Rep*, 9:442–447.

Lenaerts, M. *Headache in Children*. Emedicine. Available: http://www.emedicine.com/oph/topic334.htm#section~treatment 2000, updated 2005.

Lenaerts, M, Bastings, E, Sianard-Gainko, J, et al (1996). Sodium valproate in severe migraine and tension–type headache patients: an open study of long–term efficacy and correlation with blood levels. *Acta Neurol Belg*, 96:126–129.

Lenaerts, M and Couch, J (2004). Post–traumatic headache. *Curr Treat Options Neurol*, 6:507–517.

Lenaerts, ME (2004). Alternative therapies for tension–type headache. *Curr Pain Headache Rep*, 8:484–488.

Lenaerts, ME (2005). Pharmacoprophylaxis of tension–type headache. *Curr Pain Headache Rep*, 9:442–447.

Lenaerts, ME (2006). Burden of tension–type headache. *Curr Pain Headache Rep*, 10:459–462.

Lenaerts, ME and Gill, PS (2006). At the crossroads between tension–type headache and fibromyalgia. *Curr Pain Headache Rep*, 10:463–466.

Lenssinck, ML, Damen, L, Verhagen, AP, et al (2004). The effectiveness of physiotherapy and manipulation in patients with tension–type headache: a systematic review. *Pain*, 112:381–388.

Linde, K, Witt, CM, Streng, A, et al (2007). The impact of patient expectations on outcomes in four randomized controlled trials of acupuncture in patients with chronic pain. *Pain*, 128:264–271.

Lipchick, GL, Holroyd, KA, Talbot, F, et al (1997). Pericranial muscle tenderness and exteroceptive suppression of temporalis muscle activity: a blind study of chronic tension–type headache. *Headache*, 37:368–376.

Lipton, RB, Scher, AI, Kolodner, K, et al (2002). Migraine in the United States: Epidemiology and patterns of health care use. *Neurology*, 58:885–894.

Lipton, RB, Stewart, WF, Cady, R, et al (2000). Sumatriptan for the Range of Headaches in Migraine Sufferers: Results of the Spectrum Study. *Headache*, 40:783–791.

Locker, D, Slade, G (1988). Prevalance of symptoms associated with temporomandibular disorders in a canadian population. *Community Dent. Oral Epidemiol.*, 16:310–313.

Lyngberg, AC, Rasmussen, BK, Jorgensen, T, et al (2005a). Has the prevalence of migraine and tension–type headache changed over a 12–year period? A Danish population study. *Eur J Epidemiol*, 20:243–249.

Lyngberg, AC, Rasmussen, BK, Jørgensen, T, et al (2005b). Secular changes in health care utilization and work absence for migraine and tension–type headache: a population based study. *Eur J Epidemiol*, 20:1007–1014.

Manias, P, Tagaris, G, and, Karageorgiou K (2000). Acupuncture in headache: a critical review. *Clin J Pain*, 16:334–339.

Martinez-Martin, P, Raffaelli, E Jr., Titus, F, et al. (2001). The Co-operative Study Group. Efficacy and safety of metamizol versus acetylsalicylic acid in patients with moderate episodic tension–type headache: a randomized, double–blind, placebo– and active–controlled, multicenter study. *Cephalalgia*, 21:604–610.

Materazzo, F, Cathcart, S, and Pritchard, D (2000). Anger, depression, and coping interactions in headache activity and adjustment: a controlled study. *J Psychosom Res*, 49:69–75.

Mathew, NT (1981). Prophylaxis of migraine and mixed headache. A randomized controlled trial. *Headache*, 21:105–109.

Mathew, NT (1987). Transformed or evolutional migraine. *Headache*, 27:305–306.

Mathew, NT, Stubits E, and Nigam MR (1982). Transformation of migraine into daily headache; analysis of factors. *Headache*, 22:66–68.

Mauskop, A, Altura, BT, Cracco, RQ, et al (1993). Serum ionized magnesium levels in patients with tension–type headache. In *Tension–type Headache: Classification, Mechanisms and Treatment* (J Olesen and J Schoenen, eds.), pp. 137–140. Raven Press, New York.

Maytal, J, Young, M, Schechter, A, et al (1997). Pediatric migraine and the International Headache Society (IHS) criteria. *Neurology*, 48:602–607.

McCrory, D, Penzian, D, Hasselblad, V, et al (2001). *Behavioral and physical treatments for tension–type and cervicogenic headache.* Foundation for chiropractic education and research: Des Moins, IA.

Mehlisch, DR, Weaver, M, and Fladung, B (1998). Ketoprofen, acetaminophen, placebo in the treatment of tension headache. *Headache*, 38:579–589.

Melchart, D, Linde, K, Fischer, P, et al (2001). Acupuncture for idiopathic headache. *Cochrane Database Syst Rev*, (1):CD001218.

Melchart, D, Streng, A, Hoppe, A, et al (2005). Acupuncture in patients with tension–type headache: randomized, controlled trial. *BMJ*, 13:376–382.

Melchart, D, Weidenhammer, W, Streng, A, et al (2006). Acupuncture for Chronic Headaches—An Epidemiological Study. *Headache*, 46:632–641.

Melis, PM, Rooimans, W, Spierings, EL, et al (1991). Treatment of chronic tension–type headache with hypnotherapy: a single–blind time controlled study. *Headache*, 31:686–689.

Mense, S (1993). Nociception from skeletal muscle in relation to clinical muscle pain. *Pain*, 54:241–289.

Merikanagas, K, Merikangas, J, and Angst, J (1993). Headache syndromes and psychiatric disorders: association and familial transmission. *J Psychiatr*, 27:197–210.

Merikangas, KR, Stevens, DE, Angst, J (1994). Psychopathology and headache syndromes in the community. *Headache*, 34:S17–S22.

Milovanovic, M, Jarebinski, M, and Martinovic, Z (2007). Prevalence of primary headaches in children from Belgrade, Serbia. *Eur J Paediatr Neurol*, 11:136–141. Miner JR, Smith SW, Moore J, et al (2007). Sumatriptan for the treatment of undifferentiated primary headaches in the ED. *Am J Emerg Med*, 25:60–64.

Mitsikostas, DD and Thomas, AM (1999). Comorbidity of headache and depressive disorders. *Cephalalgia*, 19:211–217.

Moerk, H and Jensen, R (2000). Prognosis of tension–type headache: a 10–year follow–up study of patients with frequent tension–type headache. *Cephalalgia*, 20:434.

Mongini, F, Ciccone, G, Deregibus, A, et al (2004). Muscle tenderness in different headache types and its relation to anxiety and depression. *Pain*, 112:59–64.

Murros, K, Kataja, M, Hedman, C, et al (2000). Modified–release formulation in chronic tension–type headache. *Headache*, 40:633–637.

Nash, JM (2003). Psychologic and behavioral management of tension–type headache: treatment procedures. *Cur Headache and Pain Rep*, 7:475–481.

Nash, JM (2003). Psycologic and behavioral management of tension–type headache: Treatment procedures. *Curr Pain Headache Rep*, 2:209–215.

Ottmann, R and Lipton, RB (1994). Comorbidity of migraine and epilepsy. *Neurology*, 44:2105–2110.

Østergaard, S, Russell, MB, Bendtsen, L, et al (1997). Comparison of first degree relatives and spouses of people with chronic tension headache. *BMJ*, 314:1092–1093.

Packman, D, Packman, E, Doyle, G, et al. (2000). Solubilized ibuprofen: evaluation of onset, relief and safety of a novel formulation in the treatment of episodic tension–type headache. *Headache*, 40:561–567.

Padberg, M, de Bruijn, SF, de Haan, RJ, et al. Treatment of chronic tension–type headache with botulinum toxin: a double–blind, placebo–controlled clinical trial. *Cephalalgia* 24:675–680.

Palermo, TM, Valenzuela, D, and Stork, PP (2004). A randomized trial of electronic versus paper pain diaries in children: impact on complkiance, accuracy and acceptability. *Pain*, 107:213–219.

Pfaffenrath, V, Diener, HC, and Isler, H (1994). Efficacy and tolerability of amitriptilinoxide in the treatment of chronic tension–type headache: a multi–center controlled study. *Cephalalgia*, 14:149–155.

Pfaffenrath, V, Hummelsberger, J, Pöllmann, W, et al (1991). MMPI personality profiles in patients with primary headache syndromes. *Cephalalgia*, 11:263–268.

Pfaffenrath, V and Isler, H (1993). Evaluation of the nosology of chronic tension–type headache, *Cephalalgia*, 13:60–62.

Pielsticker, A, Haag, G, Zaudig, M, et al (2005). Impairment of pain inhibition in chronic tension–type headache. *Pain*, 118:215–223.

Pilley, JR, Mohlin, B, Shaw, WC, et al (1997). A survey of craniomandibular disorders in 500 19-years-olds. *Eur J Orthod*, 19:57–70.

Pop, PHM, Gierveld, CM, Karis, HAM, et al (2002). Epidemiological aspects of headache in a workplace setting and the impact on the economic loss. *Eur J Neurol*, 9:171–174.

Pryse-Phillips, W, Findlay, H, Tugwell, P, et al (1992). A Canadian population survey on the clinical, epidemiologic and societal impact of migraine and tension–type headache. *Can J Neurol Sci*, 19:333–339.

Puca, F, Genco, S, Prudenzano, MP, et al (1999). Psychiatric comorbidity and psychosocial stress in patients with tension–type headache from headache centers in Italy. The Italian Collaborative Group for the Study of Psychopathological Factors in Primary Headaches. *Cephalalgia*, 19:159–164.

Raines, JC, Penzien, DB, McCrory, DC, et al. Behavioral headache treatment: history, review of the empirical literature, and methodological critique. *Headache*, 45: S92–S109.

Rasmussen, BK (1995). Epidemiology of headache. *Cephalalgia*, 15:45–68.

Rasmussen, BK (1999). Epidemiology and socio–economic impact of headache. *Cephalalgia*, 19(Suppl. 25):20–23.

Rasmussen, BK, Jensen, R, and Olesen, J (1991a). A population–based analysis of the diagnostic criteria of the International Headache Society. *Cephalalgia*, 11:129–134.

Rasmussen, BK, Jensen, R, Schroll, M, et al (1991b). Epidemiology of headache in a general population: a prevalence study. *J Clin Epidemiol*, 44:1147–1157.

Rasmussen, BK, Jensen, R, Schroll, M, et al (1992). Interrelations between migraine and tension–type headache in the general population. *Arch Neurol*, 49:914–918.

Robinson, RL, Birnbarm, AG, Morley, MA, et al (2003). Economic cost and epidemiological characteristics of patients with fibromyalgia claims. *J Rheumatol*, 30:1318–1325.

Romanek, K, Holroyd, KA, Cottrell, C, et al (2005). Patterns of impairment, psychiatric comorbidity, and headache beliefs differ in migraine and tension–type headache. *Headache*, 45:776–790.

Rossi, P, Di Lorenzo, G, Faroni, J, et al (2006). Use of complementary and alternative medicine by patients with chronic tension–type headache: results of a headache clinic survey. *Headache*, 46:622–631.

Rozen, TD (2003). New daily persistent headache. *Curr Pain Headache Rep*, 7:218–223.

Russell, MB (2005). Tension–type headache in 40–year–olds: a Danish population–based sample of 4000. *J Headache Pain*, 6:441–447.

Russell, MB, Levi, N, Saltyte-Benth, J, et al (2006). Tension–type headache in adolescents and adults: a population based study of 33,764 twins. *Eur J Epidemiol*, 21:153–160.

Russell, MB, Saltyte-Benth, J, and Levi, N (2006). Are infrequent episodic, frequent episodic and chronic tension–type headache inherited? A population–based study or 11,199 twin pains. *J Headache Pain* 7:119–126.

Sandrini, G, Antonaci, F, Pucci, E, et al (1994). Comparative study with EMG, pressure algometry and manual palpation in tension–type headache and migraine. *Cephalalgia*, 14:451–457.

Saper, J, Lake, AE 3rd, and Cantrell, DT (2002). Chronic daily headache prophylaxis with tizanidine: a double–blind, multi–center outcome study. *Headache*, 42:470–482.

Scher, AI, Lipton, RB, and, Stewart WF (2003). Habitual snoring as a risk factor for chronic daily headache. *Neurology*, 60:1366–1368.

Schoenen, J (2004). Tension–type headache and fibromyalgia: what's common, what's different? *J Neurol Sci*, 25:S157–S159.

Schoenen, J, Bottin, D, Hardy, F, et al (1991). Cephalic and extracephalic pressure pain thresholds in chronic tension–type headache. *Pain*, 47:145–149.

Schoenen, J, Lenaerts, M, and Gerard, P (1993). Inhibition of temporal second exteroceptive suppression produced by single or long–lasting electrical stimuli and noxious thermal stimuli in peripheral limbs: Effects of naloxone. In Tension–type Headache: Classification, Mechanisms And Treatment (J Olesen, J Schoenen, eds.), pp. 181–185. Raven Press, New York.

Schoenen, J, Sianard-Gainko, J, and Lenaerts, M (1991). Blood magnesium levels in migraine. *Cephalalgia*, 11:97–99.

Schmidt-Hansen, PT, Svensson, P, Bendtsen, L, et al (2007). Increased muscle pain sensitivity in patients with tension–type headache. *Pain*, 129:112–121.

Schmidt-Wilcke, T, Leinich, E, Straube, A, et al (2005). Gray matter decrease in patients with chronic tension–type headache. *Neurology*, 65:1483–1486.

Schwartz, BS, Stewart, WF, and, Lipton RB. Lost workdays and decreased work effectiveness associated with headache in the workplace. *J Occup Environ Med*, 39:320–327.

Schwartz, BS, Stewart, WF, Simon, D, et al (1998). Epidemiology of tension–type headache. *JAMA*, 279:381–383.

Silberstein, SD, Lipton, RB, and Sliwinski, M (1996). Classification of daily and near–daily headaches: field trial of revised HIS criteria. *Neurology*, 47:871–875.

Silberstein, SD, Stark, SR, Lucas, SM, et al (2005). Botulinum toxin type a for the prophylactic treatment of chronic daily headache: a randomized double-blind, placebo-controlled trial. *Mayo Clin Proc*, 80(9):1126–1137.

Silva, HM Jr., Garbelini, PR, Teixeira, SO, et al (2004). Effect of episodic tension–type headache on the health–related quality of life in employees of a Brazilian public hospital. *Arq Neuropsiquiatr*, 62:769–773.

Singh, NN and Misra, S (2002). Sertraline in chronic tension–type headache. *J Assoc Physicians India*, 50:873–878.

Siniatchkin, M, Riabus, M, and Hasenbring, M (1999). Coping styles of headache sufferers. *Cephalalgia*, 19:165–173.

Sjaastad, O and Spierings, EL (1984). "Hemicrania continua": another headache absolutely responsive to indomethacin. *Cephalalgia*, 4:65–70.

Spierings, EL, Ranke, AH, and Honkoop, PC (2001). Precipitating and aggravating factors of migraine versus tension–type headache. *Headache*, 41:554–558.

Steiner, TJ and Lange, R (1998). Ketoprofen (25 mg) in the symptomatic treatment of episodic tension–type headache: double–blind placebo controlled comparison with of acetaminophen (1,000 mg). *Cephalalgia*, 18:38–43.

Torelli, P, Jensen, R, and Olesen, J (2004). Physiotherapy for tension–type headache: a controlled study. *Cephlalagia*, 24:29–36.

Tomkins, GE, Jackson, JL, O'Malley, PG, et al (2001). Treatment of chronic headache with antidepressant: a meta–analysis. *Am J Med*, 111:54–63.

Trautmann, E, Lackschewitz, H, and Kröner-Herwig, B, et al (2006). Psychological treatment of recurrent headache in children and adolescents—a meta–analysis. *Cephalalgia*, 26:114–126.

Ulrich, V, Gervil, M, and Olesen, J (2004). The relative influence of environment and genes in episodic tension–type headache. *Neurology*, 62:2065–2069.

Ulrich, V, Gervil, M, Kyvik, KO, et al (1999). Evidence of a genetic factor in migraine with aura: a population–based Danish twin study. *Ann Neurol*, 45:242–246.

Urlich, V, Russell, MB, Jensen R, et al (1996). A comparison of tension–type headache in migraineurs and non–migraineurs: a population–based study. *Pain*, 67:501–506.

van Ettekoven, H and Lucas, C (2006). Efficacy of physiotherapy including a craniocervical training programme for tension–type headache; a randomized clinical trial. *Cephalalgia*, 26:983–991.

Verhagen, AP, Damen, L, Berger, MY, et al (2005). Conservative treatments of children with episodic tension–type headache. A systematic review. *J Neurol*, 252:1147–1154.

Vernon, H, McDermaid, CS, and Hagino, C (1999). Systematic review of randomized clinical trials of complementary/alternative therapies in the treatment of tension–type and cervicogenic headache. *Complement Ther Med*, 7:142–155.

Walach, H, Lowes, T, Mussbach, D, et al (2001). The long–term effects of homeopathic treatment of chronic headaches: one year follow–up and single case time series analysis. *Br Homeopath J*, 90:63–72.

Wallash, TM (1993). Transcranial Doppler ultrasonic findings in episodic and chronic tension–type headache. In *Tension–type Headache: Classification, Mechanisms And Treatment* (J Olesen and J Schoenen, eds), pp. 173–175. Raven Press, New York.

Wang, SJ (2003). Epidemiology of migraine and other types of headache in Asia. *Curr Neurol Neurosci Rep*, 3:104–108.

Wang, SJ, Fuh, JL, Lu, SR, et al (2000). Chronic daily headache in Chinese elderly: prevalence, risk factors, and biannual follow–up. *Neurology*, 54:314–319.

Wang, SJ, Fuh, JL, Lu, SR, et al (2007). Outcomes and predictors of chronic daily headache in adolescents. A 2–year longitudinal study. *Neurology*, 68:591–596.

Wang, SJ, Fuh, JL, Young, YH, et al (2001). Frequency and predictors of physician consultations for headache. *Cephalalgia*, 21:25–30.

Wang, SJ, Liu, H, Fuh, J, et al (1999). Comorbidity of headaches and depression in the elderly. *Pain*, 82:239–243.

White, KP, Nielson, WR, Harth, M, et al (2002). Chronic widespread musculoskeletal pain with or without fibromyalgia: psychological distress in a representative community adult sample. *J Rheumatol*, 29:588–594.

Wittrock, DA (1997). The comparison of individuals with tension–type headache and headache–free controls on frontal EMG levels: a meta–analysis. *Headache*, 37:424–432.

Wittrock, DA and Myers, TC (1998). The comparison of individuals with recurrent tension–type headache and headache–free controls in appraisal and coping with stressors: a review of the literature. *Ann Behav Med*, 20:118–134.

Wöber-Bingöl, C, Wöber, C, Karwautz, A, et al (1995). Diagnosis of headache in childhood and adolescence: a study in 437 patients. *Cephalalgia*, 15:13–21.

Wober, C, Holzhammer, J, Zeitlhofer, J, et al (2006). Trigger factors of migraine and tension–type headache: experience and knowledge of the patients. *J Headache Pain*, 7:188–195.

Wu J, Lin Q, McAdoo DJ, et al. Nitric oxide contributes to central sensitization following intradermal injection of capsaicin. *Neuroreport*, 9:589–592.

Xue, CC, Dong, L, Polus, B, et al (2004). Electroacupuncture for tension–type headache on distal acupoints only: a randomized, controlled, crossover trial. *Headache*, 44:333–341.

Yunus, MB (2005a). The concept of central sensitivity syndromes. In *Fibromyalgia and Other Central Pain Syndromes* (D Wallace, D Clauw, eds) pp. 29–44. Lippincott Williams & Wilkins: Philadelphia.

Yunus, MB (2005b). Symptoms and signs of fibromyalgia syndrome: an overview. In *Fibromyalgia and Other Central Pain Syndromes.* (D Wallace, D Clauw, eds) pp. 125–132. Lippincott Williams & Wilkins: Philadelphia.

Yunus, MB, Arslan, S, and Aldag, JC (2002). Relationship between fibromyalgia features and smoking. *Scand J Rheumatol*, 31:301–305.

Yunus, MB, Masi, AT, and Aldag, JC (1989). A controlled study of primary fibromyalgia syndrome: clinical features and association with other functional syndromes. *J Rheumatol*, 19:62–71.

Zhao, C and Stillman, M (2003). New developments in the pharmacotherapy of tension–type headache. *Expert Opin Pharmacother*, 4:2229–2237.

13 Chronic Daily Headache Including Transformed Migraine, Chronic Tension-type Headache, and Medication Overuse Headache

Stephen D Silberstein, Richard B Lipton, and Joel R Saper

INTRODUCTION

Chronic daily headache (CDH) is an umbrella term for headache disorders that occur very frequently. Although the classification remains intensely debated, the consensus is that the term CDH refers to headache disorders, including headaches associated with medication overuse, which are experienced 15 or more days a month. Our approach to classifying frequent headaches consists of first defining whether it is a primary or secondary entity and then subclassifying primary CDH on the basis of average daily headache duration (⩾4 hours or >4 hours). Primary CDH is not related to a structural or systemic illness and probably reflects an intrinsic brain disturbance (Silberstein and Lipton, 2001). This approach is reviewed in the broader context of headache diagnosis in Chapter 2.

In clinic-based studies in the United States, approximately 80% of patients have CDH (Mathew et al., 1982; Mathew et al., 1987; Rapoport, 1988). In population-based studies around the world, 4%–5% of the general population have primary CDH, and 0.5% have severe headaches on a daily basis (Scher et al., 1998; Castillo et al., 1999; Wang et al., 2000). In population samples, chronic tension-type headache (CTTH) is the leading cause of primary CDH (Rasmussen, 1992). Patients with CDH account for the greatest number of consultations in headache subspecialty practices (Silberstein et al., 1994).

Patients with CDH frequently overuse medication, which may play a role in initiating or sustaining the pattern of pain (Saper and Jones, 1986). Anxiety, depression, and other psychological disturbances may accompany the headaches (Silberstein et al., 1994).

Secondary CDH has an identifiable underlying cause, although the secondary process may provoke a preexisting primary headache entity, such as migraine. An example of this would be medication overuse headache (MOH), which principally serves to aggravate the preexisting migraine. Other causes of secondary CDH include head trauma, cervical spine disorders, vascular disorders, nonvascular intracranial disorders, temporomandibular joint disorders, sinus infections (Brain, 1963; Rapoport, 1988; Lake et al., 1990; Mathew, 1991; Lake et al., 1993), chronic meningitis, and idiopathic intracranial hypertension (IIH) (Mathew, 1982; Mathew et al., 1982; Saper, 1983; Mathew et al., 1987; Olesen et al., 1993). IIH is easily diagnosed when papilledema is present, but some patients with IIH do not have papilledema, in which case the disorder can mimic primary CDH. Cervicogenic headache is a unilateral pain disorder that does not switch sides, occurs mainly in women, and may be associated with ipsilateral blurred vision, tinnitus, lacrimation, tingling, difficulty swallowing, photophobia, arm pain, and, when more severe, nausea and anorexia (Sjaastad et al., 1983; Sjaastad, 1990). Certain focal dystonias of the head and neck (pharyngeal dystonia, spasmodic torticollis, mandibular dystonia, lingual dystonia, and segmental craniocervical dystonia) are often accompanied by daily headache.

Once secondary headache (including MOH) has been excluded, primary daily- or almost-daily-headache sufferers are subdivided into two groups based on headache duration. When the headache duration is less than 4 hours, the differential diagnosis includes cluster headache, paroxysmal hemicrania, idiopathic stabbing headache, hypnic headache, and SUNCT (short-lasting unilateral neuralgiform headache attacks with conjunctival injection and tearing). When the headache duration is greater than 4 hours, the major primary disorders to consider are chronic migraine (CM), hemicrania continua (HC), CTTH, and new daily persistent headache (NDPH) (Table 13–1) (Silberstein et al., 1994). [CTTH was included in the first International Headache Society (IHS) classification and inappropriately equated to CDH.] (Headache Classification Committee of the International Headache Society, 1988). Currently CM, NDPH, and HC are the primary CDH disorders that are included in the second IHS classification (ICHD-2) (Headache Classification Committee, 2004) (Table 13–1). Transformed migraine (TM) is similar, but not identical, to CM.

In this chapter, we discuss the classification and treatment of primary CDH of long duration, highlighting the four categories outlined earlier (Headache Classification Committee, 2004). We will comment and, when appropriate, provide alternate criteria. We will also discuss the role of medication overuse in the development and treatment of these disorders, as well as their mechanisms and treatment.

TABLE 13–1 Chronic Daily Headache.

Primary chronic daily headache

- Headache duration >4 hours or more
  - Chronic migraine (previously transformed migraine)
  - Chronic tension-type headache
  - New daily persistent headache
  - Hemicrania continua
- Headache duration less than 4 hours
  - Cluster headache
  - Paroxysmal hemicranias
  - Hypnic headache
  - Idiopathic stabbing headache
  - SUNCT

Secondary chronic daily headache

- Medication overuse headache (MOH)
- Posttraumatic headache
- Cervical spine disorders
- Headache associated with vascular disorders [arteriovenous malformation, arteritis (including giant cell arteritis), dissection, and subdural hematoma]
- Headache associated with nonvascular intracranial disorders [intracranial hypertension, infection (EBV, HIV), neoplasm]
- Other (temporomandibular joint disorder; sinus infection)

Source: Modified from Silberstein et al. (1994).

HISTORIC WEAKNESSES OF IHS CLASSIFICATION OF CDH

Many studies have identified weaknesses in the original criteria mandated by the IHS to classify CDH (Headache Classification Committee of the International Headache Society, 1988), one of the most common disorders seen in headache centers (Saper, 1990; Messinger et al., 1991; Solomon et al., 1992b; Mathew, 1993; Pfaffenrath and Isler, 1993; Silberstein, 1993; Sanin et al., 1994). These studies showed that CDH was not easily classified within the old IHS system (Messinger et al., 1991; Solomon et al., 1992b; Mathew, 1993; Pfaffenrath and Isler, 1993; Sanin et al., 1994). When originally classified, the headaches were placed in the CTTH group. But because the daily headaches often evolved from episodic migraine and the patients had many migrainous features, it was inappropriate to classify them as CTTH. The headaches were too frequent to permit them being classified as migraine (Solomon et al., 1992b).

Migraine and tension-type headache (TTH) have long been considered distinct entities, and the ICHD-2 continues this separation (Headache Classification Committee of the International Headache Society, 1988; Headache Classification Committee, 2004). However, many clinicians and epidemiologists now believe that the TTH that migraineurs experience is, often, a milder form of migraine (Silberstein, 1993). In nonmigraineurs, it is perhaps a distinct entity; but as headache frequency increases, the clinical distinction between migraine and TTH becomes blurred. Moreover, as migraine becomes more frequent, headaches often decrease in severity and associated migrainous features decline in prominence. The headaches occur daily or almost every day, and occasional full-blown migraine attacks may be superimposed on these background headaches. Saper used the term "progressive migraine" for this disorder, and referred to the condition as complex headache syndrome because of the presence of comorbidities (Saper and Winters, 1982; Saper, 1983). Saper credits John Graham with being one of the first physicians to note the transition from intermittent to daily headache. Mathew referred to this disorder as transformed migraine (Mathew et al., 1982), a term that was readily accepted. An older term was "mixed or combined headache" (Saper, 1990; Solomon et al., 1992b). The IHS did not use these terminologies to describe headaches that progressed or transformed in frequency, and therefore there was no appropriate classification within the first IHS classification formulation for this phenomenon. From at least the late 1970s and early 1980s, the entity was recognized by US experts. Nevertheless, at least in the United States it was a common problem in headache subspecialty practices (Silberstein, 1993). Although the first classification did not include the entity, the second IHS classification (Headache Classification Committee, 2004) now uses the term chronic migraine, which varies somewhat from TM (see later).

In fact, several studies illustrated the fact that the original IHS system did not adequately classify or even recognize many of the patients seen in subspecialty centers, particularly in the United States. Messinger et al. (1991), using the IHS criteria and questionnaire data from two surveys, attempted to classify a clinic-based sample of 410 subjects who had a headache history of more than 2 years. They were unable to classify 35.9% of the patients. Overall, only 9.1% had CTTH, but approximately 86% of these patients with CTTH had two or more migrainous features. Solomon et al. (1992b) evaluated 100 consecutive patients who presented to a tertiary headache center with CDH. Most (61%) had continuous headache; 39% had intermittent headache defined by pain-free intervals of at least 1 hour at least 4 days a week. More than 50% overused acute medication. While two-thirds of these patients met the criteria for CTTH, many had migrainous features. One-third of the patients could not be classified as CTTH because they had too many migrainous features. Many of these headaches would be classifiable as migraine were it not for their daily occurrence. Many patients could not be classified in the old IHS system [except as "headache of the tension-type not fulfilling above (other) criteria"]. The authors pointed out that the IHS criteria did not take into account the historical features of CDH before it becomes daily. Is CDH preceded by episodic migraine or TTH, or do the headaches begin de novo? Past history is an essential part of the headache diagnosis. Solomon and Lipton concluded that the IHS criteria should be modified to include TM (CDH evolving from migraine), and that subtypes with and without medication overuse should be distinguished both for TM and CTTH. They did not propose specific diagnostic criteria for these disorders.

In a less selected sample, Sanin et al. (1994) attempted to validate the IHS criteria in a headache clinic population. They randomly selected the clinical records of 400 patients and classified them using the IHS criteria. More than 55% of the patients had more than one diagnosis, and 37.7% had CDH. One hundred and ten patients were diagnosed with CTTH; 90% of them also suffered from migraine. Sanin et al. concluded that most patients in their clinic had more than one IHS diagnosis, that CTTH occurring alone is rare, and that chronic headache classification needed revision. Pfaffenrath and Isler (1993) investigated the IHS criteria for CTTH in a sample of 211 subjects participating in a clinical trial of antidepressant treatment. Fifty-six percent of patients had daily headache. The remaining 44% experienced headaches on an average of 18 days per month. More than two-thirds met the two major IHS criteria for CTTH (bilateral pain, 79%; pressure or tightening, 72%). Fifty-nine percent met all the IHS criteria for CTTH. However, many symptoms of migraine were also reported: unilateral headache, 20%; throbbing, 28%; anorexia, 39%; osmophobia, 25%; phonophobia, 60%; nausea, 53%; and increased pain with physical activity, 48%. In total, half of the patients failed to meet one or more of the criteria of migraine. Many patients experienced the symptoms of migraine with headaches of mild intensity. These studies suggested that the IHS criteria needed to be revised with respect to the classification of daily headache.

Despite being ignored by the IHS classification process, several studies and reports supported the existence of headache evolution or progression, most widely referring to it as transformed migraine (Saper and VanMeter, 1980; Mathew et al., 1982; Saper and Winters, 1982). Mathew (1993) reported a series of patients with distinct attacks of migraine, whose headaches evolved over the years into a daily or near-daily problem. The majority of women had menstrual aggravation of headache (Saper and VanMeter, 1980; Mathew et al., 1982; Saper and Winters, 1982; Saper, 1983). Patients had features of both migraine and TTH. Most (90%) had migraine without aura. These patients had more triggers, gastrointestinal symptoms, and family history of headaches than patients with CTTH (Mathew, 1993). Most overused acute medications. Stopping the overused medication frequently resulted in distinct headache improvement (Saper and VanMeter, 1980).

Saper (1983) found that 80% of his patients with CDH had prior episodic migraine, with onset between the ages of 26 and 41 years. These patients were typically women. They were frequently clinically depressed and had superimposed acute bouts of migraine. Many of them overused abortive headache medications, and had significant long-term improvement after detoxification.

Sandrini et al. (1993) classified 90 consecutive outpatients with CDH, who attended a clinic in Italy. Most (75%) had CDH evolving from migraine, while 16.7% began de novo and 7.7% had evolved from episodic tension-type headache (ETTH). They differentiated two subsets of patients with CDH evolving from migraine. TM referred to those patients who had distinct bouts of migraine that evolved into CDH with the disappearance of typical migraine attacks. Migraine with interparoxysmal headache was defined as recurrent bouts of migraine with a constant, low-severity headache between attacks.

Silberstein et al. (1990) studied 300 patients who had chronic refractory headache and were admitted to an inpatient unit. Most (216) had CDH associated with acute medication overuse. A subset of these patients (50) who overused medication were followed for 2 years. Most had TM (74%), some had NDPH (24%), and only 2% had CTTH with a diagnosis of prior ETTH. Most patients (80%) reverted to episodic headache after detoxification, suggesting that both TM and NDPH associated with medication overuse are perpetuated by drug overuse.

Based upon these and other observations, Silberstein and Lipton concluded that: (1) The IHS classification was not comprehensive, for there was a large subset of patients with daily headache who were not well classified; (2) daily headache is often TM; in this area, the IHS criteria for CTTH may not be valid; and (3) CDH is often associated with medication overuse, but may occur without it. They recommended revising the IHS criteria for chronic, frequent primary headache disorders, and proposed adding several headache types to the 1988 IHS classification (Silberstein et al., 1994). They defined CDH as a group of several distinct types of primary headaches. CDH includes all of the primary headache disorders with daily or near-daily headaches that last more than 4 hours a day untreated. CDH was subdivided into TM, CTTH evolved from ETTH, NDPH, and HC.

Silberstein and Lipton proposed operational criteria for TM in 1994, including it as a subset of migraine (Table 13–2). Its diagnosis depended on a history of IHS-defined migraine and the presence of head pain lasting more than 4 hours a day on at least 15 days a month. They elected not to require particular characteristics for the daily or near-daily headaches, in part because these headaches are pleiomorphic; daily headaches may be unilateral or bilateral, mild to severe in intensity, with or without associated migrainous features. They originally required a history of transformation, that is, a period when migraine headaches increased in frequency while the prominence of associated migrainous features decreased. Some patients with TM continue to have superimposed episodic bouts of full-blown migraine, but others find that their acute migraine headaches disappear. Some find that their migraine headaches disappear completely. For this reason, Silberstein and Lipton did not originally use the continuing

Table 13–2 Original Proposed Criteria for Transformed Migraine.

1.8 Transformed Migraine (TM)

A. History of episodic migraine meeting any IHS criteria 1.1 to 1.6
B. Daily or almost daily (more than 15 days/month) head pain for more than 1 month
C. Average headache duration of 4 hours/day (if untreated)
D. History of increasing headache frequency with decreasing severity of migrainous features over at least 3 months
E. At least one of the following
  1. There is no suggestion of one of the disorders listed in groups 5–11
  2. Such a disorder is suggested, but it is ruled out by appropriate investigations
  3. Such disorder is present, but first migraine attacks do not occur in close temporal relation to the disorder

1.8.1 Transformed Migraine with medication overuse

1.8.2 Transformed Migraine without medication overuse

occurrence of superimposed migraine attacks as part of their definition.

According to the Silberstein and Lipton criteria, TM was subdivided into two categories, one with and one without medication overuse, using a consensus of published reports to define medication overuse. They recommended field-testing their proposed revisions to the IHS criteria to determine whether they served the intended purposes. They prospectively assessed (in a headache subspecialty center) the comprehensiveness of the IHS criteria with and without the addition of the original criteria for TM. They then determined whether subjects could provide the information necessary to assign diagnoses using the revised criteria. They identified subjects who could not be classified, and recommended modifications based on the results of the field tests (Silberstein et al., 1996).

Silberstein and Lipton argued that the existing data and authoritative experience confirm that the old IHS criteria were not comprehensive: they were unable to classify 43% of daily headache sufferers. [This result is concordant with the previous studies (Messinger et al., 1991; Solomon et al., 1992b) conducted at subspecialty centers.] They estimated that 25% of patients still could not be classified. Some patients had difficulty remembering the characteristics of their prior headaches, that is, whether their headaches had escalated, when they had escalated, and how long the process of escalation took. They therefore modified the definition of TM to include subjects with either a history of IHS migraine, a history of escalation more than 3 months, or a current headache that, except for duration, met the IHS criteria for migraine (Table 13–3). This allowed the use of both historical and current features of the headache,

Table 13–3 Silberstein–Lipton (Revised) Criteria for Chronic Migraine.

1.8 Chronic migraine

A. Daily or almost daily (more than 15 days/month) head pain for more than 1 month
B. Average headache duration of more than 4 hours/day (if untreated)
C. At least one of the following:
  1. History of episodic migraine meeting any IHS criteria 1.1 to 1.6
  2. History of increasing headache frequency with decreasing severity of migrainous features over at least 3 months.
  3. Headache at some time meets IHS criteria for migraine 1.1 to 1.6 other than duration
D. Does not meet criteria for new daily persistent headache (4.7) or hemicrania continua (4.8)
E. At least one of the following:
  1. There is no suggestion of one of the disorders listed in groups 5–11
  2. Such a disorder is suggested, but it is ruled out by appropriate investigations
  3. Such a disorder is present, but first migraine attacks do not occur in close temporal relation to the disorder

Source: Modified from Silberstein *et al.* (1994).

which are crucial to the diagnosis. Using the 1995 Silberstein–Lipton criteria, 15.3% of patients had CTTH, 78% had TM, none had NDPH, and 6.7% had none of these disorders. To avoid more than one diagnosis for a single headache type, they imposed hierarchical diagnostic rules: patients could not be diagnosed with CTTH if they met the criteria for TM. The purpose of their effort was to make the IHS criteria more comprehensive by providing a place for patients with TM.

CM VERSUS TRANSFORMED MIGRAINE

As if it were not sufficiently complicated, the new IHS classification includes an entity called CM, which is similar, but not identical, to TM (Silberstein et al., 1996). It includes only the third IHS criterion for migraine. For the purpose of simplicity, in this chapter we will call TM by the name CM, the term currently used by the IHS.

Many studies have described the process of an evolution or progression of headache (Mathew, 1982; Mathew et al., 1982; Saper, 1983; Mathew et al., 1987; Olesen et al., 1993; Silberstein et al., 1996), which is similar to transformational migraine as described by Mathew (1982). Patients with TM often had a past history of episodic migraine that began in their teens or twenties (Saper, 1983; Mathew et al., 1987; Silberstein et al., 1996). Most patients with this disorder are women, 90% of whom have a history of migraine without aura. Patients often report a process of transformation or progression characterized by headaches that become more frequent over months to years, with the associated symptoms of photophobia, phonophobia, and nausea becoming less severe and less frequent (Mathew, 1982; Saper, 1983; Mathew, 1987). Patients often develop (or transform into) a pattern of daily or nearly-daily headaches that phenomenologically resemble a mixture of TTH and migraine. That is, the pain is often mild to moderate and is not always associated with photophobia, phonophobia, or gastrointestinal features. Other features of migraine, including unilaterality, gastrointestinal symptoms, and aggravation by menstruation and other trigger factors, may persist. Many patients experience attacks of full-blown migraine superimposed on a background of less severe headaches. Eighty percent of patients with TM have depression (Saper, 1983; Mathew, 1993), which often lifts when the pattern of medication overuse and daily headache is interrupted. The term CM is now being used by the IHS, in part because a history of transformation is frequently missing. CM is classified as a subset of migraine.

Silberstein and Lipton's revised criteria for TM (Table 13–3) provided three alternative diagnostic links to migraine: (1) a prior history of IHS migraine; (2) a clear period of escalating headache frequency with decreasing severity of migrainous features; or (3) current superimposed attacks of headaches that meet all the IHS criteria for migraine except duration (Silberstein et al., 1996). Bigal et al. (2003) used the Silberstein–Lipton criteria to compare the features of TM patients with (TM+) and without (TM−) a history of migraine in a preventive trial of TM. The groups were similar in age (42.5 versus 44.2 years), gender (86.4% versus 78.3% female), monthly migraine days (13.6 versus 12.6), Migraine Disability Assessment Scale grades, and Beck Depression Inventory (BDI) scores. The groups differed in time of onset (10.6 versus 17.5 years). This suggests that they have the same disorder and supports the Silberstein–Lipton criteria for TM. The difference between the groups is the longer duration of TM−, suggesting that these patients may have forgotten their history of migraine.

THE RELATIONSHIP OF CM (TM) TO MOH

Migraine often transforms into CDH as a result of medication overuse (MOH), but transformation can occur without overuse (Mathew et al., 1982; Mathew et al., 1990). Approximately 80% of patients with CDH seen in subspecialty clinics overuse symptomatic medication (Mathew et al., 1982; Saper, 1983; Mathew, 1987; Mathew et al., 1987; Bigal et al., 2002). Headache frequency often increases when medication use increases. In many, but not all, cases, stopping the overused medication results in distinct headache improvement, although it may take days to weeks. Many patients have significant long-term improvement after detoxification.

Using the 1998 IHS criteria, a diagnosis of headache induced by substance use or exposure requires that the headaches remit completely after the overused medication is discontinued (Headache Classification Committee of the International Headache Society, 1988). This criterion was impractical to apply because, according to the criteria, the diagnosis was impossible to establish until the overused medication was discontinued (Silberstein et al., 1994). The 2004 IHS criteria attempted to get around this issue by using the term probable CM (see below).

The ICHD-2 (Headache Classification Committee, 2004) considers CM to be a subset of migraine (Table 13–4). Its diagnosis originally required migraine headache to occur on 15 or more days a month for more than 3 months without medication overuse. The requirement that the daily headache must meet the criteria for migraine without aura for 15 or more days a month was a concern. Even episodic migraine does not always meet IHS migraine criteria throughout the attack. Bigal et al. (2002) applied alternative diagnostic approaches to 638 patients with CDH in a specialty care practice. Patients were classified according to both the Silberstein–Lipton and the 2004 IHS classification systems. Patients were predominantly female (65.0%), with ages ranging from 11 to 88 years. Using the Silberstein–Lipton classification, they found eight different diagnoses. The most common diagnosis was TM (87.4%), followed by NDPH (10.8%). Six patients had CTTH. Using the IHS criteria, they found 14 different diagnoses. Migraine was found in 576 patients (90.2%). CTTH occurred in 621 patients (97.3%), with only 10 (1.57%) having this as the sole diagnosis. They concluded that both systems allow for the classification of most patients with CDH when daily headache diaries are available.

TABLE 13–4 Original IHS Criteria for Chronic Migraine (Headache Classification Committee of the International Headache Society, 1988).

A. Headache fulfilling criteria C and D for 1.1 *Migraine without aura* on 15 days or more permonth for more than 3 months
B. Not attributed to another disorder

Source: The ICHD-2 (Headache Classification Commitee, 2004).

The main difference is that the IHS classification is cumbersome and requires multiple diagnoses. They found that the Silberstein–Lipton system is easier to apply and more parsimonious.

Because of these problems, the ICHD-2 criteria for CM were revised (Olesen et al., 2006). They now require that migraine or treatment with a triptan or ergot occur on at least 8 days a month, and that headache is present on at least 15 days a month (Table 13–5). It must not be attributable to another disorder including HC, NDPH, or medication overuse. When medication overuse is present (and the headache worsens with overuse), the diagnosis is now MOH. [The original unwieldy IHS rule was to code these patients according to the antecedent migraine subtype plus probable CM plus probable MOH. If criteria for CM are still fulfilled 2 months after medication overuse has ceased, diagnose CM plus the antecedent

TABLE 13–5 Revised IHS Criteria for Chronic Migraine (REF).

A. Headache (tension-type and/or migraine) on 15 or more days per month for at least 3 months
B. Occurring in a patient who has had at least five attacks fulfilling criteria B–D for 1.1 *Migraine without aura*
C. On 8 or more days per month for at least 3 months headache has fulfilled C1 and/or C2 below, that is, has fulfilled criteria for pain and associated symptoms of migraine without aura
    1. Has at least two of a–d
        (a) unilateral location
        (b) pulsating quality
        (c) moderate or severe pain intensity
        (d) aggravation by or causing avoidance of routine physical activity (e.g., walking or climbing stairs)

    and at least one of a or b
        (a) nausea and/or vomiting
        (b) photophobia and phonophobia
    2. treated and relieved by triptan(s) or ergot before the expected development of C1 above
D. No medication overuse and not attributed to another causative disorder

migraine subtype and discard the diagnosis of probable MOH. If CM criteria are no longer fulfilled, change the diagnosis to MOH plus the antecedent migraine subtype and discard the diagnosis of probable CM (Headache Classification Committee, 2004).] The revised ICHD-2 CM criteria are easier to use, but many still prefer the Silberstein–Lipton criteria.

Many researchers have used the Silberstein–Lipton criteria to study the clinical characteristics of TM. Krymchantowski et al. (1999) retrospectively evaluated 215 patients with CDH seen in a headache clinic. Subjects included 158 women and 57 men aged 12–83 years, mean age 35 years, who had clear-cut prior IHS migraine attacks (with and/or without aura). Most met the Silberstein–Lipton criteria for TM. All had daily moderate pain and some had intermittent attacks of severe headache; 46.5% had bilateral pain, 37.1% hemicranial pain, 12.1% diffuse pain, and 26.5% other pain locations. Approximately 41% had throbbing pain; 36.2% had tightening pain, 17.2% a combination of throbbing and dull pain, 4.2% burning pain, and 7.4% other types of headache.

Monzón et al. (1999) classified and analyzed the clinical features of 164 consecutive patients with CDH (headache at least 15 days a month during the previous 6 months). CDH had evolved from a previous headache in 151 cases: migraine in 118 (72%) (TM) and ETTH in 33 (20%). CDH was unremitting from onset in 13 cases (8%) (NDPH). Most patients had nonpulsating, bilateral pain of moderate intensity with few associated symptoms. Sixty-five percent overused analgesics or ergots; 18% were men and 82% were women.

DIFFERENTIATING CM FROM OTHER CDHs

CDH refers to a set of primary headache disorders (mainly CM and CTTH, but also NDPH and HC); however, the diagnosis requires that the headaches are not attributable to another disorder, the most common of which is MOH. Causes of frequent headaches include prior trauma (chronic posttraumatic headache), cervical spine disorders, vascular disorders, chronic meningitis, IIH, temporomandibular joint disorder, and sinus infection (Bousser and Russell, 1997; Silberstein and Lipton, 2001).

Intracranial hypertension is readily diagnosed when papilledema is present, but if it is absent, intracranial hypertension can mimic CDH. Intracranial hypertension may be idiopathic (IIH), with no clear identifiable cause, or symptomatic; underlying etiologies for the latter include venous sinus occlusion, a mass lesion, meningitis, trauma, radical neck dissection, hypoparathyroidism, vitamin A intoxication, systemic lupus, renal disease, or drug side-effects (nalidixic acid, danazol, steroid withdrawal). Intracranial hypertension from cerebral venous outflow obstruction can be caused by chronic otitis, head trauma, tumors, hypercoagulable states, or cerebral edema (Wall et al., 2001). Increased intracranial pressure consequent to venous outflow hypertension can also occur without obstruction when patients have arteriovenous malformations, cardiac failure, and pulmonary failure.

Increased intracranial pressure is not always associated with either headache or papilledema, and there is no direct correlation between the degree of pressure elevation and the presence of headache. IIH, although more common in obese women, can also occur in nonobese women and in men. The presence of transient visual obscurations and intracranial noises provide clues to the diagnosis. Cerebral venous thrombosis may be difficult to diagnose. The typical features of cerebral venous thrombosis may be absent; that is, there is no history of new onset seizures, no focal neurologic deficits, no change of consciousness, no cranial nerve palsies, no bilateral cortical signs, and no evidence of papilledema on funduscopic examination.

CDH associated with elevated CSF pressure is easily diagnosed when papilledema is present, but not when it is absent. Secondary intracranial hypertension can mimic primary CDH (see Chapter 18). This issue was further studied by Mosek et al. (1999), who prospectively measured the CSF opening pressure of 24 patients who had CDH without papilledema. The average CSF opening pressure was 170 $\pm$ 41 mm, and five patients (21%) had an opening pressure of greater than 200 mm CSF. Patients with CDH had a mean CSF opening pressure that was 13 mm higher than nonheadache patients ($p = 0.05$), after adjusting for body mass index, age, sex, and various nonheadache disorders. The odds of having a CSF opening pressure greater than

200 mm CSF was five times greater for patients with CDH than nonheadache patients. These observations suggest that increased intracranial pressure may be comorbid with CDH in some patients.

Spontaneous intracranial hypotension (often due to a spontaneous CSF leak) typically presents as a daily headache with a positional component. However, it can be missed, as the postural components may disappear soon after onset or over time. Occasionally, orthostatic features are absent. Patients may notice that their headaches begin after arising and gradually worsen during the day (Mathew, 1991). CSF hypotension may begin suddenly, with a thunderclap presentation. Infectious causes, including fungal (coccidiomycosis), bacterial (Lyme, tuberculosis), and parasitic (neurocysticercosis) causes, should be considered in high-risk patients. Sphenoid sinusitis can present as an intractable headache that is unresponsive to analgesics and interferes with sleep (Chapter 24). It often occurs without associated nasal symptoms. Obstructive sleep apnea can present with daily headaches upon awakening. It should be considered when patients have a snoring history, large neck size, or are obese. Cervical spine, temporomandibular joint, or dental pathology must be considered when chronic cranial, nuchal, or facial pain is present. Cervicogenic headache (Sjaastad et al., 1983) is a unilateral pain disorder that does not switch sides (Sjaastad, 1990), occurs mainly in women, and may be associated with ipsilateral blurred vision, tinnitus, lacrimation, tingling, difficulty swallowing, photophobia, arm pain, and, when more severe, nausea and anorexia. "Neck triggers" and reduced cervical range of motion are characteristic. As it is uncertain whether cervicogenic headache is an independent entity or migraine or TTH with a cervical trigger (Pfaffenrath and Kaube, 1990), its classification is uncertain.

Magnetic resonance imaging (MRI) plus magnetic resonance venogram (MRV) (with gadolinium if needed) are the neuroimaging procedures of choice for patients suspected of having a secondary cause for CDH, since many of these disorders remain undetected even with contrast-enhanced CT. Special attention must be paid to sinus disorders, particularly the sphenoid sinus (see Chapter 24). With a normal physical examination and absence of red flags or worrisome historical features, secondary causes of CM can usually be eliminated (Gladstone et al., 2003).

Once secondary headache has been excluded, frequent headache sufferers are subdivided into two groups, based on headache duration. When headache duration is less than 4 hours, the differential diagnosis includes cluster headache, chronic paroxysmal hemicrania, idiopathic stabbing headache, hypnic headache, and other miscellaneous headache disorders. When the headache duration is greater than 4 hours, the major primary disorders to consider are CM, HC, CTTH, and NDPH (Table 13–1) (Silberstein et al., 1994).

Several authors have examined the relative frequency of some of these conditions in patients with CDH. Mathew et al. (1987) found that 77% of patients with CDH had what they called TM. Solomon et al. (1992a) found that most of their patients with CDH had TM. Sandrini et al. (1993) classified 90 consecutive patients with CDH who attended an outpatient clinic in Italy. Most had CDH evolving from migraine (75.0%); 16.7% had CDH that had begun de novo, and 7.7% had CDH that had evolved from ETTH. They differentiated two subsets of patients with CDH evolving from migraine. TM referred to those patients who had distinct bouts of migraine that evolved into CDH with the disappearance of typical migraine attacks. "Migraine with interparoxysmal headache" was defined as recurrent bouts of migraine with a constant, low-severity headache between attacks. This can also be described as coexistent migraine and CTTH. If the frequent headache disorder does not last longer than 4 hours, the diagnosis of one of the trigeminal autonomic cephalgias (TACs) should be considered.

CTTH is described by the IHS as: "A disorder evolving from ETTH, with daily or very frequent episodes of headache lasting minutes to days. The pain is typically bilateral, pressing or tightening in quality and of mild to moderate intensity, and does not worsen with routine physical activity. There may be mild nausea, photophobia or phonophobia" (Pfaffenrath and Isler, 1993). Episodic migraine and CTTH can coexist. Guitera et al. (1999b) have suggested, based on population-based epidemiologic data, that coexistent CTTH and episodic migraine can coexist if, and only if, the current CTTH has no migrainous features and there is a remote history of migraine.

The introduction of CM into ICHD-2 creates a problem in the differential diagnosis between CM and CTTH. Both diagnoses require headache (meeting the criteria for migraine or TTH) on at least 15 days a month. Therefore, it is theoretically possible for a patient to have both these diagnoses. In the Silberstein–Lipton criteria, the diagnosis of one disorder takes precedence over the diagnosis of another (Saper, 1983; Mathew et al., 1987; Silberstein et al., 1996). They suggested that a putative diagnosis of CTTH has not met criteria for HC, NDPH, or CM. This would handle the difficulty of the small group of patients who fulfill the IHS diagnostic criteria for both CM and CTTH. This would be possible when two (and only two) of the four pain characteristics are present and headaches are associated with mild nausea. These cases are most likely CM and have been shown to have elevated levels of calcitonin gene-related peptide (CGRP) (a marker for migraine). They should be coded as CTTH and episodic migraine only if the daily baseline headache has no migrainous features. If the daily baseline headache is migrainous, they should be coded as CM, despite what the new IHS criteria state.

NDPH is characterized by the relatively abrupt onset of an unremitting primary CDH (Vanast, 1986; Li and Rozen, 2002). The IHS now includes NDPH in its classification. NDPH requires the absence of a history of evolution from migraine or ETTH. In the absence of rapid development, it is coded as CTTH or CM. NDPH may be associated with medication overuse or not. A diagnosis of NDPH takes precedence over CM and CTTH. The evaluation of NDPH (as with any new-onset headache) should include neuroimaging. Two disorders can mimic NDPH: spontaneous intracranial hypotension (often due to a spontaneous CSF leak) and intracranial hypertension (due to IIH or even cerebral venous sinus thrombosis). The evaluation of NDPH (as with any new-onset headache) should include neuroimaging, specifically brain MRI with and without gadolinium (to look for diffuse pachymeningeal enhancement associated with spontaneous CSF leaks) and MRV (to diagnose venous sinus thrombosis). If these tests are negative, a lumbar puncture should be considered, especially if the patient is treatment-refractory. The lumbar puncture can rule out an indolent infection and determine CSF pressures.

HC (Newman et al., 1993; Peres, Silberstein, et al., 2001) is an indomethacin-responsive headache disorder characterized by a continuous, moderately severe, unilateral headache that varies in intensity, waxing and waning without disappearing completely (Bordini et al., 1991). Some patients have photophobia, phonophobia, and nausea. The IHS now includes HC in its headache classification. It is described as a "...persistent strictly unilateral headache responsive to indomethacin" (Headache Classification Committee, 2004). It differs from CM in that it must be unilateral and must respond to indomethacin.

CHRONIC TENSION-TYPE HEADACHE

Daily headaches may also develop in patients with a history of ETTH. CTTH (Table 13–6) now requires head pain for 15 days a month for only 3

TABLE 13–6 IHS Criteria for Chronic Tension-type Headache.

A. At least 10 episodes fulfilling criteria B–F. Number of days with such headache ⩾15 days per month for at least 3 months period. (=180 days per year).
B. Headache lasts hours or may be continuous
C. At least two of the following pain characteristics:
  1. Pressing or tightening quality
  2. Mild or moderate severity (may inhibit but does not prohibit activities)
  3. Bilateral location
  4. No aggravation by walking stairs or similar routine physical activity
D. Both of the following:
  1. No more than one of the following: Photophobia, phonophobia, or mild nausea
  2. No moderate or severe nausea and no vomiting
E. Use of analgesics or other acute medication on = 10 days per month.
F. Not attributed to another disorder

2.2.1 Chronic tension-type headache associated with the disorder of pericranial muscles
2.2.2 Chronic tension-type headache unassociated with the disorder of pericranial muscles

months (before it was 6 months); many patients have daily headache. Problems with the new 2004 IHS classification of CTTH still exist. Although the pain criteria are identical to episodic TTH, the IHS allows one of *mild* nausea (but not *moderate or severe nausea or vomiting*), photophobia, or phonophobia. The presence of *mild* nausea is consistent with the IHS diagnosis of CTTH, but not ETTH. We believe that mild nausea or mild photophobia and phonophobia are not compatible with the diagnosis of CTTH. The need to include any migrainous features in the IHS definition of CTTH may be a result of the practice of including CM under the rubric of CTTH. CM is now classified separately, and there may be no need to include migrainous features in the diagnostic criteria for CTTH. Migraine and CTTH may coexist with the caveat that the non-migrainous headaches have no migrainous features. Castillo et al. have suggested, on the basis of population-based epidemiological data, that CTTH and migraine can coexist if, and only if, the current headache has no migrainous features and there is a remote history of migraine (Castillo et al., 1999).

CTTH may develop in patients with a history of ETTH. The headaches of CTTH are often diffuse or bilateral, and frequently involve the posterior aspect of the head and neck. In contrast to patients with CM, patients with CTTH do not have prior or coexistent episodic migraine, and most features of migraine are absent.

CTTH that has evolved from ETTH presupposes prior evidence of ETTH. Diagnostic confidence increases if ETTH frequency increases to meet the criteria of CTTH. Although the IHS definition of CTTH contains no explicit headache duration, available evidence does not support a critical value. (We arbitrarily suggested 4 hours to separate out cluster headache and the other shorter-duration daily headaches.) One could argue that CTTH could begin without preceding ETTH, analogous to chronic cluster (i.e., unrelenting from onset—NDPH). However, cluster headache includes a series of episodic attacks, not a constant headache. CTTH, unremitting from onset, is now classified as NDPH.

CTTH is etiologically and biologically heterogeneous. Pfaffenrath and Isler (1993) proposed alternative modifications of the CTTH criteria to allow some migrainous features, such as pulsatile pain, predominantly one-sided pain location, photophobia and phonophobia, mild nausea, and anorexia, but not severe nausea or vomiting. They recognized that some patients with primary CDH could not be classified within the 1984 IHS system. They advocated expanding the CTTH group, instead of expanding the migraine group. Because of the arguments outlined earlier that tie TM to migraine, we prefer to expand the migraine group. The IHS elected to expand migraine and add CM in their new criteria.

Russell et al. (1999) evaluated CTTH in a family study of 122 probands and 377 first-degree relatives. Sensitivity, specificity, predictive values, and chance-corrected agreement rate for the diagnosis of CTTH were 68%, 86%, 53% (PV+), 92% (PV−), and 0.48, respectively. The low sensitivity of CTTH assessed by proband report indicates that a clinical interview of family members is necessary. Clinically interviewed parents, siblings, and children had a 2.1- to 3.9-fold increased risk of CTTH compared with the general population. The proband's gender did not influence the risk of CTTH among first-degree relatives. The significantly increased familial risk, with no increased risk found in spouses, suggests that a genetic factor is involved in CTTH.

The introduction of CM into the ICHD-2 creates a problem in the differential diagnosis between CM and CTTH. Both diagnoses require headache (meeting the criteria for migraine or TTH) on at least 15 days a month for at least 3 months. Therefore, it is theoretically possible for a patient to have both these diagnoses. This would be possible when two (and only two) of the four pain characteristics are present and headaches are associated with mild nausea. These cases are most likely CM, and have been shown to have elevated levels of CGRP (a marker for migraine). They should be coded as CTTH and episodic migraine only if the daily baseline headache has no migrainous features (Ashina et al., 2000).

NEW DAILY PERSISTENT HEADACHE

NDPH, first described by Vanast in 1986 (Vanast, 1986), is characterized by the relatively abrupt onset of an unremitting primary CDH. He believed it was a benign form of CDH that spontaneously improved. However, NDPH is likely to be a heterogeneous disorder. NDPH may also be one of the most treatment-refractory of all headache disorders. NDPH is unique: the daily headache develops abruptly, over less than 3 days, and typically the patient has no prior headache history. It can continue for years without any sign of alleviation despite aggressive treatment. Some cases may reflect a postviral syndrome (Vanast, 1986). Patients with NDPH are generally younger than those with TM (Vanast, 1986).

NDPH has been included in the ICHD-2 (Table 13–7) as a subtype of CTTH. It is not clear whether or not NDPH is etiologically related to TTH. We cannot accept the IHS classification of NDPH as a subtype of CTTH, since it is typically associated with migrainous symptoms (Li and Rozen, 2002; Takase et al., 2004). We (Silberstein–Lipton) proposed alternative criteria for NDPH (Li and Rozen, 2002). We have modified our original criteria, but continued to define NDPH by its mode of presentation. We changed "Acute onset (developing over less than 3 days) of constant unremitting headache" to "Acute onset (developing over less than 3 days) of new and *near*-constant unremitting headache," so as to include patients who have short pain-free intervals. We also eliminated "Headache is constant in location." To be consistent with the new ICHD-2, we use the term "Not attributed to another disorder" (Silberstein–Lipton criteria Table 13–8). NDPH requires the absence of a history of evolution from migraine or ETTH. Excluding all patients with a history of ETTH is problematic, as almost 70% of men and 90% of women have had a TTH in the past. We allow a diagnosis of NDPH in patients with migraine or ETTH if these disorders do not increase in frequency to give rise to NDPH. A diagnosis of NDPH takes precedence over TM and CTTH.

Three NDPH case series exist. Vanast (1986) noted a female predominance (26 women and 19 men). Women had an earlier age of onset than men. Pain was constant in 72% of the patients. The location of pain was temporal in 9 of 45 patients, temporal plus other areas in 14 patients, occipital and extra sites in 20 patients, and holocranial in five patients. "Migrainous" associated symptoms were common: nausea in 55%, vomiting in 12%, photophobia in 34%, and phonophobia in 37%.

Li and Rozen performed a retrospective chart review at the Jefferson Headache Center using the original Silberstein–Lipton NDPH criteria, and

TABLE 13–7 IHS Criteria for New Daily Persistent Headache.

A. Headache for more than 3 months fulfilling criteria B–D
B. Headache is daily and unremitting from onset or less than 3 days from onset
C. At least two of the following pain characteristics:
    1. Bilateral location
    2. Pressing/tightening (non-pulsating) quality
    3. Mild or moderate intensity
    4. Not aggravated by routine physical activity such as walking or climbing stairs
D. Both of the following
    1. No more than one of photophobia, phonophobia, or mild nausea
    2. Neither moderate or severe nausea or vomiting
E. Not attributed to another disorder

TABLE 13–8 Silberstein–Lipton Proposed Criteria for New Daily Persistent Headache.

A. Average headache frequency more than 15 days/month for more than 1 month
B. Average headache duration more than 4 hours/day (if untreated). Frequently constant without medication but may fluctuate.
C. No history of tension-type headache or migraine, which increases in frequency and decreases in severity in association with the onset of NDPH (more than 3 months).
D. Acute onset (developing over less than 3 days) of new and **near**-constant unremitting headache
E. Does not meet criteria for hemicrania continua
F. Not attributed to another disorder

Source: Modified from Silberstein et al. (1994)

found 40 women and 16 men, 82% of whom were able to pinpoint the exact day their headache started. Age of onset ranged from 12 to 78 years; headache onset occurred in relation to an infection or flu-like illness in 30% of patients, to extracranial surgery (e.g., hysterectomy) in 12%, and to a stressful life event in 12%. More than 40% of patients could not identify any precipitating event. The duration of daily headache ranged from 1.5 to 24 hours; 79% of the headaches were continuous. Baseline average pain intensity was moderate (4–6 out of 10 on a visual analog pain scale) in 61% of patients, while 21% experienced severe pain (≥7 out of 10) all of the time. Headache location was bilateral in 64% of patients. Almost 60% of patients had some occipital-nuchal pain; 44% had retro-orbital pain, and 18% had holocranial pain. Headache was throbbing in 55% of patients and pressure-like in 54%. Nausea occurred in 68% of patients, photophobia in 66%, phonophobia in 61%, and lightheadedness in 55%. Aura-type symptoms were present in some patients and included visual photopsias in 9% and zigzag lines in 5%. NDPH appears to predominantly affect women, and is marked by a continuous daily headache with associated migrainous symptoms (Li and Rozen, 2002).

Using the new IHS criteria, Takase et al. found that 13 of 30 patients had nausea, photophobia, or pulsating pain, suggesting the migrainous nature of this disorder (Takase et al., 2004). There was a male predominance (17 men and 13 women). Age of onset ranged from 13 to 73 years. All patients had severe headache. Headache was present throughout the entire day, with little if any headache-free time.

Some patients state that they had a flu-like illness when their headache began. Some authors have linked Epstein–Barr virus (EBV) infection with NDPH. Diaz-Mitoma et al. (1987) identified EBV in oropharyngeal secretions in 20 of 32 patients with NDPH compared with 4 of 32 age- and gender-matched controls. Li and Rozen (2002) tested EBV titers in seven patients, five of whom had positive titers, indicating past but not active infection. Santoni and Santoni-Williams (1993) found evidence of systemic infection (Salmonella, adenovirus, toxoplasmosis, herpes zoster, EBV, and *Escherichia coli* urinary tract infections) in 108 patients.

Infection is not the only presumed cause of NDPH. Although 40%–60% of patients with NDPH have no recognized trigger, a stressful life event has been reported in a subset of patients. Stewart et al. (2001) documented that stressful life events are a risk factor for CDH in the general population.

NDPH also occurs in children. Mack identified 41 children with NDPH, 15 of whom had headache onset during a viral infection (Mack, 2003). Sixty percent had a positive EBV titer. Headaches began after mild head injury in eight of the remaining children, after a surgical procedure in three, and during high altitude camping in one. Five patients reported no inciting event.

Laboratory and neuroimaging studies of patients with NDPH are usually normal. EBV titer elevations have been identified, but their significance is unknown. Cerebrospinal fluid (CSF) data, when available, appears to be normal in adults with NDPH. Rozen et al. (2004) reported a low and almost non-existent CSF protein level in four of four adolescent patients with NDPH.

NDPH can be extremely disabling. Many consider primary NDPH to be the most treatment-refractory of all headache disorders. Patients with NDPH often overuse medications, but, unlike patients with MOH, stopping the overuse does not relieve their pain. In contrast, the self-limited form of NDPH has a good prognosis, as patients appear to improve without any intervention. Vanast (1986) found that 30% of the men with NDPH were headache-free at 3 months, and 86% were headache-free at 2 years. Thirty percent of women were pain-free at 3 months, while 73% were pain-free at 2 years. The refractory form of NDPH can continue unabated for years to decades, even with aggressive treatment.

HEMICRANIA CONTINUA

HC was once thought to be a rare headache disorder, but many cases have been reported (Peres, Silberstein, et al., 2001). It is an indomethacin-responsive headache disorder characterized by a continuous, moderately-severe, unilateral headache that varies in intensity, waxing and waning without disappearing completely. Exacerbations of pain are often associated with autonomic disturbances, such as ptosis, miosis, tearing, and sweating. HC may alternate sides, although this is rare (Bordini et al., 1991). HC is frequently associated with jabs and jolts (idiopathic stabbing headache). It is not triggered by neck movements, but tender spots in the neck may be present. Some patients have photophobia, phonophobia, and nausea.

Medina and Diamond were probably the first to describe HC (Medina and Diamond, 1981). The term "hemicrania continua" was coined by Sjaastad and Spierings in 1984 (1984). They reported two patients, a woman aged 63 years and a man aged 53 years, who developed a strictly unilateral headache that was continuous from onset and absolutely responsive to indomethacin. In 1983, Boghen and Desaulniers described a patient with a similar headache that they called "background vascular headache responsive to indomethacin" (Boghen and Desaulniers, 1983).

HC may be more common than is currently believed. Prevalence of primary CDH in the general population is 4%, and HC may represent a sizable group of these patients. Epidemiologic studies may not have identified HC because indomethacin trials were not undertaken in suspected cases. However, unilateral headache was found in 42% of CTTH and 61% of patients with CM (Scher et al., 1998). HC has been reported in different countries and races. HC is seen in noncaucasian populations (Joubert, 1991). The first Japanese case was reported in 2002 (Ishizaki et al., 2002). Wheeler also reported HC in African–Americans (Wheeler, 2002).

Although the disorder almost invariably has a prompt and enduring response to indomethacin, the requirement that a therapeutic response to indomethacin is an essential diagnostic criterion (Table 13–9) in the ICHD-2 is problematic for several reasons. It effectively excludes the diagnosis of HC from epidemiologic studies if patients were never treated with indomethacin or if another agent helped. Treatment response is generally not a part of IHS case definitions of headache disorders. Cases have been described that did not respond to indomethacin but meet the phenotype; for this reason, alternate means of diagnosis have been suggested. HC exists in continuous and remitting forms. In the remitting variety, distinct headache phases last weeks to months, with prolonged pain-free remissions (Iordanidis and Sjaastad, 1989; Pareja et al., 1990; Newman et al., 1993). In the continuous variety, headaches occur on a daily, continuous basis, sometimes for years. The continuous variety can be subclassified into (1) an evolutive, unremitting form that arises from the remitting form (Sjaastad and Tjorstad, 1987; Sjaastad and Antonaci, 1993) and (2) an unremitting form characterized by continuous headache from the onset (Zukerman et al., 1987). Fifteen percent of patients have the remitting form, 32% have the evolutive form, and 53% have the unremitting form. A chronic form evolving to a remitting form (Pareja, 1995), a bilateral case, and a patient whose attacks alternated sides (Newman et al., 1993) have all been described. HC takes precedence over the diagnosis of other types of primary CDH. Many patients with this disorder overuse acute medication; it must be differentiated from TM.

Table 13–9 IHS Diagnostic Criteria for Hemicrania Continua.

A. Headache for more than 3 months fulfilling criteria B–D
B. All of the following characteristics
   1. Unilateral pain without side-shift
   2. Daily and continuous without pain-free periods
   3. Moderate intensity but with exacerbation of severe pain
C. At least one of the autonomic features occurs during exacerbation and ipsilateral to the side of pain.
   1. Conjuctival lacrimation and/or lacrimation
   2. Nasal congestion and/or rhinorrha
   3. Ptosis and/or miosis
D. Complete response to therapeutic doses of indomethacin
E. Not attributed to another disorder

One of the essential features of HC is unilateral headache; however, some bilateral (Pasquier et al., 1987) or alternating side (Newman et al., 1992; Peres and Young, 2003) cases have been reported. Ekbom (1974) reported side alternation in 10% of episodic cluster patients. Bilateral cases of chronic paroxysmal hemicrania (Pollmann and

Pfaffenrath, 1986) and of cluster headache have been reported in the literature, and a mechanism of failed contralateral suppression was proposed by Young and Rozen (1999). Bilateral HC may be underdiagnosed, since one would not consider HC in a patient who presents with bilateral CDH. Hannerz (2000) reported an indomethacin test performed in a population of CDH patients with bilateral headaches who met diagnostic criteria for TTH. An absolute response was found in three patients. There may be a subgroup of patients with bilateral chronic headache who respond to indomethacin in the group of patients otherwise diagnosed as having CTTH or even NDPH and chronic (transformed) migraine.

Associated symptoms present in HC can be divided into three main categories: (1) autonomic symptoms, (2) "jabs and jolts," and (3) migrainous features. Autonomic symptoms consist of conjunctival injection, tearing, rhinorrhea, nasal stuffiness, eyelid edema, and forehead sweating. These symptoms are not as prominent in HC as they are in cluster headache and chronic paroxysmal hemicrania. Patients with HC have described symptoms of ocular discomfort, at times premonitory. Some patients report a feeling of sand in the eye, which may be specific for HC (Pareja, 1999). Peres et al. (Peres, Silberstein, et al., 2001) found autonomic symptoms more common in the exacerbation period compared with the baseline in HC. Seventy-five percent of patients had at least one autonomic symptom. Jabs-and-jolts syndrome is described as a sharp pain that lasts less than 1 minute; it occurs in patients with tension-type, migraine, and cluster headache or in headache-free individuals, and responds to indomethacin. Jabs-and-jolts pain occurs in HC, more frequently in the exacerbation periods. Jabs-and-jolts syndrome is described in 26% of HC cases reported in the literature. Peres et al. (Peres, Silberstein, et al., 2001) found it in 41% of cases. Its prevalence in the general population is 30%. Because of its low sensitivity and specificity, it should not be part of the diagnostic criteria for HC.

Migrainous features (nausea, vomiting, photophobia, and phonophobia) are common in HC, particularly in the exacerbation period (Peres, 2002). The association between HC and visual auras was recently described (Peres, Siow, et al., 2002). Evers et al. (1999) reported a patient with HC and attacks of hemiparesis, with a familial history of hemiplegic migraines. Pasquier et al. (1987) reported a patient with unilateral paresthesias. Little is known about the natural history of HC during pregnancy and reproductive life events. Hemicrania postpartum, a new HC variant, has been recently reported (Spitz and Peres, 2004).

The relative rarity of HC has made it difficult to study its pathophysiology. Pain pressure thresholds are reduced in patients with HC, as they are in patients with chronic paroxysmal hemicrania (Antonaci et al., 1994). In contrast, orbital phlebography is relatively normal compared with patients with chronic paroxysmal hemicrania (Antonaci, 1994), although this area is controversial (Bovim et al., 1992). Pupillometric studies have shown no clear abnormality in HC (Antonaci et al., 1992), and studies of facial sweating have shown modest changes similar to those seen in chronic paroxysmal hemicrania (Antonaci, 1991).

Neuroimaging findings are unique in HC. Matharu et al. (2004) studied seven patients with HC. Positron emission tomography (PET) showed significant activation of the contralateral posterior hypothalamus and ipsilateral dorsal rostral pons. In addition, there was activation of the ipsilateral ventrolateral midbrain, which extended over the red nucleus (RN), the substantia nigra (SN), and the bilateral pontomedullary junction. No obvious intracranial vessel dilation was seen. Posterior hypothalamic activation is seen in TACs, such as cluster headache. Unlike the TACs, the posterior hypothalamic activation was contralateral, not ipsilateral, to the pain. In migraine, the brainstem is activated contralateral to the side of headache, but in HC it is ipsilateral. The activation pattern demonstrated in HC mirrors the overlapping clinical phenotype.

The differential diagnosis of HC includes other CDHs that can also be strictly unilateral. All patients who have strictly unilateral headaches should undergo an indomethacin trial to rule out a diagnosis of HC. The continuous form of HC should be differentiated from other primary CDH disorders (TM, CTTH, and NDPH) by an indomethacin test. HC is also classified as a TAC. HC is differentiated from cluster headache and chronic paroxysmal hemicrania primarily by its continuous moderate pain and the lack of autonomic features between the painful exacerbations. Chronic paroxysmal hemicrania does not have the continuous baseline headache found in HC; headache duration is shorter (2–45 minutes), and frequency is usually greater than five a day. It is precipitated by neck movement, a feature that is not found in HC. Autonomic symptoms are more prominent in chronic paroxysmal hemicrania and cluster headache than they are in HC.

Secondary cases have been reported. One patient had a mesenchymal tumor in the sphenoid bone, in which the response to indomethacin faded after 2 months (Antonaci and Sjaastad, 1992); another had HIV (Brilla et al., 1998); and another had a 2.5 cm adenocarcinoma lung mass (Eross et al., 2002).

HC-like headache associated with internal carotid artery dissection may respond to indomethacin. Ashkenazi et al. (2007) described a patient with traumatic internal carotid artery dissection, who presented with a clinical picture mimicking HC that initially responded to indomethacin. D'Alessio et al. (2004) reported two patients with a classical phenotype of HC, including indomethacin responsiveness, who had large extracranial vascular malformation. In one case, the headache disappeared after embolization of the malformation. The other went into sustained remission after indomethacin treatment, leaving open the question of a causal relation between the headache and the vascular lesion. These cases suggest HC; but if there is a need for escalating doses of indomethacin or loss of indomethacin's efficacy, they should be treated with suspicion and the patient reevaluated.

Espada et al. (1999) studied the prognosis of five men and four women [eight continuous, one remitting, with a mean age of onset of 53.3 years (range 29–69)] who had HC that was diagnosed using Goadsby and Lipton's draft diagnostic criteria (Goadsby and Lipton, 1997). All nine patients had initial relief with indomethacin (mean daily dose 94.4 mg; range 50–50). They were able to follow eight patients. Indomethacin could be discontinued after 3, 7, and 15 months, respectively, and patients remained pain-free. Three patients discontinued treatment because of side-effects and had headache recurrence; two had relief with aspirin. Two other patients continue to take indomethacin with partial relief. Pareja et al. (2001) studied HC and chronic paroxysmal hemicrania patients and found that 42% of patients experienced a decrease of up to 60% in the dose of indomethacin required to maintain a pain-free state; 23% of patients reported gastrointestinal complaints that were relieved with ranitidine.

DRUG OVERUSE AND MEDICATION OVERUSE (REBOUND) HEADACHE

MOH was previously called rebound headache, drug-induced headache, and medication-misuse headache. Patients with frequent headaches often overuse analgesics, opioids, ergotamine, and triptans (Katsarava et al., 1999). Medication overuse is a biobehavioral disorder (Saper et al., 2005), and may be a response to both chronic pain or, in headache-prone patients, medication overuse, which can induce the headache. In addition, medication overuse can make headaches refractory to prophylactic medication (Diamond and Dalessio, 1982; Wilkinson, 1988; Saper, 1987a; Saper, 1989; Mathew, 1990; Mathew et al., 1990). Although stopping the acute medication may result in withdrawal symptoms and a period of increased headache, subsequent headache improvement occurs usually but not always (Rapoport et al., 1986; Saper and Jones, 1986; Andersson, 1988; Baumgartner et al., 1989; Saper, 1989). Many patients with primary CDH, who were withdrawn from ergotamine and analgesics and given no further therapy, no longer had daily headaches, although about 40% still had episodic migraine attacks (Dichgans et al., 1984; Rapoport, 1988).

Definition and Classification of MOH

In 1988, the IHS used the term "drug-induced headache" for MOH (Headache Classification Committee of the International Headache Society, 1988). This terminology has been criticized because the single intake of several drugs, such as nitrates, may also lead to headache. To emphasize the regular intake of drugs as the basis of this headache form, the new term, "medication-overuse headache," was introduced in the 2004 IHS classification (Headache Classification

Committee, 2004). The ICHD-2 further extended the definition according to the clinical symptoms caused by different drugs (Table 13–10, including D). However, the first ICHD-2 classification of MOH was confusing. It stated that a diagnosis of headache attributed to a substance becomes definite only when the headache resolves or greatly improves after exposure to the substance is terminated. In the case of MOH, an arbitrary period of 2 months after overuse cessation was stipulated by the IHS; if the diagnosis was definite, improvement must occur in that time frame. Before cessation, or pending improvement within 2 months after cessation, the diagnosis of probable MOH was used. If improvement did not then occur within the 2-month period, the MOH diagnosis was discarded. Patients with a preexisting primary headache, who developed a new type of headache or whose migraine or TTH was made markedly worse during medication overuse, were given the diagnosis of both the preexisting headache and probable MOH.

Table 13–10 New IHS Criteria for Headache Attributed to Medication Overuse (Headache Classification Committee of the International Headache Society, 1988).

A. Headache present on more than 15 days/month
B. Regular overuse for more than 3 months of one or more acute/symptomatic treatment drugs as defined under subforms of 8.2.
   1. Ergotamine, triptans, opioids, **or** combination analgesic medications on 10 days or more per month on a regular basis for more than 3 months
   2. Simple analgesics **or** any combination of ergotamine, triptans, analgesics opioids on 15 days or more per month on a regular basis for more than 3 months without overuse of any single class alone
C. Headache has developed or markedly worsened during medication overuse
D. Headache resolves or reverts to its previous pattern within 2 months after discontinuation of overused medication)[a]

[a] Eliminated in the latest revision (Headache Classification Committee, 2006).

Source: The ICHD-2 (Headache Classification Commitee, 2004).

General dissatisfaction with the ICHD-2 diagnostic criteria has led to its revision. MOH could not be diagnosed until the overuse was discontinued and the patient improved. Some patients do not improve after withdrawal, and may or may not become responsive to prophylactic medication. Other patients do not improve after discontinuation of medication overuse. For these reasons "*Headache resolves or reverts to its previous pattern within 2 months after discontinuation of overused medication*" has been eliminated in the most recent version of the ICHD-2 criteria (Headache Classification Committee, 2006). The diagnosis of probable MOH and probable CM (or probable CTTH) no longer has to be made when a patient has medication overuse. The default diagnosis is now MOH (Table 13–10).

It was believed that rebound headaches occurred if usage days exceeded 2–3 days a week, week after week, month after month (Saper, 1983), emphasizing frequency and reliability of use. According to the ICHD-2, overuse is now defined in terms of treatment days per month and, as previously described, emphasizes frequency and regularity of days per week. For example, the diagnostic criterion of use on 10 or more days a month (15 for simple analgesics) translates into two to three treatment days every week. Bunching treatment days and going for long periods without medication intake, as practiced by some patients, is much less likely to cause MOH. The amount of use that constitutes overuse depends on the drug. Ergotamine-overuse headache requires intake on 10 or more days a month on a regular basis for three or more months. The headache is often daily and constant. Triptan-overuse headache is usually frequent, intermittent, and migrainous. Triptan intake (any formulation) on 10 or more days a month may increase migraine frequency to that of CM. Evidence suggests that this occurs sooner with triptan overuse than with ergotamine overuse (Diener and Dahlof, 1999; Limmroth et al., 2002). Medication overuse fulfills the criteria for physical dependency (Saper and Jones, 1986).

In American subspecialty centers, most patients with drug-induced headache have a history of episodic migraine that has been converted into CDH (MOH) as a result of medication overuse (Kudrow, 1982; Diener et al., 1984; Mathew et al., 1987; Rapoport, 1988; Mathew, 1990; Mathew et al., 1990; Rasmussen et al., 1992). In European headache centers, 5%–10% of the patients have drug-induced headache (Kudrow, 1982; Diener et al., 1984; Mathew et al., 1987; Rapoport, 1988; Mathew, 1990; Mathew et al., 1990; Rasmussen et al., 1992; Diener and Tfelt-Hansen, 1993). Patients with CM, TTH, HC, and NDPH may overuse symptomatic medications. Drug-induced primary CDH, or as Isler (1988) has termed it, "painkiller headache," has been reported since the seventeenth century, with occurrences reaching epidemic proportions in Switzerland after World War II.

The epidemiology of MOH is uncertain, since some cases are drug-induced and some are just associated with drug overuse. In European headache centers, 5%–10% of patients have drug-induced headache. One series of 3000 consecutive headache patients reported that 4.3% had drug-induced headaches (Micieli et al., 1988). Experiences in the United Kingdom (Goadsby, personal communication) suggest that drug-associated headache is more common than the literature suggests. In American specialty headache clinics, as many as 80% of patients who presented with primary CDH used analgesics on a daily or near-daily basis (Rapoport, 1988). In some headache clinics, a smaller percentage, although still a majority, are reported to have the problem (Solomon et al., 1992a). In India, in contrast, medication overuse is less common (Ravishankar, 1997).

Diener and Dahlöf (1993) summarized 29 studies that included 2612 patients with chronic MOH. Migraine was the primary headache in 65% of patients, TTH in 27%, and mixed or other headaches (i.e., cluster headache) in 8%. Women had more drug-induced headache than men (3.5:1; 1533 women, 442 men). This ratio is slightly higher than one would expect because of the usual migraine frequency gender differences. The mean duration of primary headache was 20.4 years. The mean admitted time of frequent drug intake was 10.3 years in one study, and the mean duration of daily headache was 5.9 years. Results from headache diaries show that the number of tablets or suppositories taken daily averaged 4.9 (range 0.25–25). Patients averaged 2.5–5.8 different pharmacologic components simultaneously (range 1–14) (Diener and Dahlof, 1999).

Patients attending an outpatient neurology clinic in Austria reported taking, on average, 6.3 different headache pain drugs (Schnider et al., 1994). Of these patients, 26.5% reported using both prescription and over-the-counter medications; 31.3% used over-the-counter medications only, and 27.7% used prescription drugs only. Acetaminophen (average dose 500 mg) was the most frequently used analgesic. Most patients attending a London migraine clinic used multiple medications (Silberstein and Saper, 1993). Acetaminophen, again, was the most commonly used analgesic (34.9%), followed by aspirin (22.9%).

In a cross-sectional survey carried out in Tromsø in 1986–1987, 19,137 men and women (aged 12 –56 years) from the general population were asked about their drug use more than the preceding 14 days. On average, 28% of the women and 13% of the men had used analgesics. The most significant predictor of analgesic use was headache; a lesser association was found with infections. Drug use in women was associated with symptoms of depression. Drug use in men was associated with sleeplessness. Higher drug use was associated with smoking and high coffee consumption, but not with frequent alcohol intake (Eggen, 1993).

In a representative sample of the Swiss population, 4.4% of men and 6.8% of women took analgesics at least once a week; 2.3% took them daily (Gutzwiller and Zemp, 1986). Analgesic dependency was more frequent than the dependence on tranquilizers, hypnotics, and stimulating drugs in psychiatric inpatients in Switzerland (Kieholz and Ladewig, 1981). In Germany, possibly 1% of the population take up to 10 pain tablets every day (Schwarz et al., 1985).

In the United States, 20.2% of a national sample survey of 20,468 individuals reported "severe headache"; 62.6% of the women and 74.6% of the men used over-the-counter medications, while prescription drugs were used by 34.5% of the women and 21.3% of the men. Over-the-counter analgesic use was greater than prescription medication use among migraineurs, as well as among those suffering from undefined severe headache (Celentano et al., 1992). This could be either a cause or a result of the severe headache.

A random telephone survey of 24,159 households in Canada produced a sample of 1573 households with one or more eligible headache sufferers. Ninety percent of the IHS-diagnosed migraineurs reported using over-the-counter drugs, and 44% reported using prescription drugs. In this sample, 1.5% of migraineurs had rebound headache resulting from ergotamine tartrate or analgesic overuse. Drug-induced rebound headache is a major public health problem in both the clinic and the community (Robinson, 1993).

Clinical Features of MOH

Wilkinson et al. (2001) and Bahra et al. (2003) have shown that when migraine-prone patients take frequent opioid medication for non-headache reasons, headaches will escalate and MOH will occur, and that discontinuing daily low-dose caffeine frequently results in withdrawal headache (Silverman et al., 1992). Nonetheless, analgesic rebound headache has not been demonstrated in placebo-controlled trials. In a controlled study of caffeine withdrawal, 64 normal adults (71% women) with low-to-moderate caffeine intake (the equivalent of about 2.5 cups of coffee a day) were given a 2-day caffeine-free diet and either placebo or replacement caffeine. Under double-blind conditions, 50% of the patients who were given placebo had a headache by day two, compared with 6% of those given caffeine. Nausea, depression, and flu-like symptoms were common in the placebo group. This study is relevant since caffeine is frequently used by headache sufferers for pain relief, often in combination with analgesics or ergotamine. The study is a model for short-term caffeine withdrawal, but does not demonstrate the long-term consequences of detoxification. In a community-based telephone survey of 11,112 subjects in Lincoln and Omaha, Nebraska, 61% reported daily caffeine consumption, and 11% of the caffeine consumers reported symptoms upon stopping coffee (Potter et al., 2000). A group of those who reported withdrawal were assigned to one of three regimes: abrupt caffeine withdrawal, gradual withdrawal, and no change. One-third of the abrupt-withdrawal group and an occasional member of the gradual-withdrawal group had symptoms that included headache and tiredness.

The actual dose limits and the time needed to develop rebound headaches have not been defined in rigorous studies, and the relationship of drug half-life to rebound development is not known. Our clinical knowledge is derived from observing patterns of medication use in patients who present with rebound headaches. Because there may be large individual differences in susceptibility to rebound headaches, anecdotal data must be generalized cautiously. Overuse was believed to occur when patients took three or more simple analgesics daily more often than 5 days a week, triptans or combination analgesics containing barbiturates, sedatives, or caffeine more often than 3 days a week, or opioids or ergotamine tartrate more often than 2 days a week (Diamond and Dalessio, 1982; Saper, 1987a; Wilkinson, 1988; Mathew, 1990; Mathew et al., 1990). These limits served in part as the basis of the ICHD-2 definitions.

Specific limits are necessary to prevent analgesic, ergotamine, and triptan overuse. Wilkinson (1988), Saper and Jones (1986), Mathew et al. (1987), and Scholz et al. (1988) compared ergotamine intake in patients with and without primary CDH. In the groups without primary CDH, the maximum ergotamine intake was 24 mg a month. However, one patient with primary CDH consumed only 7 mg of ergotamine a month. The frequency of days of ergotamine use (treatment days per week) was emphasized as the most important variable, not the daily or monthly total dose (Saper, 1983; Saper and Jones, 1986). Rebound headache can develop when patients take as little as 0.5–1 mg of ergotamine three times a week (Saper, 1987b; Wilkinson, 1988; Baumgartner et al., 1989; Silberstein, 1993).

Scholz et al. (1988) studied simple analgesic consumption in patients with and without rebound headache. Patients with rebound headache consumed between 1200 and 1500 mg of analgesics a day. Increased caffeine, but not codeine, consumption was correlated with the development of primary CDH. Barbiturate consumption was significantly higher in patients with primary CDH (60–500 mg a day; mean 160 mg a day) than in those without primary CDH (mean >60 mg a day). All of the triptans, selective 5-HT_1 agonists that are effective in acute migraine treatment, have been reported to induce rebound headache

(Diener et al., 1991; Catarci et al., 1994; Gaist et al., 1996; Diener and Silberstein, 2006; Obermann et al., 2006). Kaţsarava et al. (1999) reported the first cases and the specific clinical features of drug-induced headache after the frequent use of zolmitriptan and naratriptan. All patients remained responsive to triptans. Six patients had never previously used triptans or ergotamine derivatives, but developed drug-induced headache within 6 months of taking the drug. Four patients consumed 7.5–10 mg of zolmitriptan or 10–12 mg of naratriptan weekly. The weekly dosages necessary to initiate drug-induced headache with the centrally penetrant triptans may be lower than with ergotamines or sumatriptan, and the time of onset might be shorter. Increasing attack frequency can be the first sign that drug-induced headache is developing. We recommend limiting the use of triptans to 3 days a week.

Many patients with CDH overuse acute medication and can develop psychological dependence, tolerance, and abstinence syndromes (Mathew et al., 1990). MOH may be a biobehavioral disorder (Saper et al., 2005). Medication overuse may be responsible, in part, for the transformation of episodic migraine or ETTH into daily headache and for the perpetuation of the syndrome (Saper, 1983). However, medication overuse, by definition, is not the sine qua non of CM or CTTH. In the presence of acute medication overuse, the default diagnosis is MOH. Many patients develop CM or CTTH without overusing medication, and others continue to have daily headaches long after the overused medication has been discontinued. Medication overuse is usually motivated by a patient's desire to treat the headaches (Kaiser, 1999). However, some headache patients may overuse combination analgesics to treat a mood disturbance (Saper, 2006; Saper and Lake, 2006). Medication overuse rarely represents a form of primary substance abuse. Certain personality types may have a predilection for certain types of medication overuse, and patients with personality disorders are likely to overuse opioids (Lake et al., 2006).

A prospective study of 98 patients investigated the pharmacologic features, such as mean critical duration until onset of MOH, mean critical monthly intake frequencies, and mean critical monthly dosages, as well as specific clinical features of MOH after overuse of different acute headache drugs. In this study, triptan overuse far outnumbered ergot overuse. This reflects the fact that, despite high costs, triptans have become widely used (and overused), and suggests that with the exception of opioid use in the United States they are about to become the most important group to cause MOH. Unlike patients who suffer from MOH after ergot or analgesic overuse, migraine patients (but not TTH patients) with triptan-induced headache did not describe the typical tension-type daily headache but rather a migraine-like daily headache (a unilateral, pulsating headache with autonomic disturbances) or a significant (and pure) increase in migraine attack frequency. Furthermore, the delay between the frequent medication intake and the development of daily headache was shortest for triptans (1.7 years), longer for ergots (2.7 years), and longest for analgesics (4.8 years). The intake frequency (single dosages per month) was lowest for triptans (18 single dosages per month), higher for ergots (37 single dosages per month), and highest for analgesics (114 single dosages per month). Hence, triptans not only cause a different spectrum of clinical features, but are able to cause MOH faster and with lower dosages than other substance groups (Limmroth et al., 2002).

Some doubted the existence of drug-induced headache (Fisher, 1988). When Fisher (1988) failed to find analgesic rebound headache in patients who were using analgesics for arthritis, he attempted to refute the concept. His work has been reinterpreted to suggest that headache-prone patients are especially vulnerable to the rebound phenomenon. As mentioned earlier, headache-prone patients often develop daily headaches if they are put on analgesics for a nonheadache indication (Lance et al., 1988; Bowdler et al., 1990). Bahra et al. found that 8 of 103 patients (7.6%) attending a rheumatology-monitoring clinic developed CDH with regular analgesic use. All had a history of migraine, which preceded CDH in seven patients and began about the same time as CDH in one patient. Regular use of analgesics preceded the onset of daily headache in five patients by a mean of 5.4 years (range, 2–10 years). Individuals with primary headache, specifically migraine, are predisposed to developing

CDH in association with the regular use of analgesics (Bahra et al., 2000).

In addition to exacerbating the headache disorder, drug overuse has other serious effects. The overuse of acute drugs may interfere with the effectiveness of preventive headache medications. Prolonged use of large amounts of medication may cause renal or hepatic toxicity in addition to tolerance, habituation, or dependence. Tolerance refers to the decreased effectiveness of the same dose of an analgesic, often leading to the use of higher doses to achieve the same degree of effectiveness. Tolerance reflects receptor hyposensitivity (Mao et al., 2002). Habituation and dependence are, respectively, the psychological and physical need to repeatedly use drugs.

PSYCHIATRIC COMORBIDITY OF CDH

Anxiety, depression, panic disorder, and bipolar disease are more frequent in migraineurs than in nonmigraine control subjects (Merikangas et al., 1990; Breslau and Davis, 1993). Since CM is a complication of migraine, one would expect to find psychiatric comorbidity in CM. In clinic-based samples, depression occurs in 80% of patients with CM. The Minnesota Multiphasic Personality Inventory (MMPI) was abnormal in 61% of patients with primary CDH, compared with 12.2% of patients with episodic migraine. Pateints with primary CDH had significantly higher Zung and BDI scores than did migraine controls (Saper, 1987b; Mathew et al., 1990; Mathew, 1990; Mathew, 1991). Comorbid depression often improves when the cycle of daily head pain is broken. Mongini et al. (1997) found that several MMPI and State and Trait Anxiety Index 2 scores decreased after headache improvement occurred, but 12 of 20 patients continued to have a conversion Vs configuration on the MMPI. Many previous studies do not clearly differentiate between CDH subtypes.

Mitsikostas and Thomas (1999) found that patients with headache had significantly higher average Hamilton rating scores for anxiety and depression (17.4 and 14.2, respectively) than did nonheadache controls (6.8 and 5.7, respectively). High headache attack frequency, a long history of headaches, and female gender correlated to the Hamilton rating elevation for both anxiety and depression. Patients with CTTH, mixed headache, or drug abuse headache had the highest Hamilton rating scores for depression and anxiety.

Verri et al. (1998) found current psychiatric comorbidity in 90% of patients with primary CDH, 81% of migraineurs, and 83% of patients with chronic low back pain (no significant differences). Generalized anxiety disorders were the most common in each group (primary CDH 69.3%, $p \leqslant 0.001$; migraine 59.5%, $p \leqslant 0.05$; chronic low back pain 65.7%, $p \leqslant 0.001$). The most common mood disorder in primary CDH was major depressive disorder (25%). This was significantly more frequent than dysthymia ($p \leqslant 0.001$) and significantly more frequent ($p \leqslant 0.05$) in primary CDH than in patients with chronic low back pain. Somatoform disorders (including somatization, conversion disorder, and hypochondriasis) were found in 5.7% of patients with primary CDH, always concomitant with anxiety and mood disorders.

Psychiatric comorbidity is a predictor of intractability. The MMPI was abnormal in 100% of patients with primary CDH who failed to respond to aggressive management (31% of the primary CDH group), compared with 48% of the responders. Physical, emotional, or sexual abuse, parental alcohol abuse, and a positive dexamethasone suppression test also correlated highly with a poor response to aggressive management (Saper and VanMeter, 1980). Curioso et al. (1999) found that 31 of 69 (45%) patients with primary CDH had an adjustment disorder, 16 (23%) had major depression, 12 (17%) were dysthymic, 6 (9%) had generalized anxiety disorder, 1 (2%) was bipolar, and 3 (4%) were normal. The risk of a bad outcome after treatment was significantly greater for patients with major depression than those without. Pateints with primary CDH who have major depression or have abnormal BDI scores have worse outcomes at 3–6 months compared with patients who are not depressed.

Monzon and Lainez (1998), using the Medical Outcomes Study Short Form (SF-36) questionnaire, found that patients with primary CDH had significantly worse scores in physical functioning, role functioning (physical), bodily pain, general health perceptions, and mental health than migraineurs (Solomon et al., 1993).

Using the SF-36, Guitera et al. (1999a) analyzed CDH's impact on quality of life in a population sample of 1883 individuals, 4.7% of whom met the CDH criteria established by Silberstein et al. (1996). Eighty-nine healthy subjects and 89 episodic migraineurs were control groups. All the concepts evaluated by the Medical Outcome Short Form (SF-36) were significantly reduced in the CDH patients compared with the healthy subjects. There were no significant differences in quality of life between TM patients and CTTH patients. TM patients had a general reduction in quality of life compared with episodic migraine patients (significant for vitality and general and mental health). CDH patients who overused analgesics scored significantly lower than non-overusers in physical role and bodily pain. The impact of CDH on quality of life depends on the chronicity of the headache disorder rather than on the severity of a given attack. The impact is worse when analgesic overuse is present. CDH patients who overused analgesics scored significantly lower than did nonoverusers in physical role and bodily pain.

Puca et al. (1999) evaluated psychopathologic symptoms and psychiatric disorders in 234 adult patients with CDH (184 women and 50 men, mean age 43.05 ± 12.90 years). The Structured Clinical Interview for the Diagnostic and Statistical Manual of Mental Disorders-IV edition and the Symptom Check List 90R were used. At least one psychiatric disorder (anxiety disorder 45%, mood disorder 33%) was detected in 66% of the sample CDH patients. The prevalence of psychopathologic symptoms was more than 78%. At least one psychosocial stress factor was found in 42% of cases, and 64% of the whole sample overused symptomatic drugs.

Wang et al. (2001) looked at the quality of life of 901 headache patients in Taiwan using the SF-36. Using the Silberstein–Lipton CDH criteria, TM was diagnosed in 310 patients and CTTH in 231; 193 had episodic migraine. The patients with TM had the worst SF-36 scores. The scores of those with CTTH and those with migraine were similar.

Juang et al. (2000) investigated the frequency of depressive and anxiety disorders in 261 consecutive CDH patients seen in a headache clinic. CDH subtypes were classified according to the Silberstein–Lipton criteria. A psychiatrist evaluated the patients according to the structured Mini-International Neuropsychiatric Interview to assess the comorbidity of depressive and anxiety disorders. Mean age was 46 years, and 80% of the patients were women. TM was diagnosed in 152 patients (58%) and CTTH in 92 (35%). Seventy-eight percent of patients with TM had psychiatric comorbidity, including major depression (57%), dysthymia (11%), panic disorder (30%), and generalized anxiety disorder (8%). Sixty-four percent of patients with CTTH had psychiatric diagnoses, including major depression (51%), dysthymia (8%), panic disorder (22%), and generalized anxiety disorder (1%). The frequency of anxiety disorders was significantly higher in patients with TM after controlling for age and sex. Both depressive and anxiety disorders were significantly more frequent in women. These results demonstrate that women and patients with TM are at higher risk of psychiatric comorbidity. In their most recent review of 276 consecutive patients treated on an inpatient unit, almost all of whom suffered from CDH, Lake et al. (Lake et al., 2006), found a striking presence of psychiatric comorbidity, including anxiety, depression, and cluster B personality disorders (borderline, narcissistic, antisocial).

CDH occurs in children. Guidetti et al. (Guidetti and Galli, 1999) examined the characteristics of childhood- and adolescent-onset CDH and the prevalence of psychiatric comorbidity. Eighty-six CDH patients (60 girls, 26 boys; mean age 12.3 years; SD + 2.1 years, range 7–18 years) were compared with 100 controls (60 girls, 40 boys; mean age 10.7 years; SD + 2.6 years; range 4–18 years). Sixty-four patients had migraine and 36 had ETTH. All subjects underwent clinical interviews and psychometric testing. CDH was diagnosed using the Silberstein criteria (Silberstein et al., 1996): CTTH was present in 40% of patients, TTH plus intermittent migraine attacks in 35%, and mixed forms in 25%. Psychiatric comorbidity was present in 90% of CDH patients, 67% of migraine patients, and 25% of TTH patients.

OTHER COMORBIDITIES

Fibromyalgia (FM) and TM are common chronic pain disorders. Peres et al. (Peres, Young, et al., 2001) estimated the prevalence of FM in 101 TM patients and analyzed its relationship to depression, anxiety, and insomnia. They enrolled 101 consecutive TM patients seen at a headache clinic in Sao Paulo. All had normal neuroimaging and clinical examinations. TM was diagnosed according to the 1996 Silberstein–Lipton criteria (Silberstein et al., 1996). FM was diagnosed according to the American College of Rheumatology diagnostic criteria (Mathew et al., 1982). FM was diagnosed in 35.6% of cases. Patients with FM had more insomnia, were older, and their headaches were more incapacitating than patients without FM. The mean BDI score was 21.1. Fifty-seven patients (87.7%) had at least mild depression. Forty-four patients (67.7%) had state score more than 46, and 51 patients (78.5%) had trait score more than 46. The BDI scores correlated to pain intensity ($p = 0.002$) and state and trait anxiety scores ($p > 0.001$). Depression, as measured by the BDI scores, was also associated with FM ($p = 0.007$), insomnia ($p = 0.043$), and disability ($p = 0.05$). Predictors of FM in patients with TM included insomnia (odds ratio (OR) 10.05, 95% confidence interval (CI), 9.03–13.55) and depression (OR 6.8, 95% CI, 4.91–8.68).

Fatigue is a common, frequently reported symptom in many disorders, including headache. Peres et al. (Peres, Zukerman, et al., 2002) determined the prevalence of fatigue in 63 TM patients from the Sao Paulo headache clinic. TM was diagnosed using the Silberstein–Lipton criteria. FM was diagnosed according to the 1990 diagnostic criteria established by the American College of Rheumatology (Wolfe et al., 1990). The Fatigue Severity Scale (FSS) (Krupp et al., 1989) (cut-off of 27 defined fatigue) and the Chalder fatigue scale (Chalder et al., 1993) (Likert scoring) (Morriss et al., 1998) were used. The Chalder fatigue scale has two parts, physical and mental fatigue. Items related to mental fatigue include difficulty concentrating, problems thinking clearly, difficulty finding the correct word, and memory problems. Those related to physical fatigue include tiredness, need to rest more, sleepiness, drowsiness, lack of energy, and weakness or decreased muscle strength. Fifty-three patients (84.1%) had FSS scores greater than 27. Forty-two patients (66.7%) met the criteria for chronic fatigue syndrome established by the Centers for Disease Control. Thirty-two patients (50.8%) met the modified criteria of the Centers for Disease Control, in which headache was eliminated as a criterion of chronic fatigue syndrome. BDI scores correlated with FSS, mental and physical fatigue scores. Trait anxiety scores also correlated with fatigue scales. Women had higher FSS scores than men, $p > 0.05$. Physical fatigue was associated with FM, $p > 0.05$. Fatigue as a symptom and chronic fatigue syndrome as a disorder were both common in TM patients.

EPIDEMIOLOGY OF CDH

In population-based surveys using the Silberstein–Lipton criteria, primary CDH occurred in 4.1% of Americans, 4.35% of Greeks, 3.9% of elderly Chinese, and 4.7% of Spaniards. Population-based estimates for the 1-year period prevalence of CTTH are 1.7% in Ethiopia (Tekle Haimanot et al., 1995), 3% in Denmark (Rasmussen, 1995), 2.2% in Spain (Castillo et al., 1999), 2.7% in China (Wang et al., 2000), and 2.2% in the United States (Scher et al., 1998).

Scher et al. (1998), using a validated computer-assisted telephone interview, ascertained the prevalence of CDH in 13,343 individuals aged 18–65 years in Baltimore County, Maryland. Those reporting 180 or more headaches a year were classified as having frequent headache. Three mutually exclusive subtypes of frequent headache were identified: TM, CTTH, and unclassified frequent headache. The overall prevalence of CDH was 4.1% (5.0% women, 2.8% men; 1.8:1 women to men ratio). In both men and women, prevalence was highest in the lowest educational category. More than half (52% women, 56% men) met criteria for CTTH (2.2%), almost one-third (33% women, 25% men) met criteria for TM (1.3%), and the remainder (15% women, 19% men) were unclassified (0.6%). Overall, 30% of women and 25% of men who were frequent headache sufferers met IHS criteria for migraine (with or without aura). On the basis of chance, migraine and CTTH would co-occur in 0.22% of the population; the fact that TM occurred in 1.3% of this population would suggest that their co-occurrence is more than random.

Castillo et al. (1999) sampled 2252 subjects older than 14 years of age in Cantalucia, Spain.

Overall, 4.7% had CDH. Using the criteria of Silberstein et al. (1994), none had HC, 0.1% had NDPH, 2.2% had CTTH, and 2.4% had TM. Nineteen percent of CTTH patients and 31.1% of TM patients had a history of acute medication overuse. Eight patients had a previous history of migraine without aura and now had primary CDH with the characteristics of TTH only. These headaches met the criteria of CM but could have been migraine and coincidental CTTH.

In August 1993, Wang et al. (2000) looked at the characteristics of primary CDH in a population of elderly Chinese (more than 65 years of age) in two townships on Kinmen Island. Seventy-seven percent of the eligible population (1533/2003) participated. Sixty patients (3.9%) had CDH. Significantly more women than men had primary CDH (5.6% and 1.8%, $p < 0.001$). Of the patients with primary CDH, 42 (70%) had CTTH (2.7%), 15 (25%) had CM (1%), and 3 (5%) had other CDH. Only 23% of patients had consulted a physician for headache in the previous year.

Lu et al. (2001) conducted a two-stage population-based headache survey among subjects aged 15 years or more in Taipei, Taiwan. Subjects who had had CDH in the past year were identified, interviewed, and followed up. CDH was defined as headache frequency of more than 15 days a month, with a duration of more than 4 hours a day. Of the 3377 participants, 108 (3.2%) fulfilled the criteria for CDH, with a higher prevalence in women (4.3%) than men (1.9%). TM was the most common subtype (55%), followed by CTTH (44%). Thirty-four per cent of the CDH subjects overused analgesics.

TABLE 13–11 Risk Factors for CDH.

1. High headache frequency
2. Female gender
3. Obesity (BMI more than 30)
4. Snoring
5. Stressful life events
6. High caffeine consumption
7. Acute medication overuse
8. Depression
9. Head trauma
10. History of migraine
11. Less than a high school education

Risk Factors for CDH

Wang et al. (2000) ascertained that significant risk factors for CDH (Table 13–11) included analgesic overuse (OR = 79), a history of migraine (OR = 6.6), and a Geriatric Depression Scale-Short Form score of 8 or above (OR = 2.6). At follow-up, patients with persistent primary CDH had a significantly higher frequency of analgesic overuse (33% versus 0%, $p = 0.03$) and major depression (38% versus 0%, $p = 0.04$).

Granella et al. (1998) found that risk factors that were associated with the evolution of migraine without aura into TM included head trauma (OR 3.3), analgesic use with every attack (OR 2.8), and long duration of oral contraceptive use.

Scher et al. (2003) described the factors that predict CDH onset and remission in an adult population. CDH was more common in women [OR 1.65 (1.3–2.0)], those previously married [OR 1.5 (1.2–1.9)], with obesity (BMI > 30) [OR 1.27 (1.0–1.7)], and those with less education. Obesity, high baseline headache frequency, high caffeine consumption, habitual daily snoring, and stressful life events were significantly associated with new-onset CDH (Scher et al., 2002). Having less than a high school education was associated with a three-fold increased risk of CDH [OR 3.56 (2.3–5.6)].

Bigal et al. (2002), in a clinic-based study, looked for risk factors associated with CDH and its subtypes. TM without MOH (in comparison with episodic migraine) was associated with allergies, asthma, hypothyroidism, hypertension, and daily caffeine consumption.

Zwart et al. (2003) examined the relationship between analgesic use at baseline and the subsequent risk of chronic pain (15 days or more per month) and the risk of analgesic overuse in a population-based study. In total, 32,067 adults reported the use of analgesics from 1984 to 1986 and at follow-up 11 years later (1995–1997). The risk ratios (RR) of chronic pain and of analgesic overuse in the different diagnostic groups (i.e., migraine, nonmigrainous headache, and neck pain) were estimated in relation to analgesic consumption at baseline. Individuals who reported use of analgesics daily or weekly at baseline showed significant increased risk for having chronic pain at follow-up. The risk was most evident for CM (RR = 13.3, 95% CI: 9.3–19.1), intermediate for chronic nonmigrainous headaches (RR = 6.2, 95% CI: 5.0–7.7), and lowest for chronic neck pain (RR = 2.4, 95% CI: 2.0–2.8). Among the subjects with chronic pain associated with analgesic overuse, the RR was 37.6 (95% CI: 21.3–66.4) for CM, 14.4 (95% CI: 10.4–19.9) for chronic nonmigrainous headaches, and 7.1 for chronic neck pain (95% CI: 5.5–9.2). The RR for chronic headache (migraine and nonmigrainous headache combined) associated with analgesic overuse was 19.6 (95% CI: 14.8–25.9) compared with 3.1 (95% CI: 2.4–4.2) for those without overuse. Analgesic overuse strongly predicts chronic pain and chronic pain associated with analgesic overuse 11 years later, especially among those with CM.

(For more details see Chapter 4 "Epidemiology")

PATHOPHYSIOLOGY OF CDH

The trigeminal nucleus caudalis (TNC) of the trigeminal complex, the major relay nucleus for head and face pain, receives nociceptive input from cephalic blood vessels and pericranial muscles (via the trigeminal and upper cervical nerves), as well as inhibitory and facilitatory suprasegmental input. The trigeminal nerve has three divisions: ophthalmic, mandibular, and maxillary. Anterior pain-producing structures are innervated by the ophthalmic (first) division. Posterior regions are subserved by the upper cervical nerves (Messlinger and Burstein, 1999). Afferent processes of the trigeminal nerve converge to form the sensory root of the trigeminal nerve, entering the brain stem at the pontine level and terminating in the trigeminal brain stem nuclear complex. The trigeminal brain stem nuclear complex is composed of the principal trigeminal nuclei and spinal trigeminal nuclei (subdivided into the nucleus oralis, the subnuclear interpolaris, and the nucleus caudalis). The brain stem spinal trigeminal nucleus is analogous to the dorsal horn of the spinal canal, the first synapse in the central nervous system.

Most spinothalamic and trigeminothalamic tract neurons that originate from the dorsal horn and project to ventroposterior lateral and ventroposterior medial nuclei have wide dynamic-range characteristics (Sweatt et al., 2002). The trigeminothalamic tract is analogous to the spinothalamic tract. Second-order neurons from the trigeminal spinal nuclei form the trigeminothalamic tract and project to other midbrain structures, as well as to the thalamic tract.

Most ventroposterior medial nuclei, some with wide dynamic-range characteristics, respond to low-threshold stimuli (Messlinger and Burstein, 1999). Recent evidence suggests that central pain facilitatory neurons (on-cells) are present in the ventromedial medulla. In addition, neurons in the TNC can be sensitized as a result of intense neuronal stimulation.

Pain has three spatiotemporal characteristics: (1) as pain intensity increases, the area in which it is experienced often enlarges (radiation); (2) the pain may outlast the evoking stimulus; and (3) repeated nociceptive stimuli may increase the perceived pain intensity, even without increased input (sensitization) (Woolf and Mitchell, 2001). Pain has both sensory and affective dimensions. In addition to being physically unpleasant, pain is associated with negative emotional feelings shaped by context, anticipations, and attitudes (Sweatt et al., 2002). Pain unpleasantness is in series with pain sensation intensity.

Pain in Migraine

Migraine is a primary brain disorder, a form of neurovascular headache in which neural events result in the dilation of blood vessels, neuronal activation, and pain. Migraine most likely results from a dysfunction of the trigeminal nerve and its central connections that normally modulate sensory input. Components involved include: (1) the cranial blood vessels and meninges; (2) the trigeminal innervation of the vessels and meninges; (3) the reflex connections of the trigeminal system with the cranial parasympathetic outflow; and (4) local and descending pain modulation. The key pathway for the pain is trigeminovascular input from the meningeal vessels. Brain imaging studies suggest that important modulation of the trigeminovascular nociceptive input stems from the dorsal raphe nucleus, locus coeruleus, and nucleus raphe magnus (Goadsby et al., 2002).

Although the source of pain in CDH is unknown and may depend on the subtype of CDH, recent work suggests several mechanisms that could contribute to the process: (1) increased peripheral nociceptive activation (perhaps due to chronic neurogenic inflammation) and activation of silent nociceptors; (2) peripheral sensitization; (3) altered sensory neuron excitability due to changes in ion-channel expression/phosphorylation/accumulation in primary afferents; (4) central sensitization of TNC neurons due to post-translational changes in ligand- and voltage-gated ion-channel kinetics, altering excitability and strength of their synaptic inputs; (5) phenotype modulation due to alterations in the expression of receptors/transmitters/ion channels in peripheral and central neurons; (6) synaptic reorganization modification of synaptic connections caused by cell death or sprouting; (7) decreased pain modulation due to loss of local and descending input (Woolf and Mitchell, 2001); or (8) a combination of these.

Peripheral Mechanisms

Although the brain itself is largely insensate, pain can be generated by large cranial vessels, proximal intracranial vessels, or dura mater. The central convergence of the ophthalmic division of the trigeminal nerve and the branches of C2 nerve roots explain the typical distribution of migraine pain over the frontal and temporal regions and the referral of pain to the parietal, occipital, and high cervical regions (Goadsby et al., 2002). During a migraine attack, an inflammatory process (neurogenic inflammation) occurs in the meninges, at the site of the nerve terminal. Trigeminal nerve activation is accompanied by the release of vasoactive neuropeptides, including CGRP, substance P (SP), and neurokinin A from the nerve terminals. These mediators produce mast cell activation, sensitization of the nerve terminals, and extravasation of fluid into the perivascular space around the dural blood vessels. Intense neuronal stimulation causes induction of c-fos (an immediate early gene product) in the TNC of the brainstem. SP and CGRP further amplify the trigeminal terminal sensitivity by stimulating the release of bradykinin and other inflammatory mediators from nonneuronal cells (Moskowitz, 1992). Inflammatory mediators increase the responsiveness of and turn on silent, or sleeping, nociceptors. Neurotropins, such as nerve growth factor (NGF), are synthesized locally and can also activate mast cells and sensitize nerve terminals (Montalcini et al., 1995). Bradykinin and kallidin, both acting through the B_1 and B_2 receptors, can activate primary afferent nociceptors (Rang and Urban, 1995). Prostaglandins and nitric oxide (a diffusible gas that acts as a neurotransmitter) (Edelman and Gally, 1992) are both endogenous mediators that can be produced locally and can sensitize nociceptors.Cortical spreading depression (the cause of the aura) can activate the trigeminal system. Repeated episodes of neurogenic inflammation may chronically sensitize the pain pathways and contribute to the development of daily headache.

Sarchielli et al. (2001) measured CSF levels of NGF, CGRP, and SP in patients with TM both with and without medication overuse. Higher NGF, CGRP, and SP levels were found in CSF in both groups of patients compared with controls. A correlation was found between NGF and SP levels. All levels correlated with the duration of the disorder. This study suggests the involvement of NGF and chronic activation of the trigeminal vascular system in TM. NGF production could arise from peripheral trigeminal nerve terminals as well as the TNC and pain facilitating pathways. Ashina et al. (2000) compared interictal plasma levels of CGRP of patients with chronic TTH and healthy control subjects. Patients whose usual headache quality was throbbing had a higher interictal plasma CGRP level than control subjects ($p = 0.002$), whereas plasma CGRP level was normal in 22 patients with pressing headaches ($p = 0.36$). This strongly suggests that the patients with an elevated CGRP level had TM, and that the trigeminal vascular system is activated as part of the process of TM.

Sensitization in Migraine

Selby and Lance observed that during migraine attacks patients complain of increased pain with stimuli that would ordinarily be non-nociceptive (Selby and Lance, 1960). These stimuli include hair-brushing, wearing a hat, and resting the head on a pillow. This phenomenon of pain being produced by nonpainful stimuli is referred to as allodynia. In a series of now-classic experiments, Burstein et al. (2000) explored allodynia development in patients with migraine. He measured pain thresholds for hot, cold, and pressure stimuli, both within the region of spontaneous pain and outside it. He found that as an attack progressed in a selected group of migraine sufferers, cutaneous allodynia developed in the region of pain and then outside it (extracephalic locations). He found that 33 of 42 patients (79%) developed allodynia. Allodynia began over the first half of the attack in those who eventually developed it.

Peripheral Sensitization

Sensitization of nociceptors results in an increased spontaneous neuronal discharge rate. Neurons show increased responsiveness to both painful and nonpainful stimuli. The receptor fields expand and, as a result, pain is felt over a greater part of the dermatome. This results in hyperalgesia (increased sensitivity to pain) and cutaneous allodynia. An example of this is sunburn, with increased sensitivity to temperature (i.e., a warm shower feels painfully hot).

How does sensitization occur? Tissue injury and inflammation result in the release of inflammatory mediators, such as prostaglandin E2, bradykinin, and NGF. These substances act on G-protein-coupled receptors or tyrosine kinase receptors expressed on nociceptor terminals. This activates intracellular signaling pathways, resulting in phosphorylation of receptors and ion channels. Phosphorylation changes the threshold and kinetics of the nociceptor terminals, producing increased sensitivity and excitability that results in peripheral sensitization (Julius and Basbaum, 2001). Transcriptional or translational regulation can also contribute to peripheral sensitization. NGF-induced activation of p38 mitogen-activated protein kinase in primary sensory neurons after peripheral inflammation increases the expression and peripheral transport of TRPV1 [a member of the (transient receptor potential) TRP family], exacerbating heat hyperalgesia (Ji et al., 2002). [The TRP superfamily consists of cation channels related to the product of the *Drosophila trp* (for transient receptor potential) gene. The vanilloid receptor 1 (VR1) forms a distinct subgroup of the TRP family of ion channels. Members of the vanilloid receptor family (TRPV) are activated by a diverse range of stimuli, including heat, protons, lipids, phorbols, phosphorylation, changes in extracellular osmolarity and/or pressure, and depletion of intracellular Ca^{2+} stores. However, VR1 remains the only channel activated by vanilloids such as capsaicin.]

The normal rhythmic pulsation of the meninges, which are innervated by peripheral trigeminal neurons, can mediate the throbbing pain that migraineurs experience. With the increase in intracranial neuronal sensitivity that migraine patients experience, the normal rhythmic pulsation is interpreted as painful. Bendtsen, Jensen, and Olesen (1996) have found evidence for sensitization in CTTH patients. Pericranial myofascial tenderness, evaluated by manual palpation, was considerably higher in patients than in controls ($p > 0.00001$). The stimulus–response function from highly tender muscle was qualitatively different than from normal muscle, suggesting that myofascial pain may be mediated by low-threshold mechanosensitive afferents projecting to sensitized dorsal horn neurons.

Central Sensitization

Central sensitization needs to be differentiated from windup, which is an immediate activity-dependent plasticity characterized by a progressive increase in action potential output from dorsal horn neurons during a conditioning train of repeated low-frequency C-fiber nociceptor stimuli (Battaglia and Rustioni, 1988). It results in increased synaptic efficacy, that is, enhanced responses in the conditioning nociceptor pathway (homosynaptic potentiation) (Battaglia and Rustioni, 1988). C-fiber activation elicits slow synaptic potentials that last several hundred milliseconds (Murase et al., 1986; Sivilotti et al., 1993). Windup results from the summation of these slow synaptic potentials at relatively low afferent input frequencies. This produces a cumulative depolarization that leads to removal of the voltage-dependent Mg^{2+} channel blockade in N-methyl-D-aspartic acid (NMDA) receptors. Thus the action potential progressively increases in response to each stimulus in a train of inputs as a result of increased glutamate sensitivity (Thompson et al., 1990).

Morphine pretreatment and NMDA receptor antagonists block windup, mediated by NMDA and tachykinin receptors. It may be the trigger to long-lasting neuronal sensitization. Neurons that exhibit windup are less sensitive to opioids than the neurons that do not exhibit this phenomenon (Post and Silberstein, 1994). Windup is accompanied by calcium entry via NMDA channels. The increased intracellular calcium induces translocation (from cytosolic to membrane-bound form) and activation of protein kinase C and phosphorylation of the NMDA channel, which relieves the Mg^{+2} block on the ion channel (Price et al., 1994). The increased calcium may also be responsible for the induction of the two early gene products, c-fos and c-jun, which can alter other peptides, proteins, and receptors (Price et al., 1994). This results in increased glutamate sensitivity. NGF and inflammatory cytokines may change the phenotype of sensory neurons, making them more sensitive to nociception (Woolf, 1995). NGF increases the synthesis, transport, and neuronal content of SP and CGRP. It also regulates two ion channels in sensory neurons: the capsaicin receptor ion channel and the tetrodotoxin-resistant Na^{+} channel (Dray et al., 1994).

Central sensitization, in contrast, refers to an activity- or use-dependent increase in the excitability of nociceptive neurons in the CNS as a result of, and outlasting, a short barrage of nociceptor input. This can take up to 60 minutes to develop. Sensitization results from the activation of multiple intracellular signaling pathways in dorsal horn neurons by the neurotransmitter (glutamate) and the neuromodulators (SP, brain-derived neurotrophic factor, and ephrin-B ligands). Central sensitization is characterized by increased spontaneous discharge rate, reductions in threshold and increased responsiveness to both noxious and nonnoxious peripheral stimuli, and expanded receptive fields of CNS nociceptive neurons (Woolf, 1983; Woolf and Wall, 1986; Cook et al., 1987). Most dorsal horn neuronal input is subthreshold—the synaptic strength is too weak to evoke an action potential output (Woolf and King, 1989). After induction of central sensitization, the same input can activate dorsal horn neurons as a result of increases in synaptic efficacy (Woolf and King, 1990). This is called homosynaptic potentiation. In addition, additional inputs from non-stimulated A–B afferents become activated (Simone et al., 1989; Woolf and King, 1990). This is called heterosynaptic facilitation, because the Aβ fibers are not the ones that were activated by the nociceptive conditioning stimuli (C fibers must be activated to produce central sensitization). As a result of central sensitization, low-threshold sensory fibers activated by innocuous stimuli, such as light touch, can activate normally high-threshold nociceptive secondary sensory neurons in the dorsal horn. The increased excitability of CNS neurons results in a reduction in pain threshold (tactile allodynia).

If the stimulus is maintained, central sensitization persists. It can outlast the stimulus for several hours (Woolf and Wall, 1986). Clinically, central sensitization contributes to pain hypersensitivity in the skin, muscle, joints, and viscera (Sarkar et al., 2000). Cutaneous allodynic pain is referred to the periphery, but it arises from within the CNS. Does sensitization play a role in headache? Brief chemical irritation of the dura with a cocktail (inflammatory soup) of four inflammatory mediators (histamine, serotonin, bradykinin, and prostaglandin E2) made meningeal perivascular neurons pain-sensitive for a period of 1–2 hours (Strassman et al., 1996). This peripheral sensitization can explain the intracranial hypersensitivity (i.e., the worsening pain during coughing, bending over, or any head movement) and the throbbing pain of migraine (Anthony and Rasmussen, 1993).

Brief dural chemical irritation may also result in central sensitization with changes in the central trigeminal neurons that receive convergent input from the dura and the skin. Their threshold decreases and their excitability increases in response to brushing and heating of the periorbital skin—stimuli to which they showed only minimal or no response before chemical stimulation (Burstein et al., 1998). In addition, the threshold of cardiovascular responses to facial and intracranial stimuli is reduced (Yamamura et al., 1999).

Central sensitization results in muscle tenderness and cutaneous allodynia in patients with migraine. Most migraineurs exhibit cutaneous allodynia inside and outside their pain-referred areas during migraine attacks. Burstein et al. (1998) studied the development of cutaneous allodynia during migraine by measuring the pain thresholds in the head and forearms of a patient at several points during the migraine attack and by comparing the pain thresholds in the absence of an attack (Burstein et al., 2001). (Studies in animals show that peripheral nociceptors became sensitized and mediated the symptoms of cranial hypersensitivity approximately 30 minutes after their initial activation.) The barrage of impulses then activated second-order neurons and initiated their sensitization, mediating the development of cutaneous allodynia on the ipsilateral head. Many patients had periorbital cutaneous allodynia ipsilateral to the headache. Patients with allodynia were significantly older than those without cutaneous allodynia, hinting at a possible correlation between age and sensitization. These findings provide a neural basis for the pathophysiology of migraine pain and suggest a basis for continued head pain.

Gallai et al. (2003) found elevated CSF levels of glutamate and nitrite [a nitric oxide (NO) metabolite] in TM patients with and without medication overuse. The increase in CSF nitrite, a marker for NO production, was accompanied by an increase in cGMP. CGRP, SP, and, to a lesser extent, neurokinin A were also elevated in patients compared with controls. NO plays a crucial role in animal models of sensitization. Its formation is triggered by glutamate receptor activation.

Does central sensitization play a role in headache? In animal models of head pain, there is good evidence for c-fos activation in the trigeminal NC. In the NC superior dorsal horn, c-fos is a marker for nociceptive stimulation and may be a signal for the adaptive responses of the nervous system to insult (Mungliani and Hunt, 1995). This may produce long-lasting neuronal sensitization with increased activation of the trigeminal vascular system.

Evidence now exists that central sensitization, defined by the presence of cutaneous allodynia, exists in CDH, including TM with and without medication overuse. Shukla et al. (2003) studied dynamic mechanical (brush) allodynia (BA) in headache patients in an inpatient setting. This study demonstrated that mechanical dynamic BA is common in hospitalized CDH patients. Of a total of 78 patients, most of whom had TM, 32 (41%) experienced BA. Allodynia was more common and more severe in V1, indicating the role of central sensitization in its development. Allodynia was significantly more common in patients with unilateral headaches, and was usually ipsilateral to the headache.

Creach et al. (2003) compared heat-pain thresholds in patients with TM with and without medication overuse and patients with episodic migraine. Extracranial, but not face, allodynia was more common in both TM groups (39.5% versus 12.1%). Using a questionnaire, Sobrino (2003) found that 56.3% of TM patients had cutaneous allodynia in their pain-referred areas.

Bendtsen, Jensen, and Olesen (1996) found evidence for sensitization in patients with CTTH. Pericranial myofascial tenderness, evaluated by manual palpation, was considerably higher in patients than in controls ($p < 0.00001$). The stimulus–response function from highly tender muscle was qualitatively different from normal muscle, suggesting that myofascial pain may be mediated by low-threshold mechanosensitive afferents projecting to sensitized dorsal horn neurons.

Pain Modulation

The mammalian nervous system contains networks that modulate nociceptive transmission. The trigeminal brain stem nuclear complex receives monoaminergic, enkephalinergic, and peptidergic projections from the regions known to be important in the modulation of nociceptive systems. A descending inhibitory neuronal network extends from the frontal cortex and hypothalamus through the periaqueductal gray (PAG) to the rostral ventromedial medulla (RVM) and the medullary and spinal dorsal horn. The RVM includes the nucleus raphe magnum and the adjacent reticular formation and projects to the outer laminae of the spinal and medullary dorsal horn. Electrical stimulation or injection of opioids into the PAG reduces nociresponsive neuron activity. The PAG receives projections from the insular cortex and the amygdala (Messlinger and Burstein, 1999). Stimulation of the RVM can result in inhibition and/or facilitation of nociceptive and non-nociceptive input. The RVM is a relay in descending modulation of nociception (Porreca et al., 2002). RVM stimulation at relatively high current intensities is both antinociceptive (in the tail-flick test) and responsible for decreased responses of dorsal horn neurons. By contrast, lower-current intensity stimulation at the same sites are facilitatory (Zhuo and Gebhart, 1990; Zhuo and Gebhart, 1992; Zhuo and Gebhart, 1997). Excitatory neurotransmitters (e.g., glutamate, neurotensin) microinjected into the RVM replicated the effects of stimulation, facilitating and inhibiting spinal nociception at lower and higher doses, respectively (Zhuo and Gebhart, 1992; Zhuo and Gebhart, 1997; Urban and Gebhart, 1997; Urban et al., 1999a). Microinjection of NMDA into the RVM facilitated the tail-flick reflex in a dose-dependent manner, an effect blocked by an NMDA receptor antagonist (Urban et al., 1999b).

Antinociception can be measured by nociceptive reflex inhibition. In the RVM and PAG, three classes of neurons have been identified (Fields et al., 1991). "Off-cells" pause immediately before the nociceptive reflex, whereas "on-cells" are activated. Neutral cells show no consistent changes in activation (Messlinger and Burstein, 1999). On-cells and off-cells fire in a reciprocating pattern; tail-flick latency was longer during periods of increased off-cell activity and shorter when on-cells were active. Opioids activate off-cells and inhibit on-cells; nociceptive reflexes are inhibited. Naloxone-precipitated opioid withdrawal increases on-cell activity (Bederson et al., 1990; Kim et al., 1990). This is abolished by intra-RVM injection of lidocaine (Kaplan and Fields, 1991; Heinricher and Roychowdhury, 1997). Thus, off-cell activity suppresses nociception, whereas on-cell activity enhances the response to noxious stimuli. On- and off-cell activity is modulated by 5-HT_1 receptor agonists (Messlinger and Burstein, 1999). Off- and on-cells (descending inhibitory and facilitatory pathways) project from the RVM through both dorsal and ventral parts of the spinal cord to the spinal dorsal horn (Porreca et al., 2002).

Opioids can paradoxically induce pain and decrease tolerance to nociception. This is mechanistically similar to the abnormal pain that follows peripheral nerve injury. Both are less responsive to the antinociceptive effects of morphine and are reversed by NMDA antagonists (Ma and Woolf, 1995). Both activate the RVM descending pain facilitation pathways. Increased RVM facilitation may be mediated by pronociceptive peptide cholecystokinin (CCK). CCK exists throughout the brain and spinal cord. Immunoreactivity is seen in the PAG and RVM. CCK can contribute to RVM neuron excitability. Intra-RVM CCK produces reversible thermal and tactile hypersensitivity (Kovelowski et al., 2000), and prevents both the activation of off-cells and the antinociception produced by systemic morphine (Heinricher et al., 2001). Conversely, microinjection of a CCK antagonist into the RVM blocks thermal and tactile hypersensitivity in rats with peripheral nerve injury (Kovelowski et al., 2000). CCK antagonists also enhance morphine-induced antinociception and reverse morphine tolerance (Dourish et al., 1990). The RVM produces descending facilitation by elevating spinal dynorphin expression (Vanderah et al., 2000). Dynorphin acts as an endogenous pronociceptor mediator, resulting in enhanced release of CGRP and SP (Draisci et al., 1991; Arcaya et al., 1999; Gardell et al., 2002). Dynorphin upregulation is blocked by lesions in the RVM descending pathways. The lesions also block enhanced CGRP release and abnormal pain. Antibodies to dynorphin also block CGRP release in model systems (Gardell et al., 2002).

Opioid analgesic tolerance is a pharmacological phenomenon that occurs after prolonged opioid administration, in part due to the activation of the NMDA receptor (NMDAR). Excess activation of NMDARs can lead to neurotoxicity. Mao et al. (2002) showed that spinal neuronal apoptosis was induced in rats that are made tolerant to morphine administered through intrathecal boluses or continuous infusion. The apoptotic cells were predominantly located in the superficial spinal cord dorsal horn. Most apoptotic cells expressed glutamic acid decarboxylase, a key enzyme for the synthesis of the inhibitory neurotransmitter GABA. This was associated with increased nociceptive sensitivity to heat stimulation. Morphine-induced neuronal apoptosis was modulated by spinal glutamatergic activity. Prolonged morphine administration resulted in the upregulation of the proapoptotic caspase-3 and Bax proteins, but downregulation of the antiapoptotic Bcl-2 protein in the spinal cord dorsal horn. Coadministration with morphine of a pan-caspase inhibitor or a relatively selective caspase-3 inhibitor blocked morphine-induced neuronal apoptosis. These results suggest that opioid-induced neurotoxicity depletes inhibitory GABA interneurons, a mechanism that may have clinical implications in opioid therapy and substance abuse and may account for refractoriness in CM.

The RVM modulates the activity of the TNC and dorsal horn neurons. Increased on-cell activity in the brain stem's pain modulation system could enhance the response to both painful and nonpainful stimuli. Opioid withdrawal results in increased firing of the on-cells, decreased firing of the off-cells, and enhanced nociception (Bederson et al., 1990; Fields et al., 1991). Descending facilitatory influences could contribute to chronic pain states and the development and maintenance of hyperalgesia (Urban and Gebhart, 1999). Headache may be caused, in part, by enhanced neuronal activity in the nucleus caudalis as a result of enhanced on-cell and decreased off-cell activity. Other conditioned stimuli associated with pain and stress also can turn on the pain system and may account, in part, for the association between pain and stress (Fields et al., 1991). CDH may result, in part, from enhanced neuronal activity in the TNC as a result of enhanced on-cell and decreased off-cell activity. Overuse of acute medication (analgesics, opioids, barbiturates, ergotamine-containing compounds, or triptans) can contribute to the transformation of episodic migraine into TM (Post and Silberstein, 1994). Drug-induced primary CDH has been defined as owing to a rebound effect, wherein migraine medication withdrawal triggers the next headache, which in turn leads to the consumption of more drug (Saper and VanMeter, 1980; Saper, 1983; Saper and Jones, 1986). This produces a self-promoting and sustaining cycle, resulting in more frequent drug use and drug-induced primary CDH. Continued high fluctuating doses could result in resetting the pain control mechanisms in susceptible individuals, perhaps by enhancing on-cell activity, enhancing central sensitization through NMDA receptors, or blocking adaptive antinociceptive changes. Formulations of drugs that maintain sustained, nonfluctuating levels might avoid the development of drug-induced headache (Post and Silberstein, 1994). Chronic opioid use has clearly been shown to activate RVM pain facilitation. Opioid-induced neurotoxicity by depleting inhibitory GABA interneurons may result in headache intractability (Mao et al., 2002).

Compensatory adaptive changes associated with frequent headaches (if they occur) may not be enough to allow continued drug effectiveness. If tolerance has decreased drug effectiveness, a drug holiday could renew the response (Post and Silberstein, 1994). Drug overuse may, in part, prevent the occurrence of antinociceptive adaptive changes. The analgesic washout period could be a result of the time required for the system to reset. The failure of preventive drugs could result from the lack of endogenous antinociceptive agents. A similar phenomenon occurs in contingent tolerance in the seizure kindling model.

Clinical strategies based on these concepts might be used to reverse tolerance in the long-term treatment of CDH. Switching a patient to a drug that has a different mechanism of action and does not show cross-tolerance or discontinuing the ineffective drug and reintroducing it later may be effective for some migraine or TM patients.

PET in primary headaches, such as migraine (Weiller et al., 1995) and cluster (May, Bahra, et al., 1998) headache, has demonstrated activations (as measured by increased cerebral blood flow) in brain areas associated with pain, such as the cingulate cortex, insulae, frontal cortex, thalamus, basal ganglia, and cerebellum. These areas are similarly activated when head pain is induced by injecting capsaicin into the forehead of volunteers (May, Kaube, et al., 1998). Cortical (but not brainstem) activation is reversed by sumatriptan, as is the headache. This area of the brainstem is rich in opioids and includes the pain control centers (Ren and Dubner, 2002). Dihydroergotamine (DHE) and centrally penetrant triptans selectively bind to this area of the brainstem. This area of the brainstem may integrate the phenomenon we call migraine, or it could be activated as a result of the migraine attack. If the first explanation is correct, ongoing activity in this area of the brainstem could produce recurrent or daily headache. If this area is responsible for controlling pain, then its failure to activate could explain ongoing headache activity. Acute migraine medications may induce daily headache by preventing the development of adaptive changes and perhaps by maintaining brainstem activation (Weiller et al., 1995).

Manjit et al. (2003) reported eight patients with the IHS diagnosis of CM who showed a marked beneficial response to implanted bilateral suboccipital stimulators. Stimulation evoked local paraesthesia, the presence of which was a criterion of pain relief. On stimulation, the headache began to improve instantaneously and was completely suppressed within 30 minutes. When the stimulation was switched off, the headache recurred instantly and peaked within 20 minutes. PET scans were performed using rCBF as a marker of neuronal activity. Each patient was scanned in the following three states: (1) stimulator at optimum settings: patient pain-free but with paresthesia; (2) stimulator off: patient in pain and no paresthesia; (3) stimulator partially activated: patient with intermediate levels of pain and paresthesia. There were significant changes in rCBF in the dorsal rostral pons, anterior cingulate cortex (ACC), and cuneus, correlated to pain scores, and correlated to stimulation-induced paresthesia scores in the ACC and left pulvinar. The activation pattern in the dorsal rostral pons is highly suggestive of a role for this structure in the pathophysiology of CM. The localization and persistence of activity during stimulation is exactly consistent with a region activated in episodic migraine and with persistent activation of that area after successful treatment. The dorsal rostral pons may be a locus of neuromodulation by suboccipital stimulation. In addition, suboccipital stimulation modulated activity in the left pulvinar.

Welch et al. (1999) used high-resolution magnetic resonance techniques to map the transverse relaxation rates R2 (1/T2), R2′ (1/T2∗–1/T2), and R2∗ (1/T2∗) in the brain, particularly the PAG, RN, and SN. These measures are sensitive to free iron: R2′ is a measure of non-heme iron in tissues. They evaluated patients with TM, patients with episodic migraine, and nonmigraine controls. Mean R2′ and R2∗ values in the PAG significantly increased in both the episodic migraine and TM patients. The value increased with disease duration. A decrease in mean R2′ and R2∗ values in the RN and SN of only the TM group was observed; they attributed this to the CBF changes due to head pain. Aurora et al. (Aurora, 2003) reported normalization of SN and RN, but not PAG R2′ values after detoxification. These fascinating findings await replication.

Contingent negative variation (CNV) is the surface negative slow wave potential elicited in expectancy conditions. It represents the excitability of cortical pyramidal neurons. Migraine patients have enhanced negativity and reduced habituation compared with nonmigraine controls. Siniatchkin et al. (1998) have shown that patients with CDH also have reduced habituation, but significantly lower amplitude than episodic migraine patients. This suggests the presence of a common mechanism in these disorders. CDH patients may have lost the compensatory mechanism that is present in episodic patients, leading to chronification and lower negativity of the slow wave. Post suggested the kindling model for epilepsy as a model for nonepileptic progressive disorders, such as mania. Post and Silberstein (1994) suggested that spontaneous recurrent migraine headaches might be analogous to the low levels of electrical stimulation in the kindling model in the process of headache transformation. Preventive migraine treatment could provide a dual benefit by preventing the occurrence of episodes and blocking the sensitization process that could lead to syndrome progression.

In primary CDH, hypersensitivity of neurons in the TNC may be a result of supraspinal facilitation. Peripheral nociceptors may be hypersensitive as a result of sensitization. The vascular nociceptor may be hypersensitive in CM; and the myofascial nociceptor may be hypersensitive in CTTH associated with a disorder of the pericranial muscles. Less myofascial nociceptor hypersensitivity and a general increase in nociception may be present in CTTH not associated with a disorder of the pericranial muscles. CTTH and CM may result from a defective interaction between endogenous nociceptive brainstem activity and peripheral input. Physical or psychologic stress or nonphysiologic working positions can increase nociception that could trigger or sustain an attack in an individual with altered pain modulation. Emotional mechanisms may also reduce endogenous antinociception. Long-term potentiation of nociceptive neurons and decreased activity in the antinociceptive system could cause primary CDH. Sensitization of the TNC neurons can result in normally nonpainful stimuli becoming painful, producing trigger spots, an overlap in the symptoms of migraine and TTH, and activation of the trigeminal vascular system.

Clinical strategies based on these concepts might be used to reverse tolerance in the long-term treatment of migraine or TM. Switching a patient to a drug that has a different mechanism of action and does not show cross-tolerance or discontinuing the ineffective drug and reintroducing it later may be effective in some migraine or TM patients.

CTTH

Jensen and Olesen (1996) used sustained teeth-clenching to trigger TTH in 58 patients with frequent, but not daily, CTTH or ETTH and 58 matched controls. Within 24 hours, 69% of patients (more than would be expected) and 17% of controls developed TTH. Shortly after clenching, electromyography (EMG) amplitude was significantly increased in the trapezius but not in the temporal muscle, and tenderness (which was increased at baseline in the headache patients) further increased only in the patients who subsequently developed headache. Mechanical pain thresholds remained unchanged in the group that developed headache, but increased in the group that did not develop headache. Pain tolerance decreased in the patients who developed headache, was unchanged in the remaining patients, and increased in controls, suggesting that headache patients do not effectively activate their antinociceptive system. This study clearly shows that peripheral mechanisms alone cannot explain TTH, but they could act as a trigger for a central process. Tenderness, not muscle contraction, correlates to headache development. Tenderness may have a central cause or it may be a result of muscle contraction causing activation and chemical sensitization on myofascial mechanoreceptors and their afferent fibers.

Exteroceptive suppression is the inhibition of voluntary EMG activity of the temporalis muscle induced by trigeminal nerve stimulation (Schoenen et al., 1987). There are two successive periods of ES (ES1 and ES2) (silent periods). ES2, a multisynaptic reflex subject to limbic and other modulation, was originally reported to be absent in 40% of patients with CTTH and reduced in duration in 87%, whereas ES1, an oligosynaptic reflex, was normal (Pritchard, 1989; Makashima and Takahashi, 1991; Paulus et al., 1992). More recent studies have not confirmed these findings. Zwart and Sand (1995) found normal ES2 values in a small blinded study of 11 patients with CTTH. Bendtsen et al. and Lipchich et al. did not find abnormalities in ES2 in blinded studies of patients with CTTH (Bendtsen, Jensen, Brennum, et al., 1996; Lipchik et al., 1996; Lipchik et al., 1997). Measures of ES2's duration depend on tricky methodologic variables, level of arousal. ES2 may be absent in more headache-prone patients (Nakashima and Takahashi, 1991; Paulus et al., 1992).

Schoenen et al. (1987) measured the ES2, pain threshold, EMG activity, anxiety scores, and response to biofeedback in 32 women with CTTH, and found an abnormal EMG in 62.5% of the patients if three different muscles and three states were tested. The EMG was abnormal in only 40% if only one muscle and one state were tested. A decreased pain threshold was found in half the patients tested in one of three muscles, but in only 34% if only one muscle was tested. ES2 duration was reduced in 87% of patients.

Schepelmann et al. (1998) compared ES2 values in patients with FM syndrome to patients with CTTH and controls. The duration of ES2 ($\pm$SD) in FM syndrome patients was 30.6 $\pm$ 7.5 ms and was not significantly different from the control group (33.1 $\pm$ 7.8 ms), whereas it was significantly shortened in CTTH patients (22.9 $\pm$ 11.5 ms).

Lipchik et al. (1996) evaluated masseter ES2 suppression and tenderness in the pericranial muscles of young adults with CTTH, ETTH, migraine without aura, migraine with aura, and controls. Pericranial muscle tenderness better distinguished diagnostic subgroups and better distinguished recurrent headache sufferers from controls than did masseter ES2. CTTH sufferers had the highest pericranial muscle tenderness and controls exhibited the lowest tenderness ($p < 0.01$). The association between pericranial muscle tenderness and CTTH was independent of the intensity, frequency, or chronicity of headaches. Pericranial muscle tenderness may be present early in the development of tension headache, while ES2 suppression may only emerge later.

An adequate pain stimulus induces two pain sensations: the first is acute, short-lasting, and well localized and the second is longer lasting and less localized. The second pain intensity increases with repeat stimulation and is enhanced in chronic headaches (Fusco et al., 1997). Fusco et al. (1997) examined second pain in subjects with ETTH, CDH, migraine without aura, and controls using percutaneous electrical shock. Second pain intensity was significantly greater in the group of patients with CDH compared with other groups.

Fusco et al. (1999) evaluated the effect of dextromethorphan and Mg^{2+} on temporal summation of second pain in seven patients with TM and five with other chronic headaches. They used a sequence of four electrical shocks delivered on the medial forearm at 3-second intervals. Pain intensity was measured with a visual analog scale. The stimulus was repeated 1 hour after a 100-mg oral dose of dextromethorphan, 10 minutes after the end of a slow intravenous infusion of Mg^{2+}, or both. First-pain intensity did not change. The exaggerated temporal summation of second pain in chronic headache was confirmed. Dextromethorphan significantly decreased this. Mg^{2+} alone had no effect, but it did increase dextromethorphan's effect. Pharmacologic modulation of NMDA receptors may improve chronic headaches.

Ashina et al. (1999b) measured trapezius muscle hardness in 20 CTTH patients and 20 healthy controls. The patients were examined on 2 days, one with headache and one without headache. Pericranial myofascial tenderness (manual palpation) and muscle hardness (using a meter) were measured in 30 healthy controls and five patients outside of headache. Muscle hardness on days with headache did not differ significantly from muscle hardness on days without headache. Muscle hardness positively correlated to the local tenderness score recorded from the trapezius muscle on days both with and without headache. The total tenderness score on days with headache was significantly higher than the total tenderness score on days without headache. There was a significant difference between the total tenderness score recorded in patients without headache, 15 $\pm$ 11, and controls, 4 $\pm$ 4 ($p = 0.002$). Muscle hardness was significantly higher in patients on days without headache than in controls. The authors found that muscle hardness and tenderness are permanently altered in CTTH, and are not only a consequence of actual pain. The positive correlation between muscle hardness and tenderness supports the clinical observation that tender muscles are harder than normal muscles.

Sakai et al. (1995) found that pericranial muscle hardness was significantly greater in women than in men. In TTH patients, the trapezius muscles were significantly harder in patients than they were in normal subjects. Posterior neck muscle hardness was also significantly greater in patients than in normal subjects. There was no significant difference in muscle hardness between ETTH and CTTH. Muscle hardness was reduced in patients who displayed clinical improvement.

Reduced Achilles tendon pain thresholds were found in half of CTTH patients when compared with headache-free controls (Schoenen et al., 1991). Biofeedback moderately but significantly increased the pain threshold, perhaps by normalizing limbic input to the brainstem pain modulating system. Increased EMG activity or decreased pain thresholds were found in 72% of the patients (Schoenen et al., 1991), consistent with a diagnosis of "CTTH associated with disorder of pericranial muscles," but these findings were not present in the remaining 28% of patients, consistent with a diagnosis of "CTTH unassociated with such disorder." Headache severity, anxiety, ES2, and response to biofeedback did not differ between these two groups, suggesting that their separation may be artificial or a consequence of the headache.

Lassen et al. (1997) discovered that nitroglycerin, an NO donor, can induce headache in CTTH patients. In a randomized, double-blind, crossover trial, 16 CTTH patients (who never had migraine) and 16 healthy volunteers received an IV infusion of nitroglycerin (0.5 μg/kg/minutes for 20 minutes) or placebo on nonheadache days. The primary end point was the difference between the area under the headache curve [AUC (duration times intensity)] recorded on an active day and on a placebo day. In patients, the median AUC on a nitroglycerin day (2221) was significantly higher than on a placebo day (730) ($p = 0.008$). Peak pain intensity occurred 8 hours after nitroglycerin infusion. On a nitroglycerin day, the median AUC in patients (2221) was also significantly higher than in controls (43) ($p = 0.0001$). This study suggests that NO may play an important role in the pathophysiology of CTTH.

Ashina et al. (1999a) randomized 16 CTTH patients in a double-blind, crossover-designed trial to either intravenous infusions of 6 mg/kg L-NMMA (NG-Monomethyl-L-Arginine.Monoacetate) or placebo on 2 days, separated by at least 1 week. Trapezius muscle hardness (measured with a meter) and pericranial myofascial tenderness (evaluated by a standardized validated manual palpation) were recorded at baseline and at 60 and 120 minutes after beginning the infusion. Compared with baseline, muscle hardness and tenderness were significantly reduced at 60 and 120 minutes. Placebo had no significant effect. Compared with placebo, the summary score of muscle hardness was significantly reduced, while tenderness showed a nonsignificant reduction after treatment with L-NMMA. Increased muscle hardness in CTTH patients may reflect sensitization of second-order neurons due to prolonged nociceptive input from myofascial tissues. The decrease in muscle hardness after treatment with L-NMMA may be caused by decreased central sensitization.

Nociception from pericranial myofascial tissues may play a major role in the pathophysiology of TTH. Increased myofascial tenderness is the most prominent abnormal finding in patients with CTTH. There is increased muscle hardness and a positive correlation between muscle hardness and tenderness in CTTH. CTTH sufferers also exhibit signs of increased CNS sensitivity. Pressure pain detection and tolerance thresholds to mechanical stimuli are decreased. and pain perception is qualitatively altered. CTTH may be due to sensitization at the level of the spinal dorsal horn/trigeminal nucleus induced by prolonged nociceptive input from pericranial myofascial tissues (Ashina, 2004).

TREATMENT

Overview

Patients with CDH can be difficult to treat, especially when the disorder is complicated by medication overuse, comorbid psychiatric disease, low frustration tolerance, and physical and emotional dependency (Mathew et al., 1987; Saper, 1987b). We recommend the following steps. First, exclude secondary headache disorders; second, diagnose the specific primary headache disorder (CM, CTTH, HC, or NDPH); and third, identify comorbid medical and psychiatric conditions and exacerbating factors, especially medication overuse. Limit acute medications (with the possible exception of the long-acting NSAIDs). Patients should be started on preventive medication (to decrease reliance on acute medication), with the explicit understanding that the drugs may not become fully effective until medication overuse has been eliminated (Silberstein and Saper, 1993). Some patients need to have their headache cycle terminated (Silberstein and Saper, 1993). Patients require education and continuous support during this process. Outpatient detoxification options, including outpatient infusion in an ambulatory infusion unit, are available. If outpatient treatment proves difficult or is dangerous, hospitalization may be required (Zed et al., 1999; Silberstein and Lipton, 2001).

In some cases, CDH reverts to episodic headache when preventive medication is initiated and acute medications limited. In other cases, there may be only moderate or no improvement. Zeeberg et al. described the treatment outcomes in patients withdrawn from medication overuse. They studied 337 outpatients who were diagnosed with MOH and treated and dismissed from the Danish Headache Centre in 2002 and 2003. A 46% decrease in headache frequency from the first visit to dismissal occurred ($p < 0.0001$). Patients with no improvement 2 months after complete drug withdrawal ($N = 88$) subsequently responded to pharmacologic and/or non-pharmacologic prophylaxis, with a 26% decrease in headache frequency as measured from the end of withdrawal to dismissal. At dismissal, 47% of patients were on prophylaxis. In this population, about half of MOH patients benefit from drug withdrawal alone (Zeeberg et al., 2006).

Patients can have severe exacerbations of their migraine during detoxification. Thus patients, even if they are on preventive medication, often need additional treatment (which we call *headache terminators)* to break the cycle of CDH and/or help with the exacerbation that occurs when overused medications are discontinued. Terminators can be given orally, by suppository, or by injection, and some can be given intravenously repetitively. The route of administration depends on both the setting and the intensity of treatment.

Patients need education and continuous support during this process. Disturbances in mood and function are common and require management with behavioral methods of pain management and supportive psychotherapy. Treatment of coexistent psychiatric illness is often necessary before CM comes under control. Chronobiologic interventions, such as encouraging regular habits of sleep, exercise, and meals, are often useful (Silberstein and Saper, 1993).

Psychophysiologic therapy involves reassurance, counseling, stress management, relaxation therapy, biofeedback, and cognitive behavioral therapy. The use of traditional acupuncture is controversial and has not proved more effective than placebo (Tavola et al., 1992). Physical therapy consists of modality treatments (heat, cold packs, ultrasound, and electrical stimulation); improvement of posture through stretching, exercise, and traction; trigger point injections; occipital nerve blocks; and a program of regular exercise and stretching (Silberstein, 1984). It has been our experience that treating painful trigger areas in the neck can result in improvement of intractable CDH.

Patients who are overusing acute medication may not become fully responsive to acute and preventive treatment for 2–10 weeks after medication overuse is eliminated, and some may never fully respond. Withdrawal symptoms include severely exacerbated headaches accompanied by nausea, vomiting, agitation, restlessness, sleep disorder, and (rarely) seizures. Barbiturates, opioids, and benzodiazepine, unless replaced with long-acting derivatives, must be tapered to avoid a serious withdrawal syndrome. The washout period may last 3–8 weeks; once it is over, considerable headache improvement frequently occurs (Raskin, 1986; Baumgartner et al., 1989; Mathew et al., 1990; Silberstein et al., 1990).

Outpatient treatment in an ambulatory infusion unit and home treatment options are available. If outpatient treatment proves difficult or is dangerous, hospitalization may be required (Saper, Silberstein, et al., 1999; Lake et al., 2006). Diener et al. (1988) were able to detoxify only 1.5% of 200 patients on an outpatient basis. Hering and Steiner (1991), in contrast, successfully used outpatient detoxification in 37 of 46 patients who were taking simple analgesics or ergotamine. A recent consensus paper by the German Migraine Society recommends outpatient withdrawal for highly motivated patients who do not take barbiturates or tranquilizers with their analgesics. Inpatient treatment is recommended for patients who fail outpatient treatment, have high depression scores, or take tranquilizers, codeine, or barbiturates (Diener et al., 1992). Hospitalization may be necessary for severe dehydration, for which inpatient parenteral therapy may be necessary; diagnostic suspicion (confirmed by appropriate diagnostic testing) of organic etiology; prolonged, unrelenting headache with associated symptoms, such as nausea and vomiting, which, if allowed to continue, would pose a further threat to the patient's welfare; status migraine; dependence on analgesics, ergots, opiates, barbiturates, or tranquilizers; pain that is accompanied by serious adverse reactions or complications from therapy wherein continued use of such therapy aggravates or induces further illness; pain that occurs in the presence of significant medical disease but appropriate treatment of headache symptom aggravates or induces further illness; failed outpatient detoxification, for which inpatient pain and psychiatric management may be necessary; or treatment requiring co-pharmacy with drugs that may cause a drug interaction, thus necessitating careful observation (monoamine oxidase inhibitors and β-blockers). We have proposed guidelines for hospitalization (Table 13–12).

Acute Pharmacotherapy

Choice of acute treatment depends upon the diagnosis. CM patients, who by definition are not overusing acute medication, can treat acute migrainous headache exacerbations with antimigraine drugs, including triptans and DHE, or NSAIDs. These drugs must be strictly limited to prevent superimposed MOH that will complicate treatment and require detoxification. The risk of MOH is much lower for DHE and triptans than for analgesics, opioids, and ergotamine. CTTH and NDPH can be treated with nonspecific headache medications, and HC can be treated with supplemental doses of indomethacin.

Preventive Pharmacotherapy

Patients with very frequent headaches should be treated primarily with preventive medications, with the explicit understanding that their medications may not become fully effective until the overused medication has been eliminated. It may take 3–6 weeks for treatment effects to develop. However, some patients remain refractory (Saper, Lake, et al., 1999).

The following principles guide the use of preventive treatment: (1) from among the first-line drugs, choose preventive agents based on their adverse event (AE) profiles, comorbid and

Table 13–12 Criteria for Hospitalization.

I. Emergency or Urgent Admission:

A. Certain migraine variants (e.g., hemiplegic migraine, suspected migrainous infarction, basilar migraine with serious neurologic symptoms such as syncope, confusional migraine, etc.)
  1. When a diagnosis has not been established during a previous similar occurrence
  2. When a patient's established outpatient treatment plan has failed

B. Diagnostic suspicion of infectious disorder involving CNS (e.g., brain abscess, meningitis) with initiation of appropriate diagnostic testing

C. Diagnostic suspicion of acute vascular compromise (e.g., aneurysm, subarachnoid hemorrhage, carotid dissection) with initiation of appropriate diagnostic testing

D. Diagnostic suspicion of a structural disorder causing symptoms requiring an acute setting (e.g., brain tumor, increased intracranial pressure) with initiation of appropriate diagnostic testing

E. Low cerebrospinal fluid headache when an outpatient blood patch has failed and an outpatient treatment plan has failed or there is no obvious cause.

F. Medical emergency presenting with a severe headache.

G. Severe headache associated with intractable nausea and vomiting producing dehydration or postural hypotension, or unable to retain oral medication, and unable to be controlled in an outpatient setting or with admission to observation status

H. Failed outpatient treatment of an exacerbation of episodic headache disorder with:
  1. Failure to respond to "rescue" or backup medications or
  2. Failure to respond to outpatient treatment with IV DHE on a schedule of a minimum of twice daily

II. Nonemergent Admission:

A. Coexistent psychiatric disease documented by psychologic or psychiatric evaluation with sufficient severity of illness such that a failure to admit could pose a health risk to the patient or impair the implementation of outpatient treatment

B. Coexistent or risk of disease (e.g., unstable angina, unstable diabetes, recent transient ischemic attack, myocardial infarction in the past 6 months, renal failure, hypertension, age more than 65 years) necessitating monitoring for treatment of headache significant enough to warrant admission

C. Severe chronic daily headaches involving chronic medication overuse when there is:
  1. Daily use of potent opioids and/or barbiturates
  2. Daily use of triptans, simple analgesics, or ergotamine in a patient with a documented failed trial of withdrawal of these medications

D. Impaired daily functioning (e.g., threatened relationships, many lost days at work or school due to headache), with a failure to respond to 2 days of outpatient treatment with IV DHE, IV neuroleptics, or IV corticosteroids on a schedule of a minimum of twice daily or equivalent treatment

coexistent conditions, and specific indications (e. g., indomethacin for HC); (2) start at a low dose; (3) gradually increase the dose until you achieve efficacy, the patient develops side-effects, or the ceiling dose for the drug in question is reached; (4) treatment effects develop over weeks and treatment may not become fully effective until rebound is eliminated; (5) if one agent fails and if all other things are equal, choose an agent from another therapeutic class; (6) prefer monotherapy, but be willing to use combination therapy; (7) communicate realistic expectations (Silberstein and Lipton, 1994).

Most preventive agents used for primary CDH have not been examined in well-designed double-blind studies. Table 13–13 summarizes an assessment of the efficacy, safety, and evidence for a number of agents (Silberstein and Saper, 1993).

Antidepressants are attractive agents for use in primary CDH, since many patients have comorbid depression and anxiety. The most widely used tricyclic antidepressants are nortriptyline (Aventyl, Pamelor), amitriptyline (Elavil), which has been effective in many but not all studies (Lance and Curran, 1964; Diamond and Baltes, 1971; Couch et al., 1976; Pluvinage, 1978; Holland et al., 1983; Pfaffenrath et al., 1986; Bussone et al., 1991; Holroyd et al., 1991; Gobel et al., 1994; Pfaffenrath et al., 1994; Bonuccelli et al., 1996; Cerbo et al., 1998; Mitsikostas et al., 1997) and doxepin (Sinequan) (Morland et al., 1979). In an open-label study of 82 nondepressed patients with either ETTH or CTTH, Cerbo et al. (1998) found that amitriptyline (25 mg a day) significantly reduced ($p < 0.05$) analgesic consumption and the frequency and duration of headache in CTTH, but not in ETTH. Descombes et al. (2001) assessed the effects of amitriptyline and sudden analgesic withdrawal on headache frequency and quality of life in patients suffering from MOH related to analgesic abuse. Seventeen nondepressed patients with MOH were included in a 9-week, parallel-group, randomized, double-blind, placebo-controlled study. After abrupt analgesic withdrawal, amitriptyline or an active placebo (trihexyphenidyl) was started. The primary efficacy variable was headache frequency recorded on a headache diary in the last 4 weeks of each treatment. Headache

TABLE 13–13 Summary of Prophylactic Drugs for Use in Chronic Daily Headache.

Drug	*Clinical efficacy*	*Adverse events*	*Clinical evidence**
Antidepressants			
Amitriptyline	+++	++	+++
Doxepin	+++	++	++
Fluoxetine	++	+	+++
Anticonvulsants			
Divalproex	+++	++	++
Topiramate	++	++	+++
Topiramate	++++	++	+++
Beta Blockers			
Propranolol, Nadolol, etc.	++	+	+
Calcium Channel Blockers			
Verapamil	++	+	+
Miscellaneous			
Methysergide	+++	+++	+

Source: Modified from Tfelt-Hansen and Welch (2000)

Note: All categories are rated from + to ++++ based on a combination of published literature and clinical experience.

*Ratings of +++ for clinical evidence indicate at least one double-blind, placebo-controlled study. A rating of ++ indicates open well-designed studies, and + indicates ratings based on clinical experience. A rating of ++++ requires at least two double-blind placebo-controlled trials.

frequency decreased by 45% in the amitriptyline group and by 28% in the trihexyphenidyl group. Amitriptyline enhanced all dimensions of quality of life, and significantly improved emotional reaction and social isolation. Fluoxetine (Prozac), a selective serotonin reuptake inhibitor, is coming into wider use for daily headaches; evidence from a double-blind study demonstrates its efficacy in CDH (Bussone et al., 1991; Saper et al., 1994). The combination of fluoxetine and amitriptyline was not more effective than amitriptyline alone. Krymchantowski et al. (2002) evaluated the efficacy and tolerability of combined treatment with amitriptyline (20 mg BID) and fluoxetine (20 mg BID), compared with amitriptyline alone for CDH due to TM. Thirty-nine patients, 26 women and 13 men, aged 20–69 years, who fulfilled the Silberstein/Lipton criteria for TM, were prospectively studied. The mean difference between the initial and final (9 weeks) headache index was 513.5 ($p < 0.0005$) for group 1 and 893 ($p < 0.0017$) for group 2. Fluvoxamine appears to be effective (Manna et al., 1994) and may have analgesic properties (Palmer and Benfield, 1994). Other selective serotonin reuptake inhibitors, including paroxetine (Foster and Bafaloukos, 1994) and monoamine oxidase inhibitors, may have a therapeutic role, but this has not been proven to date (Langemark and Olesen, 1994). Venlafaxine, a selective serotonin and norepinephrine reuptake inhibitor, may be effective for migraine, but no data exist for CDH (see Chapter 11—Migraine treatment).

Beta-blockers (propranolol, nadolol) remain a mainstay of therapy for migraine (Silberstein and Saper, 1993) and are used for primary CDH (Mathew, 1981; Pfaffenrath et al., 1986). Clinicians fear that β-blockers may exacerbate depression; however, this issue is controversial (Bright and Everitt, 1992). Beta-blockers are relatively contraindicated in patients who have asthma and Raynaud's disease.

Calcium channel blockers are very well tolerated (Silberstein and Saper, 1993); anecdotal evidence supports their use for CM. Verapamil (Calan) is the most widely prescribed agent in this family. Diltiazem (Cardizem) and nifedipine (Procardia) may also be considered. Flunarizine (Lake et al., 1993; Silberstein and Saper, 1993) is widely used in Canada and Europe, but is not available in the United States.

Antiepileptic Drugs

The anticonvulsant, divalproex sodium (Depakote) (Jensen et al., 1994), is effective in migraine prevention, as shown in four double-blind placebo-controlled studies (Hering and Kuritzky, 1992; Jensen et al., 1994; Klapper, 1995; Mathew et al., 1995). Smaller open studies support its utility in CM (Mathew and Ali, 1991). In an open-label study, Edwards et al. (1999) assessed the possible benefit of sodium valproate in 20 consecutive CDH patients whose headaches were refractory to multiple standard treatments. Eleven (55%) had a response (mild or no headaches within 1–4 weeks). The doses ranged from 375 to 1500 mg a day. Two patients (10%) discontinued medication due to side-effects (nausea and difficulty thinking). Frietag et al. (2001) assessed the safety and efficacy of divalproex sodium in the long-term treatment of CDH in a retrospective chart review of 642 patients treated with divalproex sodium for CDH. The mean improvement was 47%, with an improvement in migraine of about 65%. At least 50% reduction in headache frequency was reported by 93 of the 138 patients who received treatment with divalproex sodium only. Approximately 35% of the patients experienced AEs, none of which were severe. Gabapentin, structurally related to γ-aminobutyric acid (GABA), is effective in a number of chronic pain conditions. Wessely et al. (1987) reported only in abstract form, did not find it effective in episodic migraine. Mathew et al. (2001) studied gabapentin in the prophylaxis of episodic migraine. Patients were titrated weekly from 900 (end of week 1) to 2400 mg/day (end of week 4). Intent-to-treat analysis showed that 36% of patients on gabapentin and 16.1% of patients receiving placebo had at least a 50% reduction in the 4-week migraine rate. The most frequently reported AEs were asthenia, dizziness, somnolence, and infection.

Spira et al. (Spira and Beran, 2003) studied gabapentin in the treatment of CDH in a placebo-controlled study. Gabapentin was significantly superior to placebo for the primary efficacy variable for CDH prophylaxis: 9.1% difference in headache-free rates. Other measures were also significantly better with gabapentin, including headache-free days/month, severity, and quality of life. However, this study had limitations. First, they did not subclassify CDH. The study preceded the new IHS criteria, but did not use the Silberstein–Lipton criteria for the diagnosis of CDH subtypes. Second, the study did not take into account acute medication overuse, which is a major confounding factor in both treatment and interpretation of treatment results. Third, although their results were significant, they were modest (9.1% difference in headache-free days) and may not be clinically important. Future CDH studies require subset analysis and control for acute medication overuse (Silberstein, 2003).

Topiramate, a D-fructose derivative, is effective in episodic migraine. In two large, double-blind, placebo-controlled, multicenter trials, topiramate, both 100 and 200 mg, was effective in reducing migraine attack frequency by 50% in half of the patients (Brandes et al., 2003; Mathew et al., 2003; Silberstein et al., 2004). Topiramate works by blocking voltage-gated Na^+ channels. It also modulates the action of GABA on $GABA_A$ receptors by increasing GABA-induced chloride currents (White et al., 2000). Topiramate has antagonistic properties at the AMPA/kainate subtype of glutamate receptors. It inhibits the activity of L-type high voltage-activated calcium channels (HVACCs) (Zhang et al., 2000). It also selectively inhibits carbonic anhydrase (CA) II and IV isozymes that may be important in its anticonvulsant action. Paresthesias can occur; however, they are mild and often transient; when bothersome, they can be controlled with potassium supplementation (Silberstein, 2002). The reported incidence of renal calculi is about 1.5%, representing a two to four-fold increase over the estimated occurrence in the general population. Patients taking topiramate often lose rather than gain weight.

Shuaib et al. (1999) treated 37 patients who had more than 10 migraine headaches a month with topiramate (25–100 mg a day) in an open-label study. Most patients had CDH in addition to migraine; all had failed previous preventive treatment. Over a 3- to 9-month follow-up, 11 patients (30%) had an excellent result (headache frequency decreased by more than 60%), 11 patients had a good result (headache frequency decreased 40%–60%), three patients discontinued therapy due to side-effects, and eight patients had no improvement. This uncontrolled study suggests that topiramate may be useful for CM.

Silberstein et al. (2007) evaluated the efficacy and safety of topiramate (100 mg/day) compared with placebo for the treatment of CM. This was a randomized, placebo-controlled, parallel group, multicenter study consisting of 16 weeks of double-blind treatment. Subjects aged 18–65 years with 15 or more headache days per month, at least half of which were migraine/migrainous headaches, were 1:1 randomized to either topiramate 100 mg/day or placebo. Concomitant preventive migraine treatment was not allowed, and acute headache medication use was not to exceed 4 days per week during the double-blind maintenance period. The intent-to-treat population included 306 of 328 randomized subjects who provided at least one efficacy assessment. Topiramate treatment resulted in a statistically significant mean reduction of migraine/migrainous headache days (topiramate –6.4 versus placebo –4.7, $p = 0.010$) and migraine headache days relative to baseline (topiramate –5.6 versus placebo –4.1, $p = 0.032$). Discontinuations due to AEs occurred in 18 (10.9%) topiramate subjects and 10 (6.1%) placebo subjects. There were no serious AEs or deaths. Topiramate treatment at daily doses of approximately 100 mg resulted in statistically significant mprovements compared with placebo in migraine/migrainous and migraine headache days. Safety and tolerability of topiramate was consistent with experience in previous clinical trials.

Saper et al. (2002), using a placebo-controlled, double-blind format, demonstrated that tizanidine, an alpha adrenergic agonist, was effective as an adjunctive agent for the treatment of CDH.

Other Medications

The ergot derivative, methysergide, (Silberstein, 1998) was the first migraine preventive drug approved by the Food and Drug Administration. The usual initial dose of methysergide is 2 mg BID. It can be increased to a maximum of 8 mg a day (2 mg four times a day). It is no longer available in the United States.

NSAIDs can be used for both symptomatic and preventive headache treatment. Naproxen sodium is effective in prevention at a dose of one or two 275-mg tablets BID (Miller et al., 1987). Other NSAIDs that are effective include tolfenamic acid, ketoprofen, mefenamic acid, fenoprofen, and ibuprofen (Johnson and Tfelt-Hansen, 1993; Mylecharane and Tfelt-Hansen, 1993). Aspirin was found to be effective in one study (Kangasniemi et al., 1983) and equal to placebo in another (Scholz et al., 1987). We believe that the short-acting NSAIDs, such as ibuprofen and aspirin, cause MOH and hence their use should be limited. The potential of MOH with the other NSAIDs is uncertain. Indomethacin is the drug of choice for HC, and the response to this medication defines the disorder. In patients with strictly unilateral headaches, we give indomethacin, a therapeutic trial to rule out HC, but we otherwise limit the use of NSAIDs.

Fontes-Ribeiro et al. (1999) treated 78 CTTH patients (65 evaluable) with L-5-hydroxytryptophan 5HTP (100 mg) or placebo three times a day for 8 weeks, after a washout period of 2 weeks and with a follow-up period of more 2 weeks. Only analgesic drugs were permitted. There was a trend toward reduction in the number of headache days and headache intensity, but this was not statistically significant due to the high placebo effect (about 30%). The decrease in analgesic consumption was statistically significant. During the 2 weeks of follow-up, there was a significant decrease in the number of headache days (a postdrug effect).

Although monotherapy is preferred, it is sometimes necessary to combine preventive medications. Antidepressants are often used with β-blockers or calcium channel blockers, and divalproex sodium may be used in combination with any of these medications. Pascual et al. (2003) found that combining a β-blocker and sodium valproate could lead to increased benefit for patients with migraine previously resistant to either alone. Fifty-two patients (43 women) with a history of episodic migraine with or without aura, and previously unresponsive to β-blockers or sodium valproate in monotherapy, were treated with a combination of propranolol (or nadolol) and sodium valproate in an open-label fashion. Fifty-six percent had greater than 50% reduction in migraine days. This open trial supports the practice of combination therapy. Controlled trials are needed to determine the true advantage of this combination treatment in episodic and CM.

New Treatments

Open trials and small placebo-controlled trials have suggested that CDH may improve following injection with botulinum toxin A [Botox (BTX-A)]; whether this is due to paralysis of muscles or to unknown mechanisms is uncertain (Gobel et al., 1999; Smuts et al., 1999).

Mauskop (1999) used botulinum toxin to treat 12 refractory CDH patients (5 men, 7 women) who overused acute medications almost daily. Injections were given into the frontalis, temporalis, glabellar and, when occipital pain was present, the spinus erectus muscles. Six to eleven points were injected with 50–100 U of botulinum toxin type A (BTX-A). Only one patient obtained good relief; she has had repeated injections. The most likely potential cause of the low efficacy of botulinum toxin in this group of patients is acute medication overuse. Eross and Dodick (2002) evaluated the effect of BTX-A (25–100 units) on reducing disability in 47 patients with either episodic or CM. A decrease in migraine-associated disability was reported in 58% of all patients on using a well-validated tool that is used to assess migraine-related disability (the Migraine Disability Assessment Scale questionnaire). Episodic migraine patients ($n = 12$) appeared to demonstrate the most benefit, with 75% reporting a decrease in migraine frequency compared with 53% of CM patients.

Ondo and colleagues (Ondo and Derman, 2002) conducted a randomized, double-blind, placebo-controlled, parallel clinical trial that examined the effect of BTX-A treatment on patients with CDH, including CTTH and TM. Sixty patients who had headache more than 15 days each month were enrolled and randomized to receive, based upon the "follow-the-pain" rationale, either 200 units of BTX-A or matching placebo and at 12 weeks, if the patient consented, a second open-label BTX-A injection. Following the first injection, patients treated with BTX-A had significantly fewer headache days from week 8–12 compared with placebo. In addition, 10% of patients treated with BTX-A reported a dramatic improvement and 24% reported a marked improvement compared with 3% and 7%, respectively, in the placebo-treated group. At week 24, patients who had received two BTX-A injections had significantly fewer headache days over the second 12-week period than those who had received one injection (40 versus 19 days, $p < 0.05$)

Mathew et al. evaluated the safety and efficacy of BTX-A for the prophylactic treatment of CDH in an 11-month, randomized, double-blind, placebo-controlled study. Following a 30-day screening period and a 30-day, single-blind, placebo-response period to identify placebo responders, eligible patients from both the placebo responder and placebo nonresponder groups were injected with BTX-A or placebo every 90 days and assessed every 30 days for 9 months, a period encompassing three treatment cycles. The primary efficacy measure was the change from baseline in the frequency of headache-free days in a 30-day period for the placebo nonresponder group at day 180, the chosen efficacy time point. The secondary efficacy measure was the proportion of patients with a decrease from baseline of 50% or more in the frequency of headache days per 30-day period for the placebo nonresponder group at day 180. The change from baseline in the frequency of headaches (per 30-day period), the proportion of patients with a decrease from baseline of 50% or greater in the frequency of headaches per 30-day period, acute medication use, and AEs were also assessed. Of 571 patients assessed over the baseline period, 355 were enrolled and randomized. At the end of the placebo run-in period, 279 patients (79%) were classified as placebo nonresponders and 76 patients (21%) as placebo responders. Subsequently, patients were randomized within each group to receive either BTX-A or placebo. In the placebo nonresponder stratum, the mean number of headache-free days at baseline was 5.8 ($\pm$4.7) for BTX-A- versus 5.5 ($\pm$4.7) for placebo-treated patients. At day 180, placebo nonresponders treated with BTX-A had an improved mean change from baseline of 6.7 headache-free days per 30-day period compared with a mean change from baseline of 5.2 headache-free days for placebo-treated patients. The between-group difference of 1.5 headache-free days favored BTX-A treatment, although the difference between the groups was not statistically significant. However, a statistically significant difference was observed at day 180, end point for the secondary efficacy measure. A significantly higher percentage of BTX-A patients had a decrease from baseline of 50% or greater in the frequency of headache days per 30-day period at day 180 (32.7% versus15.0%, $p = 0.027$). Also, the mean change from baseline in the frequency of headaches per 30-day period at day 180 was –6.1 for BTX-A patients versus –3.1 for the placebo patients ($p = 0.013$). Only 4 of 173 BTX-A-treated patients (2.3%) discontinued the study due to AEs. The majority of treatment-related AEs were transient and mild to moderate in severity.

BTX-A treatment resulted in patients having, on average, approximately seven more headache-free days compared with baseline. Although at the primary time point (day 180) the BTX-A treatment resulted in a 1.5 between-group difference compared with placebo, this difference was not statistically significant. The treatment met secondary efficacy outcome measures, including the percentage of patients experiencing a 50% or more decrease in the frequency of headache days, in addition to statistically significant reductions in headache frequency. BTX-A was also well tolerated in patients with CDH (Mathew et al., 2005).

Dodick et al. assessed the efficacy and safety of BTX-A for headache prevention in CDH patients without the confounding factor of concurrent prophylactic medications in a subgroup analysis of the Mathew study. Of the 355 patients in the study, 228 (64%) were not taking preventive medication and were included in this analysis (117 received BTX-A,111 received placebo injections). After two injection sessions, the maximum change in the mean frequency of headaches per 30 days was –7.8 in the BTX-A group compared with only –4.5 in the placebo group ($p = 0.032$), a statistically significant between-group difference of 3.3 headaches. The between-group difference favoring BTX-A treatment continued to improve to 4.2 headaches after a third injection session ($p = 0.023$). In addition, BTX-A treatment at least halved the frequency of baseline headaches in more than 50% of patients after three injection sessions compared with baseline. Statistically significant differences between BTX-A and placebo were evident for the change from baseline in headache frequency and headache severity for most time-points from day 180 through day 270. Only five patients (four patients receiving BTX-A treatment; one patient receiving placebo) discontinued the study due to AEs, and most treatment-related events were transient and mild to moderate in severity. BTX-A was an effective and well-tolerated prophylactic treatment in migraine patients with CDH who are not using other prophylactic medications (Dodick et al., 2005; Mathew et al., 2005).

Silberstein et al. studied the safety and efficacy of 0 U, 50 U, 100 U, 150 U (five sites), 86 Usub and 100 Usub (three sites) BTX-A (in a fixed site/fixed dose protocol) for the prophylaxis of CTTH. Three hundred patients (62.3% female; mean age 42.6 years) enrolled. For the primary end point, the mean change from baseline in the number of TTH-free days per month, there was no statistically significant difference between placebo and four BTX-A groups, but a significant difference favouring placebo versus BTX-A 150 was observed (4.5 versus 2.8 tension headache-free days/month; $p = 0.007$). All treatment groups improved at day 60. Although efficacy was not demonstrated for the primary end point, at day 90, more patients in three BTX-A groups had 50% or more decrease in TTH days than did placebo ($p = 0.024$). Most treatment-related AEs were mild or moderate, and transient. BTX-A was safe and well tolerated in the study (Silberstein et al., 2006).

Silberstein et al. evaluated the safety and efficacy of three different doses of BTX-A as preventive CDH treatment in a randomized, double-blind, placebo controlled study. Seven hundred and two patients were enrolled and randomized. They were injected with BTX-A (in a fixed site/fixed dose protocol) at 225 U, 150 U, 75 U, or placebo, and returned for additional masked treatments at day 90 and day 180. Patients were assessed every 30 days for 9 months. The primary efficacy end point, the mean change from baseline in the frequency of headache-free days at day 180 for the placebo nonresponder group, was not met. Mean improvements from baseline at day 180 of 6.0, 7.9, 7.9, and 8.0 headache-free days per month were observed in the placebo nonresponder group treated with BTX-A at 225 U, 150 U, 75 U, or placebo, respectively ($p = 0.44$). An a priori-defined analysis of headache frequency revealed that BTX-A at 225 or 150 U had significantly greater least squares mean changes from baseline than placebo at day 240 (–8.4, –8.6, and –6.4, respectively; $p = 0.03$ analysis of covariance). Although the primary efficacy end point was not met, all groups responded to treatment. The 225 U and 150 U groups experienced a greater decrease in headache frequency than the placebo group at day 240. The placebo response was higher than expected. BTX-A was safe and well tolerated. Further study of BTX-A for preventive treatment of CDH appears warranted (Silberstein, Stark, et al., 2005). Although some studies suggest that efficacy and anecdotal reports are generally positive, doubt exists in the expert community, and more studies are required.

Opioid Maintenance

The role of maintenence opioids (daily scheduled opioid therapy) for intractable CM is controversial (Harden, 2002). Some argue that chronic opioid medication is justified (Ziegler, 1997) and useful (Robbins, 1999) when patients have truly intractable headache or alternate treatments are contraindicated (as in the senior population). Until recently, long-term studies of effectiveness, sequelae over several years, predictors of long-term benefit, comparisons of pain-related outcome measures, and prevalence of problematic drug behavior were not available. Saper et al. (2004) reported the results of a treatment program of 160 sequential patients who were followed for 3–5 years. Seventy of the 160 remained on opioids for at least a 3-year period and qualified for inclusion in the efficacy analysis. The primary clinical efficacy variable was percentage improvement in the severe headache index (frequency X severity of severe headaches/week). Only 41 of the original 160 patients (26%) had more than 50% improvement. Fifty percent of patients exhibited problem drug behavior (dose violations, lost prescriptions, multisourcing); the most common of these was dose violation. Most patients (74%) either failed to show significant improvement or were discontinued from the program for clinical reasons. This study showed that a low percentage of patients had demonstrated efficacy, and there was an unexpectedly high prevalence of misuse. Daily scheduled opioid therapy did offer significant benefit for a select group of intractable headache patients. Subsequent follow-up with many of the "benefited" patients suggests to the authors that no more than 15% of the original 160 actually did well, and that several of those reporting improvement had (via collateral information gathering) fared much more poorly than initially reported. Recently, Saper and Lake (2006) have recommended against opioid maintenance, except in rare circumstances. Guidelines have been provided (Saper and Lake, 2006).

Breaking the Headache Cycle

Patients often need *headache terminators* to break the cycle of daily headache and/or help with the exacerbation that occurs when overused medications are discontinued. Terminators are given orally, by suppository, or by injection, and some [DHE, neuroleptics (prochlorperazine, chlorpromazine, and droperidol), corticosteroids, valproate sodium, magnesium, and ketorolac] can be given repetitively intravenously. Outpatient home terminators include long-acting NSAIDs, Cox-2 inhibitors, short courses of corticosteroids and typical (e.g., prochlorperazine suppositories) and atypical (e.g., olanzapine) neuroleptics. We also teach patients to self-inject DHE [subcutaneous or intramuscular DHE (0.25–1 mg)], ketorolac, and droperidol.

One of the original headache terminators is DHE. Patients who are not good candidates for DHE or do not respond to it can use repetitive intravenous neuroleptics, such as chlorpromazine, droperidol, prochlorperazine, and/or corticosteroids. Refractory patients can be given these agents to supplement repetitive intravenous DHE (Silberstein et al., 1990). In the infusion and inpatient units, we typically insert a heplock and administer IV fluids and parenteral medications via that route. Our typical hydration mixture is D5W in 0.5 normal saline at a rate of 100–200 ml/hour, which is 3–4 l/day.

Repetitive intravenous DHE was effective in eliminating intractable headache in 89% of patients within 48 hours (with or without acute medication overuse). Silberstein et al. (1990) also found that repetitive intravenous DHE was effective in eliminating prolonged migraine, cluster headache, and CM with or without medication overuse.

Repetitive intravenous DHE is often coadministered with metoclopramide (Raskin, 1986), which helps control nausea and is an effective antimigraine drug in its own right. Following 10 mg of intravenous metoclopramide, DHE 0.5 mg is administered intravenously (Fig. 13–1). Subsequent doses are adjusted based on pain relief and side-effects. Promethazine intravenously (0.15 mg/kg diluted in 50 ml of 5% dextrose or normal saline) or ondansetron (a selective 5-HT3-receptor antagonist) orally (8-mg tablet) or intravenously (4–8 mg) can be used by patients who cannot tolerate metoclopramide because of side-effects. Responsiveness may be increased by using other antiemetics and neuroleptics.

We use the neuroleptics, chlorpromazine, droperidol, haloperidol, and prochlorperazine, intravenously, intramuscularly, and by suppository, as terminators for nausea, vomiting, and pain. We also use the new atypical neuroleptics, such as olanzapine. Sixteen trials (AHCPR Technical Report) compared the efficacy of rectally and parenterally administered antiemetics. Intravenous chlorpromazine and prochlorperazine are effective in controlling intractable headache (Callaham and Raskin, 1986; Bell et al., 1990;Silberstein and Lipton, 1994; Silberstein, Saper, et al., 2001). Chlorpromazine was found to be more effective than the combination of meperidine and dimenhydrinate, and prochlorperazine was more effective than placebo in treating emergency department patients (Jones et al., 1989). Neuroleptics are locally irritating when given intravenously; they are more effective than when given intramuscularly or by suppository. We have found that intramuscular haloperidol (5 mg), droperidol (1–2.5 mg), and thiothixene (5 mg) are effective for severe migraine headache (Silberstein et al., 1990). Intravenous haloperidol and droperidol have also been used successfully.

Prochlorperazine (Compazine) administered intramuscularly, intravenously, or rectally is relatively safe and effective for the treatment of migraine headache and associated nausea and vomiting. It can be given intravenously (7.5–15 mg over 5–10 minutes) via a saline drip or "slow push" (Callaham and Raskin, 1986; Jones et al., 1989). Prochlorperazine suppositories (25 mg) are used as a rescue treatment for headache and nausea, and also as an outpatient terminator medication. They can be used daily, as often as three times a day, for several days. The drug is not as

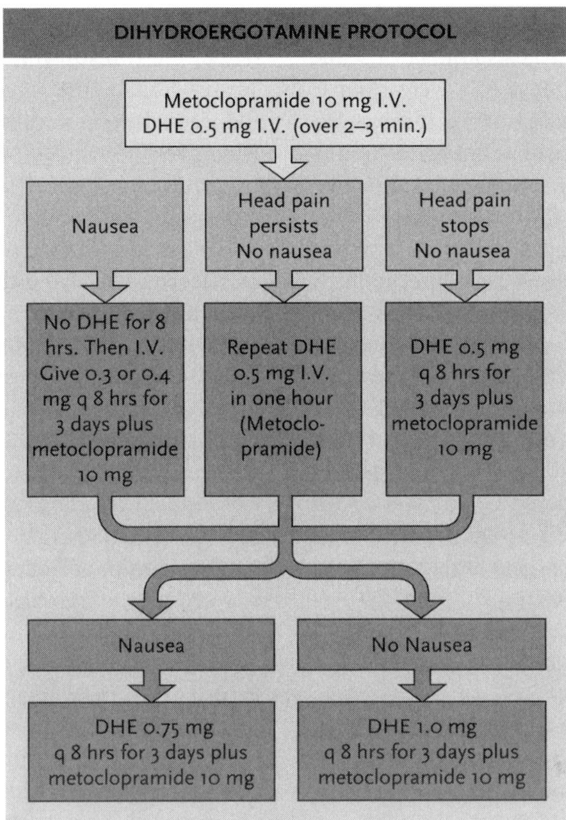

Figure 13–1 Dihydroergotamine protocol.

effective orally. Lu et al. (2000) retrospectively analyzed the data of refractory CDH in patients who received intravenous repetitive prochlorperazine. A total of 135 patients were recruited, including 95 (70%) with analgesic overuse. After intravenous prochlorperazine treatment, 121 (90%) achieved a 50% or greater reduction of headache intensity, including 85 (63%) who became headache-free. Compared with DHE, prochlorperazine seemed less effective in achieving "freedom from headache" during hospitalization, but had a similar outcome at follow-up.

Chlorpromazine (Thorazine), 10–50 mg 3–4 times a day diluted in 20–30 ml of saline, can be administered intravenously by rapid drip or "slow push" over several minutes. It can also be administered intramuscularly, rectally, or orally. The oral dose is 25–50 mg. Hypotension may result if the patient is not adequately hydrated before intravenous chlorpromazine administration.

Droperidol is a parenteral neuroleptic that was effective in a pilot study of 35 patients with status migrainosus or refractory migraine in an ambulatory infusion center. Droperidol (2.5 mg) was given intravenously every 30 minutes until either three doses were given or the patient was completely or almost headache-free (Wang et al., 1997). The success rate (headache-free or mild headache) was 88% in patients with status migrainosus and 100% in patients with refractory migraine. A double-blind, placebo-controlled, randomized, parallel-group, 22-center study (Silberstein, Young, et al., 2001) showed intramuscular droperidol to be effective for the acute treatment of migraine with or without aura. More patients in the 2.75, 5.5, and 8.25 mg treatment groups experienced a significant reduction in headache by 2 hours (moderate or severe to none or mild; 87%, 81%, and 84%, respectively) compared with placebo (57%). AEs occurring in more than 5% of patients receiving droperidol included asthenia, anxiety, akathisia, somnolence, and injection site reactions. Most AEs were mild to moderate. Patients can successfully self-inject droperidol. We now use repetitive intravenous droperidol (1–2.5 mg every 6 hours) in combination with intravenous diphenhydramine (25–50 mg). One concern with using neuroleptics is a prolonged QTc interval on EKG. This is more likely to occur with droperidol use than with chlorpromazine or prochlorperazine. It is unlikely with olanzapine. Patients who receive daily repetitive intravenous droperidol should have an EKG before their first dose of the medication and daily thereafter. A QTc that is above 450 is considered a "grey zone" (the drug should be stopped or the dose reduced) and a QTc above 500 is a "red zone" (an absolute contraindication). Bradycardia, abnormal EKG, and a change in the QTc of more than 60 ms are the other risk factors for torsades de pointes associated with prolonged QT syndrome.

Olanzapine, a thienobenzodiazepine, is a new, "atypical" antipsychotic drug. Olanzapine's properties suggest that it would be effective for headaches, with a low risk of acute extrapyramidal reactions and tardive dyskinesia. The oral dose is 5–10 mg.

Controlled studies have shown corticosteroids to be effective in the treatment of headache associated with altitude sickness (Silberstein and Lipton, 1994; Silberstein, Saper, et al., 2001). Clinical experience suggests that corticosteroids are also effective in the treatment of other headache types. Hydrocortisone or Solu-Medrol (methyl prednisolone sodium succinate) can be given intravenously in the following manner: 100 mg via a saline drip over 10 minutes every 6 hours for 24 hours; every 8 hours for 24 hours; every 12 hours for 24 hours; and then a final dose. Dexamethasone (Decadron) can be administered intravenously or intramuscularly, starting at a dose of 8–20 mg per day in divided doses, rapidly tapering over 2–3 days. Oral dexamethasone, 1.5–4 mg twice daily for 2 days with a taper over three more days, has also proven useful for less disabled migraineurs with prolonged migraine headache.

At least five different chemical classes of NSAIDs have been used for headache treatment (Pradalier et al., 1988). The major mechanism of action of NSAIDs is the differential inhibition of one of the two subtypes of the enzyme cyclooxygenase (COX1, the constitutive, and COX2, the induced form) preventing prostaglandin synthesis (Campbell, 1990). The AHCPR analyzed 33 controlled trials of NSAIDs and other nonopiate analgesics, and found that aspirin, ibuprofen, tolfenamic acid, and naproxen sodium were superior to placebo in relieving the pain of migraine. We use naproxen, indomethacin rectal suppositories, and selective COX2 inhibitors. In addition, we use intramuscular or intravenous ketorolac, especially in situations where neuroleptics, narcotics, and DHE are relatively contraindicated. When we use intravenous ketorolac, we reduce the risk of gastrointestinal bleeding or renal injury by limiting the days of use (30 mg intravenously every 8 hours, for a maximum of 3 days in a row). We do not use steroids and we give gastrointestinal protection concurrently.

We occasionally use intravenous valproic acid to treat CDH. In an open-label study, Edwards and Santarcangelo (Edwards et al., 1999) assessed the possible benefit of sodium valproate in 20 consecutive CDH patients who were refractory to multiple standard treatments. Eleven of the twenty patients (55%) had a response to mild or no headaches within 1–4 weeks. The dose ranged from 375–1500 mg a day. Two patients (10%) discontinued medication due to AEs (difficulty thinking and nausea). In a randomized, double-blind, prospective trial, Tanen et al. (2003) compared IV sodium valproate to IV prochlorperazine in the acute treatment of migraine headache in the emergency department. Patients received either 10 mg of prochlorperazine or 500 mg of valproate over 2 minutes. Prochlorperazine was statistically and clinically superior to sodium valproate for the treatment of the pain and nausea of acute migraine headache. Sodium valproate, in this study, failed to significantly reduce the pain or nausea of acute migraine headache. When we use sodium valproate, we give 250–500 mg IV push (one-time dose, occasionally may repeat; recently published protocol every 8 hours. One can give 500–1000 mg IV drip.

Propofol (2,6-diidopropylphenol) is an intravenous sedative-hypnotic agent used for induction and maintenance of anesthesia or sedation. It is the active ingredient in Diprivan, an injectable emulsion. Propofol's rapid induction of hypnosis—usually within 40 seconds of injection—occurs as a result of the rapid equilibration between the plasma and the highly perfused tissue of the brain. The half-time of the blood-brain equilibration is approximately 1–3 minutes. Krusz et al. (Krusz and Belanger, 1999) reported that intravenous propofol was effective in treating acute headache and other headaches that were refractory to the usual therapy. Mendes et al. (2002) conducted a pilot prospective study using repetitive low-dose boluses of intravenous propofol to treat patients with CDHs refractory to standard medications. A total of 21 trials were conducted on 18 patients. Over 90% of patients had at least some headache relief with no complications.

Hand and Stark (2000) retrospectively surveyed 19 consecutive inpatients, 18 with MOH and three with status migrainosus, who were treated with intravenous lignocaine infusion. The 19 patients (16 women) received 27 lignocaine infusions. An EKG was obtained before and 30–60 minutes after the infusion was started. Lignocaine was infused at a rate of 2 mg/minute by a pump device. The infusion was maintained until the patients were headache-free for a minimum of 12 hours or a maximum of 14 days. Preventive medication was permitted and was started during the hospital stay. Seven minor AEs were noted during four infusions. Eighteen patients had 22 infusions for MOH, with headache resolution in 82% of infusions (17 of the 18 patients responded at least once). The median duration was 5 days. Four patients obtained lasting relief; six returned to their regular manageable pattern of migraine (two of these patients had recurrent CDH after 6 months); four were lost to follow-up; and four had no long-term benefit. Five infusions were given to three patients with status migrainosus, with four of these infusions successfully relieving the headache. Intravenous lignocaine appears to be safe and may be useful in managing severe intractable CDH and status migrainosus. It is uncertain how much of the improvement was due to the intravenous lignocaine and how much was due to discontinuing the overused acute medication and initiating preventive medication.

Rosen et al. conducted a retrospective chart review of all patients admitted to Thomas Jefferson University Hospital who received intravenous lidocaine for CDH or chronic cluster headache. All patients had failed other aggressive inpatient treatments, such as IV DHE, antiemetics, neuroleptics, and steroidal and non-steroidal anti-inflammatory drugs (often in combination or sequentially). Patients had continuous telemetry, including continuous cardiac monitoring during treatment. Vital signs (every 8 hours) and basic blood studies (complete blood count, basic chemistry panel, magnesium and phosphate) and a daily 12-lead EKG were also obtained. After the initial laboratory work and initial EKG were determined to be within an acceptable range, a standard peripheral IV was placed and a lidocaine infusion was started, typically at a rate of 1 mg/minute for 4 hours, after which it was raised to 2 mg/minute. Some patients received doses as high as 4 mg/minute after non-toxic levels were obtained. They attempted to keep the level below the upper limit of the therapeutic range for arrhythmia (1–5 μg/ml). Lidocaine levels were obtained when indicated (e.g., before going above 3 and then 4 mg/minute) during treatment. Concurrent IV medications, including corticosteroids, NSAIDs, DHE, and anti-emetics, were given as needed. They found that 25.4% of patients exhibited a complete response, 57.1% exhibited a partial response, 3.2% worsened, and 14.3% exhibited no change during the lidocaine infusion. Although 50% of the patients experienced some AE (including hallucinations, tachycardia, tremors, hypotension, lightheadedness, phlebitis, line infection, and hypertension), none caused the treatment to be aborted. Most resolved after dose reduction (Rosen et al., 2007).

Swidan and colleagues (Swidan et al., 2005) showed that diphenhydramine delivered by intravenous infusion was as effective as DHE in a retroactive comparative study of intractable patients on an inpatient unit.

Strategies of Treatment

Outpatient

Two general outpatient strategies are in use. One approach is to taper the overused medication. The alternative strategy is to abruptly discontinue the overused drug, substitute a transitional medication to replace the overused drug, and subsequently taper the transitional drug. Serious withdrawal syndromes must be prevented. For example, if high doses of a butalbital-containing analgesic combination are abruptly discontinued, phenobarbital should be used to prevent barbiturate withdrawal syndrome. Similarly, benzodiazepines must be gradually tapered or replaced with long-acting ones. Ergotamine can be replaced with DHE, and short-acting NSAIDs with long-acting ones. Terminators are used to stop the headache cycle. Drugs used for this purpose include DHE, NSAIDs, Cox-2 inhibitors, corticosteroids, typical and atypical neuroleptics, and triptans (Diener et al., 1991; Bonuccelli et al., 1996; Drucker and Tepper, 1998). Outpatient treatment is preferred for motivated patients, but it is not always safe or effective.

Patients who do not need hospital-level care but cannot be safely or adequately treated as outpatients can be considered for ambulatory infusion treatment. Outpatient ambulatory infusion treatment is effective for migraine status and uncomplicated CDH with and without MOH. It must be done in a supervised medical setting where the patient can be monitored frequently (every 15 minutes). Under these circumstances, repetitive intravenous treatment can be given twice a day for several days in a row. Although ambulatory infusion treatment is better for many patients than outpatient treatment, major concerns still exist. Contraindications to outpatient ambulatory infusion treatment include the possibility of withdrawal symptoms occurring at night when patients are withdrawn from long-acting or potent drugs; psychiatric disorders that interfere with treatment (these patients cannot be treated aggressively as outpatients); and comorbid medical illnesses that require prolonged monitoring. No long-term observation is available, and many problems manifest themselves in an intensely monitored interactive environment.

Inpatient

The goals of inpatient headache treatment include: (1) acute medication withdrawal and rehydration; (2) pain control with parenteral therapy; (3) establishment of effective preventive treatment; (4) termination of the pain cycle; (5) patient education; and (6) establishment of outpatient methods of pain control (Saper, Lake, et al., 1999). Hospitalization is also used as a time for patient education, for introducing behavioral methods of pain control, and for adjusting an outpatient program of preventive and acute therapy.

Our (Silberstein et al., 1990) experience with more than 300 patients has shown that repetitive IV DHE is a safe and effective means of rapidly controlling intractable headache. Of 214 patients suffering from daily headache with rebound, 92% became headache-free with an average length of stay of 7.3 days. Pringsheim and Howse (1998) reported similar but less robust results (see later). Patients whose significant medical or behavioral comorbidities and/or opioid dependence are a cause of their MOH often require longer lengths of stay (Lake et al., 2006).

Hospitalization is an essential step in achieving effective control and diagnosis for a large number of otherwise intractable headache patients. The benefits of hospitalization extend beyond IV protocols and other pharmacologic manipulations and withdrawal therapies. Observing patients' behavior in their daily interactions with staff, peers, and family, as well as being able to influence their sleeping and eating patterns, have proven enormously helpful in establishing short- and long-term treatment plans (Saper, Silberstein, et al., 1999; Lake et al., 2006). Moreover, observing drug-seeking behavior, tolerance or intolerance for varying levels of pain, and the accuracy of pain reporting are additional observational assets of an inpatient treatment environment, and can serve as the foundation for subsequent outpatient care.

Various behavioral disturbances are more commonly seen in a hospital as opposed to an outpatient setting. Lake and Saper (Lake et al., 2006) recently reported the results of 276 consecutively discharged patients. Although approximately 70% were discharged feeling moderately to significantly better than upon admission, the observation was made that patients with personality disorders were much more likely to have MOH than those without, and that certain personality disorders, such as borderline personality and narcissistic personality disorders, seemed to have a predilection for opioid misuse (Saper and Lake III, 2002; Saper et al., 2005; Lake et al., 2006). The authors raise the possibility that personality disorders may serve as a predisposing factor to both MOH and certain drug-specific pursuits (Saper and Lake, 2006). The authors also speculated that the behavior of an individual, as imposed upon the treating physician, might prompt that physician to provide opioids defensively, even against his or her best judgment (Saper and Lake III, 2006).

PROGNOSIS

The "natural history" of primary CDH, and rebound headache in particular, has never been, and probably never will be, studied for ethical and technical reasons. Recognition of the rebound process is probably therapeutic in and of itself and could affect the patient's behavior or the physician's approach. Retrospective analysis suggests that there may be periods of stable drug consumption and periods of accelerated medication use. Patients treated aggressively generally improve. There are no literature reports of spontaneous improvement of rebound headache, although this may happen. We (Silberstein and Silberstein, 1992) performed follow-up evaluations on 50 hospitalized primary CDH drug overuse patients who were treated with repetitive IV DHE and became headache-free. Once detoxified, treated, and discharged, most patients did not resume daily analgesic or ergotamine use. Seventy-two percent continued to show significant improvement at 3 months, and 87% continued to show significant improvement after 2 years. This would suggest at least 70% improvement at 2 years in the initial group (35/50), allowing for patients lost to follow-up.

Our (Silberstein and Silberstein, 1992) 2-year success rate of 87% is consistent with the long-term success rates reported in the literature (Table 13–14). In a series of 23 papers (Andersson, 1975; Tfelt-Hansen and Krabbe, 1981; Isler, 1982; Dichgans et al., 1984; Henry et al., 1984; Rapoport et al., 1986; Andersson, 1988; Diener et al., 1988; Baumgartner et al., 1989; Diener et al., 1989; Schoenen et al., 1989; Lake et al., 1990; Mathew, 1990; Mathew et al., 1990; Hering and Steiner, 1991; Diener et al., 1992; Silberstein and Silberstein, 1992; Pini et al., 1996; Schnider et al., 1996; Granella et al., 1998; Monzon and Lainez, 1998; Pringsheim and Howse, 1998; Suhr et al., 1999) published between 1975 and 1999, the success rate of withdrawal therapy (often accompanied by pharmacologic and/or behavioral intervention) in patients overusing analgesics, ergotamine, or both was between 48% and 91%, with the rate being reported as 77% or higher in 10 papers (Table 13–14).

Henry et al. (1984) hospitalized, detoxified, and followed 22 primary CDH drug overuse patients for 4–24 months. Nine of fifteen patients showed marked improvement, one showed slight improvement, and five did not improve. Rapoport et al. (1986) studied 90 patients with primary CDH who discontinued analgesics. After 1 month, 30% were significantly improved; 67% were significantly improved within 2 months, 80% after 3 months, and 82% after 4 months. The authors suggested that an "analgesic washout period" exists and may be as long as 3 months for some patients.

Diener et al. (1988) hospitalized 85 patients who were overusing analgesics or various migraine drugs (including ergotamine). The length of admission was 14 days. They detoxified these patients and followed them for 10–75 months (mean 35 months) after discharge. Sixty-nine percent had at least 50% improvement; 29.4% were unchanged, and one had deteriorated. Fifty-four patients with drug-induced headache were hospitalized by Baumgartner et al. (1989) for 2 weeks. They were detoxified and started on a prophylactic drug. At an average of 16.8 months (13.6 months) after treatment and discharge, 38 patients were evaluated: 76.3% had reduced their analgesic intake and 60.5% had experienced a significant relief in headache intensity and frequency.

Lake et al. (1990) reported on 100 patients who had been hospitalized with severe refractory primary CDH frequently complicated by symptomatic medication overuse. At follow-up between 3 months and 1 year after discharge, the mean number of severe headaches was reduced by 64% and the mean number of dysfunctional days was reduced by 70%. Overall, 87% of patients reported at least 50% headache reduction.

TABLE 13–14 MOH: Long-Term Followup.

Year	Author	Drug E/A/T	No. of patients	Follow-up (months)	Positive results (%)	Relapse rate %
1975	Andersson	E	44	6	91	9
1981	Tfelt-Hansen and Krabbe	E	40	12	47.6	29
1982	Ala-Hurula	E	23	3–6	78	19
1982	Isler	A	104	1–30	77.9	58.6
1984	Dichgans	E/A	52	16	77	9
1985	Henry et al.	E/A	22	3	78	33
1986	Rapoport et al.	A	90	4	82	?
1998	Granella et al.	A	95	6	?	22
1988	Diener et al.	E/A	85	35	69	?
1988	Andersson	E	32	6	50	?
1989	Baumgartner et al.	E/A	38	16	60.5	24
1989	Diener et al.	A	139	34		
1989	Schoenen et al.	A	121	6	50	20
1990	Lake and Saper	E/A	100	3–12	87	
1990	Mathew et al.	E/A	200	3	86	?
1991	Hering and Steiner	E/A	46	6	80.4	4
1992	Silberstein and Silberstein	E/A	50	24	87	13
1996	Pini et al.	E/A/T	104	4	72	28
1996	Schnider et al.	E/A	38	60	50	39.5
1998	Pringsheim and Howse	E/A/T	132	3	56	
1999	Monzon et al.	E/A	104	12	66	?
1999	Suhr et al.	E/A/T	101	72±48		20.8
1999	Lorenzatto et al.	E/A/T	140	12	84.6%	
2005	Katsarava et al.	E/AT	96	48	96/98*	41%/45%*8

* 98 detoxified/96 had improved in 1 month ** 1 year and 4 years.

Abbreviations: A, Analgesics; E, Ergotamine tartrate; T, Triptans.

Hering and Steiner (1991) followed 46 migraineurs who developed primary CDH as a result of analgesic overuse. Six months after analgesic and ergotamine withdrawal, 37 (80.4%) were no longer overusing the agents and no longer had primary CDH.

Mathew et al. (1990; Mathew, 1990) studied 200 patients who were overusing daily symptomatic medication, 58% of whom were taking prophylactic medication without achieving a benefit. At the 3-month follow-up, if the analgesics had been discontinued and prophylactic medication started or modified, a reduction of approximately 86% in the weekly headache index was achieved, with a dropout rate of 10.3%. If symptomatic medication had been continued, only 21% improvement was achieved. It is interesting to note that merely discontinuing symptomatic medication resulted in 58% improvement.

Schnider et al. (1996) followed 38 primary CDH inpatients who had overused ergotamine and/or analgesics and were detoxified. After 5 years, 19 patients had headache eight or less days a month and 18 had no or only mild headaches. Outcome was related to headache frequency and duration of drug use. Fifteen patients (39.5%) had relapsed and were again overusing acute drugs.

Pini et al. (1996) evaluated 102 primary CDH patients who were overusing ergotamine, analgesics (including butalbital combinations), and/or sumatriptan. Patients were treated as either outpatients or inpatients based on the therapeutic schedule to be followed. Both groups showed equal improvement at 1 and 4 months in the headache index, but the outpatients had a higher relapse rate (38%) than the inpatients (25%). This suggests that the more complicated and refractory patients were admitted to the hospital.

Granella et al. (1998) looked for factors that were associated with the evolution of migraine without aura into CM. Risk factors included head trauma (OR 3.3), analgesic use with every attack (OR 2.8), and long duration of oral contraceptive use.

Pringsheim and Howse (1998) detoxified 174 inpatients who were overusing ergotamine, analgesics, and triptans and treated them with repetitive IV DHE; 132 patients were followed after 3 months by telephone. Sixty-one percent had an immediate good result. Of these, 56% continued to do well at 3 months and 5% relapsed.

Suhr et al. (1999) conducted a prospective study of 257 primary CDH patients allocated to inpatient (147) or outpatient (110) treatment, depending on the personal situation of the patient. Only 5% of the patients were headache-free at follow-up, which was up to 5 years after treatment. The total relapse to drug overuse was 20.8%, occurring in 14.0% of the outpatients and 25.0% of the inpatients. No baseline analysis of headache days a month or mean pain intensity was given, but there was no significant difference in these outcomes between groups.

Monzon et al. (1999) prospectively studied the long-term (6 and 12 months) outcome of 164 consecutive primary CDH patients and analyzed various etiologic causal factors. One hundred and eighteen patients (72%) had CM, 33 patients (20%) had CTTH, and 13 patients (8%) had NDPH. One hundred and forty-nine patients were treated with outpatient therapy, and 15 refractory patients were admitted to a comprehensive inpatient treatment. At 6 months, 54 patients had an excellent result, 64 had a good result, and 41 had a fair result; five patients continued to have CM. At 12 months, 104 patients were analyzed: 23 had an excellent result, 46 had a good result, and 28 had a fair result; seven patients continued to have CM. There were no statistically significant differences in evolution when transformation factors were analyzed. Although differences were not statistically significant, treatment was less efficacious when inpatient therapy was necessary and when patients had a history of analgesic abuse or traumatic life events. This, again, suggests that the more severe and intractable cases were admitted to the hospital.

Lorenzatto et al. (1999), using the criteria proposed by Silberstein et al. (1996), retrospectively studied 140 patients (101 women and 39 men aged 17 to 83) who had CDH, that is, they overused acute drugs. The patients were taken off acute medications and were treated with preventive medications and education. After 1 month, 23.6% of patients had more than 50% improvement in headache intensity and frequency and 56.4% had a similar improvement. Fifty percent improvement after 3 months was observed after 6 months in 70.2% of patients, after 9 months in 82.6%, and after 12 months in 84.6%.

Katsarava et al. did a prospective 4-year follow-up study of 98 MOH patients after withdrawal.

Two of ninety-eight patients did not improve 4 months after withdrawal and were excluded from the study. Of the remaining 96 patients, 78 women and 18 men, with mean age 43 years (range 23–65 years), 69 (71%) suffered from migraine, 13 (14%) from TTH, and 14 (15%) from a combination of migraine and TTH. Mean duration of primary headache was 22 years. Forty-six paitents (48%) overused analgesics, 12 (13%) overused ergots, and 38 (39%) overused triptans. Twenty-six patients (31%) relapsed within the first 6 months after withdrawal. The number of relapses increased to 32 (41%) 1 year and to 34 (45%) 4 years after withdrawal. The 4-year relapse rate was lower in patients with migraine than in those with TTH (32% versus 91%) and those with a combination of migraine and TTH (32% versus 70%), and also lower in patients overusing triptans than those overusing analgesics (21% versus 71%). Most relapses occurred within the first year after withdrawal; the long-term success of withdrawal depends on the type of primary headache and the type of overused medication. (Katsarava et al., 2005).

Why Treatment Fails

When patients fail to respond to therapy or announce that they have already tried everything and nothing will work, it is important to try to identify the reason or reasons why that treatment has failed (Table 13–15). The cause of treatment failure may be an incomplete or incorrect diagnosis (Lipton et al., 2003). For example: (1) an undiagnosed secondary headache disorder is the major source of the head pain; (2) a misdiagnosed primary headache disorder is present (e.g., HC is mistaken for CM, episodic paroxysmal hemicrania or hypnic headache is mistaken for cluster); or (3) two or more different headache disorders are present. In addition, pharmacotherapy may have been inadequate or important exacerbating factors such as medication overuse may have been missed.

PREVENTION

Headache sufferers often do not realize that excessive or frequent self-treatment may perpetuate or exacerbate their headaches. Since most headache sufferers do not seek medical advice until and unless the pain becomes frequent or intense, the opportunity for diagnosis and physician intervention to halt the cycle is often missed. Physicians need to screen CDH patients for analgesic overuse. Headache patients must be informed about the risks of analgesic overuse and rebound headache. Yet, even when patients are aware of the risks, they may still overmedicate. This requires continued vigilance on the part of the treating physician.

Because patients who overuse medication may feel ashamed and out of control, an accurate history may be difficult to obtain. To facilitate this process, the condition of medication rebound should be explained as part of the natural history of migraine. Even if the patient is not rebounding at the time, all symptomatic headache medications, with the possible exception of the long-acting NSAIDs, should be limited to prevent rebound headache.

TABLE 13–15 Why Treatment Fails.

The diagnosis is incomplete or incorrect

- An undiagnosed secondary headache disorder is present
- A primary headache disorder is misdiagnosed
- Two or more different headache disorders are present

Important exacerbating factors may have been missed

- Medication overuse (including over-the-counter)
- Caffeine overuse
- Dietary or lifestyle triggers
- Hormonal triggers
- Psychosocial factors
- Other medications that trigger headaches

Pharmacotherapy has been inadequate

- Ineffective drug
- Excessive initial doses
- Inadequate final doses
- Inadequate duration of treatment

Other factors

- Unrealistic expectations
- Comorbid conditions complicate therapy
- Inpatient treatment required

Source: Modified from Lipton et al., 2003.

Patients with drug-induced CDH, while difficult to treat, often return to a state of intermittent episodic headache after detoxification and treatment with a preventive medication.

References

Ala-Hurula, V, Myllyla, V, Hokkanen, E (1982). Ergotamine abuse: results of ergotamine discontinuation, with special reference to the plasma concentrations, *Cephalalgia*, 2(4):189–95.

Andersson, PG (1975). Ergotamine headache. *Headache*, 15:118–121.

Andersson, PG (1988). Ergotism: the clinical picture. In *Drug Induced Headache* (HC Diener and MS Wilkinson, eds.), pp. 16–19. Springer, Berlin.

Anthony, M and Rasmussen, BK (1993). Migraine without aura. In *The Headaches* (J Olesen, P Tfelt-Hansen, MA Welch, eds.), pp. 255–261. Raven Press, New York.

Antonaci, F (1991). The sweating pattern in hemicrania continua. A comparison with chronic paroxysmal hemicrania. *Funct Neurol*, 6:371–375.

Antonaci, F (1994). Chronic paroxysmal hemicrania and hemicrania continua: orbital phlebography and MRI studies. *Headache*, 34:32–34.

Antonaci, F, Sand, T, and Sjaastad, O (1992). Hemicrania continua and chronic paroxysmal hemicrania: a comparison of pupillometric findings. *Funct Neurol*, 7:385–389.

Antonaci, F, Sandrini, G, Danilov, A, et al. (1994). Neurophysiological studies in chronic paroxysmal hemicrania and hemicrania continua. *Headache*, 34:479–483.

Antonaci, F and Sjaastad, O (1992). Hemicrania continua: a possible symptomatic case, due to mesenchymal tumor. *Funct Neurol*, 7:471–474.

Arcaya, JL, Cano, G, Gomez, G, et al. (1999). Dynorphin A increases substance P release from trigeminal primary afferent C-fibers. *Eur J Pharmacol*, 366:27–34.

Ashina, M (2004). Neurobiology of chronic tension-type headache. *Cephalalgia*, 24:161–172.

Ashina, M, Bendtsen, L, Jensen, R, et al. (1999a). Possible mechanisms of action of nitric oxide synthase inhibitors in chronic tension-type headache. *Brain*, 122:1629–1635.

Ashina, M, Bendtsen, L, Jensen, R, et al. (1999b). Muscle hardness in patients with chronic tension-type headache: relation to actual headache state. *Pain*, 79:201–205.

Ashina, M, Bendtsen, L, Jensen, R, et al. (2000). Plasma levels of calcitonin gene-related peptide in chronic tension-type headache. *Neurology*, 55:1335–1340.

Ashkenazi, A, Abbas, MA, Sharma, DK, et al. (2007). Hemicrania continua-like headache associated with internal carotid artery dissection may respond to indomethacin. *Headache*, 47:127–130.

Aurora, SK (2003). Imaging chronic daily headache. *Curr Pain Headache Rep*, 7:209–211.

Bahra, A, Walsh, M, Menon, S, et al. (2000). Does chronic daily headache arise de novo in association with regular analgesic use? *Cephalalgia*, 20:294 (Abstract).

Bahra, A, Walsh, M, Menon S, et al. (2003). Does chronic daily headache arise de novo in association with regular use of analgesics? *Headache*, 43:179–190.

Battaglia, G and Rustioni, A (1988). Coexistence of glutamate and substance P in dorsal root ganglion neurons of the rat and monkey. *J Comp Neurol*, 277:302–312.

Baumgartner, C, Wessly, P, Bingol, C, et al. (1989). Long-term prognosis of analgesic withdrawal in patients with drug-induced headaches. *Headache*, 29:510–514.

Bederson, JB, Fields, HL, and Barbaro, NM (1990). Hyperalgesia during naloxone-precipitated withdrawal from morphine is associated with increased on-cell activity in the rostral ventromedial medulla. *Somatosens Mot Res*, 7:185–203.

Bell, R, Montoya, D, Shuaib, A, et al. (1990). A comparative trial of three agents in the treatment of acute migraine headache. *Ann Emerg Med*, 19:1079–1082.

Bendtsen, L, Jensen, R, Brennum, J, et al. (1996). Exteroceptive suppression of temporal muscle activity is normal in patients with chronic tension-type headache and not related to actual headache state. *Cephalalgia*, 16:251–256.

Bendtsen, L, Jensen, R, and Olesen, J (1996). Qualitatively altered nociception in chronic myofascial pain. *Pain*, 65:259–264.

Bigal, M, Lipton, RB, deGryse, R, et al. (2003). Similarity of chronic migraine patients with and without a history of migraine. *Cephalalgia*, 23:747 (Abstract).

Bigal, ME, Sheftell, FD, Rapoport, AM, et al. (2002). Chronic daily headache in a tertiary care population: correlation between the International Headache Society diagnostic criteria and proposed revisions of criteria for chronic daily headache. *Cephalalgia*, 22:432–438.

Boghen, D, and Desaulniers, N (1983). Background vascular headache: relief with indomethacin. *Can J Neurol Sci*, 10:270–271.

Bonuccelli, U, Nuti, A, Lucetti, C, et al. (1996). Amitriptyline and dexamethasone combined treatment in drug-induced headache. *Cephalalgia*, 16:197–200.

Bordini, C, Antonaci, F, Stovner, LJ, et al. (1991). "Hemicrania Continua" -a clinical review. *Headache*, 31:20–26.

Bousser, MG and Russell, RR (1997). Cerebral venous thrombosis. In *Major Problems in Neurology* (MG Bousser and RR Russell, eds.), pp. 175. Saunders, London.

Bovim, G, Jenssen, G, and Ericson, K (1992). Orbital phlebography: a comparison between cluster headache and other headaches. *Headache*, 32:408–412.

Bowdler, I, Killian, J, and Gänsslen-Blumberg, S (1990). The association between analgesic abuse and headache—coincidental or causal. *Headache*, 30:494.

Brain, WR (1963). Some unsolved problems of cervical spondylosis. *Br Med J*, 1:771–777.

Brandes, JL, Jacobs, DJ, Neto, W, et al. (2003). Topiramate in the prevention of migraine headache: a randomized, double-blind, placebo-controlled, parallel study (MIGR-002). *Neurology*, 60:A238 (Abstract).

Breslau, N and Davis, GC (1993). Migraine, physical health and psychiatric disorders: a prospective epidemiologic study of young adults. *J Psychiatric Res*, 27:211–221.

Bright, RA and Everitt, DE (1992). β-blockers and depression: evidence against association. *JAMA*, 267:1783–1787.

Brilla, R, Evers, S, Soros, P, et al. (1998). Hemicrania continua in an HIV-infected outpatient. *Cephalalgia*, 18:287–288.

Burstein, R, Cutrer, MF, and Yarnitsky, D (2001). The development of cutaneous allodynia during a migraine attack: clinical evidence for the sequential recruitment of spinal and supraspinal nociceptive neurons in migraine. *Brain*, 123:1703–1709.

Burstein, R, Yamamura, H, Malick, A, et al. (1998). Chemical stimulation of the intracranial dura induces enhanced responses to facial stimulation in brainstem trigeminal neurons. *J Neurophysiol*, 79:964–982.

Burstein, R, Yarnitsky, D, Goor-Aryeh, I, et al. (2000). An association between migraine and cutaneous allodynia. *Ann Neurol*, 47:614–624.

Bussone, G, Sandrini, G, Patruno, G, et al. (1991). Effectiveness of fluoxetine on pain and depression in chronic headache disorders. In *Headache and Depression: Serotonin Pathways as a Common Clue* (G Nappi, G Bono, G Sandrini, et al., eds), pp. 265–272. Raven Press, New York.

Callaham, M and Raskin, N (1986). A controlled study of dihydroergotamine in the treatment of acute migraine headache. *Headache*, 26:168–171.

Campbell, WB (1990). Lipid-derived autocoids: eicosanoids and platelet-activating factor. In *The Pharmacological Basis of Therapeutics* (AG Gilman, TW Rall, and P Taylor, eds), pp. 600–617. Pergamon Press, New York.

Castillo, J, Munoz, P, Guitera, V, et al. (1999). Epidemiology of chronic daily headache in the general population. *Headache*, 39:190–196.

Catarci, T, Fiacco, F, and Argentino, C (1994). Ergotamine-induced headache can be sustained by sumatriptan daily intake. *Cephalalgia*, 14:374–375.

Celentano, DD, Stewart, WF, and Lipton, RB (1992). Medication use and disability among migraineurs: a national probability sample. *Headache*, 32:223–228.

Cerbo, R, Barbanti, P, Fabbrini, G, et al. (1998). Amitriptyline is effective in chronic but not in episodic tension-type headache: pathogenic implications. *Headache*, 38:453–457.

Chalder, T, Berelowitz, G, Pawlikowska, T, et al. (1993). Development of a fatigue scale. *J Psychosom Res*, 37:147–153.

Cook, AJ, Woolf, CJ, Wall, PD, et al. (1987). Dynamic receptive field plasticity in rat spinal cord dorsal horn following C primary afferent input. *Nature*, 325:151–153.

Couch, JR, Ziegler, DK, and Hassainein, R (1976). Amitriptyline in the prophylaxis of migraine. *Arch Neurol*, 26:121–127.

Creach, C, Radat, F, Laffitau, M, et al. (2003). Cutaneous allodynia in transformed migraine with medication overuse. *Cephalalgia*, 23:656–657 (Abstract).

Curioso, EP, Young, WB, Shechter, AL, et al. (1999). Psychiatric comorbidity predicts outcome in chronic daily headache patients. *Neurology*, 52:A471 (Abstract).

D'Alessio, C, Ambrosini, A, Colonnese, C, et al. (2004). Indomethacin-responsive hemicrania associated with an extracranial vascular malformation: report of two cases. *Cephalalgia*, 24:997–1000.

Descombes, S, Brefel-Courbon, C, Thalamas, C, et al. (2001). Amitriptyline treatment in chronic drug-induced headache: a double- blind comparative pilot study. *Headache*, 41:178–182.

Diamond, S and Baltes, B (1971). Chronic tension headache treated with amitriptyline: a double blind study. *Headache*, 11:110–116.

Diamond, S and Dalessio, DJ (1982). Drug abuse in headache. In *The Practicing Physician's Approach to Headache* (S Diamond and DJ Dalessio, eds), pp. 114–121. Williams & Wilkins, Baltimore.

Diaz-Mitoma, F, Vanast, WJ, and Tyrrell, DL (1987). Increased frequency of Epstein-Barr virus excretion in patients with new daily persistent headaches. *Lancet*, 1:411–415.

Dichgans, J, Diener, HD, Gerber, WD, et al. (1984). Analgetika-induzierter dauerkopfschmerz. *Dtsch Med Wschr*, 109:369.

Diener, HC and Dahlof, CG (1999). Headache associated with chronic use of substances. In *The Headaches* (J Olesen, P Tfelt-Hansen, and KMA Welch, eds), pp. 871–878. Lippincott, Williams & Wilkins, Philadelphia.

Diener, HC, Dichgans, J, Scholz, E, et al. (1984). Analgesic-induced chronic headache: long-term results of withdrawal therapy. *J Neurol*, 236:9–14.

Diener, HC, Dichgans, J, Scholz, E, et al. (1989). Analgesic-induced chronic headache: long-term results of withdrawal therapy. *J Neurol*, 236:9–14.

Diener, HC, Gerber, WD, and Geiselhart, S (1988). Short and long-term effects of withdrawal therapy in drug-induced headache. In *Drug-induced Headache* (HC Diener and M Wilkinson, eds), pp. 133–142. Springer-Verlag, Berlin.

Diener, HC, Haab, J, Peters, C, et al. (1991). Subcutaneous sumatriptan in the treatment of headache during withdrawal from drug-induced headache. *Headache*, 31:205–209.

Diener, HC, Pfaffenrath, V, Soyka, D, et al. (1992). Therapie des medikamenten-induzierten dauerkopfschmerzes. *Münch Med Wschr*, 134:159–162.

Diener, HC and Silberstein, SD (2006). Medication overuse headache. In *The Headaches* (J Olesen, PJ Goadsby, NM Ramadan, et al., eds), pp. 971–979. Lippincott Williams & Wilkins, Philadelphia.

Diener, HC and Tfelt-Hansen, P (1993). Headache associated with chronic use of substances. In *The Headaches* (J Olesen, P Tfelt-Hansen, and KMA Welch, eds.), pp. 721–727. Raven Press , New York.

Dodick, DW, Mauskop, A, Elkind, AH, et al. (2005). Botulinum toxin type A for the prophylaxis of chronic daily headache: subgroup analysis of patients not receiving other prophylactic medications: a randomized double-blind, placebo-controlled study. *Headache*, 45:315–324.

Dourish, CT, O'Neill, MF, Coughlan, J, et al. (1990). The selective CCK-B receptor antagonist L-365,260 enhances morphine analgesia and prevents morphine tolerance in the rat. *Eur J Pharmacol*, 176:35–44.

Draisci, G, Kajander, KC, Dubner, R, et al. (1991). Up-regulation of opioid gene expression in spinal cord evoked by experimental nerve injuries and inflammation. *Brain Res* 560:186–192.

Dray, A, Urban, L, and Dickenson, A (1994). Pharmacology of chronic pain. *Trends Pharmacol Sci*, 15:190–197.

Drucker, P and Tepper, S (1998). Daily sumatriptan for detoxification from rebound. *Headache*, 38:687–690.

Edelman, GM and Gally, JA (1992). Nitric oxide: linking space and time in the brain. *Proc Natl Acad Sci USA*, 89:11651–11652.

Edwards, K, Santarcangelo, V, Shea, P, et al. (1999). Intravenous valproate for acute treatment of migraine headaches. *Cephalalgia*, 19:356 (Abstract).

Eggen, AE (1993). The Tromsø study: frequency and predicting factors of analgesic drug use in a free-living population (12–56 years). *J Clin Epidemiol*, 46:1297–1304.

Ekbom, K (1974). Clinical aspects of cluster headache. *Headache*, 13:176–180.

Eross, EJ and Dodick, DW (2002). The effects of botulinum toxin type A on disability in episodic and chronic migraine. *Neurology*, 58(7):A497 (Abstract).

Eross, EJ, Swanson, JW, and Dodick, DW (2002). Hemicrania continua: an indomethacin-responsive case with an underlying malignant etiology. *Headache*, 42:527–529.

Espada, F, Morales-Asín, F, Escalza, I, et al. (1999). Hemicrania continua: nine new cases. *Cephalalgia*, 19:442 (Abstract).

Evers, S, Bahra, A, and Goadsby, PJ (1999). Coincidence of familial hemiplegic migraine and hemicrania continua? A case report. *Cephalalgia*, 19:533–535.

Fields, HL, Heinricher, MM, and Mason, P (1991). Neurotransmitters as nociceptive modulatory circuits. *Annu Rev Neurosci*, 14:219–245.

Fisher, CM (1988). Analgesic rebound headache refuted. *Headache*, 28:666

Fontes-Ribeiro, CA (1999). L-5-hydroxytryptophan in the prophylaxis of chronic tension-type headache: a double-blind randomized placebo-controlled study. *Cephalalgia*, 19:453 (Abstract).

Foster, CA and Bafaloukos, J (1994). Paroxetine in the treatment of chronic daily headache. *Headache*, 34:587–589.

Freitag, FG, Diamond, S, Diamond, M, et al. (2001). Divalproex in the long-term treatment of chronic daily headache. *Headache*, 41:271–278.

Fusco, BM, Colantoni, O, and Giavovazzo, M (1997). Alteration of central excitation circuits in chronic headache and analgesic misuse. *Headache*, 37:486–491.

Fusco, BM, Colantoni, O, Saturnino, C, et al. (1999). Altered "second pain" in chronic headaches: pharmacological modulation. *Cephalalgia*, 19:399–400 (Abstract).

Gaist, D, Hallas, J, Sindrup, SH, et al. (1996). Is overuse of sumatriptan a problem? A population-based study. *Eur J Clin Pharmacol*, 50:161–165.

Gallai, V, Alberti, A, Gallai, B, et al. (2003). Glutamate and nitric oxide pathway in chronic daily headache: evidence from cerebrospinal fluid. *Cephalalgia*, 23:166–174.

Gardell, LR, Wang, R, Burgess, SE, et al. (2002). Sustained morphine exposure induces a spinal dynorphin-dependent enhancement of excitatory transmitter release from primary afferent fibers. *J Neurosci*, 22:6747–6755.

Gladstone, J, Eross, E, and Dodick, D (2003). Chronic daily headache: a rational approach to a challenging problem. *Semin Neurol*, 23:265–276.

Goadsby, PJ and Lipton, RB (1997). A review of paroxysmal hemicranias, SUNCT syndrome and other short-lasting headaches with autonomic features, including new cases. *Brain*, 120:193–209.

Goadsby, PJ, Lipton, RB, and Ferrari, MD (2002). Migraine-current understanding and treatment. *N Engl J Med*, 346:257–270.

Gobel, H, Hamouz, V, Hansen, C, et al. (1994). Chronic tension-type headache: amitriptyline reduces clinical headache-duration and experimental pain sensitivity but does not alter pericranial muscle activity readings. *Pain*, 59:241–249.

Gobel, H, Lindner, V, Krack, P, et al. (1999). Treatment of chronic tension-type headache with botulinum toxin. *Cephalalgia*, 19:455 (Abstract).

Granella, F, Cavallini, A, Sandrini, G, et al. (1998). Long-term outcome of migraine. *Cephalalgia*, 18:30–33.

Guidetti, V and Galli, F (1999). Chronic daily headache in children and adolescents: clinical features and psychiatric comorbidity. *Cephalalgia*, 19:389 (Abstract).

Guitera, V, Munoz, P, Castillo, J, et al. (1999a). Impact of chronic daily headache in the quality of life: a study in the general population. *Cephalalgia*, 19:412–413 (Abstract).

Guitera, V, Munoz, P, Castillo, J, et al. (1999b). Transformed migraine: a proposal for the modification of its diagnostic criteria based on recent epidemiological data. *Cephalalgia*, 19:847–850.

Gutzwiller, F and Zemp, E (1986). Der analgetikakonsum in der bevölkerung und sozioökonomische aspekte des analgetikaabusus. In *Das analgetikasyndrom* (MJ Mihatsch, ed.), pp. 197–205. Thieme, Stuttgart.

Hand, PJ and Stark, RJ (2000). Intravenous lignocaine infusions for severe chronic daily headache. *Med J Aust*, 172:157–159.

Hannerz, J (2000). Chronic bilateral headache responding to indomethacin. *Headache*, 40:840–843.

Harden, RN (2002). Chronic opioid therapy: another reappraisal. *APS Bulletin*, 12:1–12.

Headache Classification Committee (2004). The International Classification of Headache Disorders, 2nd Edition. *Cephalalgia*, 24:1–160.

Headache Classification Committee of the International Headache Society (1988). Classification and diagnostic criteria for headache disorders, cranial neuralgia, and facial pain. *Cephalalgia*, 8:1–96.

Heinricher, MM, McGaraughty, S, and Tortorici, V (2001). Circuitry underlying antiopioid actions of cholecystokinin within the rostral ventromedial medulla. *J Neurophysiol*, 85:280–286.

Heinricher, MM and Roychowdhury, SM (1997). Reflex-related activation of putative pain facilitating neurons in rostral ventromedial medulla requires excitatory amino acid transmission. *Neuroscience*, 78:1159–1165.

Henry, et al. (1984). In Migraine: Proceedings from the Fifth International Migraines, C. Rose (ed.), Symposium. London 1984, p. 197.

Henry, P, Dartigues, JF, Benetier, MP, et al. (1985). Ergotamine- and analgesic-induced headache. *Headache*, 25:273–275.

Hering, R and Kuritzky, A (1992). Sodium valproate in the prophylactic treatment of migraine: a double-blind study versus placebo. *Cephalalgia*, 12:81–84.

Hering, R and Steiner, TJ (1991). Abrupt outpatient withdrawal from medication in analgesic-abusing migraineurs. *Lancet*, 337:1442–1443.

Holland, J, Holland, C, and Kudrow, L (1983). Low dose amitriptyline prophylaxis in chronic scalp muscle contraction headache. Proceedings of the first international headache congress. Munich, September.

Holroyd, KA, Nash, JM, and Pingel, JD (1991). A comparison of pharmacologic (amitriptyline HCl) and nonpharmacologic (cognitive-behavioral) therapies for chronic tension headaches. *J Consult Clin Psychol*, 59:387–393.

Iordanidis, T and Sjaastad, O (1989). Hemicrania continua: a case report. *Cephalalgia*, 9:301–303.

Ishizaki, K, Takeshima, T, Ijiri, T, et al. (2002). [Hemicrania continua: the first Japanese case report]. *Rinsho Shinkeigaku*, 42:754–756.

Isler, H (1982). Migraine treatment as a cause of chronic migraine. In *Advances in Migraine Research and Therapy* (FC Rose, ed.), pp. 159–164. Raven Press, New York.

Isler, H (1988). Headache drugs provoking chronic headache: historical aspects and common misunderstandings. In *Drug-induced Headache* (HC Diener and M Wilkinson, eds), pp. 87–94. Springer-Verlag, Berlin.

Jensen, R, Brinck, T, and Olesen, J (1994). Sodium valproate has a prophylactic effect in migraine without aura. *Neurology*, 44:647–651.

Jensen, R and Olesen, J (1996). Initiating mechanisms of experimentally induced tension-type headache. *Cephalalgia*, 16:175–182.

Ji, RR, Samad, TA, Jin, SX, et al. (2002). p38 MAPK activation by NGF in primary sensory neurons after inflammation increases TRPV1 levels and maintains heat hyperalgesia. *Neuron*, 36:57–68.

Johnson, ES and Tfelt-Hansen, P (1993). Nonsteroidal antiinflammatory drugs. In *The Headaches* (J Olesen, P Tfelt-Hansen, and KMA Welch, eds.), pp. 391–395. Raven Press, New York.

Jones, J, Sklar, D, Dougherty, J, et al. (1989). Randomized double-blind trial of intravenous prochlorperazine for the treatment of acute headache. *JAMA*, 261:1174–1176.

Joubert, J (1991). Hemicrania continua in black patient—the importance of the non-continuous stage. *Headache*, 31:480–482.

Juang, KD, Wang, SJ, Fuh, JL, et al. (2000). Comorbidity of depressive and anxiety disorders in chronic daily headache and its subtypes. *Headache*, 40:818–823.

Julius, D and Basbaum, AI (2001). Molecular mechanisms of nociception. *Nature*, 413:203–210.

Kaiser, RS (1999). Substance abuse and headache. *41st Annual Scientific Meeting*. Boston, MA.

Kangasniemi, PJ, Nyrke, T, Lang, AH, et al. (1983). Femoxetine—a new 5HT uptake inhibitor—and propranolol in the prophylactic treatment of migraine. *Acta Neurol Scand*, 68:262–267.

Kaplan, H and Fields, HL (1991). Hyperalgesia during acute opioid abstinence: evidence for a nociceptive facilitating function of the rostral ventromedial medulla. *J Neurosci*, 11:1433–1439.

Katsarava, Z, Limmroth, V, Fritsche, G, et al. (1999). Drug-induced headache following the use of zolmitriptan or naratriptan. *Cephalalgia*, 19:414 (Abstract).

Katsarava, Z, Muessig, M, Dzagnidze, A, et al. (2005). Medication overuse headache: rates and predictors for relapse in a 4-year prospective study. *Cephalalgia*, 25:12–15.

Kieholz, P and Ladewig, D (1981). Probleme des medikamentenmissbrauches. *Schweis Arztezeitung*, 62:2866–2869.

Kim, DH, Fields, HL, and Barbaro, NM (1990). Morphine analgesia and acute physical dependence: rapid onset of two opposing, dose-related processes. *Brain Res*, 516:37–40.

Klapper, J (1995). Divalproex sodium in the prophylactic treatment of migraine. *Headache*, 35:290 (Abstract).

Kovelowski, CJ, Ossipov, MH, Sun, H, et al. (2000). Supraspinal cholecystokinin may drive tonic descending facilitation mechanisms to maintain neuropathic pain in the rat. *Pain*, 87:265–273.

Krupp, LB, LaRocca, NG, Muir-Nash, J, et al. (1989). The fatigue severity scale. Application to patients with multiple sclerosis and systemic lupus erythematosus. *Arch Neurol*, 46:1121–1123.

Krusz, JC and Belanger, J (1999). Propofol—a highly effective treatment for acute headaches. *Cephalalgia*, 19:358 (Abstract).

Krymchantowski, AV, Barbosa, JS, Lorenzatto, WS, et al. (1999). Clinical features of transformed migraine. *Cephalalgia*, 19:336–337 (Abstract).

Krymchantowski, AV, Silva, MT, Barbosa, JS, et al. (2002). Amitriptyline versus amitriptyline combined with fluoxetine in the preventative treatment of transformed migraine: a double-blind study. *Headache*, 42:510–514.

Kudrow, L (1982). Paradoxical effects of frequent analgesic use. *Adv Neurol*, 33:335–341.

Lake, AE, Saper, JR, Hamel, RL (2006). Inpatient treatment of intractable headache: outcome for 267 consecutive program completers. *Headache*, 46:893 (Abstract).

Lake, A, Saper, J, Madden, S, et al. (1990). Inpatient treatment for chronic daily headache: a prospective long-term outcome. *Headache*, 30:299–300 (Abstract).

Lake, AE, III Saper, JR, Madden, SF, et al. (1993). Comprehensive inpatient treatment for intractable migraine: a prospective long-term outcome study. *Headache*, 33(2):55–62.

Lance, F, Parkes, C, and Wilkinson, M (1988). Does analgesic abuse cause headache de novo? *Headache*, 1:61–62.

Lance, JW and Curran, DA (1964). Treatment of chronic tension headache. *Lancet*, 1:1236–1239.

Langemark, M and Olesen, J (1994). Sulpiride and paroxetine in the treatment of chronic tension-type headache. *Headache*, 34:20–24.

Lassen, LH, Ashina, M, Christiansen, I, et al. (1997). Nitric oxide synthase inhibition in migraine. *Lancet*, 349:401–402.

Li, D and Rozen, TD (2002). The clinical characteristics of new daily persistent headache. *Cephalalgia*, 22:66–69.

Limmroth, V, Katsarava, Z, Fritsche, G, et al. (2002). Features of medication overuse headache following overuse of different acute headache drugs. *Neurology*, 59:1011–1014.

Lipchik, GL, Holroyd, KA, France, CR, et al. (1996). Central and peripheral mechanisms in chronic tension-type headache. *Pain*, 64:467–475.

Lipchik, GL, Holroyd, KA, Talbot, F, et al. (1997). Pericranial muscle tenderness and exteroceptive suppression of temporalis muscle activity: a blind study of chronic tension-type headache. *Headache*, 37:368–376.

Lipton, RB, Silberstein, SD, Saper, J, and Goadsby, PJ (2003). Why headache treatment fails. *Neurology*, 60:1064–1070.

Lorenzatto, WS, Cheim, CF, Adriano, M, et al. (1999). Long-term outcome in chronic daily headache. *Cephalalgia*, 19:413 (Abstract).

Lu, SR, Fuh, JL, Chen, WT, et al. (2001). Chronic daily headache in Taipei, Taiwan: prevalence, follow-up and outcome predictors. *Cephalalgia*, 21:980–986.

Lu, SR, Fuh, JL, Juang, KD, et al. (2000). Repetitive intravenous prochlorperazine treatment of patients with refractory chronic daily headache. *Headache*, 40:724–729.

Ma, QP and Woolf, CJ (1995). Noxious stimuli induce an N-methyl-D-aspartate receptor-dependent hypersensitivity of the flexion withdrawal reflex to touch: implications for the treatment of mechanical allodynia. *Pain*, 61:383–390.

Mack, K (2003). What causes new daily persistent headache in children? *Cephalalgia*, 23:609 (Abstract).

Makashima, K and Takahashi, K (1991). Exteroceptive suppression of the masseter, temporalis and trapezius muscles produced by mental nerve stimulation in patients with chronic headaches. *Cephalalgia*, 11:23–28.

Manjit, SM, Thorsten, B, Ward, N, et al. (2003). Central neuromodulation in chronic migraine patients with suboccipital stimulators: a PET study. *Brain*, 1:220–230 (Abstract).

Manna, V, Bolino, F, and DiCicco, L (1994). Chronic tension-type headache, mood depression and serotonin. *Headache*, 34:44–49.

Mao, J, Sung, B, Ji, RR, et al. (2002). Neuronal apoptosis associated with morphine tolerance: evidence for an opioid-induced neurotoxic mechanism. *J Neurosci*, 22:7650–7661.

Matharu, MS, Cohen, AS, McGonigle, DJ, et al. (2004). Posterior hypothalamic and brainstem activation in hemicrania continua. *Headache*, 44:462–463 (Abstract).

Mathew, NT (1981). Prophylaxis of migraine and mixed headache. A randomized controlled study. *Headache*, 21:105–109.

Mathew, NT (1982). Transformed migraine. *Cephalalgia*, 13:78–83.

Mathew, NT (1987). Transformed or evolutional migraine. *Headache*, 27:305–306.

Mathew, NT (1990). Drug induced headache. *Neurol Clin*, 8:903–912.

Mathew, NT (1991). Chronic daily headache: clinical features and natural history. In *Headache and Depression: Serotonin Pathways as a Common Clue* (G Nappi, G Bono, G Sandrini, et al. eds.), pp. 49–58. Raven Press, New York.

Mathew, NT (1993). Transformed migraine. *Cephalalgia*, 13:78–83.

Mathew, NT and Ali, S (1991). Valproate in the treatment of persistent chronic daily headache. An open label study. *Headache*, 31:71–74.

Mathew, NT, Frishberg, BM, Gawel, M, et al. (2005). Botulinum toxin type A (BOTOX) for the prophylactic treatment of chronic daily headache: a randomized, double-blind, placebo-controlled trial. For the BOTOX CDH study group. *Headache*, 45:293–307.

Mathew, NT, Kurman, R, and Perez, F (1990). Drug induced refractory headache—clinical features and management. *Headache*, 30:634–638.

Mathew, NT, Rapoport, A, Saper, J, et al. (2001). Efficacy of gabapentin in migraine prophylaxis. *Headache*, 41:119–128.

Mathew, NT, Reuveni, U, and Perez, F (1987). Transformed or evolutive migraine. *Headache*, 27:102–106.

Mathew, NT, Saper, JR, Silberstein, SD, et al. (1995). Migraine prophylaxis with divalproex. *Arch Neurol*, 52:281–286.

Mathew, NT, Schmit, TJ, Jacobs, D, et al. (2003). Topiramate in migraine prevention (MIGR-001): effect on migraine frequency. *Neurology*, 60:A336 (Abstract).

Mathew, NT, Stubits, E, and Nigam, MR (1982). Transformation of episodic migraine into daily headache: analysis of factors. *Headache*, 22:66–68.

Mauskop, A (1999). Botulinum toxin in the treatment of chronic daily headaches. *Cephalalgia*, 19:453 (Abstract).

May, A, Bahra, A, Buchel, C, et al. (1998). Hypothalamic activation in cluster headache attacks. *Lancet*, 352:275–278.

May, A, Kaube, H, Buchel, C, et al. (1998). Experimental cranial pain elicited by capsaicin: a PET study. *Pain*, 74:61–66.

Medina, J and Diamond, S (1981). *Arch Neurol*, 38:705–709.

Mendes, PM, Silberstein, SD, Young, WB, et al. (2002). Intravenous Propofol in the Treatment of Refractory Headache. *Headache*, 42:638–641.

Merikangas, KR, Angst, J, and Isler, H (1990). Migraine and psychopathology: results of the Zurich cohort study of young adults. *Arch Gen Psychiatry*, 47:849–853.

Messinger, HB, Spierings, ELH, and Vincent, AJP (1991). Overlap of migraine and tension-type headache in the International Headache Society classification. *Cephalalgia*, 11:233–237.

Messlinger, K and Burstein, R (1999). Anatomy of central nervous system pathways related to head pain. In *The Headaches* (J Olesen, P Tfelt-Hansen, and KMA Welch, eds), pp. 77 Lippincott, Williams & Wilkins, Philadelphia.

Micieli, G, Manzoni, GC, Granella, F, et al. (1988). Clinical and epidemiological observations on drug abuse in headache patients. In *Drug-induced Headache* (HC Diener and M Wilkinson, eds), pp. 20–28. Springer-Verlag, Berlin.

Miller, DS, Talbot, CA, Simpson, W, et al. (1987). A comparison of naproxen sodium, acetaminophen and placebo in the treatment of muscle contraction headache. *Headache*, 27:392–396.

Mitsikostas, DD, Gatzonis, S, Thomas, A, et al. (1997). Buspirone vs amitriptyline in the treatment of chronic tension-type headache. *J Neurol Scand*, 96:247–251.

Mitsikostas, DD and Thomas, AM (1999). Comorbidity of headache and depressive disorders. *Cephalalgia*, 19:211–217.

Mongini, F, Defilippi, N, and Negro, C (1997). Chronic daily headache. A clinical and psychologic profile before and after treatment. *Headache*, 37:83–87.

Montalcini, RL, Daltos, R, Dellavalle, F, et al. (1995). Update of the NGF saga. *J Neurol Sci*, 130:119–127.

Monzon, MJ and Lainez, MJ (1998). Quality of life in migraine and chronic daily headache patients. *Cephalalgia*, 18:638–643.

Monzón, MJ, Láinez, MJA, Morales, F, et al. (1999). Clinical characteristics of chronic daily headache. *Cephalalgia*, 19:410 (Abstract).

Monzon, MJ, Lainez, MJA, Morales, F, et al. (1999). Long-term prognosis of chronic daily headache. *Cephalalgia*, 19:410 (Abstract).

Morland, TJ, Storli, OV, and Mogstad, TE (1979). Doxepin in the prophylactic treatment of mixed "vascular" and tension headache. *Headache*, 19:382–383.

Morriss, RK, Wearden, AJ, and Mullis, R (1998). Exploring the validity of the Chalder Fatigue scale in chronic fatigue syndrome. *J Psychosom Res*, 411–417.

Mosek, A, Swanson, JW, O'Fallon, WM, et al. (1999). CSF opening pressure in patients with chronic daily headache. *Cephalalgia*, 19:323 (Abstract).

Moskowitz, MA (1992). Neurogenic versus vascular mechanisms of sumatriptan and ergot alkaloids in migraine. *Trends Pharmacol Sci*, 13:307–311.

Mungliani, R and Hunt, SP (1995). Molecular biology of pain. *Br J Anaesth*, 75:186–192.

Murase, K, Ryu, PD, and Randic, M (1986). Substance P augments a persistent slow inward calcium-sensitive current in voltage-clamped spinal dorsal horn neurons of the rat. *Brain Res*, 365:369–376.

Mylecharane, EJ and Tfelt-Hansen, P (1993). Miscellaneous drugs. In *The Headaches* (J Olesen, P Tfelt-Hansen, and KMA Welch, eds.), pp. 397–402. Raven Press, New York.

Nakashima, K and Takahashi, K (1991). Exteroceptive suppression of the masseter, temporalis and trapezius muscles produced by mental nerve stimulation in patients with chronic headaches. *Cephalalgia*, 11:23–28.

Newman, LC, Lipton, RB, Russell, M, et al. (1992). Hemicrania continua: attacks my alternate sides. *Headache*, 32:237–238.

Newman, LC, Lipton, RB, and Solomon, S (1993). Hemicrania continua: 7 new cases and a literature review. *Headache*, 32:267.

Obermann, M, Bartsch, T, and Katsarava, Z (2006). Medication overuse headache. *Expert Opin Drug Saf*, 5:49–56.

Olesen, J, Tfelt-Hansen, P, and Welch, KMA (1993). *The Headaches*, Raven Press, New York.

Olesen J, Bousser MG, Diener HC, et al. (2006). Headache Classification Committee. New appendix criteria open for a broader concept of chronic migraine. *Cephalalgia*, 26:742–746.

Ondo, WG and Derman, HS (2002). Botulinum toxin A for chronic daily headache: a 60-patient, randomized, placebo-controlled, parallel design study. *Headache*, 42:431 (Abstract).

Palmer, KJ and Benfield, P (1994). Fluvoxamine: an overview of its pharmacologic properties and a review of its use in nondepressive disorders. *CNS Drugs*, 1:57–87.

Pareja, JA (1995). Chronic paroxysmal hemicrania: dissociation of the pain and autonomic features. *Headache*, 35:111–113.

Pareja, JA (1999). Hemicrania continua: ocular discomfort heralding painful attacks. *Funct Neurol*, 14:93–95.

Pareja, JA, Caminero, AB, Franco, E, et al. (2001). Dose, efficacy and tolerability of long-term indomethacin treatment of chronic paroxysmal hemicrania and hemicrania continua. *Cephalalgia*, 21:906–910.

Pareja, JA, Palomo, T, Gorriti, MA, et al. (1990). Hemicrania episodica—a new type of headache or prechronic stage of hemicrania continua. *Headache*, 30:344–346.

Pascual, J, Leira, R, and Lainez, JM (2003). Combined therapy for migraine prevention? Clinical experience with a beta-blocker plus sodium valproate in 52 resistant migraine patients. *Cephalalgia*, 23:961–962.

Pasquier, F, Leys, D, and Petit, H (1987). Hemicrania continua: the first bilateral case. *Cephalalgia*, 7:169–170.

Paulus, W, Raubuchl, O, Schoenen, J, et al. (1992). Exteroceptive suppression of temporalis muscle activity in various types of headache. *Headache*, 32:41–44.

Pazzaglia, PJ and Post, RM (1992). Contingent tolerance and reresponse to carbamazepine: a case study in a patient with trigeminal neuralgia and bipolar disorder. *J Neuropsychiat Clin Neurosci*, 4:76–81.

Peres, MF (2002). Hemicrania continua: recent treatment strategies and diagnostic evaluation. *Curr Neurol Neurosci Rep*, 2:108–113.

Peres, MF, Silberstein, SD, Nahmias, A, et al. (2001). Hemicrania continua is not that rare. *Neurology*, 57:948–951.

Peres, MF, Siow, HC, and Rozen, TD (2002). Hemicrania continua with aura. *Cephalalgia*, 22:246–248.

Peres, MF and Young, WB (2003). Side-shifting hemicrania continua with aura or chronic migraine with alternating symptoms responsive to indomethacin. *Cephalalgia*, 23:735–736.

Peres, MF, Young, WB, Kaup, AO, et al. (2001). Fibromyalgia is common in patients with transformed migraine. *Neurology*, 57:1326–1328.

Peres, MF, Zukerman, E, Young, WB, et al. (2002). Fatigue in chronic migraine patients. *Cephalalgia*, 22:720–724.

Pfaffenrath, V, Diener, HC, Isler, H, et al. (1994). Efficacy and tolerability of amitriptylinoxide in the treatment of chronic tension-type headache: a multicentre controlled study. *Cephalalgia*, 14:149–155.

Pfaffenrath, V and Isler, H (1993). Evaluation of the nosology of chronic tension-type headache. *Cephalalgia*, 13:60–62.

Pfaffenrath, V and Kaube, H (1990). Diagnostics of cervicogenic headache. *Funct Neurology*, 5:159–164.

Pfaffenrath, V, Kellhammer, U, and Pollmann, W (1986). Combination headache: practical experience with a combination of beta-blocker and an antidepressive. *Cephalalgia*, 6:25–32.

Pini, LA, Bigarelli, M, Vitale, G, et al. (1996). Headaches associated with chronic use of analgesics: a therapeutic approach. *Headache*, 36:433–439.

Pluvinage, R (1978). Le traitement des migraines et des cephalees psychogenes par l'amitriptyline. *Sem Hop*, 54:713–716.

Pollmann, W and Pfaffenrath, V (1986). Chronic paroxysmal hemicrania: the first possible bilateral case. *Cephalalgia*, 6:55–57.

Porreca, F, Ossipov, MH, and Gebhart, GF (2002). Chronic pain and medullary descending facilitation. *Trends Neurosci*, 25:319–325.

Post, RM and Silberstein, SD (1994). Shared mechanisms in affective illness, epilepsy, and migraine. *Neurology*, 44:S37–S47.

Potter, DL, Hart, DE, Calder, CS, et al. (2000). A double-blind, randomized, placebo-controlled, parallel study to determine the efficacy of topiramate in the prophylactic treatment of migraine. *Neurology*, 54:A15 (Abstract).

Pradalier, A, Clapin, A, and Dry, J (1988). Treatment review: nonsteroid antiinflammatory drugs in the treatment and long-term prevention of migraine attacks. *Headache*, 28:550–557.

Price, DD, Mao, J, and Mayer, DJ (1994). Central neural mechanisms of normal and abnormal pain states. In *Progress in Pain Research and Management* (HL Fields and JC Liebeskind, eds), pp. 61–84. IASP Press, Washington.

Pringsheim, T and Howse, D (1998). Inpatient treatment of chronic daily headache using dihydroergotamine: a long-term followup study. *Can J Neurol Sci*, 25:146–150.

Pritchard, DW (1989). EWG cranial muscle levels in headache sufferers before and during headache. *Headache*, 29:103–108.

Puca, F, Genco, S, Prudenzano, MP, et al. (1999). Psychiatric comorbidity and psychosocial stress in patients with tension-type headache from headache centers in Italy. The Italian Collaborative Group for the Study of Psychopathological Factors in Primary Headaches. *Cephalalgia*, 19:159–164.

Rang, HP and Urban, L (1995). New molecules in analgesia. *Br J Anaesth*, 75:145–156.

Rapoport, AM (1988). Analgesic rebound headache. *Headache*, 28:662–665.

Rapoport, AM, Weeks, RE, Sheftell, FD, et al. (1986). The "analgesic washout period": a critical variable evaluation in the evaluation of headache treatment efficacy. *Neurology*, 36:100–101.

Raskin, NH (1986). Repetitive intravenous dihydroergotamine as therapy for intractable migraine. *Neurology*, 36:995–997.

Rasmussen, BK (1992). Migraine and tension-type headache in a general population: psychosocial factors. *Int'l J Epidemiol*, 21:1138–1143.

Rasmussen, BK (1995). Epidemiology of headache. *Cephalalgia*, 15:45–68.

Rasmussen, BK, Jensen, R, and Olesen, J (1992). Impact of headache on sickness absence and utilization of medical services. *J Epidemiol Community Health*, 46:443–446.

Ravishankar, K (1997). Headache pattern in India: a headache clinic analysis of 1000 patients. *Cephalalgia*, 17:143–144.

Ren, K and Dubner, R (2002). Descending modulation in persistent pain: an update. *Pain*, 100:1–6.

Robbins, L (1999). Long-acting opioids for severe chronic daily headache. *Headache Quarterly*, 10:135–139.

Robinson, RG (1993). Pain relief for headaches. *Can Fam Physician*, 39:867–872.

Rosen, NL, Abbas, MA, and Silberstein, SD (2007). Effects of intravenous lidocaine in the treatment of refractory chronic daily headache (unpublished).

Rozen, T, Haynes, G, Range, C, et al. (2004). Low cerebrospinal fluid protein levels in adolescents with new daily persistent headache. *Neurology*, 62:A336 (Abstract).

Russell, MB, Stergaard, S, Endtsen, L, et al. (1999). Familial occurrence of chronic tension-type headache. *Cephalalgia*, 19:207–210.

Sakai, F, Ebihara, S, Akiyama, M, et al. (1995). Pericranial muscle hardness in tension-type headache: a noninvasive measurement method and its clinical application. *Brain*, 118:523–531.

Sandrini, G, Manzoni, GC, Zanferrari, C, et al. (1993). An epidemiologic approach to nosography of chronic daily headache. *Cephalalgia*, 13:72–77.

Sanin, LC, Mathew, NT, Bellmyer, LR, et al. (1994). The International Headache Society (IHS) headache classification as applied to a headache clinic population. *Cephalalgia*, 14:443–446.

Santoni, JR and Santoni-Williams, CJ (1993). Headache and painful lymphadenopathy in extracranial or systemic infection: etiology of new daily persistent headaches. *Intern Med*, 32:530–532.

Saper, JR (1983). *Headache Disorders: Current Concepts in Treatment Strategies*. Wright-PSG, Littleton.

Saper, JR (1987a). Ergotamine dependence. *Headache*, 27:435–438.

Saper, JR (1987b). Ergotamine dependency—a review. *Headache*, 27:435–438.

Saper, JR (1989). Chronic headache syndromes. *Neurol Clin*, 7:387–412.

Saper, JR (1990). Daily chronic headache. *Neurol Clin*, 8:891–901.

Saper, JR (2006). Approach to the intractable headache case: identifying treatable barriers to improvement. *Headache*, 12:259–284.

Saper, JR, Hamel, RL, and Lake, AE III (2005). Medication overuse headache (MOH) is a biobehavioural disorder. *Cephalalgia*, 25:545–546.

Saper, JR and Jones, JM (1986). Ergotamine tartrate dependency: features and possible mechanisms. *Clin Neuropharmacol*, 9:244–256.

Saper, JR and Lake, AE III (2002). Borderline personality disorder and the chronic headache patient: review and management recommendations. *Headache*, 42:663–674.

Saper, JR and Lake, AE III (2006). Medication overuse headache: type I and type II. *Cephalalgia*, 26:1262.

Saper, JR, Lake, AE III, Cantrell, DT, et al. (2002). Chronic daily headache prophylaxis with tizanidine: a double-blind, placebo-controlled, multicenter outcome study. *Headache*, 42:470–482.

Saper, JR, Lake, AE, Hamel, RL, et al. (2004). Daily scheduled opioids for intractable head pain: long-term observations of a treatment program. *Neurology*, 62:1687–1694.

Saper, JR, Lake, AE III, Madden, SF, et al. (1999). Comprehensive/tertiary care for headache: a 6-month outcome study. *Headache*, 39:249–263.

Saper, JR and Lake, AEI (2006). Sustained opioud therapy should rarely be administered to headache patients: clinical observations, literature review, and proposed guidelines. *Headache Currents*, 3:67–70.

Saper, JR, Silberstein, SD, Gordon, CD, et al. (1999). *Handbook of Headache Management: A Practical Guide to Diagnosis and Treatment of Head, Neck, and Facial Pain*. Lippincott Williams & Wilkins, Inc., Baltimore.

Saper, JR, Silberstein, SD, Lake, AE, et al. (1994). Double-blind trial of fluoxetine: Chronic daily headache and migraine. *Headache*, 34:497–502.

Saper, JR and VanMeter, MJ (1980). Ergotamine habituation: analysis and profile. *Headache*, 20:159 (Abstract).

Saper, JR and Winters, M (1982). Chronic "mixed" headaches: profile and analysis of 100 consecutive patients experiencing daily headache. *Headache*, 22:145–146 (Abstract).

Sarchielli, P, Alberti, A, Floridi, A, et al. (2001). Levels of nerve growth factor in cerebrospinal fluid of chronic daily headache patients. *Neurology*, 57:132–134.

Sarkar, S, Aziz, Q, Woolf, CJ, et al. (2000). Contribution of central sensitisation to the development of non-cardiac chest pain. *Lancet*, 356:1154–1159.

Schepelmann, K, Dannhausen, M, Kotter, I, et al. (1998). Exteroceptive suppression of temporalis muscle activity in patients with fibromyalgia, tension-type headache, and normal controls. *Electroencephalog Clin Neurophysiol*, 107:196–199.

Scher, AI, Lipton, RB, and Stewart, W (2002). Risk factors for chronic daily headache. *Cur Pain Headache Rep*, 6:486–491.

Scher, AI, Stewart, WF, Liberman, J, et al. (1998). Prevalence of frequent headache in a population sample. *Headache*, 38:497–506.

Scher, AI, Stewart, WF, Ricci, JA, et al. (2003). Factors associated with the onset and remission of chronic daily headache in a population-based study. *Pain*, 106:89.

Schnider, P, Aull, S, Baumgartner, C, et al. (1996). Long-term outcome of patients with headache and drug abuse after inpatient withdrawal: five-year followup. *Cephalalgia*, 16:481–485.

Schnider, P, Aull, S, and Feucht, M (1994). Use and abuse of analgesics in tension-type headache. *Cephalalgia*, 14:162–167.

Schoenen, J, Bottin, D, Hardy, F, et al. (1991). Cephalic and extracephalic pressure pain threshold in chronic tension-type headache. *Pain*, 47:145–149.

Schoenen, J, Jamart, B, Gerard, P, et al. (1987). Exteroceptive suppression of temporalis muscle activity in chronic headache. *Neurology*, 37:1834–1836.

Schoenen, J, Lenarduzzi, P, and Sianard-Gainko, J (1989). Chronic headaches associated with analgesics and/or ergotamine abuse: a clinical survey of 434 consecutive outpatients. In *New Advances in Headache Research* (FD Rose, ed.), pp. 29–43. Smith-Gordon, London.

Scholz, E, Diener, HC, Geiselhart, S, et al. (1988). Drug-induced headache: does a critical dosage exist? In *Drug-induced Headache* (HC Diener, ed.), pp. 29–43. Springer-Verlag, Berlin.

Scholz, E, Gerber, WD, Diener, HC, et al. (1987). Dihydroergotamine vs flunarizine vs nifedipine vs metoprolol vs propranolol in migraine prophylaxis: a comparative study based on time series analysis. In *Advances in*

Headache Research (E Scholz, WD Gerber, HC Diener, et al., eds), pp. 139–145. John Libbey & Co., London.

Schwarz, A, Farber, U, and Glaeske, G (1985). Daten zu analgetikakonsum und analgetikanephropathie in der bundesrepublik. *Offentiches gesundheitswesen*, 47:298–300.

Selby, G and Lance, JW (1960). Observation on 500 cases of migraine and allied vascular headaches. *J Neurol Neurosurg Psychiatry*, 23:23–32.

Shuaib, A, Ahmed, F, Muratoglu, M, et al. (1999). Topiramate in migraine prophylaxis: a pilot study. *Cephalalgia*, 19:379–380 (Abstract).

Shukla, P, Richardson, E, and Young, WB (2003). Brush allodynia in an inpatient headache unit. *Headache*, 43:542 (Abstract).

Silberstein, SD (1984). Treatment of headache in primary care practice. *Am J Med*, 77:65–72.

Silberstein, SD (1993). Chronic daily headache and tension-type headache. *Neurology*, 43:1644–1649.

Silberstein, SD (1998). Methysergide. *Cephalalgia*, 18:421–435.

Silberstein, SD (2002). Control of topiramate-induced paresthesias with supplemental potassium (Letter). *Headache*, 42:85.

Silberstein, SD (2003). Gabapentin in the treatment of chronic daily headache (Commentary). *Neurology*, 61:1637.

Silberstein, SD, Gobel, H, Jensen, R, et al. (2006). Botulinum toxin type A in the prophylactic treatment of chronic tension-type headache: a multicentre, double-blind, randomized, placebo-controlled, parallel-group study. *Cephalalgia*, 26:790–800.

Silberstein, SD and Lipton, RB (1994). Overview of diagnosis and treatment of migraine. *Neurology*, 44:6–16.

Silberstein, SD and Lipton, RB (2001). Chronic daily headache including transformed migraine, chronic tension-type headache, and medication overuse. In *Wolff's Headache and Other Head Pain* (SD Silberstein, RB Lipton, and DJ Dalessio, eds), pp. 247–282. Oxford University Press, New York.

Silberstein, SD, Lipton, RB, Dodick, DW, et al. (2007). Efficacy and safety of topiramate for the treatment of chronic migraine: a randomized, double-blind, placebo-controlled trial. *Headache*, 47:170–180.

Silberstein, SD, Lipton, RB, and Sliwinski, M (1996). Classification of daily and near-daily headaches: field trial of revised IHS criteria. *Neurology*, 47:871–875.

Silberstein, SD, Lipton, RB, Solomon, S, et al. (1994). Classification of daily and near daily headaches: proposed revisions to the IHS classification. *Headache*, 34:1–7.

Silberstein, SD, Neto, W, Schmitt, J, et al. (2004). Topiramate in the prevention of migraine headache: a randomized, double-blind, placebo-controlled, multiple-dose study. For the MIGR-001 Study Group. *Arch Neurol*, 61:490–495.

Silberstein, SD and Saper, JR (1993). Migraine: diagnosis and treatment. In *Wolff's Headache and Other Head Pain* (DJ Dalessio and SD Silberstein, eds.), pp. 96–170. Oxford University Press, New York.

Silberstein, SD, Saper, JR, and Freitag, F (2001). Migraine: Diagnosis and treatment. In *Wolff's Headache and Other Head Pain* (SD Silberstein, RB Lipton, and DJ Dalessio, eds.), pp. 121–237. Oxford University Press, New York.

Silberstein, SD, Schulman, EA, and Hopkins, MM (1990). Repetitive intravenous DHE in the treatment of refractory headache. *Headache*, 30:334–339.

Silberstein, SD and Silberstein, JR (1992). Chronic daily headache: prognosis following inpatient treatment with repetitive IV DHE. *Headache*, 32:439–445.

Silberstein, SD, Stark, SR, Lucas, SM, et al. (2005). Botulinum toxin type A for the prophylactic treatment of chronic daily headache: a randomized, double-blind, placebo-controlled trial. *Mayo Clin Proc*, 80:1126–1137.

Silberstein, SD, Young, WB, Mendizabal, J, et al. (2001). Efficacy of intramuscular droperidol for migraine treatment: a dose response study. *Neurology*, 56:A64 (Abstract).

Silverman, K, Evans, SM, Strain, EC, et al. (1992). Withdrawal syndrome after the double-blind cessation of caffeine consumption. *N Eng J Med*, 327:1109–1114.

Simone, DA, Baumann, TK, Collins, JG, et al. (1989). Sensitization of cat dorsal horn neurons to innocuous mechanical stimulation after intradermal injection of capsaicin. *Brain Res*, 486:185–189.

Siniatchkin, M, Gerber, WD, Kropp, P, et al. (1998). Contingent negative variation in patients with chronic daily headache. *Cephalalgia*, 18:565–569.

Sivilotti, LG, Thompson, SW, and Woolf, CJ (1993). The rate of rise of the cumulative depolarization evoked by repetitive stimulation of small-calibre afferents is a predictor of action potential windup in rat spinal neurones in vitro. *J Neurophysiol*, 69:1621–1631.

Sjaastad, O (1990). The headache challenge in our time: cervicogenic headache. *Funct Neurol*, 5:155–158.

Sjaastad, O and Antonaci, F (1993). Chronic paroxysmal hemicrania (CPH) and hemicrania continua: transition from one stage to another. *Headache*, 33:551–554.

Sjaastad, O, Saumte, C, and Hovdahl, H (1983). Cervicogenic headache, a hypothesis. *Cephalalgia*, 3:249–256.

Sjaastad, O and Spierings, EL (1984). Hemicrania continua: another headache absolutely responsive to indomethacin. *Cephalalgia*, 4:65–70.

Sjaastad, O and Tjorstad, K (1987). Hemicrania continua: a third Norwegian case. *Cephalalgia*, 7:175–177.

Smuts, JA, Baker, MK, Smuts, HM, et al. (1999). Botulinum toxin type A as prophylactic treatment in chronic tension-type headache. *Cephalalgia*, 19:454 (Abstract).

Sobrino, FE (2003). Cutaneous allodynia in chronic migraine. *Cephalalgia*, 23:750 (Abstract).

Solomon, GD, Skobieranda, FG, and Gragg, LA (1993). Quality of life and well-being of headache patients: measurement by the Medical Outcomes Study instrument. *Headache*, 33:351–358.

Solomon, S, Lipton, RB, and Newman, LC (1992a). Clinical features of chronic daily headache. *Headache*, 32:325–329.

Solomon, S, Lipton, RB, and Newman, LC (1992b). Evaluation of chronic daily headache-comparison to criteria for chronic tension-type headache. *Cephalalgia*, 12:365–368.

Spira, PJ and Beran, RG (2003). Gabapentin in the prophylaxis of chronic daily headache. A randomized, placebo-controlled study for the Australian Gabapentin Chronic Daily Headache Group. *Neurology*, 61:1753–1759.

Spitz, M and Peres, MF (2004). Hemicrania continua postpartum. *Cephalalgia*, 24:603–604.

Stewart, WF, Scher, AI, and Lipton, RB (2001). Stressful life events and risk of chronic daily headache: results from the frequent headache epidemiology study. *Cephalalgia*, 21:278–280.

Strassman, AM, Raymond, SA, and Burstein, R (1996). Sensitization of meningeal sensory neurons and the origin of headaches. *Nature*, 384:560–564.

Suhr, B, Evers, S, Bauer, B, et al. (1999). Drug-induced headache: long-term results of stationary versus ambulatory withdrawal therapy. *Cephalalgia*, 19:44–49.

Sweatt, JD, Weeber, EJ, and Levenons, JM (2002). Central neural mechanisms that interrelate sensory and affective dimensions of pain. *Mol Interven*, 2:393–402.

Swidan, SZ, Lake, AE III, and Saper, JR (2005). Efficacy of intravenous diphenhydramine versus intravenous DHE-45 in the treatment of severe migraine headache. *Curr Pain Headache Rep*, 9:65–70.

Takase, Y, Nakano, M, Tatsumi, C, et al. (2004). Clinical features, effectiveness of drug-based treatment, and prognosis of new daily persistent headache (NDPH): 30 cases in Japan. *Cephalalgia*, 24:955–959.

Tanen, DA, Miller, S, French, T, et al. (2003). Intravenous sodium valproate versus prochlorperazine for the emergency department treatment of acute migraine headaches: a prospective, randomized, double-blind trial. *Ann Emerg Med*, 41:847–853.

Tavola, T, Gala, C, Conte, G, et al. (1992). Traditional Chinese acupuncture in tension-type headache: a controlled study. *Pain*, 48:325–329.

Tekle Haimanot, R, Seraw, B, Forsgren, L, et al. (1995). Migraine, chronic tension-type headache, and cluster headache in an Ethiopian rural community. *Cephalalgia*, 15:482–488.

Tfelt-Hansen, P and Krabbe, AA (1981). Ergotamine. Do patients benefit from withdrawal? *Cephalalgia*, 1:29–32.

Tfelt-Hansen, P and Welch, KMA (2000). Prioritizing prophylactic treatment of migraine. In *The Headaches* (J Olesen, P Tfelt-Hansen, and KMA Welch, eds.), pp. 499–500. Lippincott Williams & Wilkins, Philadelphia.

Thompson, SW, King, AE, and Woolf, CJ (1990). Activity-dependent changes in rat ventral horn neurones in vitro: summation of prolonged afferent evoked post-synaptic depolarizations produce a D-APV sensitive windup. *Eur J Neurosci*, 2:638–649.

Urban, MO, Coutinho, SV, and Gebhart, GF (1999a). Biphasic modulation of visceral nociception by neurotensin in rat rostral ventromedial medulla. *J Pharmacol Exp Ther*, 290:207–213.

Urban, MO, Coutinho, SV, and Gebhart, GF (1999b). Involvement of excitatory amino acid receptors and nitric oxide in the rostral ventromedial medulla in modulating secondary hyperalgesia produced by mustard oil. *Pain*, 81:45–55.

Urban, MO and Gebhart, GF (1997). Characterization of biphasic modulation of spinal nociceptive transmission by neurotensin in the rat rostral ventromedial medulla. *J Neurophysiol*, 78:1550–1562.

Urban, MO and Gebhart, GF (1999). Supraspinal contributions to hyperalgesia. *PNAS*, 96:7687–7692.

Vanast, WJ (1986). New daily persistent headaches: definition of a benign syndrome. *Headache*, 26:317.

Vanderah, TW, Gardell, LR, Burgess, SE, et al. (2000). Dynorphin promotes abnormal pain and spinal opioid antinociceptive tolerance. *J Neurosci*, 20:7074–7079.

Verri, AP, Cecchini, P, Galli, C, et al. (1998). Psychiatric comorbidity in chronic daily headache. *Cephalalgia*, 18:45–49.

Wall, M, Silberstein, SD, and Aiken, RD (2001). Headache associated with abnormalities in intracranial structure or function: high cerebrospinal fluid pressure headache and brain tumor. In *Wolff's Headache and Other Head Pain* (SD Silberstein, RB Lipton, DJ Dalessio, eds.), pp. 393–416. Oxford University Press, New York.

Wang, SJ, Fuh, JL, Lu, SR, et al. (2000). Chronic daily headache in Chinese elderly: prevalence, risk factors and biannual follow-up. *Neurology*, 54:314–319.

Wang, SJ, Fuh, JL, Lu, SR, et al. (2001). Quality of life differs among headache diagnoses: analysis of SF-36 survey in 901 headache patients. *Pain*, 89:285–292.

Wang, SJ, Silberstein, SD, and Young, WB (1997). Droperidol treatment of status migrainosus and refractory migraine. *Headache*, 37:377–382.

Weiller, C, May, A, Limmroth, V, et al. (1995). Brainstem activation in spontaneous human migraine attacks. *Nat Med*, 1:658–660.

Welch, KMA, Nagesh, V, Rozell, K, et al. (1999). Functional MRI of chronic daily headache. *Cephalalgia*, 19:462–463 (Abstract).

Wessely, P, Baumgartner, C, Klinger, D, et al. (1987). Preliminary results of a double-blind study with the new migraine prophylactic drug Gabapentin. *Cephalalgia*, 7:477–478.

Wheeler, SD (2002). Hemicrania continua in African Americans. *J Natl Med Assoc*, 94:901–907.

White, HS, Brown, SD, Woodhead, JH, et al. (2000). Topiramate modulates GABA-evoked currents in murine cortical neurons by a nonbenzodiazepine mechanism. *Epilepsia*, 41:S17–S20.

Wilkinson, M (1988). Introduction. In *Drug induced headache* (HC Diener and M Wilkinson, eds.), pp. 1–2. Springer-Verlag, Berlin.

Wilkinson, SM, Becker, and WJ, Heine, JA (2001). Opiate use to control bowel motility may induce chronic daily headache in patients with migraine. *Headache*, 41:303–309.

Wolfe, F, Smythe, HA, and Yanus, MB (1990). The American College of Rheumatology 1990 criteria for the classification of fibromyalgia: report of the Multicenter Criteria Committee. *Arthritis Rheum*, 33:160–172.

Woolf, CJ (1983). Evidence for a central component of postinjury pain hypersensitivity. *Nature*, 306:686–688.

Woolf, CJ (1995). Somatic pain: pathogenesis and prevention. *Br J Anaesth*, 75:169–176.

Woolf, CJ and King, AE (1989). Subthreshold components of the cutaneous mechanoreceptive fields of dorsal horn neurons in the rat lumbar spinal cord. *J Neurophysiol*, 62:907–916.

Woolf, CJ and King, AE (1990). Dynamic alterations in the cutaneous mechanoreceptive fields of dorsal horn neurons in the rat spinal cord. *J Neurosci*, 10:2717–2726.

Woolf, CJ and Mitchell, MB (2001). Mechanism-based pain diagnosis issues for analgesic drug development. *Anesthesiology*, 95:241–249.

Woolf, CJ and Wall, PD (1986). The relative effectiveness of C primary afferent fibres of different origins in evoking a prolonged facilitation of the flexor reflex in the rat. *J Neurosci*, 6:1433–1443.

Yamamura, H, Malick, A, Chamberlin, NL, et al. (1999). Cardiovascular and neuronal responses to head stimulation reflect central sensitization and cutaneous allodynia in a rat model of migraine. *J Neurophysiol*, 81:479–493.

Young, WB and Rozen, TD (1999). Bilateral cluster headache: case report and a theory of (failed) contralateral suppression. *Cephalalgia*, 19:188–190.

Zed, PJ, Loewen, PS, and Robinson, G (1999). Medication-induced headache: overview and systematic review of therapeutic approaches. *Ann Pharmacother*, 33:61–72.

Zeeberg, P, Olesen, J, and Jensen, R (2006). Discontinuation of medication overuse in headache patients: recovery of therapeutic responsiveness. *Cephalalgia*, 26:1192–1198.

Zhang, XL, Velumian, A, Jones, OT, et al. (2000). Modulation of high voltage-activated calcium channels in dentate granule cells by topiramate. *Epilepsia*, 41: S52–S60.

Zhuo, M and Gebhart, GF (1990). Characterization of descending inhibition and facilitation from the nuclei reticularis gigantocellularis and gigantocellularis pars alpha in the rat. *Pain*, 42:337–350.

Zhuo, M and Gebhart, GF (1992). Characterization of descending facilitation and inhibition of spinal nociceptive transmission from the nuclei reticularis gigantocellularis and gigantocellularis pars alpha in the rat. *J Neurophysiol*, 67:1599–1614.

Zhuo, M and Gebhart GF (1997). Biphasic modulation of spinal nociceptive transmission from the medullary raphe nuclei in the rat. *J Neurophysiol*, 78:746–758.

Ziegler, DK (1997). Opioids in headache treatment: is there a role? *Neurol Clin*, 15:199–207.

Zukerman, E, Hannuch, SN, de Carvalho, S, et al. (1987). Hemicrania continua: a case report. *Cephalalgia*, 7:171–173.

Zwart, JA, Dyb, G, Hagen, K, et al. (2003). Analgesic use: a predictor of chronic pain and medication overuse headache: the Head-HUNT Study. *Neurology*, 61:160–164.

Zwart, JA and Sand, T (1995). Exteroceptive suppression of temporalis muscle activity: a blind study of tension-type headache, migraine, and cervicogenic headache. *Headache*, 35:338–343.

14 Trigeminal Autonomic Cephalalgias: Diagnosis and Management

Manjit S Matharu and Peter J Goadsby

The trigeminal autonomic cephalalgias (TACs) are a group of primary headache disorders characterized by unilateral head pain that occurs in association with often prominent ipsilateral cranial autonomic features (Goadsby and Lipton, 1997). The TACs include cluster headache (CH), paroxysmal hemicrania (PH), short-lasting unilateral neuralgiform headache attacks with conjunctival injection and tearing (SUNCT), and short-lasting unilateral neuralgiform headache attacks with cranial autonomic symptoms (SUNA). CH, PH, and SUNCT are currently grouped into section 3 of the revised International Classification of Headache Disorders (ICHD-II) (Headache Classification Committee of The International Headache Society, 2004) whereas SUNA is described in the appendix section. Hemicrania continua (HC) is currently not considered a TAC, being classified under Section 4, Other Primary Headaches, although one might argue for its inclusion here.

CH, PH, and SUNCT are characterized by short-lasting headaches with autonomic features. A more comprehensive list of short-lasting headaches is provided in Table 14–1. Despite their common elements, these three TACs differ in attack duration and frequency as well as the response to therapy. CH has the longest attack duration and relatively low attack frequency. PH has intermediate duration and intermediate attack frequency. SUNCT has the shortest attack duration and the highest attack frequency (Table 14–2). The importance of recognizing these syndromes resides in their excellent but highly selective response to treatment.

CLUSTER HEADACHE

CH is a strictly unilateral headache that occurs in association with cranial autonomic features. It is an excruciating syndrome and is probably one of the most painful conditions known, with female patients describing each attack as being worse than childbirth. In most patients, it has a striking circannual and circadian periodicity.

Historical Note

In 1641, Tulp gave an incomplete clinical description of a patient who probably suffered from CH (Koehler, 1993). Gerhard van Swieten gave a full description of a case of episodic CH (ECH) in 1745 (Isler, 1993). Wilfred Harris' descriptions in 1926 of what he called migrainous neuralgia were the first record of CH in the English medical literature (Lance and Anthony, 1971). The subsequent clinical description of CH by Bayard Horton and colleagues (1939) was comprehensive, except for the omission of Horner's syndrome and the male predominance of the disease. Horton and Harris are generally given credit for making the entity known to the medical world. Noting the tendency for the headache attacks to cluster in time, Kunkle and colleagues (1952) proposed the term "cluster headache."

The term CH is widely accepted now though the condition was known by a large number of names, many of which reveal the perceived views of the pathophysiology of the condition. These older names include "red migraine," "erythroprosopalgia of Bing," "ciliary neuralgia,"

TABLE 14–1 Primary Short-lasting Headaches[a].

Prominent autonomic features	*Sparse or no autonomic features*
Cluster headache	Trigeminal neuralgia
Paroxysmal hemicrania	Primary stabbing headache
SUNCT	Primary cough headache
SUNA	Primary exertional headache
	Primary headache associated with sexual activity
	Hypnic headache

[a] Short-lasting is taken to be generally <4 hours.

Abbreviations: SUNCT, short-lasting unilateral neuralgiform headache attacks with conjunctival injection and tearing; SUNA, short-lasting unilateral neuralgiform headache attacks with cranial autonomic symptoms.

"erythromelalgia of the head," "Horton's headache," "histaminic cephalalgia," "petrosal neuralgia," "sphenopalatine neuralgia," "Vidian neuralgia," "Sluder's neuralgia," "hemicrania angioparalytica," "hemicrania periodic neuralgiforms," "syndrome of hemicephalic vasodilatation of sympathetic origin," and "autonomic faciocephalalgia." Symonds (1956) used the noncommittal title of "a particular variety of headache."

TABLE 14–2 Clinical Features of the Trigeminal Autonomic Cephalalgias.

	Cluster headache	*Paroxysmal hemicrania*	*SUNCT*
Sex F:M	1:2.5–7.2	1.6–2.4:1	1:1.5
Pain type	Stabbing, boring	Throbbing, boring, stabbing	Burning, stabbing, sharp
Severity	Excruciating	Excruciating	Severe to excruciating
Site	Orbit, temple	Orbit, temple	Periorbital
Attack frequency	1/alternate day–8/day	1–40/day (>5/day for more than half the time)	3–200/day
Duration of attack	15–180 minutes	2–30 minutes	5–240 seconds
Autonomic features	Yes	Yes	Yes[a]
Migrainous features[b]	Yes	Yes	One third
Alcohol trigger	Yes	One-fifth	No
Cutaneous triggers	No	No	Yes
Indomethacin effect	—	+ +	—
Abortive treatment	Sumatriptan injection Sumatriptan or Zolmitriptan nasal spray Oxygen	Nil	Nil
Prophylactic treatment	Verapamil Methysergide Lithium Corticosteroids	Indomethacin	Lamotrigine Topiramate Gabapentin Intravenous lidocaine

Abbreviation: SUNCT, short-lasting unilateral neuralgiform headache attacks with conjunctival injection and tearing.

+ + Indicates absolute response to indomethacin.

[a] Prominent conjunctival injection and lacrimation by definition.

[b] Nausea, photophobia or phonophobia.

Epidemiology

Prevalence

CH is relatively rare, but the exact prevalence remains a matter of debate because of the remarkable variation of the estimated prevalence between 56 and 401 per 100,000 population in the various studies (Table 14–3). Recent studies suggest that the prevalence of CH may be as high as 2 per 1000 (Russell, 2004).

Sex Distribution

CH has long been recognized to predominate in men. The gender ratio has varied between 5:1 and 7.2:1 in the older large case series (Horton, 1956; Lovshin, 1961; Kudrow, 1980; Ekbom and Waldenlind, 1981; Krabbe, 1986). However, recent case series report lower male-to-female ratios, which vary between 2.5:1 and 3.5:1 (Klapper et al., 2000; Torelli et al., 2001; Bahra et al., 2002; Schurks et al., 2006). This change in the gender ratio is likely to be an ascertainment issue related to underrecognition in women rather than a real shift in female incidence.

Age of Onset

CH can begin at any age, although onset most commonly occurs between the second and fourth decades of life. The reported mean age at onset varies between 26 and 30 years in the various case series (Friedman and Mikropoulos, 1958; Ekbom, 1970a; Manzoni, Terzano, et al., 1983; Klapper et al., 2000; Bahra et al., 2002). The youngest age at onset is 3 years and the oldest 91 years (Kudrow, 1980; Seidler et al., 2006).

Clinical Features

Several of the terms relating to CH can be confusing and require defining. A *CH* or *attack* is an individual episode of pain that can last from a few minutes to few hours. A *cluster bout* or *period* refers to the duration during which recurrent cluster attacks are occurring; it usually lasts from a few weeks to months. A *remission* is the pain-free period between two cluster bouts.

CH is a disorder with highly distinctive clinical features. These features are dealt with under two major headings: *the cluster attack* and *the cluster bout.*

The Cluster Attack

Site and Laterality of Pain The pain is predominantly over the retroorbital, supraorbital, or temporal regions but can be experienced over a wide area including the forehead, jaw, cheek, upper and lower teeth, and, less commonly, the ear, nose, neck, shoulder, and other regions of the hemicranium (Bahra et al., 2002).

The pain of CH is almost always strictly unilateral, with less than 3% of patients reporting bilateral attacks (Torelli et al., 2001). In the majority of patients, the pain of CH always affects the same side of the head; however, approximately 30% of patients experience a side shift with the pain during a cluster period or from one cluster period to the next or, very rarely, within the same attack (Bahra et al., 2002). The pain is present more

TABLE 14–3 Epidemiological studies of cluster headache.

Study	*Country*	*Population sample*	*Affected*	*Prevalence (per 100,000)*
Ekbom et al. (1978)	Sweden	9803	9	92
D'Alessandro et al. (1986)	San Marino	21,792	14	69
Swanson et al. (1994)	USA	6476	26	401
Tonon et al. (2002)	San Marino	26,628	15	56
Sjaastad et al. (2003)	Norway	1838	7	381
Torelli et al. (2005)	Italy	7522	21	279

frequently on the right (47%–60%) than the left (38%–39%) (Ekbom, 1970a; Kudrow, 1980; Bahra et al., 2002; Lance and Goadsby, 2005).

Temporal Profile, Intensity and Character of Pain The attack often begins as a vague discomfort and rapidly increases to excruciating pain, reaching a maximal intensity within 9 minutes of onset in 86% of patients (Torelli and Manzoni, 2003). In the majority of patients, the pain is maintained at the maximum intensity or fluctuates slightly. In some patients, periods of repetitive peaks of pain separated by brief troughs of lesser pain characterizes the "temporal profile." The end of the attack usually comes abruptly, with rapidly decreasing pain intensity and finally free from pain. In some patients a slight discomfort or ache persists in the symptomatic area between attacks (Lance and Goadsby, 2005).

CH is arguably one of the most painful conditions in humans. Many patients who have had other pain experiences, such as renal colic and childbirth, report that the pain of CH is much worse. There are several reports of patients who have directed violent self-harm at the site of the pain or attempted suicide because of the extraordinary intensity of pain (Kudrow, 1980; Blau, 1993; Geweke, 2002; Rothrock, 2006).

The character of the pain is described as constant burning, boring, piercing, tearing or screwing (Lance and Goadsby, 2005). Patients frequently report a feeling of a "hot poker in the eye" or as if "the eye is being pushed out." A minority (38%) describe the pain as throbbing or pounding (Friedman and Mikropoulos, 1958). Sudden brief jabs of intense pain may also be experienced in the symptomatic area during the attack.

Duration and Frequency of Attacks The headache usually lasts 30 minutes to 2 hours but can range from 15 minutes to 3 hours (Kudrow, 1980; Manzoni and Sandrini, 2000). Occasional episodes may be longer-lasting, sustained for 8 hours or more (Bahra et al., 2002; Lance and Goadsby, 2005). In a prospective study of 77 attacks, total duration was less than 30 minutes in 29%, less than 45 minutes in 62%, and less than 1 hour in 78% of patients (Russell, 1981). In contrast, another case series of 230 patients reported that the mean minimum and maximum attack durations were 72 and 159 minutes, respectively (Bahra et al., 2002).

The frequency of the attacks ranges from one every alternate day to eight daily though 75%–88% of patients have one to two attacks daily (Ekbom, 1970a; Lance, 1978; Manzoni and Sandrini, 2000). The attacks tend to be less frequent (and severe) at the beginning and end of a cluster bout.

Circadian Periodicity Periodicity is a hallmark of CH. Most patients (47%–87%) state that their attacks are liable to recur at a particular time of the day or night (Ekbom, 1970a; Lance, 1978). Various attack patterns have been documented. Manzoni, Terzano, and colleagues (1983) reported that attacks peak at 1–2 AM, 1–3 PM, and 9 PM. Russell (1981) reported that 51% of the attacks begin when patients are asleep, the peak frequency being from 4 to 10 AM. Most patients report predictability of attack onset nocturnally (73%), awakening them from sleep, and less so during the day (37%) (Bahra et al., 2002).

Patients often develop attacks about 90 minutes after going to sleep, suggesting a relationship with rapid eye movement (REM) and sleep phase (Dexter and Weitzman, 1970; Manzoni et al., 1981). Furthermore, polysomnography studies show that 31%–80% of CH patients have evidence of obstructive sleep apnea (OSA), and nocturnal attacks occur during periods of oxygen desaturation with OSA associated with REM sleep (Chervin et al., 2000; Nobre et al., 2003; Graff-Radford and Newman, 2004; Nobre et al., 2005).

Associated Features The signature feature of CH is the association with cranial autonomic symptoms. Lacrimation (82%–91%) and conjunctival injection (58%–84%) are the most common symptoms followed by nasal congestion or rhinorrhea (68%–76%). Approximately one-third of the patients report drooping of the eyelid and miosis, though these symptoms are present in two thirds of patients observed by clinicians during an attack (Ekbom, 1970a; Kudrow, 1980). Forehead sweating, facial flushing, and eyelid edema are relatively rare. These cranial autonomic features are transient, lasting only for the duration of the attack, with the exception of partial Horner's syndrome; ptosis or miosis may rarely persist, especially after frequent attacks. These cranial autonomic symptoms are usually ipsilateral to the pain but occasionally occur on both sides. Cranial autonomic symptoms may not be clinically evident in 1%–7% of patients (Ekbom, 1970a; Torelli et al., 2001; Schurks et al., 2006).

Fluctuations in heart rate, blood pressure, and cardiac rhythm, including premature ventricular beats, transient episodes of atrial flutter, and first-degree atrioventricular or sinoatrial block, can also occur (Russell and Storstein, 1983). Moreover, both diastolic and systolic blood pressures may be increased (Russell and von der Lippe, 1982).

There have been several recent descriptions of the full range of typical migrainous symptoms in significant proportions of CH patients (Silberstein et al., 2000; Bahra et al., 2002). Premonitory symptoms, preceding individual attacks from minutes to hours, have been reported in 61%–65% of patients (Blau and Engel, 1998; Raimondi, 2001). These premonitory symptoms include lethargy, mood alteration (depression, elation, apathy, irritability, and anxiety), neurological involvement (disorientation, yawning, and cravings for food), and gastrointestinal upset (nausea, dyspepsia, anorexia, and hunger). Patients may also experience sensations in the area of subsequent pain including twinges, tingling, and pulsations. During the cluster attack, gastrointestinal symptoms are less common than in migraine, but approximately half of patients feel nauseated and a quarter report vomiting (Bahra et al., 2002). Similar numbers report at least one of photophobia (56%), which is often lateralized, phonophobia (43%), and osmophobia (26%). Aura symptoms have been described in association with CH (Ekbom, 1970a; Lance and Anthony, 1971; Graham, 1972; Manzoni, Terzano, et al., 1983). Recent series reported aura symptoms in 6%–23% of CH patients (Silberstein et al., 2000; Bahra et al., 2002; Schurks et al., 2006).

Behavior During An Attack In contrast to migraine, the vast majority (68%–93%) of CH patients report restlessness during an attack (Bahra et al., 2002; Schurks et al., 2006) and, therefore, this feature has been incorporated into the ICHD-II diagnostic criteria. Most patients are unable to sit still or lie down, but prefer to pace about or sit and rock back and forth (Blau, 1993). Subjects may rub or compress their head and apply hot or cold packs to the site of pain. Many individuals isolate themselves or prefer to go outdoors into the cold or fresh air during the attack (Torelli and Manzoni, 2003). Violent behavior is rare, though patients may strike their heads on the wall. Many contemplate suicide during attacks because of the torment of the excruciating pain; hence the reason CHs are often referred to as "suicide headaches."

Precipitating and Relieving Factors Alcohol, nitroglycerine (Ekbom, 1968), and histamine (Horton, 1956) can trigger a cluster attack. Alcohol induces acute attacks, usually within an hour of intake, in the vast majority of sufferers, contrasting with migraine sufferers who generally have headache some hours after alcohol intake. Alcohol triggers attacks during a cluster bout but not in a remission. Exercise, elevated environmental temperature (Blau and Engel, 1999), and the smell of volatile substances, such as solvents, varnishes and perfumes, are also recognized precipitants of acute cluster attacks. There is a preponderance of attacks beginning in sleep, with a tendency to occur during REM sleep. During the daytime, more than 70% of attacks occur when the patient is physically relaxed (Russell, 1981). Allergies, food sensitivities, reproductive hormonal changes, and stress do not appear to have any significant role in precipitating attacks.

Compression of the ipsilateral superficial temporal artery or common carotid artery has been reported to transiently relieve the pain of a cluster attack (Ekbom, 1975). Some patients report that they are able to alleviate the pain through short-lasting, intense physical activity (Black et al., 2006). Setting aside conventional medicines, nothing consistently provides relief.

The Cluster Bout

CH is classified according to the duration of the bout. Approximately 80%–90% of patients have *ECH,* which is diagnosed when they experience recurrent bouts, each with a duration of more than a week and separated by remissions lasting more than 1 month. The remaining 10%–20% of patients have *chronic CH* (CCH) in which either no remission occurs within 1 year or the remissions last less than 1 month.

Frequency, Duration and Periodicity of the Bouts in ECH Most patients with ECH have bouts with a frequency between once every 2 years and twice a year. In a series of 182 ECH patients, the remission period was between 6 months and 2 years in 82% of patients (Bahra et al., 2002). In most cases, the cluster bouts last 1–3 months, with a mean duration of 8.6 weeks (Bahra et al., 2002). Often, a striking circannual periodicity is seen with the cluster bouts that tend to occur in the same month of the year. In other patients, the cluster periods tend to recur at regular intervals that are consistently different from 12 months. Ekbom (1970b) reported that cluster bouts have a seasonal predilection, being more frequent in spring and autumn. Kudrow (1987) studied this periodicity in a large series of patients and reported that the frequency of cluster bouts increases with a gradual increase or decrease in daylight hours during the year, with two significant peaks starting 7–10 days after the longest day and the shortest day. Patients often report that this circannual periodicity becomes less evident after a few years.

Psychological Profile

Graham (1972) claimed that men with CH had a leonine appearance but were usually very insecure and had strong traits of hysteria. Other researchers claim that the personality type characteristically associated with CH is ambitious, hard driving, energetic and obsessive, but has also feelings of inadequacy and dependency (Friedman and Mikropoulos, 1958; Kudrow, 1974). In contrast, CH patients did not differ from other headache groups with regard to psychological status (Cuypers et al., 1981). Using the Minnesota Multiphasic Personality Inventory, CH patients had a personality profile similar to that observed in migraine (Andrasik et al., 1982). It may be concluded that the concept of a CH personality seems outdated and is without good evidence.

CH sufferers overindulge in nonessential consumption habits (Ekbom, 1970b; Kudrow, 1980; Manzoni, 1998). Approximately two-thirds of CH patients are smokers and another 15% ex-smokers (Bahra et al., 2002; Schurks et al., 2006). Similar, but somewhat less consistent, is the heavy use of alcohol. Although earlier reports generally indicated a tendency to alcohol abuse (Kudrow, 1974; Manzoni, Terzano, et al., 1983), some of the more recent ones showed no significant differences versus control groups [Italian Cooperative Study Group on the Epidemiology of Cluster Headache (ICECH), 1995]. A significant tendency to consume excessive amounts of coffee has also been reported, with 10% of CH male sufferers drinking more than six cups of coffee a day (Manzoni, 1999).

Past History and Comorbidities

An association of CH with sleep apnea (see section "Circadian Periodicity"), head trauma, peptic ulcer disease, and coronary disease has been reported. The association with peptic ulcer and coronary disease is predictable given the high prevalence of smoking.

Head Trauma Several case series report an association of previous head trauma with CH [Lance and Anthony, 1971; Kudrow, 1980; Italian Cooperative Study Group on the Epidemiology of Cluster Headache (ICECH), 1995; Manzoni, 1999]. These series report an incidence of previous head trauma ranging between 5% and 37%. There is often a long interval between the head trauma and the onset of the CHs. One series reported a mean latency of the 10 years (Manzoni, 1999). Furthermore, several reports described the development of CH after enucleation of the ipsilateral eye (Evers et al., 1997) or after dental extraction (Soros et al., 2001).

Considering the generally long interval of time separating the two events, it is not easy to ascribe a direct causal role for head trauma in the etiology of CH. It is possible that head trauma may damage intracranial structures hence predisposing to the subsequent development of CH. However, there is also the possibility that previous head trauma may be more frequent among CH patients because of their lifestyle, which may leave them more exposed to the risk of traumatic events.

Family History and Genetics

A review of 12 studies performed between 1947 and 1985 revealed a family history in 4% (47/1182) of patients with CH, thereby suggesting an increased familial risk (Russell, 1997). Since then four genetic epidemiological surveys have provided more complete information about familial risk (Kudrow and Kudrow, 1994; Russell et al., 1995a;

Leone et al., 2001; El Amrani, Ducros, et al., 2002). These studies suggest that the first-degree relatives have a 5–18 times higher risk, and second-degree relatives have a 1–3 times higher risk of CH than the general population. The increased familial risk of CH strongly suggests a genetic cause for the disease.

CH has been reported in five concordant monozygotic twin pairs (Eadie and Sutherland, 1966; Sjaastad and Salvesen, 1986; Couturier et al., 1991; Roberge et al., 1992; Sjaastad et al., 1993). This indicates the importance of genetic factors, although publication selection bias cannot be ruled out. In this respect, the Swedish Twin Registry and the Swedish in patient registry survey reported that two monozygotic and nine dizygotic twin pairs had all been discordant for CH for 10–31 years (Svensson et al., 2003). These data support the importance of both genetic and environmental factors.

Complex segregation analysis suggests that an autosomal dominant gene has a role in the inheritance of CH in some families (Russell et al., 1995b). Researchers investigating the importance of the familial hemiplegic migraine gene *CACN1A*, the clock gene 3092 T→C, and the nitric oxide synthase genes, *NOS1*, *NOS2A*, and *NOS3*, have not found any differences between patients with CH and control individuals (Sjostrand et al., 2001; Sjostrand et al., 2002; Rainero et al., 2005). An Italian group performed an association study between polymorphism of hypocretin/orexin pathway genes (*HCRT*, *HCRTR1*, and *HCRTR2*) and the disorder in a large cohort of CH patients (Rainero et al., 2004). A highly significant association between the 1246G > A polymorphism of the *HCRTR2* gene and CH was found. However, these results were not replicated in study of a large cohort of Danish, Italian, and British patients and control subjects (Baumber et al., 2006). It is probable that CH is a complex genetic disorder, with phenotypic and genetic heterogeneity which is compounding attempts at gene identification.

Classification and Diagnostic Criteria

The revised International Classification of Headache Disorders (ICHD-II) classification criteria for CH are listed in Table 14–4.

Differential Diagnosis

In spite of the rather characteristic clinical picture, the differential diagnosis may be difficult in some cases as each of the features of CH can be mimicked by other headaches (see Table 14–5). The main differential diagnoses to consider are as follows: symptomatic causes of CH, other TACs, migraine, and hypnic headache. The differentiation of CH from other TACs is discussed later in the chapter.

Symptomatic CH

Before a diagnosis of CH can be made, secondary headache disorders that mimic CH need to be excluded. Symptomatic CH has been described after infectious, vascular, and neoplastic intracranial lesions. Any atypical features in the history or abnormalities on neurological examination (with the exception of partial Horner's syndrome) warrant further investigations to search for organic causes. A particular issue in this regard emerging from the literature is the importance of pituitary tumors (Levy et al., 2005; Favier et al., 2007).

Migraine

Unilaterality of pain and presence of migrainous and autonomic symptoms are features common to both migraine and CH and differentiating between them can be difficult in some cases. The features that can be useful in distinguishing CH from migraine include the following: relatively short duration of headache, rapid onset and cessation, circadian periodicity, precipitation within an hour, rather than several hours, by alcohol, and clustering of attacks with intervening remissions in ECH.

Hypnic Headache

Hypnic headache typically occurs in aged persons and predominates in females. Patients are awakened from sleep by headaches that are frequently bilateral but maybe unilateral and typically not associated with autonomic features. The headaches are brief, lasting 5–180 minutes and can occur up to three times per night. Effective

TABLE 14–4 The International Classification of Headache Disorders II (ICHD-II) Diagnostic Criteria for Cluster Headache.

Cluster headache has two key forms:
Episodic: occurs in periods lasting 7 days to 1 year separated by pain free periods lasting 1 month or more
Chronic: attacks occur for more than 1 year without remission or with remissions lasting less than 1 month
Headaches must have each of:
A. At least five attacks fulfilling criteria B–E
B. Severe or very severe unilateral orbital, supraorbital, and/or temporal pain lasting 15–180 minutes if untreated
C. Headache is accompanied by at least one of the following:
  1. Ipsilateral conjunctival injection and/or lacrimation
  2. Ipsilateral nasal congestion and/or rhinorrhoea
  3. Ipsilateral eyelid oedema
  4. Ipsilateral forehead and facial sweating
  5. Ipsilateral miosis and/or ptosis
  6. A sense of restlessness or agitation
D. Attacks have a frequency from one every other day to eight per day 2
E. Not attributed to another disorder

Source: Adapted from Headache Classification Committee of The International Headache Society (Headache Classification Committee of The International Headache Society, 2004).

treatments include bedtime doses of lithium, indomethacin, or caffeine (Evers and Goadsby, 2003).

Diagnostic Workup

Given that CH mimics can be extremely difficult to dissect clinically from primary CH, some initial investigation seems appropriate. A magnetic resonance imaging (MRI) scan of the brain would be a reasonable screening investigation with dedicated pituitary views where possible Lesions listed in Table 14–5, which can be sought on their own merits.

Management

The management of CH includes offering advice on general measures to patients, treatment with abortive and preventive agents, and rarely surgery.

General Measures and Patient Education

Patients should be advised to abstain from taking alcohol during the cluster bout. Otherwise, dietary factors seem to have little importance in CH. Anecdotal evidence suggests that patients should be cautioned against prolonged exposure to volatile substances, such as solvents and oil based paints. Patients should be instructed to avoid afternoon naps as sleeping can precipitate attacks in some patients.

Abortive Treatments

The pain of CH builds up very rapidly to such an excruciating intensity that most oral agents are absorbed too slowly to cure the pain within a reasonable period of time. The most efficacious abortive medications are those that involve parentral or pulmonary administration (Table 14–6).

Triptans

Sumatriptan. Subcutaneous sumatriptan 6 mg is the drug of choice in abortive treatment of a cluster attack. A randomized, placebo-controlled, double-blind, crossover study completed in 39 patients (Ekbom et al., 1993) showed that in 74% of attacks, the severity of the headache at 15 minutes reduced in which sumatriptan was administered compared to 26% in which placebo was given. Thirty-six percent of patients were pain-free within 10 minutes of taking sumatriptan, compared to 3%

TABLE 14–5 Differential Diagnoses of Cluster Headache.

Primary headache syndromes
Paroxysmal hemicrania
SUNCT
Hemicrania continua
Migraine
Hypnic headache
Secondary causes of cluster headache
Vascular causes
Carotid artery dissection (Rosebraugh et al., 1997; Mainardi et al., 2002; Razvi et al., 2006) or aneurysm (Greve and Mai, 1988)
Vertebral artery dissection (Cremer et al., 1995) or aneurysm (West and Todman, 1991)
Pseudoaneurysm of intracavernous carotid artery (Koenigsberg et al., 1994)
Anterior communicating artery aneurysm (Sjaastad et al., 1976; Greve and Mai, 1988)
Occipital lobe arteriovenous malformation (AVM) (Mani and Deeter, 1982)
Middle cerebral artery territory AVM (Munoz et al., 1996)
AVM in soft tissue of scalp above ear (Thomas, 1975)
Frontal lobe and corpus callosum AVM (Gawel et al., 1989)
Cervical cord infarction (de la Sayette et al., 1999)
Lateral medullary infarction (Cid et al., 2000)
Frontotemporal subdural hematoma (Formisano et al., 1990)
Tumors
Pituitary tumors (Tfelt-Hansen et al., 1982; Greve and Mai, 1988; Levy et al., 2005; Negoro et al., 2005; Favier et al., 2007)
Parasellar meningioma (Hannerz, 1989)
Sphenoidal meningioma (Lefevre et al., 1984; Molins et al., 1989)
Epidermoid tumor in the prepontine (behind the dorsum sella turcica) (Levyman et al., 1991)
Tentorial meningioma (Taub et al., 1995)
High cervical meningioma (Kuritzky, 1984)
Nasopharyngeal carcinoma (Appelbaum and Noronha, 1989)
Infective causes
Maxillary sinusitis (Molins et al., 1989)
Orbito-sphenoidal aspergillosis (Heidegger et al., 1997)
Herpes zoster ophthalmicus (Sacquegna et al., 1982)
Posttraumatic or surgery
Facial trauma (Lance and Goadsby, 1998)
Following enucleation of eye (Rogado and Graham, 1979; McKinney, 1983; Prusinski et al., 1985; Evers et al., 1997)
Dental causes
Impacted wisdom tooth (Romoli and Cudia, 1988)
Following dental extraction (Soros et al., 2001)
Miscellaneous
Cervical syringomyelia and Chiari malformation (Seijo-Martinez et al., 2004)
Idiopathic intracranial hypertension (Volcy and Tepper, 2006)
Secondary headache syndromes
Tolosa–Hunt syndrome
Temporal arteritis
Raeder's paratrigeminal neuralgia (Goadsby, 2002)

Table 14–6 Abortive Management of Cluster Headache.

Good efficacy	• Oxygen 100% at 7–12 l/minutes for 15–30 minutes • Sumatriptan subcutaneous injection 6 mg (maximum twice daily for the duration of the cluster bout)
Moderate efficacy	• Sumatriptan nasal spray 20 mg or Zolmitriptan nasal spray 5 mg (maximum thrice daily for the duration of the cluster bout) • Octreotide subcutaneous injection 100 μg
Poor efficacy or unproven	• Ergotamine tablets or suppository • Intranasal lidocaine

after placebo. Sumatriptan was well tolerated and there were no serious adverse events.

A double-blind, crossover and randomized study compared sumatriptan 6 and 12 mg with placebo in 134 patients (Ekbom et al., 1993). The 12 mg dose was not more effective than the 6 mg dose and was associated with more side effects.

Two large clinical trials have been performed to assess the effects of long-term administration of subcutaneous sumatriptan. In one study (Ekbom et al., 1995), the safety and efficacy profile of subcutaneous sumatriptan 6 mg was evaluated in 138 patients in the first 3 months of a 2-year open study. They treated a maximum of two attacks each daily, comprising a total of 6353 attacks. Headache relief was obtained at 15 minutes for 96% of the attacks treated. There was no indication of any increase in the interval prior to response or increased frequency of attacks with long-term treatment. Adverse events were quantitatively similar to those seen in migraine trials and did not increase with frequent use of sumatriptan. In the second trial, (Gobel et al., 1998) subcutaneous sumatriptan, administered during a period of 1 year, was evaluated. A total of 2031 attacks in 52 patients were studied. It was highly efficacious in 88% of the patients with no evidence of tachyphylaxis or rebound headaches. The profile of adverse events was comparable to long-term migraine trials. The overall efficacy of subcutaneous sumatriptan was reported to be approximately 8% less in patients with CCH than in patients with ECH.

In summary, subcutaneous sumatriptan 6 mg is a highly effective abortive treatment for cluster headache attacks. It has a rapid effect and high response rate. In CH, unlike in migraine, subcutaneous sumatriptan can be prescribed at a frequency of twice daily, on a long-term basis, if necessary. Although generally well tolerated, sumatriptan is contraindicated in patients with ischemic heart disease or uncontrolled hypertension. Caution must be exercised in patients with CH because the disorder predominates in middle-aged men, who often have risk factors for cardiovascular disease, particularly smoking (Manzoni, 1999).

Intranasal sumatriptan is effective in CH although certainly in less number of patients and generally with a slower onset of action. A randomized, placebo-controlled, double-blind, crossover study completed in 86 patients showed that in 56% of attacks, the severity of the headache for 30 minutes reduced in which sumatriptan nasal spray was administered compared to 26% in which placebo was given (van Vliet et al., 2001). In comparison, in an open randomized crossover trial, 20 mg nasal sumatriptan was compared to 6 mg subcutaneous sumatriptan in 26 patients each of whom was treated for two attacks with the nasal and two attacks with the subcutaneous formulation. At 15 minutes only, 13% of attacks treated with the nasal formulation had been aborted compared to 94% treated with subcutaneous sumatriptan (Hardebo and Dahlof, 1998). The inferior result in the open-label study might have been affected by the lack of blinding. Open labeled studies in CH are of dubious value when the hypothesis is clear and testable with a properly controlled design.

Zolmitriptan. A double-blind, placebo-controlled trial compared the efficacy of oral zolmitriptan 5 and 10 mg for the treatment of acute attacks in ECH and CCH (Bahra et al., 2000). With headache response defined as a two-point reduction on a 5-point pain intensity scale, 30-minute response rates in ECH were 29%, 40%, and 47% following placebo, 5 and 10 mg zolmitriptan, respectively. The difference only reached statistical significance for 10 mg zolmitriptan compared to placebo. In addition, significantly more ECH patients reported mild or no pain at 30 minutes after treatment with 5 and 10 mg zolmitriptan (57% and 60%, respectively) than following placebo (42%). The response rates in CCH patients following treatment with zolmitriptan 5 or 10 mg were not significantly different from placebo. The efficacy of oral zolmitriptan in ECH is modest and does not approach the efficacy or speed of subcutaneous sumatriptan or oxygen, thereby rendering it of limited utility in clinical practice. It may be considered for patients who cannot tolerate subcutaneous or intranasal triptans and oxygen, or those who desire oral medications.

Zolmitriptan nasal spray is more effective than the oral formulation and has an efficacy comparable to nasal sumatriptan. A randomized, placebo-controlled, double-blind, crossover study of 5 and 10 mg zolmitriptan nasal spray completed in 69 patients showed the severity of the headache at *30 minutes* was reduced in 40% and 62% of attacks in which 5 and 10 mg, respectively, were administered compared to 21% in attacks treated with placebo (Cittadini et al., 2006). The response rates were higher in ECH compared to CCH.

Oxygen

Normobaric Oxygen. Oxygen inhalation is safe and clinical experience suggests it is an effective treatment of acute CH. Horton was the first to discover that 100% oxygen inhalation at the onset of attacks alleviates the CH pain (Horton, 1956). Friedman and Mikropoulos also reported on its favorable effect (Friedman and Mikropoulos, 1958). Kudrow noted a significant relief from cluster pain in 75% of 52 randomly selected out-patients treated with 100% oxygen administered through a facial mask at a rate of 7 l/minute for 15 minutes (Kudrow, 1981). Headache relief occurred in 62% of the patients within the first 7 minutes of oxygen inhalation; in 31% within 8–10 minutes, and in 7% within 10–15 minutes. The best results were obtained in ECH patients younger than 50.

Oxygen at 6 l/minute for 15 minutes was compared to air inhalation in a double-blind crossover study of 19 sufferers (Fogan, 1985). Eleven patients used both gases. Nine out of sixteen patients (56%) who used oxygen perceived a complete or substantial relief in 80% or more of their cluster attacks, compared to only 1 of 14 patients (7%) who used air.

In summary, inhalation of 100% oxygen at 7–12 l/minute is rapidly effective in relieving pain in the majority of sufferers. It should be inhaled continuously for 15–20 minutes via a non-rebreathing facial mask. Patients need to be informed that they should cover any apertures on the facemask. If oxygen inhalation is initiated as soon as the attack starts, it often aborts the attack rapidly and entirely (Kudrow, 1981) though some patients find oxygen to be completely effective if taken when the pain is at maximum intensity (Igarashi et al., 1991). Up to 25% of patients noted that oxygen simply delays the attack for minutes to hours rather than completely aborting it (Kudrow, 1981).

The great advantage with oxygen is that it has no established side effects. It can be readily combined with other abortive and preventive treatments. It can be used several times daily as opposed to subcutaneous or intranasal sumatriptan that can only be used up to a maximum of two or three times daily, respectively. The major drawback with oxygen inhalation treatment is the practical limitation imposed by the bulky equipment, and, although small portable cylinders are available, most patients find these cumbersome and inconvenient. Furthermore, it forces the patient to sit still during treatment, a behavior that is usually incompatible with the excruciating pain of CH. Some patients are unable to hold the facemask against the face as skin contact worsens the pain. Patients need to be cautioned that oxygen is a highly combustible material and fire precautions need to be observed; in particular, the danger of smoking in its presence need to be pointed out. On long-term treatment only a few responders seem to continue using oxygen, especially chronic sufferers. Gallagher and colleagues (1996) found that 76% of patients had significant relief but only

31% stayed on oxygen for subsequent headaches. Further studies are needed to investigate patients' preferences of symptomatic treatment.

Hyperbaric oxygen. Weiss and colleagues (1989) first reported the effectiveness of hyperbaric oxygen as an abortive agent in CH. Subsequently, an open trial of hyperbaric oxygen (1.3ATA) in 14 patients reported that 18 cluster attacks (12 spontaneous, and 6 induced by sublingual nitroglycerine) resolved rapidly, with complete relief achieved within a mean of 6.2 minutes (range: 30 seconds–13 minutes) (Porta et al., 1991). A small placebo-controlled study of hyperbaric oxygen (2ATA) delivered during 30 minutes demonstrated efficacy in six of seven patients within 5 to 30 minutes (Di Sabato et al., 1993). In addition, in three of six responders the cluster bout was completely interrupted whereas in the other three responders the cluster bout was partially interrupted for 3–6 days. Subsequently, hyperbaric oxygen (2.5ATA) was tested as a preventive treatment in CH. No significant effect was obtained in a double-blind placebo-controlled crossover study on 12 episodic and 4 chronic sufferers (Nilsson Remahl et al., 2002).

In summary, hyperbaric oxygen appears to be effective as an abortive agent in CH, which is not surprising considering the beneficial effect of normobaric oxygen. It would not be surprising if hyperbaric oxygen was more effective than normobaric oxygen though this need to be confirmed in a properly conducted trial. With the currently available data, there is very weak evidence for a prophylactic effect of hyperbaric oxygen in CH. The clinical utility of this treatment modality is likely to remain limited in the foreseeable future because of the lack of general availability and the other practical limitations already outlined for normobaric oxygen.

Topical Local Anesthetics Intranasal cocaine and lignocaine have been used in CH for anesthesia of the pterygopalatine (sphenopalatine) fossa region.

Cocaine. Intranasal cocaine has been reported to be effective at aborting nitroglycerine-induced cluster attacks in an open-label trial in 10 patients (Barre, 1982). The patients applied 50 mg of cocaine flakes on a cotton swab in the region of the ipsilateral pterygopalatine ganglion. Nine patients experienced 80% or more reduction in the intensity of their induced CH within $2\frac{1}{2}$ minutes.

More recently, 10% cocaine (1 ml; 50 mg per application) was reported to be effective at aborting nitroglycerine-induced cluster attacks in a double-blind, placebo-controlled study in nine patients (Costa et al., 2000). Cocaine or saline was applied using a cotton swab in the area corresponding to the pterygopalatine fossa, *under anterior rhinoscopy*. The treatment was applied *bilaterally* for 5 minutes. All patients responded to intranasal cocaine with complete cessation of pain occurring after 31.3 ± 13.1 minutes.

Cocaine does not have widespread medicinal uses because of its addictive potential; lidocaine (lignocaine) is preferentially used.

Lidocaine (Lignocaine). Kittrelle and colleagues (1985) first reported that lignocaine solution applied topically to the region of the pterygopalatine fossa alleviated the pain of the cluster attack. In an open-label trial of intranasal lignocaine 4% solution, four of five patients obtained rapid relief of nitroglycerine-induced CHs. Lignocaine was also effective in relieving spontaneous attacks. Subsequently, Hardebo and Elner (1987) reported on the use of intranasal lidocaine 4% solution in an open-label trial in 19 patients. Seven patients (37%) reported a 50% or greater response; seven patients (37%) reported a response less than 50%, and five patients (26%) reported no benefit.

Robbins (1995) reported on the use of four to six *sprays* of lidocaine 4% in the nostril ipsilateral to the painful side in an open-label trial in 30 patients. Eight patients (27%) reported moderate relief, eight patients (27%) obtained mild relief, and 14 patients (46%) stated that they had no relief from lidocaine. No patient reported excellent relief. These findings were considerably poorer than those of Kittrelle and colleagues (1985) and Hardebo and Elner (1987). This poorer efficacy reported by Robbins may, at least in part, be attributable to the formulation used; Robbins used a spray rather than the nose drops used in other studies (Kudrow and Kudrow, 1995).

Recently, 10% lidocaine was reported to be effective at aborting nitroglycerine-induced cluster attacks in a double-blind, placebo-controlled study in nine patients (Costa et al., 2000). Lidocaine or saline was applied using a cotton swab in the area corresponding to the pterygopalatine fossa, *under anterior rhinoscopy*. The treatment was applied *bilaterally* for 5 minutes. All patients responded rapidly to intranasal lignocaine with complete cessation of pain occurring after 37.0 ± 7.8 minutes. The authors partly attributed these results to bilateral application of lignocaine and to the procedure of drug administration, which involved anterior rhinoscopy. Although the 100% response rate appears to be excellent, the stated mean time to cessation of pain is unacceptably long for the majority of patients.

Ergot Derivatives

Ergotamine. Horton (1941) was the first to describe the beneficial effect of intravenous (IV) ergotamine in the abortive treatments of CH in a case report. Subsequently, Kunkle and colleagues (1952) reported the rapid termination of cluster attacks in four patients with IV ergotamine. Horton and colleagues (1948) reported "excellent" results in open-label use of oral Cafergot (ergotamine tartrate 1 mg and caffeine 100 mg) in 10 out of 14 patients. A subsequently published open trial of Cafergot suppositories reported a considerably lower response rate of 4 out of 20 patients (Magee et al., 1952). Friedman and Mikropoulos (1958) reported that oral, suppository, or IV preparations of ergotamine were "effective to a greater or lesser extent" in 30 out of 35 patients.

Kudrow noted a significant relief from cluster pain in 70% of 50 randomly selected outpatients treated with sublingual ergotamine at 15 minutes in a crossover study with 100% oxygen (Kudrow, 1981). The peak response to sublingual ergotamine occurred within 10–12 minutes of treatment. Oxygen was regarded as superior to ergotamine, especially because there were no complications and contraindications to its use.

Inhaled ergotamine, used in an open-label manner, has been reported to produce an "excellent" effect, in 11 of 13 patients (Speed, 1960). Another open-label study reported that inhaled ergotamine given to 12 patients produced relief from pain within 30 minutes in 71% of 114 attacks (Graham et al., 1960). Kudrow (1980) reported that 79 out of 100 patients obtained "significant relief" from sublingual or inhaled ergotamine preparations.

There are no well-controlled trials of ergotamine in abortive treatment of CH. Inhaled, subcutaneous, intramuscular, or IV injections of ergotamine are now not widely available. Oral or rectal ergotamine is generally too slow in onset to provide meaningful relief in a timely manner, especially when compared to the rapidity of onset of action of subcutaneous sumatriptan and high-dose oxygen. Moreover, ergotamine is a potent vasoconstrictor. It is contraindicated in patients with coronary or peripheral vascular disease, arterial hypertension, and severe disease of the liver and kidney. It cannot be used concurrently with triptans, dihydroergotamine (DHE), and methysergide.

Dihydroergotamine. Parenteral DHE has been considered to be an effective abortive agent for CH for some time (Horton, 1952; Friedman and Mikropoulos, 1958). DHE is available in injectable and intranasal formulations. Although there are no controlled trials of injectable DHE, clinical experience has demonstrated that IV administration provides prompt and effective relief of CH within 15 minutes (Dodick et al., 2000). However, given the frequency and the rapid peak intensity of cluster attacks, IV DHE is not a feasible long-term solution. The intramuscular and subcutaneous routes of administration provide slower relief, though they have the advantage that they can be self-administered.

DHE nasal spray 1 mg has been studied in a double-blind, placebo-controlled, crossover trial in 25 patients (Andersson and Jespersen, 1986). There was no difference in the headache frequency or duration, but the pain intensity was significantly reduced with DHE compared to placebo. The dosage used (1 mg) was lower than the recommended dosage for migraine (2 mg) and less than the currently available preparations of DHE nasal spray (4 mg). Therefore, DHE nasal spray at a dose of 2 or 4 mg may be more effective than 1 mg although this needs to be studied in a controlled fashion.

Somatostatin Analogs

Somatostatin. Two studies have evaluated the abortive effect of somatostatin in CH. In the first study, IV somatostatin (25 μg/minute for 20 minutes) was compared to treatment with ergotamine (250 μg intramuscularly) or placebo in a double-blind trial comprising 72 attacks in eight patients (Sicuteri et al., 1984). Infusion of somatostatin reduced the maximal pain intensity and the duration of pain significantly compared to placebo, and to a degree comparable to intramuscular ergotamine. In another randomized, double-blind study subcutaneous somatostatin was compared with ergotamine (Geppetti et al., 1985). Five patients were treated for three attacks by each of the drugs. Subcutaneous somatostatin and ergotamine were equally beneficial as regards effects on maximal pain intensity and the pain area, but somatostatin was less effective in reducing the duration of pain. This limited evidence of the beneficial effect of somatostatin needs to be explored further in properly controlled and adequately powered studies. The problem with native somatostatin as a potential abortive agent for CH is that its short half-life of several minutes necessitates an IV infusion, limiting its utility in clinical practice.

Octreotide. Octreotide, a somatostatin analog with a half-life of approximately 1.5 hours, is a potentially attractive agent as it can be given subcutaneously. A randomized, placebo-controlled, double-blind, crossover study of subcutaneous octreotide 100 μg completed in 46 patients showed that the severity of the headache at 30 minutes reduced in 52% of attacks in which octreotide was administered compared to 36% in which placebo was given (Matharu, Levy, et al., 2004). Octreotide was well tolerated and there were no serious adverse events. This was the first adequately powered and controlled study to demonstrate the effectiveness of a somatostatin analog in the treatment of acute CH attacks and proves the concept that somatostatin analogs offer a novel therapeutic approach to the treatment of acute CHs. In clinical practice, octreotide may have a particular utility in patients who are unresponsive to or intolerant of $5\text{-HT}_{1B/1D}$ agonists and oxygen and as an alternative to oxygen in patients with cardiovascular disease.

Olanzapine Olanzapine has been evaluated as a CH abortive agent in an open-label trial (Rozen, 2001). Oral olanzapine at a dose ranging from 2.5 to 10 mg was administered to 5 patients (4 with CCH and 1 with ECH). It reduced the severity of cluster pain by at least 80% in 4 of 5 patients, and 2 patients were rendered pain-free. The pain was typically alleviated within 20 minutes and the treatment response was reported to be consistent across multiple attacks. The only adverse effect was sleepiness. This result needs to be replicated in a double-blind, placebo-controlled study.

Analgesics Opiates, nonsteroidal antiinflammatory drugs (NSAIDs) and combination analgesics have no routine role in the acute management of CH. The pain of CH builds up very rapidly and to such an excruciating intensity that most oral medications are too slowly absorbed to act within a reasonable period of time. Furthermore, on prolonged treatment with high dosages, problems with habituation and toxicity may develop. In one study of 60 patients, only 21% reported significant relief of pain with oral analgesics, but 65% continued using analgesics despite their lack of effectiveness (Gallagher et al., 1996). The authors concluded that CH patients preferred to use oral analgesics for reasons that are not solely to do with the relief of pain.

A recent study reported the development of medication overuse headache in 17 patients (4%) out of a cohort of 430 CH sufferers (Paemeleire et al., 2006). These patients developed medication overuse headache in association with overuse of a wide range of monotherapies or varying combinations of simple analgesic, caffeine, opioids, ergotamine, and triptans. Remarkably, 15 of these 17 patients had a personal or family history, or both, of migraine. The other two patients gave a family history of unspecified headache. Medication withdrawal was attempted and successful in 13 patients. Hence, CH patients should be carefully monitored, especially those with a personal or family history of migraine. Acute treatments not supported by evidence, such as opiates, combination analgesics, and oral triptans should be avoided particularly in patients with a personal or family history of migraine. However, in patients who develop medication overuse headache with intranasal or subcutaneous triptans, withdrawal of these agents should only be considered if there is an effective strategy to control the problem; otherwise, it may be unethical to subject the patient to the excruciating pain of CH.

Preventive Treatments

The aim of preventive therapy is to produce a rapid suppression of attacks and to maintain that remission with minimal side effects until the cluster bout is over or for a longer period in CCH patients. Preventive therapy in CH is partly based on clinical experience as very few randomized controlled clinical trials have been performed. The preventive treatments that are commonly advocated include the following: verapamil, lithium, methysergide, ergotamine, corticosteroids, and valproic acid. Recently, several new entities have been reported to be effective preventive agents for CH. The established and emerging preventive agents are discussed below.

Verapamil Verapamil was first reported to be effective as a preventive in CH by Meyer and Hardenberg (1983). In an open trial employing verapamil at doses of 160–720 mg daily in five CCH patients, a reduction in the mean monthly frequency of headaches was reported in all patients. In a further open-label study employing verapamil at doses of 160–480 mg daily in 34 CCH patients, 79% of patients reported a decrease in frequency and severity of the headaches (Jonsdottir et al., 1987). In another open trial employing verapamil at doses of 240–600 mg daily in ECH and 120–1200 mg daily in CCH, an improvement of more than 75% was noted in 33 of 48 (69%) patients (Gabai and Spierings, 1989).

A double-blind, crossover trial comparing verapamil 360 mg daily to the then standard prophylactic drug lithium 900 mg daily, each given for 8 weeks, found equivalent effects in the 24 CCH patients who completed the trial (Bussone et al., 1990). Verapamil and lithium were superior to placebo. Verapamil caused fewer side effects and had a shorter latency period. A double-blind, placebo-controlled trial evaluated the efficacy of verapamil 360 mg daily during a 2-week period in 30 ECH patients (Leone, D'Amico, et al., 2000). Fifteen patients were randomized to the verapamil group whereas the remaining 15 patients were treated with placebo. A statistically significant reduction in headache frequency and analgesic consumption was seen in the verapamil-treated patients, with a greater reduction in the second week of treatment. At the end of 2 weeks, 80% of the verapamil-treated group showed an improvement of greater than 50% in daily headache frequency, whereas no responders were observed in the placebo group.

In summary, verapamil is the preventive drug of choice in both ECH and CCH where the bout is sufficiently long to establish a suitable dose. Clinical experience has clearly demonstrated that higher doses than those used in cardiological indications are needed. Dosages commonly employed are 240–960 mg daily in divided doses. It is unproven clinical experience that standard preparations of verapamil are more effective than the modified-release formulations (Krabbe and Steiner, 2000). Verapamil can cause cardiac arrhythmias by slowing conduction in the atrioventricular node (Singh and Nademanee, 1987). Observing for PR interval prolongation on electrocardiogram (EKG) can monitor potential development of heart block, although it is a coarse measure. There is only one formal guideline in the literature for the titration of the verapamil dose (Matharu and Goadsby, 2002b). This guideline states that a baseline EKG should be performed before starting patients on verapamil 80 mg three times daily and thereafter the total daily dose is increased in increments of 80 mg every 10–14 days. An EKG should be performed prior to each increment and at least 10 days after the last dose change. The dose is increased until the cluster attacks are suppressed, side effects intervene or the maximum dose of 960 mg daily is achieved. An audit of a cohort of patients treated using this guideline demonstrated that 18% developed arrhythmias (first- and second-degree heart block, junctional rhythm, and right bundle-branch block) and 37% developed bradycardia, of whom 4% required cessation of treatment (Cohen et al., 2006a). This study highlights the importance of careful monitoring of patients on verapamil. Constipation is the most common side effect, but dizziness, ankle swelling, nausea, and fatigue may also occur. β-Blockers should not be given concurrently.

Lithium The effectiveness of lithium in psychiatric conditions of a cyclical nature, such as manic-depressive psychosis and seasonal affective disorder, led Ekbom (1974, 1977) to try this agent in CH, in view of its striking circannual and circadian periodicity. Lithium was administered to 5 patients (3 chronic and 2 episodic) in an open-label fashion. The lithium dose was adjusted until a serum lithium concentration of 0.7–1.2

mmol/l was achieved. In all three CCH patients there was an immediate, partial remission of the headache. Withdrawal of the drug resulted in an increase in intensity and frequency of the headaches. A second period of treatment again resulted in a definite improvement. In the two ECH patients, lithium had only a slight or no effect on the headaches.

The effectiveness of lithium was subsequently suggested in several unblinded series of CH patients. Ekbom (1981) reviewed the open-trials of lithium. Collectively, in more than 28 clinical trials involving 468 patients, good to excellent results were found in 236 (78%) of 304 CCH patients. The response to lithium in patients with ECH was less robust than in CCH, with good efficacy having been obtained in 103 (63%) of a total of 164 patients treated.

Most unblinded trials used a lithium dose of 600–1200 mg daily. Lithium was often effective at serum concentrations (0.4–0.8 mEq/l) less than that usually required for the treatment of bipolar disorder. Patients who improved on lithium often showed dramatic relief within the first week (Kudrow, 1977; Mathew, 1978; Ekbom, 1981). Manzoni, Bono, and colleagues (1983) assessed the long-term therapeutic efficacy of lithium in 18 patients with CCH and reported that it appears to be durable for up to 4 years after treatment. On interruption or cessation of lithium therapy in patients with CCH, a transition to ECH has been recognized. Some patients eventually become resistant to lithium.

Lithium has also been evaluated in two randomized, double-blind trials. A double-blind, crossover trial comparing verapamil 360 mg daily to lithium 900 mg daily, each given for 8 weeks, found equivalent effects in the 24 CCH patients who completed the trial (Bussone et al., 1990). Verapamil and lithium were superior to placebo. A double-blind, placebo-controlled, randomized, parallel group trial of sustained relief lithium 800 mg daily in 27 patients (13 on lithium and 14 on placebo) with ECH assessed efficacy at 1 week after treatment was begun. Cessation of attacks within 1 week occurred in 2 patients in each group, whereas substantial improvement was noted in 6 (43%) of 14 patients on placebo and 8 (62%) of 13 patients on lithium. Lithium treatment was associated with a subjective improvement rate, but this was not statistically significant in comparison to the placebo group. The authors made an assumption at onset of the trial that the placebo response would be zero. This assumption turned out to flawed and, consequently, the study was inadequately powered to test the proposed hypothesis. Hence, it had been assumed that placebo response in prophylactic studies of CH was insubstantial. This flawed assumption was highlighted by another trial recently published (El Amrani, Massiou, et al., 2002). If nothing else, both studies teach a useful lesson for future trial designs.

In summary, lithium is an effective agent for CH prophylaxis, although the response is less robust in ECH than CCH. Most patients will benefit from dosages between 600 and 1200 mg daily. Lithium has the potential for many side effects and has a narrow therapeutic window. Side effects of lithium include weakness, nausea, thirst, tremor, slurred speech, and blurred vision. Toxicity is manifested by nausea, vomiting, anorexia, diarrhea, and neurological signs of confusion, nystagmus, ataxia, extrapyramidal signs, and seizures. Hypothyroidism and polyuria (nephrogenic diabetes insipidus) can occur with a long-term use. Polymorphonuclear leukocytosis may occur and be mistaken for occult infection. Renal and thyroid function tests need to be performed prior to and during treatment. The concomitant use of NSAIDs, diuretics, and carbamazepine is contraindicated.

Serotonergic Agonists and Antagonists

Methysergide. Methysergide is an ergot alkaloid, which is an antagonist at $5HT_{2A}$, $5HT_{2B}$, and $5HT_{2C}$ receptors and an agonist at $5HT_{1B/1D}$ receptors. It was first reported to be effective in CH by Sicuteri (1959). Subsequently, several authors confirmed this observation in open-label trials of this agent. The open-trials of methysergide were reviewed by Curran and colleagues (1967) who noted that methysergide, used at 3–12 mg/day, was effective in 329 (73%) of 451 patients with ECH and CCH.

Subsequently, Kudrow (1980) reported that, in open-label use, methysergide was effective in 50 (65%) of 77 ECH patients and 3 (20%) of 15 CCH patients but the drug appears to lose its effectiveness with repeated use in up to 20% of patients.

However, Krabbe (1989) reported a limited prophylactic benefit with methysergide, used in an open-label manner, in both ECH and CCH. The efficacy of methysergide (used at up to 12 mg/day) was examined prospectively in 42 patients (16 episodic and 26 chronic). Thirteen of the fourty two patients had good or excellent benefits, but two of these thirteen patients had severe side effects. Thus, methysergide was beneficial without side effects in 11 (26%) of 42 patients. There was no significant difference in treatment response between the episodic (25%) and chronic (27%) groups. In addition, a retrospective analysis of 164 patients treated with methysergide demonstrated a satisfactory effectiveness in only 44 (26%).

In summary, methysergide is indicated for the treatment of CH although the efficacy data from the open trials is inconsistent. It is available in Europe except Germany and Canada, but has been discontinued in USA. Doses up to 12 mg daily can be used if tolerated. To minimize side effects, patients should start with a low dose and increase the dose gradually. Common short-term side effects include nausea, vomiting, dizziness, muscle cramps, abdominal pain, and peripheral edema. Uncommon but troublesome side effects are caused by vasoconstriction (coronary or peripheral arterial insufficiency), which usually necessitate cessation of therapy with this drug. Prolonged treatment has been associated with fibrotic reactions (retroperitoneal, pulmonary, pleural, and cardiac) though these are rare (Graham et al., 1966). Ideally, the drug should only be used in patients with short cluster bouts, preferably less than 3–4 months. If prolonged use is intended then the risk of fibrotic reactions can be minimized by giving the drug for 6 months followed by a 1-month holiday before starting again. To avoid a sudden increase in headache frequency when methysergide is stopped, the patient should be weaned off during a 1-week period. Some authorities use methysergide on a continuous basis with careful monitoring, which includes auscultation of the heart and yearly echocardiogram, chest x-ray, and abdominal MRI and relevant blood tests, including biochemistry and 24-hour urine collections (Raskin, 1988). All patients receiving methysergide should remain under the supervision of the treating physician and be examined regularly for the development of visceral fibrosis or vascular complications.

Contraindications to the use of methysergide include pregnancy, peripheral vascular disorders, severe arteriosclerosis, coronary artery disease, severe hypertension, thrombophlebitis or cellulitis of the legs, peptic ulcer disease, fibrotic disorders, lung diseases, collagen disease, liver or renal function impairment, and valvular heart disease (Silberstein, 1998).

Ergotamine. Ekbom (1947) first reported the use of ergotamine tartrate for the prophylactic treatment of CH. Sixteen patients were given ergotamine at the dose of 2–3 mg/day for 1–4 weeks of whom thirteen had considerably improved. Later it was reported that a rectal suppository of ergotamine 2 mg and caffeine 100 mg or intramuscular injections in doses of 0.25–0.5 mg at bedtime were effective in preventing nocturnal attacks (Symonds, 1956). Ergotamine was widely used as the first choice prophylaxis until the efficacy of lithium and verapamil became evident.

Regular administration of ergotamine 2–4 mg/day for 2–3 weeks may be useful. If the patient has nocturnal attacks, 1–2 mg may be given at night in the form of tablets or suppositories. If the pattern of attacks is predictable, the dose can be given 30–60 minutes prior to the expected attacks. The medication needs to be carefully monitored so that the total weekly dose is not too large. Ergotamine should not be combined with DHE, methysergide, or triptans.

Dihydroergotamine. Repetitive IV DHE administered in an inpatient setting during a period of 3 days has been reported to be very useful in some patients with both ECH and CCH. In a study of 54 patients with intractable CH (23 episodic and 31 chronic) open-label use of repetitive IV DHE rendered all patients headache-free (Mather et al., 1991). At 12 months follow-up, 83% and 39% of ECH and CCH patients, respectively, remained free of headache.

Triptans. There is no controlled evidence to support the use of oral sumatriptan in CH. Sumatriptan 100 mg three times daily taken prior to an anticipated onset of an attack or at regular times does not prevent the attack and, therefore, it should not be used for CH prophylaxis (Monstad et al., 1995).

Recently, several cases have been described in whom the open-label prophylactic use of naratriptan (Eekers and Koehler, 2001; Loder, 2002; Mulder and Spierings, 2002), frovatriptan (Siow et al., 2004), and eletriptan (Wober et al., 2002; Zebenholzer et al., 2004) was effective. Double-blind, placebo-controlled studies are needed to confirm the efficacy and safety of these triptans as a preventive drug in CH.

Ergots, triptans, and methysergide. There is a considerable issue surrounding the use of ergot derivates and triptans with methysergide. This is not at all an easy subject. It is usually recommended that ergotamine or DHE should not be taken concomitantly with methysergide, whereas other vasoconstrictive agents should only be used with caution. Methysergide is an ergot derivative (Berde and Schild, 1978), but is a weak vasoconstrictor when compared with ergotamine (Garrison, 1990). It is demethylated in vivo to methylergonovine, to which it may owe some of its activity (Saxena and Den Boer, 1991). There are no reported prospective drug-interaction studies between methysergide and sumatriptan. In some of the early clinical studies with sumatriptan, methysergide continued to be used (Blakeborough et al., 1993). Eighty patients were taking either of methysergide or pizotifen, both serotonin $5HT_2$ antagonists. They had used either sumatriptan injections (n = 38) or tablets (n = 42). There was insufficient power to analyse this group but they had a similar adverse event profile (Blakeborough et al., 1993). The most worrisome case that has been reported was that of a 43 year old woman who experienced a myocardial infarction while taking methysergide and sumatriptan. (Liston et al., 1999). She had a history of migraine without aura and atypical chest pain attributed to gastroesophageal reflux. She had controlled hypertension. Coronary angiography revealed a 50% block of the left anterior descending coronary artery that was treated by stenting. In retrospect sumatriptan was contraindicated in this patient because of the ischemic heart disease, although one might argue that this was a difficult diagnostic issue. For CH we are unaware of any similar case. Thus, the combined use of ergot derivates or sumatriptan with methysergide must remain a clinical decision-based on the balance of the very considerable benefit, particularly for sumatriptan and DHE, and the concomitant use of methysergide, with each case judged on its merits.

Corticosteroids The use of corticosteroids in CH was first reported by Horton (1952) who found that cortisone at doses of 100 mg/day was effective in only 4 of 21 patients.

The effectiveness of prednisone in stopping bouts of CH was established in a double-blind trial by Jammes (1975). Couch and Ziegler (1978) reported that prednisone 10–80 mg/day employed in 19 CH patients (9 episodic and 10 chronic) provided greater than 50% relief in 14 patients (73%) and complete relief in 11 (58%) patients. Recurrence of headaches was reported in 79% of patients when the prednisone dose was tapered. Kudrow (1980) reported that, of 77 episodic cluster patients unresponsive to methysergide, prednisone relieved 77% and partially improved 12%. Prednisone was also found to provide marked relief in 40% of CCH patients and was more effective than methysergide in this patient group. In some European countries, prednisone has been discontinued and instead prednisolone is used, with response rates comparable to those reported for prednisone (unpublished observations)

Dexamethasone at a dose of 4 mg twice daily for 2 weeks followed by 4 mg/day for 1 week has also been shown to be effective (Anthony and Daher, 1992).

In summary, corticosteroids (prednisone, prednisolone, and dexamethasone) are highly efficacious and the most rapid-acting of the prophylactic agents. As in other disorders, the use of corticosteroids is contraindicated by a past history of tuberculosis or psychotic disturbance. Furthermore, caution has to be exercised in their use because of the potential for serious side effects. In this regard, bony problems with steroid use have been reviewed, and the shortest course of prednisolone reported to be associated with osteonecrosis of the femoral head is a 30-day course. Furthermore, courses of adrenocorticotrophic hormone have produced osteonecrosis after 16 days, and dexamethasone after 7 days (Mirzai et al., 1999). Thus, a tapering course of prednisolone or prednisone for 21 days is prudent. Unfortunately, relapse almost invariably occurs as the dose is tapered. For this reason, steroids are used as an initial therapy in conjunction with preventives, until the latter are effective.

Valproic acid Hering and Kuritzky (1989) evaluated the effectiveness of sodium valproate (valproic acid) as preventive therapy in 15 patients with CH in an open-label clinical trial. Thirteen patients with ECH received sodium valproate between 600 and 2000 mg/day for up to 6 months and the two with the chronic subtype received 600–1200 mg/day. Sodium valproate was effective in 11 of the 15 patients (73%). In 9 patients, it controlled the pain completely, and in the remaining 6 patients, including the 2 with CCH, it afforded 72%–85% improvement. Apart from mild nausea in three patients, sodium valproate was generally well tolerated.

In another open-label trial, sodium valproate was administered at variable doses to 26 patients with ECH or CCH (Freitag et al., 2000). The 21 patients with CCH received a mean daily dose of 850 mg/day for a mean period of 11.1 months. The five patients with ECH were treated at a mean dose of 826 mg/day. With prophylaxis, the 28-day CH frequency decreased by a mean of 58.6% and 53.9% among ECH and CCH patients, respectively. Five patients experienced adverse events of rash, hair loss, tiredness, nausea, and tremor.

A retrospective study examined the clinical efficacy and safety profile of sodium valproate used as monotherapy and polytherapy for prophylaxis in CH (Gallagher et al., 2002). The authors reviewed the medical notes of 49 CH patients. Sodium valproate (500–1500 mg/day) was administered as monotherapy in 13 patients and in combination with another prophylactic treatment in 36 patients. Seventy-three percent of patients (11 on monotherapy and 25 on polytherapy) showed improvement, though the extent of improvement was not quantified. Twenty-two percent of patients reported side effects.

El Amrani, Massiou, and colleagues (2002b) have reported the results of a double-blind, placebo-controlled, parallel group study of sodium valproate (1000–2000 mg/day) in the prophylaxis of CH. Ninety-six patients were included, 50 in the sodium valproate group (37 episodic, 11 chronic, and 2 unspecified) and 46 in the placebo group (36 episodic, 6 chronic, and 3 unspecified). After a 7-day run-in period, patients were treated for 2 weeks. The primary end-point was an at least 50% reduction in the number of attacks per week between the run-in period and the last week of treatment. There was no significant difference between the two groups, with improvement in 50% of the active treatment group and 62% in the placebo group. However, the two groups were imbalanced in that the mean duration of previous cluster bouts in the patients with ECH was shorter in the placebo group (62.4 days) compared to the treatment group (78.3 days). Consequently, the high success rate observed in the placebo group was probably attributable to the spontaneous remission of the cluster bout in addition to a true placebo response. The authors remarked that no valid conclusion about the efficacy of sodium valproate in the prophylaxis of CH could be drawn because of this methodological issue.

Topiramate Recently, five open-label studies have been reported on the efficacy of topiramate in the preventive treatment of CH (Wheeler and Carrazana, 1999; Forderreuther et al., 2002; Mathew et al., 2002; Lainez et al., 2003; Leone et al., 2003). These studies have tried topiramate in a total of 89 patients: 56 patients with ECH, 32 with CCH, and, 1 with cluster-tic syndrome. A moderate or marked effectiveness has been reported in 44 of these patients (49%). The dose of topiramate used in these studies ranged from 25 to 250 mg daily. Two of the studies reported that treatment with topiramate was associated with rapid improvement, usually within 1–4 weeks (Wheeler and Carrazana, 1999; Lainez et al., 2003). Data on adverse effects was available in 77 patients, of whom 44 (57%) reported some side effects. Thirty three patients reported mild side effects whereas eleven reported significant or intolerable side effects, usually at doses higher than 100 mg daily.

These favorable preliminary reports need to be followed up by properly controlled studies. In the interim, topiramate appears to be a reasonable treatment option in patients with otherwise refractory CH though its use may be limited by its side effect profile. Somnolence, dizziness, cognitive symptoms, and ataxia are commonly reported. Mood changes, psychosis, weight loss, and glaucoma have also been reported. Paresthesias and nephrolithiasis can occur because of the weak carbonic anhydrase inhibition of the drug.

Gabapentin Gabapentin was first reported to be effective as a prophylactic agent in two case reports of CH (Ahmed, 2000; Tay et al., 2001). Subsequently, Leandri and colleagues (2001) tried gabapentin 900 mg/day in an open-label fashion in eight patients with ECH and four with CCH. All patients were rendered pain-free within 8 days of initiating therapy. Patients with ECH discontinued gabapentin after 60 days of treatment without recurrence of the attacks. The four patients with CCH remained pain-free at follow-up of 4 months. These early reports also need to be confirmed by a placebo-controlled study of gabapentin in CH. The only side effect reported was drowsiness in two patients. This astonishingly high response rate needs to be reproduced in controlled trials.

Melatonin Melatonin is a sensitive surrogate marker of circadian rhythm in humans and is under the control of the suprachiasmatic nucleus (Brzezinski, 1997). Serum melatonin levels are reduced in patients with CH, particularly during a cluster bout (Waldenlind et al., 1987; Leone et al., 1995). Based on these observations, the striking circadian periodicity of CH, and the importance of the hypothalamus in the pathogenesis of this disorder (May, Bahra, et al., 1998) the efficacy of melatonin has been evaluated as a prophylactic agent in CH.

Leone and colleagues (1996) performed a double-blind pilot study of melatonin versus placebo in the prophylaxis of CH. Twenty patients with CH (eighteen episodic, and two chronic) participated in study. Patients with ECH entered the study between the second and tenth day of their cluster bout. After a run-in period of 1 week without prophylactic treatment, patients were randomized to receive 10 mg melatonin or placebo for 2 weeks. The authors found that, compared to the run-in period, there was a reduction in the mean number of daily attacks and a strong trend toward reduced analgesic consumption in the melatonin group but not in the placebo group. Five patients in the melatonin group responded to the treatment, with cessation of CHs after 5 days of treatment. No patient in the placebo group responded.

Recently, Peres and Rozen (2001) reported two CCH patients inadequately managed on verapamil 640 mg daily who were rendered pain-free with add-on therapy with melatonin 9 mg daily. The authors concluded that melatonin could be an adjunctive treatment for CH prophylaxis, although double-blind, placebo-controlled trials are necessary to confirm this view.

Leuprolide The utility of leuprolide (a synthetic slow-release gonadotropin-releasing hormone analogue) as a prophylactic agent in CH was investigated in a single-blind, placebo-controlled, randomized, parallel study in 60 men with CCH (Nicolodi et al., 1993). Thirty patients were administered a single dose of leuprolide 3.75 mg intramuscularly, and the remaining thirty patients were administered placebo. Leuprolide was found to induce a significant decrease of pain intensity and attack duration and frequency. The maximum effect induced by leuprolide was a 63% decrease of the pain intensity, and the mean duration of the attacks decreased from 94 minutes/day to 9.4 minutes/day. Twelve of thirty leuprolide-treated subjects reported resolution of pain 17 days after drug administration, whereas no effect was reported in four subjects. The remaining leuprolide-treated subjects reported a general benefit that increased over time. The therapeutic benefits of leuprolide began after 10 days and peaked at 21–30 days after treatment. The mean duration of improvement was 3.25 months. At relapse, a second dose of leuprolide induced a similar amelioration. The main side effect of active treatment was decrease in libido in 6 (20%) of 30 patients. Endocrinological measurements during treatment demonstrated an initial increase followed by a marked decrease of testosterone and luteinizing hormone.

Despite relatively good controlled evidence for the efficacy of leuprolide, it is rarely used in clinical practice.

Intranasal capsaicin and civamide Intranasal capsaicin was first reported to be beneficial as a prophylactic agent in CH by Sicuteri and colleagues (1989). In this open-label preliminary study, capsaicin 300 μg was applied once daily for 5 consecutive days into both nostrils of CH patients. The number of spontaneously occurring attacks was significantly reduced in the 60 days after the end of capsaicin treatment. The group subsequently reported their findings in 45 (35 episodic, 10 chronic) CH patients (Sicuteri et al., 1990). Out of 35 patients 12 with ECH received the vehicle only; this was considered as a placebo. A significant reduction in the number of attacks was observed during the observation period of 60 days. In the 23 ECH patients treated with capsaicin, 13

(57%) had complete disappearance of the attacks while 5 (22%) had a 75% reduction in the number of attacks. In the 10 CCH patients 7 (70%) displayed transient benefit, being rendered pain-free for a period of 28–40 days following treatment, while the remaining three patients derived no benefit from treatment. Intranasal capsaicin produces an intense burning sensation, lacrimation and rhinorrhoea that last for approximately 20 minutes (though these symptoms progressively decrease and disappear after five to eight applications). Consequently, placebo-controlled studies are not easily performed as patients are readily unblinded.

In a double-blind, placebo-controlled study in 13 patients, 7 patients were treated with capsaicin 0.025% twice daily for 7 days in the nostril ipsilateral to the pain while the 6 control patients received camphor 3% to simulate the painful irritation associated with topical capsaicin (Marks et al., 1993). The capsaicin-treated group experienced significantly less severe headaches over the 8 days following treatment in comparison to the 7 days during treatment. This improvement was not observed in the placebo-treated group.

In an attempted single-blind study designed to verify the difference in efficacy of treatment with nasal capsaicin, depending on the side of application, 26 ECH patients received capsaicin on the symptomatic side while 26 patients were treated on the nonsymptomatic side (Fusco et al., 1994b). Seventy percent of the episodic patients, treated on the ipsilateral side, experienced a significant ecrease in the number of attacks for 50–60 days after treatment compared with the attack frequency before treatment and compared with the patients treated on the nonsymptomatic side. In addition, 18 CCH patients alternately received both ipsilateral and contralateral treatments. Application of capsaicin on the symptomatic side had a temporary beneficial effect in most patients, but attacks occurred within 40 days in all patients. No benefit was seen with contralateral application.

Fusco and colleagues (1994a) performed an open-label study to determine the reproducibility of the therapeutic effect of intranasal capsaicin. The authors carried out a 2-year follow-up study on 25 patients with CH (17 episodic, 8 chronic) who had had a complete disappearance of their attacks with the first treatment of intranasal capsaicin. In the 17 ECH patients, 7 (41%) entered a remission or had a substantial decrease of the pain attacks on further treatment, 4 (24%) displayed benefit with one more treatment but further repetitions did not produce appreciable results, 4 patients (24%) showed no benefit with repetition and 2 patients did not experience any bouts over the follow-up period. In the eight patients with CCH, further treatment with intranasal capsaicin was effective in four patients but the pain-free periods lasted no longer than 40 days.

In summary, intranasal capsaicin applied ipsilateral to the symptomatic side appears to be effective in significant proportions of both ECH and CCH sufferers though the effect appears to be transient, especially in the chronic group. In addition, a significant proportion of patients are refractory to repeated treatment. The intense local irritation caused by intranasal capsaicin deters patients from using this drug.

As topical treatment with civamide (zucapsaicin), a capsaicin analog, is better tolerated than with capsaicin, a small trial of intranasal preparation of civamide has been conducted in CH. In a multicenter, vehicle-controlled study patients with ECH were treated for 7 days with either civamide 0.025% (25 μg) or placebo in a volume of 100 μl (Saper et al., 2002). Eighteen patients received civamide, ten recieved placebo and all were evaluated in a 20-day posttreatment period. While the number of headaches was reduced in the first 7 days (−60% versus −26%), the overall effect at day 20 was not significant. Nasal burning was common in the civamide group. The authors concluded that intranasal civamide is only modestly effective in ECH.

Other Drugs Various other drugs, including nimodipine (Meyer and Hardenberg, 1983; de Carolis et al., 1987; de Carolis et al., 1988), nifedipine (Meyer and Hardenberg, 1983; Jonsdottir et al., 1987), methylergometrine (Tfelt-Hansen et al., 1985), pizotifen (Sicuteri et al., 1967; Ekbom, 1969; Speight and Avery, 1972), baclofen (Hering-Hanit and Gadoth, 2001), botulinum toxin (Evers et al., 2002), chlorpromazine (Caviness and O'Brien, 1980), histamine "desensitization" (Diamond et al., 1986), transdermal clonidine (D'Andrea et al., 1995) and testosterone replacement therapy (Stillman, 2006), have been reported to be effective in open-label or small, poorly controlled studies. Properly controlled trials are needed to verify the efficacy of these agents.

Summary The literature on open studies is difficult to judge for various reasons: in most studies measures of efficacy are not adequately defined; true response rate is impossible to determine without knowledge of the placebo response; and the remitting nature of ECH makes it difficult to determine the effect of an intervention. In addition, there is probably a publication bias involved in that positive results are more likely to be published then negative ones. If the true success rates were as impressive as indicated by the published results, prophylactic treatment of CH would be an easy task, which it often is not (Tfelt-Hansen, 1999). Current CH prophylaxis regimes, though based to some extent on the data available in the literature, draw heavily on clinical experience given the dearth of properly controlled trials. We outline our approach to preventive management of CH below; it is, of necessity, a mixture of evidence and experience.

Preventive treatments can be divided into short-term preventives, suitable for rapidly controlling the attack frequency but not for prolonged use; and long-term therapies that are required for prolonged medical management of CH (see Table 14–7).

Short-term prevention. Patients with either short bouts, perhaps in weeks, or in whom one wishes to control quickly the attack frequency, can benefit from short-term prevention. These medicines are distinguished by the fact that they cannot be easily used in the long-term and thus may require replacement by long-term agents in many patients. Corticosteroids and methysergide are particularly useful in this setting. Traditionally, nocturnal ergotamine was advocated for patients with predictable nocturnal attacks but with the advent of better preventive treatments, this is now rarely used in clinical practice.

Long-term prevention. Some patients with either long bouts of ECH or CCH will require preventive treatment over many months, or even years. Verapamil and lithium are particularly useful in this setting. Of the neuromodulators we find topiramate the most helpful.

Invasive treatments including surgery

Several invasive approaches have been tried in CH. The approaches attempted can be subdivided into three main groups: local blockades, neuromodulation, and destructive surgical procedures. Neuromodulatory procedures and destructive surgery are the last-resort measures in treatment-resistant patients and should only be considered when the pharmacological options have been exploited to the fullest. Patients must be carefully

Table 14–7 Preventive Management of Cluster Headache.

Short-term prevention (for episodic cluster headache)	*Long-term prevention (for prolonged bouts of episodic cluster headache or chronic cluster headache)*
Prednisolone (transitional only)	Verapamil
Methysergide	Lithium
Daily (nocturnal) ergotamine[a]	Methysergide
Verapamil	Melatonin[b]
Greater occipital nerve injection	Topiramate[c]
Melatonin[b]	Gabapentin[c]
Topiramate[c]	Valproate[d]
Valproate[d]	

[a] Patients with predictable nocturnal headaches only.

[b] Limited data.

[c] Unproven but promising.

[d] Negative data.

selected. There is an emerging distinction between destructive procedures, which have historically been the only option, and neuromodulatory procedures, which with time may be used earlier in the course of the disorder.

Greater occipital nerve blockade Anthony (1985) described the use of local anesthetic and corticosteroid injections around the greater occipital nerve (GON) homolateral to the pain. Two further open-label series have recently been reported. The first study showed that of 14 patients treated with GON injection, 4 had a good response, 5 had a moderate response and 5, no response (Peres et al., 2002). The second study reported that 13 of 22 injections yielded a complete or partial response lasting for a median of 21 days for the partial response (Afridi et al., 2006).

There has been a recent report of a double-blind placebo-controlled study of suboccipital injection with a mixture of rapid- and long-acting betamethasone in CH (Ambrosini et al., 2005). The authors studied 16 ECH and 7 CCH patients. Eleven of thirteen (85%) CH patients treated with betamethasone suboccipital injection became pain-free within 1 week compared to none of the 10 patients treated with placebo injection. This effect was maintained for at least 4 weeks in the majority of patients.

Neuromodulatory Procedures

Occipital Nerve Stimulation. Based on a promising report of GON stimulation in other headache forms (Weiner and Reed, 1999; Matharu, Bartsch, et al., 2004), and the positive effects of GON injection in CH, and a wish to avoid the potential complications of deep brain stimulation (see below), cutaneous occipital nerve stimulation (ONS) has been performed in patients with intractable CCH. One center has performed the procedure in three medically-intractable CCH patients and reports that these patients either significantly improved or were rendered pain-free with continuous stimulation (Dodick et al., 2003; Schwedt et al., 2006; Schwedt et al., 2007). Another group implanted eight medically refractory CCH patients with ipsilateral occipital nerve stimulators (ONSs) (Magis et al., 2007). One of the patients switched off his stimulator after 4 months as there was no improvement. Two patients were pain-free after a follow-up of 16 and 22 months; one of them still had occasional autonomic attacks. Three patients had around a 90% reduction in attack frequency. Two patients, one of whom had had the implant for only 3 months, had improvement of around 40%. Mean follow-up was 15·1 months (range 3–22).

Intensity of attacks tends to decrease earlier than frequency during ONS and, on average, is improved by 50% in remaining attacks. All but one patient were able to substantially reduce their preventive drug treatment. Interruption of ONS by switching off the stimulator or because of an empty battery was followed within days by recurrence and increase of attacks in all improved patients. ONS did not significantly modify pain thresholds. There were no serious adverse events.

In a medium-term follow-up, eight patients with medically intractable CCH were reported who had had electrodes for neurostimulation therapy—ONS—implanted in the suboccipital region (Burns et al., 2007). Other than the first patient who was initially stimulated unilaterally before being stimulated bilaterally, all other patients were stimulated bilaterally during treatment. At a median follow-up of 20 months (range 6–27 months for bilateral stimulation), six of eight patients reported responses that were meaningful to them sufficient to recommend ONS to similarly affected patients with CCH. Specifically, two patients noticed a marked improvement of 90% or better (90% and 95%) in their attacks. Three patients noticed a moderate improvement in their attacks 40% or better (40%, 60%, and 20%–80%) and one patient recorded a mild improvement of 25%. Improvements occurred in both frequency and severity. In each patient recording improvement the change took weeks or months, although remarkably attacks returned in days when the device malfunctioned, such as with battery depletion. Adverse events of concern were lead migrations in one patient and battery depletion requiring replacement.

CCH is a devastating illness and given the low morbidity of ONS and the relatively consistent outcomes, one might argue that this modality should be explored before deep brain stimulation. Further studies are required and the ability to blind and control such interventions is challenging; however, the consistent results from two centers and the recrudescence of attacks with technical problems suggests that this novel therapy will find a place in the treatment of CCH.

Hypothalamic Stimulation. Based on the finding of ipsilateral inferior posterior hypothalamic activation in CH, various centers have treated intractable CCH patients by electrode implantation and stimulation of this region (Schoenen et al., 2005; D'Andrea et al., 2006; Leone et al., 2006). Leone (2006) recently reviewed the results of hypothalamic deep brain stimulation in these patients. Twenty-four patients have had 26 hypothalamic implants sited; two patients had bilateral implants. Most patients achieved stable and notable pain reduction, and many became pain-free. The results at one center where 18 implants have been sited in 16 patients, with a mean follow-up of over 2 years, show that 13 patients (81%) have improved substantially, with 10 patients (63%) being rendered completely pain-free. The benefit developed gradually over 6 weeks and frequent adjustment of stimulation parameters was required. In most patients the headaches recurred when the stimulation was stopped. There are no substantial changes in hypothalamus-controlled functions during stimulation.

However, a note of caution needs to be struck about this exciting novel approach. One patient died soon after the operation due to implantation-induced intracerebral hemorrhage, and implantation was stopped intraoperatively in another patient who had a panic attack (Schoenen et al., 2005). This underlines the importance of appreciating that deep-brain stimulation procedures are associated with a small risk of morbidity and mortality.

Destructive Surgery This is a last-resort measure in treatment-resistant patients and should only be considered when the pharmacological options, and probably other surgical options also, have been exploited to the fullest. Patients must be carefully selected; since we have begun to use neurostimulation approaches none of our patients have had this treatment option. Only patients whose headaches are exclusively unilateral should be considered for surgery, as patients whose attacks have alternated sides are at risk of a contralateral recurrence after surgery. A number of procedures that interrupt either the trigeminal sensory or autonomic (cranial parasympathetic) pathways can be performed though few are associated with long-lasting results while the side effects can be devastating. The procedures that have been reported to show some success include trigeminal sensory rhizotomy via a posterior fossa approach (Kirkpatrick et al., 1993), radiofrequency trigeminal gangliorhizolysis (Mathew and Hurt, 1988), gamma knife radiotherapy (Ford et al., 1998; Donnet et al., 2005), and microvascular decompression of the trigeminal nerve with or without microvascular decompression of the nervus intermedius (Lovely et al., 1998). Complete trigeminal analgesia may be required for the best results. Complications include diplopia, hyperacusis, jaw deviation, corneal anesthesia and anesthesia dolorosa. Aggressive long-term ophthalmic follow-up is essential.

The long-term follow-up from destructive procedures is relatively small. The Mayo clinic series reported two striking findings (Jarrar et al., 2003). First, trigeminal sensory root section is associated with significant morbidity and a small risk of mortality. Secondly, the Mayo clinic series confirmed our finding that there are clearly defined patients whose attacks persist after complete trigeminal root section and continue to respond to sumatriptan (Matharu and Goadsby, 2002a).

Natural History and Prognosis

Although there is a paucity of literature on the long-term prognosis of CH, the available evidence suggests that it is a lifelong disorder in the majority of patients. In one study, about one-tenth of patients with ECH evolved into CCH whereas one-third of patients with CCH transformed into ECH (Manzoni et al., 1991). An encouraging piece of information for CH sufferers is that a substantial proportion of them can expect to develop longer remission periods as they age (Igarashi and Sakai, 1996).

PAROXYSMAL HEMICRANIA

PH responds in a dramatic and absolute fashion to indomethacin, thereby underlining the importance of distinguishing it from CH and SUNCT, which are not responsive to indomethacin (Antonaci et al., 2003; Matharu and Goadsby, 2005c).

Historical Note and Nomenclature

In 1974 Sjaastad and Dale reported the first case of PH which they described rather aptly as "a new treatable headache entity" (Sjaastad and Dale, 1974). They subsequently coined the term "chronic paroxysmal hemicrania" to describe this disorder (Sjaastad and Dale, 1974). The initial cases described were characterized by daily headaches for years without remission. Subsequently, it became apparent that not all patients experienced a chronic, unremitting course; in some patients, discrete headache bouts were separated by prolonged pain-free remissions. This remitting pattern was named episodic PH (EPH) (Kudrow et al., 1987; Blau and Engel, 1990; Coria et al., 1992; Newman et al., 1993; Goadsby and Lipton, 1997; Veloso et al., 2001; Siow, 2004).

The first edition of the International Headache Society (IHS) classification recognized and gave diagnostic criteria for chronic PH (CPH) in 1988 (Headache Classification Committee of The International Headache Society, 1988). The release of the second edition of the IHS classification in 2004 resulted in the introduction of the umbrella term "paroxysmal hemicrania" that is recognized to have both an episodic and a chronic form (Headache Classification Committee of The International Headache Society, 2004).

Epidemiology

Prevalence

PH is a relatively rare syndrome although, with increasing awareness, it is being recognized more frequently. Data on the epidemiology of PH are scarce and many cases are probably still overlooked. The incidence and prevalence of PH is not known, but the relationship compared to CH is reported to be approximately 1%–3% (Antonaci and Sjaastad, 1989). Prevalence estimates in CH among people of European descent vary from 56 per 100,000 to 381 per 100,000 (Ekbom et al., 1978; D'Alessandro et al., 1986; Tonon et al., 2002; Sjaastad and Bakketeig, 2003). Given that the prevalence of CH is approximately 2 per 1000 (Russell, 2004), the prevalence of PH would be approximately 1 per 25,000. The disorder has been reported in various parts of the world (Rapoport et al., 1981; Tehindrazanarivelo et al., 1992; Zidverc-Trajkovic et al., 2005) and affects different races (Joubert et al., 1987; Chakravarty et al., 2004).

Sex distribution

PH was originally considered to be a female disorder, although male cases clearly occur (Price and Posner, 1978; Rapoport et al., 1981). Subsequently, three retrospective surveys reported a female predominance by a sex ratio of 1.6–2.4:1 (Antonaci and Sjaastad, 1989; Newman and Lipton, 1997; Boes and Dodick, 2002). Comprehensive and methodologically well-designed epidemiological studies are required to establish the actual extent of the female preponderance in PH.

Age of onset

PH may begin at any age, although its onset usually occurs during adulthood with the reported mean age varying between 34 and 41 years (Antonaci and Sjaastad, 1989; Boes and Dodick, 2002). The youngest age at onset was 1 year and the oldest 81 years (Antonaci and Sjaastad, 1989; de Almeida et al., 2004). In one of the case series, EPH began earlier (mean 27 years) than CPH (mean 37 years) (Antonaci and Sjaastad, 1989).

Clinical Features

The clinical phenotype of PH is highly characteristic (Antonaci and Sjaastad, 1989; Goadsby and Lipton, 1997; Newman and Lipton, 1997; Russell, 1999; Boes and Dodick, 2002). Patients typically have unilateral, brief, severe attacks of pain associated with cranial autonomic features that recur several times per day.

Side, laterality, severity and character of pain

The pain is most often in the ophthalmic trigeminal distribution, but it can be extra-trigeminal. The maximum pain is most often centred on the ocular, temporal, maxillary, and frontal regions; less often, the pain involves the neck, occiput and the retro-orbital regions. The pain may occasionally radiate into the ipsilateral shoulder and arm (Antonaci and Sjaastad, 1989). The headache is strictly unilateral and without side shift in the majority of patients. The pain is typically excruciating in severity and is described as a claw-like, throbbing, aching, or boring sensation.

Duration of the individual attacks

The headache usually lasts 2–30 minutes, although we have seen much longer attacks. Two retrospective studies consisting of 84 and 74 patients, reported a mean attack duration of 21 minutes (range 2–120 minutes) and 26 minutes, respectively (Antonaci and Sjaastad, 1989; Boes and Dodick, 2002). In a prospective study of 105 attacks, the mean duration was found to be 13 minutes, with a range of 3–46 minutes (Russell, 1999). The headache has an abrupt onset and cessation. Interictal discomfort or pain is present in up to one-third of the patients (Antonaci and Sjaastad, 1989).

Associated features

Attacks of PH typically occur in association with ipsilateral cranial autonomic features. Lacrimation, conjunctival injection, nasal congestion, or rhinorrhoea frequently accompany the headache; eyelid oedema, ptosis, miosis and facial sweating are less frequently reported. Bilateral autonomic symptoms can occur. Photophobia (21%) and nausea (14%) may accompany some attacks though vomiting and phonophobia are rare (Antonaci and Sjaastad, 1989). In one study, 27 of 31 patients noted at least one migrainous feature of photophobia, nausea or vomiting during an attack (Boes and Dodick, 2002). During episodes of pain, approximately half the sufferers prefer to sit or lie still while the other half assume the pacing activity usually seen with CH (Antonaci and Sjaastad, 1989).

Frequency and periodicity of attacks

In PH the attacks occur at a high frequency. The frequency of attacks ranges from 1 to 40 daily. In two retrospective studies consisting of 84 and 74 patients, the mean attack frequency was 11 daily (range 2–40) and 6 daily, respectively (Antonaci and Sjaastad, 1989; Boes and Dodick, 2002). In a prospective study of 105 attacks in five patients, the mean attack frequency was 14 daily (range 4–38) (Antonaci and Sjaastad, 1989). The attacks occur regularly throughout the 24-hour period without a preponderance of nocturnal attacks as in CH. However, nocturnal attacks associated with REM phase of sleep have been described (Kayed et al., 1978).

Triggers

While the majority of patients report attacks that are spontaneous, approximately 10% of patients report attacks that may be precipitated mechanically, either by bending or by rotating the head. Attacks may also be provoked by external pressure against the transverse processes of C_{4-5}, C_2 root, or the GON. Alcohol ingestion triggers headaches in only 7% of patients (Antonaci and Sjaastad, 1989). In our clinical experience, cutaneous triggering, such as touching the skin, chewing, or talking, is not a feature of PH. The relationship between menstruation and PH attacks is undetermined. Birth control pills do not seem to influence the attack frequency. In some patients, the attacks have been reported to disappear or improve during pregnancy and return after delivery (Sjaastad et al., 1980; Stein and Rogado, 1980). We certainly have an experience of a typical case whose attacks proceeded unremittingly through the pregnancy. We found no helpful alternative treatment to indomethacin during that time. There is no reported effect of the menopause.

Atypical Features

Several unusual clinical features have been reported. There are four case reports of side-alternating attacks (Pelz and Merskey, 1982; Bogucki et al., 1984; Pradalier and Dry, 1984; Pareja, 1995). Furthermore, there are three cases of bilateral, short-lasting, frequent, indomethacin-responsive headaches without cranial autonomic features that have been reported as bilateral PH (Pollmann and Pfaffenrath, 1986; Bingel and Weiller, 2005; Mulder and Spierings, 2004); these cases may represent a novel indomethacin-responsive primary headache syndrome, bilateral paroxysmal cephalalgia, rather than bilateral PH (Matharu and Goadsby, 2005b). Interestingly, there are also three case descriptions of unilateral PH with no autonomic features (Bogucki et al., 1984; Pelz and Merskey, 1982; Boes et al., 1998). Disassociation between pain and autonomic features has also been reported (Pareja, 1995; Matharu and Goadsby,

2001), although these cases may have omitted to consider aural discomfort or fullness as a cranial autonomic symptom (Boes et al., 1998). There is one case report of a typical migrainous aura occurring in association with PH attacks (Matharu and Goadsby, 2001). Cases presenting with primary ear pain and a sensation of external acoustic meatus obstruction have been reported, and a case of the PH associated with red ear syndrome has been described (Boes et al., 1998). There are two case reports of primarily extra-trigeminal pain with PH (Dodick, 1998; Rossi et al., 2005).

Classification and Diagnostic Criteria

The revised International Classification of Headache Disorders (ICHD-II) classification criteria for PH are listed in Table 14–8.

PH is classified depending on the presence of a remission period. About 20% of patients have *EPH*, which is diagnosed when they experience recurrent bouts, each with a duration of more than a week and separated by remissions lasting 1 month or longer. The remaining 80% of patients have CPH, in which either no remission occurs within 1 year or the remissions last less than 1 month. Notably, in PH, the chronic form dominates the clinical presentation, in contrast to CH in which the episodic form prevails.

In EPH the typical duration of the headache bout ranges from 2 weeks to 4.5 months; remission periods range from 1 to 36 months (Newman and Lipton, 1997). EPH has been reported to stay episodic for up to 35 years (Antonaci and Sjaastad, 1989). EPH can evolve into typical CPH and vice versa. In contrast to ECH, circannual periodicity does not appear to be a feature of EPH, though three cases with seasonal onset has been described (Veloso et al., 2001; Siow, 2004; Rossi et al., 2005). Approximately one-quarter of the CPH cases evolve from EPH while the remaining three-quarters are chronic from onset (Antonaci and Sjaastad, 1989).

Differential Diagnosis

The differential diagnosis of PH includes symptomatic causes of PH, CH, and SUNCT. As one-

TABLE 14–8 The International Classification of Headache Disorders II (ICHD-II) Diagnostic Criteria for Paroxysmal Hemicrania.

Paroxysmal hemicrania has two key forms:

- *Episodic*: occurs in periods lasting 7 days to 1 year separated by pain free periods lasting 1 month or more
- *Chronic*: attacks occur for more than 1 year without remission or with remissions lasting less than 1 month

Headaches must have each of:

A. At least 20 attacks fulfilling criteria B–F
B. Attacks of severe unilateral orbital, supraorbital or temporal pain lasting 2–30 minutes
C. Headache is accompanied by at least one of the following:
   1. Ipsilateral conjunctival injection and/or lacrimation
   2. Ipsilateral nasal congestion and/or rhinorrhoea
   3. Ipsilateral eyelid oedema
   4. Ipsilateral forehead and facial sweating
   5. Ipsilateral miosis and/or ptosis
D. Attacks have a frequency above 5 per day for more than half of the time, although periods with lower frequency may occur
E. Attacks are prevented completely by therapeutic doses of indomethacin[a]
F. Not attributed to another disorder

Source: Adapted from Headache Classification Committee of The International Headache Society (Headache Classification Committee of The International Headache Society, 2004).

[a] To rule out an incomplete response, indomethacin should be used in a dose of 150 mg or more daily orally or rectally, or 100 mg or more by injection. Smaller doses are often sufficient for maintenance.

third of PH patients report interictal pain, HC needs to be considered in the differential diagnosis of these cases. The differentiation of PH from SUNCT is discussed in the section on SUNCT.

Symptomatic PH

Symptomatic PH is relatively common and can be caused by diverse pathological processes at various sites. Even cases fitting all criteria for PH including a complete response to indomethacin can have a symptomatic etiology. Symptomatic causes of PH are listed in Table 14–9. In practice we are most concerned to exclude pituitary tumor and fossa disease.

TABLE 14–9 Causes of Symptomatic Paroxysmal Hemicrania.

Vascular
Circle of Willis aneurysms (Medina, 1992)
Carotid aneurysm embolisation (Irimia et al., 2005)
Parietal arteriovenous malformation (Newman et al., 1992)
Stroke:
Middle cerebral artery (MCA) infarct (Newman et al., 1992)
Occipital infarct (Broeske et al., 1993)
Tumors
Frontal lobe tumor (Medina, 1992)
Gangliocytoma of the sella turcica (Vijayan, 1992)
Cavernous sinus meningioma (Sjaastad et al., 1995)
Petrous ridge meningioma (Boes and Dodick, 2002)
Pituitary tumor (Gatzonis et al., 1996; Boes and Dodick, 2002; Sarov et al., 2006)
Intracranial parotid carcinoma metastases (Mariano et al., 1999; Mariano da Silva et al., 2004)
Pancoast tumor (Delreux et al., 1989)
Tuber cinereum hamartoma (Pauri et al., 1993)
Miscellaneous
Collagen vascular disease (Medina, 1992)
Maxillary cyst (Gatzonis et al., 1996)
Intracranial hypertension (Hannerz and Jogestrand, 1993)
Essential thrombocythaemia (MacMillan and Nukada, 1989)
Ophthalmic herpes zoster (Giacovazzo et al., 1992)
Posttraumatic (Matharu and Goadsby, 2001)

Cluster Headache

There is a considerable overlap in the clinical phenotype of PH and CH. Both are strictly unilateral, relatively brief but frequent headaches occur in association with ipsilateral cranial autonomic features. Mistaking PH for CH is problematic since, generally, treatments for CH are not effective for PH. PH differs from CH for not having a male dominance, shorter duration of headaches that are more frequent, and the absolute response to indomethacin. The utility of sex of patients, and duration and frequency of the attack to distinguish PH from CH is limited by the considerable overlap of these characteristics in the two syndromes. We advocate that all patients diagnosed with TACs, who do not have a contraindication to the use of NSAIDs, should have a trial of indomethacin at the start of treatment to detect the indomethacin-sensitive group, at least until a reliable biological marker becomes available. The disadvantage of this approach is that the diagnostic yield will be low (as PH is comparatively rare) and will delay appropriate treatment by 1–2 weeks in CH patients, unless there is access to the Indotest (see section on "Diagnostic Workup"). The alternative approach is to consider the indomethacin trial only in patients with a high likelihood of having PH. Given both conditions have very long courses and can be challenging it is our view that the diagnosis should be secure at the outset.

Hemicrania Continua

HC is a strictly unilateral, continuous headache of mild to moderate intensity, with superimposed exacerbations of moderate to severe intensity that are accompanied by trigeminal autonomic features and migrainous symptoms. The syndrome is exquisitely responsive to indomethacin. Differentiating HC and PH, when the latter has interictal pain, can be particularly problematic. Some clinical features can help. First, interictal pain in PH is usually described as mild only, whereas background pain in HC is often moderate (although it can be mild). Second, exacerbations in PH are short-lasting, whereas those in

HC are longer-lasting, often lasting several hours. Third, the severity of pain during exacerbations is excruciating in PH whereas it is often moderate or severe in HC. Fourth, in general terms patients with PH who have interictal pain often have a personal or family history of migraine.

Diagnostic Workup

A good clinical history, a detailed neurological examination and an optimum therapeutic trial of indomethacin are all that are necessary to make a diagnosis of PH. As a relatively high number of symptomatic cases have been reported, an MRI scan of the brain, which must include dedicated views of the pituitary fossa, should be routinely performed in all patients with PH.

One therapeutic trial of oral indomethacin is initiated at 25 mg three times daily; if there is no or a partial response after 3 days, the dose is increased to 50 mg three times daily for 3 (to 10) days; if the index of suspicion is high then the dose is further increased to 75 mg three times daily for 10 days. Complete resolution of the headache is prompt, usually occurring within 1–2 days of initiating the effective dose, though we have come across a case which took 10 days to respond completely to indomethacin (unpublished observation). It is, therefore, worth considering prolonging the administration of the maximum indomethacin dose to 10 days. Injectable indomethacin 100 mg intramuscularly (indotest) has been proposed as a diagnostic test for PH. Two open-label studies of intramuscular indomethacin 100 mg in six and seven patients reported complete pain-relief for 11.1 $\pm$ 3.5 hours and 13.4 $\pm$ 7.7 hours, respectively (Antonaci et al., 1998; Matharu et al., 2006). The indotest has the advantage that the diagnosis can be rapidly established though it needs further validation at this stage, with placebo-controlled trials in PH and the other TACs. Unfortunately, intramuscular indomethacin is not available in some countries, including the United States. In patients who do not respond to an optimum trial of indomethacin, the diagnosis should be reconsidered.

Additional investigations are required when symptomatic PH is suspected. Symptomatic PH should be considered when the clinical picture is atypical, there are associated neurological signs, the indomethacin dose is escalating or treatment response is poor. A reasonably complete screen of a patient with PH, considering the associated clinical problems reported, would include an appropriate brain imaging procedure, blood count (looking for thrombocythaemia), pituitary hormone profile, vasculitis screen (looking for collagen vascular disease), lumbar puncture (should the pain become bilateral, a lumbar puncture should be performed to look for intracranial hypertension, even in the face of response to indomethacin), and a chest X-ray (looking for a Pancoast tumor).

Management

Drug Therapies

The treatment of PH is entirely preventive, as attacks are too short and intense for any acute oral treatment to be effective. Indomethacin is the treatment of choice.

Indomethacin Complete resolution of the headache is prompt, usually occurring within 1–2 days of initiating the effective dose. The typical maintenance dose ranges from 25 to 100 mg daily but may vary inter-and intra-individually between 12.5 and 300 mg daily, depending on the fluctuation in attack severity (Sjaastad, 1986). Hence, dosage adjustments may be necessary to address the clinical fluctuations seen in PH. On discontinuation, symptoms usually appear within 12 hours to 2 weeks though during active headache cycles, skipping or even delaying doses may result in the prompt reoccurrence of the headache (Sjaastad et al., 1980). In patients with EPH, indomethacin should be given for slightly longer than the typical headache bout and then gradually tapered. In patients with CPH, long-term treatment is usually necessary; however, long-lasting remissions have been reported in rare patients following cessation of indomethacin and hence drug withdrawal should be advised at least once every 6 months.

The most common serious side-effect of indomethacin is the development of peptic ulcers. Gastrointestinal side effect secondary to indomethacin may be treated with antacids, misoprostol, histamine H_2 receptor antagonists or proton pump inhibitors and should always be considered for patients who require long-term treatment. Indomethacin suppositories are occasionally helpful if gastric intolerance is a major problem, or when high doses, such as 300 mg daily, are required.

In patients who do not respond to indomethacin, the diagnosis should be reconsidered. Patients who need escalating doses of indomethacin to suppress the symptoms, become refractory to treatment with indomethacin or require a continuous, high dosage of indomethacin may have underlying pathology and need careful diagnostic evaluation for symptomatic causes.

For patients who cannot tolerate indomethacin, one faces a difficult challenge. No other drug is consistently effective in PH. Other drug therapies that have been reported to be effective in PH are reviewed below.

Other NSAIDs Numerous NSAIDs have been tried in PH but none show the consistent and exquisite response provided by indomethacin (Sjaastad, 1992). The NSAIDs that have been reported to be partially or completely effective, mainly in isolated cases, include aspirin (Antonaci and Sjaastad, 1989; Kudrow and Kudrow, 1989; Evers and Husstedt, 1996), ibuprofen (Evers and Husstedt, 1996), naproxen (Durko and Klimek, 1987; Hannerz et al., 1987; Evers and Husstedt, 1996; Mateo and Pascual, 1999), diclofenac (Pradalier and Dry, 1984; Evers and Husstedt, 1996), ketoprofen (Antonaci and Sjaastad, 1989), and piroxicam β-cyclodextrin (Sjaastad and Antonaci, 1995).

Cyclooxygenase-2 inhibitors There has been some limited success in treatment of PH with cyclooxygenase-2 (COX-2) inhibitors, rofecoxib (Lisotto et al., 2003; Chakravarty et al., 2004; Siow, 2004) and celecoxib (Mathew et al., 2000; Siow, 2004). However, prolonged use of both of these agents has recently been linked with an increased risk of myocardial infarctions and strokes, and this culminated in the withdrawal of rofecoxib from the market worldwide (Lenzer, 2005). In view of this, the available COX-2 inhibitors should be prescribed only with great caution in PH.

Calcium Channel Antagonists There are several case reports of a partial or complete response to verapamil (Schlake et al., 1990; Shabbir and McAbee, 1994; Evers and Husstedt, 1996; de Almeida et al., 2004; Zidverc-Trajkovic et al., 2005). Indeed, prior to the introduction of COX-2 inhibitors, verapamil was considered the more successful alternative drug treatment to indomethacin (Evers and Husstedt, 1996). Other calcium channel antagonists that have been reported to be effective in PH include flunarizine (Coria et al., 1992; Evers and Husstedt, 1996) and nicardipine (Coria et al., 1992).

Other Drugs Other drugs reported to be partially or completely effective in PH, mainly in isolated cases, include acetazolamide (Warner et al., 1994), prednisone (Hannerz et al., 1987; Antonaci and Sjaastad, 1989), ergotamines (Antonaci and Sjaastad, 1989), sumatriptan (Hannerz and Jogestrand, 1993; Evers and Husstedt, 1996; Pascual and Quijano, 1998), carbamazepine (Evers and Husstedt, 1996), lithium (Antonaci and Sjaastad, 1989), topiramate (Cohen and Goadsby, 2007) and botulinum toxin injections into ipsilateral temporal muscle (Gobel et al., 2001).

Surgery

Several surgical approaches have been tried in PH. The approaches attempted can be subdivided into two main groups: local blockades and invasive surgical procedures.

Local Blockades Local anaesthetic blockades of pericranial nerves, including the GON, supraorbital nerve, and less occipital nerve have been reported to be ineffectual as have stellate ganglion blocks, sphenopalatine ganglion blocks, and cervical sympathetic blocks (Antonaci and Sjaastad, 1989; Antonaci et al., 1997). However, there are three reports of complete response with local blockades. There is a case report of an EPH patient who consistently showed a complete response to GON blockades with a combination of lidocaine and methylprednisolone, but not bupivacaine (Rossi et al., 2005). There is another report of a CPH patient who had a complete response with GON block using lidocaine and methylprednisolone (Afridi et al., 2006). Another case report described complete response to repetitive sympathetic chain blocks with a combination of bupivacaine and methylprednisolone, introduced onto the C7 transverse process, but not with saline placebo. This patient subsequently had a stellate ganglionectomy that rendered him pain-free, though follow-up was limited to 15 months (Albertyn et al., 2004).

Invasive Surgery Besides the one report of benefit with stellate ganglionectomy, invasive surgical procedures, including trigeminal sensory root section, infraorbital nerve section, superficial petrosal nerve section, and sphenopalatine ganglionectomy have been reported to be ineffective (Antonaci and Sjaastad, 1989; Albertyn et al., 2004). Our unpublished experience on three cases of PH who have had ONS is that two have had sustained, that is, more than 6 month, benefit. As in CH, ONS holds promise in PH.

Natural History and Prognosis

As PH is a relatively recently described syndrome, there is a paucity of literature on its natural history and long-term prognosis. The available evidence suggests that it is a life-long condition, although none of the pediatric cases so far presented have been followed for more than 1 year and so the natural history in childhood unset is uncertain. Patients can expect sustained efficacy of indomethacin treatment without developing tachyphylaxis, though about one-quarter develop gastrointestinal side effects (Pareja et al., 2001). Indomethacin does not seem to alter the condition in the long-term, though a significant proportion of patients can decrease the dose of indomethacin required to maintain a pain-free state.

SHORT-LASTING UNILATERAL NEURALGIFORM HEADACHE ATTACKS WITH CONJUNCTIVAL INJECTION AND TEARING

SUNCT, as its name implies, is a disorder characterized by strictly unilateral, severe, neuralgic attacks centred on the ophthalmic trigeminal distribution that are brief in duration and occur in association with conjunctival injection and lacrimation.

Historical Note

SUNCT syndrome was described only relatively recently; the entity was first described in 1978 (Sjaastad et al., 1978) and more fully characterized in 1989 (Sjaastad et al., 1989). Three reviews of 21, 63 and 82 patients reported in the literature were published in 1997, 2003, and 2005, respectively (Matharu, Cohen, et al., 2003; Pareja and Sjaastad, 1997; Matharu and Goadsby, 2005a). The syndrome is now sufficiently validated and ICHD-II recognizes SUNCT syndrome as a subgroup of TACs. Recognizing the possibility that all patients with generically the same condition might not have both conjunctival injection and tearing, the classification committee of the IHS considered that SUNCT syndrome may be a subset of SUNAs with cranial autonomic features and included the latter in the appendix. We recently reported the largest single-center clinic-based cohort of 43 SUNCT and 9 SUNA patients (Cohen et al., 2006b).

Epidemiology

The prevalence and incidence of SUNCT are not known though the extremely low number of reported cases suggests that it is a rare syndrome; although perhaps no more so than PH. The disorder has a slight male predominance with a sex ratio of 1.5:1 (Cohen et al., 2006b). The typical age of onset is between 35 and 65 years, with a mean of 48 years and a range between 10 and 77 years (Matharu and Goadsby, 2005a).

Clinical Features

Site of Pain

The pain is usually maximal in the ophthalmic distribution of the trigeminal nerve, especially the orbital or retro-orbital regions, forehead, and temple (Cohen et al., 2006b). It may involve wider areas of the head and face, including the top, side and back of the head, nose, maxillary and mandibular distrubtion of the trigeminal nerve, teeth, neck and rarely, even regions such as ear (Pareja and Sjaastad, 1997; Graff-Radford, 2000) and throat (Wingerchuk et al., 2000).

Laterality of Attack

Attacks are typically strictly unilateral and side-locked. However, 20% of patient report side-alternating attacks (D'Andrea and Granella, 2001;

D'Andrea et al., 2001; Matharu, Cohen, et al., 2004; Cohen et al., 2006b). There are rare reports of attacks affecting both sides simultaneously (Pareja and Sjaastad, 1997; Sabatowski et al., 2001; Kuhn et al., 2005; Cohen et al., 2006b). There is a slight preponderance of SUNCT attacks for the right side.

Severity and Character of Pain

The intensity of the pain is generally excruciating. The pain had a neuralgic character in the vast majority of patients, being usually described as stabbing, sharp, burning, pricking, piercing, shooting, lancinating, or electric shock-like.

Duration, Frequency and Temporal Profile of Individual Attacks

Four different types of pain have been described in SUNCT syndrome: single stabs; groups of stabs; a saw-tooth pattern in which repetitive spike-like paroxysms occur without reaching the pain-free baseline between the individual spikes; and a continuous or intermittent background ache (Fig. 14–1). The mean duration of stabs is 58 seconds (range 1–600 seconds); stab groups, 396 seconds (range 10 seconds–20 minutes); and saw-tooth pattern of attacks, 1160 seconds (range 5 seconds–200 minutes).

Most patients are completely pain-free between attacks, although a significant minority (46%) has a dull interictal background ache (Cohen et al., 2006b) that can be continuous (Pareja and Sjaastad, 1997; Sabatowski et al., 2001; Black and Dodick, 2002; Matharu, Cohen, et al., 2004) or intermittent (Sesso, 2001; van Vliet et al., 2003). The interictal discomfort is usually ipsilateral to the SUNCT attacks, though can be bilateral.

The attack frequency during the symptomatic phase varies immensely between sufferers and within an individual sufferer. Attacks may be as infrequent as once a day or less to more than 60 per hour (Montes et al., 2001). In our series, the attack frequency was 2–600 attacks daily, with a mean of 59 attacks daily (Cohen et al., 2006b).

Periodicity of Attacks

As with CH and PH, SUNCT can be sub-classified according to the duration of the bout, though the ICHD-II does not recognize this distinction. About 30% of patients have *episodic SUNCT*, which is diagnosed when they experience recurrent bouts, each with a duration of less than 1 year and separated by remissions lasting more than 1 month. Sixty-three percent of patients have *chronic SUNCT* in which either no remission occurs within 1 year or the remissions last less than 1 month; 63% of these are chronic from onset (primary chronic) while 37% evolve to the chronic form from the episodic form (secondary chronic). The remaining 7% were unclassifiable in our series (Cohen et al., 2006b). In patients with episodic SUNCT, bouts last for a mean of 7.5 weeks (range 1–30 weeks) while the average remission time is 1 year (range 4 weeks–7 years).

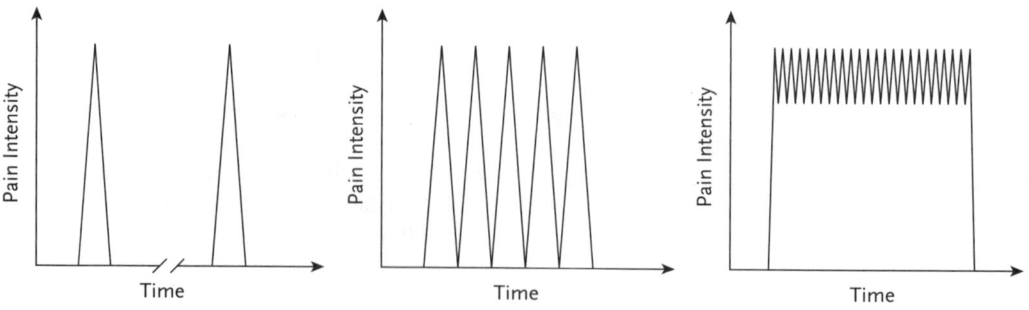

Figure 14–1 Temporal profile of SUNCT attacks (after Matharu and Goadsby, 2005a). (*A*) Single stabs; (*B*) groups of stabs; (*C*) saw-tooth pattern. SUNCT, short-lasting unilateral neuralgiform headache attacks with conjunctival injection and tearing.

SUNCT attacks occur either exclusively or predominantly during the daytime in 53% of patients, while 40% report that the attacks can occur equally during sleep and wakefulness (Cohen et al., 2006b). Only 7% of SUNCT patients reported predominantly nocturnal attacks as opposed to up to 73% of CH patients (Bahra et al., 2002; Russell, 1981).

Associated Features

By definition, all of the SUNCT patients had both ipsilateral conjunctival injection and lacrimation associated with their attacks (Headache Classification Committee of The International Headache Society, 2004). Ptosis (51%), eyelid oedema (49%), rhinorrhoea (53%), nasal congestion (40%), and facial redness (9%), or sweating (7%) are less commonly reported. Fifty-eight percent of SUNCT patients report restlessness or agitation during the attacks.

Though the current diagnostic criteria require that patients with SUNCT need to have both conjunctival injection and lacrimations, there are 11 case reports in the literature of patients who had a headache that was phenotypically similar to SUNCT and occurred in association with cranial autonomic features but did not have either one or both of conjunctival injection and lacrimation (Pareja and Sjaastad, 1997; Volcy et al., 2005; Cohen et al., 2006b). It has been proposed that a more appropriate term for the syndrome may be SUNAs (Matharu, Cohen, et al., 2003; Headache Classification Committee of The International Headache Society, 2004), of which SUNCT would be a subset. Though this will require validation by comparison of SUNCT with sizeable cohort of SUNA cases that do not have both conjunctival injection and lacrimation, some support for this notion has emerged from our case series of 43 SUNCT patients and 9 SUNA patients in which the basic phenotype and response to medications was very similar in both groups (Cohen et al., 2006b).

Nausea (2%), vomiting, photophobia (5%), phonophobia (2%), osmophobia, and worsening of pain with movement (3%) are not normally associated with SUNCT syndrome (Matharu and Goadsby, 2005a). A migrainous aura in association with SUNCT has been reported in one patient. There is a report of ipsilateral facial tingling lasting 5–10 minutes and occurring 5–15 minutes prior to the SUNCT attacks (Matharu, Cohen, et al., 2004).

Triggers

Most SUNCT patients have both spontaneous and triggered attacks, while a minority seems to exhibit exclusively spontaneous attacks (Matharu and Goadsby, 2005a). Exclusively triggered attacks are rare (Cohen et al., 2006b).

The most commonly reported triggers are touching certain trigger zones within trigeminal innervated distribution and, occasionally, even from an extra-trigeminal territory, mastication, wind blowing on the face, washing the face, brushing teeth and movements (Cohen et al., 2006b). Less common triggers included talking, blowing the nose, swallowing, REMs, coughing, sneezing, bright lights, yawning, touching the palate with the tongue, squeezing the eyes, emotional stress, laughing, loud noises, mental concentration, and physical exertion (Matharu and Goadsby, 2005a). Some patients could lessen or abort the attacks by continuously rotating their neck (Sjaastad et al., 1989; Pareja and Sjaastad, 1997).

Refractory Period

Unlike trigeminal neuralgia, SUNCT patients have generally been thought not to have a refractory period (Pareja and Sjaastad, 1997; Matharu, Cohen, et al., 2003). Our case series confirmed this general lack of a refractory period between attacks in 92% of all patients, who could experience a spontaneous attack immediately after the previous one or could trigger an attack immediately on top of the previous one (Cohen et al., 2006b). This serves as a good clinical feature to distinguish trigeminal neuralgia and SUNCT, and should be asked of all patients who are suspected to have SUNCT or trigeminal neuralgia.

Physical Examination

Generally, the neurological examination is normal in SUNCT. There are some reports of allodynia or hyperaesthesia over the ophthalmic and mandibular trigeminal divisions (Pareja and Sjaastad, 1997; Raimondi and Gardella, 1998; Graff-Radford, 2000; Sabatowski et al., 2001; Rossi et al., 2003). Trigeminal hypoesthesia has been reported in several patients (Pareja and Sjaastad, 1997; Black and Dodick, 2002; Matharu, Cohen, et al., 2004; Cohen et al., 2006b). Horner's syndrome was previously thought not to be a feature of SUNCT. However, there have been three recent descriptions of persistent Horner's syndrome in association with SUNCT (Schwaag et al., 2003; Prakash and Lo, 2004; Cohen et al., 2006b).

Classification and Diagnostic Criteria

The revised International Classification of Headache Disorders (ICHD-II) criteria for SUNCT and SUNA are listed in Tables 14–10 and Table 14–11, respectively.

Differential Diagnosis

The differential diagnosis of very brief headaches includes: SUNCT (primary and symptomatic forms); trigeminal neuralgia; primary stabbing headache and PH.

Symptomatic SUNCT

A close scrutiny of the reported cases of symptomatic SUNCT reveals that the pathological lesions occurred at two main sites: the posterior fossa and the pituitary (Table 14–12). In cases of symptomatic SUNCT secondary to pituitary tumors, it is interesting to note that the headache symptoms can precede the pituitary symptoms by 3–10 years (Ferrari et al., 1988; Massiou et al., 2002). Surgical extirpation of the pituitary lesion has proved curative in a number of cases (Levy et al., 2003; Leroux et al., 2006).

Rare cases of SUNCT have been reported in association with vascular compression of the trigeminal nerve (Ertsey et al., 2000; Gardella et al., 2001; Koseoglu et al., 2005), in contrast to trigeminal neuralgia, for which the incidence of trigeminal nerve compression is 47%–90% (Baldwin et al., 1991; Kuroiwa et al., 1996; Yang et al., 1996; Majoie et al., 1997; Love and Coakham, 2001). In our series only three patients (7%) of SUNCT had vascular compression though the laterality of the attacks and vascular compression was often discordant, raising the possibility that this is an incidental finding (Cohen et al., 2006b).

Trigeminal Neuralgia

Differentiating SUNCT from trigeminal neuralgia can be challenging in some cases, as there is a considerable overlap in the clinical phenotypes of the two syndromes. Both headaches are short-lasting, can have a high frequency of attacks and display clustering of attacks. Both are principally unilateral headaches and the trigger zones behave similarly. The usual onset is during middle or old age in both. However, there are a number of striking differences between these two syndromes, awareness of which can aid in their differentiation (Table 14–13).

Primary Stabbing Headache

Primary stabbing headache (also known as idiopathic stabbing headache) refers to brief, sharp or

Table 14–10 The International Classification of Headache Disorders II (ICHD-II) Diagnostic Criteria for Short-lasting Unilateral Neuralgiform Headache Attacks with Conjunctival Injection and Tearing (SUNCT).

Headaches must have each of:

A. At least 20 attacks fulfilling criteria B–E
B. Attacks of unilateral orbital, supraorbital or temporal stabbing or pulsating pain lasting 5–240 seconds
C. Pain is accompanied by ipsilateral conjunctival injection and lacrimation
D. Attacks occur with a frequency from 3 to 200 per day
E. Not attributed to another disorder

Source: Adapted from Headache Classification Committee of The International Headache Society (Headache Classification Committee of The International Headache Society, 2004).

TABLE 14–11 The International Classification of Headache Disorders II (ICHD-II) Diagnostic Criteria for Short-lasting Unilateral Neuralgiform Headache Attacks with Cranial Autonomic Symptoms (SUNA).

SUNA has two key forms:

- *Episodic*: occurs in periods lasting 7 days to 1 year separated by pain free periods lasting 1 month or more
- *Chronic*: attacks occur for more than 1 year without remission or with remissions lasting less than 1 month

Headaches must have each of:

A. At least 20 attacks fulfilling criteria B–E
B. Attacks of unilateral orbital, supraorbital or temporal stabbing pain lasting from 2 seconds to 10 minutes
C. Pain is accompanied by one of:
   1. Conjunctival injection and/or tearing
   2. Nasal congestion and/or rhinorrhoea
   3. Eyelid oedema
D. Attacks occur with a frequency of 1 or more per day for more than half the time
E. Not attributed to another disorder

Source: Adapted from Headache Classification Committee of The International Headache Society (Headache Classification Committee of The International Headache Society, 2004).

jabbing pain in the head that occur either as a single episode or in brief repeated volleys. The pain is usually over the ophthalmic trigeminal distribution while the face is generally spared. The pain usually lasts a fraction of a second but can persist for up to 1 minute, thereby overlapping with the phenotype of SUNCT, and recurs at irregular intervals (hours to days). These headaches are generally easily distinguishable clinically as they differ in several respects: in primary stabbing headache there is a female preponderance; the site and radiation of pain often varies between attacks; the majority of the attacks tend to be spontaneous; cranial autonomic features are absent; and the attacks commonly subside with the administration of indomethacin (Pareja et al., 1999).

Paroxysmal Hemicrania

SUNCT attacks typically last less than 5 minutes (Matharu and Goadsby, 2005c) while only exceptional attacks of PH last less than 3 minutes (Russell, 1984). SUNCT attacks tend to predominate during the daytime whereas PH attacks have a uniform distribution throughout the day and night. Most SUNCT attacks are precipitated by mechanisms acting on the trigeminal and, occasionally, even the extra-trigeminal innervated areas. Only a minority (approximately 15%) of PH patients exhibit precipitated attacks (usually with latency of 5–60 seconds) after spontaneous neck movements or after prolonged external pressure over certain sensitive areas (Sjaastad et al., 1979). In our clinical experience, cutaneous triggering, such as touching the skin, chewing or talking, is not a feature of PH. PH is exquisitely responsive to indomethacin, which is not effective in SUNCT (Matharu and Goadsby, 2005c; Cohen et al., 2006b). If there is any diagnostic uncertainty then a trial of indomethacin is warranted.

Diagnostic Workup

The association of secondary SUNCT with pituitary and posterior fossa abnormalities emphasizes the absolute need for a cranial MRI, including an adequate view of the pituitary. In addition, these patients should have a screen for basal pituitary hormone profile. We routinely perform a therapeutic trial of indomethacin to exclude an indomethacin-responsive headache.

Management

Drug Treatment

As in PH, the treatment of SUNCT is entirely prophylactic, as attacks are generally too short

TABLE 14–12 Causes of Symptomatic Short-lasting Unilateral Neuralgiform Headache Attacks with Conjunctival Injection and Tearing (SUNCT).

Posterior fossa lesions
Cerebellopontine angle arteriovenous malformations (Bussone et al., 1991; Morales et al., 1994)
Brainstem cavernous hemangioma (De Benedittis, 1996)
Posterior fossa lesion in an HIV/AIDS patient (Goadsby and Lipton, 1997)
Severe basilar impression causing pontomedullary compression in a patient with osteogenesis imperfecta (ter Berg and Goadsby, 2001)
Craniosynostosis resulting in a foreshortened posterior fossa (Moris et al., 2001) Ischaemic brainstem infarction (Penart et al., 2001)
Pontocerebellar astrocytoma (Blattler et al., 2003)
Cerebellopontine angle and frontal lobe meningiomas (Ramirez-Moreno et al., 2004)
Anomolous vertebrobasilar vascular development (Mondejar et al., 2006)
Brainstem and upper cervical lesions secondary to Devic's syndrome (Kursun et al., 2006) and multiple sclerosis (Vilisaar and Constantinescu, 2006)
Pituitary tumors
Nonfunctioning pituitary adenoma (Ferrari et al., 1988; Rocha Filho et al., 2006)
Prolactinoma (Massiou et al., 2002; Levy et al., 2003; Matharu, Levy, et al., 2003; Levy et al., 2005; Larner, 2006; Jimenez Caballero, 2007)
Acromegaly (Levy et al., 2005; Rozen, 2006)
Miscellaneous
Cavernous sinus leiomyosarcoma (Kaphan et al., 2003)
Orbital cyst (Lim and Teoh, 2003)
Intraorbital metastatic bronchial carcinoid (Black et al., 2005)
HIV-positive patient with no opportunistic infections and normal brain imaging (Barea and Forcelini, 2001)

HIV, Human immunodeficiecy virus.

AIDS, Acquired immunodeficiency syndrome.

and intense for any abortive treatment to be effective. Short-term prevention is used in the hospital with lidocaine, which arrests the problem, and long-term prevention is employed to minimize disability out of the hospital.

Short-term Prevention

IV lidocaine. IV lidocaine has been previously reported to be highly effective at completely suppressing the headaches in four patients with SUNCT, providing them with pain-free times of up to 12 hours (Matharu, Cohen, et al., 2004). A recent trial of IV lidocaine in 11 patients reported a response in all patients, albeit that the response varies from some relief to total abolition of symptoms. The longest pain-free period was 3 weeks in a patient with chronic SUNCT, 12 weeks in in a patient with chronic SUNA, and 6 months in a patient with episodic SUNCT (Cohen et al., 2005).

Long-term Prevention

Lamotrigine. Lamotrigine has been previously reported to be highly efficacious in 12 SUNCT patients (D'Andrea et al., 1999; Leone, Rigamonte, et al., 2000; D'Andrea et al., 2001; Gutierrez-Garcia, 2002; Malik et al., 2002; Chakravarty and Mukherjee, 2003; Piovesan et al., 2003). Lamotrigine, given in an open manner at 100–400 mg daily, induced a complete remission in nine patients and produced about an 80% improvement in the other three patients. Conversely, it has been reported to be ineffective in five patients (Black and Dodick, 2002; Matharu, Cohen, et al., 2004; Koseoglu et al., 2005; Sprenger et al., 2005) though the maximum dose of lamotrigine that was tried in one of these patients was only 50 mg daily. Lamotrigine had a moderate to good effect in 68% of SUNCT and 25% of SUNA patients in a recent open-label study (Cohen et al., 2005). Problems with lamotrigine include a skin reaction which may progress to Stevens–Johnson syndrome, and this necessitated the cessation of lamotrigine in at least one patient, in the literature (Rossi et al., 2003).

Topiramate. The effect of topiramate in SUNCT has been reported in nine cases. It was ineffective in three patients (Black and Dodick, 2002; Chakravarty and Mukherjee, 2003) while six patients responded completely to topiramate at 50–300 milligrams daily (Matharu and Goadsby, 2002a; Rossi et al., 2003; Matharu, Cohen, et al., 2004; Kuhn et al., 2005). Recently, in an open-label study 52% of SUNCT patients had a good response to

TABLE 14–13 Differentiating Features of SUNCT and Trigeminal Neuralgia.

Feature	*SUNCT*	*Trigeminal neuralgia*
Gender ratio (male:female)	1.5:1	1:2
Site of pain	V_1	$V_{2/3}$
Duration (seconds)	5–240	<5
Autonomic features	Prominent	Sparse or none
Refractory period	Absent	Present
Response to carbamazepine	Partial	Complete
Evidence of vascular loop on MRI	7%	47–90%

Abbreviations: SUNCT, short-lasting unilateral neuralgiform headache attacks with conjunctival injection and tearing; MRI, magnetic resonance imaging.

topiramate though the response in SUNA was less clear (Cohen et al., 2005).

Gabapentin. Gabapentin has been tried in 13 SUNCT patients. It was highly effective in three patients, completely suppressing the attacks when used at 800–2700 mg daily (Graff-Radford, 2000; Hunt et al., 2002; Porta-Etessam et al., 2002). However, it has been reported to be completely ineffective in 10 patients (Morales-Asin et al., 2000; Montes et al., 2001; Black and Dodick, 2002; Hannerz and Linderoth, 2002; Malik et al., 2002; Matharu et al., 2002; Schwaag et al., 2003; Matharu, Cohen, et al., 2004). Interestingly it was effective in 60% of SUNA cases but only 45% of SUNCT in an open-label trial (Cohen et al., 2005).

Carbamazepine. The therapeutic response to carbamazepine has been reported in 45 cases. In 30 of these 45 cases (Bouhassira et al., 1994; Pareja et al., 1995; Goadsby and Lipton, 1997; Benoliel and Sharav, 1998a; D'Andrea et al., 1999; Graff-Radford, 2000; Leone, Rigamonte, et al., 2000b; Morales-Asin et al., 2000; Montes et al., 2001; Sabatowski et al., 2001; Sesso, 2001; Black and Dodick, 2002; Gutierrez-Garcia, 2002; Hannerz and Linderoth, 2002; Malik et al., 2002; Chakravarty and Mukherjee, 2003; Piovesan et al., 2003; Rossi et al., 2003; Schwaag et al., 2003; van Vliet et al., 2003; Matharu, Cohen, et al., 2004), there was no beneficial response with the sole use of carbamazepine. However, two of these nonresponders demonstrated a partial or good response when carbamazepine was used in combination with other agents: a partial response was reported with a combination of carbamazepine, naloxone, verapamil, and lithium in one patient (Sabatowski et al., 2001) while the other patient treated with carbamazepine, in combination with IV methylprednisolone and followed by oral prednisolone, was seemingly rendered pain-free on three occasions for a variable period of time (Montes et al., 2001). In 11 of the 45 cases a partial response was reported (Pareja et al., 1995; Raimondi and Gardella, 1998; D'Andrea et al., 2001; Cohen, Matharu, and Goadsby, 2004; Prakash and Lo, 2004; Matharu, Cohen, et al., 2004), though in some patients this was variable (Hannerz and Linderoth, 2002) or transient (Becser and Berky, 1995; Black and Dodick, 2002). A complete or almost complete response was noted in four patients. One of these patients responded completely and consistently for 2 years to carbamazepine alone but thereafter required a combination of carbamazepine and verapamil to render him pain-free (Matharu et al., 2002). Another patient had substantial relief on carbamazepine and prednisolone (Raimondi and Gardella, 1998). The third patient had complete relief with some courses of treatment but this effect was inconsistent (Hannerz et al., 1992). The fourth patient responded consistently and almost completely over 10 years (Schwaag et al., 2003). However it was effective in only 39% of our series of SUNCT patients (Cohen et al., 2005), and thus is less effective than the preventives listed above.

Other drugs. Numerous pharmacological strategies have been reported to be ineffective in open-label studies including NSAIDs (indomethacin, diclofenac, ibuprofen, ketoprofen, mefenamic acid, naproxen, and piroxicam), COX-2 inhibitors (nimesulide and celecoxib), simple analgesics (acetaminophen, aspirin, metamizole), opiates (tramadol, buprenorphine, codeine, dihydrocodeine, hydrocodone, meperidine, morphine), oxygen, ergots, methysergide, β-blockers (propranolol, timolol), α-adrenoceptor agonists and antagonists (clonidine and doxazosin), histamine desensitization and receptor antagonist (cyproheptadine), calcium channel antagonists (verapamil, nifedipine, amlodipine, flunarizine and diltiazem), γ-aminobutyric acid (GABA) agonists (baclofen), benzodiazepines, tricyclic antidepressants (amitriptyline, nortriptyline, lofepramine, imipramine, and desipramine), selective serotonin reuptake inhibitor (fluoxetine), lithium, phenytoin, valproic acid, neuroleptics (pimozide, levomepromazine), central nervous system stimulants (methylphenidate, pemoline), somatostatin, angiotensin converting enzyme inhibitors (captopril, enalapril), aprotinin, tranexamic acid, omeprazole, vitamin B_{12}, and acyclovir (Matharu and Goadsby, 2005a).

Conclusion. Open-label studies and case reports clearly play an important role in the generation and testing of hypotheses. In SUNCT syndrome, several groups of pharmacological strategies have been excluded and a partial or complete effectiveness suggested with the use of lamotrigine, topiramate, gabapentin, carbamazepine, and IV lidocaine. However, the ultimate confirmation of the effectiveness of any agent in the treatment of this syndrome should come from randomized double-blind, placebo-controlled clinical trials.

On the basis of the data available in the literature and our clinical experience, we have outlined our approach to the management of SUNCT syndrome. Lamotrigine is the treatment of choice while topiramate and, perhaps, gabapentin are reasonable second line agents in patients who fail a trial of lamotrigine. It should be remembered that some patients have a useful response to carbamazepine and its use can be considered if the other agents are ineffective. When patients with SUNCT syndrome experience severe exacerbations with frequent, easily triggered, high-intensity pain attacks, acute interventions are needed because the patients are severely affected. They may not be able to eat or drink because these actions trigger attacks. In that situation, IV lidocaine can be utilized to temporarily ameliorate the attacks while conventional therapy is being optimized.

Surgery

Several surgical approaches have been tried in SUNCT syndrome. The approaches attempted can be subdivided into three main groups: local blockades, invasive procedures involving the trigeminal nerve, and hypothalamic stimulation

Local Blockades Local blockades of supraorbital nerves (Pareja et al., 1995; Hannerz and Linderoth, 2002; Piovesan et al., 2003), infraorbital nerves (Pareja et al., 1995; Hannerz and Linderoth, 2002), lacrimal nerve, orbicularis oculi muscles and the retrobulbar region (Pareja et al., 1995) have generally been reported to be ineffectual. Similarly, GON blocks have previously been reported to be ineffective in four patients (Pareja et al., 1995; Piovesan et al., 2003). However, we observed a moderate to good effect in five out of eight patients who received GON blockades with a combination of lidocaine and methylprednisolone (Cohen et al., 2005).

Invasive Surgical Procedures Involving the Trigeminal Nerve There are nine case reports of either apparently successful treatment or temporary relief of SUNCT syndrome with invasive surgical procedures involving the trigeminal nerve. The procedures that have been employed include the Janetta procedure (Lenaerts et al., 1997; Gardella et al., 2001; Schwaag et al., 2003), percutaneous trigeminal ganglion compression (Morales-Asin et al., 2000), trigeminal ganglion thermocoagulation (Piovesan et al., 2003; Matharu, Cohen, et al., 2004), retrogasserian glycerol rhizolysis and trigeminal nerve balloon compression (Hannerz and Linderoth, 2002). These procedures provided complete pain-relief though the duration of the benefit ranged from 3 months to 4.5 years. Furthermore, as the follow-up period in some of these patients was limited to less than 18 months, it is difficult to assess the actual effectiveness of the procedures given the variable nature of attack frequency in this syndrome. This is further underscored by the observation that the benefit was temporary in all reported cases with prolonged follow-up. Conversely, there are four reports of patients who were submitted to trigeminal procedures without any benefit (Black and Dodick,

2002; Hannerz and Linderoth, 2002; Matharu, Cohen, et al., 2004).

Given the uncertain efficacy of trigeminal procedures together with the potential for complications, surgery should only be considered as a last resort and only when the pharmacological options have been exploited to the fullest.

Hypothalamic Stimulation Based on the finding of ipsilateral posterior hypothalamic activation in SUNCT (see section on pathophysiology), Leone and colleagues (2004) have treated one patient with intractable SUNCT by electrode implantation and stimulation of this region. The patient was successfully treated and the procedure was well tolerated, with no significant adverse events. Nondestructive surgical treatment modalities demand further examination though caution needs to be exercised since deep brain stimulation procedures are associated with a small risk of mortality.

Natural History and Prognosis

The natural history of SUNCT syndrome is poorly understood yet. The average duration of symptoms at reporting was 7 years (Cohen et al., 2006b). The longest reported duration of SUNCT is 48 years (Pareja and Sjaastad, 1997). It appears to be a life-long disorder once it starts, though more prospective data is needed. The syndrome itself is not fatal and does not cause any long-term neurological sequelae.

PATHOPHYSIOLOGY OF TACS

The Trigemino-autonomic Reflex and Hypothalamic Activation

Any pathophysiological construct for TACs must account for the three major clinical features characteristic of the various conditions that comprise this group: trigeminal distribution pain, ipsilateral autonomic features and the curious periodicity or regularity that often marks the attack incidence. The pain-producing innervation of the cranium projects through branches of the trigeminal and upper cervical nerves to the trigeminocervical complex from whence nociceptive pathways project to higher centers. This implies an integral role for the ipsilateral trigeminal nociceptive pathways in TACs. The ipsilateral autonomic features suggest cranial parasympathetic activation (lacrimation, rhinorrhoea, nasal congestion, and eyelid oedema) and sympathetic hypofunction (ptosis and miosis). Goadsby and Lipton have suggested that the pathophysiology of the TACs revolves around the trigeminal-autonomic reflex (Goadsby and Lipton, 1997). There is considerable experimental animal literature to document that stimulation of trigeminal afferents can result in cranial autonomic outflow, the trigeminal-autonomic reflex (May and Goadsby, 1999). In fact, some degree of cranial autonomic symptomatology is a normal physiologic response to cranial nociceptive input and patients with other headache syndromes often report these symptoms (Benoliel and Sharav, 1998b). The distinction between the TACs and other headache syndromes is the degree of cranial autonomic activation, not its presence (Goadsby et al., 2001; Goadsby, 2005).

The cranial autonomic symptoms may be prominent in the TACs due to a central disinhibition of the trigeminal-autonomic reflex (Goadsby et al., 2001). Supporting evidence is emerging from functional imaging studies: positron emission tomography studies in CH (May, Bahra, et al., 1998) and PH (Matharu et al., 2006), and functional MRI studies in SUNCT syndrome (May et al., 1999; Cohen, Matharu, Kalisch, et al., 2004; Sprenger et al., 2005) have demonstrated hypothalamic activation (see Figure 14–2). Importantly, the involvement of posterior hypothalamic structures may account for the rhymicity or periodicity that is such a hallmark of these conditions. Hypothalamic activation is not seen in episodic and chronic migraine (Weiller et al., 1995; Bahra et al., 2001; Denuelle et al., 2004; Matharu, Bartsch, et al., 2004; Afridi et al., 2005a; Afridi et al., 2005b) or experimental trigeminal distribution head pain (Kupers et al., 2004; May, Kaube, et al., 1998). There are direct hypothalamic–trigeminal connections (Malick and Burstein, 1998). There is abundant evidence for a role of the hypothalamus in mediating anti-nociceptive (Wang et al., 1990; Dafny et al., 1996) and autonomic responses (Lumb and Lovick, 1993). Infact, there is direct evidence from animal experimental studies for hypothalamic activation when intracranial pain

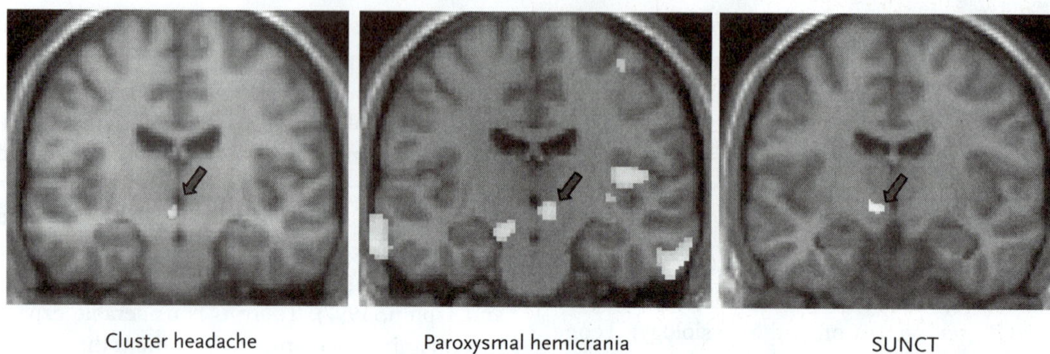

Figure 14–2 Hypothalamic activation in trigeminal autonomic cephalalgias. SUNCT, short-lasting unilateral neuralgiform headache attacks were conjunctival injection and tearing.

structures are activated (Benjamin et al., 2004). Moreover, the hypothalamic peptides Orexin A and B can elicit pro-nociceptive and anti-nociceptive effects in the trigeminal system (Bartsch et al., 2004). Hence, the TACs are probably due to an abnormality in the hypothalamus with subsequent trigeminovascular and cranial autonomic activation.

Outstanding Issues in the Pathophysiology and Nosology of TACs

There are several issues that remain unresolved in the understanding of the pathophysiology of the TACs. The nature of the hypothalamic abnormality in the TACs needs to be elucidated. Furthermore, if the defining abnormality of the TACs is hypothalamic derangement, then this raises the question as to why these syndromes have such different phenotypes and treatment responses. The hypothalamus is a complex structure with various nuclei and widespread projections to numerous central structures; it is possible that the specific substructures, neurons or biochemical pathways involved in these primary headache syndromes vary thereby explaining both, the different phenotypes and treatment responses. Nonetheless, further studies will need to seek the anatomical or functional basis of these variations. The mechanism of action of indomethacin needs to be unraveled. What special feature of the pharmacology of indomethacin accounts for its specific effect in PH? Indomethacin is a potent reversible inhibitor of prostaglandin-forming COX but its mechanism of action of indomethacin in PH appears to be independent of an effect on prostaglandin synthesis, since other NSAIDs or COX-2 inhibitors appear to have a poor, partial or inconsistent effect in these disorders (Frolich, 1997). Indomethacin lowers intracranial pressure (ICP) though the pathophysiological basis of PH is unlikely to be disordered ICP (Jensen et al., 1991; Jensen et al., 1993; Biestro et al., 1995; Slavik and Rhoney, 1999). It has been proposed that indomethacin may antagonize one or more steps in the nitric oxide pathway in the trigemino-autonomic reflex and, in this way, exert its effect on disorders characterized by activation of the cranial parasympathetic system (Dodick, 1999), though there is as yet sparse evidence for this notion. Advances in the pathophysiological understanding of the TACs are likely to lead to better treatments for these devastatingly painful syndromes.

Important nosological questions also remain unresolved. Should HC be located in section III of the International Classification of Headache Disorders? Its pathophysiology involves hypothalamic activation, and some worsenings certainly include cranial autonomic activation, while it is also indomethacin-sensitive. However, it often has prominent migrainous features and the worsenings can be without cranial autonomic activation. Moreover, other indomethacin-sensitive headaches, such as primary stabbing headache, are not TACs, and frankly never behave like the others, so indomethacin-sensitivity alone is clearly not the complete story. Are the terms episodic and chronic inappropriate? The word chronic could be applied to most of the primary headaches in the context that the disease predisposition is present over decades. Does a patient with ECH who will certainly experience years of illness, albeit with breaks, have a "chronic" illness? The classification committee will need to address these questions at some point to provide a more cohesive and face valid nomenclature for the TACs and the apparently related conditions.

CONCLUSIONS

The TACs are a group of primary headache disorders characterized by unilateral head pain that occurs in association with ipsilateral cranial autonomic features. Their phenotype usefully assembles their nosology and can be understood in terms of activation of trigeminal nociceptive afferents with a reflex activation of the cranial autonomic outflow through the facial (VIIth) cranial nerve. The TACs include CH, PH, SUNCT, and its close relative SUNA. The underlying pathophysiology includes a role for neurons in the region of the posterior hypothalamus because there is now functional imaging evidence for its involvement in each syndrome. Clinically, the syndromes can be distinguished by the frequency of attacks of pain, the length of the attacks, and very characteristic responses to medical therapy. The differentiation is important because the treatments are so distinct.

References

Afridi, S, Giffin, NJ, Kaube, H, et al. (2005a). A positron emission tomographic study in spontaneous migraine. *Arch Neurol,* 62:1270–1275.

Afridi, SK, Matharu, MS, Lee, L, et al. (2005b). A PET study exploring the laterality of brainstem activation in migraine using glyceryl trinitrate. *Brain,* 128:932–939.

Afridi, SK, Shields, KG, Bhola, R, et al. (2006). Greater occipital nerve injection in primary headache syndromes—prolonged effects from a single injection. *Pain,* 122:126–129.

Ahmed, F (2000). Chronic cluster headache responding to gabapentin: a case report. *Cephalalgia,* 20:252–253.

Albertyn, J, Barry, R, Odendaal, CL (2004). Cluster headache and the sympathetic nerve. *Headache,* 44:183–185.

Ambrosini, A, Vandenheede, M, Rossi, P, et al. (2005). Suboccipital injection with a mixture of rapid- and long-acting steroids in cluster headache: a double-blind placebo-controlled study. *Pain,* 118:92–96.

Andersson, PG and Jespersen, LT (1986). Dihydroergotamine nasal spray in the treatment of attacks of cluster headache. A double-blind trial versus placebo. *Cephalalgia,* 6:51–54.

Andrasik, F, Blanchard, EB, Arena, JG, et al. (1982). Cross-validation of the Kudrow-Sutkus MMPI classification system for diagnosing headache type. *Headache,* 22:2–5.

Anthony M (1985). Arrest of attacks of cluster headache by local steroid injection of the occipital nerve. In: Rose FC, ed. Migraine: Clinical and Research Advances. London: Karger, 169–173.

Antonaci, F, Costa, A, Ghirmai, S, et al. (2003). Parenteral indomethacin (the INDOTEST) in cluster headache. *Cephalalgia,* 23:193–196.

Antonaci, F, Pareja, JA, Caminero, AB, et al. (1997). Chronic paroxysmal hemicrania and hemicrania continua: blockades of pericranial nerves. *Funct Neurol,* 12:11–15.

Antonaci, F, Pareja, JA, Caminero, AB, et al. (1998). Chronic paroxysmal hemicrania and hemicrania continua. Parenteral indomethacin: the "indotest". *Headache,* 38:122–128.

Antonaci, F and Sjaastad, O (1989). Chronic paroxysmal hemicrania (CPH): a review of the clinical manifestations. *Headache,* 29:648–656.

Appelbaum, J and Noronha, A (1989). Pericarotid cluster headache. *J Neurol,* 236:430–431.

Bahra, A, Gawel, MJ, Hardebo, JE, et al. (2000). Oral zolmitriptan is effective in the acute treatment of cluster headache. *Neurology,* 54:1832–1839.

Bahra, A, Matharu, MS, Buchel, C, et al. (2001). Brainstem activation specific to migraine headache. *Lancet,* 357:1016–1017.

Bahra, A, May, A, and Goadsby, PJ (2002). Cluster headache: a prospective clinical study with diagnostic implications. *Neurology,* 58:354–361.

Baldwin, NG, Sahni, KS, Jensen, ME, et al. (1991). Association of vascular compression in trigeminal neuralgia versus other "facial pain syndromes" by magnetic resonance imaging. *Surg Neurol,* 36:447–52.

Barea, LM and Forcelini, CM (2001). Onset of short-lasting, unilateral, neuralgiform headache with conjunctival injection and tearing (SUNCT) after acquired human immunodeficiency virus (HIV): more than a coincidence? *Cephalagia,* 21:518.

Barre, F (1982). Cocaine as an abortive agent in cluster headache. *Headache,* 22:69–73.

Bartsch, T, Levy, MJ, Knight, YE, et al. (2004). Differential modulation of nociceptive dural input to [hypocretin] orexin A and B receptor activation in the posterior hypothalamic area. *Pain,* 109:367–378.

Baumber, L, Sjostrand, C, Leone, M, et al. (2006). A genome-wide scan and HCRTR2 candidate gene analysis in a European cluster headache cohort. *Neurology,* 66:1888–1893.

Becser, N and Berky, M (1995). SUNCT syndrome: a Hungarian case. *Headache,* 35:158–160.

Benjamin, L, Levy, MJ, Lasalandra, MP, et al. (2004). Hypothalamic activation after stimulation of the superior sagittal sinus in the cat: a Fos study. *Neurobiol Dis,* 16:500–505.

Benoliel, R and Sharav, Y (1998a). SUNCT syndrome: case report and literature review. *Oral Surg Oral Med Oral Pathol Oral Radiol Endod,* 85:158–161.

Benoliel, R and Sharav, Y (1998b). Trigeminal neuralgia with lacrimation or SUNCT syndrome? *Cephalalgia,* 18:85–90.

Berde, B and Schild, HO (1978). *Ergot Alkaloids and Related Compounds,* Springer-Verlag, Berlin.

Biestro, AA, Alberti, RA, Soca, AE, et al. (1995). Use of indomethacin in brain-injured patients with cerebral perfusion pressure impairment: preliminary report. *J Neurosurg,* 83:627–630.

Bingel, U and Weiller, C (2005). An unusual indomethacin sensitive headache: a case of bilateral episodic paroxysmal hemicrania without autonomic symptoms? *Cephalagia,* 25:148–150.

Black, DF, Bordini, CA, and Russell, D (2006). Symptomatology of cluster headaches. In *The Headaches* (3rd edn) (J Olesen, P Goadsby, N Ramadan et al., eds), pp. 789–796. Lippincott Williams & Wilkins, Philadelphia.

Black, DF and Dodick, DW (2002). Two cases of medically and surgically intractable SUNCT: a reason for caution and an argument for a central mechanism. *Cephalagia,* 22:201–204.

Black, DF, Swanson, JW, Eross, EJ, et al. (2005). Secondary SUNCT due to intraorbital, metastatic bronchial carcinoid. *Cephalalgia,* 25:633–635.

Blakeborough, P, Fowler, PA, and Ashford, EA (1993). The use of sumatriptan in patients taking migraine prophylactic agents. *Cephalalgia,* 13:163.

Blattler, T, Capone Mori, A, Boltshauser, E (2003). Symptomatic SUNCT in an eleven-year-old girl. *Neurology,* 60:2012–2013.

Blau, JN (1993). Behaviour during a cluster headache. *Lancet,* 342:723–725.

Blau, JN and Engel, H (1990). Episodic paroxysmal hemicrania: a further case and review of the literature [see comments]. *J Neurol Neurosurg Psychiatr,* 53:343–344.

Blau, JN and Engel, HO (1998). Premonitory and prodromal symptoms in cluster headache. *Cephalalgia,* 18:91–93; discussion 71–72.

Blau, JN and Engel, HO (1999). A new cluster headache precipitant: increased body heat. *Lancet,* 354:1001–1002.

Boes, CJ and Dodick, DW (2002). Refining the clinical spectrum of chronic paroxysmal hemicrania: a review of 74 patients. *Headache,* 42:699–708.

Boes, CJ, Swanson, JW, and Dodick, DW (1998). Chronic paroxysmal hemicrania presenting as otalgia with a sensation of external acoustic meatus obstruction: two cases and a pathophysiologic hypothesis. *Headache,* 38:787–791.

Bogucki, A, Szymanska, R, and Braciak, W (1984). Chronic paroxysmal hemicrania: lack of pre-chronic stage. *Cephalalgia,* 4:187–189.

Bouhassira, D, Attal, N, Esteve, M, et al. (1994). "SUNCT" syndrome. A case of transformation from trigeminal neuralgia? *Cephalalgia,* 14:168–170.

Broeske, D, Lenn, NJ, and Cantos, E (1993). Chronic paroxysmal hemicrania in a young child: possible relation to ipsilateral occipital infarction. *J Child Neurol,* 8:235–236.

Brzezinski, A (1997). Melatonin in humans. *N Engl J Med,* 336:186–195.

Burns, B, Watkins, L, and Goadsby, PJ (2007). Treatment of medically intractable cluster headache by occipital nerve stimulation: long-term follow-up of eight patients. *Lancet,* 369:1099–1106.

Bussone, G, Leone, M, Dalla Volta, G, et al. (1991). Short-lasting unilateral neuralgiform headache attacks with tearing and conjunctival injection: the first "symptomatic" case? *Cephalalgia,* 11:123–127.

Bussone, G, Leone, M, Peccarisi, C, et al. (1990). Double blind comparison of lithium and verapamil in cluster headache prophylaxis. *Headache,* 30:411–417.

Caviness, VS Jr., and O'Brien, P (1980). Cluster headache: response to chlorpromazine. *Headache,* 20: 128–131.

Chakravarty, A and Mukherjee, A (2003). SUNCT syndrome responsive to lamotrigine: documentation of the first Indian case. *Cephalalgia,* 23:474–475.

Chakravarty, A, Mukherjee, A, and Roy, D (2004). Trigeminal autonomic cephalgias and variants: clinical profile in Indian patients. *Cephalalgia,* 24:859–866.

Chervin, RD, Zallek, SN, Lin, X, et al. (2000). Timing patterns of cluster headaches and association with symptoms of obstructive sleep apnea. *Sleep Res Online,* 3:107–112.

Cid, CG, Berciano, J, Pascual, J (2000). Retro-ocular headache with autonomic features resembling "continuous" cluster headache in lateral medullary infarction [letter]. *J Neurol Neurosurg Psychiatr,* 69:134.

Cittadini, E, May, A, Straube, A, et al. (2006). Effectiveness of intranasal zolmitriptan in acute cluster headache: a randomized, placebo-controlled, double-blind crossover study. *Arch Neurol,* 63:1537–1542.

Cohen, AS and Goadsby, PJ (2007). Paroxysmal hemicrania responding to topiramate. *J Neurol Neurosurg Psychiatr,* 78:96–97.

Cohen, A, Matharu, M, and Goadsby, P (2004). SUNCT syndrome in the elderly. *Cephalalgia,* 24:508–509.

Cohen, AS, Matharu, MS, and Goadsby, PJ (2005). Suggested guidelines for treating SUNCT and SUNA [Abstract]. *Cephalalgia,* 25:1200.

Cohen, AS, Matharu, MS, and Goadsby, PJ (2006a). EKG changes associated with the use of verapamil in cluster headache. *Neurology,* 66(Suppl. 2):A131.

Cohen, AS, Matharu, MS, and Goadsby, PJ (2006b). Short-lasting unilateral neuralgiform headache attacks with conjunctival injection and tearing (SUNCT) or cranial autonomic features (SUNA)-a prospective clinical study of SUNCT and SUNA. *Brain,* 129:2746–2760.

Cohen, A, Matharu, M, Kalisch, R, et al. (2004). Functional MRI in SUNCT shows differential hypothalamic activation with increasing pain. *Cephalalgia,* 24:1098–1099.

Coria, F, Claveria, LE, Jimenez-Jimenez, FJ, et al. (1992). Episodic paroxysmal hemicrania responsive to calcium channel blockers. *J Neurol Neurosurg Psychiatr,* 55:166.

Costa, A, Pucci, E, Antonaci, F, et al. (2000). The effect of intranasal cocaine and lidocaine on nitroglycerin-induced attacks in cluster headache. *Cephalalgia,* 20:85–91.

Couch, JR Jr. and Ziegler, DK (1978). Prednisone therapy for cluster headache. *Headache,* 18:219–221.

Couturier, EG, Hering, R, and Steiner, TJ (1991). The first report of cluster headache in identical twins. *Neurology,* 41:761.

Cremer, PD, Halmagyi, GM, and Goadsby, PJ (1995). Secondary cluster headache responsive to sumatriptan. *J Neurol Neurosurg Psychiatr,* 59:633–634.

Curran, DA, Hinterberger, H, and Lance, JW (1967). Methysergide. *Res Clin Stud Headache,* 1:74–122.

Cuypers, J, Altenkirch, H, and Bunge, S (1981). Personality profiles in cluster headache and migraine. *Headache,* 21:21–24.

Dafny, N, Dong, WQ, Prieto-Gomez, C, et al. (1996). Lateral hypothalamus: site involved in pain modulation. *Neuroscience,* 70:449–460.

D'Alessandro, R, Gamberini, G, Benassi, G, et al. (1986). Cluster headache in the Republic of San Marino. *Cephalalgia,* 6:159–162.

D'Andrea, G and Granella, F (2001). SUNCT syndrome: the first case in childhood. *Cephalalgia,* 21:701–702.

D'Andrea, G, Granella, F, and Cadaldini, M (1999). Possible usefulness of lamotrigine in the treatment of SUNCT syndrome. *Neurology,* 53:1609.

D'Andrea, G, Granella, F, Ghiotto, N, et al. (2001). Lamotrigine in the treatment of SUNCT syndrome. *Neurology,* 57:1723–1725.

D'Andrea, G, Nordera, GP, and Piacentino, M (2006). Effectiveness of hypothalamic stimulation in two patients affected by intractable chronic cluster headache [Abstract]. *Neurology,* 5(Suppl. 2):140.

D'Andrea, G, Perini, F, Granella, F, et al. (1995). Efficacy of transdermal clonidine in short-term treatment of cluster headache: a pilot study [see comments]. *Cephalalgia,* 15:430–433.

de Almeida, DB, Cunali, PA, Santos, HL, et al. (2004). Chronic paroxysmal hemicrania in early childhood: case report. *Cephalalgia,* 24:608–609.

De Benedittis, G. (1996). SUNCT syndrome associated with cavernous angioma of the brain stem. *Cephalalgia,* 16:503–506.

de Carolis, P, Baldrati, A, Agati, R, et al. (1987). Nimodipine in episodic cluster headache: results and methodological considerations. *Headache,* 27:397–399.

de Carolis, P, de Capoa, D, Agati, R, et al. (1988). Episodic cluster headache: short and long term results of prophylactic treatment. *Headache,* 28:475–476.

de la Sayette, V, Schaeffer, S, Coskun, O, et al. (1999). Cluster headache-like attack as an opening symptom of a unilateral infarction of the cervical cord: persistent anaesthesia and dysaesthesia to cold stimuli. *J Neurol Neurosurg Psychiatr,* 66:397–400.

Delreux, V, Kevers, L, and Callewaert A (1989). [Paroxysmal hemicrania preceding Pancoast's syndrome (see comments)]. *Revue Neurologique,* 145:151–152.

Denuelle, M, Fabre, N, Payoux, P, et al. (2004). Brainstem and hypothalamic activation in spontaneous migraine attacks: a PET study. *Cephalalgia,* 24:782.

Dexter, JD and Weitzman, ED (1970). The relationship of nocturnal headaches to sleep stage patterns. *Neurology,* 20:513–518.

Di Sabato, F, Fusco, BM, Pelaia, P, et al. (1993). Hyperbaric oxygen therapy in cluster headache. *Pain,* 52:243–245.

Diamond, S, Freitag, FG, and Prager, J (1986). Treatment of intractable cluster headache. *Headache,* 26:42–46.

Dodick, DW (1998). Extratrigeminal episodic paroxysmal hemicrania. Further clinical evidence of functionally relevant brain stem connections. *Headache,* 38:794–798.

Dodick, D. (1999). Indomethacin responsive headache syndromes: a hypothesis on the mechanism(s) underlying the efficacy of indomethacin in these disorders. *Neurology,* 52:A210.

Dodick, DW, Rozen, TD, and Goadsby, PJ, et al. (2000). Cluster headache. *Cephalalgia,* 20:787–803.

Dodick, D, Trentman, T, Zimmerman, R, et al. (2003). Occipital nerve stimulation for intractable chronic primary headache disorders. *Cephalagia,* 23:701.

Donnet, A, Valade, D, and Regis, J (2005). Gamma knife treatment for refractory cluster headache: prospective open trial. *J Neurol Neurosurg Psychiatr,* 76:218–221.

Durko, A and Klimek, A (1987). Naproxen in the treatment of chronic paroxysmal hemicrania. *Cephalalgia,* 7:361–362.

Eadie, MJ and Sutherland, JM (1966). Migrainous neuralgia. *Med J Aust,* 1:1053–1057.

Eekers, PJ and Koehler, PJ (2001). Naratriptan prophylactic treatment in cluster headache. *Cephalalgia,* 21:75–76.

Ekbom, K (1947). Ergotamine tartrate orally in Horton's "histaminic cephalalgia"(also called Harris's "ciliary neuralgia"). *Acta Psychiatr Neurol,* 46:106–113.

Ekbom, K (1968). Nitroglycerin as a provocative agent in cluster headache. *Arch Neurol,* 19:487–493.

Ekbom, K (1969). Prophylactic treatment of cluster headache with a new serotonin antagonist, BC 105. *Acta Neurol Scand,* 45:601–610.

Ekbom, K (1970a). A clinical comparison of cluster headache and migraine. *Acta Neurol Scand,* (Suppl.):1–48.

Ekbom, K (1970b). Patterns of cluster headache with a note on the relations to angina pectoris and peptic ulcer. *Acta Neurol Scand,* 46:225–237.

Ekbom, K (1974). Litium rid kroniska symptom av cluster headache. *Opusc Med,* 19:148–156.

Ekbom, K (1975). Some observations on pain in cluster headache. *Headache,* 14:219–225.

Ekbom, K (1977). Lithium in the treatment of chronic cluster headache. *Headache,* 17:39–40.

Ekbom, K (1981). Lithium for cluster headache: review of the literature and preliminary results of long-term treatment. *Headache,* 21:132–139.

Ekbom, K, Ahlborg, B, and Schele, R (1978). Prevalence of migraine and cluster headache in Swedish men of 18. *Headache,* 18:9–19.

Ekbom, K, Krabbe, A, Micieli, G, et al. (1995). Cluster headache attacks treated for up to three months with subcutaneous sumatriptan (6 mg). Sumatriptan Cluster Headache Long-term Study Group [published erratum appears in *Cephalalgia* 1995 Oct;15(5):446]. *Cephalalgia,* 15:230–256.

Ekbom, K, Monstad, I, Prusinski, A, et al. (1993). Subcutaneous sumatriptan in the acute treatment of cluster headache: a dose comparison study. The Sumatriptan Cluster Headache Study Group. *Acta Neurol Scand,* 88:63–69.

Ekbom, K and Waldenlind, E (1981). Cluster headache in women: evidence of hypofertility(?) Headaches in relation to menstruation and pregnancy. *Cephalalgia,* 1:167–174.

El Amrani, M, Ducros, A, Boulan, P, et al. (2002). Familial cluster headache: a series of 186 index patients. *Headache,* 42:974–977.

El Amrani, M, Massiou, H, and Bousser, M (2002). A negative trial of sodium valproate in cluster headache: methodological issues. *Cephalalgia,* 22:205–208.

Ertsey, C, Bozsik, G, Afra, J, et al. (2000). A case of SUNCT syndrome with neurovascular decompression. *Cephalalgia,* 20:325.

Evers, S and Goadsby, PJ (2003). Hypnic headache: clinical features, pathophysiology, and treatment. *Neurology,* 60:905–909.

Evers, S and Husstedt, IW (1996). Alternatives in drug treatment of chronic paroxysmal hemicrania. *Headache,* 36:429–432.

Evers, S, Rahmann, A, Vollmer-Haase, J, et al. (2002). Treatment of headache with botulinum toxin A-a review according to evidence-based medicine criteria. *Cephalalgia,* 22:699–710.

Evers, S, Soros, P, Brilla, R, et al. (1997). Cluster headache after orbital exenteration. *Cephalalgia,* 17:680–682.

Favier, I, van Vliet, JA, Roon, KI, et al. (2007). Trigeminal autonomic cephalgias due to structural lesions: a review of 31 cases. *Arch Neurol,* 64:25–31.

Ferrari, MD, Haan, J, and van Seters, AP (1988). Bromocriptine-induced trigeminal neuralgia attacks in a patient with a pituitary tumor. *Neurology,* 38:1482–1484.

Fogan, L (1985). Treatment of cluster headache. A double-blind comparison of oxygen v air inhalation. *Arch Neurol,* 42:362–363.

Ford, RG, Ford, KT, Swaid, S, et al. (1998). Gamma knife treatment of refractory cluster headache. *Headache,* 38:3–9.

Forderreuther, S, Mayer, M, and Straube, A (2002). Treatment of cluster headache with topiramate: effects and side-effects in five patients. *Cephalagia,* 22:186–189.

Formisano, R, Angelini, A, De Vuono, G, et al. (1990). Cluster-like headache and head injury: case report. *Ital J Neurol Sci,* 11:303–305.

Freitag, FG, Diamond, S, Diamond, ML, et al. (2000). Divalproex sodium in the preventative treatment of cluster headache [Abstract]. *Headache,* 40:408.

Friedman, AP and Mikropoulos, HE (1958). Cluster headaches. *Neurology (Minneapolis),* 8:653–663.

Frolich, JC (1997). A classification of NSAIDs according to the relative inhibition of cyclooxygenase isoenzymes. *Trends Pharmacol Sci,* 18:30–34.

Fusco, BM, Fiore, G, Gallo, F, et al. (1994a). "Capsaicin-sensitive" sensory neurons in cluster headache: pathophysiological aspects and therapeutic indication. *Headache,* 34:132–137.

Fusco, BM, Marabini, S, Maggi, CA, et al. (1994b). Preventative effect of repeated nasal applications of capsaicin in cluster headache. *Pain,* 59:321–325.

Gabai, IJ and Spierings, EL (1989). Prophylactic treatment of cluster headache with verapamil. *Headache,* 29:167–168.

Gallagher, RM, Mueller, L, and Ciervo, CA (1996). Analgesic use in cluster headache. *Headache,* 36:105–107.

Gallagher, RM, Mueller, LL, and Freitag, FG (2002). Divalproex sodium in the treatment of migraine and cluster headaches. *J Am Osteopath Assoc,* 102:92–94.

Gardella, L, Viruega, A, Rojas, H, et al. (2001). A case of a patient with SUNCT syndrome treated with Janetta procedure. *Cephalalgia,* 21:996–999.

Garrison, JC (1990). Histamine, bradykinin, 5-hydroxytryptamine and their antagonists. In *The Pharmacological Basis of Therapeutics* (AG Gilman, TW Rall, AS Niles, et al., eds), p. 595. Pergamon Press, New York.

Gatzonis, S, Mitsikostas, DD, Ilias, A, et al. (1996). Two more secondary headaches mimicking chronic paroxysmal hemicrania. Is this the exception or the rule? *Headache,* 36:511–513.

Gawel, MJ, Willinsky, RA, and Krajewski A (1989). Reversal of cluster headache side following treatment of arteriovenous malformation. *Headache,* 29:453–454.

Geppetti, P, Brocchi, A, Caleri, D, et al. (1985). Somatostatin for cluster headache attack. In *Updating in headache* (V Pfaffenrath, PO Lundberg, and O Sjaastad, eds), pp. 302–305. Springer-Verlag, Berlin-Heidelberg-New York-Tokyo.

Geweke, LO (2002). Misdiagnosis of cluster headache. *Curr Pain Headache Rep,* 6:76–82.

Giacovazzo, M, Di Sabato, F, Gallo, MF, et al. (1992). "Chronic paroxysmal hemicrania" following ophthalmic herpes zoster. *Riv Eur Sci Med Farmacol,* 14:45–47.

Goadsby, PJ (2002). Raeder's syndrome [corrected]: paratrigeminal paralysis of the oculopupillary sympathetic system. *J Neurol Neurosurg Psychiatr,* 72:297–299.

Goadsby, PJ (2005). Trigeminal autonomic cephalalgias: fancy term or constructive change to the IHS classification? *J Neurol Neurosurg Psychiatr,* 76:301–305.

Goadsby, PJ and Lipton, RB (1997). A review of paroxysmal hemicranias, SUNCT syndrome and other short-lasting headaches with autonomic feature, including new cases. *Brain,* 120:193–209.

Goadsby, PJ, Matharu, MS, and Boes CJ (2001). SUNCT syndrome or trigeminal neuralgia with lacrimation. *Cephalalgia,* 21:82–83.

Gobel, H, Heinze, A, Heinze-Kuhn, K (2001). Botulinum Toxin A in the treatment of chronic paroxysmal hemicrania—a case report. *Cephalalgia,* 21:506.

Gobel, H, Lindner, V, Heinze, A, et al. (1998). Ribbat M, Deuschl G. Acute therapy for cluster headache with sumatriptan: findings of a one-year long-term study. *Neurology,* 51:908–911.

Graff-Radford, SB (2000). SUNCT syndrome responsive to gabapentin. *Cephalalgia,* 20:515–517.

Graff-Radford, SB and Newman, A (2004). Obstructive sleep apnea and cluster headache. *Headache,* 44:607–610.

Graham, JR (1972). Cluster headache. *Headache,* 11:175–185.

Graham, JR, Malvea, BP, and Gramm, HF (1960). Aerosol ergotamine tartrate for migraine and Horton's syndrome. *N Engl J Med,* 263:802–804.

Graham, JR, Suby, HI, LeCompte, PR, et al. (1966). Fibrotic disorders associated with methysergide therapy for headache. *N Engl J Med,* 274:360–368.

Greve, E and Mai, J (1988). Cluster headache-like headaches: a symptomatic feature? A report of three patients with intracranial pathologic findings. *Cephalalgia,* 8:79–82.

Gutierrez-Garcia, JM (2002). SUNCT syndrome responsive to lamotrigine. *Headache,* 42:823–825.

Hannerz, J (1989). A case of parasellar meningioma mimicking cluster headache. *Cephalalgia,* 9:265–269.

Hannerz, J, Ericson, K, and Bergstrand, G (1987). Chronic paroxysmal hemicrania: orbital phlebography and steroid treatment. A case report. *Cephalalgia,* 7:189–192.

Hannerz, J, Greitz, D, Hansson, P, et al. (1992). Ericson K. SUNCT may be another manifestation of orbital venous vasculitis. *Headache,* 32:384–389.

Hannerz, J and Jogestrand, T (1993). Intracranial hypertension and sumatriptan efficacy in a case of chronic paroxysmal hemicrania which became bilateral. (The mechanism of indomethacin in CPH). *Headache,* 33:320–323.

Hannerz, J and Linderoth, B (2002). Neurosurgical treatment of short-lasting, unilateral, neuralgiform hemicrania with conjunctival injection and tearing. *Br J Neurosurg,* 16:55–58.

Hardebo, JE and Dahlof, C (1998). Sumatriptan nasal spray (20 mg/dose) in the acute treatment of cluster headache. *Cephalalgia,* 18:487–489.

Hardebo, JE and Elner, A (1987). Nerves and vessels in the pterygopalatine fossa and symptoms of cluster headache. *Headache,* 27:528–532.

Headache Classification Committee of The International Headache Society (1988). Classification and diagnostic criteria for headache disorders, cranial neuralgias and facial pain. *Cephalalgia,* 1–96.

Headache Classification Committee of The International Headache Society (2004). The International Classification of Headache Disorders 2nd edition. *Cephalalgia,* 24(Suppl. 1):1–195.

Heidegger, S, Mattfeldt, T, Rieber, A, et al. (1997). Orbitosphenoidal Aspergillus infection mimicking cluster headache: a case report. *Cephalalgia,* 17:676–679.

Hering, R and Kuritzky, A (1989). Sodium valproate in the treatment of cluster headache: an open clinical trial. *Cephalalgia,* 9:195–198.

Hering-Hanit, R and Gadoth, N (2001). The use of baclofen in cluster headache. *Curr Pain Headache Rep,* 5:79–82.

Horton, BT (1941). The use of histamine in the treatment of specific types of headaches. *J Am Med Assoc,* 116:377–383.

Horton, BT (1952). Histaminic cephalgia. *J Lancet,* 72:92–98.

Horton, BT (1956). Histaminic cephalgia. Differential diagnosis and treatment:1176 patients 1937-1955. *Proc Staff Meet Mayo Clin,* 31:325–333.

Horton, BT, MacLean, AR, and Craig, WM (1939). A new syndrome of vascular headache:results of treatment with histamine. *Preliminary report Mayo Clin Proc,* 14, 257–260.

Horton, BT, Ryan, R, and Reynolds, JL (1948). Clinical observations of the use of EC110, a new agent for the treatment of headache. *Proc Staff Meet Mayo Clin,* 23:105–108.

Hunt, CH, Dodick, DW, and Bosch, EP (2002). SUNCT responsive to gabapentin. *Headache,* 42:525–526.

Igarashi, H and Sakai, F (1996). Natural history of cluster headache. *Cephalalgia,* 16:390–391.

Igarashi, H, Sakai, F, and Tazaki, Y (1991). The mechanism by which oxygen interrupts cluster headache. *Cephalalgia,* 11:238–239.

Irimia, P, Barbosa, C, and Martinez-Vila, E (2005). Paroxysmal hemicrania after carotid aneurysm embolization. *Cephalalgia,* 25:1096–1098.

Isler, H (1993). Episodic cluster headache from a textbook of 1745: van Swieten's classic description. *Cephalalgia,* 13:172–174; discussion 149.

Italian Cooperative Study Group on the Epidemiology of Cluster Headache (ICECH) (1995). Case-control study on the epidemiology of cluster headache. I: etiological factors and associated conditions. *Neuroepidemiology,* 14:123–127.

Jammes, JL (1975). The treatment of cluster headaches with prednisone. *Dis Nerv Syst*, 36:375–376.

Jarrar, RG, Black, DF, Dodick, DW, et al. (2003). Outcome of trigeminal nerve section in the treatment of chronic cluster headache. *Neurology*, 60:1360–1362.

Jensen, K, Freundlich, M, Bunemann, L, et al. (1993). The effect of indomethacin upon cerebral blood flow in healthy volunteers. The influence of moderate hypoxia and hypercapnia. *Acta Neurochir (Wien)*, 124:114–119.

Jensen, K, Ohrstrom, J, Cold GE, et al. (1991). The effects of indomethacin on intracranial pressure, cerebral blood flow and cerebral metabolism in patients with severe head injury and intracranial hypertension. *Acta Neurochir (Wien)*, 108:116–121.

Jimenez Caballero, PE (2007). SUNCT syndrome in a patient with prolactinoma and cabergoline-induced attacks. *Cephalalgia*, 27:76–78.

Jonsdottir, M, Meyer, JS, and Rogers, RL (1987). Efficacy, side effects and tolerance compared during headache treatment with three different calcium blockers. *Headache*, 27:364–369.

Joubert, J, Powell, D, and Djikowski, J (1987). Chronic paroxysmal hemicrania in a South African black. A case report. *Cephalalgia*, 7:193–196.

Kaphan, E, Eusebio, A, Donnet, A, et al. (2003). Short-lasting, unilateral, neuralgiform headache attacks with conjunctival injection and tearing (SUNCT syndrome) and tumour of the cavernous sinus. *Cephalalgia*, 23:395–397.

Kayed, K, Godtlibsen, OB, and Sjaastad, O (1978). Chronic paroxysmal hemicrania IV: "REM sleep locked" nocturnal attacks. *Sleep*, 1:91–95.

Kirkpatrick, PJ, O'Brien, MD, and MacCabe, JJ (1993). Trigeminal nerve section for chronic migrainous neuralgia. *Br J Neurosurg*, 7:483–490.

Kittrelle, JP, Grouse, DS, and Seybold, ME (1985). Cluster headache. Local anesthetic abortive agents. *Arch Neurol*, 42:496–498.

Klapper, JA, Klapper, A, and Voss, T (2000). The misdiagnosis of cluster headache: a nonclinic, population-based, Internet survey. *Headache*, 40:730–735.

Koehler, PJ (1993). Prevalence of headache in Tulp's Observationes Medicae (1641) with a description of cluster headache. *Cephalalgia*, 13:318–320.

Koenigsberg, AD, Solomon, GD, and Kosmorsky, G (1994). Psuedoaneurysm within the cavernous sinus presenting as cluster headache. *Headache*, 34:111–113.

Koseoglu, E, Karaman, Y, Kucuk, S, et al. (2005). SUNCT syndrome associated with compression of trigeminal nerve. *Cephalalgia*, 25:473–475.

Krabbe, A (1989). Limited efficacy of methysergide in cluster headache. A clinical experience. *Cephalagia*, 9 (Suppl. 10):404–405.

Krabbe, A and Steiner, TJ (2000). Prophylactic treatment of cluster headache. In *Cluster headache syndrome in general practice: Basic concepts* (O Sjaastad and G Nappi, eds), pp. 91–96. Smith-Gordon, London.

Krabbe, AA (1986). Cluster headache: a review. *Acta Neurol Scand*, 74:1–9.

Kudrow, L (1974). Physical and personality characteristics in cluster headache. *Headache*, 13:197–202.

Kudrow, L (1977). Lithium prophylaxis for chronic cluster headache. *Headache*, 17:15–18.

Kudrow, L (1980). *Cluster Headache:Mechanisms and Management*. Oxford University Press, Oxford, New York.

Kudrow, L (1981). Response of cluster headache attacks to oxygen inhalation. *Headache*, 21:1–4.

Kudrow, L (1987). The cyclic relationship of natural illumination to cluster period frequency. *Cephalalgia*, 7 (Suppl. 6):76–78.

Kudrow, L, Esperanca P, and Vijayan, N (1987). Episodic paroxysmal hemicrania? *Cephalalgia*, 7:197–201.

Kudrow, DB and Kudrow, L (1989). Successful aspirin prophylaxis in a child with chronic paroxysmal hemicrania. *Headache*, 29:280–281.

Kudrow, L and Kudrow, DB (1994). Inheritance of cluster headache and its possible link to migraine. *Headache*, 34:400–407.

Kudrow, L and Kudrow, DB (1995). Intranasal lidocaine. *Headache*, 35:565–566.

Kuhn, J, Vosskaemper, M, and Bewermeyer, H (2005). SUNCT syndrome: a possible bilateral case responding to topiramate. *Neurology*, 64:2159.

Kunkle, EC, Pfeiffer, JB, Wilhoit, WM, et al. (1952). Recurrent brief headache in "cluster" pattern. *Trans Am Neurol Assoc*, 77:240–243.

Kupers, RC, Svensson, P, and Jensen, TS (2004). Central representation of muscle pain and mechanical hyperesthesia in the orofacial region: a positron emission tomography study. *Pain*, 108:284–293.

Kuritzky, A (1984). Cluster headache-like pain caused by an upper cervical meningioma. *Cephalalgia*, 4:185–186.

Kuroiwa, T, Matsumoto, S, Kato, A, et al. (1996). MR imaging of idiopathic trigeminal neuralgia: correlation with non-surgical therapy. *Radiat Med*, 14:235–239.

Kursun, O, Arsava, EM, Oguz, KK, et al. (2006). SUNCT associated with Devic's syndrome. *Cephalalgia*, 26:221–224.

Lainez, MJ, Pascual, J, Pascual, AM, et al. (2003). Topiramate in the prophylactic treatment of cluster headache. *Headache*, 43:784–789.

Lance, JW (1978). *Mechanism and Management of Headache* (3rd edn.). Butterworths, London.

Lance, JW and Anthony, M (1971). Migrainous neuralgia or cluster headache? *J Neurol Sci*, 13:401–414.

Lance, JW and Goadsby, PJ (1998). Mechanisms and Management of Headache (6th edn.). Butterworth-Heinemann, London.

Lance, JW and Goadsby, PJ (2005). *Mechanisms and Management of Headache* (7th edn.). Elsevier Butterworth Heinemann, Philadelphia.

Larner, AJ (2006). Headache induced by dopamine agonists prescribed for prolactinoma: think SUNCT! *Int J Clin Pract*, 60:360–361.

Leandri, M, Luzzani, M, Cruccu, G, et al. (2001). Drug-resistant cluster headache responding to gabapentin: a pilot study. *Cephalalgia*, 21:744–746.
Lefevre, JP, Simmat, G, Bataille, B, et al. (1984). [Cluster headache due to meningioma. 2 cases]. *Presse Med*, 13:2323.
Lenaerts, M, Diederich, N, and Phuce, K (1997). A patient with SUNCT cured by the Janetta procedure. *Cephalalgia*, 17:461.
Lenzer, J (2005). FDA advisers warn: COX 2 inhibitors increase risk of heart attack and stroke. *BMJ*, 330:440.
Leone, M (2006). Deep brain stimulation in headache. *Lancet Neurol*, 5:873–877.
Leone, M, D'Amico, D, Frediani, F, et al. (2000). Verapamil in the prophylaxis of episodic cluster headache: a double-blind study versus placebo. *Neurology*, 54:1382–1385.
Leone M, D'Amico D, Moschiano F, et al. (1996). Melatonin versus placebo in the prophylaxis of cluster headache: a double-blind pilot study with parallel groups. *Cephalalgia*, 16:494–496.
Leone, M, Dodick, D, Rigamonti, A, et al. (2003). Topiramate in cluster headache prophylaxis: an open trial. *Cephalalgia*, 23 1001–1002.
Leone, M, Franzini, A, Broggi, G, et al. (2006). Hypothalamic stimulation for intractable cluster headache: long-term experience. *Neurology*, 67:150–152.
Leone, M, Franzini, A, D'Amico, D, et al. (2004). Hypothalamic deep brain stimulation to relieve intractable chronic SUNCT: The first case. *Neurology*, S43.003.
Leone, M, Lucini, V, D'Amico, D, et al. (1995). Twenty-four-hour melatonin and cortisol plasma levels in relation to timing of cluster headache. *Cephalalgia*, 15:224–229.
Leone, M, Rigamonte, A, Usai, S, et al. (2000). Two new SUNCT cases responsive to lamotrigine. *Cephalalgia*, 20:845–847.
Leone, M, Russell, MB, Rigamonti, A, et al. (2001). Increased familial risk of cluster headache. *Neurology*, 56:1233–1236.
Leroux, E, Schwedt, TJ, Black, DE, et al. (2006). Intractable SUNCT cured after resection of a pituitary microadenoma. *CJNS*, 33(4):411–413.
Levy, MJ, Matharu, MS, and Goadsby, PJ (2003). Prolactinomas, dopamine agonists and headache: two case reports. *Eur J Neurol*, 10:169–173.
Levy, MJ, Matharu, MS, Meeran, K, et al. (2005). The clinical characteristics of headache in patients with pituitary tumours. *Brain*, 128:1921–1930.
Levyman, C, D'Agua Filho, AdP, Volpato, MM, et al. (1991). Epidermoid tumour of the posterior fossa causing multiple facial pain—a case report. *Cephalagia*, 11:33–36.
Lim, EC and Teoh, HL (2003). Headache—it's more than meets the eye: orbital lesion masquerading as SUNCT. *Cephalalgia*, 23:558–560.
Lisotto, C, Maggioni, F, Mainardi, F, et al. (2003). Rofecoxib for the treatment of chronic paroxysmal hemicrania. *Cephalalgia*, 23:318–320.
Liston, H, Bennett, L, Usher, B Jr, et al. (1999). The association of the combination of sumatriptan and methysergide in myocardial infarction in a premenopausal woman. *Arch Intern Med*, 159:511–513.
Loder, E (2002). Naratriptan in the prophylaxis of cluster headache. *Headache*, 42:56–57.
Love, S and Coakham, HB (2001). Trigeminal neuralgia: pathology and pathogenesis. *Brain*, 124:2347–2360.
Lovely, TJ, Kotsiakis, X, and Jannetta, PJ (1998). The surgical management of chronic cluster headache. *Headache*, 38:590–594.
Lovshin, LL (1961). Clinical caprices of histaminic cephalalgia. *Headache*, 1:7–10.
Lumb, BM and Lovick, TA (1993). The rostral hypothalamus: an area for the integration of autonomic and sensory responsiveness. *J Neurophysiol*, 70:1570–1577.
MacMillan, JC and Nukada, H (1989). Chronic paroxysmal hemicrania. *N Z Med J*, 102:251–252.
Magee, KR, Westerberg, MR, and DeJong, RM (1952). Treatment of headache with ergotamine-caffeine suppositories. *Neurology*, 2:477–480.
Magis, D, Allena, M, Bolla, M, et al. (2007). Occipital nerve stimulation for drug-resistant chronic cluster headache: a prospective pilot study. *Lancet Neurol*, 6:314–321.
Mainardi, F, Maggioni, F, Dainese, F, et al. (2002). Spontaneous carotid artery dissection with cluster-like headache. *Cephalalgia*, 22:557–559.
Majoie, CB, Hulsmans, FJ, Verbeeten, B Jr., et al. (1997). Trigeminal neuralgia: comparison of two MR imaging techniques in the demonstration of neurovascular contact. *Radiology*, 204:455–460.
Malick, A and Burstein, R (1998). Cells of origin of the trigeminohypothalamic tract in the rat. *J Comp Neurol*, 400:125–144.
Malik, K, Rizvi, S, and Vaillancourt, PD (2002). The SUNCT syndrome: successfully treated with lamotrigine. *Pain Med*, 3:167–168.
Mani, S and Deeter, J (1982). Arteriovenous malformation of the brain presenting as a cluster headache—a case report. *Headache*, 22:184–185.
Manzoni, GC (1998). Gender ratio of cluster headache over the years: a possible role of changes in lifestyle. *Cephalalgia*, 18:138–142.
Manzoni, GC (1999). Cluster headache and lifestyle: remarks on a population of 374 male patients. *Cephalalgia*, 19:88–94.
Manzoni, GC, Bono, G, Lanfranchi, M, et al. (1983). Lithium carbonate in cluster headache: assessment of its short- and long-term therapeutic efficacy. *Cephalalgia*, 3:109–114.
Manzoni, GC, Micieli, G, Granella, F, et al. (1991). Cluster headache-course over ten years in 189 patients. *Cephalalgia*, 11:169–174.
Manzoni, GC, Terzano, MG, Bono, G, et al. (1983). Cluster headache-clinical findings in 180 patients. *Cephalalgia*, 3:21–30.
Manzoni, GC, Terzano, MG, Moretti, G, et al. (1981). Clinical observations on 76 cluster headache cases. *Eur Neurol*, 20:88–94.
Mariano da Silva, H, Benevides-Luz, I, Santos, A, et al. (2004). Chronic paroxysmal hemicrania as a

manifestation of intracranial parotid gland carcinoma metastasis—a case report. *Cephalalgia*, 24:223–227.

Mariano, HS, Bigal, ME, Bordini, CA, et al. (1999). Chronic paroxysmal hemicrania (CPH)to-like syndrome as a first manifestation of cerebral metastasis of parotid epidermoid carcinoma: a case report. *Cephalalgia*, 19:442.

Marks, DR, Rapoport, A, Padla, D, et al. (1993). A double-blind placebo-controlled trial of intranasal capsaicin for cluster headache [see comments]. *Cephalalgia*, 13 114–116.

Massiou, H, Launay, JM, Levy, C, et al. (2002). SUNCT syndrome in two patients with prolactinomas and bromocriptine-induced attacks. *Neurology*, 58:1698–1699.

Mateo, I and Pascual, J (1999). Coexistence of chronic paroxysmal hemicrania and benign cough headache. *Headache*, 39:437–438.

Matharu, MS, Bartsch, T, Ward, N, et al. (2004). Central neuromodulation in chronic migraine patients with suboccipital stimulators: a PET study. *Brain*, 127:220–230.

Matharu, MS, Boes, CJ, and Goadsby, PJ (2002). SUNCT Syndrome: Prolonged Attacks, Refractoriness and Response to Topiramate. *Neurology*, 58:1307.

Matharu, MS, Cohen, AS, Boes, CJ, et al. (2003). Short-lasting unilateral neuralgiform headache with conjunctival injection and tearing syndrome: a review. *Curr Pain Headache Rep*, 7:308–318.

Matharu, MS, Cohen, AS, Frackowiak, RS, et al. (2006). Posterior hypothalamic activation in paroxysmal hemicrania. *Ann Neurol*, 59:535–545.

Matharu, MS and Goadsby, PJ (2001). Post-traumatic chronic paroxysmal hemicrania (CPH) with aura. *Neurology*, 56:273–275.

Matharu, MS and Goadsby, PJ (2002a). Persistence of attacks of cluster headache after trigeminal nerve root section. *Brain*, 125:976–984.

Matharu, MS and Goadsby, PJ (2002b). Trigeminal autonomic cephalgias. *J Neurol Neurosurg Psychiatr*, 72: ii19–ii26.

Matharu, M and Goadsby, P (2005a). Short-lasting unilateral neuralgiform headache attacks with conjunctival injection and tearing (SUNCT) syndrome. In *Chronic Daily Headache for Clinicians* (PJ Goadsby, SD Silberstein, and DW Dodick, eds), pp. 89–103. Decker Inc, London.

Matharu, M and Goadsby, PJ (2005b). Bilateral paroxysmal hemicrania or bilateral paroxysmal cephalalgia, another novel indomethacin-responsive primary headache syndrome? *Cephalalgia*, 25:79–81.

Matharu, MS and Goadsby, PJ (2005c). Sudden unilateral neuralgiform pain with conjunctival injection and tearing. In *The Headaches* (J Olesen, PJ Goadsby, N Ramadan, et al., eds), pp. 823–830. Lippincott Williams & Wilkins, Philadelphia.

Matharu, MS, Levy, MJ, Meeran, K, et al. (2004c). Subcutaneous octreotide in cluster headache: randomized placebo-controlled double-blind crossover study. *Ann Neurol*, 56:488–494.

Matharu, MS, Levy, MJ, Merry, RT, et al. (2003). SUNCT syndrome secondary to prolactinoma. *J Neurol Neurosurg Psychiatr*, 74:1590–1592.

Mather, PJ, Silberstein, SD, Schulman, EA, et al. (1991). The treatment of cluster headache with repetitive intravenous dihydroergotamine. *Headache*, 31:525–532.

Mathew, NT (1978). Clinical subtypes of cluster headache and response to lithium therapy. *Headache*, 18:27–29.

Mathew, NT and Hurt, W (1988). Percutaneous radiofrequency trigeminal gangliorhizolysis in intractable cluster headache. *Headache*, 28:328–331.

Mathew, NT, Kailasam, J, and Fischer, A (2000). Responsiveness to celecoxib in chronic paroxysmal hemicrania. *Neurology*, 55:316.

Mathew, NT, Kailasam, J, and Meadors, L. (2002). Prophylaxis of migraine, transformed migraine, and cluster headache with topiramate. *Headache*, 42:796–803.

May, A, Bahra, A, Buchel, C, et al. (1998). Hypothalamic activation in cluster headache attacks. *Lancet*, 352:275–278.

May, A, Bahra, A, Buchel, C, et al. (1999). Functional magnetic resonance imaging in spontaneous attacks of SUNCT: short-lasting neuralgiform headache with conjunctival injection and tearing. *Ann Neurol*, 46:791–794.

May, A and Goadsby, PJ (1999). The trigeminovascular system in humans: pathophysiologic implications for primary headache syndromes of the neural influences on the cerebral circulation. *J Cereb Blood Flow Metab*, 19:115–127.

May, A, Kaube, H, Buchel, C, et al. (1998). Experimental cranial pain elicited by capsaicin: a PET study. *Pain*, 74:61–66.

McKinney, AS (1983). Cluster headache developing following ipsilateral orbital exenteration. *Headache*, 23:305–306.

Medina, JL (1992). Organic headaches mimicking chronic paroxysmal hemicrania. *Headache*, 32:73–74.

Meyer, JS and Hardenberg, J (1983). Clinical effectiveness of calcium entry blockers in prophylactic treatment of migraine and cluster headaches. *Headache*, 23:266–277.

Mirzai, R, Chang, C, Greenspan, A, et al. (1999). The pathogenesis of osteonecrosis and the relationships to corticosteroids. *J Asthma*, 36:77–95.

Molins, A, Lopez, M, Codina, A, et al. (1989). [Symptomatic cluster headache? Apropos of 4 case reports]. *Med Clin*, 92:181–183.

Mondejar, B, Cano, EF, Perez, I, et al. (2006). Secondary SUNCT syndrome to a variant of the vertebrobasilar vascular development. *Cephalalgia*, 26:620–622.

Monstad, I, Krabbe, A, Micieli, G, et al. (1995). Preemptive oral treatment with sumatriptan during a cluster period. *Headache*, 35:607–613.

Montes, E, Alberca, R, Lozano, P, et al. (2001). Statuslike sunct in two young women. *Headache,* 41:826–829.

Morales, F, Mostacero, E, Marta, J, et al. (1994). Vascular malformation of the cerebellopontine angle associated with "SUNCT" syndrome. *Cephalalgia,* 14:301–302.

Morales-Asin, F, Espada, F, Lopez-Obarrio, LA, et al. (2000). A SUNCT case with response to surgical treatment. *Cephalalgia,* 20:67–68.

Moris, G, Ribacoba, R, Solar, DN, et al. (2001). SUNCT syndrome and seborrheic dermatitis associated with craneosynostosis. *Cephalalgia,* 21:157–159.

Mulder, LJ and Spierings, EL (2002). Naratriptan in the preventive treatment of cluster headache. *Cephalalgia,* 22:815–817.

Mulder, LJ and Spierings, EL (2004). Non-lateralized pain in a case of chronic paroxysmal hemicrania? *Cephalalgia,* 24:52–53.

Munoz, C, Diez-Tejedor, E, Frank, A, et al. (1996). Cluster headache syndrome associated with middle cerebral artery arteriovenous malformation. *Cephalalgia,* 16:202–205.

-Negoro, K, Kawai, M, Tada, Y, et al. (2005). A case of postprandial cluster-like headache with prolactinoma: dramatic response to cabergoline. *Headache,* 45:604–606.

Newman, LC, Herskovitz, S, Lipton, RB, et al. (1992). Chronic paroxysmal headache: two cases with cerebrovascular disease. *Headache,* 32:75–76.

Newman, CN and Lipton, RB (1997). Paroxysmal Hemicranias. In *Headache* (PJ Goadsby and SD Silberstein, eds), pp. 243–250. Butterworth-Heinemann, Boston, Oxford.

Newman, LC, Lipton, RB, and Solomon, S (1993). Episodic paroxysmal hemicrania: 3 new cases and a review of the literature. *Headache,* 33:195–197.

Nicolodi, M, Sicuteri, F, and Poggioni, M. (1993). Hypothalamic modulation of nociception and reproduction in cluster headache. I. Therapeutic trials of leuprolide [see comments]. *Cephalalgia,* 13:253–257.

Nilsson Remahl, AI, Ansjon, R, Lind, F, et al. (2002). Hyperbaric oxygen treatment of active cluster headache: a double-blind placebo-controlled cross-over study. *Cephalalgia,* 22:730–739.

Nobre, ME, Filho, PF, and Dominici, M (2003). Cluster headache associated with sleep apnoea. *Cephalalgia,* 23:276–279.

Nobre, ME, Leal, AJ, Filho, PM (2005). Investigation into sleep disturbance of patients suffering from cluster headache. *Cephalalgia,* 25:488–492.

Paemeleire, K, Bahra, A, Evers, S, et al. (2006). Medication-overuse headache in patients with cluster headache. *Neurology,* 67:109–113.

Pareja, JA (1995). Chronic paroxysmal hemicrania: dissociation of the pain and autonomic features. *Headache,* 35:111–113.

Pareja, JA, Caminero, AB, Franco, E, et al. (2001). Dose, efficacy and tolerability of long-term indomethacin treatment of chronic paroxysmal hemicrania and hemicrania continua. *Cephalagia,* 21:869–938.

Pareja, JA, Kruszewski, P, and Caminero, AB (1999). SUNCT syndrome versus idiopathic stabbing headache (jabs and jolts syndrome). *Cephalalgia,* 19:46–48.

Pareja, JA, Kruszewski, P, and Sjaastad, O (1995). SUNCT syndrome: trials of drugs and anesthetic blockades. *Headache,* 35:138–142.

Pareja, JA and Sjaastad, O (1997). SUNCT syndrome. A clinical review. *Headache,* 37:195–202.

Pascual, J and Quijano, J (1998). A case of chronic paroxysmal hemicrania responding to subcutaneous sumatriptan [letter]. *J Neurol Neurosurg Psychiatr,* 65:407.

Pauri, F, Tilia, G, Cisternino, M, et al. (1993). Tuber cinereum hamartomas mimicking chronic paroxysmal hemicrania. *Ital J Neurol Sci,* 14(Suppl. 7):132.

Pelz, M and Merskey, H (1982). A case of pre-chronic paroxysmal hemicrania. *Cephalalgia,* 2:47–50.

Penart, A, Firth, M, and Bowen, JR (2001). Short-lasting unilateral neuralgiform headache with conjunctival injection and tearing (SUNCT) following presumed dorsolateral brainstem infarction. *Cephalalgia,* 21:236–239.

Peres, MF and Rozen, TD (2001). Melatonin in the preventive treatment of chronic cluster headache. *Cephalalgia,* 21:993–995.

Peres, MF, Stiles, MA, Siow, HC, et al. (2002). Greater occipital nerve blockade for cluster headache. *Cephalalgia,* 22:520–522.

Piovesan, EJ, Siow, C, Kowacs, PA, et al. (2003). Influence of lamotrigine over the SUNCT syndrome: one patient follow-up for two years. *Arq Neuropsiquiatr,* 61:691–694.

Pollmann, W and Pfaffenrath, V (1986). Chronic paroxysmal hemicrania: the first possible bilateral case. *Cephalalgia,* 6:55–57.

Porta, M, Granella, F, Coppola, A, et al. (1991). Treatment of cluster headache attacks with hyperbaric oxygen. *Cephalagia,* 11(Suppl. 11):236–237.

Porta-Etessam, J, Benito-Leon, J, Martinez-Salio, A, et al. (2002). Gabapentin in the treatment of SUNCT syndrome. *Headache,* 42:523–524.

Pradalier, A and Dry, J (1984). Chronic paroxysmal hemicrania. Treatment with indomethacin and diclofenac. *Therapie,* 39:185–188.

Prakash, KM and Lo, YL (2004). SUNCT syndrome in association with persistent Horner syndrome in a Chinese patient. *Headache,* 44:256–258.

Price, RW and Posner, JB (1978). Chronic paroxysmal hemicrania: a disabling headache syndrome responding to indomethacin. *Ann Neurol,* 3:183–184.

Prusinski, A, Liberski, PP, and Szulc-Kuberska, J (1985). Cluster headache in a patient without a ipsilateral eye. *Headache,* 25:134–135.

Raimondi, E (2001). Premonitory symptoms in cluster headache. *Curr Pain Headache Rep,* 5:55–59.

Raimondi, E and Gardella, L (1998). SUNCT syndrome. Two cases in Argentina. *Headache,* 38:369–371.

Rainero, I, Gallone, S, Valfre, W, et al. (2004). A polymorphism of the hypocretin receptor 2 gene is associated with cluster headache. *Neurology,* 63:1286–1288.

Rainero, I, Rivoiro, C, Gallone, S, et al. (2005). Lack of association between the 3092 T→C Clock gene polymorphism and cluster headache. *Cephalalgia,* 25:1078–1081.

Ramirez-Moreno, J, Fernandez-Portales, I, Garcia-Castanon, I, et al. (2004). SUNCT syndrome and neoplasms in the central nervous system. A new association. *Neurologia,* 19:326–330.

Rapoport, AM, Sheftell, FD, and Baskin, SM (1981). Chronic paroxysmal hemicrania-case report of the second known definite occurrence in a male. *Cephalalgia,* 1:67–69.

Raskin, NH (1988). *Headache.* Churchill Livingstone, New York.

Razvi, SS, Walker, L, Teasdale, E, et al. (2006). Cluster headache due to internal carotid artery dissection. *J Neurol,* 253:661–663.

Robbins, L (1995). Intranasal lidocaine for cluster headache. *Headache,* 35:83–84.

Roberge, C, Bouchard, JP, Simard, D, et al. (1992). Cluster headache in twins. *Neurology,* 42:1255–1256.

Rocha Filho, PA, Galvao, AC, Teixeira, MJ, et al. (2006). SUNCT syndrome associated with pituitary tumor: case report. *Arq Neuropsiquiatr,* 64:507–510.

Rogado, AZ and Graham, JR (1979). Through a glass darkly. *Headache,* 19:58–62.

Romoli, M and Cudia, G (1988). Cluster headache due to an impacted superior wisdom tooth: case report. *Headache,* 28:135–136.

Rosebraugh, CJ, Griebel, DJ, DiPette, DJ (1997). A case report of carotid artery dissection presenting as cluster headache. *Am J Med,* 102:418–419.

Rossi, P, Cesarino, F, Faroni, J, et al. (2003). SUNCT syndrome successfully treated with topiramate: case reports. *Cephalalgia,* 23:998–1000.

Rossi, P, Di Lorenzo, G, Faroni, J, et al. (2005). Seasonal, extratrigeminal, episodic paroxysmal hemicrania successfully treated with single suboccipital steroid injections. *Eur J Neurol,* 12:903–906.

Rothrock, J (2006). Cluster: a potentially lethal headache disorder. *Headache,* 46:327–327.

Rozen, TD (2001). Olanzapine as an abortive agent for cluster headache. *Headache,* 41:813–816.

Rozen, TD (2006). Resolution of SUNCT after removal of a pituitary adenoma in mild acromegaly. *Neurology,* 67:724.

Russell, D (1981). Cluster headache: severity and temporal profiles of attacks and patient activity prior to and during attacks. *Cephalalgia,* 1:209–216.

Russell, D (1984). Chronic paroxysmal hemicrania: severity, duration and time of occurrence of attacks. *Cephalalgia,* 4:53–56.

Russell, MB (1997). Genetic epidemiology of migraine and cluster headache. *Cephalalgia,* 17:683–701.

Russell, D (1999). Paroxysmal hemicrania. In *Cluster Headache & Related Conditions* (J Olesen and PJ Goadsby, eds), pp. 27–36. Oxford University Press, Oxford, New York.

Russell, MB (2004). Epidemiology and genetics of cluster headache. *Lancet Neurol,* 3:279–283.

Russell, MB, Andersson, PG, and Thomsen, LL (1995a). Familial occurrence of cluster headache. *J Neurol Neurosurg Psychiatr,* 58:341–343.

Russell, MB, Andersson, PG, Thomsen, LL, et al. (1995b). Cluster headache is an autosomal dominantly inherited disorder in some families: a complex segregation analysis. *J Med Genet,* 32:954–956.

Russell, D and Storstein, L (1983). Cluster headache: a computerized analysis of 24 h Holter ECG recordings and description of ECG rhythm disturbances. *Cephalalgia,* 3:83–107.

Russell, D and von der Lippe, A (1982). Cluster headache: heart rate and blood pressure changes during spontaneous attacks. *Cephalalgia,* 2:61–70.

Sabatowski, R, Huber, M, Meuser, T, et al. (2001). SUNCT syndrome: a treatment option with local opioid blockade of the superior cervical ganglion? A case report. *Cephalalgia,* 21:154–156.

Sacquegna, T, D'Alessandro, R, Cortelli, et al. (1982). Cluster headache after herpes zoster ophthalmicus. *Arch Neurol,* 39:384.

Saper, JR, Klapper, J, Mathew, NT, et al. (2002). Intranasal civamide for the treatment of episodic cluster headaches. *Arch Neurol,* 59:990–994.

Sarov, M, Valade, D, Jublanc, C, et al. (2006). Chronic paroxysmal hemicrania in a patient with a macroprolactinoma. *Cephalalgia,* 26:738–741.

Saxena, PR and Den Boer, MO (1991). Pharmacology of antimigraine drugs. *J Neurol,* 238:S28–S35.

Schlake, HP, Bottger, IG, Grotemeyer, KH, et al. (1990). Single photon emission computed tomography (SPECT) with 99mTc-HMPAO (hexamethyl propyleneamino oxime) in chronic paroxysmal hemicrania—a case report. *Cephalalgia,* 10:311–315.

Schoenen, J, Di Clemente, L, Vandenheede, M, et al. (2005). Hypothalamic stimulation in chronic cluster headache: a pilot study of efficacy and mode of action. *Brain,* 128:940–947.

Schurks, M, Kurth, T, de Jesus, J, et al. (2006). Cluster headache: clinical presentation, lifestyle features, and medical treatment. *Headache,* 46:1246–1254.

Schwaag, S, Frese, A, Husstedt, IW, et al. (2003). SUNCT syndrome: the first German case series. *Cephalalgia,* 23:398–400.

Schwedt, T, Dodick, D, Hentz, J, et al. (2007). Occipital nerve stimulation for chronic headache-long-term safety and efficacy. *Cephalalgia,* 27:153–157.

Schwedt, TJ, Dodick, DW, Trentman, TL, et al. (2006). Occipital nerve stimulation for chronic cluster headache and hemicrania continua: pain relief and persistence of autonomic features. *Cephalalgia,* 26:1025–1027.

Seidler, S, Marthol, H, Pawlowski, M, et al. (2006). Cluster headache in a ninety-one-year-old woman. *Headache,* 46:179–180.

Seijo-Martinez, M, Castro del Rio, M, Conde, C, et al. (2004). Cluster-like headache: association with cervical syringomyelia and Arnold-Chiari malformation. *Cephalalgia*, 24:140–142.

Sesso, RM (2001). SUNCT syndrome or trigeminal neuralgia with lacrimation and conjunctival injection? *Cephalalgia*, 21:151–153.

Shabbir, N and McAbee, G (1994). Adolescent chronic paroxysmal hemicrania responsive to verapamil monotherapy. *Headache*, 34:209–210.

Sicuteri, F (1959). Prophylactic and therapeutic properties of 1-methylysergic acid butanolamide in migraine. *Int Arch Allergy*, 15:300–307.

Sicuteri, F, Fanciullacci, M, Nicolodi, M, et al. (1990). Substance P theory: a unique focus on the painful and painless phenomena of cluster headache. *Headache*, 30:69–79.

Sicuteri, F, Franchi, G, Del Biancho, PL (1967). An antaminic drug, BC 105, in the prophylaxis of migraine. *Int Arch Allergy*, 31:78–84.

Sicuteri, F, Fusco, BM, Marabini, S, et al. (1989). Beneficial effect of capsaicin application to the nasal mucosa in cluster headache. *Clin J Pain*, 5:49–53.

Sicuteri, F, Geppetti, P, Marabini, S, et al. (1984). Pain relief by somatostatin in attacks of cluster headache. *Pain*, 18:359–365.

Silberstein, SD (1998). Methysergide. *Cephalalgia*, 18:421–435.

Silberstein, SD, Niknam, R, Rozen, TD, et al. (2000). Cluster headache with aura. *Neurology*, 54:219–221.

Singh, BN and Nademanee, K (1987). Use of calcium antagonists for cardiac arrhythmias. *Am J Cardiol*, 59:153B–162B.

Siow, H (2004). Seasonal episodic paroxysmal hemicrania responding to cyclooxygenase-2 inhibitors. *Cephalalgia*, 24:414–415.

Siow, HC, Pozo-Rosich, P, and Silberstein, SD (2004). Frovatriptan for the treatment of cluster headaches. *Cephalalgia*, 24:1045–1048.

Sjaastad, O (1986). Chronic paroxysmal hemicrania. In *Handbook of Clinical Neurology*, Vol 48. (P Vinken, G Bruyn, H Klawans, et al., eds), pp. 257–266. Elsevier, Amsterdam.

Sjaastad, O (1992). *Cluster Headache Syndrome*. W.B.Saunders, London.

Sjaastad, O and Antonaci, F (1995). A piroxicam derivative partly effective in chronic paroxysmal hemicrania and hemicrania continua. *Headache*, 35: 49–50.

Sjaastad, O, Apfelbaum, R, Caskey, W, et al. (1980)Chronic paroxysmal hemicrania (CPH). The clinical manifestations. A review. *Upsala J Med Sci*, (Suppl. 31):27–33.

Sjaastad, O and Bakketeig, LS (2003). Cluster headache prevalence. Vaga study of headache epidemiology. *Cephalalgia*, 23:528–533.

Sjaastad, O and Dale, I (1974). Evidence for a new (?) treatable headache entity. *Headache*, 14:105–108.

Sjaastad, O, Egge, K, Horven, I, et al. (1979). Chronic paroxysmal hemicranial: mechanical precipitation of attacks. *Headache*, 19:31–36.

Sjaastad, O, Horven, I, and Vennerod, AM (1976). A new headache syndrome? Headache resembling cluster headache headache), with recurring bouts of homolateral retrobulbar partial factor XII deficiency, bleeding tendency and a convulsive episode. *Headache*, 16:4–10.

Sjaastad, O, Russell, D, Horven, I (1978). Multiple neuralgiform, unilateral headache attacks associated with conjunctival injection and appearing in clusters. A nosological problem. Proceedings of the Scandinavian Migraine Society, p. 31.

Sjaastad, O and Salvesen, R (1986). Cluster headache: are we only seeing the tip of the iceberg? *Cephalalgia*, 6:127–129.

Sjaastad, O, Saunte, C, Salvesen, R, et al. (1989). Short-lasting unilateral neuralgiform headache attacks with conjunctival injection, tearing, sweating, and rhinorrhea. *Cephalalgia*, 9:147–156.

Sjaastad, O, Shen, JM, Stovner, LJ, et al. (1993). Cluster headache in identical twins. *Headache*, 33:214–217.

Sjaastad, O, Stovner, LJ, Stolt-Nielsen, A, et al. (1995). CPH and hemicrania continua: requirements of high indomethacin dosages—an ominous sign? *Headache*, 35:363–367.

Sjostrand, C, Giedratis, V, Ekbom, K, et al. (2001). CACNA1A gene polymorphisms in cluster headache. *Cephalalgia*, 21:953–958.

Sjostrand, C, Modin, H, Masterman, T, et al. (2002). Analysis of nitric oxide synthase genes in cluster headache. *Cephalalgia*, 22:758–764.

Slavik, RS and Rhoney, DH (1999). Indomethacin: a review of its cerebral blood flow effects and potential use for controlling intracranial pressure in traumatic brain injury patients. *Neurol Res*, 21:491–499.

Soros, P, Frese, A, Husstedt, IW, et al. (2001). Cluster headache after dental extraction: implications for the pathogenesis of cluster headache? *Cephalagia*, 21:619–622.

Speed, WG (1960). Ergotamine tartrate inhalation: a new approach to the management of recurrent vascular headaches. *Am J Med Sci*, 240:327–331.

Speight, TM and Avery, GS (1972). Pizotifen (BC-105); a review of its pharmacological properties and its therapeutic efficacy in vascular headaches. *Drugs*, 3:159–203.

Sprenger, T, Valet, M, Platzer, S, et al. (2005). SUNCT: bilateral hypothalamic activation during headache attacks and resolving of symptoms after trigeminal decompression. *Pain*, 113:422–426.

Stein, HJ and Rogado, AZ (1980). Headache rounds. Chronic paroxysmal hemicrania: two new patients. *Headache*, 20:72–76.

Stillman, MJ (2006). Testosterone replacement therapy for treatment refractory cluster headache. *Headache*, 46:925–933.

Svensson, D, Ekbom, K, Pedersen, NL, et al. (2003). A note on cluster headache in a population-based twin register. *Cephalalgia*, 23:376–380.

Swanson, JW, Yanagihara, T, Stang, PE, et al. (1994). Incidence of cluster headaches: a population-based study in Olmsted County, Minnesota. *Neurology,* 44:433–437.

Symonds, CP (1956). A particular variety of headache. *Brain,* 79:217–232.

Taub, E, Argoff, CE, Winterkorn, JM, et al. (1995). Resolution of chronic cluster headache after resection of a tentorial meningioma: case report [see comments]. *Neurosurgery,* 37:319–321; discussion 321–2.

Tay, BA, Ngan Kee, WD, and Chung, DC (2001). Gabapentin for the treatment and prophylaxis of cluster headache. *Reg Anesth Pain Med,* 26:373–375.

Tehindrazanarivelo, AD, Visy, JM, and Bousser, MG (1992). Ipsilateral cluster headache and chronic paroxysmal hemicrania: two case reports. *Cephalalgia,* 12:318–320.

ter Berg, JW and Goadsby, PJ (2001). Significance of atypical presentation of symptomatic SUNCT: a case report. *J Neurol Neurosurg Psychiatr,* 70:244–246.

Tfelt-Hansen, P (1999). Prophylactic pharmacotherapy of cluster headache. In *Cluster Headache & Related Conditions* (J Olesen and PJ Goadsby, eds), pp. 257–263. Oxford University Press, Oxford, New York.

Tfelt-Hansen, P, Bredberg, U, Eyjolfsdottir, GS, et al. (1985). Kinetics of methysergide and its main metabolite, methylergometrine, in man. *Cephalagia,* 5(Suppl. 3):54–55.

Tfelt-Hansen, P, Paulson, OB, and Krabbe, AA (1982). Invasive adenoma of the pituitary gland and chronic migrainous neuralgia. A rare coincidence or a causal relationship? *Cephalalgia,* 2:25–28.

Thomas, AL (1975). Periodic migrainous neuralgia associated with an arteriovenous malformation. *Postgrad Med J,* 51:460–462.

Tonon, C, Guttmann, S, Volpini, M, et al. (2002). Prevalence and incidence of cluster headache in the Republic of San Marino. *Neurology,* 58:1407–1409.

Torelli, P, Beghi, E, and Manzoni, GC (2005). Cluster headache prevalence in the Italian general population. *Neurology,* 64:469–474.

Torelli, P, Cologno, D, Cademartiri, C, et al. (2001). Application of the International Headache Society classification criteria in 652 cluster headache patients. *Cephalalgia,* 21:145–150.

Torelli, P and Manzoni, GC (2003). Pain and behaviour in cluster headache. A prospective study and review of the literature. *Funct Neurol,* 18:205–210.

van Vliet, JA, Bahra, A, Martin, V, et al. (2001). Intranasal sumatriptan is effective in the treatment of acute cluster headache—a double-blind placebo-controlled crossover study. *Cephalalgia,* 21:270–271.

van Vliet, JA, Ferrari, MD, and Haan, J (2003). SUNCT syndrome resolving after contralateral hemispheric ischaemic stroke. *Cephalagia,* 23:235–237.

Veloso, GG, Kaup, AO, Peres, MF, et al. (2001). Episodic paroxysmal hemicrania with seasonal variation: case report and the EPH-cluster headache continuum hypothesis. *Arq Neuropsiquiatr,* 59:944–947.

Vijayan, N (1992). Symptomatic chronic paroxysmal hemicrania [see comments]. *Cephalalgia,* 12:111–113.

Vilisaar, J (2006), Constantinescu CS. SUNCT in multiple sclerosis. *Cephalalgia,* 26: 891–893.

Volcy, M and Tepper, SJ (2006). Cluster-like headache secondary to idiopathic intracranial hypertension. *Cephalalgia,* 26:883–886.

Volcy, M, Tepper, SJ, Rapoport, AM, et al. (2005). Short-lasting unilateral neuralgiform headache attacks with cranial autonomic symptoms (SUNA)—a case report. *Cephalalgia,* 25:470–472.

Waldenlind, E, Gustafsson, SA, Ekbom, K, et al. (1987). Circadian secretion of cortisol and melatonin in cluster headache during active cluster periods and remission. *J Neurol Neurosurg Psychiatr,* 50:207–213.

Wang, Q, Mao, LM, and Han, JS (1990). Naloxone-reversible analgesia produced by microstimulation of the arcuate nucleus of the hypothalamus in pentobarbital-anesthetized rats. *Exp Brain Res,* 80:201–204.

Warner, JS, Wamil, AW, and McLean, MJ (1994). Acetazolamide for the treatment of chronic paroxysmal hemicrania. *Headache,* 34:597–599.

Weiller, C, May, A, Limmroth, V, et al. (1995). Brain stem activation in spontaneous human migraine attacks. *Nat Med,* 1:658–660.

Weiner, R and Reed, KL (1999). Peripheral neurostimulation for control of intractable occipital neuralgia. *Neuromodulation,* 2:217–221.

Weiss, LD, Ramasastry, SS, and Eidelman, BH (1989). Treatment of a cluster headache patient in a hyperbaric chamber. *Headache,* 29:109–110.

West, P and Todman, D (1991). Chronic cluster headache associated with a vertebral artery aneurysm. *Headache,* 31:210–212.

Wheeler, SD and Carrazana, EJ (1999). Topiramate-treated cluster headache. *Neurology,* 53:234–236.

Wingerchuk, DM, Nyquist, PA, Rodriguez, M, et al. (2000). Extratrigeminal short-lasting unilateral neuralgiform headache with conjunctival injection and tearing (SUNCT): new pathophysiologic entity or variation on a theme? *Cephalalgia,* 20:127–129.

Wober, C, Vigl, K, and Wessely, P (2002). Eletriptan for short-term prophylaxis of cluster headache. *Cephalagia,* 22:584.

Yang, J, Simonson, TM, Ruprecht, A, et al. (1996). Magnetic resonance imaging used to assess patients with trigeminal neuralgia. *Oral Surg Oral Med Oral Pathol Oral Radiol Endod,* 81:343–350.

Zebenholzer, K, Wober, C, Vigl, M, et al. (2004). Eletriptan for the short-term prophylaxis of cluster headache. *Headache,* 44:361–364.

Zidverc-Trajkovic, J, Pavlovic, A, Mijajlovic, M, et al. (2005). Cluster headache and paroxysmal hemicrania: differential diagnosis. *Cephalalgia,* 25:244–248.

15 Other Primary Headaches

Lawrence C Newman, Brian M Grosberg, and David W Dodick

Recognition of primary headache disorders that are less common than migraine, tension-type headache, and others discussed in this text is important, as the sufferers may be disabled, often misdiagnosed and therefore inappropriately treated. Although included under the rubric of *other primary headaches*, all of the disorders listed within this classification have secondary mimics.

International Classification of Headache Disorders (ICHD-II) criteria for these disorders, the diagnosis of the primary headache can only be given after secondary causes have been excluded. Furthermore, the proper treatment of these disorders is predicated upon establishing the correct diagnosis; some of the conditions described in this chapter respond dramatically to therapy with indomethacin but not to agents typically prescribed for the other more common primary headaches. This chapter reviews the epidemiology, clinical features, and treatment options for several of these less common disorders.

PRIMARY STABBING HEADACHE

Lansche (1964) provided the first cogent description of primary stabbing headache (PSH) in a series of patients observed with fleeting bouts of pain to the eye; this disorder was referred to as "ophthalmodynia periodica." These patients, many of them migraine sufferers, experienced sudden, unprovoked, ultrashort paroxysms of severe pain that occurred either as a single stab or a series of stabs. Since then, PSH has been recognized in the literature by alternative designations, including "ice pick headache," "sharp short-lived headache," "jabs and jolts syndrome," and "idiopathic stabbing headache" (Sjaastad et al., 1979; Raskin and Schwartz, 1980; Mathew, 1981; Pareja et al., 1996).

PSH is thought to be a rare disorder, but its brevity and coexistence with other headache disorders, such as migraine, cluster headache, tension-type headache, hemicrania continua (HC), cervicogenic headache, and chronic paroxysmal hemicranias, make it difficult to determine its true prevalence (Raskin and Schwartz, 1980; Drummond and Lance, 1984; Sjaastad, 1992; Young and Silberstein, 1993; Pareja et al., 1996). Some reports suggest that it occurs in approximately 40% of migraineurs (Raskin, 1986; Piovesan et al., 2001). Estimates in the literature from population-based studies indicate that the lifetime prevalence of PSH is less than 1%–2% (Rasmussen, 1994, 1995; Monteiro, 1995). The disorder usually begins in adulthood. The age at onset ranges from 12 to 70 years, with a mean of approximately 47 years (Pareja et al., 1996). PSH has a female predominance with a sex ratio that has ranges from 1.49:1 to 6.6:1 (Pareja et al., 1996; Sjaastad et al., 2001). The diagnostic criteria for this primary headache disorder are listed in Table 15–1.

PSH is characterized by spontaneous, paroxysmal attacks of fleeting head pain. The pain is moderate to severe in intensity and usually maximal in the ophthalmic distribution of the trigeminal nerve, particularly the orbital region (Pareja et al., 1996). Less commonly affected sites of pain include the facial, temporal, parietal, retroauricular and occipital regions of the head (Martins et al., 1995; Pareja et al., 1996). Attacks are typically unilateral, but may be bilateral, and vary in location. The pain is often sharp, pricking, or stabbing in nature. Individual attacks are very brief and generally last between 1 and 10 seconds, with more than two-thirds of reported attacks lasting 1 second (Pareja et al., 1996). The frequency of attacks is quite variable, ranging from 1 attack per year to 50 attacks

TABLE 15–1 Diagnostic Criteria for this Primary Stabbing Headache.

Description

Transient and localized stabs of pain in the head that occur spontaneously in the absence of organic disease of underlying structures of the cranial nerves

Diagnostic criteria

A. Head pain occurring as a single stab or a series of stabs and fulfilling criteria B and C
B. Exclusively or predominantly felt in the distribution of the first division of the trigeminal nerve
C. Stabs last for up to a few seconds and recur with irregular frequency ranging from one to many per day
D. No accompanying symptoms
E. Not attributed to another disorder[a]

[a] History and physical and neurological examinations do not suggest any of the disorders listed in groups 5–12 and/or neurological examinations do suggest such disorder but it is ruled out by appropriate investigations, or such disorder is present but attacks do not occur for the first time in close temporal relation to the disorder.

daily. Most attacks are distributed throughout the day and evening and may recur at irregular intervals. In one study, chronic attacks (>80% of days) occurred in 14% of 38 patients followed over a 1-year period (Pareja et al., 1996). Accompanying autonomic phenomena are generally absent. Rarely, conjunctival hemorrhage and monocular visual loss have been reported with PSH (Pareja et al., 1996; Zakaria et al., 2000).

The differential diagnosis of PSH includes other recurrent, short-lived primary headaches such as the trigeminal autonomic cephalalgias (TACs), particularly short-lasting unilateral neuralgiform headaches with conjunctival injection and tearing (SUNCT), cough headache, exertional headache, headache associated with sexual activity, hypnic headache (HH), and trigeminal neuralgia. Though the TACs enter into the differential diagnosis of short-duration primary headaches, the absence of autonomic features, such as lacrimation, ptosis, rhinorrhea, and conjunctival injection, excludes these disorders. Similarly, cough, sexual, exertional, and HH are excluded by the absence of robust trigger factors such as cough, sex, exercise, and sleep. Trigeminal neuralgia is excluded by the lack of trigger points, and trigeminal neuralgia affects the trigeminal distribution alone in less than 4% of patients. Secondary causes of stabbing headache reported in the literature include intracranial structural lesions such as meningiomas and .pituitary tumors, temporal arteritis, cerebrovascular diseases, cranial, and ocular trauma, herpes zoster, and, possibly, intraocular pressure elevation (Raskin and Schwartz, 1980; Pareja et al., 1996; Mascellino et al., 2001; Levy et al., 2003).

Acute treatment of PSH is impractical because of the brevity and repetitive nature of attacks. Indomethacin given prophylactically provides complete or partial improvement in most, but not all cases (Medina and Diamond, 1981; Pareja et al., 1996; Dodick, 2004). The usual effective dose ranges from 25 to 150 mg per day. In patients unable to tolerate indomethacin, success has been reported with melatonin, in doses ranging from 3 to 12 mg daily, and gabapentin 400 mg BID (Rozen, 2003a; Franca et al., 2004).

PRIMARY COUGH HEADACHE

Primary cough headache is uncommon, with a lifetime prevalence of approximately 1% (Rasmussen and Olesen, 1992). Primary cough headache typically affects men over the age of 40; the mean age of onset is 67 years (Pasqual, 2005). The headache is of sudden onset, occurring within seconds of coughing, but may also be precipitated by sneezing, straining, or other Valsalva maneuvers. The pain is usually described as sharp, stabbing, or splitting in nature, moderate to severe intensity, and is often bilateral and maximal in the vertex, frontal, occipital, or temporal regions. The headache typically lasts from 1 second to 30 minutes; however, some sufferers may continue to experience a dull ache for several hours afterward (ICHD II; Diamond, 1982). These headaches are not accompanied by neurological symptoms, and nausea and vomiting are absent. The criteria for primary cough headache are listed in Table 15–2.

Although the precise etiology is unknown, it has been hypothesized that these headaches may be the result of a sudden increase in intracranial venous pressure with subsequent traction on pain sensitive structures from downward displacement

TABLE 15–2 Criteria for Primary Cough Headache.

Previously used terms: Benign cough headache, Valsalva-maneuver headache

Description

Headache precipitated by coughing or straining in the absence of any intracranial disorder

Diagnostic criteria

A. Headache fulfilling criteria B and C
B. Sudden onset, lasting one second to 30 minutes
C. Brought on by and occurring only in association with coughing, straining and/or Valsalva maneuver
D. Not attributed to another disorder[a]

[a] Cough headache is symptomatic in approximately 40% of cases and the large majority of these present Arnold–Chiari malformation type I. Other reported causes of symptomatic cough headache include carotid or vertebrobasilar diseases and cerebral aneurysms. Diagnostic neuroimaging plays an important role in differentiating secondary cough headache from 4.2 Primary cough headache.

of cerebellar tonsils (Wang et al., 2000). Hypersensitivity of the pressure receptors of the venous vasculature has also been suggested as a potential mechanism for the production of this type of headache (Raskin, 1997). In a small series, patients with primary cough headache were found to have reduced volume of the posterior fossa (Chen et al., 2004).

The diagnosis of primary cough headache should be suspect when the patient is young and when the headache is unilateral, lasts longer than 30 minutes, or is associated with other neurological symptoms. Secondary cough headache has been described in patients with Chiari malformation, brain tumor—both malignant and benign (meningioma/acoustic neuroma), cerebral aneurysm, and carotid or vertebrobasilar disease (Pascual et al., 1996). Approximately one-half of all cases of cough headache are due to secondary causes (Pascual et al., 1996). Neuroimaging therefore is mandatory to distinguish the secondary causes from the primary form.

Indomethacin is the treatment of choice in those patients who frequently experience cough headache and the sustained release formulation (75 mg QD or BID) is often the best choice. A positive response to indomethacin may be seen in secondary cases and is therefore not diagnostic of primary cough headache. Response to treatment with other agents including naproxen, acetazolamide, methysergide, dihydroergotamine, propanolol, and topiramate have also been reported (Raskin, 1988a; Calandre et al., 1996; Medrano et al., 2005). In a small case series, lumbar puncture with removal of 40 ml of cerebrospinal fluid (CSF) provided prompt relief (Raskin, 1995).

PRIMARY EXERTIONAL HEADACHE

The prevalence of exertional headaches in the general population is approximately 10% (Sjaastad and Bakketeig, 2003). Similar to primary cough headache, primary exertional headache has a male predominance, however, it differs from primary cough headache in that it occurs in a younger population, with a mean age of onset of 24 years (Pascual et al., 1996). Patients often have a personal or family history of migraine (Pascual et al., 1996).

Although cough and exertional headache are often linked as "valsalva maneuver headaches," they remain distinct entities in the ICHD-II classification. The headache is of sudden onset and often bilateral in location, but unlike cough headache, the pain is often pulsatile and of longer duration (5 minutes to 48 hours). The headache is often accompanied by nausea, vomiting, photophobia, and phonophobia (Pascual et al., 1996). Primary exertional headache may be precipitated by a variety of physical exercises, such as swimming, or weight-lifting, as well as by straining or bending over (Dalessio, 1974; Paulson, 1983; Indo and Takahashi, 1990). Predisposing factors include high temperature and humidity, high altitude, hypoglycemia, and ingestion of caffeine and alcohol-containing beverages (Dalessio, 1974).

The ICHD-II criteria for primary exertional headache are listed in Table 15–3.

As in cough headache, neuroimaging to rule out a posterior fossa or craniocervical junction abnormality should be undertaken in a patient presenting with new exertional headache, particularly when the headache is unilateral (Pascual et al., 1996). In addition to unilaterality, secondary exertional headache often begins later in life, lasts

Table 15–3 The ICHD-II Criteria for Primary Exertional Headache.

Description

Headache precipitated by any form of exercise

Diagnostic criteria

A. Pulsating headache fulfilling B and C
B. Lasting 5 minutes to 48 hours
C. Brought on by and occurring only during or physical exertion
D. Not attributed to another disorder[a]

[a] On first occurrence of this headache type it is mandatory to exclude subarachnoid hemorrhage and arterial dissection.

longer (24 hours to weeks) and in cases of subarachnoid hemorrhage (SAH), the headache is associated with neurological features such as meningismus. Other secondary causes include Chiari malformation, subdural hematoma, neoplasm (primary and metastatic) and platybasia (Pascual et al., 1996). A "first-ever" presentation of exertional headache requires a work-up to rule out SAH or arterial dissection (ICHD-II).

The pathophysiology of primary exertional headache is unknown, but it is theorized that venous or arterial distention following exercise, (especially in a warm environment) may play a role by the release of vasoactive peptides leading to downstream neurogenic inflammation (Buzzi et al., 1995).

The treatment of primary exertional headache need not always consist of medications. When the headaches are mild or slow to build in intensity, patients may benefit from a gradually increasing exercise routine. A warm-up period may prevent these headaches (Lambert and Burnet, 1985). Pharmacotherapy may be given on a prophylactic or acute basis. Beta-adrenergic blockers, in typical antimigraine doses, have demonstrated benefit; however, these agents often interfere with exercise tolerance (Evans and Pascual, 2000). Because this disorder is often self-limited with most cases lasting 3–6 months, discontinuing therapy after 6 months and reevaluating the patient is advisable. Treatment with indomethacin 25–250 mg daily, or employing naproxen or ergotamine before exercise may be helpful (Diamond and Medina, 1979; Raskin ,1988a; Pascual et al., 1996).

PRIMARY HEADACHES ASSOCIATED WITH SEXUAL ACTIVITY

The exact prevalence of headache attributed to sexual activity is unknown, possibly because of the reluctance of patients to report their sexual experiences (Kritz, 1970). The lifetime prevalence has been reported to be approximately 1%; studies in subspecialty headache clinics report that 0.2%–1.3% of all patients report these headaches (Rasmussen and Olesen, 1992; Frese et al., 2003).

Headaches with sexual activity affect men more often than women. These headaches have also been referred to as benign sex headache, coital cephalalgia, benign vascular sexual headache, or benign orgasmic headaches. As they are not solely precipitated during sexual intercourse (similar headaches provoked by masturbation and during nocturnal emissions have been reported), or orgasm, the ICHD-II has classified these as primary headaches associated with sexual activity (Lance 1976; Robbins, 1994; Jacome, 1998). Three varieties of these headaches were described in the first edition of the ICHD (Headache Classification Committee of the International Headache Society, 1988); a dull type, an explosive type, and a postural type. In ICHD-II, however, these subtypes are not classified as such. Rather, primary headache associated with sexual activity is now separated into preorgasmic and orgasmic headaches. These criteria are listed in Table 15–4.

Preorgasmic headache (previously classified as the dull subtype) occurs in approximately 20% of patients with primary headache associated with sexual activity. These headaches resemble tension-type headaches in that they are characterized by a generalized dull ache involving the head and neck. Some patients describe an awareness of tightness of the muscles of the jaw and neck occurring during sexual activity. Preorgasmic headaches are bilateral, beginning as sexual excitement builds, and can be prevented or reduced by deliberate muscle relaxation.

Orgasmic headaches (previously called the explosive subtype) are the most common, accounting for approximately 75% of cases. It is estimated that 50% of these sufferers also have preexisting migraine (Silbert et al., 1991). These headaches begin abruptly, at the moment of orgasm, and may be caused by an increase in blood pressure.

TABLE 15–4 Institute for Advanced Studies (IHS) Criteria of Primary Headache Associated with Sexual Activity.

Description

Headache precipitated by sexual activity, usually starting as a dull bilateral ache as sexual excitement increases and suddenly becoming intense at orgasm, in the absence of any intracranial disorder

Preorgasmic headache

A. Dull ache in the head and neck associated with awareness of neck and/or jaw muscle contraction and fulfilling criterion B
B. Occurs during sexual activity and increases with sexual excitement
C. Not attributed to another disorder

Orgasmic headache

A. Sudden severe ("explosive") headache fulfilling criterion B
B. Occurs at orgasm
C. Not attributed to another disorder[a]

[a] On first onset of orgasmic headache it is mandatory to exclude conditions such as subarachnoid hemorrhage.

The pain is excruciatingly severe; most often described as explosive or throbbing, and may be frontal, occipital, or generalized. On occasion, this type of headache may be associated with nausea and vomiting. These headaches typically last from 1 minute to 3 hours.

The pathophysiology of these headaches is uncertain. Some investigators believe that the preorgasmic form is related to tension-type headache (Silbert et al., 1991; Lance 1992; Pascual et al., 1996), and the orgasmic form has been likened to primary exertional headache and may therefore also be owing to short-lived increases in intracranial pressure (Queiroz, 2001). Others speculate that the orgasmic form is a variant of migraine (Silbert et al., 1991).

The postural variety is the least common subtype affecting approximately 5% of sufferers. This headache resembles the headache that follows lumbar puncture in that it worsens with sitting or standing and is relieved by recumbency. It may be caused by a rent in the dura that spontaneously develops during sexual activity. This rare subtype is no longer included in the ICHD classification of headaches associated with sexual activity. Instead, these headaches are now classified as headaches attributed to spontaneous low CSF pressure.

The diagnosis of primary headache associated with sexual activity is predicated upon the exclusion of secondary causes such as SAH, arterial dissection, and lesions of the posterior fossa, CSF pathways, and cervical spine (Selwyn, 1985; Pascual et al., 1996). The mainstay of treatment of the primary forms of headaches associated with sexual activity is reassurance, both of the patient and their partner. For most patients, these are self-limited disorders; however, the course may be unpredictable. Headaches often recur during several sexual encounters over a brief period of time and never return again, whereas other patients experience them at infrequent intervals throughout their lifetime. Headache recurrence has been reported when patients resumed sexual activity within several days after an attack (Porter and Jancovic, 1981; Edis and Silbert, 1988; Kim, 1992; Lance, 1992), so advising patients to refrain from sex for a week following an attack might be prudent. Often patients with the preorgasmic subtype can lessen the severity of an impending attack by stopping the sexual activity as soon as the headache begins or by assuming a more passive role. In general, acute treatment following an attack is of little or no benefit (Frese et al., 2004). Preemptive treatment with indomethacin 50–100 mg taken 30–60 minutes before sexual activity may prevent attacks, as can naratriptan 2.5 mg or ergotamine tartrate taken 2 hours before (Kumar and Reuler, 1993; Pascual et al., 1996; Evans and Pascual, 2000). For patients who suffer from frequent, recurrent episodes preventive strategies should be employed. Indomethacin 25 mg TID with meals often prevents attacks. Other options for prophylaxis include β-blockers such as propranolol 40–240 mg daily, metoprolol 25–50 mg, and atenolol 25–50 mg. Caution is recommended however as these drugs may cause impotence and interfere with sexual function (Porter and Jancovic, 1981; Silbert et al., 1991; Kumar and Reuler, 1993; Frese et al., 2004). One patient has been reported in whom treatment with the calcium channel blocker, diltiazem 60 mg TID, was successful (Akpunonu and Ahrens, 1991), although the use of verapamil for this syndrome was ineffective in one patient (Evans and Pascual, 2000).

THE HH SYNDROME

The HH is a rare, recurrent, sleep-related, primary headache disorder that usually begins after 50 years of age. Raskin first described the disorder in 1988 (Raskin, 1988b); more than 90 cases have been subsequently reported (Newman et al., 1990; Dodick et al., 1998; Newman and Mosek, 2006). In the largest case series, HH was diagnosed in 0.07%–0.1% of all headache patients assessed annually at a specialty clinic reflecting the rarity of this syndrome (Dodick et al., 1998; Evers et al., 2003).

HH usually begins late in life with a mean age at onset of 61 ± 10 years (range 30–83 years). A report of a 9-year-old girl with probable HH has been reported, although the headache frequency did not meet International Headache Society (IHS) criteria (Grossberg et al., 2004). The condition is more prevalent in women (65%) than in men. Table 15–5 lists the ICHD-II criteria for HH.

HHs occur at a consistent time each night, usually between 1:00 and 3:00 AM, and may on rare instances occur during a daytime nap (Gould and Silberstein, 1997a; Newman and Mosek, 2006). The headaches begin abruptly, are diffuse and throbbing, and spontaneously resolve in 15–180 minutes. Rarely, the headache is hemicranial (Gould and Silberstein, 1997a, 1997b; Dodick et al., 1998; Ivanez et al., 1998; Evers et al., 2003). The pain in HH is usually localized anteriorly. On occasion it involves the occiput or radiates into the neck.

The duration of an untreated attack varies among patients. Usually the pain resolves within 1–2 hours (range 15–180 minutes), but longer attacks of up to 10 hours have been reported. The frequency of attacks is high. More than four attacks per week occurred in 70% of the cases and about half of them had daily attacks (range one per week to six per night) (Newman and Mosek, 2006). Associated autonomic symptoms accompany the pain in approximately 8% of sufferers (Evers and Dodick, 2005), and nausea, photophobia, and phonophobia may rarely be present.

Reports of probable secondary HH have been described. In one, the patient had a 9-month history of typical HH, but also reported brief episodes of giddiness. A brain magnetic resonance imaging (MRI) revealed a large posterior-fossa meningioma. Following tumor resection, there was complete resolution of the headache (Peatfield and Mendozza, 2003). Following an ischemic stroke involving the midrostral upper pons, a 72-year-old man developed HH (Moon et al., 2003). In another report, HH-like headaches occurred in the setting of intracranial hypotension. Headaches remitted following a spinal blood patch (Freeman et al., 2004).

The exact pathophysiological mechanisms of HH have not yet been elucidated. It has been postulated that HH may be the result of a chronobiological disorder, serotonin, and melatonin dysregulation, or a disturbance of rapid eye movement (REM) sleep.

Raskin hypothesized that HH results from a disturbance of the mammalian biological pacemaker of the brain residing within the suprachiasmatic nuclei (SCN) (Raskin, 1988b). Dysfunction of this "biological clock" that generates circadian rhythms has been linked to other phasic disorders such as bipolar illness, cluster headaches, and jet lag. A disturbance of the regulating system of the SCN could account for the clock-like regularity of headaches in HH.

Neuronal pathways exist between the SCN and the pain-modulating systems of the midbrain

Table 15–5 Institute for Advanced Studies (IHS) Criteria for Hypnic Headache.

Description

Attacks of dull headache that always awaken the patient from sleep

Diagnostic criteria

A. Dull headache fulfilling criteria B–D
B. Develops only during sleep, and awakens patient
C. At least two of the following characteristics:
   1. Occurs >15 times per month
   2. Lasts ⩾15 minutes after waking
   3. First occurs after age of 50 years
D. No autonomic symptoms and no more than one of nausea, photophobia or phonophobia
E. Not attributed to another disorder[a]

[a] Intracranial disorders must be excluded. Distinction from one of the trigeminal autonomic cephalgias is necessary for effective management.

periaqueductal gray matter and dorsal raphe nuclei. These pathways and the mammalian biological pacemaker are serotonergically modulated. Lithium carbonate, the agent most frequently reported to treat successfully this disorder, affects serotonin metabolism by down-regulating serotonin receptors thereby increasing serotonin release (Treiser et al., 1981).

Dysregulation of melatonin has also been suggested as a putative mechanism of the syndrome. Melatonin is the main product of the pineal gland and is a marker of circadian rhythm. Melatonin modulates many neurobiological functions such as cerebral vascular tone, serotonin neurotransmission, and inhibition of prostaglandin E_2 synthesis (Ivanez et al., 1998). With age, there is a decrease in the activity of the hypothalamic-pineal axis with a subsequent diminution of nocturnal secretion of melatonin. Lithium indirectly causes a rise in nocturnal melatonin levels by increasing serotonin production and tryptophan absorption, both melatonin precursors (Chazot et al., 1987; Lewis et al., 1990; Leone et al., 1995). Furthermore, melatonin therapy has been reported to abolish attacks in some patients with HH (Dodick, 2000; Evers and Goadsby, 2003).

In that the headaches of HH occur exclusively during sleep, often during a dream, several investigators have postulated that the syndrome is a disorder of REM sleep. REM sleep is associated with decreased levels of serotonin, increases in cerebral blood flow, and dramatic reductions in the activity of the neurons within the dorsal raphe and locus ceruleus (Somers et al., 1993), an ideal setting for headache occurrence. In most of the patients with HH who have had polysomnographic studies, attacks were associated with REM sleep (Porter and Jancovic, 1981; Morales-Asin et al., 1998; Dodick, 2000; Evers et al., 2003; Evers and Goadsby, 2003; Pinessi et al., 2003), however, non-REM related HHs have also recently been reported (Manni et al., 2004; Vieira-Dias et al., 2001).

It is probable, given the differences in medication response (see below) and in polysomnographic studies, that more than one pathophysiological mechanism is responsible for HH. Further investigations using sleep studies and functional neuroimaging are necessary to better understand this syndrome.

Lithium was the first treatment reported to be effective for HH (Raskin, 1988b; Newman et al., 1990; Evers and Goadsby, 2003; Newman and Mosek, 2006). Treatment is initiated with 300 mg at bedtime and can be increased to 600 mg at bedtime within a week. Renal and thyroid function should be assessed before initiating therapy, and periodically during treatment. Serum lithium concentrations should be monitored as well to avoid toxicity. Side effects include tremor, diarrhea, increased thirst, and polyuria.

Although lithium has higher efficacy rates than other medications, it is often poorly tolerated. By reassuring the patients of the benign nature of the headache, some will choose to delay usage of medications (Dodick et al., 1998). Other agents that have been reported to effectively treat HH include bedtime doses of caffeine (40–60 mg tablet, or as a cup of coffee) (Fischer, 1984; Dodick et al., 1998; Evers and Goadsby, 2003), flunarizine 5 mg (Fischer, 1984; Newman et al., 1990; Evers and Goadsby, 2003), melatonin (Dodick, 2000) and indomethacin 25–75 mg (Fischer, 1984; Dodick et al., 1998; Jones and Dodick, 2000; Evers and Goadsby, 2003). Indomethacin appears to be of utility for patients in whom attacks are strictly unilateral (Dodick et al., 2000).

PRIMARY THUNDERCLAP HEADACHE

Primary thunderclap headache (PTCH) is a rare and poorly understood disorder characterized by a severe headache that rapidly reaches peak intensity. The term thunderclap headache (TCH) was introduced by Day and Raskin (1986) in their report of a patient with a rapidly progressive secondary headache attributed to an unruptured cerebral aneursym. Recently, the IHS applied the term PTCH (Table 15–6) to primary headache disorders of rapid onset (Headache Classification Committee of the International Headache Society, 2004). In developing these criteria, the second edition of the ICHDs acknowledged that the evidence supporting the existence of this entity is inadequate. Consequently, an expedient and exhaustive search is strongly recommended to exclude any underlying secondary cause.

Patients with PTCH sometimes have a prior history of migraine; in others, it may presage the development of migraine. PTCH is often described as the worst headache of the patient's

Table 15–6 Diagnostic Criteria for Thunderclap Headache.

A. Severe head pain fulfilling criteria B and C
B. Both of the following characteristics:
   1. Sudden onset, reaching maximum intensity in <1 minute
   2. Lasting from 1 hour to 10 days
C. Does not recur regularly over subsequent weeks or months[a]
D. Not attributed to another disorder[b]

[a] Headache may recur within the first week after onset.

[b] Normal cerebrospinal fluid (CSF) and normal brain imaging are required.

life. The pain begins abruptly and rapidly intensifies, reaching a climax of pain within 1 minute. The pain is most commonly occipital in location, but may involve any region of the head or neck. Associated symptoms may include photophobia, phonophobia, neck stiffness, nausea, and/or vomiting. Attacks typically last several hours, but may linger at a lower level for weeks. Repeated bouts of PTCH may occur within the first two weeks or, less commonly, over the following months to years. In both instances, the attacks may begin spontaneously while at rest or be precipitated by exertion, vigorous exercise, bathing in hot water, hyperventilation, or sexual activity. Valsalva-related maneuvers appear to be a provoking factor in up to one-third of patients with PTCH (Dodick, 2002). The majority of patients have a normal neurological examination, although focal deficits have been rarely reported (Slivka and Philbrook, 1995).

PTCH is both a diagnosis of inclusion as certain features must be present, and a diagnosis of exclusion in that secondary causes must be eliminated. The differential diagnosis includes SAH, intracerebral hemorrhage, cerebral venous sinus thrombosis, arterial dissection, pituitary apoplexy, hypertensive encephalopathy, spontaneous intracranial hypotension, and posterior leukoencephalopathy (Schwedt et al., 2006).

According to ICHD-2 criteria, CSF and brain imaging must be normal. Diagnostic testing should include an emergent noncontrast CT of the brain and a lumbar puncture to exclude SAH. If the results of these studies are normal or inconclusive, further neuroimaging with cerebral MRI, magnetic resonance angiography (MRA), magnetic resonance venogram (MRV), and if necessary, MRI of the cervical arteries should be performed (Schwedt et al., 2006). The ICHD-2 criteria make no mention of the need for angiography. In some patients, MRA or four-vessel angiography may be necessary to exclude an unruptured aneurysm or arteriovenous malformation. Some patients with PTCH have angiographic evidence of segmental vasospasm (Day and Raskin, 1986; Slivka and Philbrook, 1995; Dodick et al., 1999; Chen et al., 2006). In these patients, central nervous system vasculitis should be considered in the differential diagnosis (see Chapter 31 on Emergency Headaches).

Since PTCH is usually a self-limited disorder, there are no treatment recommendations. Long-term follow up in patients with PTCH and unruptured aneurysms thus far has not revealed a tendency to bleed (Widjicks et al., 1988; Harling et al., 1989), but this remains controversial (Takeuchi et al., 1996). Recurrent TCH with vasospasm leading to stroke has been reported (Strum and Macdonell, 2000); nimodipine may lessen the risk (Nowak et al., 2003; Lu et al., 2004; Chen et al., 2006).

HEMICRANIA CONTINUA

HC is another primary headache disorder that is responsive to treatment with indomethacin. The disorder was first described in 1981 (Medina and Diamond, 1981) and officially named in 1984 (Sjaastad and Spierings, 1984). There are now more than 100 reports of HC in the literature. HC was not included in the first edition of the ICHDs (Headache Classification Committee of the International Headache Society, 1988). Because of the presence of autonomic features that accompany the painful exacerbations, HC was considered to be one of the trigeminal autonomic cephalgias (TAC) (Goadsby and Lipton, 1997). However, the ICHD-II includes HC within the other primary headaches section. Diagnostic criteria for HC are listed in Table 15–7.

Although considered rare, some have reported HC to be a more common cause of refractory, unilateral, chronic daily headache (CDH) in headache subspecialty clinics than previously

Table 15–7 Diagnostic Criteria for Hemicrania Continua (HC).

- A. Headache for >3 months fulfilling criteria B–D
- B. All of the following characteristics:
  1. Unilateral pain without side-shift
  2. Daily and continuous, without pain-free periods
  3. Moderate intensity, but with exacerbations of severe pain
- C. At least one of the following autonomic features occurs during exacerbations and ipsilateral to the side of pain:
  1. Conjunctival injection and/or lacrimation
  2. Nasal congestion and/or rhinorrhoea
  3. Ptosis and/or miosis
- D. Complete response to therapeutic doses of indomethacin
- E. Not attributed to another disorder[a]

[a] History and physical and neurological examinations do not suggest any of the disorders listed in groups 5–12, or history and/or physical and/or neurological examinations do suggest such disorder but it is ruled out by appropriate investigations, or such disorder is present but headache does not occur for the first time in close temporal relation to the disorder.

recognized (Peres et al., 2001). The disorder demonstrates a female predominance with a female to male ratio of approximately 2:1. The age of onset ranges from 11 to 58 years (mean 34 years). Clinically, HC is characterized by a unilateral, continuous headache of mild to moderate intensity. Patients usually describe this baseline discomfort as dull, aching, or pressing and it is not associated with other symptoms. The pain is maximal in the ocular, temporal, and maxillary regions. Superimposed on this background discomfort, exacerbations of more severe pain, lasting 20 minutes to several days are experienced by the majority of sufferers. Although significantly more intense than the baseline pain, these painful exacerbations usually do not reach the level experienced by cluster headache sufferers. During these excerbations, one or more autonomic symptoms (ptosis, conjunctival injection, lacrimation, and nasal congestion) occur ipsilateral to the pain. These exacerbations may occur at any time and frequently awaken the patient from sleep. Migrainous symptoms, such as nausea, vomiting, photophobia, and phonophobia may also accompany the exacerbations of pain, and a single patient with HC with associated aura has been reported (Peres et al., 2002). Many patients report PSH (stabs and jabs), and a feeling of sand or an eyelash in the affected eye (foreign body sensation) (Newman et al., 2001). Most patients experience strictly unilateral headaches without side shift, although three patients in whom attacks alternated sides (Newman et al., 1992; Marano et al., 1994; Newman et al., 2004) and three bilateral cases have been described (Pasquier et al., 1987; Iordanidis and Sjaastad, 1989; Trucco et al., 1992).

Two temporal profiles of HC exist: an episodic form with distinct headache phases separated by pain-free remissions, and a chronic form in which headaches persist without remissions (Sjaastad and Antonaci, 1993; Newman et al., 1994; Goadsby and Lipton, 1997). HC is chronic from onset in 53% of patients; evolves from an episodic pattern in 35%, although in 12% it begins and remains episodic (Peres et al., 2001). A typical presentations of HC, one in whom an initially chronic course evolved into the episodic form, and another with episodic HC with a clear seasonal pattern have been described (Pareja, 1995; Peres et al., 2001) as has a new variant of HC termed HC postpartum (Spitz and Peres, 2004).

HC is frequently misdiagnosed as another primary headache syndrome. If the physician focuses on the ipsilateral autonomic features that accompany the painful exacerbations, the disorder may be incorrectly diagnosed as cluster headache. Similarly, by focusing on the associated photophobia, phonophobia, nausea, and vomiting that may occur during exacerbations, HC may be misdiagnosed as migraine. HC is distinguished from cluster and migraine by the presence of a continuous baseline headache of mild to moderate severity, a lack of robust autonomic symptoms and signs, even during exacerbations, and a lack of exacerbations with circadian periodicity. Differentiaing HC from unilateral chronic migraine can be very difficult. A response to indomethacin is the clinical feature that best distinguishes these two disorders.

Organic mimics of HC have been reported: a mesenchymal tumor involving the sphenoid bone, clinoid process, and skull base created symptoms of HC (Goadsby and Lipton, 1997).

HC-like headaches were also reported in a patient with human immunodeficiency virus (Brilla et al., 1998), adenocarcinoma of the lung (Eross et al., 2002), and by a C7 disc herniation (Sjaastad et al., 1995). The diagnosis of HC may be masked by medication overuse headache (Young and Silberstein, 1993); with discontinuation of the overused agents, the clinical features of HC may become more evident.

The pathophysiology of this disorder is not known; some investigators believe it is a subtype of migraine, whereas others believe it is more closely related to the TAC. Migrainous features are often experienced by patients with HC, and a patient with HC and familial hemiplegic migraine has been reported (Evers et al., 1999). Functional brain imaging, it was hoped, would clarify our understanding of this disorder, but rather than showing that HC belongs to one group or the other, it appears HC is a distinct headache syndrome. Scans of patients with HC reveal activation of the contralateral posterior hypothalamus and ipsilateral dorsal rostral pons, as well as activation of the ipsilateral ventolateral midbrain, extending over the red nucleus and substantia nigra and the bilateral pontomedullary junction (Matharu and Goadsby, 2005). Although these areas have been previously demonstrated to be the sites of activation in the TAC's and migraine; contralateral brainstem activation in migraine, ipsilateral hypothalamic activation in SUNCT and cluster; in HC the findings are reversed.

Indomethacin is the treatment of choice for HC and response to therapy with indomethacin is necessary for establishing the diagnosis (ICHD-II). Therapy is usually initiated at a dose of 25 mg TID and increased to 50 mg TID in 1 week if there is no response or only partial benefit. Headache resolution is usually prompt; occurring within 1–2 days after the effective dosage is reached, although response may take as long as 2 weeks. A more rapid way to establish the diagnosis has been described. The "indotest" consists of a 50 mg intramuscular injection of indomethacin; pain relief occurs within 2 hours if the patient has HC (Antonaci et al., 1998). Unfortunately, parenteral indomethacin is not available in the United States. Maintenance with doses ranging from 25 to 100 mg usually suffices; however at times doses as high as 300 mg daily may be required.

Dosage adjustments are occasionally necessary to treat the clinical fluctuations that are sometimes seen with HC; nighttime dosing with sustained-release indomethacin often prevents nocturnal exacerbations. During the active headache cycle, patients report that skipping or even delaying doses of indomethacin may result in the prompt reemergence of symptoms. In patients suffering from the episodic form of HC, indomethacin should be given for slightly longer than the usual headache phase and then gradually tapered. In patients with the chronic subtype, long-term indomethacin dosing is required. The gastrointestinal side effects of indomethacin can be mitigated with antacids, histamine (H2) receptor antagonists, or proton pump inhibitors. These agents should always be considered for those patients requiring long-term therapy. Although the ICHD-II requires indomethacin responsiveness as a diagnostic criterion, other agents have been reported to induce a partial response. These include naproxen, paracetamol, paracetamol with caffeine, ibuprofen, piroxicam (Goadsby and Lipton, 1997), rofecoxib (Peres and Zuckerman, 2000), celecoxib (Peres and Silberstein, 2002), and melatonin (Rozen, 2003b). Patients who have otherwise met criteria for HC but failed to respond to indomethacin or other agents have been described (Kuritzky, 1992; Pasqual, 1995). This has been termed "indomethacin-resistant hemicrania continua" but as such would not meet ICHD-II criteria for the disorder.

NEW DAILY PERSISTENT HEADACHE

New daily persistent headache (NDPH) was first described by Vanast (1986) in a series of patients who developed daily unremitting headaches from onset, without a precipitating factor or a prior headache history. These headaches were typically bilateral, continuous and associated with photophobia, phonophobia, nausea, and vomiting. The disorder was felt to be self-limited as the headache improved over time without treatment in these patients. Since then, 86 cases have been reported in the literature (Li and Rozen, 2002; Takase et al., 2004). On the basis of these reports and the recent resurgence of interest by neurologists in this disorder, NDPH was added to the 2004 edition of the ICHDs (Headache Classification Committee of the International Headache Society, 2004). The diagnostic criteria for NDPH are indicated in Table 15–8. Since the literature on NDPH is very sparse, the current criteria may not accurately reflect the entire spectrum of clinical features seen in everyday practice; many patients with NDPH may have migraine features.

Although NDPH has become a more widely recognized entity, it remains a rare disorder. The relative frequency of NDPH in studies of CDH sufferers in specialty care ranges from 10.8% to 21.1% (Gladstein and Holden, 1996; Bigal et al., 2002; Koenig et al., 2002). It may account for a higher proportion of CDH in adolescents than in adults (Bigal et al., 2004). By contrast, population-based studies, such as the one by Castillo and colleagues (1999), found that only 0.1% of 2252 subjects in Spain had NDPH. NDPH most commonly affects persons in the second to fifth decade of life, although it may begin at any age. The age at onset ranged from 12 to 78 years. NDPH has a slight female predominance, with a sex ratio of 1.5:1 (Vanast, 1986; Li and Rozen, 2002; Takase et al., 2004). A family history of NDPH was not found in any of the reported cases.

Table 15–8 Diagnostic Criteria for New Daily Persistent Headache (NDPH).

A. Headache for >3 months fulfilling criteria B–D
B. Headache is daily and unremitting from onset or from <3 days from onset[a]
C. At least two of the following pain characteristics:
   1. Bilateral location
   2. Pressing/tightening (nonpulsating) quality
   3. Mild or moderate intensity
   4. Not aggravated by routine physical activity such as walking or climbing stairs
D. Both of the following:
E. No more than one of photophobia, phonophobia or mild nausea
   1. Neither moderate or severe nausea nor vomiting
F. Not attributed to another disorder[b]

[a] Headache may be unremitting from the moment of onset or very rapidly build up to continuous and unremitting pain. Such onset or rapid development must be clearly recalled and unambiguously described by the patient. Otherwise code as 2.3 Chronic tension-type headache.

[b] History and physical and neurological examinations do not suggest any of the disorders listed in groups 5–12 (including 8.2 Medication-overuse headache and its subforms), or history and/or physical and/or neurological examinations do suggest such a disorder but it is ruled out by appropriate investigations, or such disorder is present but headache does not occur for the first time in close temporal relation to the disorder.

The most striking clinical feature of NDPH is its spontaneous and rapid development as well as its persistence from onset or within 3 days of onset. A clear recall of such an onset is necessary to establish the diagnosis of NDPH. In one study, 82% of patients were able to identify the exact day their headache began (Li and Rozen, 2002). With the exception of some cases in which headache onset occurred in close relation to an infection or flu-like illness, extracranial surgery or a stressful life event, no specific precipitating events were identified (Li and Rozen, 2002). The headache of NDPH can have associated features suggestive of either migraine or tension-type headache. The pain is typically bilateral and involves the occipital-nuchal regions in the majority of patients; retro-orbital and holocranial pain occur less often. The pain is most frequently described as a throbbing, pressure-like, stabbing, achy, or tightening sensation that ranges from mild to excruciating in severity. Migrainous symptoms, such as photophobia, phonophobia, nausea, and vomiting, may accompany the headache. Other less commonly associated symptoms may include lightheadedness, neck pain, blurred vision, and vertigo (Rozen, 2003c).

Although originally described as a benign disorder, a wider spectrum of clinical phenotypes has been recently recognized, including a debilitating form of NDPH. Therefore, it appears that there may be two subtypes of NDPH: a self-limited form, which typically resolves spontaneously within several months without treatment, and a refractory form, which is associated with an inconsistent and suboptimal treatment response regardless of the therapeutic modality employed (Rozen, 2003c).

Despite extensive investigations, the cause of NDPH is unknown. Two studies have found elevated Epstein–Barr virus (EBV) titers in these patients, suggesting an infectious etiology

(Diaz-Mitoma et al., 1987; Santoni and Santoni-Williams, 1993). NDPH may be a virally mediated autoimmune disorder with continuous neurogenic inflammation of the trigeminovascular system. Stressful life events have also been implicated as a potential etiologic factor (Rozen and Jensen, 2006).

The diagnosis of NDPH is one of exclusion, following normal neuroimaging, lumbar puncture, and blood studies. Two of the most common identifiable secondary causes of NDPH are spontaneous CSF leaks and cerebral venous sinus thrombosis. Other causes that should be considered include pseudotumor cerebri, carotid or vertebral artery dissection, cervical facet syndrome, SAH, sphenoid sinusitis, posttraumatic headache, chronic subdural hematoma, temporal arteritis, neoplasm, chronic meningitis, postinfectious headache, and hypothyroidism (Goadsby and Boes, 2002; Evans, 2003; Bigal et al., 2005; Rozen and Jensen, 2006).

There is currently insufficient clinical information to support specific recommendations for acute or preventive medical therapy in the treatment of NDPH. Medications typically employed in the treatment of other headache disorders produce varying, generally unsatisfactory, results (Rozen, 2003c). Prophylactic medications that have been tried with anecdotal benefit include topirimate, gabapentin, tizanidine, baclofen, amitriptyline, valproic acid, fluvoxamine, paroxetine, and phenelzine (Goadsby and Boes, 2002; Rozen, 2003c; Takase et al., 2004). Indeed, no medication has been reported to show significant or consistent benefit in this population of patients.

NUMMULAR HEADACHE

Pareja and colleagues (2002, 2004) recently described two separate case series of nummular headache. Based largely on their reports, the disorder was included in the appendix of the second edition of the ICHDs (ICHD-2) (Headache Classification Committee of the International Headache Society, 2004), indicating the need for further study (Table 15–9). Since then nearly 50 cases have been reported in the English language literature (Cohen, 2005; Evans and Pareja, 2005; Seo and Park, 2005; Dach et al., 2006; Grosberg et al., 2006; Mathew et al., 2006; Trucco et al., 2006).

TABLE 15–9 Nummular Headache.

Previously used terms: Coin-shaped cephalalgia

Description

Pain in a circumscribed area of the head in the absence of any lesion of the underlying structures

Diagnostic criteria

A. Mild to moderate head pain fulfilling criteria B and C
B. Pain is felt exclusively in a rounded or elliptical area typically 2–6 cm in diameter
C. Pain is chronic and either continuous or interrupted by spontaneous remissions lasting weeks to months
D. Not attributed to another disorder

Nummular headache is thought to be a rare disorder, but its true prevalence and incidence are unknown. In one hospital series, the incidence of nummular headache was 6.4/1,00,000/year (Pareja et al., 2004). Nummular headache has a female predominance with a gender ratio of 2.5:1. The age at onset ranges from 13 to 72 years, with a mean age of 42 years. The duration of symptoms before diagnosis ranged from 1 month to 50 years. With the exception of some cases in which headache onset occurred in close relation to sinus surgery or head trauma, no specific precipitating events have been identified (Grosberg et al., 2006).

Nummular headache is a benign headache syndrome characterized by focal and well-circumscribed head pain of mild, moderate or severe intensity (Pareja et al., 2002; Pareja et al., 2004; Dach et al., 2006; Grosberg et al., 2006). Many patients experience superimposed exacerbations of pain, lasting from seconds to days (Pareja et al., 2002; Pareja et al., 2004; Cohen, 2005; Dach et al., 2006; Grosberg et al., 2006; Mathew et al., 2006). Infrequently, exacerbations may be precipitated by touching the symptomatic area (Pareja et al., 2004; Mathew et al., 2006), by valsalva maneuvers or by changes in weather (Grosberg et al., 2006). The character of the pain has been described as pressure-like, sharp, stabbing, achy, throbbing, burning, stinging, or itching. The attacks are typically strictly unilateral and side-locked; however, in three patients the pain was simultaneously experienced on both sides of the head (Pareja et al., 2004; Evans and Pareja, 2005;

Dach et al., 2006). The pain is present slightly more frequently on the right side than the left in patients with side-locked attacks. The pain in nummular headache is usually localized to the parietal region and less often involves the occipital, temporal, or frontal region. The site and size of the affected area are typically discrete and fixed within a rounded, elliptical, oval or, rarely, bean-shaped area (Pareja et al., 2002; Grosberg et al., 2006). As a result, the patient can often delineate the outline of the affected region with a finger. Sensory phenomena, such as paresthesias, hyperesthesias, and dysesthesias are frequently reported in the region of pain. In most patients, photophobia, phonophobia, nausea, vomiting, or other autonomic features did not accompany the headaches.

There are two major temporal patterns of nummular headache (Pareja et al., 2002; Grosberg et al., 2006). The chronic type, by far the most common, is characterized by either continuous pain that evolved from episodic pain, continuous pain since onset or long-lasting bouts of pain occurring on 15 or more days per month. The episodic type is characterized by bouts of pain, which occur on less than 15 days per month, lasting from 30 minutes up to 6 days. The frequencies of these attacks are variable, occurring bi-weekly to as often as 4–6 times per day. Short-lived periods of spontaneous remission with return to the previous pattern were observed in one series of patients (Pareja et al., 2002); only one patient had spontaneous and complete relief from pain after 1 month (Grosberg et al., 2006). Symptoms presented during daytime in all but a few patients who reported nocturnal pain with frequent or occasional awakenings (Pareja et al., 2004; Grosberg et al., 2006).

A diagnosis of primary nummular headache is made only after alternative causes have been excluded. An initial diagnostic work-up should include a complete neurological examination (including careful inspection and palpation of the scalp and the pericranial muscles, nerves and arteries), laboratory tests, and neuroimaging studies. To date, only one report of probable secondary nummular headache has been described in a patient with Marfan's syndrome (Garcia-Pastor et al., 2002). This patient presented with a 2-month history of focal, circumscribed pain in the right frontal region. An angiogram of the right external carotid artery revealed a fusiform aneurysm. The pain completely resolved following surgical resection of the abnormal vessel.

The pathogenesis of nummular headache is unclear. In a provisional conceptual model, the pain is thought to stem from a peripheral source, probably from any of the epicranial tissues, including the skull, all layers of the scalp, vessels, and nerves (Pareja, 2005). Recent evidence suggests that nummular headache may be associated with a local increase in pain sensitivity to mechanical stimulation within the symptomatic area (Fernandez-de-las-Penas et al., 2006). Furthermore, pericranial tenderness does not seem to be related to nummular headache (Fernandez-de-las-Penas et al., 2007). The absence of a therapeutic response to treatment with local anesthesia in several cases, along with the fact that some cases cross the midline argues against a focal neuropathy as the cause of the pain.

Initial reports of nummular headache suggested that the low level of pain associated with the disorder did not necessitate treatment and, if required, was typically responsive to conventional analgesics (Pareja et al., 2004). However, contrary to these reports and the current ICHD-2 criteria for nummular headache, patients may experience intense pain and require prophylactic therapy (Cohen, 2005; Grosberg et al., 2006). Recently, several agents have been suggested to be partially or completely effective in some case reports, including gabapentin (Evans and Pareja, 2005; Trucco et al., 2006), tricyclic antidepressants (Grosberg et al., 2006) and botulinum toxin (Seo and Park, 2005; Mathew et al., 2006).

References

Akpunonu, BE and Ahrens, J. (1991). Sexual headaches: case report, review, and treatment with calcium channel blocker. *Headache*, 31:141–145.

Antonaci, F, Pareja, JA, Caminero, AB, et al. (1998). Chronic paroxysmal hemicrania and hemicrania continua. Parenteral indomethacin: the "indotest". *Headache*, 38:122–128.

Bigal, ME, Lipton, RB, Tepper, SJ, et al. (2004). Primary chronic daily headache and its subtypes in adolescents and adults. *Neurology*, 63:843–847.

Bigal, ME, Rapoport, AM, Sheftell, FD, et al.(2005). The woman with never-ending headaches. In *Advanced Therapy of Headache* (2nd edn) (RA Purdy, AM Rapoport, FD Sheftell, SJ Tepper, eds), pp. 109–111. BC Decker, Hamilton.

Bigal, ME, Sheftell, FD, Rapoport, AM, et al. (2002). Chronic daily headache in a tertiary care population: correlation between the International Headache Society diagnostic criteria and proposed revisions of criteria for chronic daily headache. *Cephalalgia*, 22:432–438.

Brilla, R, Evers, S, Soros, P, et al. (1998). Hemicrania continua in an HIV-infected outpatient. *Cephalalgia*, 18:287–288.

Buzzi, MG, Bonamini, M, and Moskowitz, MA (1995). Neurogenic model of migraine. *Cephalalgia*, 15:277–280.

Calandre, L, Hernandez-Lain, A, Lopez-Valdes, E, et al. (1996). Benign Valsalva's maneuver-related headache: an MRI study of six cases. *Headache*, 36:251–253.

Castillo, J, Munoz, P, Guitera, V, et al. (1999). Epidemiology of chronic daily headache in the general population. *Headache*, 39(3):190–196.

Chazot, G, Claustrat, B, Brun, J, et al. (1987). Effects of the patterns of melatonin and cortisol in cluster headache of a single administration of lithium at 7:00 p.m. daily over one week: a preliminary report. *Pharmacopsychiatry*, 20:222–223.

Chen, SP, Fuh, JL, Lirng, JF, et al. (2006). Recurrent primary thunderclap headache and benign CNS angiopathy: spectra of the same disorder? *Neurology*, 67:2164–2169.

Chen, YY, Ling, JF, Sealfon, S, et al. (2004). Primary cough headache is associated with posterior fossa crowdedness: a morphometric MRI study. *Cephalalgia*, 24:694–699.

Cohen, GL. (2005). Nummular headache: What denomination? *Headache*, 45:1417–1418.

Dach, F, Speciali, J, Eckeli, A, et al. (2006). *Cephalalgia*, 26 (10):1234–1237.

Dalessio, DJ (1974) Effort migraine. *Headache*, 14:53.

Day, JW and Raskin, NH (1986). Thunderclap headache: symptom of unruptured cerebral aneurysm. *Lancet*, 2:1247–1248.

Diamond, S (1982). Prolonged benign exertional headache: its clinical characteristics and response to indomethacin. *Headache*, 22:96–98.

Diamond, S and Medina, JL (1979). Benign exertional headache: successful treatment with indomethacin. *Headache*, 19:249.

Diaz-Mitoma, R, Vanast, WJ, and Tyrell, DL (1987). Increased frequency of Epstein-Barr virus excretion in patients with new daily persistent headaches. *Lancet*, 1:411–415.

Dodick, DW (2000). Polysomnography in hypnic headache syndrome. *Headache*, 40:748–752.

Dodick, DW (2004). Indomethacin responsive headache syndromes. *Curr Pain Head Reports*, 8:19–28.

Dodick DW (2002). Thunderclap headache. Current Pain Headache Rep; 6:226–232.

Dodick, DW, Brown, RD, Britton, JW, et al. (1999). Nonaneurysmal thunderclap headache with diffuse, multifocal, segmental, and reversible vasospasm. *Cephalalgia*, 19:1–6.

Dodick, DW, Jones, JM, and Capobianco, DJ (2000). Hypnic headache: another indomethacin-responsive headache syndrome? *Headache*, 40:830–835.

Dodick, DW, Mosek, AC, and Campbell, JK (1998). The hypnic ("alarm clock") headache syndrome. *Cephalalgia*, 18:152–156.

Drummond, PD and Lance, JW (1984). Clinical diagnosis and computer analysis of headache symptoms. *J Neurol Neurosurg Psychiatr*, 47:128–133.

Edis, RH and Silbert, PL (1988). Sequential benign sexual headache and exertional headache. *Lancet*, 1:993.

Eross, EJ, Swanson, JW, and Dodick, DW (2002). Hemicrania Continua: An Indomethacin-Responsive Case With an Underlying Malignant Etiology. *Headache*, 42:527–529.

Evans, RW (2003). New daily persistent headache. *Curr Pain Head Reports*, 7:303–307.

Evans, RW and Pareja, JA (2005). Nummular headache. *Headache*, 45(2):164–165.

Evans, RW and Pascual, J (2000). Orgasmic headaches: clinical features, diagnosis and management. *Headache*, 40:491–494.

Evers, S, Bahra, A, and Goasby, PJ (1999). Coincidence of familial hemiplegic migraine and hemicrania continua? A case report. *Cephalalgia*, 19:533–535.

Evers, S and Dodick, DW (2005). Hypnic Headache. In *Chronic Daily Headache for Clinicians* (PJ Goadsby, SD Silberstein, and DW Dodick, eds), pp. 109–115. BC Decker, Inc, London.

Evers, S and Goadsby, PJ (2003). Hypnic headache: clinical features, pathophysiology, and treatment. *Neurology*, 60(6):905–909.

Evers, S, Rahmann, A, Schwaag, S, et al. (2003). Hypnic headache—The first Geman cases including polysomnography. *Cephalalgia*, 23:20–23.

Fernandez-de-las-Penas, C, Cuadrado, ML, Barriga, FJ, et al. (2006). Local decrease of pressure pain threshold in nummular headache. *Headache*, 46:1195–1198.

Fernandez-de-las-Penas, C, Cuadrado, ML, Barriga, FJ, et al. (2007). Pericranial tenderness is not related to nummular headache. *Cephalalgia*, 27:182–186.

Fischer, CM (1984). Painful states: a neurological commentary. *Clin Neurosurg*, 31:32–53.

Franca, Jr. MC, Costa, ALC, and Maciel, Jr. JA (2004). Gabapentin-responsive idiopathic stabbing headache. *Cephalalgia*, 24:993–996.

Freeman, WD, Brazis, PW, Capobianco, DJ, et al. (2004). Hypnic headache and intracranial hypotension. *Headache*, 44:498.

Frese, A, Eikermann, A, Frese, K, et al. (2003). Headache associated with sexual activity. Demography, clinical features, and comorbidity. *Neurology*, 61:796–800.

Frese, A, Frese, K, Schwaag, S, et al. (2004). Prophylactic treatment and course of the disease in headache associated with sexual activity. In *Preventive pharmacotherapy of headache disorders* (J Olesen, S Silberstein, and P Tfelt-Hansen, eds), pp. 50–54. Oxford University Press, Oxford.

Garcia-Pastor, A, Guillem-Mesado, A, Salinero-Paniagua, J, et al. (2002). Fusiform aneurysm of the scalp: an unusual cause of focal headache in Marfan syndrome. *Headache*, 42:908–910.

Gladstein, J and Holden, EW (1996). Chronic daily headache in children and adolescents: a 2-year prospective study. *Headache*, 36:349–351.

Goadsby, PJ and Boes, C. (2002). New daily persistent headaches. *J Neurol Neurosurg Psychiatr*, 72(Suppl. II):ii6–ii9.

Goadsby, PJ and Lipton, RB (1997). A review of paroxysmal hemicranias, SUNCT syndrome and other short-lasting headaches with autonomic feature, including new cases. *Brain*, 120:193–209.

Gould, JD and Silberstein, SD (1997a). Unilateral hypnic headache: a case study. *Neurology*, 49:1749–1751.

Gould, JD and Silberstein, SD (1997b). Unilateral hypnic headache: a case study. *Cephalalgia*, 17:310.

Grosberg, BM, Solomon, S, and Lipton, RB (2006). Nummular headache and the International Classification of Headache Disorders (ICHD-2). *Headache*, 46(5):899.

Grossberg, BM, Lipton, RB, Solomon, S, et al. (2004). Hypnic headache in childhood? *Headache*, 44:497.

Harling, DW, Peatfield, RC, Van Hille, PT, et al. (1989). Thunderclap headache: is it migraine? *Cephalalgia*, 9:87–90.

Headache Classification Committee of the International Headache Society. (1988). Classification and diagnostic criteria for headache disorders, cranial neuralgias and facial pain. *Cephalalgia*, 8(Suppl. 7):1–96.

Headache Classification Committee of the International Headache Society. (2004). The International Classification of Headache Disorders: 2nd edition. *Cephalalgia*, 24(Suppl. 1):9–160.

Indo, T and Takahashi, A (1990). Swimmer's headache. *Headache*, 30:485–487.

Iordanidis, T and Sjaastad, O (1989). Hemicrania continua:a case report. *Cephalalgia*, 9:301–303.

Ivanez, V, Soler, R, and Barreiro, P (1998). Hypnic headache syndrome: a case with good response to indomethacin. *Cephalalgia*, 18:225–226.

Jacome, DE (1998). Masturbatory-orgasmic extracephalgic pain. *Headache*, 38:138–141.

Jones, JM and Dodick, DW (2000). Hypnic headache: another indomethacin responsive headache syndrome? *Headache*, 40:412.

Kim, JS (1992). Swimming headache followed by exertional and coital headaches. *J Korean Med Sci*, 7:276–279.

Koenig MA,, Gladstein J, McCarter RJ, Hershey AD, Wasiewski W. Chronic Daily Headache in Children and Adolescents Presenting to Tertiary Headache Clinics. Headache *2002*; 42: 491–500.

Kritz, K (1970). Coitus as a factor in the pathogenesis of neurological complications. *Cesk Neurol Neurochir*, 33:162–167.

Kumar, KL and Reuler, JB (1993). Uncommon headaches: Diagnosis and treatment. *J Gen Int Med*, 8:333–341.

Kuritzky, A (1992). Indomethacin-resistant hemicrania continua. *Cephalalgia*, 12:57–59.

Lambert, RW and Burnet, DL (1985). Prevention of exercise induced migraine by quantitative warm-up. *Headache*, 25:317–319.

Lance, JW (1976). Headaches related to sexual activity. *J Neurol Neurosurg Psychiatr*, 39:1226–1230.

Lance, JW (1992). Benign coital headache. *Cephalalgia*, 12:339.

Lansche, RK (1964). Ophthalmodynia periodica. *Headache*, 4:247–249.

Leone, M, Lucini, V, D'Amico, D, et al. (1995). Twenty-four hour melatonin and cortisol plasma levels in relation to timing of cluster headache. *Cephalalgia*, 15:224–229.

Levy, MJ, Matharu, MS, Goadsby, PJ (2003). Prolactinomas, dopamine agonists and headache: two case reports. *Eur J Neurol*, 10:169–171.

Lewis, AJ, Kerenyi, NA, and Feuer, G (1990). Neuropharmacology of pineal secretion. *Drug Metab Drug Interact*, 8:247–312.

Li, D and Rozen, TF (2002). The clinical characteristics of new daily persistent headache. *Cephalalgia*, 22:66–69.

Lu, SR, Liao, YC, Fuh, JL, et al. (2004). Nimodipine for treatment of primary thunderclap headache. *Neurology*, 62(8):1414–1416.

Manni, R, Sances, G, Terzaghi, M, et al. (2004). Hypnic headache: PSG evidence of both REM- and NREM-related attacks. *Neurology*, 62:1411–1413.

Marano, E, Giampiero, V, Gennaro, DR, et al. (1994). "Hemicrania continua": a possible case with alternating sides. *Cephalalgia*, 14:307–308.

Martins, IP, Parreira, E, and Costa, I (1995). Extratrigeminal ice-pick status. *Headache*, 35:107–110.

Mascellino, AM, Lay, CL, and Newman, LC (2001). Stabbing headache as the presenting manifestation of intracerebral meningioma: a report of two patients. *Headache*, 41:599–601.

Matharu, MS and Goadsby, PJ (2005). Functional brain imaging in hemicrania continua: implications for nosology and pathophysiology. *Curr Pain Headache Rep*, 4:133–140.

Mathew, NT (1981). Indomethacin responsive headache syndromes. *Headache*, 21:147–150.

Mathew, NT, Kailasam, J, and Meadors, L (2006). Nummular headache responds to botulinum toxin type a (BoNTA): experience in four cases. *Cephalalgia*, 26:1378.

Medina, JL and Diamond, S (1981). Cluster headache variant: spectrum of a new headache syndrome. *Arch Neurol*, 38:705–709.

Medrano, V, Jmallada, J, Sempere, AP, et al. (2005). Primary cough headache responsive to topiramate. *Cephalalgia*, 25:627–628.

Monteiro, JM. (1995). Cefaleias Estudio epidemiologico e clinico de uma populacao urbana. Thesis. University of Porto, Porto.

Moon, HS, Chung, CS, Kim, HY, et al. (2003). Hypnic headache syndrome: report of a symptomatic case. *Cephalalgia*, 23:673–674.

Morales-Asin, F, Mauri, JA, Iniguez, C, et al. (1998). The hypnic headache syndrome: report of three new cases. *Cephalalgia*, 18:157–158.

Newman, LC, Goadsby, P, Lipton, RB (2001). Cluster and related headaches. In *Headache*. Medical Clinics of North America (NT Mathew, ed.), pp. 997–1016. WB Saunders, Philadelphia.

Newman, LC, Lipton, RB, Russell, M, et al. (1992). Hemicrania continua:attacks may alternate sides. *Headache*, 32:237–238.

Newman, LC, Lipton, RB, and Solomon, S (1990). The hypnic headache syndrome: a benign headache disorder of the elderly. *Neurology*, 40:1904–1905.

Newman, LC, Lipton, RB, and Solomon, S. (1994). Hemicrania continua: ten new cases and a review of the literature. *Neurology*, 44:2111–2114.

Newman, LC and Mosek, AC (2006). The Hypnic Headache Syndrome. In *The Headaches* (3rd Ed). (J Olesen, PJ Goadsby, NM Ramadan, P Pfelt-Hansen, and KMA Welch, eds), pp. 847–850. Lippincott Williams & Wilkins, Philadelphia.

Newman, LC, Spears, RC, and Lay, CL (2004). Hemicrania continua: a third case in which attacks alternate sides. *Headache*, 44(8):821–823.

Nowak, DA, Rodiek, SO, Henneken, S, et al. (2003). Reversible segmental cerebral vasoconstriction (Call-Fleming syndrome): are calcium channel inhibitors a potential treatment option? *Cephalalgia*, 23:218–222.

Pareja, JA (1995). Hemicrania continua:remitting stage evolved from the chronic form. *Headache*, 35:161–162.

Pareja, JA (2005). Nummular headache: What denomination? A Rebuttal. *Headache*, 45:1418.

Pareja, JA, Caminero, AB, Serra, J, et al. (2002). Numular headache: a coin-shaped cephalalgia. *Neurology*, 58:1678–1679.

Pareja, JA, Pareja, J, Barriga, FJ, et al. (2004). Nummular headache: a prospective series of 14 new cases. *Headache*, 44:611–614.

Pareja, JA, Rujiz, J, Deisla, C, et al. (1996). Idiopathic stabbing headache (jabs and jolt syndrome). *Cephalalgia*, 16:93–96.

Pasqual, J (1995). Hemicrania continua. *Neurology*, 45:2302–2303.

Pasqual, J (2005). Primary cough headache. *Curr Pain and Head Reports*, 4:124–128.

Pascual, J, Iglesias, F, Oterino, A, et al. (1996). Exertional and sexual headaches: an analysis of 72 benign and symptomatic cases. *Neurology*, 46:1520–1524.

Pasquier, F, Leys, D, and Petit, H (1987). Hemicrania continua:the first bilateral case. *Cephalalgia*, 7:169–170.

Paulson, GW (1983). Weightlifter's headache. *Headache*, 23:193–194.

Peatfield, RC and Mendoza, ND (2003). Posterior fossa meningioma presenting as hypnic headache. *Headache*, 43:1007–1008.

Peres, MF and Silberstein, SD (2002). Hemicrania continua responds to cyclooxygenase-2 inhibitors. *Headache*, 42:530–531.

Peres, MF, Siow, HC, and Rozen, TD (2002). Hemicrania continua with aura. *Cephalalgia*, 22:246–248.

Peres, MFP, Silberstein, SD, and Nahmias, S (2001). Hemicrania continua is not that rare. *Neurology*, 57:948–951.

Peres, MF and Zuckerman, E (2000). Hemicrania continua responsive to rofecoxib. *Cephalalgia*, 20:130–131.

Pinessi, L, Rainero, I, Cicolin, A, et al. (2003). Hypnic headache syndrome: association of the attacks with REM sleep. *Cephalalgia*, 23:150–154.

Piovesan, EJ, Kowacs, PA, Lange, MC, et al. (2001). Prevalence and semiologic aspects of the idiopathic stabbing headache in a migraine population. *Arq Neuropsiq*, 59 (2-A):201–205.

Porter, M and Jancovic, J (1981). Benign coital cephalalgia. Differential diagnosis and treatment. *Arch Neurol*, 38:710–712.

Queiroz, LP (2001). Symptoms and therapies: exertional and sexual headaches. *Curr Pain Headache Rep*, 5:275–278.

Raskin, NH (1986). Icecream, icepick and chemical headaches. In *Handbook of Clinical Neurology*, Vol. 48. (FC Rose, ed.), pp. 441–448. Elsevier Science Publishing, Amsterdam.

Raskin, NH (1988a). The hypnic headache syndrome. *Headache*, 28:534–536.

Raskin, NH (1988b). The indomethcin-responsive sydromes, In *Headache* (NH Raskin, ed.), pp. 255–268. Churchill Livingstone, New York.

Raskin, NH (1995). The cough headache syndrome: treatment. *Neurology*, 45:1784.

Raskin, NH (1997). Short-lived head pains. *Neurol Clin*, 15:143–152.

Raskin, NH and Schwartz, RK (1980). Icepick-like pain. *Neurology*, 30:203–205.

Rasmussen, BK (1994). Epidemiology of headache. Thesis. Copenhagen, Kobenhavns, Universitet.

Rasmussen, BK (1995). Epidemiology of headache. *Cephalalgia*, 15:45–68.

Rasmussen, BK and Olesen, J (1992). Symptomatic and nonsymptomatic headaches in a general population. *Neurology*, 42:1225–1231.

Robbins, L (1994). Masturbatory-orgasmic extracephalgic pain. *Headache*, 34:214–216.

Rozen, TD (2003c). New daily persistent headache. *Curr Pain and Head Reports*, 7:218–223.

Rozen, TD (2003b). Melatonin as a treatment for indomethacin responsive headaches. *Headache*, 43:591.

Rozen, TD (2003a). Melatonin as treatment for idiopathic stabbing headache. *Neurology*, 61:865–866.

Rozen TD, Jensen R. New daily persistent headache. In: Olesen J, Goadsby PJ, Ramadan NM, Tfelt-Hansen P, Welch KM, editors. The Headaches. 3rd ed. Philadelphia: Lippincott Williams and Wilkins, 2006.

Santoni JR, Santoni-Williams CH (1993). Headache and painful lymphadenopathy in extracranial or systemic infection: etiology of new daily persistent headaches, *Intern Med*, 32:530–533.

Selwyn DL (1985). A study of coital related headaches in 32 patients, *Cephalalgia*, 5(suppl 3):300–301.

Seo M, Park S (2005). Botulinum toxin in nummular *headache, Cephalalgia*, 25(10):991.

Silbert PL, Edis RH, Stewart-Wynn EG, Gubbay SS (1991). Benign vascular sexual headache and exertional headache: inter-relationships and long term prognosis. J Neurol, *Neurosurg Psychiat*, 54:417–421.

Sjaastad O, Egge K, Horven I, Kayed K, Lund-Roland L, Russel D, Slordhal Conradi I (1979). Chronic paroxysmal hemicrania. Mechanical precipitation of attacks, *Headache*, 19:31–36.

Sjaastad O, Spierings ELH (1980). Hemicrania continua: another headache absolutely responsive to indomethacin, *Cephalalgia*, 4:65–70.

Sjaastad O (1992). Cluster headache syndrome. Philadelphia, PA: WB Saunders.

Sjaastad O, Antonaci F (1993). Chronic paroxysmal hemicrania (CPH) and hemicrania continua: transition from one stage to another, *Headache*, 22:551–554.

Sjaastad O, Pettersen H, Bakketeig LS (2001). The Vaga study; epidemiology of headache I: The prevalence of ultrashort paroxysms, *Cephalalgia*, 21:207–215.

Sjaastad O, Bakketeig LS (2003). Exertional headache - II. Clinical features Vågå study of headache epidemiology, *Cephalalgia*, 23: 803–807.

Slivka A, Philbrook B (1995). Clinical and angiographic features of thunderclap headache, *Headache*, 35:1–6.

Somers VK, Dyken ME, Mark AL & Abboud FM (1993). Sympathetic-nerve activity during sleep in normal subjects, *New England Journal of Medicine*, 328:303–307.

Strum JS, Macdonell RA (2000). Recurrent thunderclap headache associated with reversible intracerebral vasospasm causing stroke, *Cephalalgia*, 20:132–135.

Takeuchi T, Kasahara E, Iwasaki M, Kojima S (1996). Necessity for searching for cerebral aneurysm in thunderclap headache patients who show no evidence of subarachnoid hemorrhage: investigation of 8 minor leak cases on operation [Japanese], *No Shinkei Geka*, 24:437–441.

Takase Y, Nakano M, Tatsumi C, Matsuyama T (2004). Clinical features, effectiveness of drug-based treatment and prognosis of new daily persistent headache (NDPH): 30 cases in Japan, *Cephalalgia*, 24:955–959.

Treiser SL, Cascio CS, O'Donohue TL, Thoa NB, Jacobowitz DM & Kellar KJ (1981). Lithium increases serotonin release and decreases serotonin receptors in the hippocampus, *Science*, 213;1529–1537.

Trucco M, Antonaci F, Sandrini G (1992). Hemicrania continua: a case responsive to piroxicam-beta-cyclodextrin, *Headache*, 32:39–40.

Trucco M, Mainardi F, Perego G, Zanchin G (1992). Nummular headache: first Italian case and therapeutic proposal, *Cephalalgia*, 26:354–356.

Young WB, Silberstein SD (1993). Hemicrania continua and symptomatic medication overuse, *Headache*, 33:485–487.

Vanast WJ (1986). New daily persistent headaches definition of a benign syndrome, *Headache*, 26:318.

Vieira-Dias M, Esperanca P (2001). Hypnic Headache: Report of Two Cases, *Headache*, 41: 726–727.

Wang SJ, Fuh JL, Lu SR (2000). Benign cough headache is responsive to acetazolamide, *Neurology*, 55: 149–150.

Widjicks EF, Kerkhoff H, van Gigjn J (1988). Long-term follow-up of 71 patients with thunderclap headache mimicking subarachnoid haemorrhage, *Lancet*, 2:68–70.

Zakaria A, Graber M, Davis P (2000). Idiopathic stabbing headache associated with monocular visual loss, *Arch Neurol*, 57:745–746.

III Diagnosis and Treatment of Secondary Headache Disorders

16 Headaches Associated with Head Trauma

William B Young, Russell C Packard, and Zaza Katsarava

Postconcussive headache (PCH) is a new headache that follows a blunt or open injury to the head or brain (Headache Classification Committee, 2004). Postconcussion syndrome is a constellation of symptoms that may follow a mild to moderate closed head injury. Symptoms of postconcussion syndrome include headache, depression, irritability, memory impairment, alcohol intolerance, dizziness or vertigo, attention and concentration difficulties, and loss of libido.

DEFINITIONS

Concussion, minor head injury, and minor traumatic brain injury are difficult to define, compared with moderate or severe injury, in which structural damage is evident. The American Congress of Rehabilitation Medicine defined minor traumatic brain injury as "a traumatically induced physiological disruption of brain function" with at least one of the following: (1) any period of loss of consciousness; (2) any memory loss for events just before or after the accident; (3) any alteration in mental state at the time of the accident; and (4) focal neurologic deficits that may or may not be transient (Packard, 1999). The injury should not result in a loss of consciousness of more than 30 minutes, an initial Glasgow coma scale (GCS) score of less than 13 (after 30 minutes), or posttraumatic amnesia exceeding 24 hours. The International Headache Society (IHS) still uses 8 hours as the amnesia period.

For many years, a concussion was considered to be a brief, reversible brain injury with transient loss of consciousness. Loss of consciousness is no longer required (Evans, 1996; Rizzo and Tranel, 1996). In this chapter, we consider concussion a minor traumatic brain injury. In sports, the American Academy of Neurology defined concussion as a "trauma-induced alteration in mental status that may or may not involve loss of consciousness." These definitions allow a range of severity and treatment protocols to be considered when evaluating patients and athletes with concussion (Packard, 1999).

The diagnostic criteria established by the IHS (Headache Classification Committee, 2004) for acute PCH with significant head trauma or confirmatory signs include the following: (1) significance of head trauma documented by at least one of the following: (a) loss of consciousness more than 30 minutes, (b) GCS less than 13, (c) posttraumatic amnesia more than 48 hours, (d) abnormal brain imaging or skull fracture; (2) headache occurs less than 7 days after regaining consciousness (or after trauma if there has been no loss of consciousness); and (3) headache disappears within 3 months after regaining consciousness (or after trauma if there has been no loss of consciousness) (Headache Classification Committee, 2004).

The IHS diagnostic criteria for acute PCH with mild head injury include loss of consciousness more than 30 minutes, GCS more than 13, symptoms and signs diagnostic of concussion headache within 2 days of trauma, and headache.

The IHS criteria require the headache to continue for 3 months after injury to be considered chronic PCH. The IHS definitions of chronicity are variable and somewhat arbitrary. Since most patients with PCH improve in the first 6 months after the injury, it has been suggested that 6 months or more should define chronicity in PCH, which would be in line with the definition of chronic pain (Packard and Ham, 1993). In place of the IHS criteria, many papers use the International Classification of Diseases 10 (ICD-10) criteria.

POSTCONCUSSION SYNDROME

A syndrome that occurs following head trauma (usually sufficiently severe to result in loss of consciousness) and includes a number of disparate symptoms, such as headache, dizziness, fatigue, irritability, difficulty in concentration and performing mental tasks, impairment of memory, insomnia, and reduced tolerance to stress, emotional excitement, or alcohol.

DSM-IV

The Diagnostic and Statistical Manual IV (DSM-IV) criteria are (1) history of traumatic brain injury causing "significant cerebral concussion;" (2) cognitive deficit in attention and/or memory; (3) at least three of eight symptoms (e.g., fatigue, sleep disturbance, headache, dizziness, irritability, affective disturbance, personality change, apathy) that appear after injury and persist for three months; (4) symptoms that begin or worsen after injury; (5) interference with social role functioning; and (6) exclusion of dementia due to head trauma and other disorders that better account for the symptoms. Criteria 3 and 4 require symptom onset or worsening to be contiguous to the head injury, distinguishable from preexisting symptoms, and exist for a minimum duration of 3 months.

EPIDEMIOLOGY

The IHS recognizes acute headache as part of the syndrome of postwhiplash headache but does not recognize a chronic version of this disorder. Persons with chronic headache after whiplash injury may be considered to have chronic PCH if they meet one of the applicable definitions.

According to the Centers for Disease Control and Prevention, in 2003 falls (32%) we the most frequent cause of traumatic brain injury, with motor vehicle accidents second (19%), followed by struck by/against events (18%), other (11%), and assaults (10%). The annual rate of traumatic brain injury in emergency department visits was 420 per 1,00,000 in 2003, down slightly from the figure in the year 1998, but the number of hospitalization cases increased slightly to 290,000 per year (Rutland-Brown et al., 2006). Many of these patients suffer from postconcussion syndrome and have additional somatic and neuropsychologic symptoms. Since many patients with mild head injuries who subsequently develop PCH are never hospitalized, it is difficult to estimate the true burden of the disorder. Patients with mild head injury, defined as a GCS score of 13–15, are hospitalized at a rate of approximately 200/1,00,000 per year (Kraus et al., 1994). PCH develops in 30%–80% of these patients (Elkind, 1992; Evans, 1992). Seventy-nine to ninety percent of patients who have postconcussion symptoms also have headache (Gfeller et al., 1994).

The term whiplash refers to the sequence of extension, flexion, and lateral motions of the neck that follows impact, with or without direct trauma to the head. Ninety-seven percent of patients who seek help from a physician after whiplash have headaches (Machado et al., 1988). The symptomatology that follows whiplash is remarkably similar to that experienced by patients following head injury. In addition to neck pain, headaches, dizziness, paresthesias, and cognitive and psychologic sequelae are extremely common. Since whiplash injuries usually do not lead to hospitalization, its incidence is even more difficult to calculate than that of head injury or PCH; however, it has been estimated to be approximately 1 million cases per year in the United States (O'Neill et al., 1972; Foreman and Croft, 1995).

CLINICAL FEATURES

Symptoms of postconcussion syndrome (Table 16–1) may develop immediately or be delayed (or not initially recognized) following trauma. Head, neck, and shoulder pain usually begins within 24–48 hours of the injury, while local occipital tenderness occurs immediately. Neuralgic symptoms can develop in the frontal or occipital region months after the injury. The IHS criteria for PCH (Table 16–2) require headache onset within 1 week of head injury or of regaining consciousness. However, in clinical practice it is often difficult to determine when the headache actually started, since head pain may be mild and other pains

TABLE 16–1 Sequelae of Mild Head Injury.

Headaches
Tension-type
Migraine
Cluster
Low cerebrospinal fluid pressure
Occipital neuralgia
Idiopathic intracranial hypotension
Supraorbital and infraorbital neuralgia
Cervicogenic
Temporomandibular joint syndrome or dysfunction
Local neuroma
Mixed
Cranial nerve symptoms and signs
Dizziness
Vertigo
Tinnitus
Hearing loss
Blurred vision
Diplopia
Convergence insufficiency
Light and noise sensitivity
Diminished taste and smell
Psychologic and somatic complaints
Irritability
Anxiety
Depression
Personality change
Fatigue
Sleep disturbance
Decreased libido
Decreased appetite
Rare sequelae
Subdural and epidural hematoma
Seizures
Transient global amnesia
Tremor
Dystonia
Other
Seizure-like spells

(particularly neck pain) more prominent. Furthermore, patients may develop chronic headaches as long as 24 months after the trauma. These late-onset headaches are similar clinically to chronic PCH. Brenner (1944) found that 6% of patients who had mild head injury had headaches that began within 16 months after discharge, while Cartlidge and Shaw (1981) found that 12% had late-acquired headache, both 6 and 24 months after discharge. These late-onset headaches (which do not meet IHS criteria for PCH) are more prevalent than would be expected by chance. Lipton found that a history of head injury is a risk factor for the development of episodic to chronic headache (Scher et al., 2002). Why these headaches begin late is uncertain. Their relationship to the preceding injury is highly controversial and difficult to establish with certainty. Some late-onset headaches may be due to a traumatically lowered headache susceptibility that is not manifest until other factors ultimately push the patient over a headache threshold. The IHS criteria that state that PCH must begin within 7 days following injury or regaining consciousness may not have physiologic validity but instead may represent an arbitrary but reasonable compromise to establish causality for disability, compensation, litigation, and insurance purposes (Headache Classification Committee, 2004).

A variety of pain patterns that resemble the primary headache disorders may develop after head injury (Table 16–1). The most frequently seen pattern resembles tension-type headache (TTH) and occurs in 85% of patients. It is characterized by generalized, persistent, bilateral, mild-to-moderate pain (Mandel, 1989). The headaches may be exacerbated by very mild physical or mental activity (Kelly, 1988). In one study (DeBenedittis and DeSantis, 1983), headaches were mild in 30% of patients, moderate in 52%, and severe in 18%, and the pain was occipital in 51% of patients, frontal in 44%, and generalized in 11% of patients. The studies do not make clear the frequency of the headaches, their tempo, and their associated symptoms. Haas (Haas, 1995) used the IHS criteria for primary headache disorders to categorize 30 PCH patients. Eight patients' headaches were classified as migraine, 12 as chronic TTH, two as analgesic abuse headache, seven as "probable analgesic abuse headache," and one was unclassifiable. Couch et al., (2000) compared 106 patients with posttraumatic chronic daily headache to a similar number of idiopathic chronic daily headache patients and found no significant differences among 19 headache characteristics.

Table 16–2 IHS criteria for posttraumatic headache. (Headache Classification Committee, 2004.)

5.1 Acute and chronic posttraumatic headache (IHS criteria)

5.1.1 With significant head trauma and/or confirmatory signs

Diagnostic criteria

A. Significance of head trauma documented by at least one of the following:
   1. Loss of consciousness;
   2. Posttraumatic amnesia lasting more than 10 minutes;
   3. At least two of the following exhibit relevant abnormality: clinical neurologic examination, X-ray of skull, neuroimaging, evoked potentials, spinal fluid examination, vestibular function test, neuropsychologic testing.

B. Headache occurs less than 14 days after regaining consciousness (or after trauma, if there has been no loss of consciousness).

C. Headache disappears within 8 weeks after regaining consciousness (or after trauma, if there has been no loss of consciousness) (acute) or continues more than 8 weeks (chronic).

5.1.2 With minor head trauma and no confirmatory signs

Diagnostic criteria

A. Head trauma that does not satisfy 5.1.1 A.

B. Headache occurs less than 14 days after injury.

C. Headache disappears within 8 weeks after injury.

An otherwise typical migraine with or without aura may be triggered by impact (Haas and Lourie, 1988). Alternatively, a pattern of recurring migraine-like headaches may begin some time after a head injury (Evans, 1992; Packard and Ham, 1996). In one study (Weiss et al., 1991), 35 patients (27 women and 8 men) had newly acquired migraine with or without aura, beginning within a few days of mild head injury or whiplash injury. Most patients experienced two or three attacks per week. Amitriptyline or propranolol was dramatically effective in 71% of patients. Some patients have PCH with features of migraine and TTH that closely resembles chronic (transformed) migraine (Saper, 1983).

Neuralgic pain that occurs in the frontal or occipitocervical region may be associated with other headache types. Researchers (Evans, 1992; Gfeller et al., 1994) have found cluster headache-like syndrome in up to 10% of patients. These headaches may not undergo remissions. Packard and Ham (Packard and Ham, 1996) found them to be quite rare.

The symptoms of postconcussion syndrome may be unreported. Only 59% of patients who were hospitalized with head injury complained spontaneously of headache; the rest required prompting or direct questioning. At 6 months, only 33% of patients with headache after head injury volunteered this information. Similar percentages of spontaneous complaints of dizziness were noted, while the percentages of patients reporting symptoms of depression, anxiety, and irritability were much smaller (Cartlidge and Shaw, 1981).

RARE TYPES OF PCH

A cerebrospinal fluid (CSF) leak through a dural root sleeve tear or a cribriform plate fracture may cause orthostatic headache. Idiopathic intracranial hypertension (pseudotumor) with and without papilledema has been reported as a consequence of head injury (Silberstein and Marcelis, 1990).

Dysautonomic cephalalgia, a rare type of PCH that occurs following injury to the anterior area of the carotid sheath, was described by Vijayan (1977). This severe, unilateral headache is localized to the frontotemporal area and is associated with ipsilateral pupillary dilation and increased facial sweating.

Temporomandibular joint injury may occur in conjunction with mild head injury. Symptoms include jaw pain with mastication or prolonged talking, incomplete jaw opening, clicking or lateral movements (which by themselves are not clinically relevant), and pain on palpation of the jaw joint or the muscles of mastication. Many experts believe that actual temporomandibular joint injury at the time of head injury or whiplash injury is rare. Temporomandibular joint dysfunction is thought to be a trigger for headache.

Trauma may also cause a fracture of the styloid process and symptoms that resemble Eagle's syndrome: unilateral pain in the throat or neck or referred pain in the shoulder, chest, tongue, eye, cheek, temporomandibular joint, or ear. The pain is usually dull and continuous, but it may be neuralgic. There may be a foreign body sensation in the throat. Symptoms of carotid artery insufficiency may also occur. The fracture should be visualized radiographically (Montalbetti et al., 1995; Wong et al., 1995).

NONHEADACHE SYMPTOMS

Most patients who have postconcussion syndrome complain of impaired memory and difficulty concentrating (Rimel et al., 1981b). A survey of high school and university students demonstrated that those with self-reported head injury had more cognitive and emotional symptoms than those without such injury (Segalowitz and Lawson, 1995). Some patients have neurocognitive deficits and an inability to process information (Gronwall and Wrightson, 1974). Many have difficulty processing different stimuli simultaneously and appear absentminded because they must devote full concentration to the task at hand. If the information-processing capacity is overtaxed, the patient will appear forgetful (Andrasik and Wincze, 1994). Patients with head injury often appear distracted due to their inability to disregard irrelevant stimuli. Other frequently reported symptoms include anger, depression, and personality changes. Irritability, which may be immediate or delayed, is commonly reported after traumatic brain injury (Kim et al., 1999). Constitutional abnormalities include changes in appetite, alterations in sexual drive, weight loss or gain, and menstrual irregularities. Patients may meet the criteria for posttraumatic stress disorder (Hickling et al., 1992) (Table 16–2) with uncertain frequency (Jensen and Nielson, 1990; Sbordone and Liter, 1995). Posttraumatic stress disorder often requires aggressive intervention (Sbordone and Liter, 1995).

Both nonspecific dizziness and episodic and positional vertigo are common among patients with postconcussion syndrome (Lidvall et al., 1974). Sleep disturbances, including insomnia and daytime drowsiness, are frequent. Nonrestorative sleep and hypersomnolence are common complaints, with polysomnographic studies showing increased fragmentation of nocturnal sleep (Prigatano et al., 1982). Seizure-like events may occur, although few events appear to be epileptic and the electroencephalograph is usually normal. Nonspecific staring episodes, nonvestibular dizziness, and periodic loss of consciousness have been reported. Epilepsy or true syncope is rare. Narcolepsy-like or cataplexy-like spells, episodic disorientation, and fugue-like states can occur (Lankford et al., 1994; Silberstein et al., 1995). The attacks are more common when there has been a loss of consciousness at the time of the initial injury (Lake et al., 1995).

CONTROVERSIES SURROUNDING THE DIAGNOSIS OF PCH AND POSTCONCUSSION SYNDROME

Patients with postconcussion syndrome are often told, either by physicians, insurers, or employers, that they are embellishing or malingering, that they have a primary psychiatric disorder, or that their condition is not related to their injury. This belief is not substantiated, however, since: (1) patients with chronic PCH rarely engage in such behavior; (2) in many studies the presence of litigation does not appear to influence outcome; (3) patients are not cured by a verdict (Packard, 1992); and (4) symptoms of litigants are similar to those of nonlitigants (Davis and Luxon, 1995). Nonetheless, physicians are often placed in a position of justifying an accurate diagnosis of posttraumatic syndrome.

Miller (Miller, 1961b) published a series of lectures in the *British Medical Journal* in which he ascribed chronic postconcussion syndrome to a desire for compensation or a desire not to work. These arguments continue to be used today. Lidvall et al., (1974), however, conducted a prospective study that demonstrated that poor work adjustment did not predict postconcussion syndrome, but that patients with postconcussion syndrome subsequently demonstrated poor work adjustment.

Mittenberg et al. (1992) demonstrated that a control population identified the symptoms of postconcussion syndrome from a checklist in a similar manner to patients who complained of postconcussion syndrome. He concluded that the symptoms of postconcussion syndrome are due to the fact that patients expect to experience these symptoms, suggesting that education and reassurance of a favorable prognosis are adequate treatments and that some patients should be treated for anxiety. Alternatively, these findings suggest that most people are familiar with postconcussion syndrome, perhaps because they have experienced the symptoms following a minimal concussion or because they have heard about head injuries sustained by sports figures. The crux of postconcussion syndrome may be the organic magnification or persistence of symptoms commonly experienced by normal individuals, thus accounting for the easy recognizability of these symptoms by controls.

The fact that sports injuries rarely cause postconcussion syndrome leads to the suggestion that postconcussion syndrome occurs because of the opportunity for gain. However, the velocities and forces experienced during most sports injuries are much less than those that result from motor vehicle accidents and falls, which are the injuries that commonly cause postconcussion syndrome. In sports injuries, the head is often fixed, whereas in automobile accidents the head is freely mobile, which results in more severe damage. Nonetheless, persistent cognitive deficits are common in sports concussion (Denny-Brown, 1945). Similarly, the observation that seemingly trivial injuries can cause severe disability has led some to conclude that the disability does not have a physiologic basis. There are other disease states in which minor injuries cause severe pain. For example, incomplete peripheral nerve injuries are often excruciatingly painful, whereas nerve transections are usually painless. In some cases, a skull fracture may dissipate the energy of impact and protect the brain from an injury that could lead to postconcussion syndrome, producing fewer symptoms in a population that superficially appears more injured.

One of the arguments used against the organicity of postconcussion syndrome is that patients do not have abnormal studies and there are no abnormal signs on examination. Many neurologic diseases, such as migraine with aura, have no abnormal signs on examination. Several paraclinical studies show group differences between uninjured mild head injury patients without chronic postconcussion syndrome and postconcussion syndrome patients (see below). They do not yet have the sensitivity to distinguish individuals with "organic" PCH from those with psychological or other causes of PCH.

One possible cause for the symptoms of postconcussion syndrome is misattribution. The symptoms of postconcussion syndrome are common in new-injured individuals, including those with depression (Iverson, 2006), and in an arbitrary group of healthy university students (Wang et al., 2006). A careful history, including a review of prior medical records and a tight definition of postconcussion syndrome with new headache starting very shortly after injury should keep the physician from this error in most cases.

Work factors have been hypothesized to cause prolonged disability. Miller (1961a, 1961b) stated that unskilled workers and less intelligent persons suffer more prolonged disability due to postconcussion syndrome. Jobs that require certain cognitive skills are particularly difficult for patients suffering from postconcussion syndrome. Laborers whose jobs depend upon sustained physical effort and mental vigilance have particular difficulty performing their jobs, whereas patients whose jobs allow more flexibility and do not require physical activity may be better able to cope with the disability. Patients who blame their employer as a large impersonal body had more symptoms than those who did not. This has been attributed to be "clear evidence of nervous and emotional factors at work in the production of symptoms" (Rutherford et al., 1977). The other possibility—that patients who are anxious, depressed, irritable, and have more symptoms due to their postconcussion syndrome are more likely to blame others—was not addressed. Many kinds of brain injuries, including stroke and neurodegenerative disease, produce psychiatric symptoms. Chronic pain by itself can induce depression and abnormal behavior; this does not mean that organic pathology does not exist. Having a disabling illness that is not accepted by medical professionals, employers, and family is a legitimate cause of anxiety, depression, and abnormal behaviors.

A study (Obelieniene et al., 1998) of Lithuanian automobile accident victims failed to show an increased incidence of headache or neck pain years after injury. This finding was attributed to the fact that insurance was not available to compensate Lithuanian accident victims for lost work, and to the general lack of recognition of postconcussion headache/postconcussion syndrome in the community. In contrast to Lithuania, a recent study from Sweden showed that, 7 years later, a motor vehicle accident with a whiplash injury is associated with a four-fold risk of headache compared with controls (Berglund et al., 2001). Postconcussion headache/postconcussion syndrome is recognized across many cultures in the Americas, Europe, and Asia.

RISK FACTORS

Age, gender, and certain mechanical factors are risks for a poor outcome after head injury or whiplash injury. Compared with men, women have a 1.9-fold increased risk of PCH (Jensen et al., 1990) and postconcussion syndrome (Fenton, 1996; Bazarian et al., 1999). Increasing age is associated with a less rapid and less complete recovery (Bohnen et al., 1992; McClelland et al., 1994; Fenton, 1996). One study found that children under 15 years of age may develop acute, but not chronic, PCH (Keshavan et al., 1981). Jensen and Nielson (1990), however, found that the risk of PCH did not vary with age. In addition to the force of impact, mechanical factors are important. If the head is rotated, increased stress is put on the cervical structures and more rotational forces are applied to the brain; thus, PCH is more likely if the head is inclined or rotated prior to impact. A rear-end collision and an unprepared occupant are other factors that increase the likelihood of postconcussion syndrome (Mendelson, 1982).

The relationship between the severity of the injury and the severity of postconcussion syndrome has not been conclusively established. In general, the headache's persistence does not correlate with the duration of unconsciousness or the presence of posttraumatic amnesia, skull fracture, electroencephalogram (EEG) abnormalities, or bloody CSF (DeBenedittis and DeSantis, 1983). Some authors have found an inverse relationship between the severity of the injury and the severity of the PCH (Yamaguchi, 1992; Couch and Bearss, 2001). In one study, the initially hospitalized mild head injury patients had similar symptoms to patients who were discharged from the emergency room. However, *hospitalized* patients recovered more quickly. These findings could support the concept that more severe mild head injury causes less PCH and postconcussion syndrome, although other explanations are possible (Barrett et al., 1994).

On the other hand, a study found that patients who had lost consciousness had more depression and anger-control problems than patients who did not lose consciousness (Lake et al., 1995). Duration of posttraumatic amnesia has also been correlated with persistence of postconcussion syndrome (Bazarian et al., 1999) and the presence of retrograde amnesia. Diplopia, anosmia, and the presence of central nervous system abnormality at 24 hours correlating with the persistence of symptoms 6 weeks after injury suggests that a subset of patients with more severe injury have worse outcomes (Rutherford, 1989). This difference suggests that more research using prospectively followed, stratified patient samples is needed before definitive conclusions can be reached.

Radanov et al. (1995) studied patients 7 days and again 2 years after whiplash injury. Patients who had high multiple-symptom scores shortly after their injury had a significantly greater chance of having symptoms 2 years after the injury. Patients who were still disabled 2 years after their injury had higher multiple-symptom scores at the initial examination compared with patients who were symptomatic but not disabled after 2 years. In persons presenting to the Emergency Department, duration of posttraumatic amnesia, headache, dizziness, and nausea are risk factors for chronic PCH (DeKruijk et al., 2002). Radanov believes that patients with more severe injuries have higher initial-symptom scores and worse outcomes. Alternatively, individual vulnerability could lead to a greater number of initial symptoms and a poorer long-term outcome, regardless of the severity of the initial injury.

Authorities have speculated that a history of prior headache increases the risk for PCH. Jensen found that pretraumatic migraine was not a risk factor for developing PCH after hospitalization for cerebral concussion (Jensen and Nielson, 1990). This study suffered from recall bias since the patients were interviewed 9–12 months after the injury. Weiss et al. (1991) reported that 31% of patients who developed migraine-like attacks following mild head or neck trauma had a history of migraine in first-degree relatives. The authors suggested that head or neck trauma triggers the migraine process in susceptible individuals. In another study in which patients were interviewed immediately following whiplash injury, pretraumatic headache was a significant risk factor for developing PCH (Radanov et al., 1995). Early headache, occurring within 24 hours of injury, is a strong risk factor for postconcussion syndrome at 6 weeks (Wilkinson and Gilchrist, 1980).

Lack of education was not a risk factor for acute postconcussion syndrome; unskilled laborers were more likely to develop chronic symptoms (Lidvall et al., 1974). Likewise, socioeconomic status may predict employment 3 months after minor head injury. Business managers and executives (in Rimel's study) were more likely than unskilled laborers to be employed 3 months after injury. Higher education also predicted continued employment. These studies do not differentiate between the premorbid effect of lack of education, poor motivation to return to a menial job, poor resources to adjust to the effects of the injury, or employer intolerance (Rimel et al., 1981b).

Preexisting psychopathology may influence the clinical evolution of postconcussion syndrome. In one study, patients and their relatives were interviewed within 1 month of head injury to assess for premorbid psychopathology. The patient's psychologic state prior to the injury correlated with the subjective symptomatology. However, physical and social dysfunction correlated with the severity of the injury, not with preexisting factors (Keshavan et al., 1981). In another study, patients with pretraumatic emotional problems had higher scores on scales of cognitive and emotional-vegetative dysfunction after mild head injury (Bohnen et al., 1992). Disability was not measured. These studies suggested that preexisting psychopathology influenced how symptoms are reported rather than impacting on disability.

In contrast, McClelland (1994) found no difference in premorbid personality adjustment between chronic postconcussion syndrome sufferers and patients whose symptoms resolved. Likewise, Lidvall et al. (1974) found no differences in pretraumatic neuroticism or adjustment to work between similarly injured patients who developed postconcussion syndrome and those who did not. Fenton (1996) found no differences between premorbid social adjustment, life events, and chronicity of symptoms. These studies have methodologic problems: their psychologic assessments were retrospective and the methods used to ascertain preexisting psychopathology were often not well described.

Using the Freiburg Personality Inventory, Radanov (Radanov et al., 1995) assessed patients shortly after whiplash injury. Scores on the nervousness, depression, openness, neuroticism, and masculinity scales did not correlate with outcome 2 years after injury. In contrast, poor well-being scale scores correlated with the persistence of symptoms, but not with disability, among patients who were symptomatic 2 years after injury (Sturzenegger, 1991).

PATHOPHYSIOLOGY

Postconcussion syndrome is probably not a single pathologic entity, but a group of traumatically induced disorders with overlapping symptoms. The cognitive, sleep, and psychologic deficits these patients exhibit are manifestations of brain injury. Headache is mainly a manifestation of brain dysfunction, with occasional contributions from persistent musculoskeletal injuries.

Neck, jaw, and scalp tissue injuries may contribute to acute PCH; pain originating from these areas can be referred to the head. Most of these injuries heal completely and cannot, by themselves, account for chronic PCH or the associated neurocognitive symptoms of PCH. However, soft tissue or skeletal injuries may initiate or trigger a transformation process in headache-prone patients similar to the process by which daily intermittent migraine or TTH evolves into chronic daily headache. Postconcussion headache patients have more upper cervical segment joint dysfunction, less endurance of neck flexor muscle, and a higher incidence of moderately tight neck musculature, yet the neck range of motion is normal (Treleaven et al., 1994). These findings could be due to adaptive, and sometimes maladaptive, phenotypic central nervous system changes similar to the phenomenon of central sensitization that is observed in experimental models of chronic pain. One model, based upon the kindling phenomenon in experimental epilepsy (Post and Silberstein, 1994), could explain the evolution of peripheral injuries into chronic centrally maintained pain. Nerve or musculoskeletal injuries could induce windup and sensitization, which could ultimately result in permanently altered neuronal function. Because these changes occur postsynaptically as well as presynaptically, neuronal function may be altered at distant brain sites involved in the production or experience of pain (Post and Silberstein, 1994).

As a result of head injury or whiplash, shear forces are applied to the brain; this can result in diffuse axonal injury that can be elicited histologically. In experimental models, direct impact is not necessary to produce significant diffuse axonal injury (Gennarelli, 1993). Diffuse axonal injury is most common in the corpus callosum, internal capsule, fornices, dorsolateral midbrain, and pons (Blumbergs et al., 1989). Gennarelli et al. (1975) suggested that there is a continuum of diffuse axonal injury that varies from functional abnormalities alone to structural lesions that become increasingly severe and result in widespread injury. Immunohistochemical studies demonstrate similar, although less severe, histological findings in the rat fluid percussion model in mild head injury compared with moderate head injury. These changes are delayed in mild injury (Gennarelli et al., 1975). The relevance and extent of diffuse axonal injury in human mild head injury is not fully elucidated. One report indicates that diffuse axonal injury occurs in concussive mild head injury (Blumbergs et al., 1994).

Because of unsynchronized rotations that may develop between the cerebral hemispheres and the cerebellum (Elson and Ward, 1994), axons in the upper brainstem may be particularly vulnerable to diffuse axonal injury. Evidence of brainstem vulnerability in humans comes from a demonstration of midbrain hemorrhage on magnetic resonance imaging (MRI) in a patient with mild head injury (Servadei et al., 1994). Brainstem axons that are sheared in diffuse axonal injury are responsible for control of arousal, vigilance, and sleep (Goodman, 1994). Serotonergic and adrenergic projection fibers are postulated to play a central role in pain modulation (Weiller et al., 1995); when both are injured, head pain results. Reactive synaptogenesis, a process of axonal sprouting that restores synaptic contact on denuded dendrites, has been demonstrated in at least one model of head injury (Erb and Povlishock, 1991). This could account for both physiologic improvement through appropriate healing and new or worsening symptoms as aberrant connections are made. Evidence for synaptogenesis in human head injury is awaited.

Head injury usually involves a combination of translational and rotational forces. Restricted rotation makes it more difficult to produce a concussion in animals (Elson and Ward, 1994). Rotational forces occur even when movement is primarily translational (see below). In studies using windows in cadaver skulls, the brain has been demonstrated to lag behind the skull, due to inertia, when the head is accelerated. As a result of the translational force, the brain is compressed near the point of impact, while negative pressures develop opposite to the site of impact.

Experimental models of head injury have advanced several observations. Gennarelli's angular acceleration model, which uses subhuman primates, demonstrates axonal changes in the brainstem (Jane et al., 1985) similar to the human autopsy cases of minor head injury (Povlishock and Coburn, 1989). In this model, diffuse axonal injury is a major finding of severe head injury and is probably the cause of coma (Gennarelli et al., 1975). In the cat fluid percussion model of experimental brain injury, a hydraulic pressure pulse, lasting milliseconds, creates a physiologic response similar to that seen in moderate or mild human head injury. Based on microscopic changes observed after this type of head injury, Povlishock speculated that stretching or compression, not shearing, is the cause of axonal injury in this model and possibly in human head injury (Povlishock and Coburn, 1989). Finally, a fluid percussion pulse injury in rats causes loss of cholinergic neurons in the forebrain, but not in the brainstem (Schmidt and Grady, 1995). The relevance of these findings to human head injury is unknown.

Finite element modeling is a computerized structural analysis technique used to study the effect of various acceleration forces on the brain. Finite element modeling has shown that rotational brain movements occur even when the motion of the head is primarily translational. It has also shown that various brain compartments have different rotations. Shear stress in the brainstem is influenced by a number of factors, including pressure release at the foramen magnum, motion of the medulla due to neck motion, the influence of individually rotating cerebral hemispheres and the cerebellum, the proximity of the brainstem to the skull, and restraint provided by the tentorium (Ward, 1982; Elson and Ward, 1994).

As it does in severe head injury, abnormal cerebrovascular autoregulation may have a role in postconcussion syndrome. Forty-eight hours after minor head injury, 28% of patients and none of the controls had poorly functioning or absent autoregulation (Junger et al., 1997). There was no correlation with the GCS score. Since long-term clinical outcomes were not studied, the role of this observation in chronic PCH or postconcussion syndrome is unknown.

A series of neurochemical changes occurs with experimental head injury (Table 16–3)(Packard and Ham, 1997). The relevance of these alternatives to human head injury and the role of such changes in the evolution of postconcussion syndrome are unknown. However, an altered chemical or electrical environment could account for immediate impact headache or aura. It could result in cellular injury and in postconcussion syndrome. The similarity between the biochemical changes of migraine headaches and those that are seen after head injury suggest a shared physiology and possibly a role for similar treatment strategies (Packard, 1999).

The effectiveness of treatments such as repetitive intravenous dihydroergotamine in PCH suggests a similar or shared mechanism with the primary headache disorders. This could be due to a "final common pathway" of symptom expression, including trigeminovascular activation (McBeath and Nanda, 1994; Young et al., 1994).

Many authors uphold the "psychogenesis" of chronic PCH and postconcussion syndrome, but few point out specific mechanisms to account for it. Duckro et al. (1995) used a "path analysis," a directional multiple regression analysis, to

TABLE 16–3 A Comparison of Biochemical Changes in Mild Head Injury and Migraine Headache.

Mild Head Injury	*Migraine*
Increased extracellular K^+ and intracellular Na^+, Ca^{2+} and Cl^-	Increased extracellular K^+ and intracellular Na^+, Ca^{2+} and Cl^-
Excessive release of EAAs (primarily glutamate)	Excessive release of EAAs (glutamate and aspartate)
Accumulation of platelet-derived 5-HT in CNS	Excessive firing of dorsal raphe leads to increased 5-HT release and depletion of available 5-HT pool
Increased levels of endogenous opioids (findings mixed)	B-endorphin content may be reduced in headache-free periods; high MET-endorphin levels during attacks
Decline in intracellular and total brain Mg	Deficiency of Mg levels between and during attacks
Influx of extracellular Ca^{2+} in compromised axolemmas	Increase in intracellular ratio Ca^{2+}/Mg^{2+} ratio
Nitric oxide may be converted to free oxygen radical, potentially leading to tissue injury	Nitric oxide may be involved in migraine pathogenesis; at the vascular endothelium, it is a potent vasodilator; in the spinal cord it is pronociceptive

Abbreviations: CNS, central nervous system; EAAs, excitatory amino acids; MET, metabolic equivalent.

examine the relationship between posttraumatic pain, disability, depression, and anger. He concluded that depression might cause disability, and that expressed and unexpressed anger contribute to depression.

Kelly (1988) posited that nonvalidation of cognitive and physically painful symptoms by medical, legal, and employment authorities leads to an anxiety/depressive reaction that results in the persistence of originally organic symptoms. He relied on the now outdated concept that emotional tension is a principal cause of persistent headache.

It is likely that at least two processes occur in patients with PCH or postconcussion syndrome. The first process is likely due to diffuse axonal injury and correlates with the acceleration/deceleration forces. When more severe, it is associated with abnormalities on MRI, positron emission tomography, single photon emission computed tomography (SPECT), S100, and certain neuropsychologic tests. A challenge to this hypothesis is the observation that patients with severe closed head injury do not report as many symptoms as those with less severe injuries. It could be argued, however, that symptoms of postconcussion syndrome and PCH are only masked by coexisting illnesses and manifestations of the sequelae of severe head injury. Clinical improvement of diffuse axonal injury may occur over several months, with normalization or amelioration of the radiologic tests. Also neuropsychologic testing may indicate full recovery but tests for attention may still be abnormal.

A second process may be responsible for many of the symptoms that persist after minor head injury. A preexisting vulnerability may be necessary for the chronic posttraumatic symptoms to manifest, since preexisting headache is a risk factor in some patients. A mechanism similar to the kindling model of epilepsy, or, perhaps, aberrant connections made by injured axons may underlie this mechanism and explain most of the symptoms of chronic postconcussion syndrome and PCH. Additional factors, perhaps psychologic, may influence the expression of symptoms caused by the second process.

For most patients with postconcussion syndrome, the clinical history of new-onset or changed headache after an injury associated with new cognitive, emotional, and sleep disturbances is so characteristic that once intracranial pathology is excluded, confirmatory tests are not required in order to proceed with treatment. Unfortunately, tests are often conducted for medicolegal reasons, increasing patients' anxiety and self-doubt when they are negative. Negative test results are often used to indicate no abnormality. However, no test has the specificity or sensitivity to make or exclude a diagnosis in a particular individual. Similarly, if postconcussion syndrome is not a single entity but a syndrome derived from several pathologic processes initiated by head trauma, no single test would be expected to diagnose the same in all patients.

TESTING

Although many studies have attempted to establish the extent of the head injury and the diagnosis of postconcussion syndrome, no test reliably distinguishes patients with postconcussion syndrome from normal controls or from patients with primary headache disorders.

COMPUTED TOMOGRAPHY AND MRI

Few studies specifically evaluate brain imaging in postconcussion syndrome. Most series included patients with head injury who might have required neurosurgical intervention. When specifically looking at a group of head injury patients, no MRI abnormalities were found among the subgroup of patients with postconcussion syndrome (Kraus et al., 1994). On the other hand, Levin et al. (1987) found MRI abnormalities within several weeks of injury in 17 of 20 hospitalized patients with mild or moderate head injury. MRI was clearly superior to computed tomography (CT) in identifying these abnormalities, which were located in the white matter or at the gray/white-matter junction. Levin et al. (Levin et al., 1992) studied patients who were admitted with mild to moderate head injury and found that a reduction of the mean parenchymal lesion size occurred with the passage of time. Most of the resolutions occurred within the first month, and lesions that were present at 1 month remained at 3 months. Patients who had abnormal MRI had more cognitive deficits than did patients who had normal MRI. In the absence of pathologic confirmation, one cannot speculate that these lesions represent diffuse axonal injury with resolving edema. Hughes et al. (2004) found MRI abnormalities in 26 of 80 hospitalized mild traumatic brain injury patients. These findings did not influence return to work in a followup questionnaire. We also speculate that the MRI changes resolve with resolution of the edema when the diffuse axonal injury is less severe, whereas the changes are permanent when the diffuse axonal injury is more severe.

Mittle (1994) obtained MRI on 20 consecutively hospitalized head injury patients. These studies were reviewed by two blinded readers. The readers concurred that diffuse axonal injury was present in 30% of patients. One radiologist diagnosed diffuse axonal injury in 20% of patients, indicating that even MRI may not always provide an unequivocal diagnosis. These MRI findings may not be characteristic of head injury patients who were not hospitalized. Nevertheless, diffuse axonal injury of a severity that does not produce MRI abnormalities could still be present.

There are no prospective studies that establish the value of brain imaging in patients with PCH or postconcussion syndrome. In the acute setting, it is prudent to image all patients who have mild behavioral abnormalities, abnormal findings on clinical examination, or a GCS score of less than 15 because of the risk of subsequent deterioration. With subacute or chronic postconcussion syndrome, there is little information to guide the clinician. Neuroimaging should be guided by findings on clinical examination, by the medical history, and by the history of symptom evolution or resolution.

FUNCTIONAL IMAGING

SPECT observes the physiologic behavior of the brain. It can contribute information about the spatial distribution of radiolabeled ligands and the time course of ligand uptake and washout. It is analyzed by CT analysis. SPECT has been used to study head injury patients, but has not been used specifically in PCH or postconcussion syndrome. In the acute phase of head injury, technetium-99m hexamethylpropyleneamineoxine SPECT is more useful than CT in identifying brain lesions and demonstrating abnormalities of function when CT cannot. It shows more lesions than CT and is helpful in predicting outcome (Abdel-Dayem et al., 1994). One study of 20 patients with head injury revealed technetium-99m hexamethylpropyleneamineoxine SPECT abnormalities in 60% of patients, whereas only 25% had abnormalities on CT (Gray et al., 1992). Another study examined 12 patients with mild-to-moderate head injury 1–9 years after the injury. In this study, 10 patients had abnormal technetium-99m hexamethylpropyleneamineoxine SPECT, while CT was abnormal in only 6 (Krelina et al., 1989). Another study showed that the number of lesions on SPECT correlates with the extent of disability (Newton et al., 1992).

Abnormal sites on imaging studies include the basal ganglia and thalamus in 55% of patients, the frontal lobes in 23%, the temporal lobes in 13%, the parietal lobes in 4%, and the insular and occipital regions together in 5% (Abdel-Dayem et al., 1998). Another study showed significant orbitofrontal hypoperfusion in 67% of patients with posttraumatic anosmia. By contrast, there were no group differences in other brain regions and individual abnormalities were infrequent (Varney and Bushnell, 1998). Anosmia may be a marker for orbitofrontal brain injury.

Masdeu (1995) suggests that two types of lesions may be seen on SPECT: circumscribed areas of hypoperfusion that represent contusion, and diffuse occipitotemporal hypoperfusion that represents multiple small contusions or diffuse axonal injury. The Academy of Neurology's Therapeutics and Technology Assessment Subcommittee has determined the use of SPECT for the evaluation of head trauma to be "investigational" based on Class II evidence (one or more well designed clinical studies) (American Academy of Neurology, 1996).

Using xenon-inhalation cerebral blood flow, Ramadan et al. studied the correlation between headache disability and cerebral blood flow. Both the emotional subscale score and the function subscale score of a headache disability inventory correlated with the mean asymmetry score (Ramadan et al., 1995). The same investigators reported that patients with chronic PCH have lower mean initial slope indices, significant regional interhemispheric flow differences, and more interhemispheric asymmetries compared with migraineurs and nonheadache controls (Gilkey et al., 1997). The authors concluded that the cerebral blood flow findings are indicators of neurovascular instability that persists months to years after the initial head injury.

Like SPECT, position emission tomography examines physiologic activity within the brain. In head trauma, positron emission tomography has revealed widespread abnormalities in cerebral glucose metabolism (Alavi et al., 1987; George et al., 1989) and areas of diminished perfusion that tend to improve with clinical recovery (George et al., 1989). One study showed that these areas of perfusion abnormality corresponded to the areas of abnormality that had been identified by neuropsychologic testing (Rao et al., 1984).

One month after head injury, patients with minor traumatic brain injury and control subjects showed different brain activation patterns in response to increasing working memory processing loads. Patients with minor traumatic brain injury had significantly more cognitive symptoms but performed as well as controls on a neuropsychological battery, differing only in response speed, sample reaction time, and distractibility tasks of the continuous performance test. The presence of headache was not commented on (Rao et al., 1984).

ELECTROENCEPHALOGRAPHY

Routine electroencephalography is usually of little value in evaluating postconcussion syndrome in patients with head injury. While it may be abnormal immediately after injury, it often normalizes within minutes to weeks. Persistent findings that were once considered abnormal are now considered normal variants, having the same incidence as the general population (Schoenhuber and Gentilini, 1989).

Quantitative electroencephalography may or may not be useful in head injury. In one small study, quantitative electroencephalography showed a statistically significant increase in both slow and fast activity over the temporal region of the skull. However, the author concluded that this test offers little benefit to the patient with PCH, since there is a great deal of variability within the PCH group and these findings are common in both PCH and control patients (Hughes and Robbins, 1990). Another study examined the ability of power spectrum analysis to discriminate between 608 head injury patients and 108 age-matched controls, and found that head injury could be discriminated from age-matched controls with more than 90% accuracy (Thatcher et al., 1989). In one study the generators of abnormal slow waves on quantitative EEG correlated with reduced focal perfusion on SPECT (Korn et al., 2005). No correlation was made between the symptoms of PCH or postconcussion syndrome and abnormal test results. Therefore, the predictive value of this study is uncertain at this time. In general, these studies indicate that PCH patients, as a group, differ from nonheadache controls. But unlike the study of Ramadan et al. (1995), they cannot reliably differentiate an individual PCH patient from a patient with an idiopathic headache.

MAGNETIC SOURCE IMAGING

Magnetic source imaging combines MRI and magnetoencephalography. One study showed abnormalities in 5% of a normal control group, 10% of an asymptomatic mild-head-injury group, and 65% of a group of patients with persistent symptoms ($p < 0.01$). These abnormal findings improve as the patient improves. Like the xenon cerebral blood flow studies of Ramadan and Gilkey (1997), this study demonstrates an organic abnormality in patients with postconcussion syndrome.

EVOKED POTENTIALS AND ELECTRONYSTAGMOGRAPHY

Short latency somatosensory evoked potentials are not of value in testing patients with head injury or postconcussion syndrome (Bricolo and Turella, 1990). On the other hand, brainstem auditory evoked potentials have been found to be abnormal in 10%–20% of patients with head injury and postconcussion syndrome. The more prolonged the unconsciousness, the greater the incidence of abnormalities (Schoenhuber and Gentilini, 1989). The brainstem auditory evoked potentials can either improve or deteriorate from 2 days to 1 month after injury (Geets and Louette, 1983). Symptomatic dizziness does not correlate with brainstem auditory evoked potential abnormalities. While the brainstem auditory evoked potential separates groups of postconcussion syndrome patients from groups of controls, it is of no value in distinguishing an individual with postconcussion syndrome from one without postconcussion syndrome.

The P300 is an event-related potential manifested by a positive cortical potential that occurs after an infrequent stimulation to which the patient is attending, such as a loud sound in a train of soft sounds. It has been correlated with cognitive functions, such as memory information delivery and decision making, and decreases in amplitude with drowsiness or inattention. Studies of P300 in head injury have yielded mixed results. One study demonstrated significant abnormalities of P300 amplitude and latency in 20 head injury patients compared with 20 control subjects (Pratap-Chand et al., 1988). Another study (Werner and Vanderzant, 1991) found an abnormal response in only 1 of 18 patients. More recently, Kobylare and colleagues found a correlation between an abnormal P300 and an abnormal MRI (Kobylare et al., 1995). An interesting study demonstrated that hearing accident-related words (i.e., "stressful") produced a significantly larger P300 than hearing neutral words in patients with mild head injury, but not in nonhead injury controls. The P300 amplitude difference correlated with the patient's two-way state anxiety score (Granovsky et al., 1998). The role this study may play in evaluating head injury is uncertain.

Electronystagmogram is abnormal in 40%–50% of patients with head injury or "whiplash" in clinic-based studies. Toglia (1969) examined 150 patients who complained of vestibular symptoms following either head injury or whiplash injury. Spontaneous, latent, and positional nystagmus were searched for. Bithermal caloric tests and rotational tests were performed when possible. Abnormal caloric tests (including both canal paresis and directional preponderance) were found in 63% of whiplash patients and 68% of head injury patients. Abnormal rotatory tests were found in 9 of 16 whiplash patients (56%) and 20 of 24 head injury patients (83%). Rowe and Carlson (1980) studied 19 patients with postconcussive dizziness following head injury and found 11 patients (58%) had abnormalities consisting of latent or positional nystagmus or caloric-induced nystagmus. None of Rowe and Carlson's patients who had abnormal brainstem auditory evoked potentials (three standard deviations) had normal electronystagmograms. Conversely, most patients with abnormal electronystagmograms had normal brainstem auditory evoked potentials. This suggests that the electronystagmogram may be more sensitive than the brainstem auditory evoked potential. More recently, Mallinson and Longridge (1998) found electronystagmogram abnormalities in patients with whiplash injury and mild head injury, but not in whiplash injury alone, although symptoms of dizziness were similar in both groups.

Computerized dynamic posturography was studied in a referral population of dizzy patients after whiplash injury, alone or with mild head injury. Both groups had positive findings, although the type of posturography abnormality was different between groups (Mallinson and Longridge, 1998).

BLOOD TESTING: S-100

The S-100 is a marker of brain injury in head trauma and correlates with the GCS on admission (Herrmann et al., 1999). In hospitalized mild-head-injury patients, S-100 was detectable in 28% of patients, 36% of whom had contusions on MRI. In patients with detectable S-100 levels, there was a trend toward impaired neuropsychological functioning on measures of attention, memory, and information-processing speed (Ingebrigtsen et al., 1999). Correcting for muscle injury improves the predictive value (Bazarian et al., 2006).

NEUROPSYCHOLOGIC TESTING

Neuropsychologic testing in head injury often shows marked early abnormalities that improve or resolve with time. These include information processing, auditory vigilance, reaction time, sustained divided and distributed attention, visual and verbal memory, design fluency imagination, and analytic capacity. Eisenberg reported that tests of design fluency and verbal memory improved and normalized over 1–3 months in parallel with MRI findings (Eisenberg, 1989). The paced auditory serial addition test is a widely used test of information processing that is often abnormal shortly after head injury. Patients are presented with a random series of digits at intervals of either 1–2 or 2–4 seconds (same interval for entire test), and are asked to add the most recently presented number to the one before. The score is expressed as the percentage correct at each rate or as the mean correct response per second. It has been given serially over 8 weeks postinjury and demonstrates cognitive recovery to normal. Paced auditory serial addition test recovery, however, was delayed in head injury patients with postconcussion syndrome compared with a nonpostconcussion syndrome control group (Gronwall and Wrightson, 1974).

Within 8 weeks of head injury, a test of auditory vigilance in which patients had to detect the rare instances in which the interval between elements in a string of numbers was longer than in the others showed normalization (McCarthy, 1977). However, "recovered" head injury patients performed more poorly than normal controls at simulated high altitude (Ewing et al., 1980), demonstrating that deficits may reappear under physiologic stress. Several measures of reaction time, which are believed to be indicators of attention deficits, are also impaired in patients with head injury at various times after injury, although recovery was demonstrated in one study of mild head injury patients 10 years after injury compared with twin controls (Dencker and Lofving, 1958). In a test of selective attention devised by Gentilini et al. (1989), head injury patients were significantly slower but not less accurate than controls 3 months after injury. Tests of sustained and divided attention, again devised by Gentilini et al. (1989), showed significant differences from controls at 1 month, but were inconclusive 3 months after injury. On the other hand, Bohnen demonstrated that patients with mild head injury and postconcussion syndrome performed less well on a test of sustained attention than mild head injury controls (without postconcussion syndrome) 12–34 months after injury (Bohnen et al., 1995). Gentilini et al. (1989) demonstrated that tests of distributed attention showed deficits 1 and 3 months after head injury. The authors pointed out that the most sensitive tools for revealing cerebral dysfunction test the function of the greatest number of cortical and subcortical areas simultaneously (Gentilini et al., 1989). Chan (2002) found that patients with chronic PCH have a persisting deficit in attention performance compared to normal controls, which persists after emotional performance is controlled. In contrast, cognitive symptoms were accounted for by depression (Suhr and Gunstad, 2002). Only one study (Bohnen's) has been shown to distinguish PCH or postconcussion syndrome from mild head injury alone (Gentilini et al., 1989).

Keidel et al. (1992) performed repeated neuropsychologic tests on 30 patients with postconcussion syndrome after whiplash injury. Attention and concentration deficits recovered within 6 weeks. Visual memory, imagination, and analytic capacity recovered within the next 6 weeks. Verbal memory abstraction, cognitive selectivity, and information-processing speed took more than 12 weeks to recover (Keidel et al., 1992). These findings demonstrate a hierarchy of functional recovery occurring over a period of greater than 12 weeks after apparently mild injury.

Ham (Ham et al., 1994) studied patients with PCH and compared them with patients with chronic "combination headache" and low-back pain, and with pain-free controls. PCH patients had the highest scale elevations on the Symptom Checklist 90-Revised, a brief screen for somatic and psychologic symptoms that are broken down into nine primary "dimensions" or scales. Elevations were significant on all scales except the hostility and phobic anxiety scale. PCH patients scored significantly higher than pain-free controls in the Beck Depression Inventory, but did not differ significantly from other pain groups. State anxiety, a measure of acute anxiety, was significantly higher in PCH than controls and other pain states, but trait anxiety, a measure of anxious personality structure, differed significantly only from controls. Mean headache severity was higher (but not significantly) in the PCH group than in the control headache group. These findings suggest that PCH patients exhibit more psychopathology than individuals with other headache types and normal controls. On some tests, patients with PCH had more psychopathology than patients with low-back pain. In general, these tests do not demonstrate any specific pattern to the psychopathology (Ham et al., 1994).

DIAGNOSIS

The diagnosis of PCH and postconcussion syndrome is established by symptoms consistent with this syndrome and trauma-related onset. The IHS criteria for PCH require the headache to occur within 14 days after regaining consciousness (or after the trauma if there is no loss of consciousness). There are no IHS criteria for late-onset PCH. The IHS differentiates between acute PCH, which lasts less than 8 weeks, and chronic PCH, which lasts longer (Table 16–4). A worsening of a preexisting headache disorder does not qualify as PCH. A substantial difference between headache features before and after injury must be present for the designation of PCH.

Other physiologic or psychologic disorders must be meticulously excluded. The differential diagnosis includes, among others, subdural or epidural hematoma, CSF hypotension, cerebral vein thrombosis, cavernous sinus thrombosis, cervical or carotid artery dissection, cerebral hemorrhage, epilepsy, and hydrocephalus.

Many patients diagnosed with postconcussion syndrome are portrayed as malingerers or are thought to profoundly embellish their symptoms. Most experts believe this is rare. Binder (1986) suggests that the diagnosis of malingering should be actively made by surreptitiously observing a patient performing a task he stated he could not accomplish. Simulators have been shown to perform worse on sensorimotor tests (Heaton et al., 1978) and memory tests (Benton and Spreen, 1961) than would be expected. Performance that is significantly worse than chance on a forced choice memory test can be interpreted as the deliberate production of wrong answers. Such a result may not distinguish between malingering and conversion reactions (Binder, 1990). If a patient is suspected of malingering, the clinician should actively search for other clues, such as antisocial or borderline personality, poor work record, prior claims for injury, random test performance, and excessive endorsement of symptoms (Ruff and Willie, 1993).

Table 16–4 DSM Posttraumatic Stress Disorder.

Person exposed to traumatic event
Traumatic event persistently reexperienced
Persistent avoidance of stimuli associated with trauma and numbing of general responsiveness
Persistent symptoms of increased arousal
Duration of the disturbance is more than 1 month
Disturbance causes clinically significant distress or impairment in social, occupational, or other important areas of functioning

Source: Abstracted from *Diagnostic and Statistical Manual IV* (American Psychiatric Association, 1994).

TREATMENT

Patients with postconcussion syndrome are often distressed and misunderstood, and they require an objective and comprehensive treatment approach. Treating them inappropriately may create pathologic resentment and disability that is refractory to treatment. The comprehensive approach to treatment utilizes medications, physical modalities, and biofeedback or counseling. Medina (1992) found that 85% of patients had returned to work after being treated aggressively in individualized programs that included medication, biofeedback, stress management, exercise, and neuromuscular relaxation.

In the absence of any known remediable mechanism, treatment should be directed at the identifiable components of postconcussion syndrome. Headache is treated as if it had arisen as a primary headache disorder. Cervical and soft tissue injury should be identified and treated. Anxiety and depression should be meticulously identified and addressed. Cognitive dysfunction should also be addressed.

Few studies have evaluated specific drug treatments for PCH and few have looked at which headache responds to which drugs. Most have involved the use of the antidepressant, amitriptyline. In an uncontrolled study, Tyler et al. (1980) found amitriptyline effective in 90% of PCH patients, not distinguishing between various headache patterns of PCH. The dose of amitriptyline varied from 75 to 250 mg. Saran (1988) used amitriptyline in two groups of psychiatrically hospitalized patients with depression, one with PCH, the other with idiopathic headaches. Outcome was based on average daily headache intensity calculated from a headache calendar. Amitriptyline, at an average dose of 175 mg a day, was effective for the uninjured patients but not for the postconcussion syndrome patients. This study is likely to have selected a particularly intractable subgroup of postconcussion syndrome patients and may not apply to all patients with PCH. Depression in patients with postconcussion syndrome is relatively resistant to tricyclic antidepressant treatment.

Other antidepressants, including imipramine, doxepin, nortriptyline, selective serotonin reuptake inhibitors, venlafaxine, and mirtazapine may be effective in PCH (unpublished observation). Donepezil is used for the cognitive symptoms of major head injury but it has not been studied after minor head injury or postconcussion syndrome.

Acute medications are widely used for patients with postconcussion syndrome. One must be on the lookout for analgesic and ergotamine overuse. Sumatriptan is effective for the migrainous exacerbation of PCH, but not for the baseline headache (Gawel et al., 1993). Repetitive intravenous dihydroergotamine is effective for PCH that meets the criteria of chronic daily headache (McBeath and Nanda, 1994; Young et al., 1994) and appeared to improve cognitive function in one study (Young et al., 1994). Intravenous chlorpromazine has been effective in acute PCH (Herd and Ludwig, 1994). Patients with daily or near-daily headache should use preventive medications preferentially and limit their use of acute medications.

In the presence of true epilepsy, anticonvulsant therapy is indicated. Divalproex sodium is our drug of first choice if the patient has PCH and a seizure disorder. The many other spells seen in this population rarely respond to anticonvulsant treatment.

Biofeedback and psychotherapy or behavior modification may be helpful for many patients. Biofeedback enables the patient to recognize muscle tension and bring it under voluntary control. A recent study (Ham and Packard, 1996) found that biofeedback enabled 53% of patients to moderately increase their ability to relax and cope with pain, and 80% of patients felt that it was at least moderately helpful.

Occipital nerve blocks may be effective for PCH (Hecht, 2004). Four patients with a Tinel sign over the occipital nerve responded to greater occipital nerve block with pain relief that lasted up to 2 months (Yi et al., 2005).

If a whiplash type of injury has occurred, or if there is significant persistent neck pain with a suggestive physical examination, cervical zygoapophyseal joint pain should be searched for and treated if identified. Lord et al., (1996) found the prevalence of zygoapophyseal joint pain in patients with chronic neck pain after whiplash injury to be 60%. Among patients with whiplash injury who rated their headaches more severe than their neck pain, the incidence of C2-3 zygoapophyseal joint pain (based upon diagnostic blocks) was 50% (Lord et al., 1996). When initially successful, the benefits of radiofrequency neurotomy last an average of 422 days, and repeat procedures are successful (McDonald et al., 1999).

Physical modalities, such as physical therapy and exercise, chiropractic treatment, and massage, have been beneficial for some patients, particularly when headache is related to or occurs in association with cervical trauma. Cold, heat, electrotherapy, and cervical orthoses have been used successfully, particularly in the acute stage, to improve functioning. In one open study, manual therapy was more successful than cold packs in relieving chronic postconcussion syndrome (Jensen et al., 1990). After the initial, acute phase, exercise programs are important to prevent deconditioning with a decrease in the overall level of functioning.

Behavior modification or cognitive therapy is often helpful in providing support and education and improving the patient's ability to cope. Patients with more severe psychopathology may need long-term psychotherapy. Medication may be valuable to treat anxiety and depression. Cognitive retraining exercises, counseling, adaptive strategy programs, and vocational rehabilitation are useful treatments for neurocognitive dysfunction. Alexander (1995) suggests that programs that allege to treat attention and memory problems are of uncertain value in head injury in general and are inappropriate for mild head injury. Cognitive behavioral therapy may be a helpful supplement to the treatment of posttraumatic headache (Gurr and Coetzer, 2005).

OUTCOME

Prognostic studies have used various definitions of head injury, different study designs, and varying subject characteristics. Results have varied, making it difficult to accurately ascertain the prognosis of patients presenting at various stages of postconcussion syndrome. At 1 month after mild head injury, 31% (Munderhoud et al., 1980) to 90% (Denker, 1944) of patients had headache. At 2–3 months postinjury, 32% (Denny-Brown, 1945) to 78% (Rimel et al., 1981b) of patients had headache. One year after injury, the range was 8% (Rutherford et al., 1978) to 35% (Dencker and Lofving, 1958). Two to four years after injury, three studies show that 20%–24% of patients have persistent headache. Dizziness, memory problems, and irritability are less likely to be noted within the first few months of injury but are more likely to persist (Evans, 1994). As in mild head injury, persons with headache after moderate to severe head injuries show a pattern of improvement and then stabilize by 6 months posthospitalization (Walker et al., 2005).

Approximately one-third of patients are unable to return to work after head injury (Rutherford et al., 1978). In one study, 34% of previously employed patients who were admitted to a hospital had not returned to work 3 months after injury. Older patients with higher levels of education and employment, greater income, and higher socioeconomic status were more likely to return to work (Rimel et al., 1981b).

Patients with mild traumatic brain injury have 1.8 times the risk of behavioral discharge from the armed services compared to the total discharge population. Mild and moderate head injury patients have 2.6 and 5.4 times the risk of discharge for alcohol and drug abuse, respectively, compared with the total population (Rimel et al., 1981a). An alternate explanation for these findings could be that the behavioral abnormalities are the risk factor for mild head injury [although previous studies (see risk factors) in other populations have failed to show that behavioral abnormalities have such a strong effect on outcome].

CONCLUSION

Chronic PCH and postconcussion syndrome are common and frequently disabling conditions. There is no specific symptom cluster or reliable diagnostic test to unequivocally establish a diagnosis, however, there are several accepted definitions. The diagnosis is thus most reliably made by establishing the onset of symptoms soon after injury. The absence of a generally accepted mechanism for the genesis of chronic symptoms has led to an unfortunate skepticism about the validity of these symptoms, which has hindered the development of more effective treatments. The search for better treatment should continue; if new treatments can be based on interfering with a putative mechanism of symptom genesis (i.e., windup, kindling, aberrant reinnervation, neurochemical cascade), they may provide insight into the causes of postconcussion syndrome. Relying on "psychogenesis" as the sole explanation of the syndrome feeds into a culture that could be harmful to individuals who have already been injured.

References

Abdel-Dayem, HM, Abu-Judeh, H, Kumar, M, et al. (1998). SPECT brain perfusion abnormalities in mild or moderate traumatic brain injury. *Clin Nucl Med*, 23:309–317.

Abdel-Dayem, HM, Masdeu, J, and O'Connell, R (1994). Brain perfusion abnormalities following minor/moderate closed head injury: comparison between early and late imaging in two groups of patients. *Eur J Nucl Med*, 21:750.

Alavi, A, Fazekas, T, Alves, W, et al. (1987). Positron emission tomography in the evaluation of head injury. *J Cereb Blood Flow Metab*, 7:646.

Alexander, MP (1995). Mild traumatic brain injury: pathophysiology, natural history, and clinical management. *Neurology*, 45:1253.

American Academy of Neurology (1996). Assessment of brain SPECT. Report of the therapeutics and technology assessment subcommittee of the American Academy of Neurology. *Neurology*, 46:278.

American Psychiatric Association (1994). *Diagnostic and Statistical Manual of Mental Disorders*. American Psychiatric Press,Washington.

Andrasik, F and Wincze, JP (1994). Emotional and psychologic aspects of mild head injury. *Semin Neurol*, 14:60.

Barrett, K, Ward, AB, Boughey, A, et al. (1994). Sequelae of minor head injury: the natural consciousness and followup. *J Accid Emerg Med*, 11:79.

Bazarian, JJ, Beck, C, Blyth, B, et al. (2006). Impact of creatine kinase correction on the predictive value of S-100B after mild traumatic brain injury. *Restor Neurol Neurosci*, 24:163–172.

Bazarian, JJ, Wong, T, Harris, M, et al. (1999). Epidemiology and predictors of post-concussive syndrome after minor head injury in an emergency population. *Brain Inj*, 13:173–189.

Benton, AL and Spreen, O (1961). Visual memory test: the simulation of mental incompetence. *Arch Gen Psychiatry*, 4:79.

Berglund, A, Alfredsson, L, Jensen, I, et al. (2001). The association between exposure to a rear-end collision and future health complaints. *J Clin Epidemiol*, 54:851–856.

Binder, LM (1986). Persisting symptoms after mild head injury: a review of the postconcussive syndrome. *J Clin Exp Neuropsychol*, 8:323–346.

Binder, LM (1990). Malingering following minor head trauma. *Clin Neuropsychol*, 4:25.

Blumbergs, PC, Jones, NR, and North, JB (1989). Diffuse axonal injury in head trauma. *J Neurol Neurosurg Psychiatry*, 52:838–841.

Blumbergs, PC, Scott, G, Manavis, J, et al (1994). Staining of amyloid precursor protein to study axonal damage in mild head injury. *Lancet*, 344:1055.

Bohnen, N, Twinjnstra, A, and Jolles, J (1992). Posttraumatic and emotional symptoms in different subgroups of patients with mild head injury. *Brain Inj*, 6:481–487.

Bohnen, NI, Jolles, J, Twijnstra, A, et al. (1995). Late neurobehavioural symptoms after mild head injury. *Brain Inj*, 9:27.

Brenner, C and Friedman, AP (1944). Posttraumatic headache. *J Neurosurg*, 1:379–391.

Bricolo, AP and Turella, GS (1990). Electrophysiology of head injury. In *Handbook of Clinical Neurology* (R Braakman, ed.), pp. 181–206. Elsevier, New York.

Cartlidge, N and Shaw, D (1981). *Head Injury*, (N Cartlidge and D Shaw, eds.), pp. 95–154. WB Saunders, Philadelphia.

Chan, RC (2002). Attentional deficits in patients with persisting postconcussive complaints: a general deficit or specific component deficit? *J Clin Exp Neuropsychol*, 24:1081–1093.

Couch, JR and Bearss, C (2001). Chronic daily headache in the posttraumatic syndrome: relation to extent of head injury. *Headache*, 41:559–564.

Couch, JR, Samuel, S, Leviston, T, et al. (2000). Can head injury by itself produce the syndrome of chronic daily headache. American Headache Society 42nd Annual Scientific Meeting, June 23–25.

Davis, RA and Luxon, LM (1995). Dizziness following head injury: a neurotologic study. *J Neurol*, 242:222.

DeBenedittis, G and DeSantis, A (1983). Chronic posttraumatic headache: clinical, psychopathologic features and outcome determinants. *J Neurosurg Sci*, 27:177.

DeKruijk JR, Leffers P, Menheere PP, Meerhoff S, Rutten J, Twijnstra A (2002). Prediction of post-traumatic complaints after mild traumatic brain injury: early symptoms and biochemical markers. *J Neurol Neurosurg Psychiatry*, 73:727–732.

Dencker, SJ and Lofving, BA (1958). A psychometric study of identical twins discordant for closed head injury. *Acta Psychiatr Neurol Scand*, 122:119–126.

Denker, PG (1944). The postconcussion syndrome: prognosis and evaluation of the organic factors. *NY State J Med*, 44:379–384.

Denny-Brown, D (1945). Disability arising from closed head injury. *JAMA*, 127:429–436.

Duckro, PN, Chibnall, JT, and Tomazic, TJ (1995). Anger, depression, and disability: a path analysis of relationships in a sample of chronic posttraumatic headache patients. *Headache*, 35:7–9.

Eisenberg, HM (1989). CT and MRI finding in mild to moderate head injury. In *Mild Head Injury* (HL Levin, HM Eisenberg, and Benton AL, eds.), p. 133. Oxford University Press, New York.

Elkind, AH (1992). Posttraumatic headache. In *The Practicing Physician's Approach to Headache* (S Diamond and DJ Dalessio, eds.), pp. 146–161. Williams and Wilkins, Baltimore.

Elson, LM and Ward, CC (1994). Mechanisms and pathophysiology of mild head injury. *Seminars Neurol*, 14:8–18.

Erb, DE and Povlishock, JT (1991). Neuroplasticity following traumatic brain injury: a study of GABAergic terminal loss and recovery in the cat dorsal lateral vestibular nucleus. *Exp Brain Res*, 83:253–267.

Evans, RW (1992). The postconcussion syndrome and the sequelae of mild head injury. *Neurol Clin*, 10:815–847.

Evans, RW (1994). The postconcussion syndrome: 130 years of controversy. *Semin Neurol*, 14:32.

Evans, RW (1996). The postconcussion syndrome and the sequelae of mild head injury. In *Neurology and Trauma* (RW Evans, ed.), W.B.Saunders, Philadelphia.

Ewing, R, McCarthy, D, Gronwall, D, et al. (1980). Persisting effects of minor head injury observable during hypoxic stress. *J Clin Neuropsychol*, 2:147.

Fenton, GW (1996). The postconcussional syndrome reappraised. *Clin Electroencephalog*, 27:174–182.

Foreman, S and Croft, A (1995). *Whiplash Injuries: The Cervical Acceleration/Deceleration Syndrome*. Williams & Wilkins, Baltimore.

Gawel, MJ, Rothbart, P, and Jacobs, H (1993). Subcutaneous sumatriptan in the treatment of acute episodes of posttraumatic headache. *Headache*, 33:96–97.

Geets, W and Louette, N (1983). EEG et potentials évoqués du tronc cérébral dans 125 commotions récentes. *Electroencephalogr Neurophysiol Clin*, 13:253.

Gennarelli, TA (1993). Mechanisms of brain injury. *J Emerg Med*, 1:5–11.

Gennarelli, TA, Thibault, LE, Adams, JH, et al. (1975). Diffuse axonal injury and traumatic coma in the primate. In *Trauma of the Central Nervous System* (RG Dacey, et al., eds.), p. 169. Raven, New York.

Gentilini, TM, Michelli, P, and Schoenhuber, R (1989). Assessment of attention in mild head injury. In *Mild Head Injury* (HS Levin, HM Eisenberg, and AL Benton, eds.), p. 163. Oxford University Press, New York.

George, JK, Alavi, Z, Zimmerman, RA, et al. (1989). Metabolic (PET) correlates of anatomic leads (CT/MRI) produced by head trauma. *J Nucl Med*, 30:802 (Abstract).

Gfeller, JD, Chibnall, JT, and Duckro, PN (1994). Postconcussion symptoms and cognitive functioning in posttraumatic headache patients. *Headache*, 34:503–507.

Gilkey, SJ, Ramadan, NM, Aurora, TK, et al. (1997). Cerebral blood flow in chronic posttraumatic headache. *Headache*, 37:583–587.

Goodman, JC (1994). Pathologic changes in mild head injury. *Semin Neurol*, 14:19.

Granovsky, Y, Sprecher, E, Hemli, J, et al. (1998). P300 and stress in mild head injury patients. *Electroencephalogr Clin Neurophysiol*, 108:554–559.

Gray, BG, Ichise, M, and Chung, D (1992). Technetium-99m-HMPAO SPECT in the evaluation of patients with remote history of traumatic brain injury: a comparison with X-ray computed tomography. *J Nucl Med*, 33:52–58.

Gronwall, D and Wrightson, P (1974). Delayed recovery of intellectual function after minor head injury. *Lancet*, 2:605–609.

Gurr, B and Coetzer, BR (2005). The effectiveness of cognitive-behavioral therapy for post-traumatic headaches. *Brain Inj*, 19:481–491.

Haas, DC (1995). Classification of chronic posttraumatic headache. *Cephalalgia*, 15:162.

Haas, DC and Lourie, T (1988). Trauma-triggered migraine: an explanation for common neurologic attacks after mild head injury. *Neurosurg*, 68:181–188.

Ham, LP, Andrasik, F, Packard, RC, et al. (1994). Psychopathology in individuals with posttraumatic headaches and other pain types. *Cephalalgia*, 14:118.

Ham, LP and Packard, RC (1996). A retrospective, follow-up study of biofeedback-assisted relaxation therapy in patients with posttraumatic headache. *Biofeedback and Self Regul*, 21:93–104.

Headache Classification Committee (2004). The International Classification of Headache Disorders, 2nd Edition. *Cephalalgia*, 24:1–160.

Heaton, RK, Smith, HH, Lehman, RA, et al. (1978). Prospects for faking believable deficits on neuropsychologic testing. *J Consult Clin Psychol*, 46:892.

Hecht, JS (2004). Occipital nerve blocks in postconcussive headaches: a retrospective review and report of ten patients. *J Head Trauma Rehabil*, 19:58–71.

Herd, A and Ludwig, L (1994). Relief of posttraumatic headache by intravenous chlorpromazine. *J Emerg Med*, 12:849–851.

Herrmann, M, Curio, N, Jost, S, et al. (1999). Protein S-100B and neuron specific enolase as early neurobiochemical markers of the severity of traumatic brain injury. *Restorative Neurol Neurosci*, 14:109–114.

Hickling, EJ, Blanchard, EB, Silverman, DJ, et al. (1992). Motor vehicle accidents, headaches, and posttraumatic stress disorder. *Headache*, 32:147.

Hughes, DG, Jackson, A, Mason, DL, et al. (2004). Abnormalities on magnetic resonance imaging seen acutely following mild traumatic brain injury: correlation with neuropsychological tests and delayed recovery. *Neuroradiology*, 46:550–558.

Hughes, JR and Robbins, LD (1990). Brain mapping in migraine. *Clin Electroencephalog*, 21:14.

Ingebrigtsen, T, Waterloo, K, Jacobsen, EA, et al. (1999). Traumatic brain damage in minor head injury: relation of serum S-100 protein measurements to magnetic resonance imaging and neurobehavioral outcome. *Neurosurg*, 45:468–475.

Iverson, GL (2006). Misdiagnosis of the persistent postconcussion syndrome in patients with depression. *Arch Clin Neuropsychol*, 21:303–310.

Jane, JA, Steward, O, and Gennarelli, TA (1985). Axonal degeneration induced by experimental noninvasive minor head injury. *J Neurosurg*, 62:96.

Jensen, OK and Nielson, FF (1990). The influence of sex and pretraumatic headache on the incidence and severity of headache after injury. *Cephalalgia*, 10:285–293.

Jensen, OK, Nielsen, FF, and Vosmar, L (1990). An open study comparing manual therapy with the use of cold packs in the treatment of posttraumatic headache. *Cephalalgia*, 10:241–250.

Junger, EC, Newell, DW, Grant, GA, et al. (1997). Cerebral autoregulation following minor head injury. *J Neurosurg*, 86:425–432.

Keidel, M, Yaguez, L, Wilhelm, H, et al. (1992). Prospective followup of neuropsychologic deficiency after cervicocephalic acceleration trauma. *Neurologische Klinik and Poliklinik, Universitat Essen Nervenarzt*, 63:731.

Kelly, R (1988). Headache after cranial trauma. In *Headache: Problems in Diagnosis and Management* (A Hopkins, ed.), p. 219. Saunders, London.

Keshavan, MS, Channabasavanna, SM, and Reddy, GN (1981). Posttraumatic psychiatric disturbances: patterns and predictors of outcome. *Br J Psychiatry*, 138:157–160.

Kim, SH, Manes, F, Kosier, T, et al. (1999). Irritability following traumatic brain injury. *J Nerv Mental Dis*, 187:327–335.

Kobylare, EJ, Dunford, J, Jabbari, B, et al. (1995). Auditory event-related potentials in head injury patients. *Neurology*, 45:358.

Korn, A, Golan, H, Melamed, I, et al. (2005). Focal cortical dysfunction and blood-brain barrier disruption in patients with Postconcussion syndrome. *J Clin Neurophysiol*, 22:1–9.

Kraus, JF, McArthur, DL, and Silberman, TA (1994). Epidemiology of mild brain injury. *Seminars Neurol*, 14:1–7.

Krelina, M, Reid, R, and Ballinger, J (1989). Regional cerebral blood flow in patients with remote close-head injuries. *Can J Neurol Sci*, 2:279 (Abstract).

Lake, AE, Branca, B, Lutz, T, et al. (1995). Comorbid symptoms in chronic posttraumatic headache. I: comparison to intractable migraine. II: relationship to severity of injury and litigation. *Headache*, 35:302 (Abstract).

Lankford, DA, Wellman, JJ, and O'Hara, C (1994). Posttraumatic narcolepsy in mild to moderate closed head injury. *Sleep*, 17:S25–S28.

Levin, HS, Amparo, E, and Eisenberg, HM (1987). Magnetic resonance imaging and computerized tomography in relation to the neurobehavioral sequelae of mild and moderate head injuries. *J Neurosurg*, 66:706–713.

Levin, HS, Williams, DH, Eisenberg, HM, et al. (1992). Serial MRI and neurobehavioral findings after mild to moderate head injuries. *J Neurol Neurosurg Psychiatry*, 55:255.

Lidvall, HF, Linderoth, B, and Norlin, B (1974). Causes of the postconcussional syndrome. *Acta Neurol Scand*, 40:1–143.

Lord, SM, Barnsley, L, Wallis, BJ, et al. (1996). Chronic cervical zygoapophyseal joint pain after whiplash: a placebo-controlled prevalence study. *Spine*, 21:1737–1744.

Machado, EB, Michet, CJ, Ballard, DJ, et al. (1988). Trends in incidence and clinical presentation of temporal arteritis in Olmsted County, Minnesota, 1958–1985. *Arthritis Rheum*, 31:745–749.

Mallinson, AI and Longridge, NS (1998). Dizziness from whiplash and head injury: differences between whiplash and head injury. *Am J Otol*, 19:814–818.

Mandel, S (1989). Minor head injury may not be "minor". *Postgrad Med J*, 85:213–215.

Masdeu, JC, Abdel-Dayhem, H, and VanHeertum, RL (1995). Head trauma: use of SPECT. *J Neuroimag*, 5:53.

McBeath, JG and Nanda, A (1994). Use of dihydroergotamine in patients with postconcussion syndrome. *Headache*, 34:148–151.

McCarthy, D. (1977). *Memory and Vigilance after Concussion*. University of Auckland, Auckland.

McClelland, RJ, Fenton, GW, and Rutherford, W (1994). The postconcussional syndrome revisited. *J R Soc Med*, 87:508–510.

McDonald, GJ, Lord, SM, and Bogduk, N (1999). Long-term followup of patients treated with cervical radiofrequency neurotomy for chronic neck pain. *Neurosurgery*, 45:61.

Medina, JL (1992). Efficacy of an individualized outpatient program in the treatment of chronic posttraumatic headache. *Headache*, 32:180–183.

Mendelson, G (1982). Not "cured by a verdict". *Med J Aust*, 2:132–134.

Miller, H (1961a). Accident neurosis: lecture I. *BMJ*, 1:918.

Miller, H (1961b). Accident neurosis: Lecture II. *BMJ*, 1:992.

Mittenberg, W, DiGiulio, D, Perrin, S, et al. (1992). Symptoms following mild head injury: expectation as etiology. *J Neurol Neurosurg Psychiatry*, 55:200.

Mittle, RL, Grossman, RI, Hiehl, JF, et al. (1994). Prevalence of MR evidence of diffuse axonal injury in patients with mild head injury and normal head Ct findings. *Am J Neuroradiol*, 15:1583.

Montalbetti, L, Ferrandi, D, Pergami, P, et al. (1995). Elongated styloid process and Eagle's syndrome. *Cephalalgia*, 15:80.

Munderhoud, JM, Boclens, ME, and Huizenga, J (1980). Treatment of minor head injuries. *Clin Neurol Neurosurg*, 82:127–140.

Newton, MR, Greenwood, RJ, Britton, KF, et al. (1992). A study comparing SPECT with CT and MRI after closed head injury. *J Neurol Neurosurg Psychiatry*, 55:92.

O'Neill, B, Haddon, W, Kelley, AB, et al. (1972). Automobile head restraints: frequency of neck claims in relation to the presence of head restraints. *Am J Public Health*, 62:403.

Obelieniene, D, Bovim, G, Schrader, H, et al. (1998). Headache after whiplash: a historical cohort study outside the medicolegal context. *Cephalalgia*, 18:559–564.

Packard, RC (1992). Posttraumatic headache: permanency and relationship to legal settlement. *Headache*, 32:496–500.

Packard, RC (1999). Epidemiology and pathogenesis of posttraumatic headache. *J Head Trauma Rehabil*, 14:9–21.

Packard, RC and Ham, LP (1993). Posttraumatic headache: determining chronicity. *Headache*, 33:133–134.

Packard, RC and Ham, LP (1996). Incidence of cluster-like posttraumatic headache: an inconsistency. *Headache Q*, 7:139.

Packard, RC and Ham, LP (1997). Pathogenesis of posttraumatic headaches and migraine: a common headache pathway? *Headache*, 37:142–152.

Post, RM and Silberstein, SD (1994). Shared mechanisms in affective illness, epilepsy, and migraine. *Neurology*, 44:S37–S47.

Povlishock, JT and Coburn, TH (1989). Morphopathologic change associated with mild head injury. In *Mild Head Injury* (HS Levin, HM Eisenberg, and AL Benton, eds.), Chapter 4, pp. 37–53, Oxford University Press, New York.

Pratap-Chand, R, Sinniah, M, and Salem, FA (1988). Cognitive evoked potential (P300): a metric for cerebral concussion. *Acta Neurol Scand*, 78:185.

Prigatano, GP, Stahl, ML, Orr, WC, et al. (1982). Sleep and dreaming disturbances in closed head injury patients. *J Neurol Neurosurg Psychiatry*, 45:78.

Radanov, BP, Sturzeneger, M, and DiStefano, G (1995). Long-term outcome after whiplash injury: a 2-year followup considering features of injury mechanism and somatic, radiologic, and psychosocial findings. *Medicine*, 74:281.

Ramadan, NM, Norris, LL, and Shultz, LR (1995). Abnormal cerebral flood flow correlates with disability to chronic posttraumatic headache. *J Neuroimaging*, 5:68 (Abstract).

Ramadan, NM, Schultz, LL, and Gilkey, SJ (1997). Migraine prophylactic drugs: proof of efficacy, utilization, and cost. *Cephalalgia*, 17:73–80.

Rao, N, Turski, PA, Polcyn, RE, et al. (1984). ^{18}F Positron emission computed tomography in closed head injury. *Arch Phys Med Rehab*, 65:780.

Rimel, RW, Giordani, B, Barth, JT, et al. (1981a). Disability caused by minor head injury. *Neurosurgery*, 9:221–228.

Rimel, RW, Giordani, B, Barth, JT, et al. (1981b). Disability caused by minor head injury. *Neurosurgery*, 9:221–228.

Rizzo, M and Tranel, D (1996). *Head Injury and Postconcussion Syndrome*. Churchill Livingstone, New York.

Rowe, MJ and Carlson, C (1980). Brainstem auditory evoked potentials in postconcussion dizziness. *Arch Neurol*, 37:679.

Ruff, MR and Willie, T (1993). Malingering and malingering-like aspects of mild closed head injury. *J Head Trauma Rehab*, 8:60.

Rutherford, WH (1989). Postconcussion symptoms. In *Mild Head Injury* (HS Levin, HM Eisenberg, AZ Beriton, eds.), p. 217. Oxford University Press, New York.

Rutherford, WH, Merrett, JD, and McDonald, JR (1977). Sequelae of concussion caused by minor head injuries. *Lancet*, 1:1–4.

Rutherford, WH, Merrett, JD, and McDonald, JR (1978). Symptoms of one year following concussion from minor head injuries. *Injury*, 10:225–230.

Rutland-Brown, W, Langlois, JA, Thomas, KE, et al. (2006). Incidence of traumatic brain injury in the United States, 2003. *J Head Trauma Rehabil*, 21:544–548.

Saper, JR (1983). *Headache Disorders: Current Concepts in Treatment Strategies*. Wright-PSG, Littleton.

Saran, A (1988). Antidepressants not effective in headache associated with minor closed head injury. *Int J Psychiatry Med*, 18:75–83.

Sbordone, RJ and Liter, JC (1995). Mild traumatic brain injury does not produce posttraumatic stress disorder. *Brain Inj*, 9:405.

Scher, AI, Lipton, RB, and Stewart, W (2002). Risk factors for chronic daily headache. *Cur Pain Headache Rep*, 6:486–491.

Schmidt, RH and Grady, MS (1995). Loss of forebrain cholinergic neurons following fluid-percussion injury: implications for cognitive impairment in closed head injury. *J Neurosurg*, 83:496.

Schoenhuber, R and Gentilini, M (1989). Neurophysiologic assessment of mild head injury. In *Mild Head Injury* (HS Levin, HM Eisenberg, and AL Benton, eds.), p. 142–150. Oxford University Press, New York.

Segalowitz, SJ and Lawson, S (1995). Subtle symptoms associated with self-reported mild head injury. *J Learn Disabil*, 28:309.

Servadei, P, Vergoni, G, Pasini, A, et al. (1994). Diffuse axonal injury with brainstem localization: report of a case in a mild head injured patient. *J Neurosurg Sci*, 38:129.

Silberstein, SD, Lipton, RB, Saper, JR, et al. (1995). Headache and facial pain: part A. *Continuum*, 1:8.

Silberstein, SD and Marcelis, J (1990). Pseudotumor cerebri without papilledema. *Headache*, 30:304.

Sturzenegger, M (1991). Ultrasound findings in spontaneous carotid artery dissection. *Arch Neurol*, 48:1057–1063.

Suhr, JA and Gunstad, J (2002). Postconcussive symptom report: the relative influence of head injury and depression. *J Clin Exp Neuropsychol*, 24:981–993.

Thatcher, RW, Walker, RA, Gerson, I, et al. (1989). EEG discriminate analyses of mild head trauma. *Electroencephalogr Clin Neurophysiol*, 73:94–106.

Toglia, JU (1969). Dizziness after whiplash injury of the neck and closed head injury. In *The Late Effects of Head Injury* (WF Walker, WF Caveness, and M Critchley, eds.), p. 72. Thomas, Springfield.

Treleaven, J, Jull, G, and Atkinson, L (1994). Cervical musculoskeletal dysfunction in postconcussional headache. *Cephalalgia*, 14:273–279.

Tyler, GS, McNeely, HE, and Dick, ML (1980). Treatment of posttraumatic headache with amitriptyline. *Headache*, 20:213.

van der, NJ, van Zomeren, AH, Sluiter, WJ, et al. (1999). One year outcome in mild to moderate head injury: the predictive value of acute injury characteristics related to complaints and return to work. *J Neurol Neurosurg Psychiatry*, 66:207–213.

Varney, NR and Bushnell, D (1998). NeuroSPECT findings in patients with posttraumatic anosmia: a quantitative analysis. *J Head Trauma Rehabil*, 13:63–72.

Vijayan, N (1977). A new posttraumatic headache syndrome. *Headache*, 17:19–22.

Walker, WC, Seel, RT, Curtiss, G, et al. (2005). Headache after moderate and severe traumatic brain injury: a longitudinal analysis. *Arch Phys Med Rehabil*, 86:1793–1800.

Wang, Y, Chan, RC, and Deng, Y (2006). Examination of postconcussion-like symptoms in healthy university students: relationships to subjective and objective neuropsychological function performance. *Arch Clin Neuropsychol*, 21:339–347.

Ward, CC (1982). Finite element modeling of the head and neck. In *Impact Injury of the Head and Spine* (R Ewing, et al., eds.), p. 421. Thomas, Springfield.

Weiller, C, May, A, Limmroth, V, et al. (1995). Brainstem activation in spontaneous human migraine attacks. *Nat Med*, 1:658–660.

Weiss, HD, Stern, BJ, and Goldbert, J (1991). Posttraumatic migraine: chronic migraine precipitated by minor head or neck trauma. *Headache*, 31:451–456.

Werner, RA and Vanderzant, CW (1991). Multimodality evoked potential testing in acute mild closed head injury. *Arch Phys Med Rehabil*, 72:31.

Wilkinson, M and Gilchrist, E (1980). Posttraumatic headache. *Ups J Med Sci*, 31:48.

Wong, E, Lee, G, and Mason, DT (1995). Temporal headaches and associated symptoms relating to the styloid process and its attachments. *Ann Acad Med*, 24:124.

Yamaguchi, M (1992). Incidence of headache and severity of head injury. *Headache*, 32:422.

Yi, X, Cook, AJ, Hamill-Ruth, RJ, et al. (2005). Cervicogenic headache in patients with presumed migraine: missed diagnosis or misdiagnosis? *J Pain*, 6:700–703.

Young, WB, Hopkins, MM, Janyszek, B, et al. (1994). Repetitive intravenous DHE in the treatment of refractory posttraumatic headache. *Headache*, 34:297 (Abstract).

17 Headache Associated with Vascular Disorders

Hans-Christoph Diener and David W Dodick

INTRODUCTION

Many vascular disorders of the brain present with headache as the leading or an important symptom. Headache in vascular conditions presents acutely and with neurological signs and symptoms. The temporal relationship between the onset of headache and neurological symptoms and signs helps to make the correct diagnosis.

In most vascular disorders such as ischemic or hemorrhagic stroke, headache is overshadowed by focal signs or overlooked because of disorders of consciousness. In conditions such as subarachnoid hemorrhage (SAH) or arteritis, headache is usually the most prominent symptom. In a number of other diseases that may lead to both headache and stroke [dissection, cerebral venous thrombosis (CVT), and temporal arteritis] headache is often an initial warning symptom. It is therefore crucial to recognise the association of headache with these vascular disorders to initiate appropriate treatment.

Headache because of vascular disorders can occur in patients who have a prior history of a recurrent primary headache disorder such as migraine. Although tension-type headache is ubiquitous in the general population and secondary headaches may recapitulate the symptoms associated with a patient's prior headaches, including migraine, patients are usually able to differentiate the new headache from prior migraine or tension-type headaches. The headaches associated with vascular disorders is usually hyperacute with an intensity that peaks rapidly, does not respond to conventional analgesics or the patient's usual therapy, persists and progresses in severity, or becomes associated with other neurological signs or symptoms. This chapter describes the different headaches attributed to vascular diseases and follows the International Classification of Headache Disorders revised diagnostic criteria (International Headache Society, 2004).

HEADACHE ATTRIBUTED TO ISCHEMIC STROKE OR TRANSIENT ISCHEMIC ATTACK

Diagnostic criteria according to IHS are:

A. Any new acute headache fulfilling criterion C;
B. Neurological signs and/or neuroimaging evidence of a recent ischemic stroke or transient ischemic attack (TIA);
C. Headache develops simultaneously with or in very close temporal relationship to signs or other evidence of ischemic stroke.

The headache associated with TIAs ischemic stroke is accompanied by focal neurological signs and/or alterations in consciousness. In contrast to migraine aura, neurological symptoms are present within seconds and do not evolve slowly or develop in succession (i.e., visual symptoms followed by sensory symptoms). Headache is usually of moderate intensity and has no specific or defining characteristics (Gorelick et al., 1986; Arboix et al., 1994).

In a large series including patients with both TIAs and cerebral infarctions, Fisher found headache in 31% of patients with internal carotid stenosis or occlusion (proven by pathologic or angiographic examination), independent of whether they had TIAs, a minor stroke, or a major neurological deficit (Fisher, 1968a). In patients with basilar territory infarctions or TIAs, headache was reported in 44% and 35%, respectively. In the Harvard Cooperative Stroke Registry, headache occurred at the onset of the ictus in 9% of patients with cerebral embolism, in 12% of those with large artery thrombosis, and in 3% of patients with lacunar infarcts (Mohr et al., 1978). Headache preceding the ischemic event occurred in 10% of patients with large artery thrombosis, in 5% with embolic infarcts, and in 6% with lacunar infarcts, whereas the figures for headache following the event were 9%, 11%, and 2%, respectively. Edmeads found headache in 25% of prospectively evaluated patients with either TIAs or ischemic infarcts admitted to the stroke unit of a university medical center (Edmeads, 1979). In a large prospective study including 867 patients with ischemic and hemorrhagic stroke, Jorgensen and colleagues indicated that headache occurred in 25% of the patients with ischemic stroke (Jorgensen et al., 1994). It was more frequent when the vertebrobasilar circulation was involved (37%), compared to 26% of the patients who experienced headache in associated with carotid territory ischemia. Predictors of headache in ischemic stroke are infarctions in the distribution of the posterior circulation, absence of history of hypertension, female sex, history of migraine, and younger age (Tentschert et al., 2005; Mitsias et al., 2006).

Although more common with basilar- than carotid-territory TIA, headache is very rarely a prominent symptom of TIA. The differential diagnosis between TIA with headache and an attack of migraine with aura may be particularly difficult. The mode of onset is crucial: the focal deficit is typically sudden in a TIA and more frequently evolves over 15–60 minutes in an aura. Furthermore, positive phenomena (fortifications) are far more common in migrainous aura than in TIA whereas negative phenomena are more usual in TIA (Fisher, 1968b). In addition, different aura symptoms (visual, sensory, and language) may occur sequentially as opposed to TIA where all symptoms occur simultaneously. Headache in patients with ischemic stroke can be treated with acetaminophen, which does not interact with the coagulation system.

Headache evolving after systemic or local thrombolysis is suggestive of a hemorrhagic complication. In these cases, immediate brain computed tomography (CT) is required. Delayed headache in patients with TIA or stroke may be caused by the intake of dipyridamole used for secondary stroke prevention (Diener et al., 1996; Theis et al., 1999; Lindgren et al., 2004). Patients with preexisting migraine are more likely to develop dipyridamole-induced headache than nonmigraneurs (Kruuse et al., 2006). The headache usually resolves within a few days, although in some instances the headache persists and the medication must be discontinued. It can be partially avoided by starting with half of the usual dose (Chang et al., 2006).

HEADACHE ATTRIBUTED TO NON-TRAUMATIC INTRACRANIAL HEMORRHAGE

Headache Attributed to Intracerebral Hemorrhage

Diagnostic criteria:

A. Any new acute headache fulfilling criterion C;
B. Neurological signs or neuroimaging evidence of recent nontraumatic intracerebral hemorrhage;
C. Headache develops simultaneously with or in very close temporal relation to intracerebral hemorrhage.

Headache is more frequent and more severe in hemorrhagic than ischemic stroke (Gorelick et al., 1986). It is usually overshadowed by focal neurological deficits or a decrease in the level of consciousness. Headache can be the only symptom in cerebellar hemorrhage. Headache is present in 70% of cerebral hemorrhages (Caplan, 1988). Headache attributed to intracerebral hemorrhage is more often because of associated subarachnoid blood and to local compression than to intracranial hypertension (Melo et al., 1996). Headache in intracerebral hemorrhage can present as thunderclap headache (Dodick, 2002; Schwedt et al., 2006).

Headache Attributed to SAH

Diagnostic criteria:

A. Severe headache of sudden onset fulfilling criteria C and D;

B. Neuroimaging [CT or MRI (magnetic resonance imaging) T2or fluid attenuated inversion recovery (FLAIR)] or cerebrospinal fluid (CSF) evidence of non-traumatic SAH with or without other clinical signs;
C. Headache develops simultaneously with hemorrhage;
D. Headache resolves within 1 month.

SAH is by far the most common cause of severe and incapacitating headache of abrupt onset (thunderclap headache) and any patient with headache of abrupt onset or thunderclap headache should be evaluated for SAH (van Gijn, 1992). However, it may be less severe and without associated signs and in 70% of cases occurs in isolation (Linn et al., 1994). A prospective hospital-based study of sudden onset headache by Landtblom and colleagues showed that 11% of patients had SAH whereas in a community-based prospective study of 148 patients with sudden onset headache, Linn and colleagues reported that 37 (25%) had SAH (Linn et al., 1994; Landtblom et al., 2002). The most common cause (85%) of SAH is rupture of an intracranial aneurysm. Approximately 10% of nonaneurysmal SAH is because of perimesenphalic (pretruncal) SAH, which invariably is associated with a very favorable prognosis. Less common causes of SAH include trauma, transmural arterial dissection, arteriovenous malformations (AVMs), dural arteriovenous fistula, mycotic aneurysm, and cocaine abuse.

The headache of SAH is often associated with nuchal rigidity and accompanied by nausea, vomiting, disturbances of consciousness (Linn et al., 1998). Loss of consciousness occurs in a third of patients with SAH (Blousse et al., 1992; Afridi and Goadsby, 2003). Other associated symptoms include seizures (6%–9%), delirium (16%), stroke (caused by intracerebral hematoma), visual disturbances (because of intraocular hemorrhage), nausea, vomiting, dizziness, neck stiffness, and photophobia (Calabrese et al., 1992; Calabrese, 2001; Brown et al., 2005). The abrupt onset of headache in temporal relationship with physical activity or sexual intercourse is a key feature, though exertion and intercourse may be associated with benign primary headache disorders and the headache associated with SAH can occur during rest (Pascual et al., 1996; Landtblom et al., 2002). The headache usually persists for days and it is rare to resolve within 2 hours.

SAH is a serious condition with 50% mortality and despite advances in imaging and treatment, 10% of patients die before reaching a hospital, one third of survivors remain dependent, and 25%–50% are initially misdiagnosed (Edlow and Caplan, 2000). In patients who present with headache as the only symptom, physical findings may be subtle. Neck stiffness and subhyaloid retinal hemorrhages may be present in up to 25% of patients, but patients often guard against movement of their head because of the intensity of the pain and fundoscopic examination may be difficult because of photophobia.

Diagnosis is confirmed by CT scan without contrast or MRI (FLAIR sequences) that have a sensitivity of more than 98% in the first 24 hours. The sensitivity of CT scanning declines with time, falling to 50% within 1 week. Therefore, imaging should be done as soon as possible after the onset of symptoms (Morgenstern et al., 1998). FLAIR MRI sequences have superior sensitivity compared to CT scanning between 3–40 days after the ictus. If imaging is negative, equivocal or technically inadequate, a lumbar puncture must be performed (Sidman et al., 1996). In addition to routine assessment of cell counts, protein, glucose, and visual inspection for xanthochromia, analysis by spectrophotometry should also be done if available. Spectrophotometry is more sensitive after the first 12 hours of hemorrhage with a sensitivity of more than 95% that persists for up to 2 weeks after SAH (Vermeulen et al., 1989). All patients with SAH should undergo conventional angiography in search of a ruptured aneurysm.

SAH is an emergency and requires immediate hospitalisation in a hospital equipped with an intensive care unit, neurosurgery, neurology and interventional neuroradiology. Headache in SAH is treated with acetaminophen or codeine. In refractory cases, opioids can be used. The dose should however not compromise the evaluation of the patient's level of consciousness. The presence of severe sudden headache referred as sentinel headache before SAH indicates a group of patients with a very high risk of early rebleeding (Beck et al., 2006).

HEADACHE ATTRIBUTED TO UNRUPTURED VASCULAR MALFORMATION

Headache Attributed to Saccular Aneurysm

Diagnostic criteria:

A. Any new acute headache including thunderclap headache and/or painful third nerve palsy fulfilling criteria C and D;
B. Neuroimaging evidence of saccular aneurysm;
C. Evidence exists of causation by the saccular aneurysm;
D. Headache resolves within 72 hours;
E. SAH, intracerebral hemorrhage and other causes of headache ruled out by appropriate investigations.

The prevalence of unruptured cerebral aneurysms varies from 0.4% to 6.0% depending on the method of diction. In a systematic review of 23 studies involving 56,304 patients, the prevalence of intracranial aneurysms was between 0.4% and 3.6% on retrospective and prospective autopsy studies, respectively whereas in retrospective and prospective angiography studies, the prevalence was between 3.7% and 6.0%, respectively (Rinkel, 1998). Headache is reported by approximately 20% of patients with unruptured cerebral aneurysm (Raps et al., 1993, Weir, 2002). However, based on the prevalence of aneurysms in the general population, the headache and aneurysm may be unrelated—the aneurysm may be entirely coincidental, and this applies to patients who present with thunderclap headache without SAH present on CT or within CSF (Day and Raskin, 1986; Dodick, 2002). The differentiation between an unrelated sudden severe headache and a "sentinel" headache may however be very difficult. Sentinel headaches, which occur in up to 43% of patients who suffer a SAH within days or weeks, are most likely because of a minor leak of blood into the subarachnoid space and are frequently overlooked or misdiagnosed because patients do not seek medical attention or if they do, there is no abnormality on neurological examination (Polmear, 2003).

Headache occurrence depends on the size and the location of the aneurysm and lacks distinguishing or specific features. However, a classic warning sign (signalling impending rupture or progressive enlargement) is headache concomitant with acute third nerve palsy with retro-orbital pain and a dilated pupil, indicating an aneurysm of the posterior communicating cerebral artery distal carotid artery (Fig. 17–1). The prognosis depends on the size of the aneurysm. The rupture rate is 0.05% per year in aneurysms less than 10 m and 1% per year for aneurysms more than 10 mm (Wiebers et al., 2003). The guiding principle should be that any patient with a sudden and severe headache (thunderclap headache) should prompt appropriate noninvasive investigations [Magnetic resonance angiography (MRA) or CT angiography], even in the absence of SAH, and if the index of suspicion is high or the noninvasive images are technically inadequate, conventional angiography should be performed.

Headache Attributed to AVM

Diagnostic criteria:

A. Any new acute headache fulfilling criteria C and D;
B. Neuroimaging evidence of AVM;
C. Evidence exists of causation by the AVM;
D. Headache resolves within 72 hours;
E. SAH, intracerebral hemorrhage and other causes of headache ruled out by appropriate investigations.

The prevalence of headache in AVMs is 15 % (Brown et al., 2005). A few cases have been reported on the association of AVM with headaches such as cluster headache (Mani and Deeter, 1982; Hindfelt Olivecrona, 1991; Muoz et al., 1996), chronic paroxysmal hemicrania (CPH) and short-lasting unilateral neuralgiform headache with conjunctival injection and tearing (SUNCT). Most of these cases had atypical features. There is no good evidence of a relationship between AVM and these primary headaches when they are typical.

Migraine with aura has been reported in up to 58% of women with AVM. A strong argument in favor of a causal relationship is the overwhelming correlation between the side of the headache or of the aura and the side of the AVM. AVMs may cause attacks of migraine with aura (symptomatic

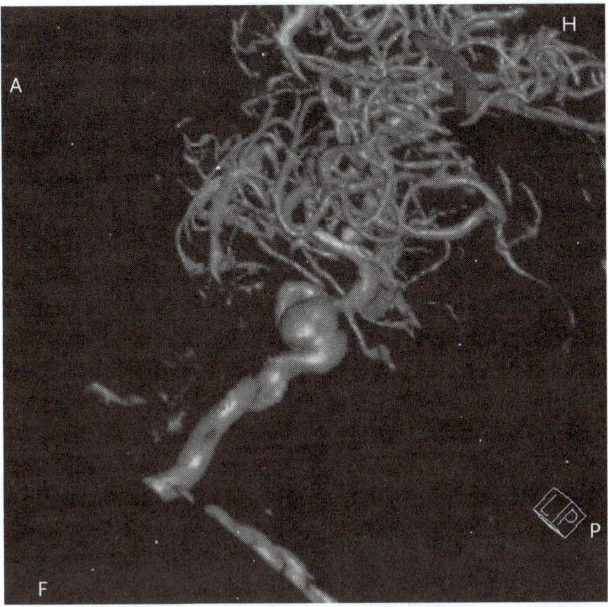

Figure 17–1 Unruptured aneurysm causing headache. Forty-two-year-old woman presents with mild left retro-orbital headache that progresses over 24 hours (10/10 pain intensity) and diplopia because of a partial left third nerve palsy. Computed tomography (CT) and cerebrospinal fluid (CSF) normal but angiogram demonstrates 11 cm cavernous carotid aneurysm.

migraine). Yet in large AVM series, migraine as a presenting symptom is rare, much less common than hemorrhage, epilepsy, or focal deficits.

Headache Attributed to Dural Arterio-Venous Fistula

Diagnostic criteria:

A. Any new acute headache fulfilling criterion C;
B. Neuroimaging evidence of dural arteriovenous fistula;
C. Evidence exists of causation by the fistula;
D. SAH, intracerebral hemorrhage and other causes of headache ruled out by appropriate investigations.

There are no prospective studies on headache with dural arteriovenous fistula. The most common symptom is pulsatile tinnitus (Chung et al., 2002). Headache may occur with complications of the fistula such as cerebral venous sinus thrombosis or hemorrhage with other signs of intracranial hypertension. Internal and external carotid-cavernous fistulae lead to painful ophthalmoplegia.

Headache Attributed to Cavernous Angioma

Diagnostic criteria:

A. Any new acute headache fulfilling criterion C;
B. Neuroimaging evidence of cavernous angioma;
C. Evidence exists of causation by the cavernous angioma;
D. SAH, intracerebral hemorrhage and other causes of headache ruled out by appropriate investigations.

Cavernous malformations are circumscribed lesions that consist of packed, enlarged, capillary-like vessels without intervening brain parenchyma. They are angiograpically "occult." Clinical presentations range from asymptomatic lesions discovered incidentally on neuroimaging (MRI), seizures, and hemorrhage (Fig. 17–2). There is no good study devoted to headache associated with these malformations. Headache has been demonstrated as the only complaint in up to 30%

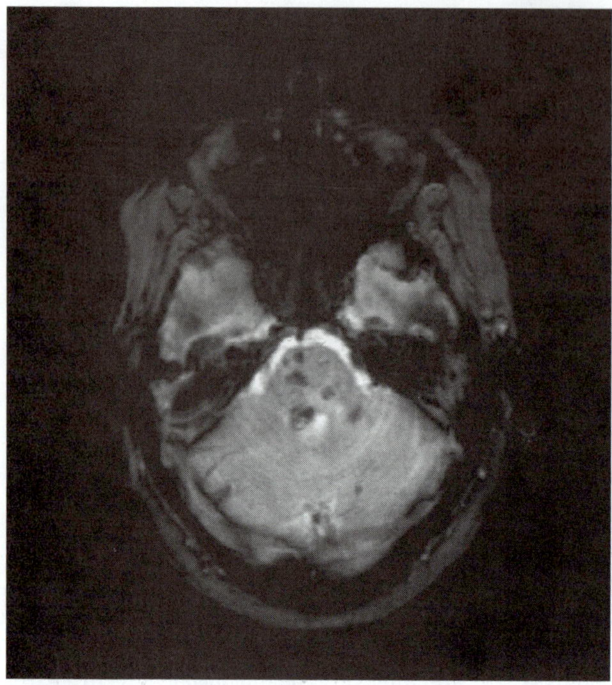

Figure 17–2 Cavernous malformations in the brainstem in a 56-year-old patient presenting with new onset migraine.

of cases (Simard et al., 1986; Robinson et al., 1991). In other studies, up to 44% of patients harboring single or multiple lesions had no symptoms. Recently, two cases of brainstem cavernous malformations presenting as migraine were described (Afridi and Goadsby, 2003; Katsarava et al., 2003). Headache is otherwise reported as a consequence of cerebral hemorrhage because of cavernous angioma.

HEADACHE ATTRIBUTED TO ARTERITIS

Headache Attributed to Giant Cell Arteritis

Diagnostic criteria:

A. Any new persisting headache fulfilling criteria C and D;
B. At least one of the following:
   1. Swollen tender scalp artery with elevated erythrocyte sedimentation rate (ESR) and/or C-reactive protein (CRP);
   2. Temporal artery biopsy demonstrating giant cell arteritis (GCA).
C. Headache develops in close temporal relation to other symptoms and signs of GCA;
D. Headache resolves or greatly improves within 3 days of high-dose steroid treatment.

GCA, formally called temporal arteritis or Horton's disease, usually presents with headache as the most prominent symptom (Murray, 1977; Huston et al., 1978; Ward et al., 2004; Ward and Levin, 2005). The incidence of GCA is between 8 and 36/1,00,000 per year with a female preponderance of 3:1 (Machado et al., 1988; Baldursson et al., 1994). New headache or change in pattern of a long-standing primary headache in any patient older than 50 years is suggestive of GCA (Solomon and Cappa, 1987). The headache may occur in any location and is not necessarily present in or confined to the temporal regions, despite its name and involvement of the temporal artery. The pattern may be intermittent or constant and may mimic many common primary headache disorders such as migraine without aura, tension-type headache. Even scintillations may occur from retinal ischemia and be mistaken for aura (Caselli et al, 1988; Campbell and Caselli, 1991; Ward et. al., 2005). Temporal or occipital artery tenderness is invariably present but may be absent in up to one third of patients. More typical than any headache feature is the associated symptoms that accompany the headache. Jaw claudication is highly characteristic and occurs in 40% of patients. Tongue claudication is also associated with GCA occurring in 4% of patients. Scalp sensitivity, ameurosis, polymyalgia, are also features which should be elicited to support the diagnosis. About half of the patients have symptoms of polymyalgia rheumatica (Hamilton et al., 1971). Untreated GCA may lead to visual loss, either as an early symptom or following repeated attacks of amaurosis fugax. In addition to the clinical picture increased ESR and CRP are indicative. The ESR is elevated in approximately 97% of patients with GCA and CRP may be even more sensitive and has become increasingly used to monitor disease activity (Campbell and Caselli, 1991). Other common laboratory abnormalities include a normochromic microcytic anemia, thrombocytosis, and elevations of plasma a-2 globulins. Temporal artery biopsy is suggested.

Headache responds usually within 24–48 hours to treatment with prednisone in doses between 40 and 80 mg/day. In most patients long term is necessary to prevent visual loss (see Chapter 26 for details).

Headache Attributed to Primary Central Nervous System Angiitis

Diagnostic criteria:

A. Any new persisting headache fulfilling criteria D and E;
B. Encephalic signs of any type (e.g., stroke, seizures, disorders of cognition or consciousness);
C. Central nervous system (CNS) angiitis proven by cerebral or meningeal biopsy or suspected on angiographic signs in the absence of systemic arteritis;
D. Headache develops in close temporal relation to encephalic signs;
E. Headache improves within 1 month of steroid and/or immunosuppressive treatment.

Primary CNS angiitis, also called isolated CNS angiitis or granulomatous CNS angiitis leads to headache in 50%–80% of cases (Moore, 1989). The headache is nonspecific and the diagnosis is only suspected when other signs are present such as focal neurological deficits, seizures, aphasia, altered cognition, memory disturbances, or disorders of consciousness (Calabrese et al., 1992). The absence of both headache and CSF pleocytosis makes CNS angiitis unlikely. The diagnosis is based on clinical symptoms, laboratory changes, CT angiography or MRA, or conventional catheder angiography. In some cases the diagnosis depends on the results of a biopsy of brain and dura (Moore and Richardson, 1998).

The pathogenesis of the headache can be because of the inflammation, stroke (ischemic or hemorrhagic), or SAH. Headache usually improves with treatment of the underlying condition, initially with prednisone, followed by immunosuppressive therapy with cyclophosphamide when required.

CAROTID OR VERTEBRAL ARTERY PAIN

Headache or Facial or Neck Pain Attributed to Arterial Dissection

Diagnostic criteria:

A. Any new headache, facial pain or neck pain of acute onset, with or without other neurological symptoms or signs and fulfilling criteria C and D;
B. Dissection demonstrated by appropriate vascular and/or neuroimaging investigations;
C. Pain develops in close temporal relation to and on the same side as the dissection;
D. Pain resolves within 1 month.

Headache with or without neck pain can be the only manifestation of cervical artery dissection in 15% of cases with carotid or vertebral artery dissection (Biousse et al., 1992). Headache is the most frequent symptom (50%–100% of cases) together with Horner's syndrome or transient and permanent cerebral ischemia (Biousse et al., 1994; Sturzenegger, 1995; Schievink, 2001). Headache and facial pain are usually ipsilateral to the dissected internal carotid artery. Headache and neck pain are typical for vertebral artery dissection. Headache is usually severe and persistent and can mimic migraine (Ramadan et al., 1991), cluster headache (Lai et al., 2005) or thunderclap headache (Schwedt et al., 2006). In vertebral artery dissection the headache and neck pain can be constant or intermittent (de Sousa et al., 2005). Headache usually precedes the onset of TIA or cerebral ischemia and therefore requires early diagnosis and treatment. Diagnosis is based on MRI with axial T1-weighted sections, MRA, Duplex sonography or conventional angiography (Zetterling et al., 2000; Schwedt et al., 2006). Intracranial carotid artery dissection is characterized by severe ipsilateral headache with a high risk of severe stroke or SAH (Ohkuma et al., 2002). Migraine appears to be a risk factor for dissection (Lucas, 2005).

Headache should be treated with drugs that do not produce a procoagulant effect or vasoconstriction, such as ergots or triptans. Treatment options include etaminophen, aspirin, and opioids. Although there is a lack of controlled clinical trials, acute dissection of carotid or vertebral arteries is treated with intravenous heparin followed by oral anticoagulation for 3–6 months (Schievink, 2001; Beletsky et al., 2003). This approach, however, is not evidence based.

Post-endarterectomy Headache

Diagnostic criteria:

A. Acute headache with one of the following sets of characteristics and fulfilling criteria C and D:
   1. diffuse mild pain;
   2. unilateral cluster-like pain occurring once or twice a day in attacks lasting for 2–3 hours;
   3. unilateral pulsating severe pain.

B. Carotid endarterectomy has been performed;

C. Headache, in the absence of dissection, develops within 1 week of surgery;

D. Headache resolves within 1 month after surgery.

Three subforms of headache have been described after carotid endarterectomy. The most frequent (up to 60% of cases) is a diffuse, mild isolated headache occurring in the first few days after surgery. It is a benign self-limited condition. The second type (reported in up to 38% of cases) is a unilateral cluster-like pain with attacks, lasting for 2–3 hours, occurring once or twice a day. It resolves in approximately 2 weeks. The third type is part of the rare hyperperfusion syndrome with a unilateral pulsating and severe pain occurring after an interval of 3 days after surgery. It often precedes a rise in blood pressure and the onset of seizures or neurological deficits on about postoperative day seven. Urgent treatment is required because these symptoms can herald cerebral hemorrhage. Hyperperfusion syndromes can also be observed after angioplasty and stenting (Abou-Chebl et al., 2004).

Carotid or Vertebro-basilar Artery Angioplasty Headache

Diagnostic criteria:

A. Any new acute headache fulfilling criteria C and D;

B. Extracranial or intracranial angioplasty has been performed;

C. Headache, in the absence of dissection, develops during or within a week of angioplasty;

D. Headache resolves within 1 month.

Percutaneous transluminal angioplasty (PTA) and stenting are presently performed in patients not suitable for endarterectomy or in patients with recurrent TIA or minor strokes and intracranial stenosis. Data on headache are still scarce and headache is not mentioned in two recently published randomized trials (Mas et al., 2006; The Space Collaborative Group, 2006). In a small series of 53 patients, cervical pain occurred in 51% of patients and head pain in 33% during balloon inflation. The headache mostly disappeared within seconds of balloon deflation. In another series of intracranial angioplasty in awake patients, headache was the most common adverse event(Abou-Chebl et al., 2006). Headache as part of a hyperperfusion syndrome may also occur after carotid angioplasty and stenting (McCabe et al., 1999).

Headache Attributed to Intracranial Endovascular Procedures

Diagnostic criteria:

A. Unilateral severe localised headache of abrupt onset and fulfilling criteria C and D;

B. Intracranial angioplasty or embolisation has been performed;
C. Headache develops within seconds of the procedure;
D. Headache resolves within 24 hours after the end of the procedure.

A very specific subtype of headache has been reported after balloon inflation or embolisation of an AVM or aneurysm. It is a severe pain of abrupt onset, localised in specific areas according to the artery involved, occurring within a few seconds of the procedure and disappearing rapidly.

Headache Attributed to CVT

Diagnostic criteria:

A. Any new headache, with or without neurological signs, fulfilling criteria C and D;
B. Neuroimaging evidence of CVT;
C. Headache (and neurological signs if present) develops in close temporal relation to CVT;
D. Headache resolves within 1 month after appropriate treatment.

Headache is the most frequent symptom of CVT (present in 80%–90% of cases) and it is also the most frequent initial symptom (Masuhr et al., 2004). The headache associated with CVT has no specific characteristics. Most often it is diffuse, progressive, severe, and associated with other signs of intracranial hypertension such as papilledema, nausea, and vomiting. It can also be unilateral and sudden, and sometimes very misleading, mimicking migraine, primary thunderclap headache, low CSF pressure headache, or SAH. Headache can be the only manifestation of CVT (Cumurciuc et al., 2005; Ravishankar, 2006). In the majority of cases it is associated with focal signs (neurological deficits or seizures) and/or signs of intracranial hypertension or cavernous sinus syndrome (Ehtisham and Stern, 2006).

Given the absence of specific characteristics, any recent persisting headache should raise suspicion, particularly in the presence of an underlying prothrombotic condition such as pregnancy (Lanska and Kryscio, 1998) or a young women on hormonal oral contraception. Diagnosis is based on MRI plus MR venography (MRV), CT scan plus CT angiography, or catheter angiography. Investigations for predisposing prothrombotic states (e.g., anticardiolipin antibody, factor V leiden mutation, protein C or protein S deficiency) and underlying diseases (e.g., malignancy, Bechet's disease) should unsue. Treatment should be started as early as possible and includes symptomatic treatment, heparin followed oral anticoagulation for at least 6 months of and, whenever identified, treatment of the underlying cause.

HEADACHE ATTRIBUTED TO OTHER INTRACRANIAL VASCULAR DISORDER

Cerebral Autosomal Dominant Arteriopathy with Subcortical Infarcts and Leukoencephalopathy

Diagnostic criteria:

A. Attacks of migraine with aura, with or without other neurological signs;
B. Typical white matter changes on MRI T2WI;
C. Diagnostic confirmation from skin biopsy evidence or genetic testing (Notch 3 mutations).

Cerebral autosomal dominant arteriopathy with subcortical infarcts and leukoencephalopathy (CADASIL) is a autosomal dominant small vessel disease of the brain characterized by migraine with aura, lacunar infarctions, subcortical dementia, and psychiatric manifestations (Chabriat et al., 1995a, 1995b; Hutchinson et al., 1995; Joutel et al., 1996; Ruchoux and Maurage, 1997). Spoardic cases have been described (Joutel et al., 2000).

Migraine with aura is present in one third of the cases (Dichgans et al., 1998). Migraine with aura is usually the first manifestation of the disease and appears at a mean age of 30 (Chabriat et al., 1995b). Attacks are typical of migraine with aura except for an unusual frequency of prolonged auras. MRI is abnormal with severe white matter changes on T2 weighted imaging (Vahedi et al., 2004; Gladstone and Dodick, 2005). Characteristic lesions may be seen in the anterior temporal lobes and external capsule (Fig. 17–3). The diagnosis may be confirmed by a skin biopsy with electron

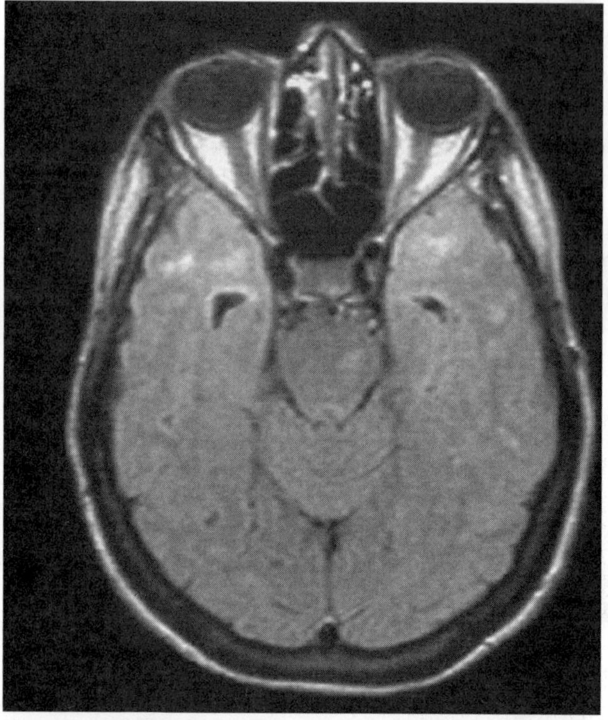

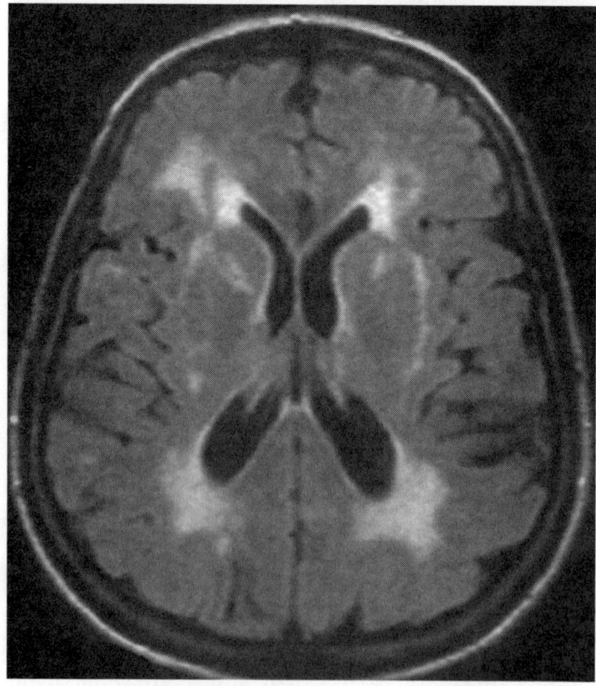

Figure 17–3 Thirty-eight-year-old woman with cerebral autosomal dominant arteriopathy with subcortical infarcts and leukoencephalopathy (CADASIL) after presenting with migraine with aura. The axial fluid attenuated inversion recovery (FLAIR) sequence illustrates the anterior temporal lobe white matter hyperintensities often seen in this disease. The second axial FLAIR magnetic resonance imaging (MRI) image also demonstrates the linear lesions along the external capsule, in addition to the more extensive periventricular and subcortical white matter hyperintensity.

microscopy demonstrating the pathogpneumonic granular osmiophilic basement membrane deposits or by genotyping which demonstrates a mutation within the *notch* 3 gene. (Joutel et al., 1997). CADASIL is an excellent model to study the pathophysiology of migraine with aura and the relationships between migraine and ischemic stroke.

Mitochondrial Encephalopathy, Lactic Acidosis and Stroke-like episodes

Diagnostic criteria:

A. Attacks of migraine with or without aura;
B. Stroke-like episodes and seizures;
C. Genetic abnormality [3243 point mitochondrial DNA mutation in the tRNA Leu gene or other DNA MELAS (mitochondrial encephalopathy, lactic acidosis, and stroke-like episodes) point mutation].

Migraine-like attacks are frequent in MELAS (Montagna et al., 1988 and Koo et al., 1993). The headache responds to sumatriptan suggesting that it has a pathophysiology similar to migraine (Iizuka et al., 2003). This has led to the hypothesis that mitochondrial mutations could play a role in migraine with aura. The 3243 mutation was not detected in two groups of subjects with migraine with aura (Klopstock et al., 1996; Ojaimi et al., 1998). In fact, in another study, none of the nine point mutations reported in patients with MELAS (A3243G, C3256T, T3271C, T3291C, A5814G, T8356C, T9957C, G13513A, and A13514G) or three secondary Leber's Hereditary Optic Neuropathy (LHON) mutations (T4216C, A4917G, and G13708A) were found among 10 patients with migraine associated with prolonged aura (Rozen, 2004). The authors concluded that migraine with prolonged aura is not an oligosymptomatic form of MELAS and is not related to secondary LHON mutations. The significance of a tRNA A4336G variant found in one patient is unknown.

Headache Attributed to Benign (or Reversible) Angiopathy of the CNS

Diagnostic criteria:

A. Diffuse, severe headache of abrupt or progressive onset, with or without focal neurological deficits, and/or seizures and fulfilling criteria C and D;
B. "Strings and beads" appearance on angiography and SAH ruled out by appropriate investigations;
C. One or both of the following:
   1. Headache develops simultaneously with neurological deficits and/or seizures;
   2. Headache leads to angiography and discovery of "strings and beads" appearance.
D. Headache (and neurological deficits, if present) resolves spontaneously within 2 months.

This is a poorly understood condition characterised clinically by a severe headache at onset (Calabrese, 1995, 1999, 2001, 2003). The headache can be abrupt, mimicking SAH or thunderclap headache, or progressive rapidly over hours or more slowly over days (Chen et al., 2006). Severe headache can be the only symptom of this condition. Other possible symptoms include fluctuating focal neurological deficits and sometimes seizures. Angiography is, by definition, abnormal, with alternating segments of arterial constriction and dilatation (Woolfenden et al., 1998; Jolly et al., 2004).

This disorder has recently been referred to as reversible cerebral vasoconstriction syndrome (RCVS) because the outcome is not always benign, angiopathy implies primary pathology within the blood vessels, and a variety of disorders all describing the same entity have been reported in the literature with varying eponyms or syndromic names often based on the patient's medical history, time of onset of symptoms or the specialty of the physician caring for the patient (Calabrese et al., 2007). Previous syndromes or eponyms include benign angiopathy of the CNS, migrainous vasospasm, Call–Fleming syndrome, postpartum angiopathy, and drug-induced vasculitis as reports of this syndrome have been described in patients with a history of migraine, during the puerperium, during sexual intercourse, and after exposure to certain drugs such as ergotamine, triptans, selective serotonin reuptake inhibitors, pseudoephedrine, cocaine, amphetamines, methylenedioxymethamphetamine (ecstasy), and bromocriptine (Schwedt et al., 2006). RCVS must be considered in patients who present with

Table 17–1 Clinical and Imaging Features that Distinguish Reversible Cerebral Vasoconstriction Syndrome (RCVS) from Primary Angiitis of the Central Nervous System (PACNS).

Variable	*RCVS*	*PACNS*
Onset	Acute (seconds–minutes)	Subacute–chronic
Headache	Acute, severe often thunderclap	Insidious, progressive
CSF	Normal, near normal	Abnormal in >95%
CT/MRI	Normal, PRES, watershed stroke	Abnormal in >90% WMHIs and cortical/sibcortical infarctions
Angio	Multiple stenoses; reversible	Cut-off, luminal irreg; often irrevesible

Abbreviations: CSF, cerebrospinal fluid; CT/MRI, computed tomography/magnetic resonance imaging; PRES, posterior reversible encephalopathy syndrome; WMHIs, white matter hyperintensities.

sudden severe (thunderclap) headache, reversible vasoconstriction of one or more arteries of the circle of Willis and normal or near-normal cerebrospinal-fluid. Neurological symptoms or signs may include alteration in the level of consciousness, motor and sensory deficits, seizures, visual disturbances, ataxia, speech abnormalities, nausea, and vomiting. Stroke has been described in up to 50% of patients.

Patients with RCVS are often confused as having primary CNS vasculitis or primary angiitis of the CNS (PACNS). The distinguishing features (Table 17–1) are important to recognize to institute appropriate treatment with calcium channel blockers and avoid the unnecessary use of immunosuppressive drugs. Brain MRI in patients with PACNS typically reveals multifocal lesions in the deep white matter and cortical infarctions in the distribution of separate vascular territories. In contract, brain MRI in patients with RCVS is either normal, or demonstrates changes consistent with posterior reversible encephalopathy syndrome, especially in the setting of acute or malignant hypertension, or cerebral infarctions in a watershed distribution (Fig. 17–4).

The treatment of RCVS is nimodipine or verapamil. Vasoconstrictive agents should be avoided and hypertension treated judiciously so as to avoid hypotension and cerebral hypoperfusion, especially in the distribution of a severely

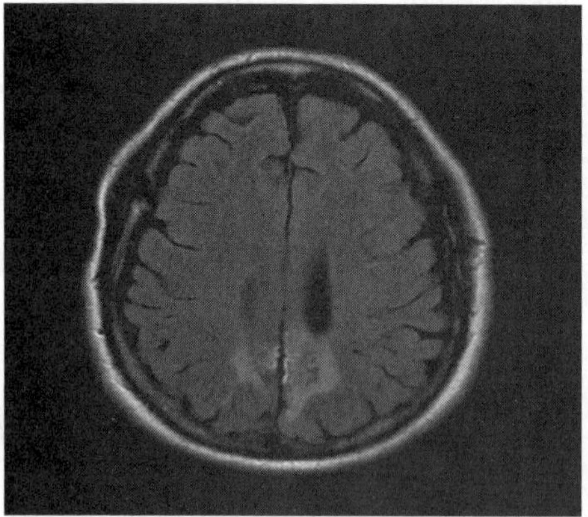

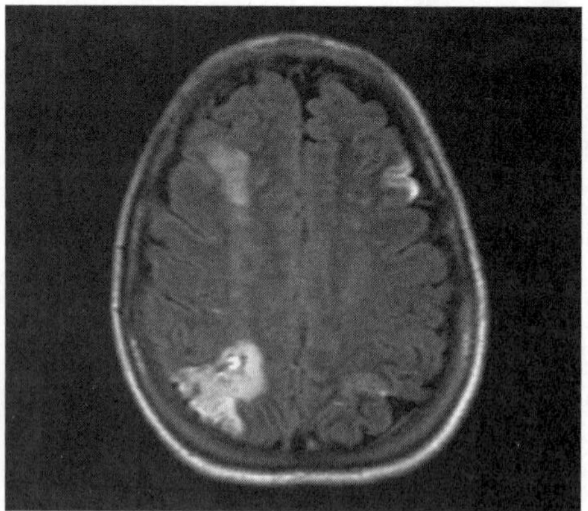

Figure 17–4 Fluid attenuated inversion recovery magnetic resonance imaging (FLAIR MRI) features of (*A*) reversible cerebral vasoconstriction syndrome (RCVS) and (*B*) primary angiitis of the central nervous system (PACNS). Note the presence of bilateral symmetric posterior occipital watershed infarctions in a patient with RCVS who had severe spasm in the basilar artery. Note the absence of any other imaging abnormalities in contract to the MRI of a patient with PACNS demonstrating diffuse white matter hyperintensites and multiple cortical infarctions in difference vascular territories.

constricted vessel. The headache can be treated with simple analgesics such as acetaminophen or opioids.

Headache Attributed to Pituitary Apoplexy

Diagnostic criteria:

A. Severe acute retro-orbital, frontal or diffuse headache accompanied by at least one of the following and fulfilling criteria C and D:
   1. Nausea and vomiting;
   2. Fever;
   3. Diminished level of consciousness;
   4. Hypopituitarism;
   5. Hypotension;
   6. Ophthalmoplegia or impaired visual acuity.

B. Neuroimaging evidence of acute hemorrhagic pituitary infarction;

C. Headache develops simultaneously with acute hemorrhagic pituitary infarction;

D. Headache and other symptoms and/or signs resolve within 1 month.

This rare clinical syndrome is an acute, life-threatening condition, characterised by spontaneous hemorrhagic or ischemic infarction of the pituitary gland. The leading symptom is severe headache not responding to analgesics. The prevalence of headache as the initial symptom is between 75% and 100% (Rolih and Ober, 1993; Elsässer-Imboden et al., 2005; Dubuisson et al., 2007). In most cases bleeding occurs into a preexisting adenoma. In rare cases this might happen in patients with a normal hypophysis. This condition can lead to acute pituitary failure. Pituitary hemorrhage can be a cause of thunderclap headache (Dodick and Wijdicks, 1998; Schwedt et al., 2006). Additional symptoms include visual loss, ophthalmopligia, nausea and vomiting (Gsponer et al., 1999). Magnetic resonance imaging is more sensitive than CT scan for detecting intrasellar pathology.

References

Abou-Chebl, A, Krieger, DW, Bajzer, CT, et al. (2006). Intracranial angioplasty and stenting in the awake patient. *J Neuroimaging*, 16(3):216–223.

Abou-Chebl, A, Yadav, JS, Reginelli, JP, et al. (2004). Intracranial hemorrhage and hyperperfusion syndrome following carotid artery stenting: risk factors, prevention, and treatment. *J Am Coll Cardiol*, 43 (9):1596–1601.

Afridi, S and Goadsby, P (2003). New onset migraine with a brain stem cavernous angioma. *J Neurol Neurosurg Psychiatr*, 74(5):680–682.

Arboix, A, Massons, J, Oliviers, M, et al. (1994). Headache in acute cerebrovascular disease: a prospective clinical study in 240 patients. *Cephalalgia*, 14:37–40.

Baldursson, O, Steinsson, K, Bjornsson, J, et al. (1994). Giant cell arteritis in Iceland. An epidemiological and histopathologic analysis. *Arthritis Rheum*, 37:1007–1012.

Beck, J, Raabe, A, Szelenyi, A, et al. (2006). Sentinel headache and the risk of rebleeding after aneurysmal subarachnoid hemorrhage. *Stroke*, 37(11):2733–2737.

Beletsky, V, Nadareishvili, Z, Lynch, J, et al. (2003). Cervical arterial dissection. Time for a therapeutic trial? *Stroke*, 34:2856–2860.

Biousse, V, D'Anglejan-Chatillon, J, Massiou, H, et al. (1994). Head pain in non-traumatic carotid artery dissection: a series of 65 patients. *Cephalalgia*, 14:33–36.

Biousse, V, Woimant, F, Amarenco, P, et al. (1992). Pain an the only manifestation of internal carotid artery dissection. *Cephalalgia*, 12:314–317.

Brown, R, Flemming, K, Meyer, F, et al. (2005). Natural history, evaluation, and management of intracranial vascular malformations. *Mayo Clin Proc*, 80 (2):269–281.

Calabrese, LH (1995). Vasculitis of the central nervous system. *Rheum Dis Clin North Am*, 21(4):1059–1076.

Calabrese, LH (1999). Angiographically defined primary angiitis of the CNS: is it really benign? *Neurology*, 52 (6):1302; author reply 1302–1303.

Calabrese, L. (2001). Primary angiitis of the central nervous system: the penumbra of vasculitis. *J Rheumatol*, 28(3):465–466.

Calabrese, LH. (2003). Clinical management issues in vasculitis. Angiographically defined angiitis of the central nervous system: diagnostic and therapeutic dilemmas. *Clin Exp Rheumatol*, 21(6 Suppl. 32):S127–S130.

Calabrese, L, Furlan, A, Gragg, L, et al. (1992). Primary angiitis of the central nervous system: diagnostic criteria and clinical approach. *Cleve J Med*, 59:293–306.

Calabrese, LH, Dodick, DW, Schwedt, TJ, et al. (2007). Narrative review: reversible cerebral vasoconstriction syndromes. *Ann Intern Med*, 146:34–44.

Campbell JK and Caselli, RJ (1991). Headache and other craniofacial pain. In *Neurology in Clinical Practice: Principles of Diagnosis and Management* (WG Bradley, RB Daroff, GM Fenichel, and CD Marsden, eds.), pp. 1507–1561. Butterworth-Heinemann, Philadelphia, PA.

Caplan, L (1988). Intracerebral hemorrhage revisited. *Neurology*, 38:624–627.

Caselli, RJ, Hunder, GG, and Whisnant, JP (1988). Neurologic disease in giant cell (temporal) arteritis. *Neurology*, 38:352–359.

Chabriat, H, Tournier-Lasserve, E, Vahedi, K, et al. (1995a). Autosomal dominant migraine with MRI white-matter abnormalities mapping to the CADASIL locus. *Neurology*, 45:1086–1091.

Chabriat, H, Vahedi, K, Iba-Zizen, MT, et al. (1995b). Clinical spectrum of CADASIL: a study of 7 families. *Lancet,* 346:934–939.
Chang, YJ, Ryu, SJ, and Lee, TH. (2006). Dose titration to reduce dipyridamole-related headache. *Cerebrovasc Dis,* 22(4):258–262.
Chen, SP, Fuh, JL, Lirng, JF, et al. (2006). Recurrent primary thunderclap headache and benign CNS angiopathy: spectra of the same disorder? *Neurology,* 67(12):2164–2169.
Chung, SJ, Kim, JS, Kim, JC, et al. (2002). Intracranial dural arteriovenous fistulas: analysis of 60 patients. *Cerebrovasc Dis,* 13:79–88.
Cumurciuc, R, Crassard, I, Sarov, M, et al. (2005). Headache as the only neurological sign of cerebral venous thrombosis: a series of 17 cases. *J Neurol Neurosurg Psychiatr,* 76(8):1084–1087.
Day, JW and Raskin, NH (1986). Thunderclap headache: symptom of unruptured cerebral aneurysm. *Lancet,* 2:1247–1248.
de Sousa, JE, Halfon, MJ, Bonardo, P, et al. (2005). Different pain patterns in patients with vertebral artery dissections. *Neurology,* 64:925–926.
Dichgans, M, Mayer, M, and Uttner, I, (1998). The phenotypic spectrum of CADASIL: clinical findings in 102 cases. *Ann Neurol,* 44(5):731–739.
Diener, HC, Cuhna, L, Forbes, C, et al. (1996). European Stroke Prevention Study 2. Dipyridamole and acetylsalicylic acid in the secondary prevention of stroke. *J Neurol Sci,* 143:1–13.
Dodick, DW (2002). Thunderclap headache. *J Neurol Neurosurg Psychiatr,* 72:6–11.
Dodick, DW and Wijdicks, EF (1998). Pituitary apoplexy presenting as a thunderclap headache. *Neurology,* 50 (5):1510–1511.
Dubuisson, AS, Beckers, A, and Stevenaert, A (2007). Classical pituitary tumour apoplexy: clinical features, management and outcomes in a series of 24 patients. *Clin Neurol Neurosurg,* 109(1):63–70.
Edlow, JA and Caplan, LR (2000). Avoiding pitfalls in the diagnosis of subarachnoid hemorrhage. *N Engl J Med,* 342:29–36.
Edmeads, J (1979). The headaches of ischemic cerebrovascular disease. *Headache,* 19:345–349.
Ehtisham, A and Stern, BJ (2006). Cerebral venous thrombosis: a review. *Neurologist,* 12(1):32–8.
Elsässer-Imboden, PN, De Tribolet, N, Lobrinus, A, et al. (2005). Apoplexy in pituitary macroadenoma: eight patients presenting in 12 months. *Medicine,* 84:188–196.
Fisher, CM (1968a). Headache in cerebrovascular disease. In *Handbook of Clinical Neurology* (PJ Vinken and GW Bruyn, eds.), pp. 124–126. Elsevier, Amsterdam.
Fisher, CM (1968b). Migraine accompaniments versus arteriosclerotic ischemia. *Trans Am Neuol Assoc,* 93:211–213.
Gladstone, JP and Dodick, DW (2005). Migraine and cerebral white matter lesions: when to suspect cerebral autosomal dominant arteriopathy with subcortical infarcts and leukoencephalopathy (CADASIL). *Neurologist,* 11(1):19–29.
Gorelick, PB, Hier, DB, Caplan, LR, et al. (1986). Headache in acute cerebrovascular disease. *Neurology,* 36:1445–1450.
Gsponer, J, De Tribolet, N, Deruaz, JP, et al. (1999). Diagnosis, treatment, and outcome of pituitary tumors and other abnormal intrasellar masses. Retrospective analysis of 353 patients. *Medicine (Baltimore),* 78 (4):236–269.
Hamilton, CR, Shelly, WM, and Tumulty, PA (1971). Giant cell arteritis. Including temporal arteritis and polymyalgia rheumatica. *Medicine (Baltimore),* 50:1–27.
Hindfelt, B and Olivecrona, H (1991)Cerebral arteriovenous malformation and cluster-like headache. *Headache,* 31:514–517.
Huston, KA, Hunder, GG, Lie, JT, et al. (1978). Temporal arteritis: a 25 year epidemiologic, clinical and pathologic study. *Ann Intern Med,* 88:162–167.
Hutchinson, M, Oriordan, J, Javed, M, et al. (1995). Familial hemiplegic migraine and autosomal dominant arteriopathy with leukoencephalopathy (CADASIL). *Ann Neurol,* 38:817–824.
Iizuka, T, Sakai, F, Endo, M, et al. (2003). Response to sumatriptan in headache of MELAS syndrome. *Neurology,* 61(4):577–578.
International Headache Society (2004). The International Classification of Headache Disorders: 2nd Edition. *Cephalalgia,* 24(Suppl. 1):9–160.
Jolly, M, Curran, JJ, and Ellman, M (2004). Benign angiopathy of the central nervous system. *J Clin Rheumatol,* 10(2):80–82.
Jorgensen, HS, Jespersen, HF, Nakayama, H, et al. (1994). Headache in stroke: the copenhagen stroke study. *Neurology,* 44:1793–1797.
Joutel, A, Corpechet, C, Ducros, A, et al. (1996). Notch3 mutations in CADASIL, a hereditary adult-onset condition causing stroke and dementia. *Nature,* 383:707–710.
Joutel, A, Corpechot, C, Vayssière, C, et al. (1997). Characterization of Notch3 mutations in CADASIL patients. *Neurology,* 48:1729–1730.
Joutel, A, Dodick, DD, Parisi, JE, et al. (2000). De novo mutation in the Notch3 gene causing CADASIL. *Ann Neurol,* 47(3):388–391.
Katsarava, Z, Egelhof, T, Kaube, H, et al. (2003). Symptomatic migraine and sensitization of trigeminal nociception associated with contralateral pontine cavernoma. *Pain,* 105:381–384.
Klopstock, T, May, A, Seibel, P, et al. (1996). Mitochondrial DNA in migraine with aura. *Neurology,* 46:1735–1738.
Koo, B, Becker, LE, Chuang, S, et al. (1993). Mitochondrial encephalomyopathy, lactic acidosis, stroke-like episodes (MELAS): clinical, radiological, pathological and genetic observations. *Ann Neurol,* 34:25–32.
Kruuse, C, Lassen, LH, Iversen, HK, et al. (2006). Dipyridamole may induce migraine in patients with migraine without aura. *Cephalalgia,* 26(8):925–933.

Lai, SL, Chang, YY, Liu, JS, et al. (2005). Cluster-like headache from vertebral artery dissection: angiographic evidence of neurovascular activation. *Cephalalgia,* 25 (8):629–632.

Landtblom, AM, Fridriksson, S, Boivie, J, et al. (2002). Sudden onset headache: a prospective study of features, incidence and causes. *Cephalalgia,* 22:354–360.

Lanska, DJ and Kryscio, RJ (1998). Stroke and intracranial venous thrombosis during pregnancy and puerium. *Neurology,* 51:1622–1628.

Lindgren, A, Husted, S, Staaf, G, et al. (2004). Dipyridamole and headache—a pilot study of initial dose titration. *J Neurol Sci,* 223(2):179–184.

Linn, FHH, Rinkel, GJE, Algra, A, et al. (1998). Headache characteristics in subarachnoid hemorrhage and benign thunderclap headache. *J Neurol Neurosurg Psychiatr,* 65:791–793.

Linn, FHH, Wijdicks, EFM, van der Graf, Y, et al. (1994). Prospective study of sentinel headache in aneurysmal subarachnoid haemorrhage. *The Lancet,* 344:590–593.

Lucas, C (2005). Headache from idiopathic cervical artery dissection: time-course and follow-up. *Rev Neurol (Paris),* 161(6–7):703–705.

Machado, EBV, Michet, CJ, Ballard, DJ, et al. (1988). Trends in incidence and clinical presentation of temporal arteritis in Olmsted County, Minnesota. *Arthritis Rheum,* 31:745–749.

Mani, S and Deeter, J. (1982). Arteriovenous malformation of the brain presenting as a cluster headache—a case report. *Headache,* 22:184–185.

Mas, JL, Chatellier, G, Beyssen, B, et al. (2006). EVA-3S Investigators. Endarterectomy versus stenting in patients with symptomatic severe carotid stenosis. *N Engl J Med,* 355:1660–1671.

Masuhr, F, Mehraein, S, and Einhäupl, K (2004). Cerebral venous and sinus thrombosis. *J Neurol,* 251:11–23.

McCabe, D, Brown, M, and Clifton A (1999). Fatal cerebral reperfusion hemorrhage after carotid stenting. *Stroke,* 30:2483–2486.

Melo, TP, Pinto, AN, and Ferro, JM (1996). Headache in intracerebral hematomas. *Neurology,* 47:494–500.

Mitsias, PD, Ramadan, NM, Levine, SR, et al.(2006). Factors determining headache at onset of acute ischemic stroke. *Cephalalgia,* 26(2):150–157.

Mohr, J, Caplan, L, Melski, J, et al.(1978). The Harvard Cooperative Stroke Registry: a prospective registry. *Neurology,* 28:754–762.

Montagna, P, Gallassi, R, Medori, R, et al. (1988). MELAS syndrome: characteristic migrainous and epileptic features and maternal transmission. *Neurology,* 38:751–754.

Moore, PM (1989). Diagnosis and management of isolated angiitis of the central nervous system. *Neurology,* 39:167–173.

Moore, P and Richardson, B (1998). Neurology of the vasculitides and connective tissue diseases. *J Neurol Neurosurg Psychiatr,* 65(1):10–22.

Morgenstern, LB, Luna-Gonzales, H, Huber, JC, et al. (1998). Worst headache and subarachnoid hemorrhage: prospective, modern computed tomography and spinal fluid analysis. *Ann Emerg Med,* 32:297–304.

Muoz, C, Diez-Tejedor, E, Frank, A, et al. (1996). Cluster headache syndrome associated with middle cerebral artery arteriovenous malformation. *Cephalalgia;* 16:202–205.

Murray, TJ (1977). Temporal arteritis. *J Am Geriatr Soc,* 25:450–453.

Ohkuma, H, Suzuki, S, and Ogane K (2002). Dissecting aneurysms of intracranial carotid circulation. *Stroke,* 33:941–947.

Ojaimi, J, Katsabanis, S, Bower S, et al. (1998). Mitochondrial DNA in stroke and migraine with aura. *Cerebrovasc Dis,* 8:102–106.

Pascual, J, Iglesias, F, Oterino, A, et al. (1996). Cough, exertional, and sexual headaches: an analysis of 72 benign and symptomatic cases. *Neurology,* 46;1520–1524.

Polmear, A (2003). Sentinel headaches in aneurysmal subarachnoid haemorrhage: what is the true incidence? A systematic review. *Cephalalgia,* ;23:935–941.

Ramadan, NM, Tietjen, GE, Levine, SR, et al. (1991). Scintillating scotoma associated with internal carotid artery dissection. *Neurology,* 41:1084–1087.

Raps, E, Rogers, J, Galetta, D, et al. (1993). The clinical spectrum of unruptured intracranial aneurysms. *Arch Neurol,* 50:265–268.

Ravishankar, K (2006). Incidence and pattern of headache in cerebral venous thrombosis. *J Pak Med Assoc,* 56 (11):561–564.

Rinkel, GJ, Djibuti, M, Algra, A, Van Gijn, J (1998). Prevalance and risk of rupture of intracranical aneurysms: a systematic review. *Stroke,* 29(1):251–256.

Robinson, J, Awad, I, and Little, J (1991). Natural history of the cavernous angioma. *J Neurosurg,* 75 (5):709–714.

Rolih, CA and Ober, KP (1993). Pituitary apoplexy. *Endocrinol Metab Clin North Am,* 22(2):291–302.

Rozen, TD, Shanske, S, Otaequi, D, et al. (2004). Study of mitochondrial DNA mutations in patients with migraine with prolonged aura. *Headache,* 44:674–677.

Ruchoux, MM and Maurage, CA (1997). CADASIL: cerebral autosomal dominant arteriopathy with subcortical infarcts and leukoencephalopathy. *J Neuropathol Exp Neurol,* 56:947–964.

Schievink, WI (2001). Spontaneous dissection of the carotid and vertebral arteries. *N Engl J Med,* 344:898–906.

Schwedt, TJ, Matharu, MS, and Dodick, DW (2006). Thunderclap headache. *Lancet Neurol,* 5(7):621–631.

Sidman, R, Connolly, E, and Lemke, T (1996). Subarachnoid hemorrhage diagnosis: lumbar puncture is still needed when the computed tomography scan is normal. *Acad Emerg Med,* 3(9):827–831.

Simard, M, Garcia-Bengochea, F, Ballinger, WJ, et al. (1986). Cavernous angioma: a review of 126 collected and 12 new clinical cases. *Neurosurgery,* 18 (2):162–172.

Solomon, S and Cappa, K (1987). The headache of temporal arteritis. *J Am Geriatr Soc,* 35:163–165.

Sturzenegger, M (1995). Spontaneous internal carotid artery dissection: early diagnosis and management in 44 patients. *J Neurol,* 242:231–238.

Tentschert, S, Wimmer, R, Greisenegger, S, et al. (2005). Headache at stroke onset in 2196 patients with ischemic stroke or transient ischemic attack. *Stroke,* 36(2):e1–e3.

The Space Collaborative Group (2006). 30 day results from the SPACE trial of stent-protected angioplasty versus carotid endarterectomy in symptomatic patients: a randomised non-inferiority trial. *Lancet,* 368(9543):1239–1247.

Theis, JGW, Deichsel, G, and Marshall, S (1999). Rapid development of tolernace to dipyridamole-associated headaches. *Br J Clin Pharmacol,* 48:750–755.

Vahedi, K, Chabriat, H, Levy, C, et al. (2004). Migraine with aura and brain magnetic resonance imaging abnormalities in patients with CADASIL. *Arch Neurol,* 61:1237–1240.

van Gijn, J (1992). Subarachnoidal haemorrhage. *Lancet,* 339:653–655.

Vermeulen, M, Hasan, D, Blijenberg, BG, et al. (1989). Xanthochromia after subarachnoid haemorrhage needs no revisitation. *J Neurol Neurosurg Psychiatr,* 52:826–828.

Ward, TN and Levin, M (2005). Headache in giant cell arteritis and other arteritides. *Neurol Sci,* 26(Suppl. 2): s134–s137.

Ward, TN, Levin, M, and Wong RL (2004). Headache Caused by Giant Cell Arteritis. *Curr Treat Options Neurol,* 6(6):499–505.

Weir B (2002). Unruptered intracranial aneurysms: a review. *J Neurosurg,* 96(1):3–42.

Wiebers, DO, Whisnant, JP, Huston, J, et al. (2003). Unruptured intracranial aneurysms: natural history, clinical outcome, and risks of surgical endovascular treatment. *Lancet,* 362:103–110.

Woolfenden, AR, Tong, DC, Marks, MP, et al. (1998). Angiographically defined primary angiitis of the CNS: is it really benign? *Neurology,* 51(1):183–188.

Zetterling, M, Carlstrom, C, and Konrad, P (2000). Internal carotid artery dissection. *Acta Neurol Scand,* 101:1–7.

18 Headache Associated with Abnormalities in Intracranial Structure or Function: High-cerebrospinal-fluid-pressure Headache and Brain Tumor

Deborah I Friedman, Michael Wall, and Stephen D Silberstein

INTRODUCTION

Headache is one of the most common clinical manifestations of altered intracranial pressure (ICP). Any disruption of cerebrospinal fluid (CSF) production, flow, or absorption may lead to alterations in ICP and produce headaches. Severe headaches may accompany conditions of high or low ICP, which may be iatrogenic or pathological in origin. Some disorders produce unique symptoms that aid in their diagnosis, for example, the cough headache associated with hindbrain abnormalities such as Chiari malformations. The International Headache Society (IHS) (Headache Classification Committee of the International Headache Society, 2004) classifies these disorders as "Headache associated with nonvascular intracranial disorder" (Table 18–1). Patients may have worsening of a preexisting headache or may develop a new form of headache (including migraine, tension-type headache, or cluster headache) in close temporal relationship to a nonvascular intracranial disorder. Causality is not necessarily implied.

THE CEREBROSPINAL FLUID

Galen first described the ventricular cavities in the second century, but it was left to Contugno, in 1764, to describe the CSF. Magendie, in 1825, named the CSF and discovered, between the fourth ventricle and the subarachnoid space, the foramen that bears his name (Fishman, 1992). Dandy's work supported the view that the CSF originated from the choroid plexus and the perivascular spaces of the brain. Key and Retzius demonstrated that the CSF passes from the subarachnoid space through the Pacchionian bodies into the cerebral venous sinuses (Fishman, 1992). Lumbar puncture (LP) was introduced by Quinke in 1891. Using a percutaneous needle with a stylet, he measured the components of CSF and its pressure in normal and disease states. Bier first described post-LP headache in 1898, when he injected cocaine into his own subarachnoid space and developed a violent postdural headache (Morewood, 1993). Schaltenbrand (1938) was the first to describe spontaneous ICH using the term spontaneous aliquorrhea.

The major source of CSF is the choroid plexus; however, some CSF is formed in extrachoroidal sites. The estimated rate of CSF formation in humans is 0.37 ml/min, which represents a formation rate of 500 ml/day. The total CSF volume is renewed every 6–8 h. The arachnoid villi, located within the calvarium and spinal column, are sites of CSF resorption. In addition, the lymphatic networks penetrating the cribriform plate may be a major outflow pathway for cranial CSF in humans and other species (Johnston, 2004).

The average lumbar CSF pressure in adults, measured in the lateral recumbent position, is 150 mm of CSF, with a range of 70–200 mm (Milhorat, 1972; Fishman, 1992; Neville and Egan, 2005). Corbett and Mehta (1988) recorded CSF pressures between 200 and 250 mm of CSF in normal nonobese controls, suggesting that values

TABLE 18–1 Headache Associated with Nonvascular Intracranial Disorder.

1. Headache attributed to high cerebrospinal fluid pressure
2. Headache attributed to low cerebrospinal fluid pressure
3. Headache attributed to noninfectious inflammatory disease
4. Headache attributed to intracranial neoplasm
5. Headache attributed to intrathecal injection
6. Headache attributed to epileptic seizure
7. Headache attributed to Chiari malformation type I
8. Syndrome of transient headache and neurological deficits with cerebrospinal fluid lymphocytosis (HaNDL)
9. Headache attributed to other nonvascular intracranial disorder

in this range are nondiagnostic. However, normal values for CSF pressure in adults and children have not been firmly established and there is some controversy over the upper and lower limits used to define various diseases. When CSF pressure falls below 50–90 mm of CSF, symptoms of intracranial hypotension occur. At times the CSF pressure is not measurable and CSF can only be obtained by aspiration (Milhorat, 1972; Gamache et al., 1987; Fishman, 1992). If simultaneous pressures are taken from the cerebral ventricles, the cisterna magna, and the lumbar sac during a change from the recumbent to the erect posture, there is a significant change in pressure throughout the system. The pressure rises to 375–565 mm in the lumbar sac, becomes 0 at the level of the cisterna magna, and can fall to − 85 mm of CSF in the ventricles (Freemont-Smith and Kubie, 1929; Loman, 1934; Loman et al., 1935; VonStorch et al., 1937; Milhorat, 1972). Normal CSF pressure may rise to 500 mm CSF or more during routine daily activity. Performing a Valsalva maneuver during a LP elevates the CSF pressure into the pathological range (up to 470 mm CSF) in normotensive patients (Neville and Egan, 2005).

Transmitted venous pressure is the most important of the factors that determine CSF pressure (Table 18–2) (Milhorat, 1972). ICP can be elevated by any of the mechanisms of Table 18–3. A mass lesion can produce elevated ICP when it: (1) reaches a critical size; (2) obstructs the intracranial venous system producing increased venous pressure; or, (3) obstructs the CSF pathways. According to the Monro–Kellie doctrine, any increase in intracranial volume leads to increased ICP; since an adult's skull has rigid walls, it forms a closed chamber, with a small exit, the foramen magnum, providing the only outlet for CSF into the vertebral canal.

INTRACRANIAL HYPERTENSION

Intracranial hypertension may be either: (1) idiopathic, with no clear identifiable cause, or (2) secondary to a particular cause, including venous sinus occlusion, a mass lesion, meningitis, trauma, radical neck dissection, hypoparathyroidism, vitamin A intoxication, renal disease, or drug side effects (tetracyclines, tretinoins, human growth hormone, corticosteroid withdrawal) (Digre and Corbett, 2001). Intracranial venous outflow obstruction can be caused by chronic otitis, head trauma, tumors, hypercoagulable states, and cerebral edema (Johnston et al., 1991). Extracranial venous outflow obstruction occurs with surgical ligation and further compression of venous outflow. Cranial venous outflow hypertension can

TABLE 18–2 Factors Determining CSF Pressure.

1. CSF secretion pressure
2. CSF absorption rate
3. Intracranial arterial pressure
4. Intracranial venous pressure
5. Brain bulk
6. Hydrostatic pressure
7. Presence of intact/surrounding coverings
8. Lymphatic drainage

TABLE 18–3 Mechanisms for Elevated Intracranial Pressure.

1. Increased CSF production or secretion pressure
2. Decreased CSF absorption
3. Increased venous pressure
4. Obstruction of normal CSF flow
5. Increase in brain bulk
   Mass lesion/cerebral edema
6. Impaired CSF lymphatic drainage
7. Increased bulk or pressure in dura
8. Combination of above

also occur without obstruction in patients with arteriovenous malformations, cardiac failure, and pulmonary failure. Increased ICP is not always associated with either headache or papilledema, and there is no direct correlation between the degree of pressure elevation and the presence of headache. Postulated mechanisms for headache with intracranial hypertension are listed in Table 18–4.

Although increased CSF pressure is not necessary for headache development, it clearly plays a role in some patients with CNS neoplasms, acute obstructive hydrocephalus, and idiopathic intracranial hypertension (IIH). The rate of the change in pressure may be critical. Sudden increases in ICP by tumors obstructing the foramen of Monro or the cerebral aqueduct may cause abrupt, severe headache associated with gait disturbance, syncope, incontinence, or visual obscurations.

INTRACRANIAL TUMORS

Mass lesions can produce headaches by several mechanisms, including traction on pain-sensitive intracranial structures, impediment of CSF flow, or directly increasing ICP by mass effect. There are no characteristic features of "brain tumor" headaches. However, an intracranial mass should be suspected in any patient with the new onset of headaches over age 50 years, a crescendo pattern of headaches, a change in the pattern or intensity of a previous headache disorder, new headaches in the setting of immunosuppression or known malignancy, and any headache with papilledema, focal neurological symptoms or signs.

Headaches are initially present in 20% of patients with brain tumors and rise to approximately 60% during the disease (Jaeckle, 1993). Headache is a rare initial symptom in patients with pituitary tumors, craniopharyngiomas, or cerebellopontine angle tumors (Lavyne and Patterson, 1987; Jaeckle, 1991). It is a very common initial symptom with infratentorial tumors (other than cerebellopontine angle tumors), occurring in 80%–85% of patients (Northfield, 1938; Kunkle, Pfeiffer, et al., 1942). Elevation of ICP is not necessary for headache production. In one older, pre-CT series of 72 brain tumor patients, headache occurred in those patients without elevated ICP as often as it did in those with increased ICP (Lavyne and Patterson, 1987).

Brain tumor headaches are usually bilateral, but they can be ipsilateral to the tumor (Lavyne and Patterson, 1987; Jaeckle, 1991). The location of the tumor may influence the location and character of the headache. Frontal and periorbital headache is common in supratentorial tumors because of irritation of trigeminal sensory afferents. Supratentorial tumors that impinge on structures innervated by the ophthalmic division of the fifth cranial nerve usually produce frontotemporal headache. A convexity meningioma may distort the adjacent middle meningeal artery and cause pain, which may be referred to the ipsilateral frontotemporal region. Posterior fossa masses may compress the ninth and tenth cranial nerves and produce occipitonuchal pain. A posterior fossa

TABLE 18–4 Mechanisms for Headache with Increased Intracranial Pressure.

1. Traction on pain-sensitive intracerebral vessels (venous sinuses and arteries at the base of the brain)
2. Transient herniation of hippocampal gyri
3. Traction on cranial or cervical nerves, or elevation of intracranial pressure
4. Distention or traction on the dura

tumor may also impinge upon the seventh cranial nerve, producing a headache that is referred to the ipsilateral ear.

Metastatic brain tumors may invade the meninges (meningeal carcinomatosis) and produce generalized headache and other signs of meningeal irritation. Occasionally, brain tumors produce a migraine-like headache, but rarely with a visual aura. Nausea and/or vomiting accompany the headache in 50% of patients. The classic, mild, early-morning, frontal headache that resolves within 30–60 min after waking is *uncommon* in brain tumor patients (Forsyth and Posner, 1993). The severe headaches that patients with tumors experience can be aggravated by Valsalva, change in position, or exertion, and probably result from sudden increases in ICP or traction on pain-sensitive structures such as the dura, cranial nerves, or large venous sinuses (Ray and Wolff, 1940).

The features associated with the headache of brain tumor are increased ICP, large tumor size and amount of midline shift, and a prior history of headache (Forsyth and Posner, 1993). Increased ICP (mostly from posterior fossa and leptomeningeal tumors) usually produces headaches. Headache is more commonly an isolated symptom in patients who have multiple metastases than in persons with single lesions.

The presence of large tumor size and degree of midline shift for causing headache is congruent with the observation in intracranial stimulation experiments (Kunkle, Bronson, et al., 1942) that brain tumor headaches result from traction on intracranial pain-sensitive structures. Traction by the tumor mass may distort pain-sensitive structures or act distantly by causing brain displacement or hydrocephalus.

One pre-CT/MRI series looked at the characteristic headache features of 221 patients who had brain tumors, only 60% of whom had headache (Rushton and Rooke, 1962). Tumor location had no significant bearing on the presence or absence of headache. Pain intensity was mild to moderate in 63% of patients and severe in 37%. The headaches were intermittent in 85%, throbbing in 15%, aggravated by changing position in 20%, by coughing or exertion in 25%, and on the side of the tumor in 30%. Five patients had exertional headaches. Half of the patients had nausea or vomiting. Twenty-five percent had headache during sleep, on arising, or both. Increased ICP was observed in 42% of patients with headache and in 6% of patients without headache.

In a survey of 778 patients with cerebral tumor, headache was the earliest or principal symptom in 54%. No difference in headache frequency was noted between rapidly growing and slow-growing tumors. The headache can occur intermittently and mimic migraine (Heyck, 1968).

Patients who have a history of headaches are more likely to have headaches if they have a brain tumor. In many cases this headache is similar in character to the prior headache, but it is often more severe, more frequent, or associated with neurological signs or symptoms (Vazquez-Barquero et al., 1994). In one series, only 8% of patients with brain tumors had headache as their first and isolated clinical manifestation at the time of diagnosis (Vazquez-Barquero et al., 1994). Thirty-one percent eventually experienced headache, but only one of the original patients continued to have headache as an isolated symptom. The prevalence of headache as an initial symptom of brain tumor has decreased in many series due to earlier detection by neuroimaging.

Boiardi et al. (2004) evaluated 1253 brain tumors patients seen at the "Carlo Besta" Neurological Institute. Metastatic brain tumors were frequently accompanied by headache and in 22% this was the first symptom. In medulloblastoma patients, headache occurred as a presenting symptom in 16% of cases but was very soon accompanied by vertigo and ataxia. In all the other cases, headache was confirmed in no more than 12% as an isolated sign, in the absence of any other neurological manifestation. The brain tumor headache was nonspecific and there are no significant correlations between progressive headache and the size of the tumor. The most common type of "brain tumor headache" was tension-type seen in 77% of patients, and described as severe, worse in the morning and accompanied by nausea and vomiting in only 17% of cases.

There is a significant overlap between the headache of brain tumor and that of migraine or tension type headache. A headache of recent onset, a headache that has changed in character or a headache accompanied by a neurological sign or symptom that cannot be easily explained by the aura of migraine requires a thorough evaluation, particularly if the headache is severe or occurs with nausea or vomiting. Morning or nocturnal headache associated with vomiting and increased headache frequency can be seen with both migraine and brain tumor.

In other space occupying lesions such as subdural hematomas and brain abscesses, headache is an earlier and more frequent symptom. Of McKissock's (1960) 216 patients with chronic subdural hematoma, 81% had headache; only 11% of acute and 53% of subacute subdural hematoma patients had headache. The difference in headache prevalence between tumor and subdural hematoma is believed to be due to the more rapid evolution and greater extent of the hematomas. The lesser occurrence of headache in acute and subacute subdural hematomas compared with chronic subdural hematoma may be due to the underlying traumatic cerebral changes in the former, affecting consciousness early and making it difficult to elicit a history of headache.

In brain abscesses, a progressively severe, intractable headache is common. In published clinical series, headache was present in 70%–90% of patients (Britt, 1985) (Fig. 18–1). The higher headache prevalence in patients with abscesses, compared to those with tumors, may be due to the faster evolution, the associated meningeal reaction, surrounding edema, and the occasional low grade fever that may accompany an abscess (see Chapter 20).

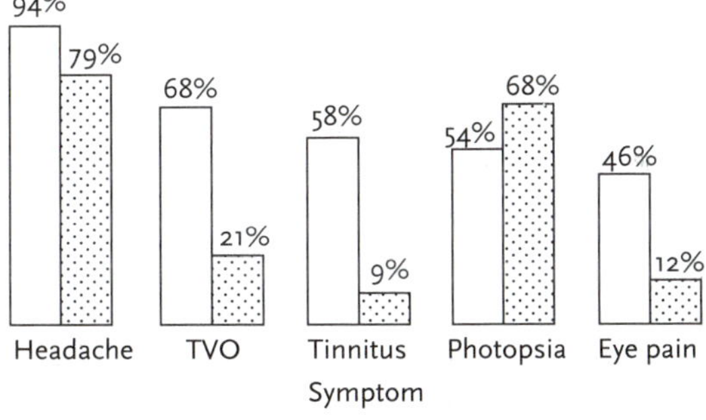

Figure 18–1 Frequency in percent of symptoms of patients with IIH compared with a control group. ICN, intracranial noises (pulse synchronous tinnitus); TVO, transient visual obscurations. (Reprinted from Giuseffi et al., 1991 with permission.)

PEDIATRIC BRAIN TUMORS

Headaches are a more common symptom of brain tumors in children (over 90%) than in adults (60%), due in part, perhaps, to the greater prevalence of posterior fossa tumors in children (Zulch et al., 1974). The following characteristics occur frequently: headache that awakens the child from sleep or is present on awakening, severe or prolonged headache, increased severity or frequency of headache, and increased frequency of vomiting. Most children (94%) with headache also had neurological signs. In 96%, diagnostic clues appeared within 4 months of the onset of headache (Honig and Charney, 1982).

The Childhood Brain Tumor Consortium published their retrospective record review on the incidence of headache in children with CNS tumors. The overall incidence of headache was 62%, ranging from 70% with infratentorial lesions, to 58% with supratentorial tumors, to 35% in patients with spinal canal tumors, approximately the incidence of benign headache in elementary school children (Childhood Brain Tumor Consortium, 1991). Headache was typically associated with other signs or symptoms and was rarely an isolated symptom (<1%). Symptoms of intracranial tumor included reduced academic performance, difficulty walking, back or abdominal pain, bladder symptoms, increasing head circumference, and failure to thrive. Headache frequency increased through age seven and leveled off regardless of tumor location. The low percentage of headache in the very young may be due to the expansile nature of the infant skull or may be an artifact of the inability of young children to communicate the source of their discomfort.

In a series of children with posterior fossa or pineal tumors, four children developed episodic, severe hemicranial headaches associated with nausea and transient visual loss, hemisensory deficit, dysphasia, or hemiparesis 14–32 months following successful combined whole-brain radiotherapy and chemotherapy (Shuper et al., 1995). These children had no prior history of similar headaches, no family history of migraine, and no evidence of tumor recurrence. It is unclear what produced these migrainous manifestations. The occurrence of headaches in treated brain tumor patients does not necessarily mean tumor recurrence.

UNCOMMON HEADACHES IN BRAIN TUMOR PATIENTS

Paroxysmal headaches are a unique feature of some patients who have a colloid cyst of the third ventricle or other pedunculated tumor that may obstruct CSF flow. These headaches are generally sudden in onset, reaching peak intensity in seconds, and are brief. They may also resolve quickly and may be suddenly precipitated (and relieved) by changes in position. There may be brief losses of consciousness or "drop attacks." Patients may walk unsteadily between headaches.

Cough or exertional headache is a transient, severe headache precipitated by Valsalva maneuver, exercise or sexual activity. These headaches are usually brief and poorly localized. Brain tumors have been identified in 2%–11% of patients who have these types of headaches, so appropriate diagnostic and neuroimaging studies are warranted in all patients being evaluated for cough or exertional headache (Symonds, 1956; Cutrer, 2004).

Headaches may be caused by base-of-skull metastasis. Five distinct syndromes have been defined according to location (Greenberg et al., 1981). These include: (1) orbital syndrome, (2) parasellar syndrome, (3) gasserian ganglion syndrome, (4) jugular foramen syndrome, and (5) occipital condyle syndrome. The orbital syndrome results from orbital metastases and consists of a dull supraorbital ache. It may be followed by diplopia, proptosis, and, in its later stages, deteriorating visual acuity. The parasellar syndrome is caused by metastasis to the sella turcica. The tumor (metastases) erodes into the cavernous sinus and produces unilateral frontal headache, periorbital edema, ocular paresis, and ophthalmic trigeminal sensory loss. The gasserian ganglion syndrome is characterized a dull ache in the cheek, jaw, or forehead and occasional trigeminal neuralgia-like pain. Loss of sensation is present in the V_2 and V_3 sensory distribution. Jugular foramen metastases produce a unilateral, dull, aching, retroauricular pain, hoarseness, and dysphagia. Occipital condyle metastases cause severe, unilateral, occipital headaches that are aggravated by neck flexion. Patients may also complain of dysarthria and dysphagia. Ipsilateral tongue atrophy is also commonly seen.

IDIOPATHIC INTRACRANIAL HYPERTENSION

IIH, also called pseudotumor cerebri, is characterized by elevated CSF pressure without ventriculomegaly. It is most commonly occurs in obese women in the childbearing years. Its primary presenting symptom, present in more than 90% of cases, is headache. The disorder is characterized by the symptoms and signs of increased ICP in an alert and oriented patient, but without localizing neurological findings (Table 18–5) (Friedman and Jacobson, 2002). Neurodiagnostic studies show no evidence of deformity or obstruction of the ventricular system, intracranial mass or abnormal enhancement. The CSF is normal except for increased CSF pressure (greater than 250 mm of CSF) (Corbett and Mehta, 1983). In addition, no secondary cause of generalized intracranial

TABLE 18–5 Criteria for the Diagnosis of Idiopathic Intracranial Hypertension.

1. If symptoms are present, they may only reflect those of generalized intracranial hypertension or papilledema
2. If signs are present, they may only reflect those of generalized intracranial hypertension or papilledema
3. Documented elevated cerebrospinal fluid pressure measured by lumbar puncture in the lateral decubitus position (>250 mm CSF in adults)
4. Normal cerebrospinal fluid composition
5. No evidence of hydrocephalus, mass, structural, or vascular lesion on MRI or contrast-enhanced CT scan for typical patients, and MRI and MR venography for all others
6. Patient is awake and alert

hypertension is present (Table 18–6). The common signs and symptoms of increased ICP are headache, transient episodes of visual loss (transient visual obscurations), pulse synchronous tinnitus, diplopia due to sixth cranial nerve paresis, and papilledema with its associated loss of sensory visual function.

Table 18–6 Differential Diagnosis of Idiopathic Intracranial Hypertension (IIH).

Highly likely causes and associations

Decreased flow through arachnoid granulations
- Scarring from previous inflammation (e.g., meningitis, sequel to subarachnoid hemorrhage)

Obstruction to venous drainage
- Venous sinus thromboses
  - Hypercoagulable states
  - Contiguous infection (e.g., middle ear or mastoid, otitic hydrocephalus)
- Bilateral radical neck dissections
- Superior vena cava syndrome
- Increased right heart pressure

Exogenous Agents
- All-trans-retinoic acid (for acute promyelocytic leukemia)
- Corticosteroid withdrawal
- Human growth hormone replacement in children
- Hypervitaminosis A
- Isotretinoin
- Leuprorelin acetate (LH-RH analogue)

Endocrine disorders
- Addison's disease
- Hypoparathyroidism
- Obesity/recent weight gain
- Polycystic ovarian syndrome

Nutritional disorders
- Hyperalimentation in deprivation dwarfism

Arteriovenous malformations and dural shunts

Orthostatic edema

Probable causes and associations

Anabolic steroids (may cause venous sinus thrombosis)

Chlordecone (kepone)

Table 18–6 (continued)

Ketoprofen or indomethacin in Bartter syndrome

Obstructive sleep apnea

Systemic lupus erythematosis

Thyroid replacement therapy in hypothyroid children

Tetracycline, minocycline, doxycycline

Turner's syndrome

Uremia

Possible causes

Amiodarone

Diphenylhydantoin

Iron deficiency anemia

Lithium carbonate

Nalidixic acid

Norplant system

Sarcoidosis

Sulfa antibiotics

Causes frequently cited that are unlikely causes

Corticosteroid intake

Hyperthyroidism

Hypovitaminosis A

Menarche

Menstrual irregularities

Multivitamin intake

Oral contraceptive use

Pregnancy

Note: Cases must meet the diagnostic criteria of IIH (Table 18–5) except that a secondary cause is found. The table lists the etiologies of intracranial hypertension that meet the diagnostic criteria for IIH except a cause is associated. The highly likely category is a list of cases with many reports of the association with multiple lines of evidence. Probable causes have reports with some convincing evidence. Possible causes have suggestive evidence or are common conditions or medications with intracranial hypertension as a rare association. Also listed are some frequently cited but poorly documented or unlikely causes; three case–control studies suggest this group of associations are not valid.

Epidemiology

The annual incidence of IIH is 0.9/1,00,000 persons, 3.5/1,00,000 in females 15–44 years of age and 19.3/1,00,000 in obese females ages 20–44 years (Durcan et al., 1988; Radhkrishnan et al., 1993). With the epidemic of obesity in America and the western world, the incidence of IIH has essentially doubled over the past 15–20 years, with an alarming increase among obese young men (Garrett, et al., 2004; Jacobs, et al., 2004). These studies are corroborated by a 350% increase in shunting procedures for IIH between 1998 and 2002 (Curry, et al., 2005). More than 90% of IIH patients are obese and more than 90% are women. The mean age at the time of diagnosis is approximately 30 years. Studies from urban centers suggest that African–Americans may be at increased risk (Galvin and VanStavern, 2004).

Studies of conditions associated with IIH are mostly uncontrolled and retrospective. This has led to erroneous conclusions because investigators have reported chance and spurious associations with common medical conditions and medications. In addition, many case reports exist of associations with IIH where the cases do not meet the diagnostic criteria for IIH. A critical review of these associations can be found elsewhere (Digre and Corbett, 2001) (Table 18–6).

Any disorder that causes decreased flow through the arachnoid granulations or obstructs the venous pathway from the granulations to the right heart is accepted as a cause of intracranial hypertension. Arteriovenous malformations or dural fistulae with high flow may overload venous return and result in elevation of ICP.

Although corticosteroid withdrawal, human growth hormone supplementation in children, thyroid replacement therapy in hypothyroid children, Addison's disease, and hypoparathyroidism are clearly associated with IIH, links to other endocrine abnormalities remain unproven. For example, corticosteroid use has been associated with many suspected cases of IIH; however, none fulfills the diagnostic criteria for IIH.

Several other purported associations with IIH have been refuted by controlled studies (Williams, 1976; Digre and Corbett, 1988; Giuseffi et al., 1991) The association of pregnancy, irregular menses, and oral contraceptives has been shown to be due to chance. In a case–control study, no association was found between IIH and multivitamin, oral contraceptive, corticosteroid, or antibiotic use (Ireland et al., 1990). However, case reports associating some drugs appear convincing: tetracyclines, nalidixic acid, vitamin A, isotretinoin, and anabolic steroids (Digre and Corbett, 2001).

A case–control study found strong associations between IIH and obesity and weight gain during the 12 months before diagnosis (Giuseffi et al., 1991). In this study, there was no evidence that IIH was associated with any other medical condition, with pregnancy, or with consumption of any medications. In summary, other than obesity and recent weight gain, many conditions associated with IIH are common disorders of women in childbearing years and the reported associations are likely due to chance.

Pathogenesis

CSF homeostasis is disrupted in IIH and the most popular hypothesis is that IIH is a syndrome of reduced CSF absorption. Reduced conductance to CSF outflow may be due to dysfunction of the absorptive mechanism of the arachnoid granulations. ICP then must rise for CSF to be absorbed. There are conflicting results regarding development of any brain edema (Sahs and Joynt, 1956) but it is likely that brain edema does not occur (Wall et al., 1995). Malm et al. (1992) believe, but it is not yet certain, that increased CSF pressure in IIH is a result of either a rise in venous sagittal sinus pressure secondary to extracellular edema causing venous obstruction or a low conductance for CSF reabsorption producing a compensatory increase in CSF pressure.

Cerebral venous hypertension is associated with IIH. King et al. (1995) evaluated nine IIH patients with cerebral venography and manometry. Elevated venous pressure was found in the superior sagittal and proximal transverse sinuses, which dropped at the level of the lateral third of the transverse sinus. The abnormality, not as well demonstrated on venography, resembled mural thrombosis. Two patients with intracranial hypertension possibly associated with minocycline use were not found to have venous hypertension.

The same investigators performed an elegant study confirming the reciprocal relationship between cerebral venous pressure and CSF pressure (King, et al., 2002). Twenty-one patients with confirmed IIH underwent digital subtraction internal and external carotid angiography, dural sinus venography, and manometry. Immediately afterward, eight of these patients underwent lateral C1–2 puncture, and their CSF pressure was recorded before and after 20–25 ml of CSF was removed, after which the cerebral venous pressure measurement was repeated. Control subjects consisted of patients with other diagnoses or those who were suspected of having IIH but the diagnosis was later proven incorrect. Nineteen of the twenty-one IIH patients showed a large pressure gradient across the transverse venous sinus. Lowering of the ICP by removal of CSF produced a pressure drop within the transverse sinus between 12 and 41 mm Hg in six patients. The pressure drop in the other two patients was 4 and 6 mm Hg; both patients had only a small drop in CSF pressure after the cervical puncture. The drop in pressure in the proximal transverse sinus was most dramatic in patients with the highest pressures before the cervical puncture.

Several studies have demonstrated transverse venous sinus stenosis on magnetic resonance venography (MRV). In most cases, the stenosis resolves after a CSF drainage procedure (Farb, et al., 2003). These studies suggest that increased venous pressure, and venous sinus stenosis, result from, rather than cause, increased ICP in IIH (Corbett and Digre, 2002).

IIH Symptoms

The symptoms most commonly reported by IIH patients in a case–control study of outpatients were headache (94%), transient visual obscurations (68%), pulse-synchronous tinnitus (58%), photopsia (54%), and retrobulbar pain (44%) (Giuseffi et al., 1991). The frequency of these symptoms compared to controls is found in Fig. 18–1. Diplopia (38%), visual loss (30%), and retrobulbar pain on eye movement (22%) were less common accompaniments of IIH and were not reported by any of the control subjects. Of these common symptoms, all except headache and photopsia occurred much more frequently in cases than controls.

A retrospective study of 52 patients with IIH presenting to a tertiary care emergency department described headache in 48 patients, associated with dizziness, nausea, or visual complaints (Jones, et al., 1999). Twenty-seven percent of patients had atypical features such as paresthesias, neck or back pain, unilateral headache, vertigo and nystagmus; these patients were not diagnosed at their initial visit to the emergency department. Papilledema was not detected initially in 21% of patients and described as unilateral in 12%.

Headache

A prospective study characterized the headache profile of the IIH patient as severe daily, pulsatile headaches that gradually increased in intensity (Wall, 1990) (Table 18–7). Nausea was common and vomiting less common. Most of those with headache reported it was the worst head pain ever and was different from previous headaches. The headache commonly awakened the patient. Postural aggravating factors were uncommon. The pain usually lasted hours. The headaches of IIH were not specific, and may have migrainous features. Radicular pain was occasionally reported. Although uncommon, the presence of retrobulbar pain accentuated by eye movements or pain radiating in a nerve root distribution, possibly from dilation of spinal nerve root sleeves, may aid in separation of this headache syndrome. Neck stiffness was found in approximately half of patients;

TABLE 18–7 The Frequency of Symptoms Associated with Headache in Cases and Controls (Wall, 1990).

Symptom	*Cases (%)*	*Controls (%)*
Most severe	91	1
Different from previous	85	1
Radicular pain	19	0
Vomiting	36	3
One-sided	62	9
Awaken patient	62	13
Nausea	60	14
Neck stiffness	51	13
Pulsatile	79	38
Retro-orbital pain	47	15
On eye movement	23	0
Last longer than 1 h	85	53
Generalized	47	25
Intensity slowly increases	70	54
Focal	49	75

in some cases, neck and shoulder pain may be more severe than head pain.

The mechanism of IIH-related head pain is uncertain and may be related to central venous hypertension or the effect of intracranial hypertension on the dura. Intracranial hypertension produced by CSF infusion in humans can cause pulsatile pain that is usually frontal or temporal in location. It may be associated with vomiting. More commonly, however, the infusion provoked variable headache responses (Fay, 1940). In 20 IIH patients monitored using an intraventricular catheter, 13 patients had plateau waves and eight had plateau-like waves. Neither type of wave was related to headache or, for that matter, any change in clinical symptoms (Johnston and Paterson, 1974). Therefore, the trigger for headache related to raised ICP is unknown.

Transient Visual Obscurations

Visual obscurations are episodes of transient blurred vision that usually last less than 30 seconds and are followed by restoration of vision. They are often provoked by arising from a stooped or seated position. Visual obscurations occur in approximately three quarters of IIH patients (Wall and George, 1991). The attacks may be monocular or binocular. They are not correlated with the degree of intracranial hypertension or with the extent of disc edema (Hayreh, 1977). The cause of these episodes is thought to be transient ischemia of the optic nerve head due to increased tissue pressure (Sadun et al., 1984). Visual obscurations do not appear to be associated with poor visual outcome (Rush, 1980; Corbett, 1983; Wall and George, 1991).

Pulse-synchronous Tinnitus

Pulse-synchronous tinnitus (also called pulsatile intracranial noises) occurs in approximately two-third of patients with IIH, and is often not mentioned until the patient is specifically asked about the symptom. The sound is often unilateral with neither side predominating. In patients with intracranial hypertension, jugular compression ipsilateral to the sound eliminates it. Sismanis found pulsatile tinnitus in each of 20 patients studied with IIH (Sismanis, 1987). It was synchronous with the heartbeat. He reported the sound to disappear immediately, but temporarily, following LP. He attributed the noise to transmission of intensified vascular pulsations via CSF under high pressure to the walls of the venous sinuses. The periodic compressions were thought to convert the laminar blood flow to turbulent flow.

Other Symptoms

Less common symptoms of IIH include parethesias, arthalgias, back and leg pain, and ataxia (Round and Keane, 1988). Young children with IIH may have irritability, strabismus, and a stiff neck as prominent features (Lessell, 1992). Uncommonly, unilateral facial paresis and torticollis occur in children. It is not unusual for children to have asymptomatic papilledema discovered on a routine eye exam; once intracranial pathology has been excluded, these children may be closely observed without specific treatment if they have normal visual function, as the papilledema tends to be self-limited.

IIH Signs

Papilledema

Papilledema is the hallmark sign of IIH. It is usually bilateral but may be unilateral or asymmetrical (Huna-Baron, et al., 2001). The timing of the development of papilledema in patients with IIH relative to symptom onset is somewhat variable, and repeated examinations may be needed. Dilated examination of the ocular fundus using indirect ophthalmoscopy and/or slit lamp bimicroscopy is necessary to be certain there is no optic disc edema.

The recognition of early papilledema can be difficult. The earliest sign of papilledema is optic disc elevation. Unfortunately, this sign may also occur as a normal variant. The earliest objective signs of papilledema are (1) edema in the peripapillary region obscuring the details of the adjacent nerve fiber layer (Fig. 18–2), (2) coarsening and irregularity of this nerve fiber layer, (3) loss of spontaneous venous pulsations after previous documentation of their presence, and (4) associated choroidal folds (Fig. 18–2). When the presence of papilledema is difficult to determine, repeated

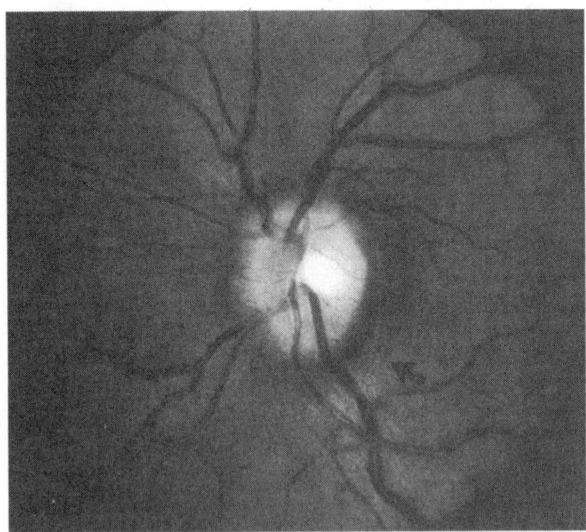

Figure 18–2 Optic disc with early papilledema showing a characteristic "c-shaped halo" with a temporal gap surrounding the disc. Also, note the choroidal folds (arrowhead).

examinations and serial optic disc stereo photographs are useful.

Papilledema is the cause of most of the visual loss of IIH. Although there is generally a significant correlation between high-grade papilledema and atrophic papilledema and visual loss (Orcutt et al., 1984; Wall and White, 1998), in the individual patient, the severity of visual loss cannot be predicted from the severity of the papilledema. A partial explanation for this is that the amount of papilledema decreases with axonal death from compression of the optic nerve.

Ocular Motility Disturbances

Horizontal diplopia occurs in approximately one of three IIH patients and sixth nerve palsies are present in 10%–20% of patients. Motility disturbances other than sixth nerve palsies have been reported. Some of these reflect erroneous conclusions from the small vertical ocular motor imbalance known to accompany sixth nerve palsies. A diagnosis of IIH should be questioned in patients with ocular motility disturbances other than sixth nerve palsies. General ophthalmoparesis rarely occurs and suggests an underlying venous sinus thrombosis (Friedman, et al., 1998).

Pupil Examination

A relative afferent pupillary defect is a sensitive sign of a unilateral optic neuropathy; it occurs in approximately 25% of patients. It is usually absent in IIH since its existence depends on asymmetry of visual loss and the optic neuropathy of IIH is most often fairly symmetric.

Central Visual Function

Visual acuity is usually unaffected in patients with papilledema except when the condition is long-standing. Decreased visual acuity at presentation often heralds a "malignant" course and should prompt aggressive treatment. Although commonly used, Snellen acuity testing is insensitive to the amount of visual loss found by perimetry and to worsening of papilledema grade (Wall and George, 1991).

A better measure of central visual loss is contrast sensitivity testing, although it is nonspecific. As opposed to Snellen acuity, it reveals deficits in 50%–75% of eyes tested, and is the only visual parameter significantly correlating with the symptom of sustained visual loss. Color vision testing has been disappointing as a method of detecting visual loss and following patients with IIH.

Perimetry

Most patients (50%–94%) with papilledema have visual loss (Wall and George, 1991), which is asymptomatic in 25%–50% of patients. However, it is important to measure since it serves as a marker for therapeutic intervention. Perimetry (automated or kinetic Goldmann methods) is the main measure used to determine the course of therapy. Following the size of the blind spot to assess treatment efficacy is not useful, as blind spot size is influenced by refraction and accommodation.

The visual field defects found in IIH are the same types as those reported to occur in papilledema due to other causes, and are similar to those found in glaucoma. The most common defects are enlargement of the physiological blind spot, loss of inferonasal portions of the visual field (Fig. 18–3) and generalized visual field

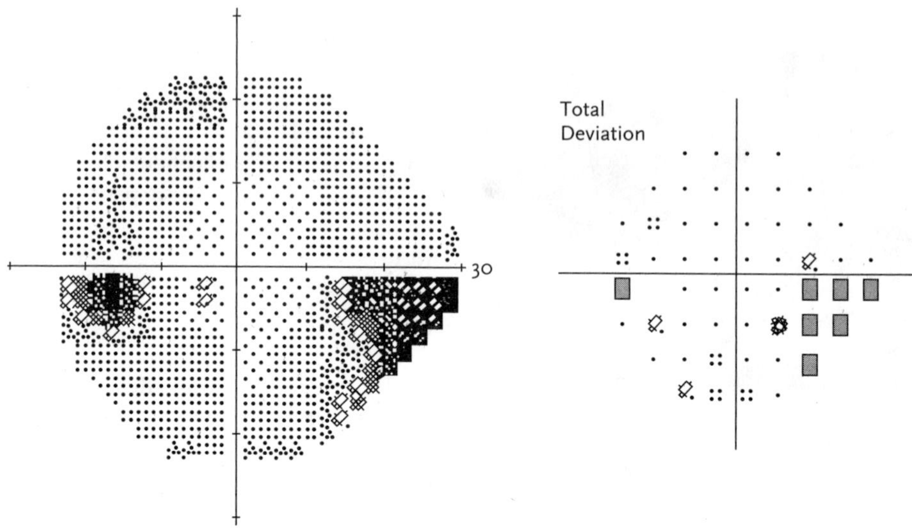

Figure 18–3 Conventional automated perimetry showing a classic inferonasal step defect.

constriction. Other defects are central, paracentral and cecocentral scotomas, arcuate scotomas, altitudinal patterns of loss and other nerve fiber bundle defects. The loss of visual field may be progressive and severe, leading to blindness. The onset of visual loss is usually gradual; however, acute severe visual loss can occur.

With treatment, there is significant improvement in the visual field in approximately 50% of patients (Wall and George, 1991). This reversibility of visual field loss in IIH is not widely appreciated. Those at risk for severe visual loss are patients with recent marked weight gain, African–Americans, postpubertal adolescent girls (Stiebel-Kalish, et al., 2006), patients with glaucoma, those with severe systemic arterial hypertension, and patients being rapidly tapered off corticosteroids.

IIH Without Papilledema

Intracranial hypertension may occasionally occur without papilledema (Spence et al., 1980; Marcelis and Silberstein, 1991; Wang et al., 1998). The clinical, historical, radiographic, and demographic characteristics are identical to patients with papilledema except for: (1) possible association with prior head trauma or meningitis; (2) extended delay in diagnosis, which requires LP in the absence of papilledema; (3) no evidence of visual loss as seen in patients with IIH with papilledema; (4) increased incidence of functional (nonorganic) visual field loss. It is rare, accounting for perhaps 1% of IIH patients in a neuro-ophthalmic practice. Patients, particularly obese women, with chronic daily headache and symptoms of increased ICP, that is, pulsatile tinnitus, a history of head trauma or meningitis, an empty sella on neuroimaging studies, or a headache that is unrelieved by standard therapy, should have a diagnostic LP.

Why there is no papilledema in these cases of intracranial hypertension is not known. Congenital or acquired optic nerve sheath defects, "chronic IIH" with resolution of papilledema, or early IIH are alternative explanations. Unless the examination has been done with slit lamp bimicroscopy, documented with fundus photos, and read by a neuro-opthalmologist, early papilledema is very easily missed.

In a case–control study conducted at a tertiary headache center, 25 consecutive patients with chronic daily headache (24 women, 1 man, 38 $\pm$ 6 years) who had IIH without papilledema were diagnosed between June 1989 and June 1996 (CSF pressure was $\geqslant$200 mm CSF on two occasions, and there was no obvious papilledema). Control subjects consisted of patients with refractory chronic daily headache who had normal CSF pressure on LP ($n = 60$, 50 women, 10 men, 36 ± 11 years). Significant predictors of IIH without papilledema in chronic daily headache patients included pulsatile tinnitus (odds ratio = 13.0) and obesity (odds ratio = 4.4) (Wang et al., 1998). Thus, a small subset of patients with chronic daily headache, who fit the stereotype of the obese female of childbearing age, may have IIH without papilledema. These patients would not have been identified without an LP (Silberstein and Corbett, 1993). This group of patients is often difficult to treat. Some may respond to CDH treatment, but the response to lowering the ICP is inconsistent and generally unsuccessful (Wang et al., 1998). Medication overuse headache must be excluded.

Therapy for IIH

The management of patients with IIH is divided into symptomatic treatment and treatment of raised ICP. Symptomatic treatment, for the most part, is treatment of headache. Most of the migraine drugs can be used to treat the headache of IIH. However, patients must be closely followed for possible weight gain associated with tricyclic antidepressants or valproic acid, peripheral edema from calcium channel blockers, and the hypotension associated with β-blockers. Topirimate may be helpful for headache treatment in IIH. However, the carbonic anhydrase inhibition of topirimate is minimal, and insufficient to lower ICP. Frequent analgesic use may complicate the clinical picture with medication overuse headaches.

Medical Treatment of IIH

Treatment of raised ICP is both medical and surgical. It is aimed at lowering of ICP. Unfortunately, all reports to date are anecdotal as there have not been any controlled clinical treatment trials for IIH. The mainstays of medical treatment are diet and diuretics. IIH can be controlled in most patients with medical therapy.

Weight Loss Weight loss is a cornerstone in the management of IIH, although there has only been one prospective study of a specific dietary regimen. Newborg reported remission of papilledema in all nine patients placed on a strict diet (Newborg, 1974). She used a low calorie rice diet with fluid and salt restriction and a total caloric intake of 400–1000 calories per day. All patients had reversal of their papilledema. Unfortunately, there was no mention of the patients' visual testing.

Kupersmith and colleagues (1998) retrospectively reviewed the charts of 56 medically treated IIH patients from two centers that had at least 6 months of follow-up. The mean time to improve one papilledema grade was approximately 4 months in patients with weight loss compared with approximately 1 year in patients without weight loss. Papilledema resolved in 28 out of 38 patients with weight loss compared with 8 out of 20 without weight loss.

Johnson et al. (1998) and coworkers retrospectively studied 15 IIH patients treated with acetazolamide and weight loss for 24 weeks. They reported 3.3% weight loss in patients having one grade of improvement in papilledema. Our experience has also been that improvement often occurs with only modest degrees of weight loss. Greer (1965), however, reported a group of six obese patients who became asymptomatic without weight loss.

Resolution of IIH in a patient following surgically induced weight loss (gastric exclusion procedure) was first reported by Amaral (Amaral et al., 1987). Sugerman et al. (1999) and coworkers performed gastric weight reduction surgery in 24 morbidly obese women with IIH. Five patients were lost to follow-up. Symptoms resolved in all but one patient within 4 months of the procedure. Two patients regained weight associated with return of their symptoms. There were many significant but treatable surgically related complications.

Many women with IIH also have orthostatic edema, with abnormal systemic retention of sodium, water or both (Friedman and Streeten, 1998). A low-salt diet and avoiding excessive fluid intake appear to be beneficial for many IIH patients. This may account for the relatively low percentage of body weight loss required for improvement in the aforementioned studies; the initial weight loss for most patients tends to be fluid.

Lumbar Punctures Repeated LPs, still occasionally used, have unproven efficacy. Reduction of CSF pressure with LP has short-lived effects; Johnston and Paterson (1974) found a return of pressure to pre-tap level after only 82 min. Also, repeated LPs to monitor therapy are prone to error since they measure CSF pressure at only one point in time. Since CSF pressure fluctuates considerably, this information has only limited clinical use for modifying treatment plans.

Corticosteroids Corticosteroids were previously used to treat IIH but are not recommended for routine use for this condition. Their mechanism of action remains unclear. The side effects of weight gain, striae, fluid retention, and acne are troublesome for obese patients and are counterproductive to dietary management. Although patients treated with steroids may initially respond well, there may be recurrence of papilledema as the dose is tapered. This may be accompanied by severe worsening of visual function.

Diuretics Acetazolamide is a carbonic anhydrase inhibitor that reduces CSF production. It appears effective in the treatment of IIH although it has never been studied prospectively. The dose needed to effectively lower ICP, as demonstrated by continuous ICP monitoring, is 2–4 g/day (Gucer and Viernstein, 1978). Acetazolamide is initiated with a dose of 250 mg twice daily and the dosage is gradually increased to 1–2 g/day. Doses as high as 4 g/day can be used if tolerated. Frequent side effects include paresthesias, altered taste sensation, and drowsiness.

Furosemide has also been used to treat IIH (Corbett, 1983). It has been well documented that furosemide can lower ICP (Roberts et al., 1987). It appears to work by both diuresis and reducing sodium transport into the brain (Buhrley and Reed, 1972). It has also been shown to effectively lower CSF pressure when combined with acetazolamide (Schoeman, 1994) although electrolyte monitoring is essential when combining diuretics. Furosemide is started at doses of 20 mg twice daily and gradually increased to a maximum dose of 40 mg p.o. TID. Potassium supplementation is often necessary.

Surgical Treatment

Optic Nerve Sheath Fenestration Current surgical therapies include various shunting and decompression procedures: lumbar or ventriculoperitoneal shunts and optic nerve sheath fenestration. Neither CSF shunting nor optic nerve sheath fenestration has been prospectively studied, and the decision to incorporate one technique over another is largely dependent on the resources available in a given location. Either treatment may fail, and some patients require multiple procedures.

Optic nerve sheath fenestration is an effective method for reversing visual loss and protecting the optic nerve from further damage (Corbett et al., 1988; Sergott et al., 1988; Kelman et al., 1992; Plotnik and Kosmorsky, 1993; Acheson et al., 1994; Goh et al., 1997). In these series, postoperative visual acuity or fields were as good as or better than preoperative studies in 88.6% of patients, with a range of 78%–100%. The major risk of the surgery is visual loss that occurs in less than 5% of patients. Post-operative visual loss can be due to traumatic optic neuropathy, anterior ischemic optic neuropathy, orbital hemorrhage, retinal artery occlusions, outer retinal ischemia, and choroidal infarcts (Plotnik and Kosmorsky, 1993; Rizzo and Lessell, 1994). Other complications are ocular motility disorders, generally self-limited, and tonic pupils. Most with experience in treating this disease have observed that the risk of operative visual loss is less when patients are treated before they have substantial visual loss and when they are treated by an experienced surgeon.

Optic nerve sheath fenestration is preferred for the patient who has progressive visual loss with mild to moderate headaches. Approximately half of patients with optic nerve sheath fenestration obtain adequate headache control, although the procedure is not recommended for treating headache alone. Since improvement in papilledema may occur in the unoperated eye and fistula formation has been demonstrated, a proposed mechanism of action of fenestration is local decompression of the subarachnoid space (Keltner, 1988).Occasional failure of the fellow eye to improve and the asymmetry of papilledema may be explained by the resistance to CSF flow produced by compartmentalization of the subarachnoid space surrounding the optic nerve in some individuals (Killer, et al., 2007), The long-term mechanism of action of optic nerve sheath fenestration is unresolved but may involve closure by scarring of the subarachnoid space in the retro-laminar optic nerve or continuous function of the fistula (Smith and Orcutt, 1986).

Shunting Procedures Lumbar subarachnoid-peritoneal shunting and related procedures, such as ventriculo-peritoneal shunting, are definitive CSF pressure-lowering procedures. Shunts are generally very effective acutely, but the majority of patients will require one or more shunt revisions (Rosenberg et al., 1993; Eggenberger et al., 1996; Burgett et al., 1997; McGirt, et al., 2004). Shunt failure frequently occurs within a year of having the procedure performed (Eggenberger, et al., 1996). The common complications are shunt occlusion and intracranial hypotension. Shunt occlusion can be accompanied by severe visual loss. Less common complications are back pain, abdominal pain, disc space infection, meningitis, disconnected tubing, and descent of the cerebellar tonsils. In one large series, lumboperitoneal shunts tended to require revision more frequently than ventriculoperitoneal shunts for shunt obstruction (McGirt, et al., 2004). Since approximately half of patients are successfully treated with a single shunt procedure, it is a viable treatment for this disease in selected patients.

Venous Sinus Stenting A case series of approximately 30 patients suggest that transverse sinus stenting with or without thrombolytic therapy may be helpful in some patients (Higgins, et al., 2003; Owler, et al., 2005). The results are inconsistent and the procedure needs further study before recommending it for routine usage. Complications of stenting include headache, transient hearing loss, transient unsteadiness, and one life-threatening acute subdural hematoma. The subdural hematoma developed during venography and stenting in a patient who also had an optic nerve sheath fenestration and external ventricular drainage. Venous re-stenosis has also occurred.

Treatment Recommendations

Patients should be educated about IIH, with an explanation of the risk of blindness as a potential outcome. A treatment decision algorithm that uses changes in visual function to determine the type of intervention is recommended (Fig. 18–4). Since symptoms and the degree of papilledema may not correlate well with loss of visual function in individual patients, treatment decisions should be based primarily on the results of perimetry.

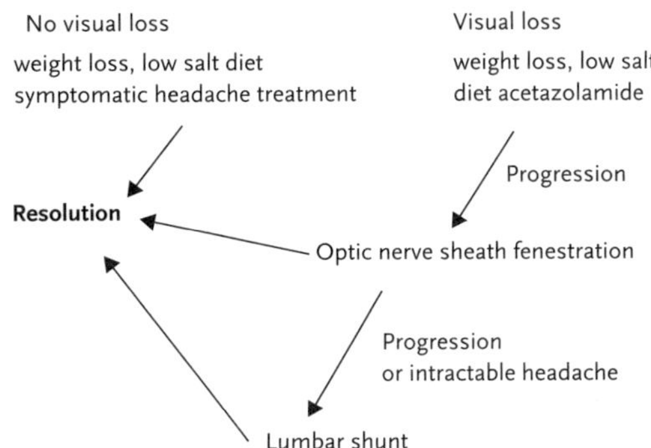

Figure 18–4 Treatment algorithm for IIH. Decisions are made for IIH therapy mainly on the results of perimetry.
Note: visual loss does not include enlargement of the blind spot unless it is compromising vision. Optic nerve sheath fenestration is preferred over steroids. (Reprinted from Wall, 1991 with permission.)

Details of treatment are beyond the scope of this monograph and can be found in other sources (Wall, 1991; Chou and Digre, 1999; Friedman, 2004). In summary, weight loss is strongly encouraged for long-term management of obese patients. The patient is asked to follow a low salt diet and avoid excessive fluid intake. A goal of 1 pound a week of weight loss for 2 months is set. This modest amount, usually approximately 5% of total body weight, may be adequate to control the disease. If visual field loss is present, acetazolamide or secondarily furosemide is used. If there is significant acuity loss at presentation, or if patients lose vision despite full medical therapy, optic nerve sheath fenestration or shunting is recommended.

If refractory headache is the main symptom, symptomatic therapy is given. Caffeine and frequent analgesic use are eliminated. If incapacitating headache remains, a shunt may be considered. However, many patients continue to experience headaches after their papilledema resolves and their ICP normalizes; they should be managed medically (Friedman and Rausch, 2002). Treatment of IIH is multifactorial and can be complex. Patients who do not respond to standard therapeutic regimens should be referred to physicians with experience treating the disease.

HEADACHES ASSOCIATED WITH COUGHING, EXERTION, AND SEXUAL ACTIVITY

Maneuvers that transiently increase ICP and intra-abdominal pressure may aggravate any type of headache, and occasionally produce headache (Williams, 1976; Van den Bergh, et al., 1987). Transient, severe head pain upon coughing, sneezing, weight lifting, bending, straining at stool, or stooping defines cough headache. Originally described by Tinel (1932b) as *"la céphalée à l'effort"* and later by Symonds (1956), cough headache mainly affects middle-aged men. It runs its course over a few years, and is uncommon: only 93 diagnoses were made at the Mayo Clinic over a 14-year period by Rooke (1968). He proposed the broader term benign exertional headache for any headache that is precipitated by exertion, has an acute onset, and is unassociated with structural central nervous system disease, thus combining cough and exertional headache. In a population-based study (Rasmussen et al., 1991), benign cough headache and benign exertional headache each had a prevalence of approximately 1%.

These nonvascular headache disorders comprise an interesting array of symptoms and diagnostic challenges. They should be considered when patients with headache do not fit the prototypes for the common headache syndromes, such as migraine and tension-type headaches. They represent an important group to recognize, since their treatments are so varied. The most recent classification of these disorders was done by IHS (Headache Classification Committee of the International Headache Society, 2004) (Tables 18–8 and 18–9). The IHS separates primary cough headache and primary exertional headache, since these entities have different clinical features, diagnostic evaluations, and treatment responses (Sands et al., 1991; Pascual et al., 1996). *It is important to exclude an intracranial abnormality in any patient experiencing any of these headache types.*

Primary cough headache. Primary cough headache is infrequent. The mean age of onset is 55, with a range of 19–78 years. It is twice as common in patients more than 40 years of age and is four times more common in men than in women (Rooke, 1968; Pascual, et al., 1996). The pain begins immediately (Symonds, 1956; Nick, 1980a) or within seconds after coughing, sneezing, or a Valsalva maneuver (lifting, straining at stool, blowing, crying, or singing) (Tinel, 1932a; Tinel, 1932b; Cutrer and Boes, 2004). The pain is severe in intensity, with a bursting, explosive, or splitting quality that lasts a few seconds or minutes. The headache is usually bilateral, with maximal pain at the vertex or in the occipital, frontal, or temporal region. Bending the head or lying down may be impossible (Mathew, 1981). The headache is not generally associated with nausea, vomiting, ptosis, lacrimation, conjunctival injection, nasal congestion or rhinorrhea, and the neurological examination is usually normal. Vomiting suggests an organic basis for the headache (Sands et al., 1991). As many as 25% of patients experience the onset of symptoms with a respiratory infection (Symonds, 1956; Rooke, 1968; Raskin, 1988). Most patients are pain-free between attacks of head pain, but in some cases the paroxysms are followed by dull, aching pain that may persist for hours; 5 of the 21 patients reported by Symonds (1956) had such additional headaches. As these patients often express their complaint as a continuous headache, they should be asked directly about the role of exertion as a trigger factor. Morphometric magnetic resonance imaging (MRI)

Table 18–8 Primary Cough Headache.

Headache precipitated by coughing or straining in the absence of any intracranial disorders
A. Sudden onset, lasting from 1 s to 30 min
B. Brought on by and occurring only in association with coughing, straining, and/or Valsalva maneuver
C. Not attributed to another disorder

May be diagnosed only after structural lesions such as posterior fossa tumor have been excluded by neuroimaging.

Table 18–9 Primary Exertional Headache.

A. Pulsating headache fulfilling criteria B and C
B. Lasting from 5 minutes to 48 hours
C. Brought on by and occurring only during or after physical exertion
D. Not attributed to another disorder

This headache commonly occurs in hot weather or high altitude.

studies showed a crowded posterior fossa in patients with primary cough headache with a lower cerebellar tonsillar tip, a shorter clivus and shorter distances from the clivus to the mid-pons and basion to the medulla than age- and sex-matched controls. The architecture of their posterior fossa may explain their predisposition for such headaches (Chen et al., 2004).

Secondary cough headache. Age at onset is significantly lower for secondary cough headache than for primary cough headache. Pascual et al. (1996) found that secondary cough headache could be precipitated by laughing, weight lifting, or acute body or head postural changes in addition to coughing. Secondary cough headache has been described with hindbrain abnormalities (i.e., Chiari malformation, platybasia), intracranial hypotension, middle and posterior fossa meningioma, midbrain cysts, basilar impression, acoustic neurinoma, unruptured posterior communicating artery aneurysm, and other brain tumors (Symonds, 1956; Rushton and Rooke, 1962; Raskin, 1978; Williams, 1980). In Pascual's series (1996), headache was the only symptom, at first, of Chiari Type I malformation in three patients; however, all patients had or eventually developed posterior fossa signs or syringomyelia. Besides beginning earlier in life than primary cough headache, secondary cough headache does not respond to indomethacin. If a patient does not respond to indomethacin, has posterior fossa signs, or is younger than 50, MRI examination with contrast-enhancement is obligatory.

Cough headache can be confused with other disorders, such as primary exertional headache, migraine precipitated by exertion, primary headache associated with sexual activity and primary thunderclap headache (Ekbom, 1986; Raskin, 1988). In fact, 40% of patients with the explosive type of primary headache associated with activity had exertional headache, suggesting a relationship between these entities (Silbert et al., 1991).

Treatment of Primary Cough Headache

Primary cough headache is almost universally responsive to indomethacin at doses of 50–250 mg daily (Mathew, 1981; Raskin, 1995). Concommitant treatment with a proton-pump inhibitor is recommended. Acetazolamide may be used if indomethacin is ineffective (Wang, et al., 2000). There are isolated cases reports of improvement with naproxen, ergonovine, intravenous dihydroergotamine, phenelzine, or naproxen in otherwise refractory patients. Therapeutic LP is occasionally helpful (Raskin, 1995) (Table 18–10).

Primary exertional headache. Primary exertional headache begins significantly earlier than benign cough headache ($p < 0.005$), by almost 40 years. It is typically throbbing, lasts from 5 minutes to 48 hours, and is provoked by physical exercise. The pain usually begins during exertion, is nonexplosive, and can be either bilateral or unilateral.

Secondary exertional headache. Secondary exertional headache is usually explosive in onset, severe, and bilateral. Twelve of Pascual et al's (1996) patients presented because of acute headache that coincided with physical exercise. Structural or vascular etiologies included subarachnoid hemorrhage, sinusitis, and brain mass.

Of the 219 cases of exertional and cough headache reviewed by Sands et al. (1991), 48 had an identifiable organic etiology (Table 18–11). Sands et al. (1991) summarizes cases of cough and exertional headache, grouping together etiologically related cases from several selected series. The group with posterior fossa space-occupying lesions includes cases with Chiari malformations and hindbrain herniation. Posttraumatic and postcraniotomy cases were also grouped together. From his review one cannot accurately estimate how many patients with exertional headache have structural disease (Tinel, 1932b; Symonds, 1956; Rooke, 1968; Nick, 1980b; Williams, 1980; Mathew, 1981; Ekbom, 1986; Ibbotson, 1987;

TABLE 18–10 Exertional, Cough, and Sex Headaches.

	Cough headache		*Exertional headache*		*Sexual headache*	
	Benign	*Symptomatic*	*Benign*	*Symptomatic*	*Benign*	*Symptomatic*
Number	13	17	16	12	13	1
Age, range	67 ± 11, 44–81	39 ± 14, 15–63	24 ± 11, 10–48	42 ± 14, 18–61	41 ± 9, 24–57	60
Sex (% men)	77%	59%	88%	43%	85%	100%
Duration	Seconds–30 minutes	Seconds–days	Minutes–2 days	1 day–1 month	1 minute–3 hours	10 days
Bilateral localization	92%	94%	56%	100%	77%	Yes
Quality	Sharp; stabbing	Bursting; stabbing	Pulsating	Explosive; pulsating	Explosive + pulsating	Explosive + pulsating
Other manifestations	No	Posterior fossa signs	Nausea, photophobia	Nausea, vomiting, double vision, neck rigidity	None	Vomiting, neck rigidity
Diagnosis	Idiopathic	Chiari Type I malformation	Idiopathic	SAH, sinusitis, brain metastases	Idiopathic	SAH

Source: Modified from Pascual et al. (1996).

Table 18–11 Etiologies for Cough and Exertional Headache in Literature.

Structural (organic)	48
Posterior fossa space-occupying lesions	18 (37.5%)
After trauma or after craniotomy	13 (27.0%)
Supratentorial space-occupying lesions	9 (18.7%)
Basilar impression/platybasia	6 (12.5%)
Syrinx	2 (4.2%)
Benign exertional headache	171
Total	219

Nightingale and Williams, 1987; Silbert et al., 1991). Exertional headache may also herald a pheochromocytoma (Paulson, et al., 1979).

Treatment of Primary Exertional Headache

Once a secondary cause is excluded, the treatment of primary exertional headache is prophylactic. Indomethacin is the medication of choice, in doses sometimes exceeding those required for primary cough headache. Propranolol, naproxen, phenelzine, and ergonovine may be effective in some patients (Cutrer and Boes, 2004).

PRIMARY HEADACHE ASSOCIATED WITH SEXUAL ACTIVITY

This headache type is precipitated by sexual activity, usually starting as a dull bilateral ache as sexual excitement increases and suddenly becoming intense at orgasm. A secondary cause must be excluded, as the differential diagnosis includes subarachnoid hemorrhage, stroke, meningitis, encephalitis, and referred cardiac pain from a myocardial infarction. Primary headache associated with sexual activity is separated into pre-orgasmic and orgasmic types. It begins later in life than primary exertional headache and earlier than primary cough headache (Table 18–12).

Pre-orgasmic headache. Pre-orgasmic headache (previously termed "dull type" or Type 1) is characterized by a dull ache in the head and neck associated with awareness of neck and/or jaw muscle contraction. It occurs during sexual activity and increases with sexual excitement (Cutrer and Boes, 2004). It is generally bilateral and occipital, and pressure-like. It is occasionally unilateral.

Orgasmic headache. Orgasmic headache (previously termed "explosive type" or Type 2) is severe and explosive with occasional throbbing and stabbing. It occurs at orgasm. The duration varies, lasting from less than 1 min to 3 h (average a half an hour). Up to one third of patients have similar episodes with other types of physical exertion.

Secondary headache associated with sexual activity. Explosive headache that occurs during coitus is usually symptomatic of a subarachnoid hemorrhage. Rooke (1968) followed 103 patients who had exertional headache but no detectable intracranial disease on initial examination. After 3 or more years of follow-up, 10 patients subsequently developed organic intracranial lesions. Thirty of the remaining ninety-three had complete headache relief within 5 years. The remainder

Table 18–12 Primary Headache Associated with Sexual Activity.

Pre-orgasmic Headache

A. Dull ache in the head and neck associated with awareness of neck and/or jaw muscle contraction and fulfilling criterion B
B. Occurs during sexual activity and increases with sexual excitement
C. Not attributed to another disorder

Orgasmic Headache

A. Sudden, severe ("explosive") headache fulfilling criterion B
B. Occurs at orgasm
C. Not attributed to another disorder

improved or were headache-free after 10 years. This pre-CT era study emphasizes the importance of careful evaluation for organic disease.

Treatment of Primary Headache Associated with Sexual Activity

Effective treatments for this headache type include propranolol (40–200 mg daily), indomethacin (25–225 mg daily), or Bellergal (Cutrer and Boes, 2004). Decreasing the intensity of sexual activity was suggested in one report (Paulson and Klawans, 1974).

References

Acheson, JF, Green, WT, and Sanders, MD (1994). Optic nerve sheath decompression for the treatment of visual failure in chronic raised intracranial pressure. *J Neurol Neurosurg Psychiatr*, 57:1426–1429.

Amaral, JF, Tsiaris, W, Morgan, T, et al. (1987). Reversal of benign intracranial hypertension by surgically induced weight loss. *Arch Surg*, 122:946–949.

Boiardi, A, Salmaggi, A, Eoli, M, et al. (2004). Headache in brain tumours: A symptom to reappraise critically. *Neurol Sci*, 25:S143–S147.

Britt, RH (1985). Brain abscess. In *Neurosurgery*, (RH Wilkins and SS Rengachary, eds), pp. 1928–1956. McGraw Hill, New York.

Buhrley, LE and Reed, DJ (1972). The effect of furosemide on sodium-22 uptake into cerebrospinal fluid and brain. *Exp Brain Res*, 14:503–510.

Burgett, RA, Purvin, VA, and Kawasaki, A (1997). Lumboperitoneal shunting for pseudotumor cerebri. *Neurology*, 49:734–739.

Chen, YY, Lirng, JF, Fuh, JL, et al. (2004). Primary cough headache is associated with posterior fossa crowdedness: A morphometric MRI study. *Cephalalgia*, 24:694–699.

Childhood Brain Tumor Consortium (1991). The epidemiology of headache among children with brain tumor: Headache in children with brain tumors. *J Neurooncol*, 10:31–46.

Chou, SY and Digre, KB (1999). Neuroophthalmic complications of raised intracranial pressure, hydrocephalus, and shunt malfunction. *Neurosurg Clin N Am*, 10:587–608.

Corbett, JJ (1983). Problems in the diagnosis and treatment of pseudotumor cerebri. The 1982 Silversides Lecture. *Can J Neurol Sci*, 10:221–229.

Corbett JJ and Digre, KB (2002). Idiopathic intracranial hypertension. An answer to, "the chicken or the egg?" *Neurology*, 58:5–6.

Corbett, JJ and Mehta, MP (1983). Cerebrospinal fluid pressure in normal obese subjects and patients with pseudotumor cerebri. *Neurology*, 33:1386–1388.

Corbett, JJ and Mehta, MP (1988). Cerebrospinal fluid pressure in normal obese subjects and patients with pseudotumor cerebri. *Neurology*, 33:1386–1388.

Corbett, JJ, Nerad, JA, Tse, DT, et al. (1988). Results of optic nerve sheath fenestration for pseudotumor cerebri. The lateral orbitotomy approach. *Arch Ophthalmol*, 106:1391–1397.

Curry, WT Jr., Butler, WE, Barker, FG II (2005). Rapidly rising incidence of cerebrospinal fluid shunting procedures for idiopathic intracranial hypertension in the United States 1888–2002. *Neurosurgery*, 57:97–108.

Cutrer, FM and Boes, CJ (2004). Cough, exertional, and sex headaches. *Neurol Clin*, 22:133–149.

Digre, KB and Corbett, JJ (1988). Pseudotumor cerebri in men. *Arch Neurol*, 45:866–872.

Digre, KB and Corbett, JJ. (2001). Idiopathic intracranial hypertension (pseudotumor cerebri): A reappraisal. *Neurologist*, 7:2–67.

Durcan, FJ, Corbett, JJ, and Wall, M (1988). The incidence of pseudotumor cerebri: population studies in Iowa and Louisiana. *Arch Neurol*, 45:875–877.

Eggenberger, ER, Miller, NR, and Vitale, S (1996). Lumboperitoneal shunt for the treatment of pseudotumor cerebri. *Neurology*, 46:1524–1530.

Ekbom, K (1986). Cough headache. In *Headache (Handbook of clinical Neurology)* (PJ Vinkin, GW Bruyn, and HL Klawans, eds), pp. 67–371. Elsevier Science Publishing, New York.

Farb, RI, Vanek, I, Scott, JN, et al. (2003). Idiopathic intracranial hypertension. The prevalence and morphology of sinovenous stenosis. *Neurology*, 60:1418–1424.

Fay, T (1940). A new test for the diagnosis of certain headaches; the cephalogram. *Dis Nerv Syst*, 1:312–315.

Fishman, RA (1992). *Cerebrospinal Fluid in Diseases of the Nervous System*. W.B. Saunders Company, Philadelphia.

Forsyth, PA and Posner, JB (1993). Headaches in patients with brain tumors. A study of 111 patients. *Neurology*, 43:1678–1683.

Freemont-Smith, F and Kubie, L (1929). Relation of vascular hydrostatic pressure and osmotic pressure to cerebrospinal fluid pressure. *Assoc Res Nerv Dis Proc*, 8:154.

Friedman, DI (2004). Pseudotumor cerebri. *Neurologic Clin N Am*, 22:99–131.

Friedman, DI, Forman, S, Levi, L, et al. (1998). Unusual ocular motility disturbances with increased intracranial pressure. *Neurology*, 50:1893–1896.

Friedman, DI and Jacobson, DM (2002). Diagnostic criteria for idiopathic intracranial hypertension. *Neurology*, 59:1492–1495.

Friedman, DI and Rausch, EA (2002). Headache diagnoses in patients with treated idiopathic intracranial hypertension. *Neurology*, 58:1551–1553.

Friedman, DI and Streeten, DH (1998). Idiopathic intracranial hypertension and orthostatic edema may share a common pathogenesis. *Neurology*, 50:1099–1104.

Galvin, JA and VanStavern, GP (2004). Clinical characterization of idiopathic intracranial hypertension at the Detroit Medical Center. *J Neurol Sci*, 223:157–160.

Gamache, FW, Patterson, RH, and Alksne, JF (1987). Headache associated with changes in intracranial pressure. In *Wolff's Headache and Other Head Pain* (DJ Dalessio, ed.), pp. 352–355. Oxford University Press, New York.

Garrett, JH, Corbett, JJ, and Braswell, R (2004). The incidence of idiopathic intracranial hypertension in Mississippi. Orlando, Florida. North American Neuro-Ophthalmology Society: 86.

Giuseffi, V, Wall, M, Siegal, PZ, et al. (1991). Symptoms and disease associations in idiopathic intracranial hypertension (pseudotumor cerebri): A case control study. *Neurology*, 41:239–244.

Goh, KY, Schatz, NJ, and Glaser, JS (1997). Optic nerve sheath fenestration for pseudotumor cerebri. *J Neuroophthalmol*, 17:86–91.

Greenberg, HS, Deck, MD, Vikram, B, et al. (1981). Metastasis to the base of the skull: clinical findings in 43 patients. *Neurology*, 31:530–537.

Greer, M (1965). Benign intracranial hypertension. VI: Obesity. *Neurology*, 15:382–388.

Gucer, G and Vierenstein, L (1978). Long-term intracranial pressure recording in management of pseudotumor cerebri. *J Neurosurg*, 49:256–263.

Hayreh, SS (1977). Optic disc edema in raised intracranial pressure. V: Pathogenesis. *Arch Ophthalmol*, 95:1553–1565.

Headache Classification Committee of the International Headache Society (2004). The International Classification of Headache Disorders, 2nd edition. *Cephalalgia*, 24(Suppl 1):1–160.

Heyck, H (1968). Examinations and differential diagnosis of headache. In *Headaches and Cranial Neuralgias* (PJ Vinken and GW Bruyn, eds), pp. 25–36. John Wiley & Sons, New York.

Higgins, JNP, Cousins, C, Owler, BK, et al. (2003). Idiopathic intracranial hypertension: 12 cases treated by venous sinus stenting. *J Neurol Neurosurg Psychiatry*, 74:1662–1666.

Honig, PJ and Charney, EB (1982). Children with brain tumor headaches. *Am J Dis Child*, 136:121–124.

Huna-Baron, R, Laudau, K, Rosenberg, M, et al. (2001). Unilateral swollen disc due to increased intrancranial pressure. *Neurology*, 56:1588–1590.

Ibbotson, S (1987). Weight-lifter's headache. *Br J Sports Med*, 21:138.

Ireland, B, Corbett, JJ, and Wallace, RB (1990). The search for causes of idiopathic intracranial hypertension: A preliminary case-control study. *Arch Neurol*, 47:315.

Jacobs, DA, Corbett, JJ, and Balcer, LJ (2004). Annual incidence of idiopathic intracranial hypertension (IIH) in the Philadephia area. Orlando, Florida. North American Neuro-Ophthalmology Society: 286

Jaeckle, KA (1991). Clinical presentations and therapy of nervous system tumors. In *Neurology in Clinical Practice* (WG Bradley, RB Daroff, GM Fenichel, et al., eds), pp. 1008–1030. Butterworth-Heinemann, Boston.

Jaeckle, KA (1993). Causes and management of headaches in cancer patients. *Oncology*, 7:27–31.

Johnson, LN, Krohel, GB, Madsen, RW, et al. (1998). The role of weight loss and acetazolamide in the treatment of idiopathic intracranial hypertension (pseudotumor cerebri). *Ophthalmol*, 105:2313–2317.

Johnston, I, Hawke, S, Kalmagyi, M, et al. (1991). The pseudotumor syndrome. *Arch Neurol*, 48:740–747.

Johnston, I and Paterson, A (1974). Benign intracranial hypertension II. CSF pressure and circulation. *Brain*, 97:301–312.

Johnson, M, Zakharov, A, Papaiconomou, C, et al. (2004). Evidence of connections between cerebrospinal fluid and nasal lymphatic vessels in humans, non-human primates and other mammalian species. *Cerebrospinal Fluid Res*, 1:1–13.

Jones, JS, Neavi, J, Freeman, MP, et al. (1999). Emergency department presentation of idiopathic intracranial hypertension. *Am J Emerg Med*, 17:517–521.

Kelman, SE, Heaps, R, Wolf, A, et al. (1992). Optic nerve decompression surgery improves visual function in patients with pseudotumor cerebri. *Neurosurg*, 1992:3–391.

Keltner, J (1988). Optic nerve sheath decompression: how does it work? Has its time come? *Arch Ophthalmol*, 106:1378–1383.

Killer, HE, Jaggi, GP, Flammer, J, et al. (2007). Cerebrospinal fluid dynamics between the intracranial and the subarachnoid space of optic nerve. Is it always bidirectional? *Brain*, 130:514–520.

King, JO, Mitchell, PJ, Thomson, KR, et al. (1995). Cerebral venography and manometry in idiopathic intracranial hypertension. *Neurology*, 45:2224–2228.

King, JO, Mitchell, PJ, Thomson, KR, et al. (2002). Manometry combined with cervical puncture in idiopathic intracranial hypertension. *Neurology*, 58:26–30.

Kunkle, EC, Bronson, SR, and Wolff, HG (1942). Studies on headache: the mechanisms and significance of the headache associated with brain tumor. *Bull NY Acad Med*, 18:400–422.

Kunkle, EC, Pfeiffer, JB, Wilholt, WM, et al. (1942). Recurrent brief headache in "cluster" pattern. *Trans Am Neurol Assoc*, 77:240–243.

Kupersmith, MJ, Gamell, L, Turbin, R, et al. (1998). Effects of weight loss on the course of idiopathic intracranial hypertension in women. *Neurology*, 50:1094–1098.

Lavyne, MH and Patterson, RH (1987). Headache and brain tumor. In *Wolff's Headache and Other Head Pain*, (DJ Dalessio, ed.), pp. 343–349. Oxford University Press, New York.

Lessell, S (1992). Pediatric pseudotumor cerebri (idiopathic intracranial hypertension). *Surv Ophthalmol*, 37:155–166.

Loman, J (1934). Components of cerebrospinal fluid pressure as affected by changes in posture. *Arch Neurol Psychiatry*, 31:679–681.

Loman, J, Myerson, A, and Goldman, D (1935). Effects of alteration of posture on cerebrospinal fluid pressure. *Arch Neurol Psychiatry*, 33:1279–1284.

Malm, J, Kristensen, B, Markgren, P, et al. (1992). CSF hydrodynamics in idiopathic intracranial hypertension: a long-term study. *Neurology*, 42:851–858.

Marceliș, J and Silberstein, SD (1991). Idiopathic intracranial hypertension without papilledema. *Arch Neurol*, 48:392–399.

Mathew, NT (1981). Indomethacin responsive headache syndromes. *Headache*, 21:147–150.

McGirt, MJ, Woodworth, G, Thomas, G, et al. (2004). Cerebrospinal fluid shunt placement for pseudotumor cerebri associated intractable headache: predictors of treatment response and an analysis of long-term outcomes. *J Neurosurg*, 101:627–632.

McKissock, W (1960). Subdural hematoma. A review of 389 cases. *Lancet*, 1:1365–1370.

Milhorat, TH (1972). *Hydrocephalus and the Cerebrospinal Fluid*. Williams and Wilkins, Baltimore.

Morewood, GH (1993). A rational approach to the cause, prevention and treatment of postdural puncture headache. *Can Med Assoc J*, 148:1087–1093.

Neville, L and Egan, RA (2005). Frequency and amplitude of elevation of cerebrospinal fluid resting pressure by the Valsalva maneuver. *Can J Ophthalmol*, 40:775–777.

Newborg, B (1974). Pseudotumor cerebri treated by rice reduction diet. *Arch Inter Med*, 133:802–807.

Nick, J (1980a). A propos d'une série de 43 cas. *Sem Hop Paris*, 56:621–628.

Nick, J (1980b). La céphalée d'effort. A propos d'une série de 43 cases. *Sem Hop Paris*, 56:621–628.

Nightingale, S and Williams (1987). Hindbrain Hernia headache, *Lancet*, 1:731–734.

Northfield, DWC (1938). Some observations on headache. *Brain*, 77:240–243.

Orcutt, JC, Page, NG, and Sanders, MD (1984). Factors affecting visual loss in benign intracranial hypertension. *Ophthalmol*, 91:1303–1312.

Owler, BK, Parker, G, Halmagyi, GM, et al. (2005). Cranial venous outflow obstruction and pseudotumor cerebri syndrome. *Adv Tech Stand Neurosurg*, 30:108–174.

Pascual, J, Igessias, F, Oterino, A, et al. (1996). Cough, exertional, and sexual headaches: An analysis of 72 benign and symptomatic cases. *Neurology*, 46:1520–1524.

Paulson, GW and Klawans, HL (1974). Benign orgasmic cephalgia. *Headache*, 13:181–187.

Paulson, GW, Zipf, RE, and Beekman, JF (1979). Pheochromocytoma causing exercise-related headache and pulmonary edema. *Ann Neurol*, 5:96–99.

Plotnik, JL and Kosmorsky, GS (1993). Operative complications of optic nerve sheath decompression. *Ophthalmol*, 100:683–690.

Powell, B (1982). Weight lifter's cephalalgia. *Ann Emerg Med*, 11:449–451.

Radhkrishnan, K, Ahlskog, JE, Cross, SA, et al. (1993). Idiopathic intracranial hypertension (pseudotumor cerebri). Descriptive epidemiology in Rochester, Minnesota, 1976 to 1990. *Arch Neurol*, 50:78–80.

Raskin, N (1978). Headaches associated with organic diseases of the nervous system. *Med Clin N Amer*, 62:459–466.

Raskin, NH (1988). The indomethacin-responsive syndromes. In *Headache*, (NH Raskin, ed.), pp. 255–268. Churchill Livingstone, New York.

Raskin, NH (1995). The cough headache syndrome: treatment. *Neurology*, 45:1784.

Rasmussen, BK, Jensen, R, Schroll, M, et al. (1991). Epidemiology of headache in a general population-a prevalence study. *J Clin Epidemiol*, 44:1147–1157.

Ray, BS and Wolff, HG (1940). Experimental studies on headache. Pain sensitive structures of the head and their significance in headache. *Arch Surg*, 41:813–856.

Rizzo, JF and Lessell, S (1994). Choroidal infarction after optic nerve sheath fenestration. *Opthalmol*, 101:1622–1626.

Roberts, PA, Pollay, M, Engles, C, et al. (1987). Effect on intracranial pressure of furosemide combined with varying doses and administration rates of mannitol. *J Neurosurg*, 66:440–446.

Rooke, ED (1968). Benign exertional headache. *Med Clin N Amer*, 52:801–808.

Rosenberg, ML, Corbett, JJ, Smith, C, et al. (1993). Cerebrospinal fluid diversion procedures in pseudotumor cerebri. *Neurology*, 43:1071–1072.

Round, R and Keane, JR (1988). The minor symptoms of increased intracranial pressure: 101 patients with benign intracranial hypertension. *Neurology*, 38:1461–1464.

Rush, JA (1980). Pseudotumor cerebri: clinical profile and visual outcome in 63 patients. *Mayo Clin Proc*, 55:541–546.

Rushton, JG and Rooke, ED (1962). Brain tumor headache. *Headache*, 2:147–152.

Sadun, AA, Currie, JN, and Lessell, S (1984). Transient visual obscurations with elevated optic discs. *Ann Neurol*, 16:489–494.

Sahs, AL and Joynt, RJ (1956). Brain swelling of unknown cause. *Neurology*, 6:791–803.

Sands, GH, Newman, L, and Lipton, R (1991). Cough, exertional, and other miscellaneous headaches. *Med Clin N Amer*, 75:733–746.

Schaltenbrand, G (1938). Neure Anschauen zor Pathophysiologie der Liquorzirkulation. *Zentralb Nforchir*, 3:290–300.

Schoeman, JF (1994). Childhood pseudotumor cerebri: clinical and intracranial pressure response to acetazolamide and furosemide treatment in a case series. *J Child Neurol*, 9:130–134.

Sergott, RC, Savino, PJ, and Bosley, TM (1988). Modified optic nerve sheath decompression provides long-term visual improvement for pseudotumor cerebri. *Arch Ophthalmol*, 106:1384–1390.

Shuper, A, Packer, RJ, and Vezina, LG (1995). Complicated migraine-like episodes in children following cranial irradiation and chemotherapy. *Neurology*, 45:1837–1840.

Silberstein, SD and Corbett, JJ (1993). The forgotten lumbar puncture. *Cephalalgia*, 13:212–213.

Silbert, PL, Edis, RH, Stewart-Wynne, EG et al. (1991). Benign vascular sexual headache and exertional headache: interrelationships and long term prognosis. *J Neurol, Neurosurg, Psychiatry*, 54:417–421.

Sismanis, A (1987). Otologic manifestations of benign intracranial hypertension syndrome: diagnosis and management. *Laryngoscope*, 97:1–17.

Smith, CH and Orcutt, JC (1986). Surgical treatment of pseudotumor cerebri. *Int Ophthalmol Clin*, 26:265–275.

Spence, JD, Amacher, AL, and Willis, NR (1980). Benign intracranial hypertension without papilledema: role of 24 hour cerebrospinal fluid pressure monitoring in diagnosis and management. *Neurosurgery*, 7:326–336.

Stiebel-Kalish, H, Kalish, Y, Lusky, M, et al. (2006). Puberty as a risk factor for less favorable visual outcome in idiopathic intracranial hypertension. *Am J Ophthalmol*, 142(2):279–283.

Sugerman, HJ, Felton, WL, Sismanis, A, et al. (1999). Gastric surgery for pseudotumor cerebri associated with severe obesity. *Ann Surg*, 229:634–640.

Symonds, C (1956). Cough headache. *Brain*, 79:557–568.

Tinel, J (1932a). La cephalee a l'effort. Syndrome de distension douloureuse des veines intracraniennes. *Medicine (Paris)*, 13:113–118.

Tinel, J (1932b). Un syndrome d'algie veineuse intracranienne. La cephalee a l'effort. *Prat Med Fr*, 13:113–119.

Van den Bergh, V, Amery, WK, and Waelkens, J (1987). Trigger factors in migraine: a study conducted by the Belgian migraine society. *Headache*, 27:191–196.

Vazquez-Barquero, A, Ibanez, FJ, and Herrera, S (1994). Isolated headache as the presenting clinical manifestation of intracranial tumor: A perspective study. *Cephalalgia*, 14:270–272.

VonStorch, T, Carmichael, A, and Banks, T (1937). Factors producing lumbar cerebrospinal fluid pressure in many in the erect position. *Arch Neurol Psychiatry*, 38:1158.

Wall, M (1990). The headache profile of idiopathic intracranial hypertension. *Cephalalgia*, 10:331–335.

Wall, M (1991). Idiopathic intracranial hypertension. *Neurol Clin*, 9:73–95.

Wall, M, Dollar, JD, Sadun, AA, et al. (1995). Idiopathic intracranial hypertension: lack of histologic evidence for cerebral edema. *Arch Neurol*, 52:141–145.

Wall, M and George, D (1991). Idiopathic intracranial hypertension: a prospective study of 50 patients. *Brain*, 114:155–180.

Wall, M and White, WN (1998). Asymmetric papilledema in idiopathic intracranial hypertension: prospective interocular comparison of sensory visual function. *Inv Ophthalmol Vis Sci*, 39:134–142.

Wang, SJ, Fuh, J-L, Lu, S-R (2000). Benign cough headache is responsive to acetazolamide. *Neurology*, 55:149–150.

Wang, SJ, Silberstein, SD, Patterson, S, et al. (1998). Idiopathic intracranial hypertension without papilledema: A case-control study in a headache center. *Neurology*, 51:245–249.

Williams, B (1976). Cerebrospinal fluid pressure changes in response to coughing. *Brain*, 99:331–346.

Williams, B (1980). Cough headache due to craniospinal pressure dissociation. *Arch Neurol*, 37:226–230.

Zulch, KJ, Mennel, HD, and Zimmerman, V (1974). Intracranial hypertension. In *Tumors of the Brain and Skull*, (PJ Vinken and GW Bruyn, eds), pp. 89–149. Elsevier, New York.

19 Headache Associated with Abnormalities in Intracranial Structure or Function: Low-cerebrospinal-fluid-pressure Headache

Bahram Mokri and Wouter I Schievink

Cerebrospinal fluid (CSF) is a circulating body fluid, sometimes referred to as the "third circulation" (Cushing, 1926). Most of the CSF is formed by the choroid plexus, which has structural and functional similarities to the distal and collecting tubules of the kidneys and maintains the compositional integrity of the CSF (Rowland et al., 1991). Only a minor portion of the CSF is secreted by the brain capillaries, entering the ventricular system through the ependyma. For many years, on the basis of data from autopsies, the CSF volume was estimated to be 150 ml. More recent volumetric studies based on magnetic resonance imaging (MRI) techniques suggest an average volume of approximately 210 ml in adults (Hogan et al., 1996; Matsumae et al., 1996). This, however, shows significant variation. Cranial CSF volume is smaller for women and for younger persons than for older persons, who have larger ventricular volumes and more generous CSF cisterns and subarachnoid spaces (Matsumae et al., 1996). Spinal CSF volume is significantly less in obese than nonobese persons (Hogan et al., 1996).

The rate of CSF formation is approximately 0.35 ml per minute, or approximately 500 ml per day. Therefore, the entire CSF volume is turned over a few times each day.

CSF is absorbed via the arachnoid villi into the cerebral venous sinuses and veins through a valve-like direct-flow mechanism termed "bulk flow" (Tripathi, 1973; Tripathi et al., 1974). Only a very minor portion of the CSF is absorbed thorough simple diffusion into the cerebral vessels.

Although increases or decreases in the rate of CSF formation have been obtained under experimental conditions in laboratory animals, human data are limited. In general, however, the rate of formation of CSF in humans is relatively constant (Fishman, 1992). There is no solid evidence to indicate that increases in CSF formation sufficient to cause intracranial hypertension occurs in any condition other than choroid plexus papilloma. The effect of increased CSF pressure (hydrocephalus, or increased intracranial pressure) on CSF formation is complex. The rate of CSF formation under these conditions can likely be reduced if the intraventricular pressure is increased to a sufficient degree for a sufficient duration (Welch, 1975), although the critical limits of pressure and duration in these situations are not clearly defined.

In the horizontal position, the lumbar, cisternal, and presumably the intracranial or vertex CSF pressures are equal, approximately 60–180 mm H_2O. In the erect posture, these pressures diverge and the vertex pressure becomes negative.

The relationship between CSF pressure and volume is exponential (Miller, 1975). In a study of induction of headache by CSF drainage in subjects in the erect posture, headache was regularly induced when 10% of the estimated total volume of the CSF was withdrawn (Kunkle et al., 1943). This caused a decrease of more than 40% in already negative vertex CSF pressure.

HISTORICAL ASPECTS

The ventricular system of the brain and its contents have been sources of curiosity for centuries

(Lyons et al., 1990). Galen, a second century Greek physician and teacher, described a gas-like "spiritus animalis," or vital spirit, filling the cerebral ventricles. This concept survived for many centuries. When Vesalius, an anatomist in Padua in the sixteenth century, described fluid within the ventricles, he was not believed. Even as late as the early nineteenth century, Romberg thought that brain cavities were filled with "humid gas." It was Francois Magendie, a French physiologist, who, in the nineteenth century, convinced others of the presence of CSF.

Lumbar puncture was introduced in the nineteenth century by Quincke (Silberstein et al., 1992). Bier experienced headaches after lumbar puncture and was the first to report them (Raskin, 1990).

Schaltenbrand, a German neurologist, in an article in German in 1938 and an article in English in 1953, emphasized two terms: "liquorrhea" and "aliquorrhea." *Liquorrhea*, a condition mimicking brain tumor, involves headaches and papilledema. This later came to be known as pseudotumor cerebri and has not been shown to be due to excess CSF production. *Aliquorrhea* is a condition associated with very low, unobtainable, or even negative CSF pressures and clinically manifested by orthostatic headache and other features that are now recognized as the clinical picture of intracranial hypotension. Recent evidence fails to show decreased CSF production, or aliquorrhea, in this condition; instead, a CSF leak is present. Before Schaltenbrand's descriptions, this syndrome had been described in the French literature as "hypotension of spinal fluid" or "ventricular collapse" (Schaltenbrand, 1953). Schaltenbrand continued to think that the cause of the syndrome was decreased CSF production; even when he discussed the appearance of the same syndrome after lumbar puncture, he speculated that lumbar puncture caused a decrease in CSF pressure and, thus, exerted a strong stimulus to the choroid plexus, causing a sudden cessation of CSF production (Schaltenbrand, 1953). He did not consider CSF leak as the cause of the clinical symptoms, including orthostatic headache. As addressed by Fishman (1992), the technology of the time would not have allowed him or his contemporaries to assess patients adequately for CSF leak.

In the United States, as early as 1940, Woltman, at the Mayo Clinic, wrote about "headaches associated with decreased intracranial pressure," stating that "occasionally an occipital or frontal headache comes on only when the patient is up and about and leaves when the patient lies down. Such a headache is often associated with low pressure of the spinal fluid. Thus, it resembles postpuncture headache."

From the 1960s to early 1990s, several publications described the clinical manifestations of the syndrome of intracranial hypotension, or CSF leak (Bell et al., 1960; Huber, 1970; Lasater, 1970; Baker, 1983; Marcelis et al., 1990; Rando et al., 1992). Furthermore, with introduction of radioisotope cisternography (Front et al., 1974; Labadie et al., 1976; Murros et al., 1983; Molins et al., 1990; Weber et al., 1991) and water-soluble myelography and computed tomography (CT)-myelography, clinicians were provided with more effective tools to discover CSF leaks.

In the early 1990s, the MRI features of intracranial hypotension and CSF leaks were recognized (Mokri et al., 1991; Sable et al., 1991; Hochman et al., 1992; Fishman and Dillon, 1993; Pannullo et al., 1993). MRI of the head and spine has revolutionized the knowledge regarding this disorder, broadened the clinical and imaging spectrum of the syndrome (Mokri, 1999), and led to detection of far more cases than was previously recognized. Many experienced clinicians have evaluated more cases of intracranial hypotension, or CSF leak, in the past decade than they had throughout all the previous years. There is little doubt that the diagnosis was missed in many patients before the advent of MRI. Some of the patients improved spontaneously, whereas others had to live with a substantially compromised quality of life and sought care from various specialists or chronic pain-management facilities.

ETIOLOGY

Systemic conditions that cause a true hypovolemic state, or reduced total body water, also can lead to decreased CSF volume. Shunt overdrainage (Table 19–1), a complication not uncommon in the practice of neurosurgery and neurology, can

TABLE 19–1 Etiology of cerebrospinal fluid (CSF) volume depletion.

A. True hypovolemic state (reduced total body water)
B. CSF shunt overdrainage
C. CSF leaks
  1. Traumatic
    a. After definite trauma (e.g., sports, motor vehicle accidents)
    b. After surgical procedure
    c. After lumbar puncture
  2. Spontaneous
    a. Unknown cause (often)
    b. Meningeal diverticulae
    c. Weak, attenuated dura
    d. Connective tissue disorders (may also relate to b and c)
      (1) Marfan syndrome
      (2) Marfanoid features
      (3) Hyperflexible joints
      (4) Retinal detachment at young age
      (5) Elastin or fibrillin abnormalities
    e. Spondylitic-dural tear
    f. "Trivial" trauma

lead to orthostatic headaches and diffuse pachymeningeal gadolinium enhancement.

Traumatic causes of CSF leak, including head or spine trauma related to various accidents, cranial or spinal surgery, lumbar puncture, or inadvertent dural tear in connection with epidural catheterization are well recognized. Posttraumatic or postsurgical leaks may lead to frank CSF otorrhea or rhinorrhea.

Spontaneous CSF leaks are the most intriguing and the most common cause of spontaneous CSF volume depletion leading to orthostatic headache and diffuse pachymeningeal gadolinium enhancement. Although the spontaneous leak may occur at the level of the skull base, in the overwhelming majority of patients it occurs at the spinal level, particularly the thoracic spine or cervicothoracic junction.

The exact cause of so-called spontaneous CSF leaks will remain unknown in the majority of the patients. However, in a significant minority, two important contributory etiologic factors are frequently suspected: (1) weakness of the meningeal sac in certain regions and (2) trivial trauma. Meningeal diverticulae, sometimes multiple, are not uncommon. Furthermore, in some patients who have had surgery to stop the leak, patches of attenuated dura of various size have been noted. Spontaneous CSF leaks have been observed in heritable disorders of the connective tissue, such as Marfan syndrome (Davenport et al., 1995). Furthermore, some patients with spontaneous CSF leaks have stigmata of connective tissue disorders, such as hyperflexible joints, marfanoid features, or retinal detachment at a young age. Abnormalities of elastin or fibrillin or both are suspected in these patients (Mokri et al., 1997, 2002; Schriver et al., 2002). Occasional dural tears resulting from spondylotic spurs on disc herniation may lead to CSF leak (Vishteh et al., 1998; Eross et al., 2002; Winter et al., 2002). Many patients report a history of trivial trauma. In some, trivial trauma likely might have started a CSF leak in the presence of an abnormality of fibrillin or elastin and of weakened and attenuated dural zones or meningeal diverticulae.

Despite speculations in the older literature (Schaltenbrand, 1938; Schaltenbrand, 1953), there is very little evidence to indicate that CSF volume depletion is ever caused by increased CSF absorption or by decreased CSF formation (Mokri, 1999).

CLINICAL MANIFESTATIONS

Headache is the main clinical feature. It is typically an orthostatic headache that is present when the patient is upright and is relieved by recumbency. It may be throbbing, but often it is nonthrobbing. The location of the headache may be occipital, bifrontal, bifrontal–occipital, or holocephalic. The variability, however, is considerable. In some patients in the early or active stages of the disease, the headache is typically orthostatic, but with chronicity the orthostatic features may diminish and the headache may take the form of lingering chronic daily headache that is often, although not invariably, worse when the patient is upright and less pronounced with recumbency.

Sometimes the headache may start as a chronic lingering headache, and after days or a few weeks, typical orthostatic headaches develop. Other patients may start with intrascapular or posterior neck pain, which may or may not be orthostatic, and after several days, typical orthostatic headaches may develop.

Sometimes the headache may have a thunderclap onset (Schievink et al., 2001) and headaches often with orthostatic features may follow. Sometimes headaches may be only exertional (Mokri et al., 2002). Rarely the postural headache may be paradoxical (present in recumbency, relieved when upright) (Mokri et al., 2004). Sometimes a second-half-of-the-day headache is noted when the headache begins late in the morning or early afternoon after the patient has been up and active for a period of time (Mokri, 2005).

In intermittent CSF leaks, the headaches, with whatever features they might have, may appear and disappear for variable periods.

A small group of patients with CSF volume depletion, whether due to CSF shunt overdrainage or to CSF leak, may have no headaches at all (Mokri, 1999).

Associated Clinical Manifestations

Although headache, and typically orthostatic headache, is often the most prominent manifestation in many patients with CSF volume depletion, many have additional clinical manifestations (Table 19–2). Occasional patients may have an unusual clinical presentation, such as stupor and encephalopathy (Beck et al., 1998) or parkinsonism, ataxia, and bulbar weakness (Pakiam et al., 1999).

Mechanism of Clinical Manifestations

The headache of CSF volume depletion is a consequence of descent of the brain. By its buoyant effect, the CSF reduces the weight of the floating brain within the cranial cavity to less than 50 g. Even at this reduced weight, the brain must be supported within the cranium. Some of the weight is shared by suspension from above, mostly by the

TABLE 19–2 Clinical Manifestations Other Than Headache in Cerebrospinal Fluid Volume Depletion.

Headache
Pain or stiff feeling of neck (sometimes orthostatic)
Interscapular pain, less commonly low back pain
Nausea with or without emesis (often orthostatic)
Horizontal diplopia due to unilateral or bilateral sixth CN palsy (Horton et al., 1994)
Diplopia due to third CN and, rarely, fourth CN palsy or a combination of these or with sixth CN palsy (Brady-McCreery et al., 2002)
Change in hearing (echoed, distant, muffled)
Visual blurring
Photophobia
Upper limb numbness, paresthesias, aches
Facial numbness or weakness
Encephalopathy (Beck et al., 1998)
Stupor (Pleasure et al., 1998)
Coma (Evans et al., 2002)
Frontotemporal dementia (Hong et al., 2002)
Parkinsonism, ataxia, bulbar manifestations (Pakiam et al., 1999)
Galactorrhea (Yamamoto et al., 1993)
Meniere's disease-like syndrome (Portier et al., 2002)
Gait unsteadiness (Nowak et al., 2003)
Upper limb radiculopathy (Albayram et al., 2002)
Trouble with bowel and bladder control (Schievink et al., 1996)
Chorea (Mokri et al., 2006)
Encephalopathy (single case report) (Pakiam et al., 1999)

Abbreviation: CN, cranial nerve.

cerebral veins ending in the sagittal sinus and, to a lesser extent, by cerebellar veins ending in the transverse and straight sinuses. Cerebellar tentorium, large vessels of the base, and skull base provide support from below. Various anchoring structures of the brain are pain-sensitive, and pain can be provoked when these structures are subjected to traction or distortion (Fay, 1937). Sinking of the brain leads to traction or distortion of these structures and, therefore, to the appearance of orthostatic headache.

The same mechanism may be responsible for the cranial nerve palsies, visual blurring or visual field defects, or even dizziness or altered hearing, which is fairly common in affected patients. Another possible mechanism for the dizziness and altered hearing, however, may be an altered pressure in the perilymphatic fluid. Stupor, encephalopathy, cerebellar size, and parkinsonism may result from compression of the diencephalon, posterior fossae, and midline structures. Various clinical manifestations and their proposed mechanisms are listed in Table 19–3.

TABLE 19–3 Presumed Mechanisms of Clinical Manifestations in Cerebrospinal Fluid (CSF) Volume Depletion.

Headaches	Sinking of the brain, stretch, and distortion of the pain-sensitive suspending structures (Fay, 1937; Rando et al., 1992; Mokri et al., 1997; Mokri and Atkinson, 2000; Miyazawa et al., 2003). Engorgement of cerebral venous sinuses and large intracranial veins also a possible contributory factor
Dizziness and change in hearing, tinnitus	Stretching of the eighth nerve or pressure changes in the perilymphatic fluid of the inner ear (Mokri et al., 1997; Portier et al., 2002; Oshiro et al., 2003)
Cranial nerve palsies	Stretching or compression or the related cranial nerves (Ferrante et al., 1998; Follens et al., 2001; Brady-McCreery et al., 2002; Warner, 2002)
Visual blurring and visual field cuts	Compression or vacular congestion of the intracranial portion of the optic nerve (Horton et al., 1994)
Upper limb symptoms	Stretching of the cervical nerve roots or irritation of the nerve root by dilated epidural venous plexus (Mokri et al., 1997; Albayram et al., 2002; Mokri, 2004)
Encephalopathy, stupor, and coma	Diencephalic compression (Beck et al., 1998; Pleasure et al., 1998; Evans et al., 2002).
Frontotemporal dementia	Compression of frontal and temporal lobes (Hong et al., 2002)
Cerebellar ataxia and parkinsonism and bulbar manifestations	Compression of posterior fossa and deep midline structures (Pakiam et al., 1999)
Gait disorder	Spinal cord venous congestion (Nowak et al., 2003), cord distortion, or deformation (Miyazawa et al., 1998; Wingerchuk et al., 2005)
Galactorrhea and increased prolactin	Distortion of the pituitary stalk (Yamamoto et al., 1993)
Chorea	Pressure or basal ganglia or their connections (Mokri et al., 2006)

Pain at different levels of the spine (cervical, thoracic, lumbar) is not uncommon. In some cases, it is tempting to use the level of the pain or the radicular symptoms as clinical indicators of the level of the leak. However, these "localizing signs" are accurate in only a small minority of patients and are "false-localizing signs" in the majority.

DIAGNOSIS

CSF Examination

The CSF opening pressure is typically very low (sometimes atmospheric or unmeasurable, very occasionally even negative). There is, however, considerable variability. In some patients, the pressure may be "low-normal," whereas some others, despite persistent symptomatic CSF leaks, may have opening CSF pressures that are consistently within the normal range (Mokri et al., 1998). Some patients with intermittent or variable leaks may have pressures that are sometimes very low, sometimes low-normal, and sometimes entirely normal.

Analysis of CSF typically reveals a clear and colorless fluid, but occasionally the fluid is xanthochromic. Some patients who have undergone multiple CSF examinations in a span of a few years have had xanthochromic fluid in some tests and clear fluid in most of them.

The CSF protein level may be normal or high. The variability is considerable. When increased, the protein concentration is often less than 100 mg/dl. However, not uncommonly, protein concentrations range from 100 to 200 mg/dl or more. Protein concentrations in the CSF have been reported to be as high as 1000 mg/dl (Mokri et al., 1997).

The CSF cell counts also show considerable variability. The CSF erythrocyte count may be normal or increased as high as several hundred. The CSF leukocyte count (typically lymphocytes) may be normal or increased. It is not unusual to find a pleocytosis with cell counts from 10 to 50/mm^3. Higher values are not rare, however, CSF pleocytosis with a cell count as high as 220/mm^3 in documented CSF leak without any evidence of meningeal infection or inflammation has been reported (Mokri et al., 1995, 1997).

Cytologic and microbiologic test results are always negative, and CSF glucose concentration is never low in proportion to plasma glucose concentration.

CT of the Head

CT of the brain is typically negative, though subdural fluid collections, increased tentorial enhancement, or small ventricular size may be seen (Pavlin et al., 1979; Sipe et al., 1981).

Because of brain sagging resulting in obliteration of the subarachnoid cisterns, head CT may occasionally be misinterpreted as showing an acute subarachnoid hemorrhage. (Schievink, Maya, and Moser, 2004)

Radioisotope Cisternography (Indium-111)

In CSF leaks, typically the radioactivity does not reach cerebral convexities, even at 24 or 48 hours. Focal extension of radioactivity beyond the dural sac may be noted, pointing to the level of the CSF leak (Fig. 19–1). Meningeal diverticula, if large enough, also may be detected by this test. Another important finding in CSF leaks is early appearance of radioactivity in the kidneys and urinary bladder within 4 hours, compared to the usual appearance between 6 and 24 hours. This finding should not be interpreted as a manifestation of increased reabsorption of the CSF causing intracranial hypotension (Molins et al., 1990; Weber et al., 1991). Rather, it is an indication of CSF leak that has led to extravasation of radioisotope in the paraspinal tissues and its early entrance into the venous system, thus its early clearance by the kidneys and early appearance in the urinary bladder.

Magnetic Resonance Imaging

It has been less than two decades since the first report on pachymeningeal gadolinium enhancement in CSF leaks appeared in the literature (Mokri et al., 1991). MRI of the head and spine has revolutionized identification, diagnosis, management, and follow-up of patients with spontaneous CSF leaks, and it has increased our overall understanding of CSF volume depletion.

Head Abnormalities

Diffuse pachymeningeal enhancement is the most common head MRI abnormality in CSF leaks

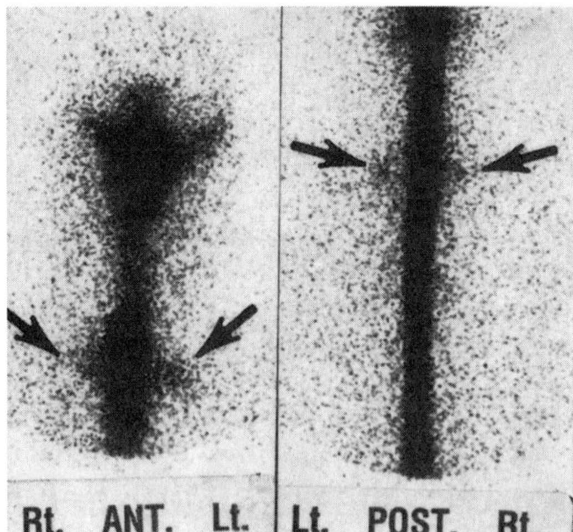

Figure 19–1 Anterior (ANT) and posterior (POST) views of upper cervical spine as noted in indium-111 cisternography, approximately 4 hours after spinal intrathecal injection of the radioisotope. The study shows extra-arachnoid accumulation of radioisotope in the upper thoracic spine, which extends laterally on both sides of the spinal canals (arrows). Note accumulation of radioisotope in the basal cisterns (upper part of the anterior view). The radioactivity never reached the cerebral convexities, even at 24 or 48 hours. (From Mokri et al., 1997. By permission of Mayo Foundation for Medical Education and Research.)

and CSF volume depletion (Table 19–4). This is limited to pachymeninges without any evidence of leptomeningeal involvement. The enhancement is both supertentorial and infratentorial (Figs. 19–2 and 19–3). It is non-nodular, linear, and typically uninterrupted (Pannullo et al., 1993; Mokri et al., 1995). It is of variable thickness, often thick and obvious, but sometimes very thin.

Descent of the brain, or "sagging" or "sinking" of the brain, is also a common finding and is manifested by descent of the cerebellar tonsils (Fig. 19–3) (which may sometimes mimic type I Chiari malformation) (Atkinson et al., 1998), decrease in the size of the prepontine cistern, inferior displacement of the optic chiasm (Fig. 19–4), effacement of perichiasmatic cisterns, and crowding of the posterior fossa.

TABLE 19–4 Abnormalities on Magnetic Resonance Imaging in Cerebrospinal Fluid Leaks.

Head
Diffuse pachymeningeal enhancement
Sinking (sagging of the brain)
Subdural fluid collections
Decrease in size of ventricles ("ventricular collapse")
Enlarged pituitary
Engorged venous sinuses
Elongation of brain stem in anteroposterior plane
Spine
Extra-arachnoid fluid (often extending to several levels)
Extradural fluid (extending to paraspinal soft tissues)
Diverticula
Level of the leak
Pachymeningeal enhancement
Engorgement of epidural venous plexus

Subdural fluid collections are usually but not always bilateral. These are thin, often measuring 2–7 mm in maximal thickness, without compression or effacement of the underlying sulci. Subdural fluid collections display variable signal intensity, depending on the composition of the fluid (protein concentration, blood) (Fig. 19–5).

In some patients, much larger subdural hematomas develop and are associated with significant mass effect (Schievink, Maya, Moser, et al., 2005). Even these hematomas can generally be managed safely with repair of the underlying spinal CSF leak without the need for hematoma evacuation. The risk of a recurrent subdural hemorrhage is high for those patients who undergo primary hematoma evacuation while leaving the spinal CSF leak untreated.

Decrease in the size of the ventricles, or "ventricular collapse," is sometimes obvious and sometimes subtle and is best noted when a head MRI obtained after recovery is compared with a previous MRI taken during the symptomatic phase (Figs. 19–3 and 19–4).

Other abnormalities noted on the MRI of the head include pituitary enlargement (Mokri et al., 1999), sometimes mimicking pituitary adenoma

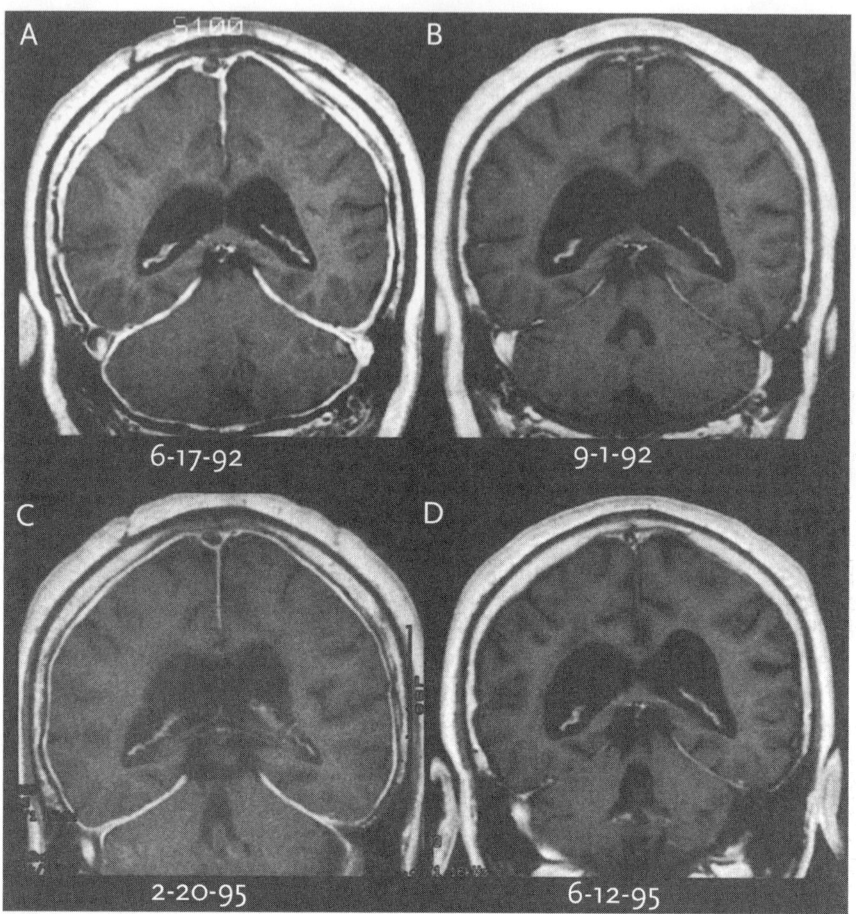

Figure 19–2 Postcontrast coronal T1-weighted magnetic resonance images through parietal lobes and fourth ventricle in a patient who had undergone shunting for normal-pressure hydrocephalus. (*A*) Image obtained after insertion of shunt shows symmetric pachymeningeal gadolinium enhancement. At this stage, the patient had significant orthostatic headaches. (*B*) After shunt revision, the ventricular system is larger, but pachymeningeal enhancement has resolved. The orthostatic headaches disappeared, but the gait disturbance related to normal-pressure hydrocephalus again increased. Cerebrospinal fluid (CSF): Shunt was revised again because of increasing ataxia and confusion. These improved, but headaches and abnormal meningeal enhancement returned. Ventricles are now slightly smaller. (*D*) Ventricles are slightly larger again, but meningeal enhancement has resolved after another shunt revision. Also note engorged and enlarged sagittal sinus in *A* and *C* (compare with *B* and *D*) during periods of shunt overdrainage. (From Mokri et al., 1997. By permission of Mayo Foundation for Medical Education and Research.)

or hyperplasia (Fig. 19–4), engorged venous sinuses (Bakshi et al., 1999) (Figs. 19–2 and 19–3), and elongation of the brain stem in the anteroposterior plane (Pakiam et al., 1999).

A minority of patients with documented spinal CSF leaks have a normal brain MRI. These patients are generally more refractory to treatment. (Schievink, Maya, and Louy, 2005).

Spine Abnormalities

Spine MRI may reveal extra-arachnoid or extradural fluid (Mokri et al., 1997; Rabin et al., 1998). This fluid may extend to the paraspinal soft tissues or present as elongated, localized collections in the epidural space within the spinal canal (Fig. 19–6C), which on axial sections appear to be

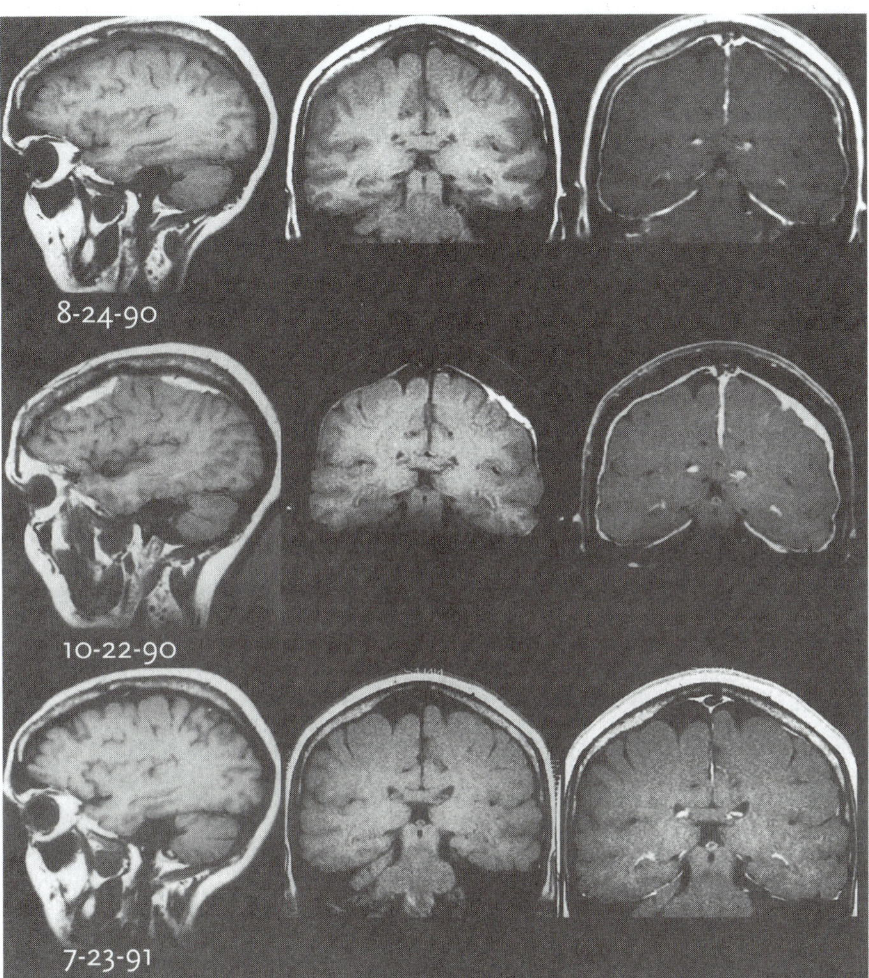

Figure 19–5 Non–contrast-enhanced T1-weighted parasagittal (left vertical row) and coronal (middle vertical row) magnetic resonance images and postcontrast T1-weighted coronal images (right vertical row) in same patient on three separate occasions. On August 24, 1990, non–contrast-enhanced images (upper horizontal row), subdural fluid collections are evident over both cerebral convexities. Diffuse pachymeningeal enhancement is noted in contrast-enhanced image. On October 22, 1990, images (middle horizontal row), while the patient was still symptomatic, extracerebral fluid collection on the right has resolved, whereas left-sided subdural collection now contains high-protein fluid or blood products and displays bright signals. The meningeal enhancement is unchanged. On July 23, 1991, images (lower horizontal row), with the headaches now resolved, the extracerebral fluid collections and abnormal meningeal enhancement have also completely resolved. (From Mokri et al., 1997. By permission of Mayo Foundation for Medical Education and Research.)

Fast Flow CSF Leaks

In such instances, by the time of postmyelogram CT scan, because of the rapidity of the leak, a substantial amount of CSF (and thus contrast) has leaked and spread across several spinal levels. Therefore, identification of the exact site of the leak becomes virtually impossible. One approach to deal with this situation is to skip the myelographic part of the study and proceed with spine CT scanning immediately after the intrathecal injection of the contrast, using a multidetector, high-speed spiral CT in order to obtain many slice images in a short period of time. This technique

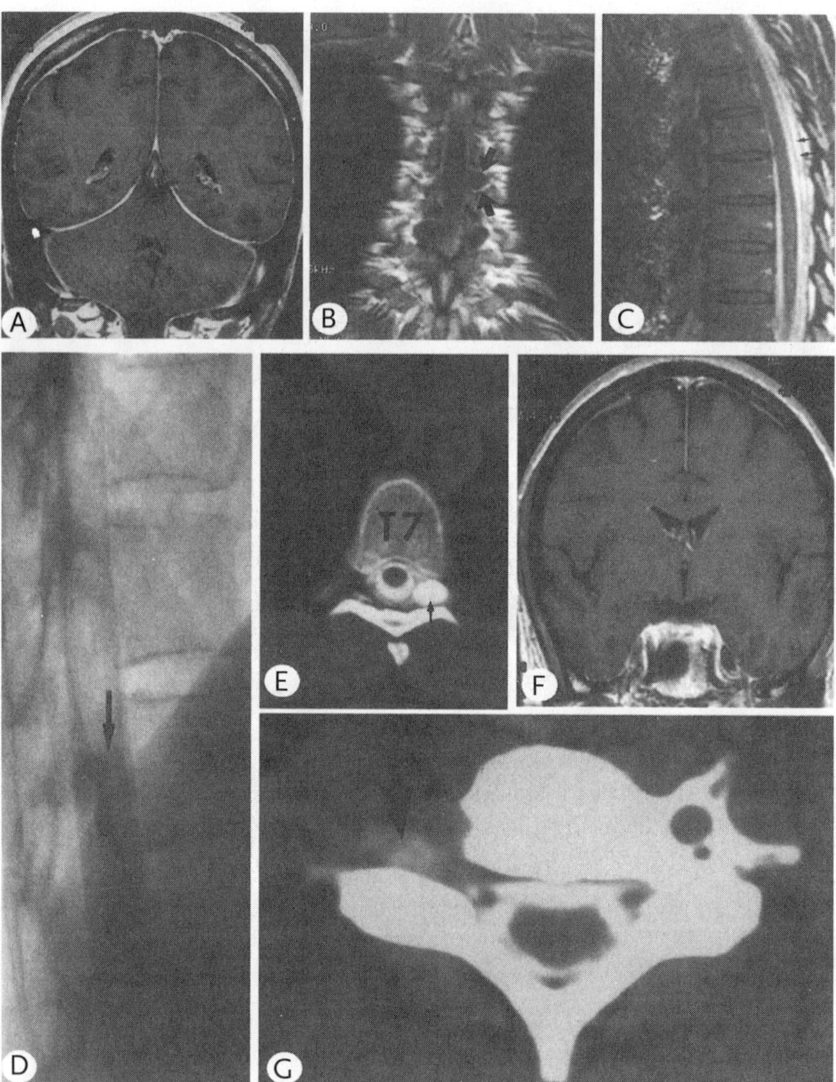

Figure 19–6 (*A*) Gadolinium-enhanced coronal magnetic resonance imaging (MRI) shows diffuse pachymeningeal enhancement. (*B*) Spine MRI shows a left T7 root sleeve diverticulum (arrows). (*C*) T2-weighted spine MRI shows subdural cerebrospinal fluid (CSF) in the posterior aspect of the thoracic canal. (*D*) and (*E*) Myelogram and computed tomography (CT)–myelogram confirm the left T7 root sleeve diverticulum (arrows) but do not show frank extravasation of CSF extradurally. (*F*) Gadolinium-enhanced coronal head MRI obtained approximately 2 months later shows resolution of pachymeningeal gadolinium enhancement. (*G*) Subsequent CT–myelogram demonstrates the site of CSF leak with contrast material exiting through the right C6 neural foramen into the soft tissues (arrow). This case not only demonstrates some of the imaging features of CSF leaks but also points to two important observations: (1) despite proven and persistent CSF leak (*G*), head MRI may fail to show pachymeningeal and gadolinium enhancement (*F*); (2) the presence of meningeal diverticulum, even when obvious and large, may not necessarily correspond to the site of CSF leak. It is important to demonstrate the site of extravasation of the fluid, which may prove to be at a level distant from a diverticulum, which would have been suspected to be the source of the leak (*E* and *G*). (From Mokri, 1999. By permission of Mayo Foundation for Medical Education and Research.)

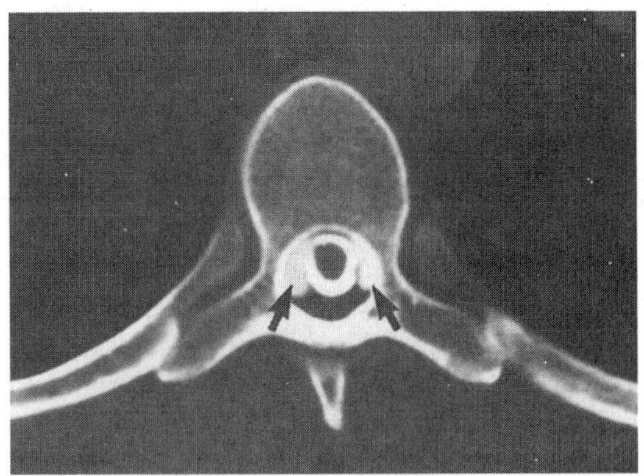

Figure 19–7 Postmyelographic computed tomographic section through thoracic level in a patient with cerebrospinal fluid leak and extra-arachnoid accumulation of contrast material. Note the accumulation of fluid on both sides, exerting a bilateral mass effect on the dural sac. These longitudinal accumulations of fluid on cross sections produce a characteristic "dog-ear" appearance (arrows). (From Mokri et al., 1997. By permission of Mayo Foundation for Medical Education and Research.)

is known as dynamic CT–myelography (Luetmer et al., 2003).

Biopsy

With the current knowledge of the clinical and imaging features of CSF volume depletion and CSF leaks, there is no justification for subjecting patients to meningeal biopsy. The information on biopsy dates back to the initial observations of meningeal enhancement on MRI, when clinicians were not confident about the association of pachymeningeal enhancement and CSF leaks or intracranial hypotension. Then, understandably, patients were vigorously investigated for various types of meningeal disease, particularly meningeal inflammation, infection, and meningeal carcinomatosis.

Meningeal biopsy has shown normal appearance of the dura on gross examination. Leptomeninges also appear normal, except in some of the long-standing cases, in which the arachnoid may appear thickened or opaque. Microscopically, the dura appears entirely normal on its epidural aspect. However, a fairly thin zone of fibroblasts and thin-walled blood vessels in an amorphous matrix is typically noted in the subdural aspect of the dura, resembling an organized hygroma. Hyperplasia of arachnoidal cells may be seen in some long-standing cases. No particular cellular infiltration or inflammatory change is noted. These pathologic findings support the notion that the dural-meningeal abnormalities represent reactive phenomena related to the changes in CSF volume or pressure (Mokri et al., 1995).

TREATMENT

Various treatments have been used for patients with spontaneous CSF leaks, but there is no definite or agreed-on standard approach. Some of these approaches are listed in Table 19–5.

Many patients, fortunately, improve spontaneously. Bed rest and increased fluid intake have been advocated. Because the majority of patients have significant orthostatic headaches, they remain recumbent. Although hydration or overhydration was recommended in some older studies (Tourtellotte et al., 1964), its effectiveness has not been definitely established. While caffeine and theophylline have been suggested as effective (Grant et al., 1989), the effectiveness of these agents is often unimpressive, and a durable beneficial effect is doubtful. The efficacy of steroids is unproven and mostly anecdotal. One might see an occasional patient who reports partial improvement with steroids, but substantial lasting effects are doubtful.

Epidural saline infusion has produced variable results (Rice et al., 1950; Usubiaga et al., 1967; Gibson et al., 1988). It can be tried with limited

TABLE 19–5 Treatment of Cerebrospinal Fluid (CSF) Leaks.

Bed rest
Caffeine
Steroids
Abdominal binder
Epidural blood patch
Continuous epidural saline infusion
Epidural infusion of dextran
Intrathecal infusion with saline or mock CSF
CSF shunting
Surgical repair

expectations in some patients in whom repeated blood patches have failed and when studies have not shown a definitive leak that can be approached surgically.

Intrathecal infusion with saline or mock CSF may become necessary as an effective temporizing measure to restore CSF volume until the CSF leak can be permanently repaired in patients who require urgent treatment, such as those with a depressed level of consciousness (Binder et al., 2002). The intrathecal infusion, however, should not be expected to actually seal the CSF leak.

Epidural blood patch is an effective technique that can be considered the treatment of choice for patients in whom conservative management has failed (Gormley, 1960; Di Giovanni et al., 1972; Crawford, 1985; Rosenberg et al., 1985; Szeinfeld et al., 1986; Seebacher et al., 1989; Geurts et al., 1990; Vakharia et al., 1997). For relieving orthostatic headache, this procedure essentially has two different modes of action; the first is the immediate effect, simply related to volume replacement (by compressing the dura); the second is the latent effect related to sealing of the dural defect. The interval between these two effects varies considerably, but sometimes (especially when the blood patch is used for headaches that occur after lumbar punctures) these two effects occur almost simultaneously. For headaches that occur after lumbar puncture, a single epidural blood patch gives relief in an overwhelming majority of patients. In the small minority who do not respond to the first epidural blood patch, a second blood patch almost always gives relief. In spontaneous CSF leaks, success is less impressive. Many patients require more than one blood patch, and in our experience, some have required as many as four to six blood patches. This difference in success rate in the two groups likely results from two factors: (1) in spontaneous CSF leaks, compared to postdural puncture leaks, the level of the epidural blood patch may be distant from the level of the leak, and this factor may render the procedure less effective; (2) in many spontaneous CSF leaks, the nature and anatomy of the leak are much different from a simple hole or rent produced by the spinal tap needle. In spontaneous CSF leaks, many of the dural defects are in the anterior aspect of the dura or in the root sleeves. In addition, the defect may not be a simple hole or a single rent but a congenitally attenuated zone or patch of the dura with the underlying arachnoid that has finally given way and is oozing CSF from one or more points. In cases such as these, blood patches fail altogether.

When epidural blood patching has failed, and the exact site of the CSF leak has been identified, percutaneous injection of fibrin glue may be considered before surgical treatment of the CSF leak. Percutaneous fibrin glue injection is a safe and minimally invasive method that has been successful in treating symptoms in about one-third of patients, thereby avoiding surgery (Schievink, Maya and Moser, 2004). The injection is performed under CT-guidance using an 18-gauge needle. Smaller gauge needles are prone to result in premature hardening of the fibrin glue mixture.

In well-selected cases, surgical CSF leak repair is effective and can be tried when conservative and less invasive approaches, such as epidural blood patching and percutaneous placement of fibrin glue have failed (Mokri et al., 1997; Schievink et al., 1998). The most straightforward scenario is when a leaking meningeal diverticulum is identified. Such diverticula can be treated with placement of a metal clip or with suture ligation. A bolster consisting of a muscle pledget may be required as well. However, surgery is not always straightforward, even when the exact site of the leak has been clearly demonstrated on preoperative imaging. Extradural CSF may be encountered intraoperatively, but no dural defect can be visualized in spite of careful exploration. Then, packing the epidural space with gel foam, fibrin glue, or muscle or a combination thereof is the only option. Also, even when the defect is visualized, the dural rent or hole may often times not be suitable for direct suturing and therefore, reinforcement with gel foam, fibrin glue, and/or muscle is necessary. This is also the best option when the nerve roots are found to be completely devoid of any dura. Intradural exploration is rarely indicated, but may allow visualization of the dural rent, particularly in patients with large CSF collections anterior to the spinal cord.

The substantial majority of the patients make a complete recovery spontaneously, with conservative management, or with more invasive measures such as epidural blood patch, epidural injection of fibrin sealant, or surgery. Overall, a complete or significant partial recovery is expected in an overwhelming majority of the patients. However, sometimes all efforts in stopping the CSF leaks fail and the patients remain substantially symptomatic. The rate of such disappointing results has not been determined, but the numbers are fortunately low.

Recurrent CSF leaks may occur within weeks, months, or years. The exact rate of recurrence is similarly unknown. However, patients with multiple meningeal diverticula and underlying disorders of connective tissue matrix may be more susceptible to recurrence either from one site or from multiple sites, although this has not been formally studied (Mokri, 2007).

Complications

The major complications of spontaneous CSF leaks include

1. Subdural hematoma, unilateral or bilateral. These are often not large or asymptomatic. However, subdural hematomas can become large, cause midline shift, lead to clinical manifestations, and create significant therapeutic challenges. (Augustin et al., 2003; de Noronha et al., 2003)
2. Cerebral venous sinus thrombosis. This is quite uncommon and should be considered when there is a change in the character of the patient's headaches. (Berrior et al., 2004) Considering the substantial variability in clinical manifestations of spontaneous CSF leaks including the features of the headache, when the headache character changes, it is rarely due to cerebral venous thrombosis.
3. Rebound intracranial hypertension. Sometimes after treatment of spontaneous CSF leaks, a rebound intracranial hypertension may develop (Mokri, 2002), that may become symptomatic. In the majority of the cases, this is self-limited. Treatment with acetozolamide has produced encouraging results.

BROADENING THE CLINICAL-IMAGING SPECTRUM OF CSF VOLUME DEPLETION

Since the recognition of MRI abnormalities in intracranial hypotension due to CSF leaks, a much larger number of patients have been identified and a broader clinical-imaging spectrum of the disorder has been recognized (Mokri, 1999). Thus far, at least four clinical-imaging syndromes in CSF volume depletion are recognized (Table 19–6). In the classic form, headache (typically orthostatic), low CSF pressure, and typical MRI abnormalities are noted. Some patients have the typical clinical manifestations and imaging abnormalities but despite documented CSF leak, have CSF opening pressures that are consistently within limits of normal (the normal-pressure group) (Mokri et al., 1998). In yet another group, despite typical clinical manifestations and documented CSF leak and low CSF pressures, the pachymeninges appear normal on MRI (Mokri, 1999). In the acephalgic group, typical MRI abnormalities are present and CSF pressure is low but headaches are curiously absent despite documented CSF volume depletion as the result of CSF leak or CSF hunt overdrainage (Hochman et al., 1999). The term "CSF volume depletion" (Mokri, 2001) or "CSF hypovolemia" (Mokri, 1999) appear to reflect this entire clinical-imaging spectrum more accurately because the term "intracranial hypotension" no longer appears to be broad enough to embrace all of the clinical and imaging variations that have emerged.

HEADACHES AFTER LUMBAR PUNCTURE

Lumbar puncture is well known to cause orthostatic headache related to CSF leak from the puncture site. These typically begin within 2 days but may be delayed for up to 2 weeks. The headaches may be dull or throbbing and are clearly positional, provoked in the upright position, and relieved with recumbency. They may be frontal, occipital, fronto–occipital, or holocephalic. Nausea and

TABLE 19–6 Clinical-imaging Syndromes in Cerebrospinal Fluid Volume Depletion.

Type I	Classic
Type II	Normal pressure
Type III	Normal meninges
Type IV	Acephalgic

neck stiffness or tightness may accompany the headache, and occasionally blurred vision, photophobia, tinnitus, change in hearing, or dizziness is reported (Raskin, 1990). Typically, the headaches resolve spontaneously within a few days. Because the diagnosis is often obvious, patients are not ordinarily subjected to neurodiagnostic techniques. Head MRI may show pachymeningeal gadolinium enhancement. Even subdural fluid collections have been reported.

Headaches occur after lumbar puncture in about one-third of patients who undergo CSF examination. In one-third of these patients, the headache is severe (in approximately 10% of the total number of patients); in one-third, it is moderate; and in one-third, it is mild (Kuntz et al., 1992). These figures are larger for patients with a history of a primary headache disorder and smaller for those without such a history.

Many investigators agree that the incidence of headaches after lumbar puncture would decrease if smaller-bore needles (e.g., 26 gauge) were used. In the usual practice of diagnostic lumbar puncture, whether in the outpatient or inpatient setting, the narrower (25–29 gauge) needles are impractical because difficulties may be encountered in inserting the needle, measuring the opening pressure, and collecting the fluid. Young female patients with a low body mass index may be at higher risk than others for development of headaches after lumbar puncture. After lumbar puncture, there is no established correlation between the CSF opening pressure, CSF composition, or position and recumbency period and the development of headache. The headache resolves spontaneously in majority of patients with or without hydration, overhydration, or caffeine. Epidural blood patch is more effective than epidural saline (Di Giovanni et al., 1972). Epidural blood patch leads to relief in approximately 90% of patients. A second epidural blood patch brings relief in almost all of the remaining cases (Vilming et al., 1993).

References

Albayram, S, Weasserman, B, Yousem, D, et al. (2002). Intracranial hypotension as a cause of radiculopathy from cervical epidural venous engorgement: case report. *AJNR Am J Neuroradiol,* 23:618–621.

Atkinson, J, Weinshenker, B, Miller, G, et al. (1998). Acquired Chiari I malformation secondary to spontaneous spinal cerebrospinal fluid leakage and chronic intracranial hypotension syndrome in seven cases. *J Neurosurg,* 88:237–242.

Augustin, J, Proust, F, Verdure, L, et al. (2003). Bilateral chronic subdural hematoma: spontaneous intracranial hypotension? *Neurochirurgie,* 49:47–50.

Baker, C (1983). Headache due to spontaneous low spinal fluid pressure. *Minn Med,* 66:325–328.

Bakshi, R, Mechtler, L, Kamran, S, et al. (1999). MRI findings in lumbar puncture headache syndrome: abnormal dural-meningeal and dural venous sinus enhancement. *Clin Imaging,* 23:73–76.

Beck, C, Rizk, L, Kiger, L, et al. (1998). Intracranial hypotension presenting with severe encephalopathy. Case report. *J Neurosurg,* 89:470–473.

Bell, W, Joynt, R, and Sahs, A (1960). Low spinal fluid pressure syndromes. *Neurology,* 10:512–521.

Berrior, S, Grabli, D, Heran, F, et al. (2004). Cerebral venous sinus thrombosis in two patients with spontaneous intracranial hypotension. *Cerebrovasc Dis,* 17:9–12.

Binder, D, Dillon, W, Fishman, R, et al. (2002). Intrathecal saline infusion in the treatment of obtundation associated with spontaneous intracranial hypotension: technical case report. *Neurosurgery,* 51:839–837.

Brady-McCreery, K, Spiedel, S, Hussein, M, et al. (2002). Spontaneous intracranial hypotension with unique strabismus due to third and fourth cranial neuropathies. *Binocul Vis Strabismus Q,* 17:43–48.

Crawford, J (1985). Epidural blood patch [letter]. *Anaesthesia,* 40:381.

Cushing, H (1926). *Studies in Intracranial Physiology and Surgery; the Third Circulation, the Hypophysics, the Gliomas* (H. Milford, ed.). Oxford University Press, London.

Davenport, R.J., S.J. Chataway and C.P. Warlow (1995). Spontaneous intracranial hypotension from a CSF leak in a patient with Marfan's syndrome. J. Neurol. Neurosurg. Psychiatry 59:516–519.

de Noronha, R, Sharrack, B, Hadjvassilioum, M, et al. (2003). Subdural haematoma: a potentially serious consequence of spontaneous intracranial hypotension. *J Neurol,* 74:752–755.

Di Giovanni, A, Galbert, M, and Wahle, W (1972). Epidural injection of autologous blood for postlumbar-puncture headache. II Additional clinical experiences and laboratory investigation. *Anesth Analg,* 51:226–232.

Dillon, W and Fishman, R (1998). Some lessons learned about the diagnosis and treatment of spontaneous intracranial hypotension [editorial]. *AJNR Am J Neuroradiol,* 19:1001–1002.

Eross, E, Dodick, D, Nelson, K, et al. (2002). Orthostatic headache syndrome with CSF leak secondary to bony pathology of the cervical spine. *Cephalalgia,* 22:439–443.

Evans, R and Mokri, B (2002). Headache in cervical artery dissections. *Headache,* 42:1061–1063.

Fay, T (1937). Mechanism of headache. *Trans Am Neurol Assoc,* 62:74–77.

Ferrante, E, Svaino, A, Briuschia, A, et al. (1998). Transient oculomotor cranial nerve palsy in spontaneous intracranial hypotension. *J Neurosurg Sci*, 42:177–179.

Fishman, R (1992). *Cerebrospinal Fluid in Diseases of the Nervous System*, (2nd edn). W.B. Saunders, Philadelphia.

Fishman, R and Dillon, W (1993). Dural enhancement and cerebral displacement secondary to intracranial hypotension. *Neurology*, 43:609–611.

Follens, I, Evans, P, and Tassignon, M (2001). Combined fourth and sixth cranial nerve palsy after lumbar puncture: a rare complication. *Bull Soc Belge Ophthalmol*, 281:29–33.

Front, D and Penning, L (1974). Subcutaneous extravasation of CSF demonstration by scinticisternography. *J Nucl Med*, 15:200–201.

Geurts, J, Haanschoten, M, van Wijk, R, et al. (1990). Post-dural puncture headache in young patients. A comparative study between the use of 0.52 mm (25-gauge) and 0.33 mm (29-gauge) spinal needles. *Acta Anaesthesiol Scand*, 34:350–353.

Gibson, B, Wedel, D, Faust, R, et al. (1988). Continuous epidural saline infusion for the treatment of low CSF pressure headache. *Anesthesiology*, 68:789–791.

Gormley, J. (1960). Current comment: treatment of post-spinal headache. *Anesthesiology*, 21:565–566.

Grant, R, Condon, B, Patterson, J, et al. (1989). Changes in cranial CSF volume during hypercapnia and hypocapnia. *J Neurol Neurosurg Psychiatry*, 52:218–222.

Haines, D, Harkey, H, and al-Mefty, O (1993). The "subdural" space: a new look at an outdated concept. *Neurosurgery*, 32:11–120.

Hochman, M and Naidich, T (1999). Diffuse meningeal enhancement in patients with overdraining, long-standing ventricular shunts. *Neurology*, 52:406–409.

Hochman, M, Naidich, T, Kobetz, S, et al. (1992). Spontaneous intracranial hypotension with pachymeningeal enhancement on MRI. *Neurology*, 42:1628–1630.

Hogan, Q, Prost, R, Kulier, A, et al. (1996). Magnetic resonance imaging of cerebrospinal fluid volume and the influence of body habitus and abdominal pressure. *Anesthesiology*, 84:1341–1349.

Hong, M, Shah, G, Adams, K, et al. (2002). Spontaneous intracranial hypotension causing reversible fronto-temporal dementia. *Neurology*, 58:1285–1287.

Horton, J and Fishman, R (1994). Neurovisual findings in the syndrome of spontaneous intracranial hypotension from dural cerebrospinal fluid leak. *Ophthalmology*, 101:244–251.

Huber, M (1970). Spontaneous hypoliquorrhea. Report on 7 personal observations [in German]. *Schweiz Arch Neurol Neurochir Psychiatr*, 106:9–23.

Kunkle, E, Ray, B, and Wolff, H (1943). Experimental studies on headache' analysis of the headache associated with changes in intracranial pressure. *Arch Neurol Psychiatry*, 49:323–358.

Kuntz, K, Kokmen, E, Stevens, J, et al. (1992). Post-lumbar puncture headaches: experience in 501 consecutive procedures. *Neurology*, 42:1884–1887.

Labadie, E, van Antwerp, J, and Bamford, C (1976). Abnormal lumbar isotope cisternography in an unusual case of spontaneous hypoliquorrheic headache. *Neurology*, 26:135–139.

Lasater, G (1970). Primary intracranial hypotension. The low spinal fluid pressure syndrome. *Headache*, 10:63–66.

Luetmer, P and Mokri, B (2003). Dynamic CT myelography: a technique for localizing high-flow spinal cerebrospinal fluid leaks. *AJNR Am J Neuroradiol*, 24:1711–1714.

Lyons, M and Meyer, F (1990). Cerebrospinal fluid physiology and the management of increased intracranial pressure. *Mayo Clin Proc*, 65:684–707.

Marcelis, J and Silberstein, S (1990). Spontaneous low cerebrospinal fluid pressure headache. *Headache*, 30:192–196.

Matsumae, M, Kinkinis, R, Morocz, I, et al. (1996). Age-related changes in intracranial compartment volumes in normal adults assessed by magnetic resonance imaging. *J Neurosurg*, 84:982–991.

Miller, J (1975). Volume and pressure in the craniospinal axis. *Clin Neurosurg*, 22:76–105.

Miyazawa, K, Chiba, A, Nishima, H, et al. (1998). Upper cervical myelopathy associated with low CSF pressure: a complication of ventriculoperitoneal shunt. *Neurology*, 50:1864–1866.

Miyazawa, K, Shiga, Y, Hasegawa, T, et al. (2003). CSF hypovolemia vs intracranial hypotension in "spontaneous intracranial hypotension syndrome." *Neurology*, 60:941–947.

Moayeri, N, Henson, J, Schaefer, P, et al. (1998). Spinal dural enhancement on magnetic resonance imaging associated with spontaneous intracranial hypotension. Report of three cases and review of the literature. *J Neurosurg*, 88:912–918.

Mokri, B (1999). Spontaneous cerebrospinal fluid leaks: from intracranial hypotension to cerebrospinal fluid hypovolemia-evolution of a concept. *Mayo Clin Proc*, 74:1113–1123.

Mokri, B (2001). The Monro-Kellie hypothesis: applications in CSF volume depletion. *Neurology*, 56:1746–1748.

Mokri, B (2002). Intracranial hypertension after treatment of spontaneous cerebrospinal fluid leaks. *Mayo Clin Proc*, 77:1241–1246.

Mokri, B (2004). Low CSF pressure syndromes. *Neurol Clin N Am*, 22:55–74.

Mokri, B (2005). Low cerebrospinal fluid volume headaches. In *Chronic Daily Headaches* (P Gondsby, S Silberstein, and D Dodick, eds), pp. 155–166, BC Decker Inc., Hamilton, London.

Mokri, B. (2007). Low cerebrospinal fluid headache. In *Neurology and Clinical Neurosciences* (A Schapira, ed.), pp. 817–824, Chapter 62. Mosby Elsevier, Philadelphia.

Mokri, B, Ahlskog, J, and Luetmer, P (2006). Chorea as a manifestation of spontaneous CSF leak. *Neurology*, 67:1490–1491.

Mokri, B, Aksamit, A, and Atkinson, J (2004). Paradoxical postural headaches in spontaneous CSF leaks. *Cephalalgia*, 24:883–887.

Mokri, B and Atkinson, J (2000). False pituitary tumor in CSF leaks. *Neurology,* 55:573–575.

Mokri, B, Atkinson, J, Dodick, D, et al. (1999). Absent pachymeningeal gadolinium enhancement on cranial MRI despite symptomatic CSF leak. *Neurology,* 53:402–404.

Mokri, B, Hunter, S, Atkinson, J, et al. (1998). Orthostatic headaches caused by CSF leak but with normal CSF pressures. *Neurology,* 51:786–790.

Mokri, B, Krueger, B, Miller, G, et al. (1991). Meningeal gadolinium enhancement in low-pressure headaches. *Ann Neurol,* 30:294–295.

Mokri, B, Maher, C, and Sencakova, D (2002). Spontaneous CSF leaks: underlying disorder of connective tissue. *Neurology,* 58:814–816.

Mokri, B, Parisi, J, Scheithauer, B, et al. (1995). Meningeal biopsy in intracranial hypotension: meningeal enhancement on MRI. *Neurology,* 45:1801–1807.

Mokri, B, Piepgras, D, and Miller, G (1997). Syndrome of orthostatic headaches and diffuse pachymeningeal gadolinium enhancement. *Mayo Clin Proc,* 72:400–413.

Molins, A, Alvarez, J, Sumalla, J, et al. (1990). Cisternographic pattern of spontaneous liquoral hypotension. *Cephalalgia,* 10:59–65.

Murros, K and Fogelholm, R (1983). Spontaneous intracranial hypotension with slit ventricles. *J Neurol Neurosurg Psychiatry,* 46:1149–1151.

Nowak, D, Radiek, S, Zinner, J, et al. (2003). Broadening of the clinical spectru: unusual presentation of spontaneous cerebrospinal fluid hypovolemia: case report. *J Neurosurg,* 98:903–907.

Oshiro, S and Fukushima, T (2003). Spontaneous intracranial hypotension manifesting as sudden deafness followed by chronic subdural hematoma. *No To Shinkei,* 55:801–805.

Pakiam, A, Lee, C, and Lang, A (1999). Intracranial hypotension with Parkinsonism, ataxia, and bulbar weakness. *Arch Neurol,* 56:869–872.

Pannullo, S, Reich, J, Krol, G, et al. (1993). MRI changes in intracranial hypotension. *Neurology,* 43:919–926.

Pavlin, D, McDonald, J, Child, B, et al. (1979). Acute subdural hematoma—an unusual sequela to lumbar puncture. *Anesthesiology,* 51:338–340.

Pleasure, S, Abosch, A, Friedman, J, et al. (1998). Spontaneous intracranial hypotension resulting in stupor caused by diencephalic compression. *Neurology,* 50:1854–1857.

Portier, F, De Minteguiaga, C, Racy, E, et al. (2002). Spontaneous intracranial hypotension: a rare cause of labyrinthine hydrops. *Ann Otol Rhinol Laryngol,* 111:817–820.

Rabin, B, Roychowdhury, S, Meyer, J, et al. (1998). Spontaneous intracranial hypotension: spinal MR findings. *AJNR Am J Neuroradiol,* 19:1034–1039.

Rando, T and Fishman, R (1992). Spontaneous intracranial hypotension: report of two cases and review of the literature. *Neurology,* 42:481–487.

Raskin, N (1990). Lumbar puncture headache: a review. *Headache,* 30:197–200.

Rice, G and Dabbs, C (1950). The use of peridural and subarachnoid injections of saline solution in the treatment of severe postspinal headaches. *Anesthesiology,* 11:17–23.

Rosenberg, P and Heavner, J (1985). In vitro study of the effect of epidural blood patch on leakage through a dural puncture. *Anesth Analg,* 64:501–504.

Rowland, L, Fink, M, and Rubin, L (1991). Cerebrospinal fluid: blood–brain barrier, brain edema, and hydrocephalus. In *Principles of Neural Science,* (3rd edn). (ER Kandel, JH Schwartz, and TM Jessell, eds), pp. 1050–1060. Elsevier, New York.

Sable, S and Ramadan, N (1991). Meningeal enhancement and low CSF pressure headache. An MRI study. *Cephalalgia,* 11:275–276.

Schaltenbrand, G (1938). Neuere Anschauungen zur Pathophysiologie der Liquorzirkulation. *Zentralbl Neurochir,* 3:290–300.

Schaltenbrand, G (1953). Normal and pathological physiology of the cerebrospinal fluid circulation. *Lancet,* 1:805–808.

Schievink, W, Maya, M, and Louy, C (2005). Cranial MRI predicts outcome of spontaneous intracranial hypotension. *Neurology,* 64:1282–1284.

Schievink, W, Maya, M, and Moser, F (2004). Treatment of spontaneous intracranial hypotension with percutaneous placement of a fibrin sealant. Report of four cases. *J Neurosurg,* 102:964–965.

Schievink, W, Maya, M, Moser, F, et al. (2005). Spectrum of subdural fluid collections in spontaneous intracranial hypotension. *J Neurosurg,* 103:608–613.

Schievink, W, Maya, M, and Tourje, J (2004). False-localizing sign of C1-2 cerebrospinal fluid leak in spontaneous intracranial hypotension. *J Neurosurg,* 100:639–644.

Schievink, W, Meyer, F, Atkinson, J, et al. (1996). Spontaneous spinal cerebrospinal fluid leaks and intracranial hypotension. *J Neurosurg,* 84:598–605.

Schievink, W, Morreale, V, Atkinson, J, et al. (1998). Surgical treatment of spontaneous spinal cerebrospinal fluid leaks. *J Neurosurg,* 88:243–246.

Schievink, W, Wijdicks, E, Meyer, F, et al. (2001). Spontaneous intracranial hypotension mimicking aneurysmal subarachnoid hemorrhage. *Neurosurgery,* 48:513–517.

Schriver, I, Schievink, W, and Godfrey, M (2002). Spontaneous spinal cerebrospinal fluid leaks and minor skeletal features of Marfan's syndrome: a microfibrillonopathy. *J Neurosurg,* 96:483–489.

Seebacher, J, Ribeiro, V, LeGuillou, J, et al. (1989). Epidural blood patch in the treatment of post dural puncture headache: a double blind study. *Headache,* 29:630–632.

Silberstein, S and Marcelis, J (1992). Headache associated with changes in intracranial pressure. *Headache,* 32:84–94.

Sipe, J, Zyroff, J, and Waltz, T (1981). Primary intracranial hypotension and bilateral isodense subdural hematomas. *Neurology*, 31:334–337.

Szeinfeld, M, Ihmeidan, I, Moser, M, et al. (1986). Epidural blood patch: evaluation of the volume and spread of blood injected into the epidural space. *Anesthesiology*, 64:820–822.

Tali, E, Ercan, N, Krumina, G, et al. (2002). Intrathecal gadolinium gadopentetate dimeglumine enhanced magnetic resonance myelography and cisternography: results of a multicenter study. *Invest Radiol*, 37:152–159.

Tourtellotte, W, Haerer, A, Heller, G, et al. (1964). *Post-lumbar Puncture Headache*. Charles C Thomas Publisher, Springfield, Illinois. pp. 6–12.

Tripathi, BJ and Tripathi, RC (1974). Vacuolar transcellular channels as a drainage pathway for cerebrospinal fluid. *J Physiol*, 239:195–206.

Tripathi, RC (1973). Ultrastructure of the arachnoid mater in relation to outflow of cerebrospinal fluid. A new concept. *Lancet*, 2:8–11.

Usubiaga, J, Usubiaga, L, Brea, L, et al. (1967). Effect of saline injections on epidural and subarachnoid space pressures and relation to postspinal anesthesia headache. *Anesth Analg*, 46:293–296.

Vakharia, S, Thomas, P, Rosenbaum, A, et al. (1997). Magnetic resonance imaging of cerebrospinal fluid leak and tamponade effect of blood patch in postdural puncture headache. *Anesth Analg*, 84:585–590.

Vilming, S and Titus, F (1993). Low cerebrospinal fluid pressure. In *The Headache*. (J Olesen, P Tfelt-Hansen, and KMA Welch, eds), pp. 687–695. Raven Press, New York.

Vishteh, A, Schievink, W, Baskin, J, et al. (1998). Cervical bone spur presenting with spontaneous intracranial hypotension. Case report. *J Neurosurg*, 89:483–484.

Warner, G (2002). Spontaneous intracranial hypotension causing a partial third cranial nerve palsy: a novel observation. *Cephalalgia*, 22:822–823.

Weber, W, Heidendal, G, and de Krom, M (1991). Primary intracranial hypotension and abnormal radionuclide cisternography. Report of a case and review of the literature. *Clin Neurol Neurosurg*, 93:55–60.

Welch, K (1975). The principles of physiology of the cerebrospinal fluid in relation to hyrocephalus including normal pressure hydrocephalus. *Adv Neurol*, 13:247–332.

Wingerchuk, D, Patel, N, Patel, A, et al. (2005). Progressive cervical myelopathy secondary to chromic ventriculoperitoneal CSF overshunting. *Neurology*, 65:171–172.

Winter, S, Maartens, N, and Amslow, P (2002). Spontaneous intracranial hypotension due to thoracic disc herniation. *J Neurosurg Spine*, 96:343–345.

Yamamoto, M, Suehiro, T, Nakata, H, et al. (1993). Primary low cerebrospinal fluid pressure syndrome associated with galactorrhea. *Intern Med*, 32:228–231.

Yoursry, I, Forderreuther, S, Moriggl, B, et al. (2001). Cervical MR imaging in postural headache: MR signs and pahtophysiological implications. *AJNR Am J Neuroradiol*, 22:1239–1250.

20 Infectious, Toxic and Metabolic Headaches

Jonathan P Gladstone and Marcelo E Bigal

INTRODUCTION

The headache disorders are divided into two broad categories by the second edition of the International Classification of Headache Disorders (ICHD-2), primary and secondary headache disorders (Headache Classification Committee, 2004). Secondary headaches are attributed to another condition such as brain tumor or head injury; for the primary disorders, the headache is not because of another condition.

The classification of all secondary headaches follows the same format:

A. A secondary disorder known to be able to cause headache has been demonstrated;
B. Headache occurs in close temporal relation to the secondary disorder and/or there is other evidence of a causal relationship;
C. Headache is greatly reduced or disappears within a specific time frame (usually 3 months, but this may be shorter for some disorders) after successful treatment or spontaneous remission of the causative disorder.

This chapter highlights secondary headaches that are attributed to infectious, toxic, and metabolic causes. These disorders are covered in chapters 8 and 9 of the ICHD-2. Medication overuse headache, which is considered a headache secondary to chronic exposure to acute headache medication(s) and is, therefore, a toxic headache, is discussed in this textbook in the chronic daily headache chapter (Chapter 12).

HEADACHES ATTRIBUTABLE TO INFECTION DISEASES

According to the ICHD-2, when a new headache occurs for the first time in close temporal relation to an infection, it should be coded as a secondary headache attributable to the infection. When there is a preexisting primary headache (e.g., migraine) which is made worse in close temporal relation to an infection, the patient could be given either the diagnosis of the preexisting primary headache *or* be given both the primary headache diagnosis and the diagnosis of headache attributed to the infection.

The ICHD-2 divides the "Headache Attributed to Infection" into four categories: (1) headache attributed to intracranial infection, (2) headache attributed to systemic infection, (3) headache attributed to human immunodeficiency virus/acquired immunodeficiency syndrome (HIV/AIDS), and (4) chronic postinfection headache. Each of these categories will be highlighted in this chapter. Headaches attributed to an extracranial infection of the head (such as ear, eye, dental, and sinus infections) are described in chapter 11 of the ICHD-2 ("Headache or facial pain attributed to disorder of the cranium, neck, eyes, ears, nose, sinuses, teeth, mouth or other facial or cranial structures") and are reviewed in chapters 21 through 23 of this text.

HEADACHE ATTRIBUTED TO INTRACRANIAL INFECTION (9.1)

Headache Attributed to Bacterial Meningitis (9.1.1)

Bacterial meningitis is a true medical emergency that requires rapid diagnosis and prompt initiation of treatment (Roos, 2000a; Tunkel et al., 2004; van de Beek et al., 2006). Headache is, frequently, the initial symptom of bacterial meningitis and, overall, it is the most common symptom of bacterial meningitis, although it is rarely present alone (van de Beek et al., 2004). The "classic triad" for bacterial meningitis consists of fever, nuchal rigidity, and change in mental status; however, this "classic triad" may be absent in up to 50% of patients with meningitis (van de Beek, 2004). Notably, infants and young children often do not complain of headache; rather, they may present with fever, bulging fontanelle (infants), drowsiness, confusion, and seizures (Saez-Llorens and McCracken, 2003) (Box 20–1).

The headache of bacterial meningitis is usually generalized but may be predominantly frontal or occipital–nuchal. The headache is typically severe and unremitting and is often associated with photophobia, phonophobia, nausea, and pain with eye movements. Pain with eye movements is a common symptom in headaches associated with fever of any etiology. The headache may be abrupt in onset ("thunderclap") or may reach maximal severity over minutes or hours. Patients with bacterial meningitis frequently report worsening of their headache with sudden movements (so-called "jolt" excentuation) (Attia et al., 1999) and often assume a flexed body posture, reflexively protecting their head and neck through spasm of the muscles of the neck and spine and by keeping their head retracted.

The pathogenesis of headache in bacterial meningitis is presumed to be because of direct stimulation of the sensory terminals located in the meninges by bacterial infection (Headache Classification Committee, 2004). Bacterial products (toxins), mediators of inflammation such as bradykinin, prostaglandins and cytokines and other agents released by inflammation not only directly cause pain but also induce sensitization of meningeal nociceptors and neuropeptide release. The septic meningeal inflammation that explains the headache of meningitis is analogous to the aseptic inflammation, that is, presumed to occur at the neurovascular junction of meningeal/dural blood vessels during migraine attacks (Moskowitz, 1990). This may account for the overlapping phenotype of both conditions.

The organisms most commonly responsible for bacterial meningitis vary with age and the immunocompetence status of the patient (van de Beek, 2006). In healthy North American adults, the most common organisms include *Neisseria meningitidis, Streptococcus pneumoniae, Haemophilus influenzae,* and *Listeria monocytogenes.* These organisms account for more than 75% of all cases. *Staphylococcus aureus* and group A Streptococci are important causes to consider in patients with head trauma, previous neurosurgical procedures, or cerebral and epidural abscesses. Pathogens to consider in patients who have had a lumbar puncture or spinal anesthesia include *Klebsiella, Proteus,* and *Pseudomonas.* In patients who are immunocompromised, receiving chemotherapy or other immunosuppressive therapy, have lymphoma, leukemia or AIDS, consideration must be given to more uncommon organisms such as *Mycobacterium tuberculosis, Candida, Cryptococcus,* and *Histoplasma.* In newborns, meningitis is usually caused by *Escherichia coli,* group B *streptococci,* or *Listeria.*

Guidelines for the diagnosis and management of bacterial meningitis were published in 2004 by the Infectious Diseases Society of America (Tunkel et al., 2004). If meningitis is clinically suspected, lumbar puncture should be performed urgently (Straus, 2006). A lumbar puncture may

Box 20–1 Headache Attributed to Bacterial Meningitis (9.1.1).

A. Headache with at least one of the following characteristics and fulfilling criteria C and D:
   1. Diffuse pain
   2. Intensity increasing to severe
   3. Associated with nausea, photophobia and/or phonophobia
B. Evidence of bacterial meningitis from examination of CSF
C. Headache develops during the meningitis
D. One or other of the following:
   1. Headache resolves within 3 months after relief from meningitis
   2. Headache persists but 3 months haven not passed since relief from meningitis

be undertaken without neuroimaging unless specific contraindications are present. Contraindications to lumbar puncture include papilledema, abnormal level of consciousness, focal neurologic deficits, immunocompromised state, history of central nervous system (CNS) disease and new-onset seizure (Tunkel et al., 2004). If clinical suspicion is high and lumbar puncture cannot be undertaken promptly, empiric treatment should be considered.

The cerebrospinal fluid (CSF) should be sent for cell count, protein, glucose, gram stain, and bacterial cultures. The typical CSF findings in acute bacterial meningitis include hypoglycorrhachia (glucose less than 40 mg/dl), increased protein (protein level greater than 45 mg/dl), and a marked pleocytosis with cell counts greater than 1000 cells/mm^3.

The headache and meningitis are best managed by analgesics, antipyretics, intravenous (IV) fluids, and immediate institution of appropriate empiric and then targeted antibiotics. The choice of initial antibiotics is determined by the age of the patient and the clinical setting (post head injury, neurosurgical procedure, previous sinus infection etc.). The interested reader is referred to the guidelines for the diagnosis and management of bacterial meningitis that were published in 2004 by the Infectious Diseases Society of America (Tunkel et al., 2004).

Headache Attributed to Lymphocytic Meningitis (9.1.2)

Lymphocytic meningitis (often referred to as "aseptic meningitis") is a syndrome that can result from a wide array of infectious and noninfectious etiologies (Connolly and Hammer, 1990; Moris and Garcia-Monco, 1999; Roos, 2000; Rothbart, 2000; Hopkins and Jolles, 2005). The syndrome consists of signs and symptoms of meningeal irritation and a CSF lymphocytic pleocytosis (usually between 10 and 1000 cells/mm). Viral meningitis is the most common cause of aseptic meningitis (Box 20–2).

The onset of a lymphocytic meningitis illness is typically acute or subacute. A prodromal flu-like illness may herald the syndrome. As for other forms of meningitis, the most common symptoms are headache, fever, and neck stiffness. The headache is often moderate-to-severe and is frequently frontal or retro-orbital in location. The headache is likely a consequence of meningeal and ependymal cell destruction and the subsequent inflammatory response. Accompanying features may include typical migraine features, such as photophobia, nausea, vomiting, as well as systemic symptoms, such as malaise and myalgias. The patient does not tend to look as toxic or ill as those patients with bacterial meningitis. Following the first few days of the illness, the course is typically one of slow, progressive improvement with a typical duration of illness ranging from several days to weeks.

Viral meningitis is estimated to affect more than 36,000 cases annually in the United States (Khetsuriani et al., 2003). The majority of cases affect children and occur in the summer and early fall. The most common viral cause of meningitis is enteroviruses accounting for 85%–95% of cases of viral meningitis in the United States. Other causes include herpex simplex virus type 2, arboviruses, measles virus, varicella-zoster virus, HIV, lyphocytic choriomeningitis virus,

Box 20–2 Headache Attributed to Lymphocytic Meningitis (9.1.2).

A. Headache with at least one of the following characteristics and fulfilling criteria C and D:
   1. Acute onset
   2. Severe intensity
   3. Nuchal rigidity, fever, nausea, photophobia and/or phonophobia
B. Examination of cerebrospinal fluid (CSF) shows lymphocytic pleocytosis, mildly elevated protein and normal glucose.
C. Headache develops in close temporal association to meningitis
D. Headache resolves within 3 months after successful treatment or spontaneous remission of infection

adenovirus, Epstein–Barr virus, and mumps (Sejvar, 2006).

CSF lymphocytosis and headache most frequently occur with viral meningitis but may be the result of a wide range of other infectious etiologies (partially treated bacterial meningitis, *Mycoplasma pneumonia, Listeria*, brucellosis, spirochete infections, rickettsial infections, tuberculosis, fungal, and parasitic infections) and noninfectious etiologies include drug-induced [nonsteroidal antiinflammatories, antibiotics, immunosuppressants, intravenous immunoglobulin (IVIG), antineoplastic agents], chemical-induced aseptic meningitis, and other medical conditions (vasculitis, sarcoidosis, collagen–vascular diseases, and meningeal carcinomatosis) (Roos, 2000).

Headache Attributed to Encephalitis (9.1.3)

Unlike meningitis, which is an inflammation of the meninges, encephalitis is an inflammation of the brain parenchyma. The inflammation is usually diffuse but can be focal (i.e., medial temporal lobes in herpes simplex encephalitis). Encephalitis typically consists of an acute febrile illness with headache accompanied by some combination of mental status changes, seizures, and/or focal neurologic signs or symptoms (Kennedy, 2004). Encephalitis is usually associated with focal signs and cognitive deficits, not with headache as a main feature. However, sometimes, especially when there is meningeal inflammation as well, or when there is associated angiitis, headache may occur early and be the only clinical symptom of encephalitis. The underlying pathogenesis of the headache likely includes meningeal irritation, increased intracranial pressure, and/or a systemic reaction to the toxic products of the infectious agent(s) (Box 20–3).

Encephalitis may be because of a primary infection (viral, bacterial, fungal, or parasitic) or may occur secondarily following a previous viral infection or vaccination. The vast majority of encephalitis cases are because of primary infection with a virus; however, although viruses are the usual presumptive cause of encephalitis, the specific agent is identifiable in only a minority of cases (Kennedy, 2004). Common causes of viral encephalitis include herpes simplex virus (HSV), other herpes viruses (varicella-zoster, Epstein–Barr), adenoviruses, influenza A, enteroviruses, and arboviruses (Japanese B encephalitis, St. Louis encephalitis, West Nile virus).

Many viral encephalitides have a characteristic geographical and seasonal incidence as is seen with arboviral infections (a common cause of viral encephalitis). These infections are transmitted through bites from infected mosquitoes and are, therefore, most common during the summer and fall months. In the United States, there are several common arthropod-borne encephalitides including St. Louis encephalitis (most commonly found along the Mississippi river in the late summer), Eastern Equine encephalitis (most commonly found in the Northeast and northern Midwest states), and West Nile virus (which has been documented throughout the United States to varying degrees).

HSV-1 is the most common cause of nonepidemic viral encephalitis and is often associated with significant morbidity (Tyler, 2004). There are approximately 2000 cases of herpes simplex

Box 20–3 Headache Attributed to Encephalitis (9.1.3).

A. Headache with at least one of the following characteristics and fulfilling criteria C and D:
   1. Diffuse pain
   2. Intensity increasing to severe
   3. Associated with nausea, photophobia, or phonophobia
B. Neurological symptoms and signs of acute encephalitis, and diagnosis confirmed by electroencephalogram (EEG), cerebrospinal fluid (CSF) examination, neuroimaging and/or other laboratory investigations
C. Headache develops during encephalitis
D. Headache resolves within 3 months after successful treatment or spontaneous remission of the infection

encephalitis yearly in the United States. HSV-1 has a predilection for the medial temporal and frontal lobes. Headache (often rapidly developing) that is moderate-to-severe, temporal or diffuse can occur in association with fever, cognitive symptoms (confusion, agitation, poor concentration, inattention), behavior or personality changes, focal neurological signs or symptoms (such as speech difficulties or hemiparesis), seizures and/or altered or decreased level of consciousness. A subacute course, consisting of headache and lethargy progressing over weeks or months has been reported.

CSF examination in herpes simplex encephalitis typically demonstrates (1) pleocytosis (usually 10–200 lymphocytes/mm^3, although neutrophils can occur early), (2) red blood cells or xanthochromia, (3) increased protein, and (4) normal glucose. In experienced laboratories, the CSF should test positive for HSV deoxyribo nucleic acid in up to 95% of cases during the first week of the illness; false negatives results can occur within the first 24–48 hours or after 10–14 days of the illness (Kennedy, 2004). Electroencephalogram (EEG) findings include periodic lateralizing epileptiform discharges (PLEDs), focal slowing, and sharp waves. The computed tomography (CT) scan is typically normal or may demonstrate unilateral or bilateral hypodensity in the temporal and/or frontal lobes. Evidence of parenchyma bleeding may be noted if there is hemorrhagic transformation. Magnetic resonance imaging (MRI) findings include increased T2, fluid attenuated inversion recovery (FLAIR) and/or diffusion-weighted signal abnormality in the inferior frontal and/or medial temporal lobes. Treatment is with IV acyclovir 10 mg/kg Q8h for 2–3 weeks (Tyler, 2004).

West Nile virus is a *Flavivirus* belonging to the Japanese encephalitis subgroup. *Flaviviruses* are small, single-stranded ribonucleic acid (RNA) viruses (Davis et al., 2006). West Nile virus is transmitted via mosquitoes to humans from infected birds (crows, ravens, blue jays). Case reports exist of transmission via blood transfusion and organ transplantation. The incubation period ranges from 3 to 14 days. Most patients infected with West Nile virus have no symptoms. Approximately 20% of infected individuals have a mild flu-like illness (fever, malaise, anorexia, myalgia, headache, and rash). In less than 1% of infected individuals, significant neurologic disorders (encephalits, meningoencephalitis, poliomyelitis-like illness) occur. To investigate for West Nile virus, serum and CSF should be obtained for IgM and IgG antibodies and polymerase chain reaction (PCR). Typically, the CSF shows lymphocytic pleocytosis with increased protein. Treatment of West Nile encephalitis is supportive; no antiviral has been demonstrated to be efficacious.

Nonviral causes of infectious encephalitis include bacterial (*M. tuberculosis*, *Mycoplasma pneuomoniae*, *L. monocytogenes*, *Borrelia burgdorferi*, leptospirosis, Brucellosis, *Legionella*, *Tropheryma whippeli*, *Treponema pallidum*), rickettsial (*Rickettsia rickettsia*, *Coxiella burnetti*, ehrlichiosis), fungal (*Cryptococcus*, aspergillosis, cocciodiomycosis) and parasitic (cerebral malaria, *Toxoplasma gondi*, trypanosomiasis). Discussing these causes in detail is beyond the scope of this chapter.

Headache Attributed to Brain Abscess

A brain abscess is a focal parenchymal brain infection that begins as a localized area of cerebritis and then develops into a collection of pus surrounded by a capsule. It is a serious, potentially life-threatening condition (Mathisen and Johnson, 1997; Calfee and Wispelwey, 2000; Bernardini, 2004; Roche et al., 2003; Kastenbauer et al., 2004) (Box 20–4).

In most case series of brain abscess, headache is the most common presenting symptom occurring in approximately 50% of patients (Kao et al., 2003; Roche, 2003; Xiao et al., 2005; Hakan et al., 2006). Other common symptoms include confusion or altered level of consciousness, nausea, vomiting, focal neurologic symptoms and signs, fever and seizures. The classic triad of headache, fever, and focal neurologic deficit is uncommon at presentation. In most cases, brain abscess presents as a rapidly or subacutely developing space-occupying lesion. Approximately 75% of patients will present with symptoms of less than 2 week's duration. Interestingly, clinical signs may develop rapidly suggesting acute meningitis or a cerebral infarction or they may evolve over weeks or months suggesting the presence of a primary or metastatic brain tumor.

There are several potential etiologies for brain abscesses: (1) spread from a contiguous focus of infection (i.e., otogenic, sinus, dental, orbit, skin,

Box 20–4 Headache Attributed to Brain Abscess (9.1.4).

A. Headache with at least one of the following characteristics and fulfilling criteria C and D:
   1. Bilateral
   2. Constant pain
   3. Intensity gradually increasing to moderate or severe
   4. Aggravated by straining
   5. Accompanied by nausea
B. Neuroimaging and/or laboratory evidence of brain abscess
C. Headache develops during active infection
D. Headache resolves within 3 months after successful treatment of the abscess

open wound, shunt), (2) hematogenous spread from a distant focus (i.e., congenital heart disease with right-to-left shunt, endocarditis, pulmonary arteriovenous malformation (AVM), septicemia), (3) consequence of traumatic head injury or neurosurgical procedure, or (4) may be cryptogenic in origin. Brain abscesses are much more common in certain predisposed/susceptible individuals (i.e., individuals with AIDS, diabetics, prolonged steroid use or other immuncompromised states) (Calfree, 2000; Roche, 2003; Kastenbauer, 2004).

Overall, the most common infecting organisms are: *Streptococcus* species (i.e., *Streptococcus milleri* which is common in abscesses arising from sinusitis or dental infections), Bacteroides species, *S. aureus*, and anaerobes. In some cases, no organism is detected. The most common etiologies vary with the age of the patient, immunological status of the patient, and presumptive underlying source of the abscess: trauma patients (*S. aureus, S. epididemis*), neurosurgical patients (*S. epididemis, S. aureus*, Gram-negative bacilli), transplant patient (*Listeria, Cryptococcus*, aspergillois, *Candida*), and immunocompromised patients (*Cryptococcus, Listeria*, aspergillosis, *Mucor, Norcardia*) (Calfree, 2000; Roche, 2003; Kastenbauer, 2004).

The most common location for brain abscesses is the frontal lobe because of its location near the frontal and ethmoid sinuses and the predeliction for hematogenous spread of septic emboli via the anterior (carotid) circulation.

Contrast-enhanced CT or MRI with gadolinium are the neuroimaging procedures of choice for suspected brain abscess. MR spectroscopy may allow differentiation between brain abscess and tumor (Bernardini, 2004). The most important investigation is CT-guided stereotactic aspiration of the brain abscess to obtain a culture of the abscess fluid or pus. Occasionally, large and superficial abscesses amenable to open evacuation of the pus under direct vision may be treated by craniotomy and evacuation of the pus. In cases when the underlying infecting organism is known and/or the abscess is inaccesible or there are multiple abscesses, nonsurgical, medical management is justified.

Lumbar puncture to obtain CSF for analysis is not recommended as raised intracranial pressure may lead to brainstem herniation and the CSF may well be sterile. In patients in whom the abscess is believed to have spread hematogenously, blood cultures are indicated.

In a patient with AIDS, a mass on neuroimaging could reflect an abscess secondary to opportunistic infections (toxoplasmosis, *Cryptococcus*, candiasis, aspergillosis, *Mycobacterium tuberculosis, Norcardia, Listeria*, etc.) or may reflect a neoplastic lesion (CNS lymphoma, glioma, Kaposi's sarcoma, or metastatic neoplasm) (American Academy of Neurology Quality Standards Subcomitee, 1998).

Brain abscess management involves prompt administration of appropriate antibiotics, surgical drainage or removal where indicated and control of perilesional edema with dexamethasone or other corticosteroids (Infection in Neurosurgery Working Party of the British Society for Antimicrobial Chemotherapy, 2000; Kastenbauer, 2004; Lu et al., 2006). Antiepileptic drugs are often necessary for seizure prophylaxis, although the efficacy of preempting seizures in patients without prior history of epilepsy has not been established. Antibiotic therapy is usually parenteral for several weeks then transitioned to several weeks or months of oral antibiotics. Antibiotic therapy should be stratified based on knowledge of the presumed/possible pathogen(s) and the antimicrobial spectrum of available agents and their penetration into abscess fluids (Infection in Neurosurgery Working Party of the British Society for Antimicrobial Chemotherapy, 2000).

Headache Attributed to Subdural Emyema

Subdural empyema is a collection of purulent material located between the dura mater and the arachnoid matter (Nathoo, 1999; Osborn and Steinberg, 2007). The vast majority of subdural empyemas are located with the cranium (most involving the frontal lobe) and a minority involve the spinal axis. Subdural empyemas are life-threatening infections that cause problems via extrinsic compression of the brain with associated increased intracranial pressure, intraparenchymal penetration, or thrombosis of the cortical veins or cavernous sinuses (Box 20–5).

Patients commonly present with headache (which may be initially focal but later generalized) and/or any combination of fever, confusion or altered level of consciousness, seizure, or focal neurologic signs or symptoms. There often is a history of recent sinusitis, otitis media, mastoiditis, meningitis, cranial surgery or trauma, sinus surgery, or pulmonary infection (Osborn and Steinberg, 2007).

In infants and young children, subdural empyema most often occurs as a complication of meningitis. In older children and adults, it occurs as a complication of paranasal sinusitis, otitis media, or mastoiditis. Infection usually enters through the frontal or ethmoid sinuses; less frequently, it enters through the middle ear, mastoid cells, or sphenoid sinus. The infection may spread intracranially through thrombophlebitis in the venous sinuses or may extend directly through the cranium and dura from an erosion of the posterior wall of the mastoid bone or frontal sinus. Direct extension also could be from an intracerebral abscess. Rarely, infection spreads hematogenously from distant foci, most commonly from a pulmonary source or as a complication of trauma, surgery, or septicemia. As such, the type of offending organism is related to the presumed source of entry of the infection. The most common causative organisms are anaerobes, aerobic streptococci, staphylococci, *H. influenzae, S. pneumoniae,* and other gram-negative bacilli (Osborn and Steinberg, 2007).

An MRI with gadolinium is the diagnostic test of choice and if unavailable a contrast-enhanced CT should be performed. Treatment of subdural empyema consists of parenteral antibiotics, immediate surgical drainage, or evacuation of the abscess and/or the primary source of infection (Greenlee, 2003).

HEADACHE ATTRIBUTED TO SYSTEMIC INFECTION (9.2)

Systemic infections may be accompanied or followed by: (1) a relatively mild headache overshadowed by malaise, fever, and systemic symptoms, (2) a prominent headache (headache that may occur with influenza), or (3) headache attributable

Box 20–5 Headache Attributed to Subdural Empyema (9.1.5).

A. Headache with at least one of the following characteristics and fulfilling criteria C and D:
   1. Unilateral or much more intense on one side
   2. Associated with tenderness of the skull
   3. Accompanied by fever
   4. Accompanied by stiffness of the neck
B. Neuroimaging and/or laboratory evidence of subdural empyema
C. Headache develops during active infection and is localised to or maximal at the site of the empyema
D. Headache resolves within 3 months after successful treatment of the empyema

TABLE 20–1 Diagnostic Criteria for Headache Attributed to Systemic Infection.

9.2 Headache attributed to systemic infection

A. Headache with at least one of the following characteristics and fulfilling criteria C and D:
  1. Diffuse pain
  2. Intensity increasing to moderate or severe
  3. Associated with fever, general malaise or other symptoms of systemic infection

B. Evidence of systemic infection

C. Headache develops during the systemic infection

D. Headache resolves within 72 hours after effective treatment of the infection

9.2.1 Headache attributed to systemic bacterial infection

A. Headache fulfilling criteria for 9.2 *Headache attributed to systemic infection*

B. Laboratory investigation discloses the inflammatory reaction and identifies the organism

9.2.2 Headache attributed to systemic viral infection

A. Headache fulfilling criteria for 9.2 *Headache attributed to systemic infection*

B. Clinical and laboratory (serology and/or polymerase chain reaction (PCR) molecular) diagnosis of viral infection

9.2.3 Headache attributed to other systemic infections

A. Headache fulfilling criteria for 9.2 *Headache attributed to systemic infection*

B. Clinical and laboratory (serology, microscopy, culture or PCR molecular) diagnosis of infection other than bacterial or viral

to meningitis or encephalitis (described in the previous sections). When meningitis or encephalitis occurs, the headache should be coded as headaches attributed to meningitis or encephalitis and not headaches attributed to systemic infection (Table 20–1).

There is significant variability in the propensity of systemic infections to cause headache. Systemic infections which frequently are accompanied by headache include viral infections (influenza, adenovirus, West Nile virus), bacterial infections (brucellosis, leptospirosis, and malaria) and other infectious agents (malaria, *Rickettsia*, *B. burgdorferi*, *Legionella penumophilia*, and *M. pneumonia*, leptospirosis) (De Marinis and Welsh, 1992).

Headaches attributed to systemic infection are relatively nonspecific without any particular characteristic or distinguishing features. In addition, systemic infections can trigger primary headache disorders such as migraine and cluster headache in susceptible individuals. Caution needs to be given when attempting to distinguish between headache attributed to a systemic infection and headache heralding meningitis or encephalitis. Accordingly, a CSF examination is necessary to exclude a CNS infection in patients with headache, symptoms of systemic infection accompanied by meningismus, focal neurologic signs, seizures, and/or altered level of consciousness.

Very little is known about the pathogenesis of headache because of systemic infection. The headache may correlate with the degree of fever or occur in the absence of fever. As such, headache occuring during systemic infection may be attributable "to direct activation of pain producing mechanisms by microorganisms or may be secondary to fever or a combinatin of both." (De marinis and Welch, 1992). Speculation exists that microrganisms may influence brain nuclei to release substances that cause headache or endotoxis may activate inflammatory and nociceptive mediators such as nitric oxide (NO), prostaglandins, and cytokines which play a role in the generation of headache (De marinis and Welch, 1992).

Treatment of headache caused by an underlying infection includes treating the underlying infection (if possible), treatment of the fever with antipyretics and treatment of associated inflammation with nonsteroidal anti-inflammatory drugs (NSAIDs).

HEADACHE ATTRIBUTED TO HIV/AIDS (9.3)

Headache is a common symptom affecting from 11% to 55% of HIV-infected individuals (Goldstein, 1990; Lipton et al., 1991; Brew, 1993; Holloway and Kieburtz, 1995; Singer et al., 1996; Mirsattari and Manitoba, 1999). Prevalence of headache increases with the degree of immunosuppresion—prevalence rates are highest in those with AIDS. The differential diagnosis of the acute and chronic headache in the patient with HIV/AIDS is broad and challenging.

Headaches in individuals affected by HIV can occur at any stage of the illness and may be related to: (1) a preexisting primary headache disorders (i.e., migraine or tension-type headache); (2) the primary HIV infection (acute illness associated with HIV seroconversion, acute, recurrent or chronic asepetic meningitis, or late-stage HIV headache without pleocytosis); (3) secondary to opportunistic infections (i.e., *Cryptococcus*, toxoplasmosis, tuberculosis, syphilis, cytomegalovirus, JC virus); (4) secondary to opportunistic neoplasms (i.e., primary or metastatic CNS lymphoma); (5) secondary to medications used to treat the HIV infection; (6) postlumbar puncture headache; (7) associated with other comorbid conditions, such as depression, or (8) associated with drug use, overuse, or withdrawal. (Khayr, 2007). Headache occurring in patients with HIV/AIDS but attributable to a specific secondary cause (i.e., infection or neoplasm) should be coded under the secondary cause (Box 20–6).

Headache may occur as part of the acute seroconversion illness following primary infection with HIV-1 in 1%–2% of all cases and may resemble acute viral meningitis. Direct correlation between the degree of viral load in the CSF or plasma with primary HIV infection and the prevalence of headache has been suggested (Tambussi et al., 2000). An acute or chronic headache accompanied by an otherwise unexplained lymphocytic pleocytosis can occur at any stage of the disease following the initial infection. New-onset chronic headaches without an identifiable etiology and without a CSF lymphocytic pleocytosis can occur in the late stages of the disease and may reflect aseptic meningitis in a lymphocyte-depleted patient (Khayr, 2007).

There is considerable variability in the location, quality, severity, and presence of associated symptoms in headache attributable to primary HIV-1 infection, and headaches secondary to opportunistic infections, making the diagnosis of headache in the HIV-infected patient particularly challenging. There are no formal guidelines for the appropriate workup for headache in the HIV-infected patients. As such, in otherwise well individuals with $CD4^{+}$ counts greater than 500 cells/mm^3, the presence of headache "red flags" (i.e., sudden-onset, first or worst headache, progressive headache, headache associated with fever, any associated neurologic signs) dictate the timing and degree of investigations (Gifford and Hecht,

Box 20–6 Headache Attributed to HIV/AIDS (9.3).

A. Headache with variable mode of onset, site and intensity fulfilling criteria C and D
B. Confirmation of human immunodeficiency virus (HIV) infection and/or of the diagnosis of acquired immunodeficiency syndrome (AIDS), and of the presence of HIV/AIDS-related pathophysiology likely to cause headache, by neuroimaging, cerebrospinal fluid (CSF) examination, electroencephalogram (EEG) and laboratory investigations
C. Headache develops in close temporal relation to the HIV/AIDS-related pathophysiology
D. Headache resolves within 3 months after the infection subsides

2001; Graham and Wippold, 2001). In patients with $CD4^+$ counts below 500 cells/mm^3, a new or chronic headache necessitates neuroimaging followed by a CSF analysis [for routine chemistry, microscopy, cytologic analyses, culture and stains for bacteria, *Mycobacterium*, viruses, fungi, cryptococcal antigen titres and Venereal Disease Research Laboratory (VDRL) titres].

HEADACHE ATTRIBUTED TO CHRONIC POSTINFECTION HEADACHE (9.4)

Chronic postbacterial meningitis headache is a new diagnostic category that has been added to the ICHD-2. In the appendix of the ICDH-2, there are proposed diagnostic criteria for chronic headache attributed to nonbacterial infectious causes. There is a paucity of data on the epidemiology and pathogenesis of postinfectious headache; however, available studies suggest that chronic headache may occur in up to 30% of patients after bacterial meningitis (Bohr et al., 1983; Neufeld et al., 1999) (Box 20–7).

HEADACHE ATTRIBUTED TO DISORDER OF HOMEOSTASIS (10.0)

In the ICHD-1 (1988), this group of headaches was referred to as "headaches associated with metabolic or systemic disease." They include the headaches attributed to as follows: (1) hypoxia and/or hypercapnia (high altitude, diving, and sleep apnea); (2) dialysis; (3) arterial hypertension; (4) hypothyroidism; (5) fasting; (6) cardiac cephalgia; (7) headache attributed to other disturbance of homeostasis.

In common, the headaches attributed to a disorder of homeostasis have all of the following:

- Symptoms, signs or both suggesting a metabolic disorders or another disorder of homeostasis;
- Laboratorial investigation confirming the disorder of the homeostasis (all these headaches require confirmation);
- The frequency or severity of headache vary as a function of the severity of the disorder with a specified time lag;
- Headache disappears in temporal relation after normalization of the homeostatic state.

Because all the headaches in the upcoming sections follow the same pattern, we will not present tables describing the diagnostic criteria of all of them. The most relevant and common will be described in better detail.

HEADACHES ATTRIBUTED TO HYPOXIA OR HYPERCAPNIA (10.1)

The ICHD-2 criteria for headache secondary to hypoxia states that headache begins within 24 hours following acute onset of hypoxia with PaO_2 <70 mmHg or in chronically hypoxic patients with PaO_2 persistently at or below these levels. The ICHD-2 comments that it is difficult to separate the effects of hypoxia and hypercapnia, a statement with which we concur.

Accordingly, an enormous number of situations or diseases that are related to acute or chronic hypoxia/hypercapnia may be associated with headache, and describing all of them is beyond the scope of this chapter. In brief, any disease that induces a hypoxic state, such as pulmonary

Box 20–7 Headache Attributed to Chronic Postmeningitis Headache (9.4.1).

A. Headache with at least one of the following characteristics and fulfilling criteria C and D:
   1. Diffuse continuous pain
   2. Associated with dizziness
   3. Associated with difficulty in concentrating and/or loss of memory
B. Evidence of previous intracranial bacterial infection from cerebrospinal fluid (CSF) examination or neuroimaging
C. Headache is a direct continuation of 9.1.1 *Headache attributed to bacterial meningitis*
D. Headache persists for >3 months after resolution of infection

diseases (asthma, chronic obstructive pulmonary disease), cardiac disease (congestive heart failure), or hematologic disorders (with significant anemia) may be associated with headache. Often, the headache is neglected by the patients because of the presence of other symptoms, or undertreated by the doctors because of therapeutic limitations.

The ICHD-2 does individualize three specific situations associated with headaches attributed to hypoxia, which are common and potentially manageable. They will be discussed in more detail herein.

High Altitude Headache (10.1.1)

The criteria required for this headache are at least two of: (1) bilateral, (2) frontal or fronto-temporal, (3) dull or pressing quality, (4) mild or moderate severity, and (5) aggravated by exercise or movement. The headache occurs at altitudes above 2500 m, within 24 hours of ascent and resolves within 8 hours of descent (Box 20–8).

Although the criteria suggest that the headache is more often bilateral, unilateral headaches can occur, and this is seen more often in migraineurs who typically experience unilateral migraine attacks (Raskin, 1988). High altitude headache is often associated with nausea, photophobia, vertigo, poor concentration and, in severe cases, impaired judgment and signs that suggest brain edema.

A recent study that used T2 and diffusion-weighted MRI to assess the pathophysiology of acute mountain sickness (AMS) investigated 22 subjects in normoxia AND after 16 hours of passive exposure to normobaric hypoxia, corresponding to a simulated altitude of 4500 m and after 6 hours recovery in normoxia. All subjects developed headache, which was associated with a mild increase in brain volume that resolved during normoxic recovery. Hypoxia was also associated with an increased T(2) relaxation time [T(2)rt] and a general trend toward an increased apparent diffusion coefficient (ADC). ADC values were consistently associated with the severity of neurologic symptoms. The authors suggested that mild extracellular vasogenic edema contributes to the generalized brain swelling observed at high altitude and may be of significance in headache attributed to altitude (Kallenberg, Bailey, et al., 2006). Furthermore, efforts to demonstrate a specific genotype associated with a predisposition to develop this headache has lead to the suggestion that low levels of messenger RNA expression of the ATP1A1 subunit of the ATPase gene may be of importance (Appenzeller, Minko, et al., 2005).

The medical treatment of the disorder involves acetazolamide, in doses higher than 250 bid (Carlsten, Swenson, et al., 2004), or steroids, such as dexamethasone.

Diving Headache (10.1.2)

More than 40% of the subjects with decompression sickness develop headache (Wirjomesito et al., 1989). Decompression sickness follows a sudden change in the pressure of ambient gases to which subjects have been acclimatized (Appenzeller, 1972). It is well established that headache in divers, while uncommon and

Box 20–8 High-altitude Headache 10.1.1.

Diagnostic criteria:

A. Headache with at least two of the following characteristics and fulfilling criteria C and D:
   1. Bilateral
   2. Frontal or frontotemporal
   3. Dull or pressing quality
   4. Mild or moderate intensity
   5. Aggravated by exertion, movement, straining, coughing or bending

B. Ascent to altitude above 2500 m

C. Headache develops within 24 hours after ascent

D. Headache resolves within 8 hours after descent

generally benign, can occasionally signify serious consequences of hyperbaric exposure such as arterial gas embolism, decompression sickness, and otic or paranasal sinus barotrauma. Inadequate ventilation of compressed gases can lead to carbon dioxide accumulation, cerebral vasodilatation, and headache (Cheshire and Ott, 2001). In patients where the headache is not obviously benign, the diagnostic evaluation should consider otic and paranasal sinus barotrauma, arterial gas embolism, decompression sickness, carbon dioxide retention, carbon monoxide toxicity, hyperbaric-triggered migraine, cervical and temporomandibular joint strain, supraorbital neuralgia, carotid artery dissection, exertional or cold stimulus headache syndromes. Focal neurologic symptoms, even in the migraineur, should not be ignored, but rather treated acutely with 100% oxygen and referred without delay to a facility with a hyperbaric chamber (Cheshire, 2004). More recently, attention has been focused on the potential relationship between patent foramen ovale (PFO) and migraine with aura, and this relationship was first suggested in scuba divers (Tobis and Azarbal, 2005). Therefore, it is prudent to screen for PFO before assigning a diagnosis of diving headache.

Symptoms can be treated acutely with 100% oxygen and, if decompression sickness is present, patients should be referred without delay to a facility with a hyperbaric chamber.

Sleep Apnea Headache (10.1.3)

The relationship between headache and sleep disorders is complex. First, sleep disturbances may trigger migraine (Poceta, 2002). Second, snoring and other sleep disorders are risk factors for migraine progression (Scher, Stewart, et al., 2003). Third, sleep apnea is a risk factor for cluster headache (Graff-Radford and Newman, 2004).

Sleep apnea can, per se, cause headache, which is better described as a daily or almost daily mild headache, that resembles chronic tension-type headache, and is more severe in the morning, resolving about 30 minutes after awakening. Other clinical symptoms of sleep apnea are usually present and the headache disappears with the treatment of the sleep-related breathing disorder (Rains and Poceta, 2006).

DIALYSIS HEADACHE (10.2)

Headache is a known emerging symptom of hemodialysis treatment (Bana, Yap, et al., 1972). About 70% of patients receiving hemodialysis complain of headache (Antoniazzi, Bigal, et al., 2003). To be classified as dialysis headache according to the ICHD-2, patients must develop headache in at least 50% of the dialysis sessions. Furthermore, headaches must resolve within 72 hours after each hemodialysis session and cease altogether after successful transplantation. However, in a prospective study, approximately one third of patients with otherwise typical dialysis headache also experienced similar headache in between the dialysis sessions (Antoniazzi, Bigal, et al., 2003). In this series, headache occurred mainly in the second half of the hemodialysis sessions (86%). Arterial hypertension (38%), arterial hypotension (12%) and changes in weight during the hemodialysis sessions (6%) were the most consistent triggers (Antoniazzi, Bigal, et al., 2002). Disequilibrium syndrome should also be considered. Furthermore, because caffeine is rapidly removed by dialysis, caffeine-withdrawal headache should be considered in patients who consume large amounts of caffeine. Treatment is symptomatic and sometimes complicated by the chronic renal insufficiency status.

HEADACHE ATTRIBUTED TO HYPERTENSION (10.4)

It is usually accepted, although the evidence to support this common acceptance is weak, that chronic mild or moderate arterial hypertension does not cause headache. It is still controversial if hypertension is a risk factor for chronic daily headache. This group of headaches will be discussed under Chapter X.[ED: Please update the chapter here.]

HEADACHE ATTRIBUTED TO HYPOTHYROIDISM (10.4)

It has been demonstrated that approximately 30% of subjects with hypothyroidism have headaches, improving after thyroid hormone replacement

(Moreau, Manceau, et al., 1998). In migraineurs with subclinical hypothyroidism, treatment of borderline hypothyroidism is sometimes followed by dramatic improvement in the control of the headache (Spierings, 2001). Furthermore, hypothyroidism was an important risk factor for new daily persistent headache in a clinic-based case control study, when the control groups were migraine [odds ratio = 16, 95% confidence interval (CI) 3.6 – 72.0] and chronic posttraumatic headache (odds ratio = 10.3, 95% CI 2.3 – 46.7) (Bigal, Sheftell, et al., 2002) (Box 20–9).

Headache attributed to hypothyroidism is a new entry to the ICHD-2 and requires a continuous, bilateral, nonpulsatile headache, in a subject with documented hypothyroidism. The headache begins within 2 months after the onset of hypothyroidism and lasts less than 3 months after its effective treatment. Headache resolves within 2 months after effective treatment of hypothyroidism.

HEADACHES ATTRIBUTED TO FASTING (10.5)

Hypoglycemia is among the most commonly reported migraine trigger. In individuals without a well-defined history of headache, prolonged fasting may also be associated with the development of headaches. This is often seen in prolonged religious fasts and has been documented as "Yom Kippur Headache" (Kundin, 1996) and "First of Ramadan Headache." (Mosek and Korczyn, 1995; Awada and al Jumah, 1999). Although hypoglycemia may be the cause with many of these headaches, fasting headache can occur in the absence of hypoglycemia, suggesting that other factors play an important role (e.g., caffeine withdrawal, duration of sleep, and circadian factors). A recent study suggested that preemptive treatment with cyclo-oxygenase 2 (COX-2) inhibitors (e.g. rofecoxib, 50 mg just before the onset of fasting) is effective in preventing or attenuating the headache associated with fasting. (Drescher and Elstein 2006). Because COX-2 inhibitors are not available in many countries, preemptive treatment with NSAIDs or long-acting triptans may be reasonable options.

THE TOXIC HEADACHES

The toxic headaches (chapter 8 of the ICHD-2) may be subdivided into three subgroups:

1. The headaches that are caused by an unwanted effect of a toxic substance (a substance that is toxic per se);
2. The headaches that happen as an unwanted effect of a normal exposure. At this point it is fundamental to differentiate the toxic headaches from the primary headaches with known triggers. For example, a migraineurs may report that alcohol triggers his or her migraine. However, a person may have a headache only when exposed to alcohol. The second situation is considered to be a toxic headache, whereas the first is a migraine with a known trigger;
3. The headaches that happen as an unwanted effect of an exposure to an experimental substance (e.g., phase 1–phase 3 studies of new medications).

For all headaches, there is a minimum dose of exposure that is required, the headache follows at least half of the exposures (and at least three times), and the headache resolves when the substance is eliminated.

Box 20–9 Headache Attributed to Hypothyroidism (10.4).

A. Headache with at least one of the following characteristics and fulfilling criteria C and D:
   1. Bilateral
   2. Nonpulsatile
   3. Continuous
B. Hypothyroidism is demonstrated by appropriate investigations
C. Headache develops within 2 months after other symptoms of hypothyroidism become evident

Furthermore, the headaches can be induced after acute and chronic exposures. The prototype of the headaches induced by chronic exposures are the medication overuse headaches (rebound headaches), which will be discussed together with the chronic daily headaches.

Discussing all of the toxic headaches in detail is beyond the scope of this chapter. Herein, we provide an overview of these headaches. The readers are referred to the ICHD-2 for a complete list of the toxic headaches, as well as a full list of references.

Herein, we discuss a few toxic headaches that exemplify the group.

The NO Donor-induced Headache

Former names of this headache include the nitroglycerine headache, dynamite headache, and hot-dog headache. Headache is the most common side effect of therapeutic use of nitroglycerin and other NO donors (Thadani and Rodgers, 2006). The ICHD-2 recognizes two subtypes of headache. An immediate and a delayed NO-donor induced headache. Both tend to be bilateral and throbbing. Furthermore, in migraineurs, NO donors are migraine triggers.

In a study where 28 migraineurs and 14 controls received 0.5 mg nitroglycerin, two types of headache developed after the nitroglycerin administration: (1) an immediate mild headache that does not fulfill the criteria for migraine and disappears spontaneously within 1 hour, occurring in both groups; (2) a typical migraine attack without aura develops several hours after the nitroglycerin administration (mean latency: 250 minutes), occurring in migraineurs only (Juhasz, Zsombok, et al., 2004).

The "hot-dog" headache syndrome consists of a NO-donor induced headache happening in susceptible individuals after eating cured meats, such as hot dogs, sausages or bacon. The NO is added to the food as a modifier (colorizer) (Henderson and Raskin, 1972; Scher and Scher, 1992).

Carbon Monoxide-induced Headache

Carbon monoxide is an odorless gas that causes a variety of symptoms at different levels of exposures. Typically, there is mild headache without gastrointestinal or neurological symptoms with carboxyhemoglobin levels in the range 10%–20%; moderate pulsating headache and irritability with levels of 20%–30%; severe headache with nausea, vomiting, and blurred vision with levels of 30%–40%. At levels greater than 40%, there are changes in consciousness (Domachevsky, Adir, et al., 2005).

In a prospective study, 100 patients referred for hyperbaric oxygen treatment of acute carbon monoxide poisoning were asked whether headache was part of their symptom complex and to describe the clinical features (Hampson and Hampson, 2002). The mean carboxyhemoglobin level was 21.3% ± 9.3%. The most common location for pain was frontal (66%), although more than one location was involved in 58% of patients. Most reported dull pain (72%). Peak intensity of pain did not correlate with the carboxyhemoglobin level. Headache improved before hyperbaric oxygen treatment in 72%, resolving entirely in 21%. Of those with residual headache, pain improved with hyperbaric oxygen in 97%, resolving entirely in 44%.

Alcohol-induced Headache

Similar to NO-donor induced headaches, the ICHD-2 codes for two forms of alcohol-induced headaches includes an immediate form (developing within 3 hours and resolving within hours), and a delayed form (the *hangover* headache) (Box 20–10).

The immediate form is much less common than the delayed form, which is considered to be one of the commonest types of headache (Rasmussen, Jensen, et al., 1991). It remains unclear whether, in addition to alcohol, other components of alcoholic beverages play a role. It also remains uncertain whether the mechanism is a delayed response to toxic effects or whether mechanisms similar to those responsible for delayed NO donor-induced headache may be involved. The headache is typically bilateral, throbbing, and aggravated by physical activity.

Alcohol is also a well-known trigger of migraine and cluster headaches.

Box 20–10 Delayed alcohol-induced headache (Hangover Headache) (8.1.4.2).

Diagnostic criteria:

A. Headache with at least one of the following characteristics and fulfilling criteria C and D:
   1. Bilateral
   2. Frontotemporal location
   3. Pulsating quality
   4. Aggravated by physical activity
B. Ingestion of a modest amount of alcoholic beverage by a migraine sufferer or an intoxicating amount by a nonmigraine sufferer
C. Headache develops after blood alcohol level declines or reduces to zero
D. Headache resolves within 72 hours

Headache Induced by Food Components and Additives

Several food components or additives are known migraine triggers, and may also induce headache in predisposed nonmigraine individuals. In such situations, the headache is considered to be secondary. Typically, these headaches are bilateral, throbbing and aggravated by physical activity.

Monosodium Glutamate-induced Headache, explains the former "Chinese-food" headache, or the "Chinese-restaurant syndrome" (Merritt and Williams, 1990). Endogenous glutamate is a major neurotransmitter. After binding to a cell membrane receptor there can be a stimulation of what can be called the NO-mediated neurotransmission pathway (NO-MNP). The activity of the enzyme that produces NO from arginine, NO synthase, and the level of NO, become elevated. NO has little activity within the cell in which it is produced, but it rapidly diffuses outside the cell and produces effects in neighboring cells. The NO-MNP can be activated to release NO in endothelial cells, which in turn acts on neighboring vascular smooth muscle cells to induce vasodilation. Therefore, exogenous, ingested glutamate, like endogenous glutamate, can lead to the same stimulation of the NO-MNP in sensitive individuals, which would then cause the symptoms of the Chinese restaurant syndrome and/or glutamate-induced asthma. (Merritt and Williams, 1990; Scher and Scher, 1992).

Aspartame, widely used as an artificial sweetener, induces headache in approximately 8% of migraineurs (Lipton, Newman, et al., 1989), and may induce headache in nonmigraineurs as well ((Blumenthal and Vance, 1997). *Sucralose,* another artificial sweetener, was recently reported as a migraine trigger (Bigal and Krymchantowski, 2006), although it has never been reported as inducing headaches in nonmigraineurs, and, although evidence is lacking, appears to induce headache less frequently than aspartame.

Many other substances, including illicit drugs, are associated with headache. For example, headache is a reported side effect of *cocaine use,* developing immediately or within 1 hour after use and is not associated with other symptoms unless there is concomitant stroke or transient ischemic attack (TIA) (Warner, 1995). *Cannabis* use is reported to cause headache associated with mouth dryness, paraesthesias, feelings of warmth and suffusion of the conjunctivae (Alvaro, Iriondo, et al., 2002).

References

Alvaro, LC, Iriondo, I, Villaverde, FJ (2002). Sexual headache and stroke in a heavy cannabis smoker. *Headache,* 42(3):224–226.

American Academy of Neurology Quality Standards Subcomittee (1998). Evaluation and management of intracranial mass lesions in AIDS. *Neurology,* 50:21–26.

Antoniazzi, AL, Bigal, ME, Bordinio, CA, et al. (2002). [Headache and hemodialysis: evaluation of the possible triggering factors and of the treatment]. *Arq Neuropsiquiatr,* 60(3-A):614–618.

Antoniazzi, AL, Bigal, ME, Bordini, CA, et al. (2003). Headache associated with dialysis: the International Headache Society criteria revisited. *Cephalalgia,* 23 (2):146–149.

Antoniazzi, AL, Bigal, ME, Bordini, CA,et al. (2003). Headache and hemodialysis: a prospective study. *Headache,* 43(2):99–102.

Appenzeller, O, Minko, T, Qualls, C, et al. (2005). Migraine in the Andes and headache at sea level. *Cephalalgia*, 25(12):1117–1121.

Attia J, Hatala R, Cook, DJ, et al. (1999). The rational clinical examination. Does this adult patient have acute meningitis? *JAMA*, 282(2):175–181.

Awada, A and al Jumah, M (1999). The first-of-Ramadan headache. *Headache*, 39(7):490–493.

Bana, DS, Yap, AU, Graham, JR, et al. (1972). Headache during hemodialysis. *Headache*, 12(1):1–14.

Bernardini, GL. (2004). Diagnosis and management of brain abscess and subdural emyema. *Curr Neurol Neurosci Rep*, 4(6):448–456.

Bigal, ME and Krymchantowski, AV (2006). Migraine triggered by sucralose—a case report. *Headache*, 46(3):515–517.

Bigal, ME, Sheftell, FD, Rapoport, AM, et al. (2002). Chronic daily headache: identification of factors associated with induction and transformation. *Headache*, 42(7):575–581.

Blumenthal, HJ and Vance, DA (1997). Chewing gum headaches. *Headache*, 37(10):665–666.

Bohr, V, Hansen, B, Kjersen, H, et al. (1983). Sequelae from bacterial meningitis and their relation to the clinical condition during acute illness, based on 667 questionnaire returns. Part II of a three part series. *J Infect*, 7:102–110.

Brew, BJ and Miller, J (1993). Human immunodeficiency virus-related headache. *Neurology*, 43:1098–1100.

Calfee, DP and Wispelwey, B (2000). Brain abscess. *Semin Neurology*, 20(3):353–360.

Carlsten, C, Swenson, ER, Ruoss, C, et al. (2004). A dose-response study of acetazolamide for acute mountain sickness prophylaxis in vacationing tourists at 12,000 feet (3630 m). *High Alt Med Biol*, 5(1):33–39.

Cheshire, WP (2004). Headache and facial pain in scuba divers. *Curr Pain Headache Rep*, 8(4):315–320.

Cheshire, WP Jr, and Ott, MC (2001). Headache in divers. *Headache*, 41(3):235–247.

de Gans, J and van de Beek, D (2002). Dexamethasone in adults with bacterial meningitis. *N Engl J Med*, 347:1549–1556.

Connolly, KJ and Hammer, SM (1990). The acute aseptic meningitis syndrome. *Infect Dis Clin North Am*, 4(4):599–622.

Davis, LE, DeBiasi, R, Goade, DE, et al. (2006). West Nile virus neuroinvasive disease. *Ann Neurol*, 60 (3):286–300.

De Marinis M, and Welch KM. (1992) Headache associated with non-cephalic infections: classification and mechanisms. *Cephalalgia*, 12 (4):197–201.

Domachevsky, L, Adir, Y, Grupper, M, et al. (2005). Hyperbaric oxygen in the treatment of carbon monoxide poisoning. *Clin Toxicol (Phila)*, 43(3):181–188.

Drescher, MJ and Elstein, Y (2006). Prophylactic COX 2 inhibitor: an end to the Yom Kippur headache. *Headache*, 46(10):1487–1491.

Gifford, Al and Hecht, FM. (2001). Evaluating HIV-infected patients with headache: who needs computed tomography? *Headache*, 41(5):441–448.

Goldstein, J. (1990). Headache and acquired immunodeficiency syndrome. *Neurol Clin*, 8:947–960.

Graham, CB and Wippold, FJ. (2001). Headache in the HIV patient: a review with special attention to the role of imaging. *Cephalalgia*, 21(3):169–174.

Graff-Radford, SB and Newman, A (2004). Obstructive sleep apnea and cluster headache. *Headache*, 44(6):607–610.

Greenlee, JE (2003). Subdural empyema. *Curr Treat Options Neurol*, 5(1):13–22.

Hakan, T, Ceran, N, Erdem, I, et al.(2006). Bacterial brain abscesses: an evaluation of 96 cases. *J Infect*, 52(5):359–366.

Hampson, NB and Hampson, LA (2002). Characteristics of headache associated with acute carbon monoxide poisoning. *Headache*, 42(3):220–223.

Headache Classification Subcommittee of the International Headache Society. The international classification of headache disorders, 2nd edn. *Cephalalgia* 2004:24 (Suppl1).

Henderson, WR and Raskin, NH (1972). "Hot-dog" headache: individual susceptibility to nitrite. *Lancet*, 2 (7788):1162–1163.

Holloway, RG and Kieburtz, KD (1995). Headache and the human immunodeficiency virus type 1 infection. *Headache*, 35:245–255.

Hopkins, S and Jolles, S (2005). Drug-induced aseptic meningitis. *Expert Opin Drug Saf*, 4(2):285–297.

Infection in Neurosurgery Working Party of the British Society for Antimicrbial Chemotherapy. (2000). The rational use of antibiotics in the treatment of brain abscess. *Br J Neurosurg*, 14(6):525–530.

Juhasz, G, Zsombok, T,Gonda, X, et al. (2004). [Nitroglycerin-induced headaches]. *Orv Hetil*, 145 (46):2323–2328.

Kao, PT, Tseng, HL, Liu, CP, et al. (2003). Brain abscess: clinical analysis of 53 cases. *J Microbiol Immunol Infect*, 36(27):129–136.

Kallenberg, KD, Bailey, M, Christ, S, et al. (2006). Magnetic resonance imaging evidence of cytotoxic cerebral edema in acute mountain sickness. *J Cereb Blood Flow Metab*, 27(5):1064–1071.

Kastenbauer, S, Pfister, HW, Wisplewey, B et al. (2004). Brain abscess. In *Infections of the Central Nervous System* (3rd Edn).(WM Scheld, RJ Whitley and CM Marra, eds), pp. 479–508. Lippincott Williams & Wilkins, Philadelphia.

Kennedy, PG (2004). Viral encephalitis: causes, differential diagnosis, and management. *JNNP*, 75 (Suppl. 1): i10–i15.

Khayr, W and Ramadan, NM (2007). Headache associated with AIDS. *Medlink*,

Khetsuriani, N, Quiroz, ES, Holman, RC, et al. (2003). Viral meningitis-associated hospitalization in the United States, 1989-1999. *Neuroepidemiology*, 22:345–352.

Kundin, JE (1996). Yom Kippur headache. *Neurology*, 47 (3):854.

Lipton, RB, Feraru, ER, Weiss, G, et al. (1991). Headache in HIV-1 related disorders. *Headache*, 31:518–522.

Lipton, RB, Newman, LC, Cohen, JS, et al. (1989). Aspartame as a dietary trigger of headache. *Headache*, 29 (2):90–92.

Lu, CH, Chang, WN, Lui, CC (2006). Strategies for the management of bacterial brain abscess. *J Clin Neurosci*, 13:976–985.

Marchioni, E, Tavazzi, E, Bono, G, et al. (2006). Headache attributed to infection: observations on the IHS classification (ICHD-II). *Cephalalgia*, 26:1427–1433.

Mathisen, GE and Johnson, JP (1997). Brain abscess. *Clin Infect Dis*, 25:763–771.

Merritt, JE and Williams, PB (1990). Vasospasm contributes to monosodium glutamate-induced headache. *Headache*, 30(9):575–580.

Mirsattari, SM and Manitoba, U (1999). Primary headaches in HIV-infected patients. *Headache*, 39:3–10.

Moreau, T, Manceau, E, Giroud-Baleydier, F, et al. (1998). Headache in hypothyroidism. Prevalence and outcome under thyroid hormone therapy. *Cephalalgia*, 18(10):687–689.

Moris, G and Garcia-Monco, JC (1999). The challenge of drug-induced aseptic meningitis. *Arch Int Med*, 159:1185–1194.

Mosek, A and Korczyn, AD (1995). Yom Kippur headache. *Neurology*, 45(11):1953–1955.

Moskowitz, MA (1990). Basic mechanisms in vascular headache. *Neurol Clin*, 8:801–815.

Nathoo, N, Nadvi, SS, and van Dellen, JR (1999). Intracranial subdural empyemas in the era of computed tomography: a review of 699 cases. *Neurosurgery*, 44:529–535.

Neufeld, MY, Treves, TA, Chistik, V, et al. (1999). Postmeningitis headache. *Headache*, 39(2):132–134.

Osborn, MK and Steinberg, JP (2007). Subdural emyema and other suppurative complications of paranasal sinusitis. *Lancet Infect Dis*, 7:62–67.

Poceta, JS (2002). Sleep-related Headache. *Curr Treat Options Neurol*, 4(2):121–128.

Rains, JC and Poceta, JS (2006). Headache and sleep disorders: review and clinical implications for headache management. *Headache*, 46(9):1344–1363.

Rasmussen, BK, Jensen, R, Schroll, M, et al. (1991). Epidemiology of headache in a general population—a prevalence study. *J Clin Epidemiol*, 44(11):1147–1157.

Roche, M, Humphreys, H, Smythe, E, et al. (2003). A twelve-year review of central nervous system bacterial abscesses: presentation and aetiology. *Clin Microbiol Infect*, 9:803–809.

Roos, KL (2000a). Acute bacterial meningitis. *Semin Neurol*, 20(3)293–306.

Roos, KL (2000b). *Mycobacterium tuberculosis* meningitis and other etiologies of the aseptic meningitis syndrome. *Semin Neurol*, 20(3):329–335.

Rothbart, HA. (2000). Viral meningitis. *Semin Neurol*, 20 (3):277–292.

Saez-Llorens, X and McCracken Jr. GH (2003). Bacterial meningitis in children. *Lancet*, 361:2139–2148.

Scher, AI, Stewart, WF, Ricca, JA, et al. (2003). Factors associated with the onset and remission of chronic daily headache in a population-based study. *Pain*, 106 (1–2):81–89.

Scher, W and BM Scher, BM (1992). A possible role for nitric oxide in glutamate (MSG)-induced Chinese restaurant syndrome, glutamate-induced asthma, "hot-dog headache," pugilistic Alzheimer's disease, and other disorders. *Med Hypotheses*, 38(3):185–188.

Sejvar, JJ (2006). The evolving epidemiology of viral encephalitis. *Curr Opin Neurol*, 19(4):350–357.

Singer, EJ, Kim, J, Fahy-Chandon, B, et al. (1996). Headache in ambulator HIV-1 infected men enrolled in a longitudinal study. *Neurology*, 47:487–494.

Spierings, EL (2001). Daily migraine with visual aura associated with an occipital arteriovenous malformation. *Headache*, 41(2):193–197.

Straus, SE, Thorpe, KE, and Holroyd-Leduc, J (2006). How do I perform a lumbar puncture and analyze the results to diagnose bacterial meningitis? *JAMA*, 296 (16):2012–2022.

Tambussi, G, Gori, A, Capiluppi, B, et al. (2000). Neurological symptoms during primary human immunodeficiency virus (HIV) infection correlate with high levels of HIV RNS in cerebrospinal fluid. *Clin Infect Dis*, 30 (6):962–965.

Thadani, U and Rodgers, T (2006). Side effects of using nitrates to treat angina. *Expert Opin Drug Saf*, 5 (5):667–674.

Tobis, MJ and Azarbal, B (2005). Does patent foramen ovale promote cryptogenic stroke and migraine headache? *Tex Heart Inst J*, 32(3):362–365.

Tunkel, AR, Hartman, BJ, Kaplan, SL et al. (2004). Practice guidelines for the management of bacterial meningitis. *Clin Inf Dis*, 39:1267–1284.

Tyler, KL (2004). Update on herpes simplex encephalitis. *Rev Neurol Dis*, 1(4):169–178.

van de Beek, D, de Gans, J, Spanjaard, L, et al. (2004). Clinical features and prognostic factors in adults with bacterial meningitis. *N Engl J Med*, 351(18):1849–1859.

van de Beek, D, de Gans, J, Tunkel, AR et al. (2006). Community-acquired bacterial meningitis in adults. *N Engl J Med*, 354(1):44–53.

Warner, EA (1995). Is your patient using cocaine? Clinical signs that should raise suspicion. *Postgrad Med*, 98 (2):173–176, 180.

Wirjosemito SA, Touhey JE, Workman WT (1989). Type II altitude decompression sickness (DCS): U.S. Air Force experiance with 133 cases. *Aviat Space Environ Med*, 60(3):256–262.

Xiao, F, Tseng, MY, Teng, LJ, et al. (2005). Brain abscess: clinical experience and analysis of prognostic factors. *Surg Neurol*. 63(5):442–449.

21 Cervicogenic Headache

Nikolai Bogduk and Thorsten Bartsch

Cervicogenic headache is among the best understood of the headaches in terms of its anatomy and physiology. Essentially it is pain referred to the head from the upper cervical spine. For this reason, it has been recognized more widely by pain specialists and manual therapists, accustomed to treating spinal pain, than by mainstream headache specialists.

Amongst headache specialists, the entity has been disputed, largely because of controversies concerning the validity of its diagnosis. Unlike other headaches, cervicogenic headache defies diagnosis by clinical features and conventional imaging. Therefore, headache specialists have lacked means of making the diagnosis. However, the diagnosis can be made using fluoroscopically guided diagnostic blocks.

DEFINITION

Cervicogenic headache is referred pain perceived in the head from a source in the upper cervical spine. The pain can be perceived in regions of the head innervated by cervical nerves (the occiput) or by the first division of the trigeminal nerve (forehead and orbit). Cervical pain might be referred to the territories of the second or third divisions of the trigeminal nerve, but evidence of this pattern of referral is sparse.

HISTORICAL BACKGROUND

Some investigators (Pearce, 1995; Haldeman and Dagenais, 2001) have traced the earliest reference to headaches and the neck to a series of lectures given by Hilton in 1860–1862. The earliest, accessible publication by an eminent authority dates back to 1913, when Gordon Holmes (1913) credited that headaches could arise from the neck. Since that time several theories have been advanced and variously refuted. [For a comprehensive review, see Bogduk (2005) and Bogduk and Bartsch (2005).]

No evidence has ever been provided for "fibrositis" (Holmes, 1913), "rheumatic headache" (Patrick, 1913; Luff, 1913; Kelly, 1942), trigger points (Travell and Rinzler, 1952; Travell, 1962), or weakened fibro-osseous insertions (Hackett, 1962; Kayfetz et al, 1963). The only diagnostic criterion for these conditions was tenderness in the upper cervical muscles, but tender points in the neck occur in many forms of headache, including migraine (Perelson, 1947; Oleson, 1978; Lous and Oleson, 1982; Langemark and Oleson, 1987), and are not indicative specifically of a cervical source of pain.

In 1926, Barré proposed that headaches could be caused by irritation of the vertebral nerve by arthritis of the cervical spine (Barré, 1926), but this mechanism has since been refuted. Electrical stimulation of the vertebral nerve does not influence vertebral blood flow (Bogduk et al, 1981). Moreover, the vertebrobasilar system is remarkably resistant even to intra-arterial injections of vasoactive agents (Bogduk et al, 1981). These physiological data support clinical opinions that there is no basis for belief in the Barré syndrome, also known as migraine cervicale (Bartschi-Rochaix, 1968; Lance, 1982). Yet, the concept continues to be promoted (Tamura, 1989).

In 1949, Hunter and Mayfield announced that occipital neuralgia could be caused by compression of the occipital nerve between the posterior arch of the atlas and the lamina of C2 (Hunter and

Mayfield, 1949), and recommended treatment by greater occipital neurectomy. It has since been shown that the greater occipital nerve cannot be injured in this way (Bogduk, 1980; Bilge, 2004). Unheeded has been a later publication, in which Mayfield was more reserved about his earlier enthusiasm for greater occipital neurectomy and its success rate (Mayfield, 1955).

Some authors have attributed headaches to cervical spondylosis (Raney and Raney, 1948; Schultz and Semmes, 1950; Brain, 1963; Wilkinson, 1971; Peterson et al, 1975; Pawl, 1977; Chirls, 1978), but no study has shown that cervical spondylosis is significantly more common in patients with headache than in asymptomatic subjects.

CONTEMPORARY CONTROVERSIES

In recent years, disputes concerning cervicogenic headache have centered on its diagnostic criteria (Bogduk, 2004c). (For a comprehensive review see Bogduk, 2005.) Neurologists in Europe have fostered diagnosis by clinical criteria (Sjaastad et al, 1983, 1990, 1998), whereas pain specialists in North America and Australia have fostered the application of controlled diagnostic blocks (Bogduk, 1984, 1997, 2004a, 2004b; Rothbart, 1996;).

The clinical criteria, proposed in 1990 and revised in 1998, defined cervicogenic headache as a unilateral headache associated with evidence of cervical involvement, in the form of provocation of pain by movement of the neck or by pressing the neck, concurrent pain in the neck, shoulder, and arm, and reduced range of motion of the neck (Sjaastad et al, 1990, 1998).

Subsequent studies showed that unilaterality was not unique to cervicogenic headache (Leone et al, 1993, 1995; D'Amico et al, 1994), nor was triggering of headache by neck movement or by pressure on the neck (Leone et al, 1998). Patients said to have cervicogenic headache have reduced pressure-pain thresholds (Bovim, 1992) and impaired muscle function (Jull et al, 1999), but their scores in these features overlap considerably those of normal subjects, so that a valid diagnostic criterion cannot be supported. Similarly, radiographic abnormalities are either lacking in patients said to have cervicogenic headache (Pfaffenrath et al, 1987; Fredriksen et al, 1989), or have a distribution that overlaps that of normal subjects (Zwart, 1997).

When tested for agreement between observers, the proposed clinical features of cervicogenic headache differ in their reliability. The most reliable were "pain starts in the neck and radiates to the fronto-temporal region," "pain radiates to the ipsilateral shoulder and arm," and "provocation of pain by neck movement" (van Suijlekom et al, 1999; 2000). Other features, such as "restricted range of motion" and "pressure pain on palpation" have low agreement.

Some authorities have proposed a less emphatic, clinical approach to diagnosis. They reduced the clinical criteria to a list of seven (Antonaci et al, 2001) (Table 21–1), and qualified the certainty of diagnosis. They proposed that "possible" cervicogenic headache could be diagnosed if patients had "unilateral headache" and "pain starting in the neck." Satisfying any three additional criteria promoted the diagnosis to "probable" cervicogenic headache. Using these operational guidelines, the authors felt that they could confidently distinguish cervicogenic headache from migraine. The clinical features most strongly indicative of cervicogenic headache were "pain radiating to the shoulder and arm," "varying duration or fluctuating continuous pain," "moderate, non-throbbing pain," and "history of neck trauma."

Nevertheless, although investigators have sought to defend the diagnostic criteria for cervicogenic headache, they have examined only the nosologic validity of the criteria, that is, the extent to which the criteria seem to distinguish cervicogenic headache from migraine and tension-type headache. No studies have established that patients who satisfy the diagnostic criteria actually have a cervical source for their pain. Fundamental to the concept of cervicogenic headache is that it constitutes pain referred to the head from a cervical source. Therefore, demonstrating such a source is essential for the diagnosis.

For this reason, advocates from North America (Rothbart, 1996) and Australia (Bogduk, 1984, 1997, 2004a, 2004b) regard response to local anesthetic blocks as essential to diagnose cervicogenic headache. They maintain that diagnostic blocks circumvent the difficulties of reliability and validity of clinical examination and provide direct evidence of a cervical source of pain.

Table 21–1 The collapsed criteria for cervicogenic headache. (Antonaci et al, 2001)

1. Unilateral headache without side-shift
2. Symptoms and signs of neck involvement:
   Pain triggered by
   - Neck movement or sustained awkward posture and/or
   - External pressure of the posterior neck or occipital region

   Ipsilateral neck, shoulder, and arm pain

   Reduced range of motion
3. Pain episodes of varying duration or fluctuating continuous pain
4. Moderate, nonexcruciating pain, usually of a nonthrobbing nature
5. Pain starting in the neck, spreading to oculo-fronto-temporal areas
6. Anesthetic blockades abolish the pain transiently provided complete anesthesia is obtained

Or sustained neck trauma a relatively short time prior to the onset

7. Various attack-related phenomena: autonomic symptoms and signs, nausea, vomiting, ispilateral edema and flushing in the periocular area, dizziness, photophobia, phonophobia, blurred vision in the ipsilateral eye

The revised criteria of the International Headache Society reflect the tension between clinical diagnosis and objective testing for cervicogenic headache (International Headache Society, 2004) (Table 21–2). They require evidence of a cervical source of pain, but the explanatory notes declare that clinical features that lack reliability or validity are not acceptable. In the absence of other evidence, controlled diagnostic blocks become the only means of establishing the diagnosis.

NEUROANATOMY

The gray matter of the pars caudalis of the spinal nucleus of the trigeminal nerve is continuous with the apical gray column of the spinal cord (Humphrey, 1952; Torvik, 1956; Kerr, 1961a; Taren and Kahn, 1962; Kaube et al, 1993; Strassman et al, 1994; Goadsby and Hoskin, 1997). Within this gray matter, no cytoarchitectonic differences distinguish trigeminal from spinal neurons, nor is there an anatomical boundary between trigeminal neurons and cervical neurons. Nevertheless, within this gray matter a nucleus can be defined. It is defined not by intrinsic features but by the afferents that it receives.

Nociceptive afferents of the trigeminal nerve descend in the spinal tract of the trigeminal nerve. They send collaterals into the pars caudalis of the spinal nucleus but continue past the dorsal horns of the upper three segments of the cervical spinal cord, into which they also send collaterals (Kerr, 1961a). This distribution defines the trigeminocervical nucleus.

The trigeminocervical nucleus is the essential structure for headache. All nociception from the head is mediated by it. It receives trigeminal afferents from the skull, meninges, nose, mouth, face, and the intracranial and extracranial blood vessels. It also receives the nociceptive afferents of the glossopharyngeal, vagus, and facial nerves. At its lower end, trigeminal afferents overlap with those of the upper three cervical segments of the spinal cord. At this level, the mechanism for cervicogenic headache operates (Fig. 21–1).

The dorsal horns of the upper three cervical segments receive descending afferents from the trigeminal nerve, and terminals from the first three cervical spinal nerves. Spinal afferents do not ascend into the pars caudalis of the trigeminal nucleus, but variously they descend or ascend to neighboring spinal cord segments (Kerr, 1961a). Within the trigeminocervical nucleus, trigeminal and spinal afferents converge on second-order neurons that they share in common. Ascending tracts from these neurons can be activated by either cervical or trigeminal afferents. This convergence allows pain to be referred between cervical and cervical afferents or between cervical and trigeminal afferents.

TABLE 21–2 Diagnostic criteria for cervicogenic headache, as proposed by the International Headache Society (2004).

Diagnostic criteria

A. Pain referred from a source in the neck and perceived in one or more regions of the head and/or face, fulfilling criteria C and D
B. Clinical, laboratory and/or imaging evidence of a disorder or lesion within the cervical spine or soft tissues of the neck known to be, or generally accepted as, a valid cause of headache[a]
C. Evidence that the pain can be attributed to the neck disorder or lesion based on at least one of the following:
   1. demonstration of clinical signs that implicate a source of pain in the neck[b]
   2. abolition of headache following diagnostic blockade of a cervical structure or its nerve supply using placebo- or other adequate controls[c]
D. Pain resolves within 3 months after successful treatment of the causative disorder or lesion

[a] Tumors, fractures, infections and rheumatoid arthritis of the upper cervical spine have not been validated formally as causes of headache, but are nevertheless accepted as valid causes when demonstrated to be so in individual cases. Cervical spondylosis and osteochondritis are NOT accepted as valid causes fulfilling criterion B. When myofascial tender spots are, the headache should be coded under 2. *Tension-type headache.*

[b] Clinical signs acceptable for criterion C1 must have demonstrated reliability and validity. The future task is the identification of such reliable and valid operational tests. Clinical features such as neck pain, focal neck tenderness, history of neck trauma, mechanical exacerbation of pain, unilaterality, coexisting shoulder pain, reduced range of motion in the neck, nuchal onset, nausea, vomiting, photophobia etc. are not unique to cervicogenic headache. These may be features of cervicogenic headache, but they do not define relationship between the disorder and the source of the headache.

[c] Abolition of headache means complete relief of headache, indicated by a score of zero on a visual analogue scale (VAS). Nevertheless, acceptable as fulfilling criterion C2 is ⩾90% reduction in pain to a level of <5 on a 100-point VAS.

PERIPHERAL ANATOMY

The connections of the trigeminocervical nucleus dictate that any of the structures innervated by the upper three cervical nerves could, in principle, be a source of referred pain to the head. The peripheral distribution of the upper three cervical nerves, therefore, predicates the possible sources of cervicogenic headache.

In general terms, the upper cervical nerves have both an intracranial and an extracranial distribution. Cervical nerves innervate the inferior surface of the tentorium cerebelli, the dura mater of the posterior cranial fossa, and the vertebral artery. This distribution accounts for most of the serious causes of pain in the differential diagnosis of cervicogenic headache. In the cervical spine, cervical nerves innervate the vertebral column and its adnexae (Fig. 21–2).

The ventral rami of the first three cervical spinal nerves innervate the sternocleidomastoid muscle and trapezius (Williams et al, 1989). The C1 and C2 ventral rami innervate the atlanto-occipital and lateral atlanto-axial joints (Lazorthes and Gaubert, 1956; Bogduk, 1981a, 1981b). The C1 dorsal ramus innervates the suboccipital muscles (Williams et al, 1989). The C2 and C3 dorsal rami innervate the posterior neck muscles and the C2–3 zygapophysial joint (Bogduk, 1982). The C1–C3 sinuvertebral nerves innervate the C2–3 intervertebral disc (Bogduk et al, 1989; Mendel et al, 1992), the transverse ligament and the alar ligament (Kimmel, 1960), and the dura mater over the clivus (Kimmel, 1960). Cervical afferents form the recurrent meningeal branches of the hypoglossal and vagus nerves (Williams et al, 1989). Sensory fibers of the vertebral nerve, which accompanies the vertebral artery, are cervical in origin (Kimmel, 1959; Bogduk et al, 1981). The sensory innervation of the extracranial portions of the internal carotid artery has not been explicitly demonstrated but is presumably also cervical in origin. To various extents, each of these structures innervated by cervical nerves has been incriminated as a source of cervicogenic headache.

PHYSIOLOGY

Over the last 40 years, the physiology of cervical pain referred to the head has been investigated

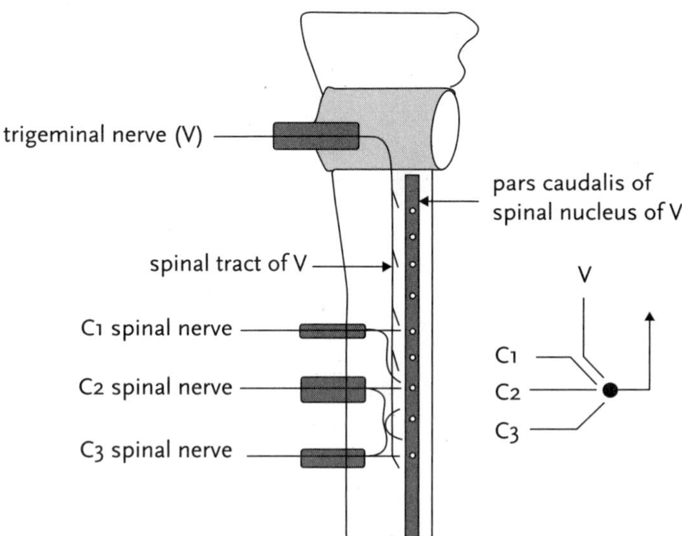

Figure 21–1 A sketch of the trigeminocervical nucleus. The nucleus is those portions of the pars caudalis of the spinal nucleus of the trigeminal nerve and the gray matter of the upper cervical spinal cord that receive trigeminal afferents. At cervical levels, the nucleus receives afferents from both the trigeminal nerve and the upper three cervical nerves. With the nucleus afferents from these sources convergence on common, second-order neurons (inset).

with increasingly sophisticated techniques in laboratory animals. In 1961, Kerr (Kerr, 1961b) provided the first evidence of convergence. He mapped the sites in the C1–2 segment of the spinal cord that responded to electrical stimulation of both the trigeminal nerve and the sensory roots of the C1 or C2 spinal nerves. Sites of convergence included the dorsal horn and the lateral cervical nucleus, but were also widespread across the segment, including the ventral horn.

Modern studies have demonstrated neurons in the lateral cervical nucleus of the cat that respond to electrical stimulation of both the superior sagittal sinus and the greater occipital nerve (Angus-Leppan et al, 1997). These studies prompted more detailed investigations of convergence between the dura mater of the skull and the greater occipital nerve.

Two complementary studies (Bartsch and Goadsby, 2002, 2003) in the rat found neurons in the C2 spinal cord that received convergent input from both trigeminal and cervical afferents. The neurons included wide-dynamic-range neurons and nociceptive-specific neurons located in laminae V and VI and laminae I and II of the dorsal horn at C2. The convergent input involved Aδ and C fibers. The trigeminal afferents were stimulated at the dura mater of the parietal bone, but had receptive fields that extended to the cutaneous territories predominantly of the ophthalmic, but also the maxillary and mandibular divisions of the trigeminal nerve. The cervical afferents were stimulated in the greater occipital nerve, but had receptive fields in the cutaneous territory of this nerve, and in the muscles that it innervates.

These studies demonstrated not only convergence but also functional interaction between trigeminal and cervical afferents (Bartsch and Goadsby, 2002, 2003). Electrical or chemical stimulation of trigeminal afferents sensitized the central neurons and increased their responses to cervical stimulation. Reciprocally, electrical or chemical stimulation of cervical afferents sensitized the neurons to trigeminal input. These observations established that either trigeminal or cervical stimulation could produce central sensitization of the trigeminocervical nucleus. Furthermore, this effect was differentially sensitive to input from different types of nerves and from different peripheral tissues.

Stimulation of C-fibers in cervical afferents produced greater and more enduring increases in central sensitization than did stimulation of

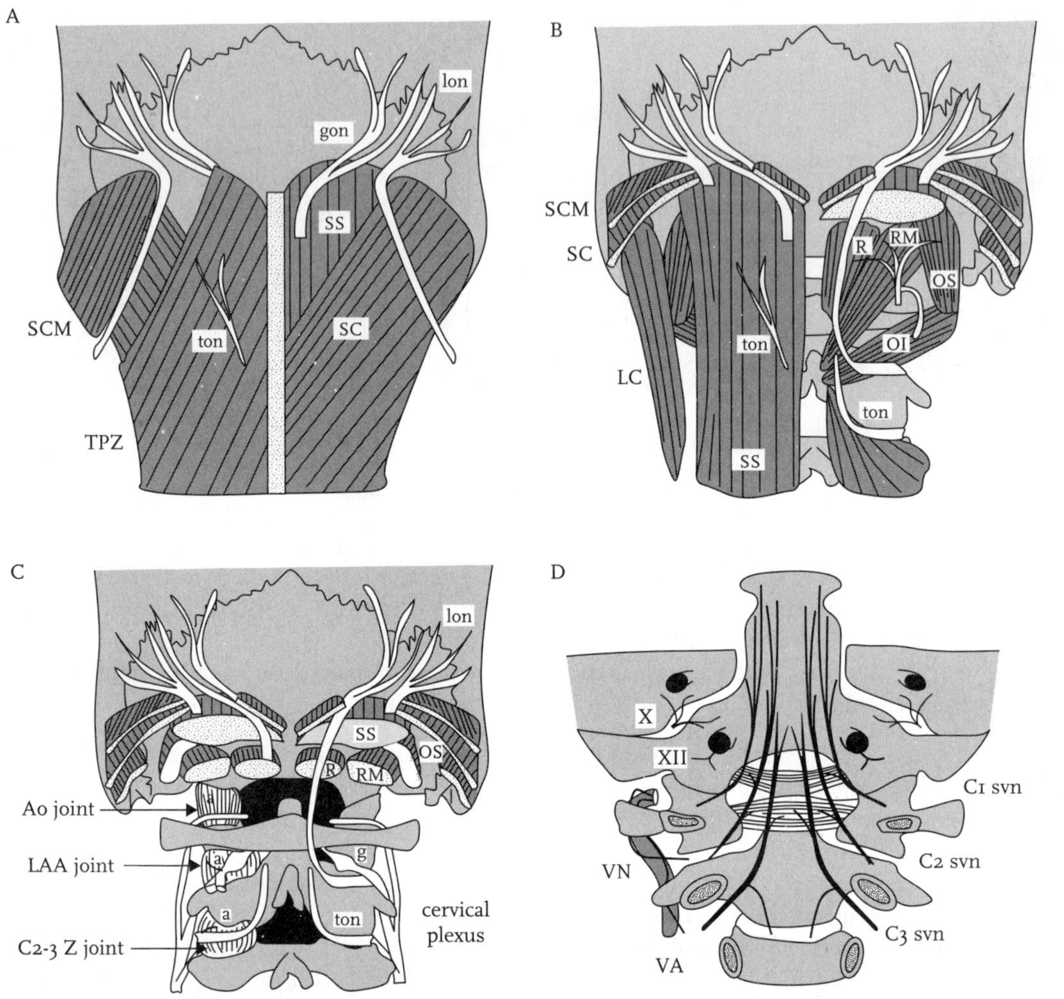

Figure 21–2 Sketches of progressively deep layers of dissection, showing the spinal structures supplied by cervical nerves. (*A*) External and superficial muscles. (*B*) deeper posterior muscles and suboccipital muscles. (*C*) The vertebrae and their synovial joints. (***D***) The sinuvertebral nerves within the vertebral canal and posterior cranial fossa. SCM: sternocleidomastoid. TPZ: trapezius; SS: semispinalis capitis; SC: splenius capitis; gon: greater occipital nerve; lon: lesser occipital nerve; ton: third occipital nerve; LC: longissimus capitis; R: rectus capitis posterior minor; RM: rectus capitis posterior major; OS: obliquus superior; OI: obliquus inferior; AO joint: atlanto-occipital joint; LAA joint: lateral atlanto-axial joint; Z joint: zygapophysial joint; svn: sinuvertebral nerve; VN: vertebral nerve; VA: vertebral artery; X: meningeal branches of the vagus nerve, from the jugular foramen; XII: meningeal branches of the hypoglossal nerve, from the hypoglossal canal.

Aδ fibers (Bartsch and Goadsby, 2002). Cervical afferent input from muscle produced a greater and longer-lasting increase in neural excitability than did cutaneous input (Bartsch and Goadsby, 2003). Conversely, stimulation of trigeminal afferents from the dura mater facilitated the response to electrical stimulation of the greater occipital nerve, and sensitized the response of cervical muscles to noxious mechanical stimulation (Bartsch and Goadsby, 2003).

These observations underscore that cervical–trigeminal interactions are reciprocal. Not only can cervical nociception facilitate trigeminal sensation, trigeminal nociception facilitates cervical perception. Consequently, the neurophysiological data support not only the referral of cervical pain to the head, but also the generation of cervical features in patients with trigeminal sources of headache. Proponents of a cervical source of headaches, therefore, need to be alert to the possibility that signs that they infer to indicate a cervical origin for pain, may instead be secondary phenomena of trigeminal origin. In experimental animals, stimulation of the dura mater increases electromyographic activity in suboccipital paraspinal muscles (Hu et al, 1995). Migraine patients may complain of neck discomfort during the premonitory phase (Giffin et al, 2003) or during their attacks (Goadsby et al, 2002) and they can exhibit hypersensitivity and increased electromyographic activity in their neck muscles (Selby and Lance, 1960; Bakal and Kaganov, 1977; Drummond, 1987).

HUMAN EXPERIMENTAL STUDIES

Studies in human volunteers have demonstrated the patterns of referred pain that can occur from cervical structures to the head. Electrical stimulation of the dorsal rootlets of C1 produces frontal headache (Kerr, 1962). Noxious stimulation of the greater occipital nerve produces headache in the ipsilateral, frontal, and parietal regions (Piovesan et al, 2001). Noxious stimulation of the suboccipital muscles of the neck produces pain in the forehead (Cyriax, 1938; Campbell and Parsons, 1944; Feinstein et al, 1954; Wolff, 1963). Noxious stimulation of the C2–3 intervertebral disc, but not lower discs, produces pain in the occipital region (Schellhas et al, 1996; Grubb and Kelly, 2000). Distending the C2–3 zygapophysial joint with injections of contrast medium produces pain in the occipital region (Dwyer et al, 1990), as does distending of the lateral atlanto-axial joint or the atlanto-occipital joint (Dreyfuss et al, 1994). In normal volunteers, all segments from the occiput to C4–5 are capable of producing the referred pain to the occiput. Referral to the forehead and orbital regions more commonly occurs from segments C1 and C2 (Campbell and Parsons, 1944).

Complementary studies in patients with headache have shown that headache can be relieved by anesthetizing structures innervated by the C1, C2, or C3 nerves. These include the C2–3 zygapophysial joint (Bogduk and Marsland, 1986, 1988; Lord et al, 1994) and the lateral atlanto-axial joint (Ehni and Benner, 1984; McCormick, 1987; Busch and Wilson, 1989; Aprill et al, 2002). The C2–3 zygapophysial joint is the most common source, followed by the lateral atlanto-axial joint, and occasionally the joint at C3–4 (Lord and Bogduk, 1996; Govind et al, 2006; Cooper et al, 2007).

From a given joint, pain can be perceived in various regions of the head, but certain trends are evident (Fig. 21–3). Pain from C2–3 tends to be perceived across the lateral occipital region and into the forehead and orbital region. Pain from C1–2 also tends to gravitate to the orbital region but more often occurs in the vertex or around the ear. Pain from C3–4 tends to focus in the suboccipital region and upper cervical spine; when it does spread to the head, it is largely restricted to the posterior regions, sparing the forehead and orbit.

CAUSES

Although various entities have been advanced as causes of cervicogenic headache, few have satisfied the International Headache Society criteria. Congenital abnormalities are only incidental findings in some patients with headache, and have not been shown to cause pain (Bogduk, 1997, 2004a, 2005; Bogduk and Bartsch, 2005). Although many practitioners favor trigger points in the neck muscles as a cause of headache, their diagnosis lacks both reliability and validity (Bogduk, 1997, 2004a, 2005; Bogduk and Bartsch, 2005). Patients with rheumatoid arthritis can develop headache when their atlanto-axial joints become involved, but the diagnosis is evident from the systemic distribution of the disease (Bogduk, 1997, 2004a, 2005; Bogduk and Bartsch, 2005). Some authors have attributed headache to osteoarthritis of the median atlanto-axial joint, but the evidence is barely circumstantial (Bogduk, 1997, 2004a, 2005; Bogduk and Bartsch, 2005).

The prevailing entities can be classified as demonstrable with a known cause, demonstrable

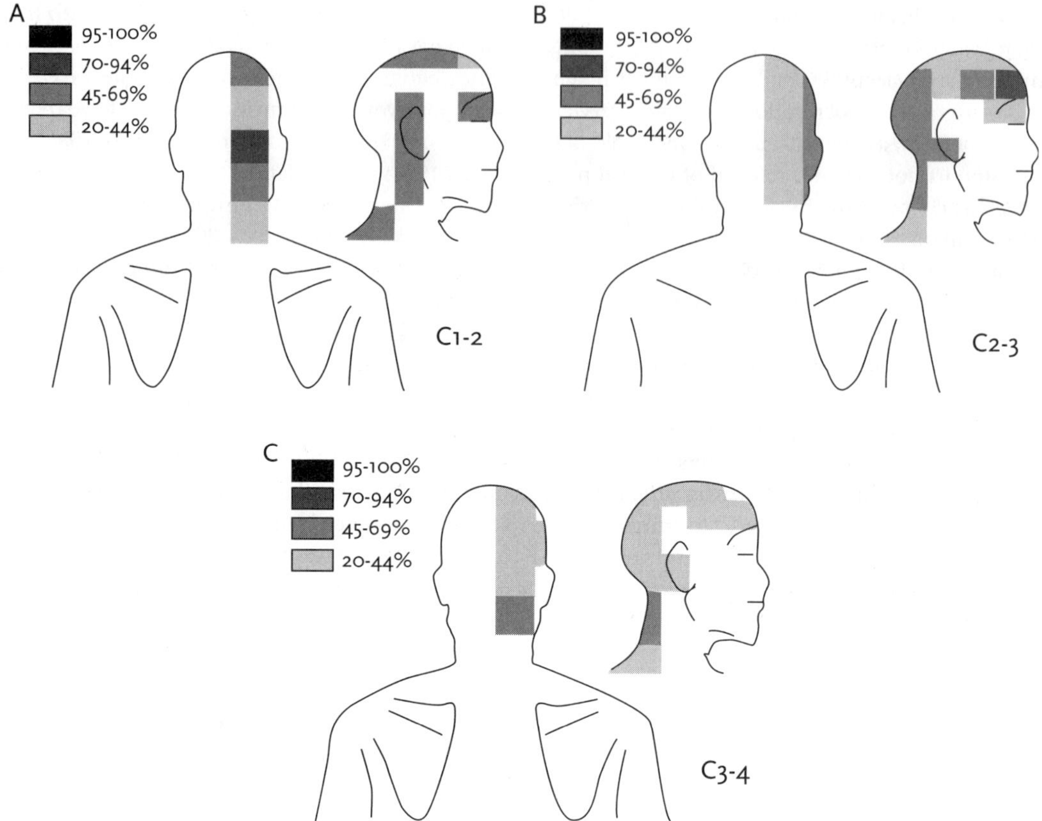

Figure 21–3 Maps of the distribution of pain in patients who were relieved of their headaches by controlled diagnostic blocks of the joints indicated. The shading reflects the proportion of patients who reported pain in the region indicated. (Based on Cooper et al., 2007.)

with no known cause, and conjectural. These can also be grouped according to neuropathic, nociceptive, and central mechanisms (Table 21–3).

Neuropathic

Neuropathic conditions are those in which the pathology affects a cervical nerve. Occipital neuralgia is one such condition, but it has to be distinguished from occipital pain.

Occipital Neuralgia

The International Headache Society defines occipital neuralgia as "paroxysmal jabbing pain in the distribution of the greater or lesser occipital nerves" (International Headache Society, 2004). Paroxysmal lancinating pain is the hallmark of neuralgia and is the essential diagnostic criterion for occipital neuralgia.

This definition does not apply to deep, aching pain in the occiput, which can arise from diseases of the posterior cranial fossa and base of skull (Sigwald and Jamet, 1968) and the upper cervical joints (Bogduk and Marsland, 1986, 1988; Lord et al, 1994). Indeed, the International Headache Society comments that occipital neuralgia must be distinguished from occipital referral of pain from the atlanto-axial or upper zygapophysial joints (International Headache Society, 2004).

Traditionally, it has been believed that occipital neuralgia is caused by irritation of the greater occipital nerve where it enters the scalp. However, there is no compelling evidence of such irritation. Lancinating occipital neuralgia has been recorded as a feature of temporal arteritis (Jundt and Mock, 1991), in which case inflammation of the occipital artery could affect the companion nerve. However, in the majority of cases of so-called occipital neuralgia no such pathology is evident. As well, anatomical studies have denied that occipital neuralgia is caused by entrapment of the greater occipital nerve where it pierces the trapezius (Bogduk, 1980). The greater occipital nerve emerges from under an aponeurosis between the trapezius and the sternocleidomastoid. At surgery, this aponeurosis could be mistaken for "scar" tissue.

There is, however, evidence that pathology can affect the C2 spinal nerve. This nerve runs behind the lateral atlanto-axial joint, resting on its capsule (Bogduk, 1981a, 1981b). Inflammatory or other disorders of the joint may result in the nerve becoming incorporated in the fibrotic changes of chronic inflammation (Jansen, Markakis, et al, 1989;). Release of the nerve relieves the symptoms. Otherwise, the C2 spinal nerve and its roots are surrounded by a sleeve of dura mater and a plexus of epiradicular veins, lesions of which can compromise the nerve. These include meningioma (Kuritzky, 1984), neurinoma (Jansen, Markakis, et al, 1989), anomalous vertebral arteries (Sharma et al, 1993), and venous abnormalities ranging from single to densely interwoven, dilated veins surrounding the C2 spinal nerve and its roots (Hildebrandt et al, 1984) to U-shaped arterial loops or angiomas compressing the C2 dorsal root ganglion (Jansen, Markakis, et al, 1989; Jansen, Bardosi, et al, 1989; Hildebrandt et al, 1984). Nerves affected by vascular abnormalities exhibit a variety of features indicative of neuropathy, such as myelin breakdown, chronic hemorrhage, axon degeneration and regeneration, and increased endoneurial and pericapsular connective tissue (Jansen, Bardosi et al, 1989).

The pain associated with these pathological changes is intermittent, lancinating pain in the occipital region associated with lacrimation and ciliary injection. This pain satisfies the criteria for occipital neuralgia, but the pathology lies in the C2 spinal nerve, not in the greater occipital nerve. Consequently, the diagnostic criterion is complete relief of pain following local anesthetic blockade of the C2, or sometimes the C3, nerve (Jansen, Markakis, et al, 1989). These blocks are performed under radiologic control and employ discrete amounts (0.6–0.8 ml) of long-acting local anesthetic to block the target nerve selectively (Jansen, Markakis, et al, 1989).

In order to distinguish this condition from occipital neuralgia, it has been referred to as "C2 neuralgia" (Bogduk, 2006). This term serves to draw attention away from the greater occipital nerve to the C2 spinal nerve, while nonetheless preserving the occipital location of the pain.

Table 21–3 The Possible Causes of Cervicogenic Headache, Tabulated by Mechanism and Whether or not the Cause and Source can be Demonstrated

Mechanism	*Demonstrable source known cause*	*Demonstrable source cause unknown*	*Conjectural, no evidence*
Neuropathic	C2 neuralgia		
Nociceptive	Aneurysms	Lateral atlanto-axial joint	
	Vertebral artery		
	Internal carotid artery	C2–3	
		Zygapophysial joint	
	Neck–tongue syndrome	C2–3 disc	
Central			Dysnociception

Nociceptive

Nociceptive causes are those in which the pathology lies in vertebral structures innervated by a cervical nerve. Currently available evidence implicates upper cervical joints as the cardinal sites of such disorders.

Neck–Tongue Syndrome

Neck–tongue syndrome is characterized by acute, unilateral, occipital pain precipitated by sudden movement of the head, usually rotation, and accompanied by a sensation of numbness in the ipsilateral half of the tongue (Lance and Anthony, 1980). The pain appears to be caused by temporary subluxation of a lateral atlanto-axial joint, whereas the numbness of the tongue arises because of impingement, or stretching, of the C2 ventral ramus against the edge of the subluxated articular process (Bogduk et al, 1981b). The numbness occurs because proprioceptive afferents from the tongue pass from the ansa hypoglossi into the C2 ventral ramus (Lance and Anthony, 1980). Neck–tongue syndrome can occur in patients with rheumatoid arthritis or with congenital joint laxity (Elisevich et al, 1984). Hypomobility in the contralateral lateral atlanto-axial joint may predispose one to the condition (Bertoft and Westerberg, 1985).

Lateral Atlanto-axial Joint Pain

Certain patients can be relieved of their headache by anesthetizing the lateral atlanto-axial joint (Ehni and Benner, 1984; McCormick, 1987; Busch and Wilson, 1989; Aprill et al, 2002). One study attributed the pain to radiographically evident osteoarthritis (Ehni and Benner, 1984), but such arthritis is not always evident. In posttraumatic cases, the responsible lesions might include capsular rupture, intra-articular hemorrhage and bruising of intra-articular meniscoids, or small fractures through the superior articular process of the axis (Schonstrom et al, 1993). In one study, the source of pain could be traced to the lateral atlanto-axial joints in 16% of patients presenting with headache, but not all patients were investigated for this condition, which suggests that 16% may be an underestimate (Aprill et al, 2002).

Discogenic Pain

There is some evidence to implicate the C2–3 intervertebral disc as a source of cervicogenic headache. Stimulation of this disc reproduces the pain suffered by some patients with headache (Schellhas et al, 1996; Grubb and Kelly, 2000). Arthrodesis of that disc has been reported to relieve headache (Schofferman et al, 2002). The nature of the causative pathology remains unknown.

Third Occipital Headache

The C2–3 zygapophysial joint is innervated by the third occipital nerve (Bogduk, 1982). This nerve crosses the joint laterally and innervates it through articular branches from its deep surface. The joint can be anesthetized by blocking the third occipital nerve under fluoroscopic guidance. Headache stemming from the C2–3 zygapophysial joint, therefore, can be relieved by third occipital nerve blocks, and accordingly has been named third occipital headache.

Initial studies describing third occipital headache were conducted using single diagnostic blocks with no controls (Bogduk and Marsland, 1986, 1988). A subsequent study used controlled diagnostic blocks and confirmed the existence of this entity (Lord et al, 1994). Moreover, that study established the prevalence of third occipital headache. In patients with neck pain after whiplash, the prevalence of third occipital headache was 27%. Amongst patients in whom headache was the dominant complaint, the prevalence was 53% [95% confidence interval (CI): 37%, 68%].

A significant feature of patients in whom third occipital nerve blocks have been positive is that all had a history of trauma. This reinforces "history of trauma" as a cardinal clinical feature for "probable" cervicogenic headache (Table 21–1). No studies have shown that third occipital headache occurs without a history of trauma.

Central Pain

The causes of primary headaches, such as migraine and tension-type headache, still remain unknown. One concept that has been invoked to explain their mechanism is dysnociception

(Olesen and Langemark, 1988). The concept postulates that disturbances occur in nuclei that regulate the trigeminocervical nucleus, resulting in disinhibition of the nucleus. As a result, the patient perceives pain because of increased activity in central trigeminocervical neurons. That activity, however, is effectively spontaneous. The cells are not activated by nociceptive activity arriving along trigeminal or cervical afferents. The source of the pain is wholly within the central nervous system.

It is possible that cervicogenic headache could be caused by such a mechanism. It has been recognized as a possibility (Bogduk, 1997; Bogduk and Bartsch, 2005), but it is no more than a theoretical concept. No actual evidence implicates such a mechanism. Nevertheless, it is a threat to other interpretations of cervicogenic headache. Various signs used to diagnose cervicogenic headache, even diagnostic blocks, might all be reflections of central hyperalgesia rather than valid features of a peripheral (and cervical) source of pain.

DIFFERENTIAL DIAGNOSIS

Since they are innervated by cervical nerves, disorders of the posterior cranial fossa can have a distribution of referred pain similar to that of cervicogenic headache. These disorders include tumors, which distend the dura mater of the posterior cranial fossa, and hemorrhage or meningitis, which irritate the dura chemically. These conditions are distinguished from cervicogenic headache by their mode of onset and by their associated features, such as neurologic signs, systemic illness, and meningismus.

Less distinctive, at onset, is headache due to dissection of either the vertebral artery or the internal carotid artery. For this reason, dissection is the cardinal differential diagnosis of cervicogenic headache.

Dissection

Headache is the most common presenting feature of internal carotid artery dissection (Biousse et al, 1994; Silbert et al, 1995), and may occur together with neck pain (Biousse et al, 1994). Headache is also the cardinal presenting feature of vertebral artery dissection. In both instances, some 60%–70% of patients present with headache, typically in the occipital region, although not exclusively so (Mokri et al, 1988; Sturzenegger, 1994; Silbert et al, 1995).

Following onset, cerebrovascular symptoms and signs typically evolve rapidly and declare the nature of the condition. Consequently, dissection is not as high in the differential diagnosis of chronic headache in the absence of cerebrovascular features.

INVESTIGATIONS

Imaging

There is no evidence that medical imaging is diagnostic of any cause of cervicogenic headache. Imaging is indicated only in patients who exhibit neurologic signs. In that context, however, imaging is used to determine the cause of the neurologic abnormality, not necessarily the cause of pain.

In patients with cardiovascular risk factors or a history of neck distortion or cervical manipulation, aneurysm needs to be considered. For this entity, magnetic resonance angiography is the appropriate investigation.

Manual Examination

Manual therapists contend that they can diagnose symptomatic joints by examining the cervical spine. Previously this belief was based on one small study that ostensibly validated manual examination of the cervical spine (Jull et al, 1988). That study, however, has now been refuted by a larger study that used more rigorous diagnostic criteria and more rigorous statistical analysis (King et al, 2007). Manual examination, therefore, lacks a foundation as a diagnostic test for cervicogenic headache.

Diagnostic Blocks

Diagnostic blocks are the mainstay of diagnosis for cervicogenic headache. Only by these means can a cervical source of pain be established in a valid manner. However, in order for blocks to be valid, they must be conducted under controlled conditions (Bogduk, 2004b).

Many studies that used diagnostic blocks in the investigation of cervicogenic headache did not implement controls (Bogduk, 2004b, 2005). Therefore, the results are uninterpretable.

Of particular concern is the common use of blocks of the greater occipital nerve. This nerve supplies no structures that are known to be a source of chronic pain. It supplies only the skin of the scalp and the occipitalis muscle. Consequently, a response to a greater occipital nerve block is not evidence of a cervical source of pain. Nor can blocks be considered to be target-specific for the nerve when they involve volumes such as 5 ml (Bovim et al, 1992) or 10 ml (Saadah and Taylor, 1987; Gawel and Rothbart, 1992) of local anesthetic (Bogduk, 2004b).

Animal studies have shown that stimulation of the greater occipital nerve facilitates responses in the trigeminocervical nucleus to noxious stimulation of the dura mater (Bartsch and Goadsby, 2002). The converse effects on this interaction have not been studied, but the prospect applies that greater occipital nerve blocks might downregulate nonspecific headache mechanisms or dysnociception, and do not imply a cervical source of pain.

Circumstantial evidence favors this interpretation. Greater occipital nerve blocks relieve pain, temporarily, in substantial proportions of patients with migraine, cluster headache, and hemicrania continua (Afridi et al, 2006). A positive greater occipital nerve block, therefore, cannot be a specific test for cervicogenic headache.

To date, in the diagnosis of cervicogenic headache, third occipital nerve blocks are the only blocks that have been subjected to controls. Consequently, C2–3 zygapophysial joint pain is the only cause of cervicogenic headache for which there are valid diagnostic data. Third occipital nerve blocks are performed under fluoroscopic guidance, using aliquots of 0.3 ml of local anesthetic (Fig. 21–4). They are controlled by using local anesthetic agents with different durations of action, on two separate occasions (Lord et al, 1994; Bogduk, 2004b).

Lateral atlanto-axial joint blocks are a complement to third occipital nerve blocks. They involve injecting local anesthetic into the cavity of the joint (Fig. 21–5), and serve either to pinpoint or to exclude a source of pain in that joint. They can be performed in a controlled fashion by first establishing that blocks of the C2–3 joint do not relieve pain.

For patients with lancinating occipital pain, C2 spinal nerve blocks are required to confirm the diagnosis. The nerve can readily be blocked, under fluoroscopic guidance, where it lies behind the lateral atlanto-axial joint (Bogduk, 1981a).

TREATMENT

In most trials of therapy for cervicogenic headache, a source of pain has not been established. Investigators have leaped from presumptive clinical diagnosis to presumptive therapy.

No drugs have been suggested, let alone proven, to be effective for cervicogenic headache. Agents such as infliximab and botulinum toxin have been explored, but no controlled studies have provided evidence of efficacy (Martelletti and van Suijlekom, 2004). Transcutaneous electrical nerve stimulation has been tried, but not in a controlled study. Reportedly, some 80% of patients obtained at least 60% reduction in their headache index, but the follow-up was of only 1 month (Farina et al, 1986).

Various forms of physical and manual therapy have been advocated for headaches believed to be of cervical origin. Most of the literature, however, consists of case reports or case series (Haldeman and Dagenais, 2001). The few randomized controlled studies provided follow-up of only 1 or 3 weeks (Vernon, 1989; Nillson, 1995; Nillson et al, 1997), and provided conflicting results (Haldeman and Dagenais, 2001).

The largest and most recent study provided encouraging results (Jull et al, 2002). It showed that treatment with manual therapy, specific exercises, or manual therapy plus exercises was significantly more effective at reducing headache frequency and intensity than was no specific care by a general practitioner. Manual therapy alone, however, was not more effective than exercises alone, and combining the two interventions did not achieve better outcomes. Some 76% of patients achieved greater than 50% reduction in headache frequency at the 7-week follow-up, and

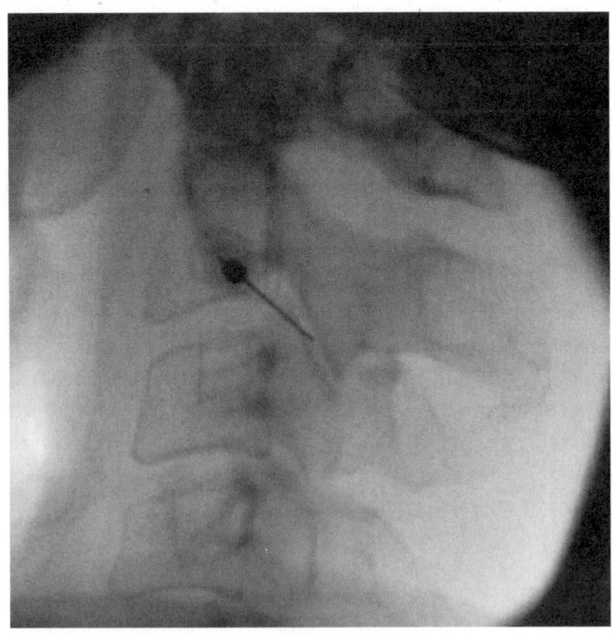

Figure 21–4 A lateral fluoroscopic image of the upper cervical spine showing a needle in place, on the C2–3 zygapophysial joint, in preparation for a third occipital nerve block.

35% achieved complete relief. At 12 months, 72% had greater than 50% reduction in headache frequency, but the proportion that had complete relief was not reported. Corresponding figures for reduction in pain intensity were not reported.

Several interventions have targeted the greater occipital nerve in patients with a clinical diagnosis of cervicogenic headache. Of 180 patients treated with an injection of 160 mg of depot methylprednisolone onto the greater occipital nerve, 169

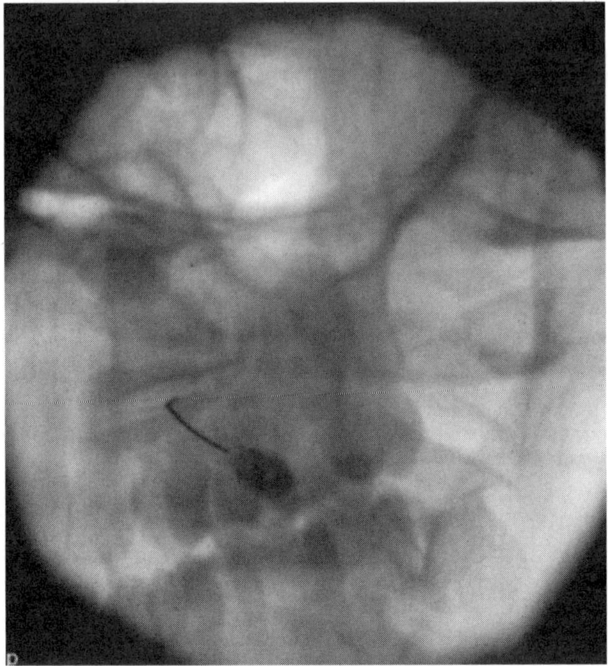

Figure 21–5 An AP fluoroscopic image of the upper cervical spine showing a needle in the left lateral atlanto-axial joint. Contrast medium in the joint creates an opaque blush that outlines the internal surface of the joint capsule.

obtained relief, but the duration of relief was only 10–77 days (Anthony, 2000). Surgical "liberation" of the nerve initially relieves headache in some 80% of cases, but the relief has a median duration of only 3–6 months (Bovim et al, 1992). Excision of the greater occipital nerve provides relief in some 70% of patients, but this has a median duration of only 244 days (Anthony, 1992).

In one study, patients were selected for surgery if they satisfied the clinical criteria for "cervicogenic headache" and obtained relief of headache from diagnostic blockade of the C2 spinal nerve (Pikus and Phillips, 1995). They underwent decompression and microsurgical neurolysis of the C2 spinal nerve, with excision of scar and ligamentous and vascular elements that compressed the nerve. Fourteen of thirty-one patients were rendered pain-free. Details on the remaining patients are incomplete, but ostensibly 51% gained what was called "adequate" relief and 11% suffered a recurrence.

Others have explored like means of treatment. One study reported that some patients could obtain relief from intra-articular injection of steroids into the C2–3 zygapophysial joint (Slipman et al, 2001). At 19 months, following such injections, 11% of patients were free of pain. A further 50% had a reduced frequency of headaches. That study, however, was not controlled. Consequently, it is not evident if the administration of steroids, or simply the act of injection into the joint, is the active component of the therapeutic effect. Nevertheless, intra-articular injection would seem to be a safe and expedient intervention that could benefit some patients.

Particularly contentious is the effectiveness of percutaneous radiofrequency neurotomy. The evidence is divided, but correlates with the diagnostic and therapeutic protocols used.

Three studies purport to show that radiofrequency neurotomy is not effective (van Suijlekom et al, 1998; Stovner et al, 2004; Haspeslagh et al, 2006). In all studies, clinical criteria were used to select patients. Diagnostic blocks were performed in one study (Stovner et al, 2004), but the results were not used as an indication for treatment. In all studies, neurotomy was performed indiscriminately at all levels from C3 to C6. In the first study, only one of fifteen patients achieved complete relief of pain (van Suijlekom et al, 1998). In the second study, outcomes were no different in patients who received active lesions from those who received sham lesions (Stovner et al, 2004). In the third study, outcomes from neurotomy were no different from those of an injection of local anesthetic onto the greater occipital nerve (Haspeslagh et al, 2006).

Three fatal technical flaws apply to these studies (Bogduk, 2004c). First, at no stage was the source of pain established. Second, the neurotomy technique used has never been validated Boguduk (2004c). Third, neurotomy was performed at segmental levels (C3–C6) that have never been incriminated as a source of headache. Jointly and severally, these flaws offend the principle of radiofrequency neurotomy.

Totally opposite results are obtained if a diagnosis is carefully established using controlled diagnostic blocks and meticulous surgical technique is used. For patients in whom diagnostic blocks indicate that the C2–3 zygapophysial joint is the source of pain, it is possible to denervate that joint percutaneously by radiofrequency neurotomy of the third occipital nerve. The procedure involves placing an electrode parallel to the nerve where it crosses the joint (Fig. 21–6), and using it to coagulate the nerve.

An early study found that radiofrequency neurotomy of the third occipital nerve did not reliably achieve relief of pain (Lord et al, 1995). The authors warned that radiofrequency neurotomy should not be adopted until technical deficiencies of the procedure had been overcome. That has now been achieved.

A subsequent study reported improvements in the technique of percutaneous radiofrequency neurotomy of the third occipital nerve (Govind et al, 2003), which improved its success rate. The revisions included holding the electrode in place during coagulation and ensuring that multiple lesions are made in order to encompass all possible locations of the nerve.

Using the revised technique, complete relief of pain could be achieved in 88% of patients. The median duration of relief was 297 days, with some patients still having continuing relief at the time of review (Govind et al, 2003). These results have been corroborated by a second, independent study (Barnsley, 2005).

For patients in whom headaches recur, relief can be reinstated by repeating the neurotomy.

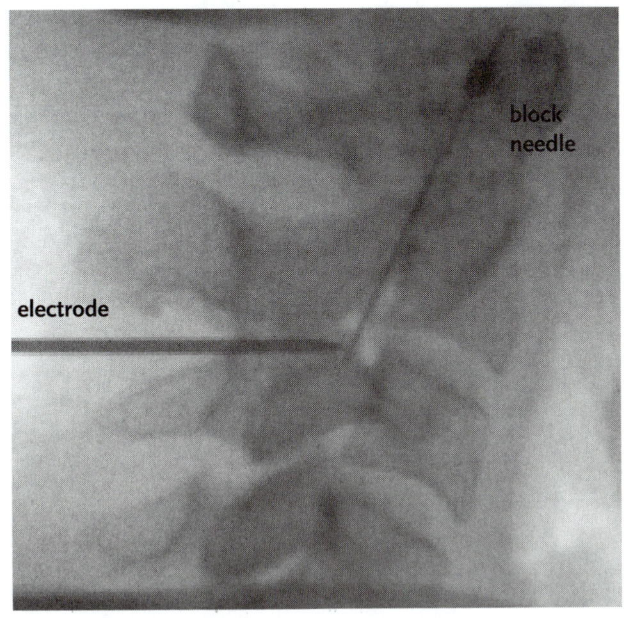

Figure 21–6 A lateral fluoroscopic image of the upper cervical spine showing an electrode in place, over the C2–3 zygapophysial joint, in preparation for a third occipital neurotomy. (A narrow gauge spinal needle lies just below the joint to provide supplementary anesthesia, if required.)

By repeating neurotomy as required, some patients have been able to maintain relief of their headache for longer than 2 years (Govind et al, 2003). A randomized, placebo-controlled trial showed that responses to radiofrequency neurotomy are not due to placebo effects (Lord et al, 1996). Its success in the treatment of third occipital headache, therefore, cannot be dismissed as a placebo effect.

For patients with pain stemming from the lateral atlanto-axial joints, intra-articular injections of corticosteroids have not been investigated, and radiofrequency neurotomy to denervate the joint is not technically possible. The one recourse is arthrodesis of the joint. The surgical literature attests to success with this procedure, albeit in small numbers of patients, with complete relief of pain lasting over 2 years (Joseph and Kumar, 1994; Ghanayem et al, 1996; Schaeren and Jeanneret, 2005).

CLINICAL PATHWAY

The primary indicator that a patient might have cervicogenic headache is pain in the occipital region or pain starting in the neck. However, even so, other forms of headache need to be considered and excluded before proceeding (Fig. 21–7). If other conditions have been excluded, a diagnosis of "possible" cervicogenic headache can be made.

The differential diagnosis includes posterior fossa lesions and dissections of either the vertebral artery or internal carotid artery. If these are possible or suspected, investigations with magnetic resonance imaging or magnetic resonance angiography are indicated. In that event, cervicogenic headache is no longer a consideration, and the patient exits the clinical pathway.

If the patient has lancinating pain, a diagnosis of occipital neuralgia can be pursued. This will entail performing C2 spinal nerve blocks to confirm the diagnosis.

A diagnosis of "probable" cervicogenic headache can be formulated if the patient has dull, aching pain that is continuous or fluctuating in intensity, associated with pain radiating into the shoulder, or a history of trauma. Such a level of diagnostic certainty can be adequate if conservative therapy is pursued.

The only conservative therapy for which there is any evidence of efficacy is manual therapy coupled with exercises. Most patients in primary care should benefit from this intervention.

Patients who do not benefit can be investigated more intensively. Since the pretest probability is highest for C2–3 zygapophysial joint pain, investigations should start with third occipital nerve blocks to test for this condition. If controlled blocks are positive, the patient can be treated with radiofrequency neurotomy. Intra-articular injection of steroids is a plausible, less destructive option, but lacks a definitive evidence base.

If C2–3 blocks are negative, the next step is to test for lateral atlanto-axial joint pain with C1–2

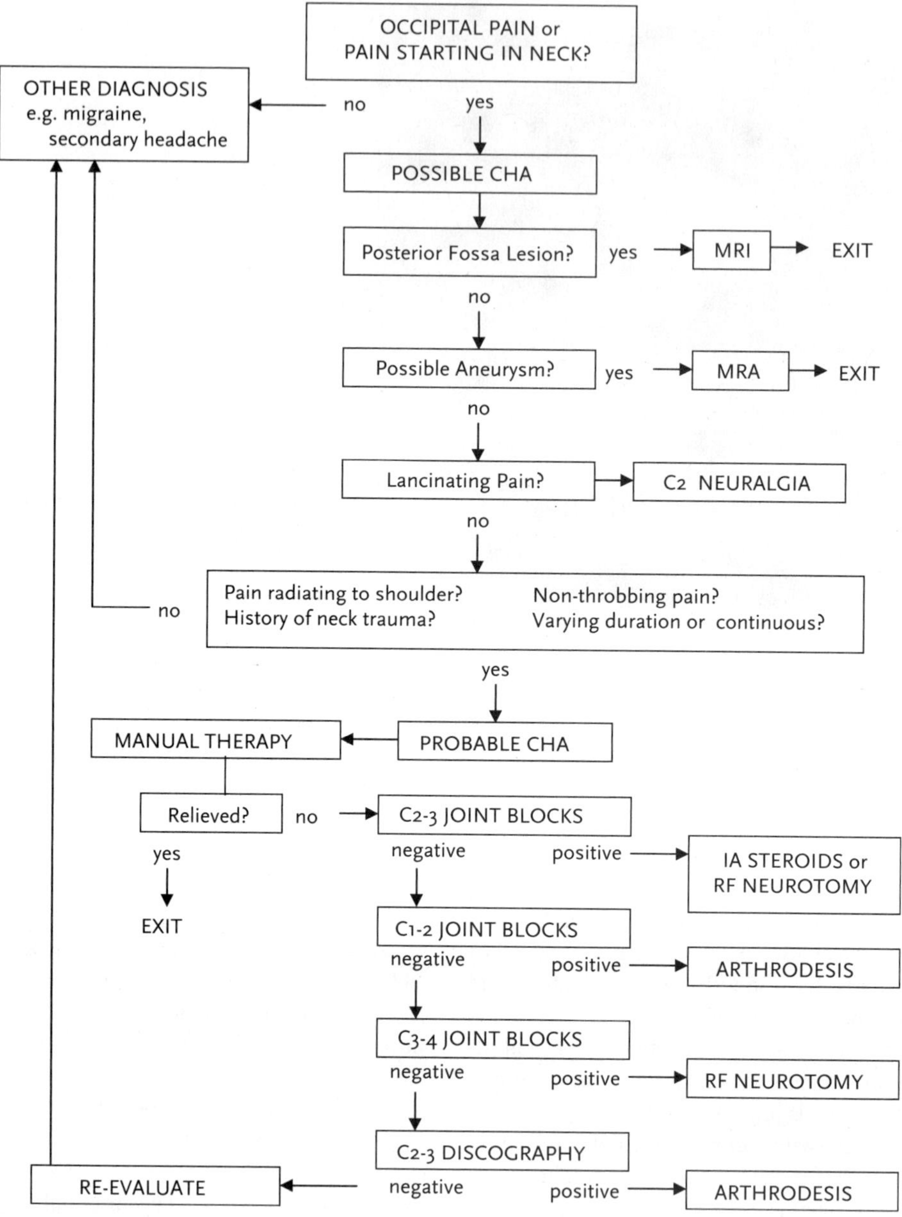

Figure 21–7 A flow chart depicted a clinical pathway for the diagnosis and management of cervicogenic headache. CHA: cervicogenic headache; MRI: magnetic resonance imaging; MRA: magnetic resonance angiography; IA steroids: intra-articular steroids; RF neurotomy: radiofrequency neurotomy.

blocks. If these are positive, treatment by arthrodesis can be considered.

If C1–2 blocks are negative, the C3–4 zygapophysial joint should be tested. If blocks are positive, treatment is possible with C3–4 medial branch radiofrequency neurotomy.

If C3–4 blocks are negative, the only remaining option is to test for C2–3 disc pain by discography. If discography is positive, treatment by arthrodesis can be considered.

If discography and blocks of the joints of the upper three cervical segments all prove negative, there are no further, established investigations to pursue. The patient and the management should be revaluated. Either the diagnosis is not cervicogenic headache, or the patient has a cervical cause of pain that cannot be pinpointed using currently available technology.

The options may be to treat the patient palliatively, by providing nonspecific pain-relief, or to enroll the patient in whatever ethics-approved study of procedures that have experimental or investigational status available. Such procedures include, but are not limited to, atlanto-occipital joint blocks, implanted greater occipital nerve stimulation, or procedures directed at suboccipital muscles as the sources of pain. Ethics-approved studies guarantee patient safety, and protect them from unwittingly becoming subjects of untested and unproven procedures.

References

Afridi, SK, Shields, KG, Bola, R, et al (2006). Greater occipital nerve injection in primary headache syndromes—prolonged effects from a single injection. *Pain*, 122:126–129.

Angus-Leppan, H, Lambert, GA, and Michalicek, J (1997). Convergence of occipital nerve and superior sagittal sinus input in the cervical spinal cord of the cat. *Cephalalgia*, 17:625–630.

Anthony, M (1992). Headache and the greater occipital nerve. *Clin Neurol Neurosurg*, 94:297–301.

Anthony, M (2000). Cervicogenic headache: prevalence and response to local steroid therapy. *Clin Exp Rheumatol*, 18(Suppl. 19):S59–S64.

Antonaci, F, Ghirmai, S, Bono, S, et al (2001). Cervicogenic headache: evaluation of the original diagnostic criteria. *Cephalalgia*, 21:573–583.

Aprill, C, Axinn, MJ, and Bogduk, N (2002). Occipital headaches stemming from the lateral atlanto-axial (C1-2) joint. *Cephalalgia* 22:15–22.

Bakal, DA and Kaganov, JA (1977). Muscle contraction and migraine headache: psychologic comparison. *Headache*, 17:208–215.

Barnsley, L (2005). Percutaneous radiofrequency neurotomy for chronic neck pain: outcomes in a series of consecutive patients. *Pain Med*, 6:282–286.

Barré, N (1926). Sur un syndrome sympathique cervicale posterieure et sa cause frequente: l'arthrite cervicale. *Revue du Neurologie*, 33:1246–1248.

Bartsch, T and Goadsby, PJ (2002). Stimulation of the greater occipital nerve induces increased central excitability of dural afferent input. *Brain*, 125:1496–1509.

Bartsch, T and Goadsby, PJ (2003). Increased responses in trigeminocervical nociceptive neurons to cervical input after stimulation of the dura mater. *Brain*, 126:1801–1813.

Bartschi-Rochaix, W (1968). Headaches of cervical origin. In *Handbook of Clinical Neurology*, Vol. 5 (PJ Vinken and GW Bruyn, eds.), pp. 192–203. Elsevier, New York.

Bertoft, ES and Westerberg, CE (1985). Further observations on the neck-tongue syndrome. *Cephalalgia*, (Suppl. 3):312–313.

Bilge, O (2004). An anatomic and morphometric study of C2 nerve root ganglion and its corresponding foramen. *Spine*, 29:485–499.

Biousse, V, D'Anglejan-Chatillon, J, Massiou, H, et al (1994). Head pain in non-traumatic carotid artery dissection: a series of 65 patients. *Cephalalgia*, 14:33–36.

Bogduk, N (1980). The anatomy of occipital neuralgia. *Clin Exp Neurol*, 17:167–184.

Bogduk, N (1981a). Local anaesthetic blocks of the second cervical ganglion: a technique with application in occipital headache. *Cephalalgia*, 1:41–50.

Bogduk, N (1981b). An anatomical basis for neck tongue syndrome. *J Neurol Neurosurg Psychiat*, 44:202–208.

Bogduk, N (1982). The clinical anatomy of the cervical dorsal rami. *Spine*, 7:319–330.

Bogduk, N (1984). Headaches and the cervical spine. An editorial. *Cephalalgia*, 4:7–8.

Bogduk, N (1997). Headache and the neck. In *Headache* (PJ Goadsby and SD Silberstein eds), pp. 369–381. Butterworth-Heinemann, Boston.

Bogduk, N (2004a). The neck and headaches. *Neurol Clin N Am*, 22:151–171.

Bogduk, N (2004b). Role of anesthesiologic blockade in headache management. *Curr Pain Headache Rep*, 8:399–403.

Bogduk, N (2004c). Editorial. Cervicogenic headache. *Cephalalgia* 24:819–820.

Bogduk, N (2005). Distinguishing primary headache disorders from cervicogenic headache: clinical and therapeutic implications. *Headache Currents*, 2:27–36.

Bogduk, N (2006). Pain of cranial nerve and cervical nerve origin other than primary neuralgias. In *The Headaches* (3rd edn) (J Olesen, PJ Goadsby, NM Ramadan, et al, eds), pp 1043–1051. Lippincott Williams & Wilkins, Philadelphia.

Bogduk, N and Bartsch, T (2005). Headaches of cervical origin: focus on anatomy and physiology. In *Chronic Daily Headache for Clinicians* (PJ Goadsby, SD Silberstein, and DW Dodick eds), pp. 369–381. BC Decker, London.

Bogduk, N, Lambert, G, and Duckworth, JW (1981). The anatomy and physiology of the vertebral nerve in relation to cervical migraine. *Cephalalgia*, 1:1–14.

Bogduk, N and Marsland, A (1986). On the concept of third occipital headache. *J Neurol Neurosurg Psychiat*, 49:775–780.

Bogduk, N and Marsland, A (1988). The cervical zygapophysial joints as a source of neck pain. *Spine*, 13:610–617.

Bogduk, N, Windsor, M, and Inglis, A (1989). The innervation of the cervical intervertebral discs. *Spine*, 13:2–8.

Bovim, G (1992). Cervicogenic headache, migraine, and tension-type headache. Pressure-pain threshold measurements. *Pain*, 51:169–173.

Bovim, G, Fredriksen, TA, Stolt-Nielsen, A, et al (1992). Neurolysis of the greater occipital nerve in cervicogenic headache. A follow up study. *Headache*, 32:175–179.

Brain, L (1963). Some unsolved problems of cervical spondylosis. *Brit Med J*, 1:771–777.

Busch, E and Wilson, PR (1989). Atlanto-occipital and atlanto-axial injections in the treatment of headache and neck pain. *Reg Anesth*, 14(Suppl. 2):45.

Campbell, DG and Parsons, CM (1944). Referred head pain and its concomitants. *J Nerv Ment Dis*, 99:544–551.

Chirls, M (1978). Retrospective study of cervical spondylosis treated by anterior interbody fusion in 505 patients performed by the Cloward technique. *Bull NY Hosp Joint Dis*, 39:74–82.

Cooper, G, Bailey, B, and Bogduk, N (2007). Cervical zygapophysial joint pain maps. *Pain Med*, 8:344–353.

Cyriax, J (1938). Rheumatic headache. *Brit Med J*, 2:1367–1368.

D'Amico, D, Leone, M, and Bussone, G (1994). Side-locked unilaterality and pain localization in long-lasting headaches: migraine, tension-type headache, and cervicogenic headache. *Headache*, 34:526–530.

Dreyfuss, P, Michaelsen, M, and Fletcher, D (1994). Atlanto-occipital and lateral atlanto-axial joint pain patterns. *Spine*, 19:1125–1131.

Drummond, PD (1987). Scalp tenderness and sensitivity to pain in migraine and tension headache. *Headache*, 27:45–50.

Dwyer, A, Aprill, C, and Bogduk, N (1990). Cervical zygapophysial joint pain patterns I: a study in normal volunteers. *Spine*, 15:453–457.

Ehni, G and Benner, B (1984). Occipital neuralgia and the C1-2 arthrosis syndrome. *J Neurosurg*, 61:961–965.

Elisevich, K, Stratford, J, Bray, G, et al (1984). Neck tongue syndrome: operative management. *J Neurol Neurosurg Psychiat*, 47:407–409.

Farina, S, Granella, F, Malferrari, G, et al (1986). Headache and cervical spine disorders: classification and treatment with transcutaneous electrical nerve stimulation. *Headache*, 26:431–433.

Feinstein, B, Langton, JBK, Jameson, RM, et al (1954). Experiments on referred pain from deep somatic tissues. *J Bone Joint Surg*, 36A:981–997.

Fredriksen, TA, Fougner, R, Tengerund, A, Sjaastad, O (1989). Cervicogenic headache. Radiological investigations concerning head/neck. *Cephalalgia*, 9:139–146.

Gawel, MJ and Rothbart, PJ (1992). Occipital nerve block in the management of headache and cervical pain. *Cephalalgia*, 12:9–13.

Ghanayem, AJ, Leventhal, M, and Bohlman, HH (1996). Osteoarthrosis of the atlanto-axial joints - long-term follow-up after treatment with arthrodesis. *J Bone Joint Surg*, 78A:1300–1307.

Giffin, NJ, Ruggiero, L, Lipton, RB, et al (2003). Premonitory symptoms in migraine: an electronic diary study. *Neurology*, 60:935–940.

Goadsby, PJ and Hoskin, KL (1997). The distribution of trigeminovascular afferents in the nonhuman primate brain Macaca Nemestrina: a c-fos immunocytochemical study. *J Anat*, 190:367–375.

Goadsby, PJ, Lipton, RB, and Ferrari, MD (2002). Migraine—current understanding and treatment. *N Engl J Med*, 346:257–270.

Govind, J, King, W, Bailey, B, et al (2003). Radiofrequency neurotomy for the treatment of third occipital headache. *J Neurol Neurosurg Psychiat*, 74:88–93.

Govind, J, King, W, Giles, P, et al (2006). Headaches and the cervical zygapophysial joints: a prevalence study. Syllabus of the 14th Annual Scientific Meeting of the International Spine Intervention Societty, Salt Lake City, July 13–15, pp. 169–171.

Grubb, SA and Kelly, CK (2000). Cervical discography: clinical implications from 12 years of experience. *Spine*, 25:1382–1389.

Hackett, GS, Huang, TC, and Raftery, A (1962). Prolotherapy for headache. *Headache*, 2:20–28.

Haldeman, S and Dagenais, S (2001). Cervicogenic headaches: a critical review. *Spine J*, 1:31–46.

Haspeslagh, SR, van Suijlekom, HA, Lame, IE, et al (2006). Randomised controlled trial of cervical radiofrequency lesions as a treatment for cervicogenic headache. *BMC Anesthesiol*, 6:1.

Hildebrandt, J and Jansen, J (1984). Vascular compression of the C2 and C3 roots—yet another cause of chronic intermittent hemicrania? *Cephalalgia*, 4:167–170.

Holmes, G (1913). Headaches of organic origin. *Practitioner*, 1:968–984.

Hu, JW, Vernon, H, and Tatourian, I (1995). Changes in neck electromyography associated meningeal noxious stimulation. *J Manipulative Physiol Ther*, 18:577–581.

Humphrey, T (1952). The spinal tract of the trigeminal nerve in human embryos between 71/2 and 81/2 weeks of menstrual age and its relation to early fetal behaviour. *J Comp Neurol*, 97:143–209.

Hunter, CR and Mayfield, FH (1949). Role of the upper cervical roots in the production of pain in the head. *Am J Surg*, 78:743–749.

International Headache Society (2004). The International Classification of Headache Disorders, 2nd edition. *Cephalalgia*, 24(Suppl. 1):115–116.

Jansen, J, Bardosi, A, Hildebrandt, J, et al (1989). Cervicogenic, hemicranial attacks associated with vascular irritation or compression of the cervical nerve root C2. Clinical manifestations and morphological findings. *Pain*, 39:203–212.

Jansen, J, Markakis, E, Rama, B, et al (1989). Hemicranial attacks or permanent hemicrania - a sequel of upper cervical root compression. *Cephalalgia*, 9:123–130.

Joseph, B and Kumar, B (1994). Gallie's fusion for atlantoaxial arthrosis with occipital neuralgia. *Spine*, 19:454–455.

Jull, G, Barrett, C, Magee, R, et al (1999). Further clinical clarification of the muscle dysfunction in cervical headache. *Cephalalgia*, 19:179–185.

Jull, G, Bogduk, N, and Marsland, A (1988). The accuracy of manual diagnosis for cervical zygapophysial joint pain syndromes. *Med J Aust*, 148:233-236.

Jull, G, Trott, P, Potter, H, et al (2002). A randomized controlled trial of exercise and manipulative therapy for cervicogenic headache. *Spine*, 27:1835–1843.

Jundt, JW and Mock, D (1991). Temporal arteritis with normal erythrocyte sediment rates presenting as occipital neuralgia. *Arthritis Rheum*, 34:217–219.

Kaube, H, Keay, KA, Hoskin, KL, et al (1993). Expression of c-fos-like immunoreactivity in the caudal medulla and upper cervical spinal cord following stimulation of the superior sagittal sinus in the cat. *Brain Res*, 629:95–102.

Kayfetz, DO, Blumenthal, LS, Hackett, GS, et al (1963). Whiplash injury and other ligamentous headache - its management with prolotherapy. *Headache*, 3:24–28.

Kelly, M (1942). Headaches, traumatic and rheumatic: the cervical somatic lesion. *Med J Aust*, 2:479–483.

Kerr, FWL (1961a). Structural relation of the trigeminal spinal tract to upper cervical roots and the solitary nucleus in the cat. *Exp Neurol*, 4:134–148.

Kerr, FWL (1961b). Trigeminal nerve volleys. *Arch Neurol*, 5:171–178.

Kerr, FWL (1962). A mechanism to account for frontal headache in cases of posterior fossa tumors. *J Neurosurg*, 18:605–609.

Kimmel, DL (1959). The cervical sympathetic rami and the vertebral plexus in the human foetus. *J Comp Neurol*, 112:141–161.

Kimmel, DL (1960). Innervation of the spinal dura mater and dura mater of the posterior cranial fossa. *Neurology* 10:800–809.

King, W, Lau, P, Lees, R, et al (2007). The validity of manual examination in assessing patients with neck pain. *Spine J*, 7:22–26.

Kuritzky, A (1984). Cluster headache-like pain caused by an upper cervical meningioma. *Cephalalgia*, 4:185–186.

Lance, JW (1982). *Mechanism and Management of Headache* (4th edn). Butterworths, London.

Lance, JW and Anthony, M (1980). Neck tongue syndrome on sudden turning of the head. *J Neurol Neurosurg Psychiat*, 43:97–101.

Langemark, M and Olesen, J (1987). Pericranial tenderness in tension headache. *Cephalalgia*, 7:249–255.

Lazorthes, G and Gaubert, J (1956). L'innervation des articulations interapophysaire vertebrales. *Comptes Rendues de l'Association des Anatomistes*, 488–494.

Leone, M, D'Amico, D, Frediani, F, et al (1993). Clinical considerations on side-locked unilaterality in long-lasting primary headaches. *Headache*, 33:381–384.

Leone, M, D'Amico, D, Grazzi, L, et al (1998). Cervicogenic headache: a critical review of the current diagnostic criteria. *Pain*, 78:1–5.

Leone, M, D'Amico, D, Moschiano, F, et al (1995). Possible identification of cervicogenic headache amongst patients with migraine: an analysis of 374 headaches. *Headache*, 35:461–464.

Lous, I and Olesen, J (1982). Evaluation of pericranial tenderness and oral function in patients with common migraine, muscle contraction headache and combination headache. *Pain*, 12:385–393.

Lord, SM and Bogduk, N (1996). The cervical synovial joints as sources of post-traumatic headache. *J Musculoskel Pain*, 4:81–94.

Lord, SM, Barnsley, L, and Bogduk, N (1995). Percutaneous radiofrequency neurotomy in the treatment of cervical zygapophysial joint pain: a caution. *Neurosurgery*, 36:732–739.

Lord, S, Barnsley, L, Wallis, B, et al (1994). Third occipital headache: a prevalence study. *J Neurol Neurosurg Psychiat*, 57:1187–1190.

Lord, SM, Barnsley, L, Wallis, BJ, et al (1996). Percutaneous radio-frequency neurotomy for chronic cervical zygapophysial-joint pain. *N Engl J Med*, 335:1721–1726.

Luff, AP (1913). The various forms of fibrositis and their treatment. *Brit Med J*, 1:756–760.

Martelletti, P and van Suijlekom, H (2004). Cervicgoenic Headache. Practical Approaches to Therapy. *CNS Drugs*, 18:793–805.

Mayfield, FH (1955). Symposium on cervical trauma. Neurosurgical aspects. *Clin Neurosurg*, 2:83–90.

McCormick, CC (1987). Arthrography of the atlanto-axial (C1–C2) joints: technique and results. *J Intervent Radiol*, 2:9–13.

Mendel, T, Wink, CS, and Zimny, ML (1992). Neural elements in human cervical intervertebral discs. *Spine*, 17:132–135.

Mokri, B, Houser, W, Sandok, BA, et al (1988). Spontaneous dissections of the vertebral arteries. *Neurology*, 38:880–885.

Nillson, N (1995). A randomized controlled trial of the effect of spinal manipulation in the treatment of cervicogenic headache. *J Manipul Physiol Ther*, 18:435–440.

Nillson N, Christensen, HW, and Hartvigsen, J (1997). The effect of spinal manipulation in the treatment of cervicogenic headache. *J Manipul Physiol Ther*, 20:326–330.

Oleson, J (1978). Some clinical features of the acute migraine attack. An analysis of 750 patients. *Headache*, 18:268–271.

Olesen, J and Langemark, M (1988). Mechanism of tension headache. A speculative hypothesis. In *Basic Mechanisms of Headache. Pain Research and Clinical Management*, Vol. 2 (J Olesen and L Edvinsson,eds), pp. 457–461. Elsevier, Amsterdam.

Patrick, HT (1913). Indurative or rheumatic headache. *JAMA*, 71:82–86.

Pawl, RP (1977). Headache, cervical spondylosis, and anterior cervical fusion. *Surg Ann*, 9:391–408.

Pearce, JM (1995). Cervicogenic headache: and early description. *J Neurol Neurosurg Psychiat*, 58:698.

Perelson, HN (1947). Occipital nerve tenderness: a sign of headache. *South Med J*, 40:653–656.

Peterson, DI, Austin, GM, and Dayes, LA (1975). Headache associated with discogenic disease of the cervical spine. *Bull Los Angeles Neurol Soc*, 40:96–100.

Pfaffenrath, V, Dandekar, R, and Pollman, W (1987). Cervicogenic headache—the clinical picture, radiological findings and hypotheses on its pathophysiology. *Headache*, 27:495–499.

Pikus, HJ, Phillips, JM (1995). Characteristics of patients successfully treated for cervicogenic headache by surgical decompression of the second cervical root. *Headache*, 35:621–629.

Piovesan, EJ, Kowacs, PA, Tatsui, CE, et al (2001). Referred pain after painful stimulation of the greater occipital nerve in humans: evidence of convergence of cervical afferences on trigeminal nuclei. *Cephalalgia*, 21:107–109.

Poletti, CE and Sweet, WH (1990). Entrapment of the C2 root and ganglion by the atlanto-epistrophic ligament: clinical syndrome and surgical anatomy. *Neurosurgery*, 27:288–291.

Raney, AA and Raney, RB (1948). Headache: a common symptom of cervical disc lesions. *Arch Neurol Psychiat*, 59:603–621.

Rothbart, P (1996). Cervicogenic headache. *Headache*, 36:516.

Saadah, HA and Taylor, FB (1987). Sustained headache syndrome associated with tender occipital nerve zones. *Headache*, 27:201–205.

Schaeren, S and Jeanneret B (2005). Atlantoaxial osteoarthritis: case series and review of the literature. *Eur Spine J*, 14:501–506.

Schellhas, KP, Smith, MD, Gundry, CR, et al (1996). Cervical discogenic pain: prospective correlation of magnetic resonance imaging and discography in asymptomatic subjects and pain sufferers. *Spine*, 21:300–312.

Schofferman, J, Garges, K, Goldthwaite, N, et al (2002). Upper cervical anterior diskectomy and fusion improves discogenic cervical headaches. *Spine*, 27:2240–2244.

Schonstrom, N, Twomey, L, and Taylor, J (1993). The lateral atlanto-axial joints and their synovial folds: an in vitro study of soft tissue injuries and fractures. *J Trauma*, 35:886–892.

Schultz, EC and Semmes, RE (1950). Head and neck pains of cervical disc origin. *Laryngoscope*, 60:338–343.

Selby, G and Lance, JW (1960). Observation on 500 cases of migraine and allied vascular headache. *J Neurol Neurosurg Psychiat*, 23:23–32.

Sharma, RR, Parekh, HC, Prabhu, S, et al (1993). Compression of the C-2 root by a rare anomalous ectatic vertebral artery. *J Neurosurg*, 78:669–672.

Sigwald, J and Jamet, F (1968). Occipital neuralgia. In *Handbook of Clinical Neurology* Vol. 5. (PJ Vinken and GW Bruyn eds), pp. 368–374. Elsevier, New York.

Silbert, PL, Makri, B, and Schievink, WI (1995). Headache and neck pain in spontaneous internal carotid and vertebral artery dissections. *Neurology*, 45:1517–1522.

Sjaastad, O, Fredriksen, TA, and Pfaffenrath, V (1990). Cervicogenic headache: diagnostic criteria. *Headache*, 30:725–726.

Sjaastad, O, Fredriksen, TA, and Pfaffenrath, V (1998). Cervicogenic headache: diagnostic criteria. *Headache*, 38:442–445.

Sjaastad, O, Saunte, C, Hovdahl, H, et al (1983). "Cervicogenic" headache. An hypothesis. *Cephalalgia*, 3:249–256.

Slipman, CW, Lipetz, JS, Plastara, CT, et al (2001). Therapeutic zygapophyseal joint injections for headache emanating from the C2-3 joint. *Am J Phys Med Rehabil*, 80:182–188.

Stovner, LJ, Kolstad, F, and Helde, G (2004). Radiofrequency denervation of facet joints C2-C6 in cervicogenic headache: a randomised, double-blind, sham-controlled study. *Cephalalgia*, 24:821–830.

Strassman, AM, Potrevbic, S, and Maciewicz, RJ (1994). Anatomical properties of brainstem trigeminal neurons that respond to electrical stimulation of dural blood vessels. *J Comp Neurol*, 346:349–365.

Sturzenegger, M (1994). Headache and neck pain: the warning symptoms of vertebral artery dissection. *Headache*, 34:187–193.

Tamura, T (1989). Cranial symptoms after cervical injury. Aetiology and treatment of the Barre-Lieou Syndrome. *J Bone Joint Surg*, 71B:283–287.

Taren, JA and Kahn, EA (1962). Anatomic pathways related to pain in face and neck. *J Neurosurg*, 19:116–121.

Torvik, A (1956). Afferent connections to the sensory trigeminal nuclei, the nucleus of the solitary tract and adjacent structures. *J Comp Neurol*, 106:51–141.

Travell, J (1962). Mechanical headache. *Headache*, 7:23–29.

Travell, J and Rinzler, SH (1952). The myofascial genesis of pain. *Postgrad Med*, 11:425–434.

van Suijlekom, JA, de Vet, HCW, van den Berg, SGM, et al. (1999). Interobserver reliability of diagnostic criteria for cervicogenic headache. *Cephalalgia*, 19:817–823.

van Suijlekom, HA, de Vet, HCW, van den Berg, SGM, et al (2000). Interobserver reliability in physical examination of the cervical spine in patients with headache. *Headache*, 40:581–586.

van Suijlekom, HA, van Kleef, M, Barendse, GAM, et al (1998). Radiofrequency cervical zygapophyseal joint neurotomy for cervicogenic headaches: a prospective study of 15 patients. *Funct Neurol*, 13:297–303.

Vernon, HT (1989). Spinal manipulation and headaches of cervical origin. *J Manipul Physiol Ther*, 12:455–468.

Wilkinson, M (1971). Symptomatology. In *Cervical Spondylosis* (2nd edn) (M Wilkinson ed.), pp. 59–67. Heineman, London.

Williams, PL, Warwick, R, Dyson, M, et al (eds) (1989). *Gray's Anatomy* (37th edn). Churchill Livingstone, Edinburgh.

Wolff, HG (1963). *Headache and Other Head Pain* (2nd edn), pp. 582–616. Oxford University Press, New York.

Zwart, JA (1997). Neck mobility in different headache disorders. *Headache* 37:6–11.

22 The Eye and Headache

James J Corbett, and Paul W Brazis

Eye pain, periorbital and retro-orbital pain, and headache or facial pain referred to the orbital region are common presenting complaints to ophthalmologists, neurologists, neurosurgeons, family practitioners, and internists. In many cases, the symptoms are magnified by the patient's concerns about possible blindness, the presence of an eye or brain tumor, or the presence of other dangerous conditions such as a cerebral aneurysm. Many patients with headache look to ocular disease as the cause of headache, given the ubiquitous belief that headaches are often the result of eye disease or the wrong glasses. In reality, the eyes are rarely the cause of common headaches (Tomsak, 1991; Martin and Soyka, 1993).

In those patients in whom eye disease is the cause of pain, the location and character of the pain, associated symptoms, and ocular signs are usually evident to the careful observer. Conjunctival injection, corneal edema, abnormal pupils, and decreased vision are the hallmark of such disorders and even the nonophthalmologist should be able readily identify and interpret these signs. A thorough examination of the eyes and visual system may uncover important clinical clues about headaches that are primarily nonocular in origin but have prominent ocular signs, such as papilledema in idiopathic intracranial hypertension (IIH) or homonymous visual field loss in stroke. Pain also may be referred to the eyes from intracranial, dental, ear, throat, vascular, or sinus disease. All patients with eye pain should undergo a thorough ophthalmologic (and neuro-ophthalmologic) examination, including evaluation of near and distance visual acuity, color vision, visual fields, pupil response (including evaluation for a relative afferent pupillary defect), intraocular pressure measurement, motility examination, eyelid exam, slit lamp biomicroscopic examination, Shirmer's test and assessment of the tear film, palpation of periocular structures, and a dilated fundus evaluation with indirect ophthalmoscopy. Examinations for trigeminal sensory loss or dysfunction, including corneal reflex testing, and facial muscle strength are also in order. In selected cases, measurement for proptosis (e.g., Hertel proptometer measurements), listening for orbital and cranial bruits, and more specialized ophthalmologic testing may be required.

The ophthalmologic and neuro-ophthalmologic examination may localize a pathologic process to specific structures affecting vision or eye motility. Further investigations can then be directed to the area affected. Thus, eye pain may be related to an ocular, optic nerve, orbital, superior orbital fissure, cavernous sinus, or intracranial process or a trigeminal neuropathy. It should be noted that in some circumstances, eye pain may occur with direct involvement of these structures with a completely normal ophthalmologic and neuro-ophthalmologic examination (e.g., eye pain with orbital metastatic disease). As discussed further on, only a high index of clinical suspicion (e.g., new eye pain in a patient with a history of cancer) and appropriately directed neuro-imaging may reveal the potentially vision- or life-threatening etiologies in these patients.

Pain in a patient with a "red or inflamed eye" is usually due to infectious or inflammatory ocular diseases affecting the cornea, conjunctiva, episclera, or sclera. These conditions are usually easily diagnosed as such by ophthalmologists. A "quiet eye" is defined clinically as one with a clear cornea without redness or irritation of the conjunctiva or sclera. Many entities that are typically associated with an inflamed eye may, in some patients, cause eye pain without remarkable signs of inflammation. This serves to further emphasize the need for a thorough examination when evaluating patients with eye pain. Various etiologies of eye pain in the "quiet eye" are outlined in Table 22–1. Because signs of intraocular inflammation can be subtle and only seen with biomicroscopy, a quiet eye when examined with a penlight may harbor significant intraocular findings. For purposes of this chapter we define the quiet eye according to what a nonophthalmologist would see. Therefore, several eye conditions would have remarkable clinical findings on complete examination, though externally, the eye appears "quiet." We have designated as "eye pain" any pain or discomfort referred by the patient to the eye itself, pain localized to the retrobulbar, orbital, retro-orbital, or periorbital regions, or headache or facial pain that is especially localized to the eye or surrounding structures.

Causes of eye pain may be divided into two groups (Brazis et al., 2002): (1) those associated with abnormal localizing ophthalmologic and neuro-ophthalmologic findings (including trigeminal neuropathies) and (2) those with a normal ophthalmologic and neurologic examinations. The latter group is further divided into the following subgroups: (1) specific short- or long-lasting headache or eye pain syndromes; (2) pain referred to the eye from other pathologic processes (secondary eye pain) sometimes caused by structures unrelated to vision; and (3) pain from orbital, superior orbital fissure, cavernous sinus, or intracranial infiltrative, neoplastic, or inflammatory disease processes with normal ophthalmologic and neuro-ophthalmologic exam. Unfortunately, in many patients, no etiology for the pain syndrome is discerned and one is left with a diagnosis of "*idiopathic eye pain*," "*eye strain*," or "*atypical facial pain*."

PAIN ASSOCIATED WITH LOCALIZING NEURO-OPHTHALMOLOGIC OR OPHTHALMOLOGIC FINDINGS

Ocular Processes

Branches of the trigeminal nerve innervate the eye and orbital tissues. The ophthalmic division (V1) divides into the frontal nerve, which innervates the conjunctiva of the lateral upper eyelid, and the nasociliary nerve, which is the sole sensory supply to the eye. Its two long ciliary nerves innervate the cornea, iris, and ciliary muscle. The many small axons that terminate as free nerve endings in the corneal stroma and epithelium make it one of the most sensitive tissues in the body. Eight to twenty short ciliary nerves innervate the sclera and uvea. The lens, vitreous, and retina do not contain pain fibers.

Several pathophysiologic mechanisms may lead to eye pain and thence to headache. These include direct, focal stimulation of cornea-scleral pain fibers by foreign bodies, abrasions, or lacerations, and more diffuse stimulation due to bullous keratopathy or severe glaucoma, or prostaglandin-mediated uveal pain. Pain, as a subjective phenomenon, varies considerably among patients. Furthermore, conditions such as herpetic keratitis are often associated with a muted pain response due to chronic damage to trigeminal nerve pain receptor fibers.

Photophobia is the clinical term used to describe an abnormal intolerance to light, usually associated with eye pain. In some cases, the reason for discomfort seems apparent, such as the pain induced with pupillary constriction in iritis. In other cases light exposure may cause the patient's vision to decrease (hemeralopia), as with cataract or cone-rod retinal dystrophies, but it is unclear why these patients frequently also describe ocular discomfort. Central mechanisms of photophobia are even less well understood. Thus, photophobia can occur in a number of very diverse clinical settings:

1. Anterior segment disorders of the eye, such as ocular surface disorders (dry eye syndrome), corneal disorders, *uveitis*, acute angle closure glaucoma, and cataract (especially posterior subcapsular cataract).
2. Vitreoretinal disorders, such as albinism, achromatopsia, retinitis pigmentosa (cone–rod dystrophy), or cancer-associated retinopathy.
3. Acquired optic neuropathies, such as optic neuritis.
4. Intracranial diseases, such as migraine, meningeal inflammation, irritation, or

TABLE 22–1 Causes of Ocular, Orbital, or Periorbital Pain in the "Quiet Eye".

Pain Associated with Localizing Ophthalmologic or Neuro-ophthalmologic Findings

1. Ocular processes
   A. Open angle glaucoma
      (1) Primary open angle glaucoma (rare)
      (2) Glaucomatocyclitic crisis (Possner–Schlossman syndrome)
      (3) Lens-induced glaucoma
         (a) Phacolytic glaucoma
         (b) Lens particle glaucoma
         (c) Phacoanaphylaxis
      (4) Intraocular tumors
      (5) Trauma
         (a) Angle recession
         (b) Hemolytic
         (c) Ghost cell
      (6) Closure of a cyclodialysis cleft
   B. Angle closure glaucoma
      (1) Primary angle closure glaucoma
      (2) Plateau iris
      (3) Lens-induced angle closure
      (4) Neovascular
      (5) Iridocorneal-endothelial (ICE) syndrome
      (6) Intraocular tumors
      (7) Ciliary block (malignant) glaucoma
      (8) Epithelial and fibrous down growth
      (9) Following intraocular surgery
      (10) Nanophthalmos
   C. Corneal disease
      (1) Dry eyes
      (2) Toxicity
      (3) Infectious keratitis
         (a) Viral keratitis (e.g., herpes simplex keratitis, varicella zoster keratitis, Epstein–Barr virus)
         (b) Bacterial
         (c) Fungal
         (d) Acanthamoeba
      (4) Meibomian gland dysfunction
      (5) Allergic keratitis (e.g., vernal keratoconjunctivitis)
      (6) Intersitial keratitis
      (7) Thygeson's superficial punctate keratitis
      (8) Superior limbic keratoconjunctivitis
      (9) Peripheral ulcerative keratitis
         (a) Mooren's ulcer
         (b) Autoimmune connective tissue disease (e.g., rheumatoid arthritis, Wegener's granulomatosis, systemic lupus erythematosus, polyarteritis nodosa, ulcerative colitis)
      (10) Recurrent corneal erosions
      (11) Corneal abrasion
      (12) Keratoconus with acute hydrops
      (13) Foreign bodies—corneal or conjunctival
      (14) Bullous keratopathy

(continued)

Table 22–1 (continued)

- D. Uveitis
  - (1) Idiopathic iridocyclitis
  - (2) Infectious iridocyclitis
    - (a) Herpes. simplex
    - (b) Herpes zoster
    - (c) Syphilis
  - (3) Lens induced
    - (a) Oversized implant
    - (b) Phacotoxic uveitis
  - (4) Sympathetic ophthalmia
  - (5) Uveitis-glaucoma-hyphema (UGH) syndrome
  - (6) Posterior uveitis
    - (a) Toxoplasmosis
    - (b) Behcet's disease
    - (c) Vogt-Koyanagi Harada's disease
    - (d) Multifocal choroiditis and panuveitis
  - (7) Endophthalmitis
    - (a) Endogenous (e.g., bacterial, fungal)
    - (b) Exogenous (e.g., trauma, postoperative)
- E. Scleritis and episcleritis
  - (1) Idiopathic
  - (2) Infectious
    - (a) Bacterial
    - (b) Fungal
    - (c) Tuberculosis
    - (d) Syphilis
    - (e) Leprosy
    - (f) Herpes simplex
    - (g) Herpes zoster
  - (3) Connective tissue disease
    - (a) Rheumatoid arthritis
    - (b) Wegener's granulomatosis
    - (c) Polyarteritis nodosa
    - (d) Systemic lupus erythematosus
    - (e) Relapsing polychondritis
    - (f) Crohn's disease
  - (4) Ocular surgery
  - (5) Sarcoidosis
- F. Intraocular tumors
  - (1) Uveal melanoma
  - (2) Metastasis
  - (3) Following radiotherapy
- G. Ocular ischemia
  - (1) Previous eye muscle surgery
  - (2) Previous scleral buckling surgery
  - (3) Sickle cell disease
- H. Suprachoroidal hemorrhage
- I. Trauma—scleral laceration or rupture

TABLE 22–1 (continued)

J. Retina/choroid process
    (1) Photocoagulation
    (2) Inflammatory disease [e.g., birdshot chorioretinopathy, acute posterior multifocal placoid pigment epitheliopathy (APMPPE)]

2. Processes affecting the optic nerve
    A. Optic neuritis
    B. Optic disk edema with a macular star (neuroretinitis)
    C. Ischemic optic neuropathy
    D. Compressive optic neuropathy
        (1) Intracranial or intraorbital benign and malignant tumors
            (a) Meningioma
            (b) Glioma
            (c) Craniopharyngioma
            (d) Pituitary adenoma
            (e) Lymphoma and leukemia
            (f) Germinoma
            (g) Sinus histiocytosis with lymphadenopathy
            (h) Nasopharyngeal cancer
            (i) Metastasis
        (2) Extramedullary hematopoiesis
        (3) Orbital fractures with bone fragment, hematoma, or edema
        (4) Pneumatocele
        (5) Inflammatory or infectious diseases (e.g., mucoceles)
        (6) Idiopathic hypertrophic cranial pachymeningitis
        (7) Primary bone diseases (e.g., osteopetrosis, fibrous dysplasia, craniometaphyseal dysplasia, Paget's disease, aneurysmal bone cyst, pneumosinus dilatans, etc.)
        (8) Vascular etiologies
            (a) Orbital hemorrhage
            (b) Orbital venous anomalies
            (c) Carotid artery and anterior communicating artery aneurysms
            (d) Supraclinoid carotid artery compression
            (e) Arteriovenous malformations
        (9) Thyroid ophthalmopathy
        (10) Iatrogenic (e.g., intracranial catheters, postoperative)
    E. Infiltrative or inflammatory optic neuropathy
        (1) Neoplastic (e.g., plasmacytoma and multiple myeloma, carcinomatous meninigitis, leukemia, lymphoma)
        (2) Infectious etiologies
            (a) Bacteria [e.g., syphilis, tuberculosis, Lyme disease, Bartonella henselae (cat scratch disease), Mycoplasma, Whipple's disease, brucellosis, beta-hemolytic streptococcus, meningococcus]
            (b) Focal infection or inflammation (e.g., paranasal sinusitis or mucocele, postinfectious, malignant otitis externa)
            (c) Fungi (e.g., aspergillus, histoplasmosis, cryptococcus, mucormycosis)
            (d) Rickettsiae (e.g., Q fever, epidemic typhus)
            (e) Protozoa (e.g., toxoplasmosis)
            (f) Parasites (e.g., toxocariasis, cysticercosis)

(continued)

TABLE 22–1 (continued)

(g) Viruses [e.g., adenovirus, hepatitis A, hepatitis B, cytomegalovirus (CMV), coxsackie B, rubella, chickenpox, herpes zoster, herpes simplex virus I, EB virus (infectious mononucleosis), measles, mumps, influenza, HTLV-1, HIV (AIDS)-related]

(3) Inflammatory diseases
(a) Churg–Strauss angiitis
(b) Contiguous sinus disease
(c) Behcet's disease
(d) Sarcoidosis
(e) Wegener's granulomatosis
(f) Systemic lupus erythematosus
(g) Sjögren's syndrome
(h) Relapsing polychondritis
(i) Polyarteritis nodosa
(j) Rheumatoid arthritis
(k) Inflammatory bowel disease

3. Orbital processes
A. Tumor
(1) Primary (including meningioma, adenoma, lacrimal gland carcinoma, neurilemmoma, melanoma, lymphoma, Hodgkin's disease)
(2) Metastatic
B. Infection (orbital cellulitis, dacroadenitis)
(1) Bacterial (e.g., septicemia, penetrating trauma, adjacent sinusitis, sinus mucocele)
(2) Viral (e.g., herpes zoster)
(3) Fungal (e.g., mucormycosis, aspergillus, Bipolaris hawaiiensis, actinomycosis)
(4) Parasites (e.g., cysticercosis, trichinosis))
C. Inflammatory and infiltrative processes
(1) Thyroid orbitopathy
(2) Orbital pseudotumor
(3) Lymphoid hyperplasia
(4) Giant cell arteritis
(5) Orbital polymyositis and giant cell myocarditis
(6) Sarcoidosis
(7) Wegener's granulomatosis
(8) Sinus histiocytosis with massive lymphadenopathy (Rosai-Dorfman disease)
(9) Erdheim-Chester disease
(10) Orbital amyloidosis
(11) Bilateral nonspecific inflammatory or Graves'-like orbitopathy with seminoma
D. Vascular
(1) Arteriovenous malformation
(2) Orbital hemorrhage
(3) Orbital venous anomalies
(4) Dural-cavernous sinus fistula
(5) Carotid-cavernous sinus fistula
E. Post-traumatic (e.g., amputation neuroma, photo-oculodynia syndrome) and postoperative (e.g., post scleral buckle procedure, postevisceration,) eye pain

4. Cavernous sinus and superior orbital fissure processes
A. Aneurysm of the internal carotid artery
B. Tumors (e.g., meningioma, pituitary adenoma, nasopharyngeal carcinoma, cavernous hemangioma, hemangiopericytoma, lymphoma, myeloma, metastasis, Waldenstrom's macroglobulinemia)

Table 22–1 (continued)

- C. Cavernous sinus thrombosis
- D. Infections (e.g., herpes zoster, aspergillus, mucormycosis)
- E. Tolosa–Hunt syndrome (idiopathic granulomatous inflammation of cavernous sinus)
- F. Inflammatory processes (e.g., sarcoidosis, Wegener's granulomatosis)
- G. Carotid-cavernous sinus or dural-cavernous sinus fistula
- H. Ischemic ocular motor nerve palsies (e.g., due to diabetes mellitus, giant cell arteritis, vasculitis, etc) (localization of process may be anywhere along course of ocular motor nerve)
- I. Neurosurgical complications
- J. Post-traumatic

5. Intracranial processes
   - A. Tumors
     - (1) Primary (e.g., pituitary adenoma, meningioma, craniopharyngioma, chondroma, lymphoma)
     - (2) Secondary (e.g., metastasis, nasopharyngeal carcinoma, carcinomatous meningitis)
   - B. Pseudotumor cerebri
   - C. Infections or inflammatory conditions (e.g., sarcoidosis, Wegener's granulomatosis)
   - D. Vascular
     - (1) Aneurysms
     - (2) Arteriovenous malformation
     - (3) Cerebral infarction, transient ischemic attacks (TIAs), or hemorrhage (e.g., ophthalmic pain with posterior cerebral artery infarction)
     - (4) Venous sinus thrombosis
     - (5) Posttraumatic (e.g., subdural hematoma)
     - (6) Pituitary apoplexy
     - (7) Cerebral vasculitis
     - (8) Hypertensive encephalopathy
   - E. Low pressure headache (intracranial hypotension)
6. Trigeminal neuropathies

   Tumors
     - (1) Primary (e.g., meningioma, schwannoma, etc)
     - (2) Secondary (e.g., metastasis, carcinomatous meningitis, squamous cell tumor of skin, nasopharyngeal carcinoma, etc)

   Post-traumatic (e.g., basal skull fracture, neurosurgical procedures)

   Infectious/inflammatory processes (e.g., aspergilloma, amyloidoma, sarcoidosis, Wegener's granulomatosis, herpetic and postherpetic neuralgia)

   Vascular (e.g., carotid aneurysm, cavernous hemangioma, dural- cavernous sinus fistula)

   Raeder's paratrigeminal syndrome

   Neuroparalytic (neurotropic) keratitis

   Isolated trigeminal neuropathy
     - (1) Systemic lupus erythematosus
     - (2) Scleroderma
     - (3) Sjogren' syndrome
     - (4) Dermatomyositis
     - (5) Rheumatoid arthritis
     - (6) Mixed connective tissue disease
     - (7) Idiopathic

(continued)

TABLE 22–1 (continued)

Pain Syndromes with a Normal Ophthalmologic and Neuro-ophthalmologic Examination

1. Primary short-lasting headache syndromes
   A. With autonomic features
      (1) Cluster headache
         (a) Episodic
         (b) Chronic
      (2) Cluster-tic syndrome
      (3) Paroxysmal hemicranias
         (a) Chronic (CPH)
         (b) Episodic
      (4) Chronic paroxysmal hemicrania (CPH)- tic syndrome
      (5) SUNCT (short-lasting unilateral neuralgiform pain with conjunctival injection and tearing) syndrome
      (6) SUNA (short-lasting unilateral neuralgiform attacks with cranial autonomic features)
   B. Without autonomic features
      (1) Trigeminal neuralgia
      (2) Sphenopalitine neuralgia
      (3) Idiopathic stabbing headache (jabs and jolts syndrome, ice-pick headache, "needle-in-the-eye" syndrome)
      (4) Valsalva maneuver headache
         (a) Cough headache
         (b) Benign exertional headache
      (5) Headache associated with sexual activity
      (6) Cold stimulus (ice cream) headache
      (7) Hypnic headache
2. Primary long-lasting headache syndromes
   A. Migraine
      (1) With aura
      (2) Without aura
   B. Tension headache and eye strain (e.g., due to uncorrected refractative error or heterophoria)
   C. Hemicrania continua (episodic and chronic)
   D. Idiopathic eye pain (includes atypical facial pain and psychogenic pain)
3. Pain referred to the eye from nonophthalmic or noncranial pathologic processes (secondary eye pain)
   A. Sinus disease (e.g., sphenoid and frontal sinusitis)
   B. Diseases of the teeth, jaw, and related structures
   C. Vascular disease
      (1) Carotodynia
      (2) Carotid artery dissection
      (3) Carotid artery occlusion or stenosis (including the ocular ischemic syndrome)
      (4) Post-carotid endarterectomy
      (5) Giant cell arteritis
   D. Eye pain with neck disease (cervicogenic headache or eye pain)
   E. Face pain with lung cancer
4. Orbital, superior orbital fissure, cavernous sinus, or intracranial infiltrative, neoplastic, or inflammatory disease processes with normal ophthalmologic and neuro-ophthalmologic exam

Source: From Brazis et al., 2002.

infection; and following intracranial trauma or surgery (Miller, 1985); and *central photophobia*, perhaps associated with thalamic injury (Cummings and Gittinger, 1981) or trigeminal dysfunction ("*central dazzle*") (Gutrecht et al., 1990).

5. Sudden exposure to light after light deprivation causing a "physiologic photophobia."
6. The fact that there are myriad clinical descriptors and classifications for *ocular inflammation* is evidence that inflammation of the eye can present in many ways, and that there are a multitude of causes (many of which are not known or understood). As with glaucoma (see below), pain is roughly proportional to the *rate* at which inflammation proceeds unchecked as well as the severity of the inflammation. In addition, pain can be caused as the end result of inflammation, such as high (inflammatory glaucoma) or low (hypotony) intraocular pressure.

Patients with acute anterior uveitis present with photophobia, eye pain, redness, lacrimation, and decreased vision in the affected eye. The eye pain may be quite severe, may be of throbbing character, and may radiate to other head and facial areas, including the teeth and sinuses. Ophthalmoscopy demonstrates cells and flares in the anterior chamber and may also reveal keratic precipitates (see Fig. 22–1). Pain usually occurs with "spill-over" inflammation into the anterior segment, which is frequently seen with toxoplasma retinochoroiditis. Most patients with uveitis have a "red eye" but some patients manifest with only eye pain. Careful slit lamp biomicroscopy may demonstrate active anterior uveitis or evidence for previous inflammation (e.g., posterior synechiae or old keratitic precipitates). *Posterior inflammation* (retinitis, choroiditis, pars planitis, *vitritis*) is more likely to present as a decline in vision, rather than pain. In some cases, inflammatory cells and debris in the vitreous (vitritis) will manifest as a decrease in the red reflex of the involved eye (Nussenblatt and Palestine, 1989).

Episcleritis is a benign, self-limited but recurrent disorder that may be nodular or simple. It is associated with relatively mild eye pain and characteristic sectoral redness, injection of the episcleral tissue, eye tenderness, and some tearing. The episcleral injection can easily be overlooked if it occurs beneath the upper or lower eyelids; therefore, careful lid retraction with complete scleral inspection is important. *Scleritis*, on the other hand, usually presents with intense, boring type pain associated with photophobia and tearing. *Necrotizing scleritis* without inflammation may not cause pain. The pain of scleritis is often localized to the eye but may radiate into the sinuses, jaw, frontal regions, or temple. Patients with anterior ocular involvement may manifest non-necrotizing, nodular, diffuse, or necrotizing forms. Anterior necrotizing scleritis with inflammation is the most severe form and present with severe pain and redness. Episcleritis and *anterior scleritis* are usually not difficult diagnoses to make using slit lamp biomicroscopy and typically shows a ciliary flush.

Posterior scleritis is often difficult to diagnose and may present with prominent eye pain or headaches that may prompt a central nervous system (CNS) evaluation until the patient complains of visual loss. The anterior sclera is commonly uninvolved and the slit lamp examination of the anterior segment may be completely normal (Benson, 1988). Patients with posterior scleritis demonstrate variable choroidal effusions, serous retinal detachments, choroidal folds, and choroidal detachments commonly associated with macular or optic disc edema.

Intraocular tumors are usually painless and most patients are asymptomatic unless the tumor involves the macula by direct extension, by causing (surrounding) overlying exudative retinal detachment, or by inducing cystoid macular edema. Patients then complain of impaired central vision, metamorphopsia, and photopsias. Some patients with either primary choroidal melanomas or metastatic tumors complain of eye pain that may be due to tumor necrosis, secondary iridocyclitis, or scleritis. Indeed we have rarely seen patients with choroidal metastatic disease in whom eye pain was their presenting complaint.

Glaucoma

Glaucoma is not a single disease, but a classification (Table 22–2) that includes many different disorders that usually (but not always) have three things in common: (1) elevated intraocular

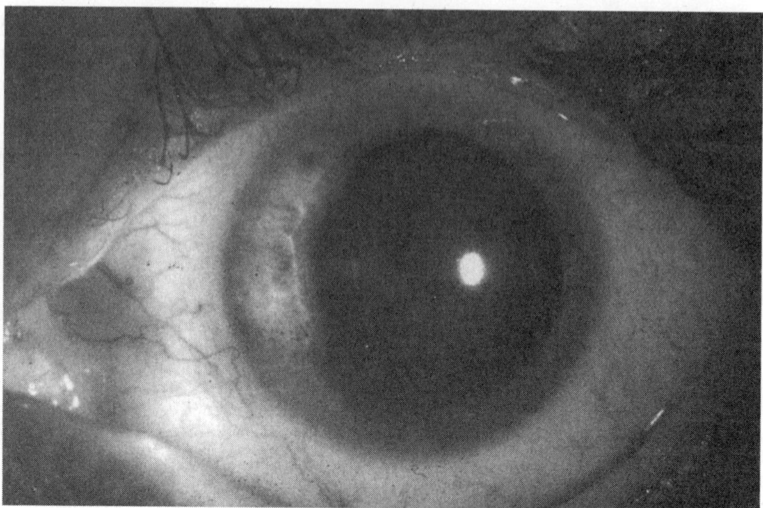

Figure 22–1 Granulomatous uveitis. A 46 year old woman reported blurred vision and mild ocular discomfort. This clinical photograph demonstrates several characteristics of granulomatous uveitis including (1) a relatively "quiet" eye (little conjunctival injection); (2) pigmented "mutton-fat" keratic precipitates (KP) adhering to the endothelium of the inferior cornea; (3) irregular pupil, as the iris is stuck to the lens capsule (posterior synechiae) from chronic inflammation.

pressure; (2) optic nerve damage manifest as an enlarged optic cup (optic disc cupping) (3) optic disc-related visual field defects. Eye pain is actually an uncommon symptom in most forms of glaucoma. However, many physicians are quick to associate glaucoma with pain because of the severe pain that occurs in a relatively uncommon (but memorable) form of glaucoma: acute angle closure glaucoma.

Open angle glaucomas are by far the most common in the United States, and a vast majority of patients in this group have *primary open angle glaucoma* (POAG). Patients with POAG have moderately elevated intraocular pressure (characteristically 22–35 mm Hg), and evidence of optic nerve "cupping" (but not pallor, see Fig. 22–2). There is a tendency to develop visual field loss. Though usually bilateral, POAG can be very asymmetric. There is a strong hereditary predisposition for the disorder. The eye does not appear to be inflamed in POAG. Patients with POAG are almost always entirely asymptomatic, with elevated intraocular pressure or optic disc cupping discovered on a routine or screening examination. The intraocular pressure in this chronic disorder elevates slowly over time, and is usually moderate—very high intraocular pressures are unusual. The absolute magnitude of the intraocular pressure is less important as a cause of pain compared to the rapidity of the pressure rise. For this reason pain is rarely seen in patients with POAG but occurs more commonly with other etiologies of secondary open angle glaucoma as outlined in Table 22–1. Most of these diseases have a more acute onset and, hence, a more rapid rise in intraocular pressure, and many of them are associated with a ciliary flush that is visible to even the neophyte observer.

In patients with severe, especially acute, head pain localized within or around the eye, *acute angle closure glaucoma* should always be considered. These patients may have associated nausea or vomiting suggesting migraine, cluster headache, or an intracranial structural lesion. In the most common form of acute angle closure glaucoma, the anterior chamber is anatomically shallow and the approach to the angle is narrow. Close apposition of the iris pupillary margin to the lens can cause a relative block to the flow of aqueous, ballooning the iris forward (iris bombe). This forward movement of the iris is sufficient to block access to the angle in predisposed eyes, driving the

TABLE 22–2 Classifying the Glaucomas..

		Findings	*Pain*
Open angle glaucomas	Primary open angle glaucoma	Normal appearing eye except for increased cupping and possible visual field defects. Intraocular pressure moderately elevated	No pain from the glaucoma, but occasionally from topical drops (especially miotics)
	Secondary open angle glaucomas (Pigment dispersion syndrome, traumatic hyphema, Pseudoexfoliation of lens, lens-induced glaucoma)	Other signs are present, but may be only evident to on ophthalmologic examination	Can have episodes of pain with acute spikes in intraocular pressure
Angle closure glaucomas	Acute primary angle closure (and secondary forms)	Red painful eye, marked elevation in pressure, see Table 22–3	Severe pain, may be confused with cluster headache
	Intermittent angle closure glaucoma	Examination may be relatively unremarkable between episodes	Intermittent
	Chronic angle closure glaucoma	Eye may appear normal except for optic disc cupping	Asymptomatic, or low-intensity brow or frontal headache
Normal tension glaucoma		Cupping and visual field loss despite normal pressure	Questionable relationship to head pain

intraocular pressure up rapidly and severely (pressures of 50–70 mmHg are not unusual). The result is an intensely painful red eye (with ciliary flush), a "steamy" edematous cornea, blurred vision, a pupil that is often mid-dilated or irregular in shape (and poorly reactive to light). (Fig. 22–3). This pupil abnormality may be mild and taken for an early compressive third nerve palsy. The intense pain may radiate widely. Misdiagnosis has led to tooth extractions (Joseph, 1999) and even laparotomies for the accompanying gastrointestinal complaints (Watson and Kirkby, 1989; Dayan, et al., 1996). Acute angle closure glaucoma often occurs in patients over 60 years of age, as the lens increases in anterior–posterior dimension from cataract, further narrowing the anatomically predisposed anterior chamber angle. The mid-dilated pupil seems most prone to cause this cascade of events, so this condition may occur in the darkness of the movie theater or as the dilating drops are wearing off after a visit to the eye doctor.

Prompt diagnosis and referral is crucial, as the condition can usually be quickly reversed by the ophthalmologist, with instantaneous relief of pain and nausea. Failure to treat can result in irreversible blindness. The fellow eye is usually likewise predisposed for an angle closure attack. Acute treatment includes the use of miotic eye drops and other pressure lowering agents. Using a laser to create a hole in the iris (laser iridotomy) is curative, as it allows an unobstructed alternate passage for the aqueous from the posterior to the anterior chamber.

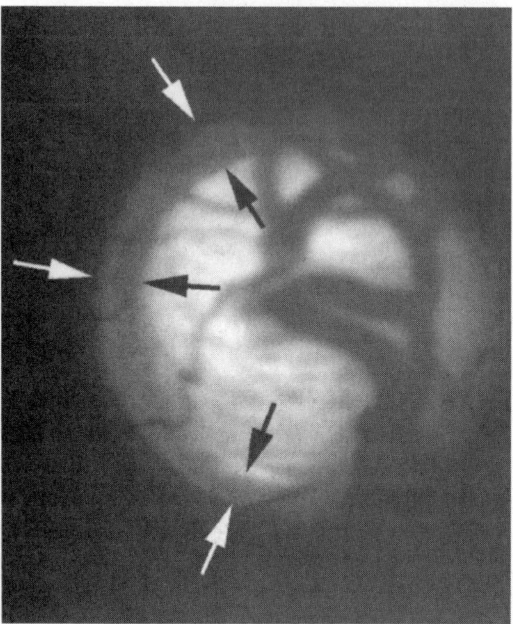

Figure 22–2 The optic disc in glaucoma. Glaucomatous optic atrophy occurs as an enlargement of the optic cup, presumably as axons in the neuroretinal rim die and drop out. An enlarged optic cup (outlined by black arrows) from primary open angle glaucoma is pictured. Note that unlike most other forms of optic atrophy that cause optic disc pallor, the neuroretinal rim (between arrowheads) in glaucoma remains a normal pink color.

Intermittent angle closure glaucoma consists of multiple, self-aborting episodes of angle closure with resultant intermittent eye pain. The typical signs and symptoms of angle closure glaucoma may not be obvious between episodes making the diagnosis difficult. Patients with intermittent angle closure may have pain episodes lasting minutes to hours. The eye may appear normal between attacks with the exception of a shallow anterior chamber angle. Shindler et al. described 11 patients who presented with headache and who were subsequently found to have occludable angles (Shindler et al., 2005). Six patients had increased optic disc cupping and 64% were initially clinically diagnosed as migraine. The headaches with glaucoma (compared to migraine headaches) were more frequent, milder, nonpulsating, of short duration, and rarely associated with nausea, vomiting, or photophobia. The average age of onset of the headaches was 54 years (versus migraine starting in adolescence). The authors emphasized two characteristic differential features from migraine: (1) the duration of the headaches was shorter than migraine (migraine $= 4 - 72$ hours; glaucoma $=$ none >4 hours and many <1 hour); and (2) the older age of onset of headaches with glaucoma (Shindler et al., 2005).

Acute angle closure glaucoma can be confused with cluster headache (Prasad et al., 1991) and

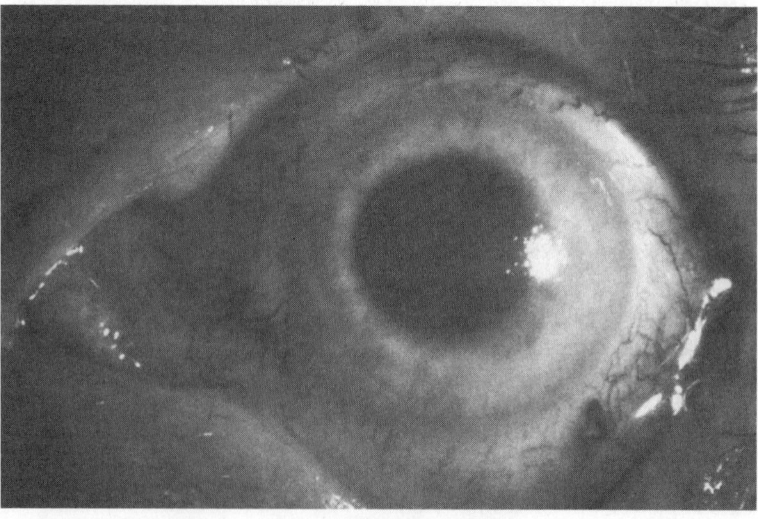

Figure 22–3 Acute angle closure glaucoma. Many typical characteristics of the appearance of an eye with acute angle closure glaucoma are seen in this clinical photograph. The cornea is edematous, as evidenced by a "steamy" a dull light reflex. The pupil is mid-dilated and somewhat irregular in shape. The conjunctiva is injected, although this finding is less impressive in this photograph than in most cases.

distinguishing these two disorders is crucial (Table 22–3). Therefore, all patients with "red eyes" or vision loss must be examined by an ophthalmologist, even when the diagnosis of cluster headache seems convincing.

In *normal tension (or low tension) glaucoma,* glaucomatous optic atrophy and progressive visual field loss occurs despite intraocular pressure measurements being normal. Its cause is unknown, and it is unclear what relationship its bears to those glaucomas with elevated intraocular pressure. An association between low tension glaucoma and headache has been proposed, but its significance is unclear (Phelps and Corbett, 1985; Ederer, 1986; Wang et al., 1997; Pradalier et al., 1998; De Marinis et al., 1999).

Optic Neuropathy

Patients with an *optic neuropathy* manifest decreased visual acuity, decreased color vision, visual field defect, an ipsilateral relative afferent pupillary defect in unilateral or bilateral asymmetric cases, light-near dissociation of the pupils in bilateral and symmetric cases, and often abnormalities of the optic disc (e.g., edema or disc atrophy, although the optic nerve may appear normal in retrobulbar optic neuropathy) (Lee and Brazis, 2003). The most common cause of an acute optic neuropathy in individuals less than 50 years of age is demyelinating or inflammatory *optic neuritis.* Periocular pain occurs in 92% of patients with typical optic neuritis and pain worsened by eye movement occurs in approximately 87% of patients (Optic Neuritis Study Group, 1991; Gerling et al., 1998). In fact, we consider the absence of pain to be atypical in patients thought to have demyelinating optic neuritis and perform further studies to investigate the cause of the optic neuropathy in these patients [e.g., orbital magnetic resonance imaging (MRI), possible lumbar puncture, etc.] (Lee and Brazis, 2003). Young patients who present with evidence of an acute unilateral optic neuropathy and eye pain are not difficult to diagnose with optic neuritis.

Optic disc edema with a macular star (ODEMS) or neuroretinitis is a heterogenous group of disorders characterized by sudden visual loss, swelling of the optic disc, peripapillary and macular exudates that may occur in a star pattern, and cells in

TABLE 22–3 Cluster Headache "Look-Alikes."

Acute angle closure glaucoma	*Cluster headache*	*Corneal erosion*
Severe unilateral headache, nausea	Severe unilateral headache, nausea	Severe, sharp, pain; nausea and vomiting unusual
Conjunctival injection is often intense, "ciliary flush" may be evident	Conjunctiva is only moderately injected	Conjunctiva is only moderately injected
Pupil usually mid-dilated and poorly reactive	Pupil may be smaller on affected side from Horner's syndrome, but reactive to light	Pupil is normal
"Protective" ptosis (orbicularis activation) only, in response to pain	True 1–2 mm ptosis from Horner's syndrome may be present	"Protective ptosis" may narrow the fissure
Cloudy cornea with "grainy" light reflex and poor vision	Clear cornea with unaffected vision	Dull cornea with decreased vision
Intraocular pressure is very elevated during the attack, (but may normalize quickly if attack has spontaneously reversed)	Intraocular pressure is normal (or slightly lower)	Intraocular pressure is normal
True emergency referral to ophthalmologist	Needs the care of an neurologist or other informed physician	Prompt referral to an ophthalmologist

the vitreous (Brazis and Lee, 1996). Eye pain, similar to that noted with optic neuritis, may be present. Although often idiopathic, ODEMS may occur on an infectious basis, especially due to syphilis, Lyme disease, cat-scratch disease, and toxoplasmosis.

As opposed to optic neuritis, pain occurs in only approximately 10%–12% of patients with *anterior ischemic optic neuropathy* (AION) (IONDT, 1995, 1996; Swartz et al., 1995; Gerling et al., 1998), and is the most common cause of acute optic neuropathy in individuals older than 55 years of age. If a patient is presumed to have AION and has pain as a prominent complaint, we consider this atypical and further investigate the patient for other etiologies of optic neuropathy (Lee and Brazis, 2003). In all patients with AION, *giant cell arteritis* (arteritic AION) should be considered as a potential etiology. All patients with AION should, thus, be queried concerning possible symptoms of giant cell arteritis, such as jaw or tongue claudication, new onset headaches or a change in a previously stable headache profile, fever, neck pain, polymyalgia rheumatica symptoms, or transient visual loss or diplopia. An erythrocyte sedimentation rate (ESR) and C-reactive protein should be obtained in all patients and if these are elevated, or the index of suspicion for giant cell arteritis is high, temporal artery biopsy is warranted. Other causes of optic neuropathy with eye pain are outlined in Table 22–1.

Orbital Processes

Mass lesions or infiltrative, infectious, inflammatory, or vascular processes involving the *orbit* may or may not be associated with eye pain. Although proptosis, conjunctival chemosis, ophthalmoplegia, or optic neuropathy are nonspecific signs of an orbital etiology, several specific orbital conditions have distinctive signs that should be recognized. For example, intermittent proptosis may occur with a *venous angioma* within the orbit and develops when the patient strains, cries, bends the head forward, hyperextends the neck, coughs, or blows the nose against a closed nostril and when the jugular vein is compressed. During these episodes, the eye may become tense and painful, the pupil may enlarge, and occasional bradycardia or syncope may develop (*oculocardiac syndrome*). Pulsation of the globe may occur with congenital sphenoid dysplasia, with orbital-cranial encephalocele, with neurofibromatosis, from orbital arteriovenous malformations or venous varices, due to tricuspid regurgitation, with arterial pulsation of the orbital vein, owing to arteriovenous fistula, or from transmission of pulsations of intracranial pressure via surgical or traumatic defects in the orbital wall. *Scirrhous carcinoma* of the breast or carcinoma of the lung, gastrointestinal tract, or prostate metastatic to the orbit may cause progressive fibrotic change, ptosis with a "glued down lid," and enophthalmos. This enophthalmos may be caused by posterior traction and tethering on the eyeball or by the tumor mass destroying the orbital wall resulting in "biologic orbital decompression."

Infiltrative and mass lesion syndromes are by far the most common manifestations of orbital metastases that produce headache (Goldberg and Rootman, 1990, Goldberg et al., 1990). However, we have seen a number of patients with orbital metastatic disease presenting with eye pain or headache as the sole manifestation of orbital involvement. The orbital or cavernous sinus metastasis may often be missed on "routine" brain neuroimaging studies that do not specifically focus upon the orbital or cavernous sinus region. Therefore, in any individual with a history of a neoplasm who complains of eye pain of recent onset, focused orbital and brain neuroimaging are recommended. MRI with specific views of the orbit and cavernous sinus with fat saturation sequences is warranted to investigate for possible metastases.

The *Tolosa–Hunt syndrome* is an idiopathic inflammatory disorder of the orbital apex or cavernous sinus that causes cranial nerve dysfunction and a painful ophthalmoplegia frequently with ipsilateral or holocranial headache. The Tolosa–Hunt syndrome is most likely the same process as orbital inflammatory pseudotumor, just more posterior in location. Both of these conditions require thorough evaluations to rule out neoplastic diseases or other known inflammatory conditions, especially sarcoidosis and orbital metastases (Table 22–1). Steroids are the mainstay of treatment for Tolosa–Hunt syndrome. Neuroimaging, preferably MRI and MR angiography and venography with "coned-down views" of the cavernous sinuses, potentially followed by other investigative procedures (e.g., lumbar puncture), is required in the investigation of all patients presenting with a cavernous sinus/superior orbital fissure syndrome and eye pain.

Vascular abnormalities of the orbit, including arteriovenous malformation, venous anomalies, dural-cavernous sinus fistula, and carotid-cavernous sinus fistula may cause eye pain. Venous anomalies of the orbit (orbital varices and lymphangiomas) typically present as orbital masses with proptosis, orbital hemorrhage, or diplopia but pain may be the major presenting feature and is present in approximately 43% of patients (Wright et al., 1997). Patients with carotid-cavernous sinus and dural-cavernous sinus fistulas usually have eyelid and facial changes (e.g., dilated periorbital vessels, chemosis, orbital congestion, and lid swelling), proptosis, subjective and objective bruits, and motility impairment, and present with a "red eye." However, some patients with low-flow dural—cavernous sinus fistulas present with eye pain, bruits, or motility impairment with mild eye redness and minimal lid swelling resembling chronic conjunctivitis (Kosmorsky et al., 1988; Brazis et al., 1994). A high index of suspicion is necessary to appropriately diagnose these "white-eye shunts." Also, in any patient with a history of eye trauma (including ocular surgery), a bleeding tendency, leukemia, or in patients taking warfarin for anticoagulation, an orbital hematoma should be considered as a potential etiology for eye pain and referred headache. Orbital imaging (e.g., CT or MRI scan) are usually diagnostic.

In general, patients with unexplained orbital signs and eye pain should undergo an imaging study directed to the orbit (e.g., orbital MRI scan with fat suppression and gadolinium contrast). The majority of conditions causing eye pain and affecting the orbit will show the characteristic abnormality on orbital imaging.

Painful Ophthalmoplegia Including Processes Affecting the Ocular Motor Nerves in the Cavernous Sinus and Superior Orbital Fissure

Small ocular deviations, especially those in which a patient can fuse with effort or with an abnormal head posture, may be associated with asthenopic symptoms. In one study, normal subjects who wore prisms to simulate an ocular muscle imbalance complained of brow ache and irritability (Eckhardt et al., 1943). In addition, chronic head positioning (like the head tilt in superior oblique palsies) can cause neck pain. Large deviations, in which fusion is not possible, are far less likely to cause headache or ocular pain. However, if patients have to keep one eye habitually closed to avoid diplopia, overworking the orbicularis can cause a tension-type headache. The use of an occluder (opaque plastic that clips onto one lens in the patient's glasses) can be a great relief when this situation occurs.

An isolated, painful peripheral *third nerve palsy* with ipsilateral or holocranial headache is most often related to an ischemic neuropathy or to a lesion in the subarachnoid portion of the nerve. Among these, compression by internal carotid-posterior communicating artery aneurysms is common. With ischemic lesions, the pupil is spared because the lesion is confined to the core of the nerve and spares peripherally situated pupillomotor fibers. By contrast, compression of the third nerve by aneurysm characteristically causes dilatation and unresponsiveness of the pupil. Sensory fibers from the ophthalmic division of the fifth cranial nerve join the oculomotor nerve within the lateral wall of the cavernous sinus (Lanzino et al., 1993). The frontal-orbital pain experienced by patients with enlarging aneurysms could thus be caused by direct irritation of the third nerve (Lanzino et al., 1993). Ischemic damage to the trigeminal fibers in the oculomotor nerve may also be the source of pain in ischemic-diabetic third nerve palsies. An oculomotor palsy may occur in association with herpes zoster ophthalmicus (HZO) (Fig. 22–4).

In the cavernous sinus, compressive lesions causing painful third nerve palsies often also involve the other ocular motor nerves and the ophthalmic branch of the trigeminal nerve (Keane, 1996). Combined oculomotor paresis and sympathetic denervation are virtually pathognemonic of a cavernous sinus lesion. Lesions in the neighborhood of the posterior clinoid process may for some time affect only the third nerve as it pierces the dura (e.g., metastatic breast and prostatic carcinoma). Lesions that begin laterally in the cavernous sinus present with retro-orbital pain first, and only later does ophthalmoparesis supervene. *Pituitary apoplexy* causes most often an oculomotor nerve deficit and involves the abducens nerve and the trochlear nerve with less frequency (McFadzean et al., 1991). Sudden onset of headache or eye pain and dysfunction of multiple ocular motor nerves on either one or both sides, with or without visual impairment, suggests the possibility of *pituitary apoplexy*. Occasionally, pituitary apoplexy may present as a painful third nerve palsy (Robinson et al., 1990). Cavernous sinus thrombosis, can also produce severe headache, usually around or behind the ipsilateral eye, typically associated with chemosis, proptosis, and ophthalmoplegia. In immunosuppressed individuals, cavernous sinus infection with mucormycosis or aspergillosis may develop.

A painful, isolated *trochlear nerve palsy* may be produced by an intracavernous internal carotid artery aneurysm (Arruga et al., 1991), a dural carotid-cavernous sinus fistula (Selky and Purvin, 1994), or a cavernous sinus meningioma (Slavin, 1987). Painful trochlear nerve palsy may also occur with HZO or oticus.

The *abducens nerve* may be damaged anywhere along its course by an ischemic neuropathy related to diabetes, collagen-vascular disease, giant cell arteritis, and parainfectious or postinfectious arteritides. Based on neurologic findings alone, it may be difficult at times to determine whether a painful sixth nerve palsy is due to a process affecting the nerve within the subarachnoid space, in the clival dura in Dorello's canal, or in the cavernous sinus. Concomitant involvement of the trigeminal nerve is more likely if the lesion is in the nerve's petrous portion. Other clinical findings may point to disease in the petrous bone, such as an external meatal discharge from chronic otitis media or mastoiditis, or deafness. An infectious or neoplastic process that spreads to the tip of the petrous bone may result in *Gradenigo syndrome,* which includes abducens nerve paresis, ipsilateral facial (usually retro-orbital) pain, and headache with deafness (Davé et al., 1997). Trauma, inferior petrosal sinus thrombosis, vascular malformations, aneurysms, and tumors may also injure the nerve at this level. Retro-orbital pain, involvement of other ocular motor nerves and, occasionally, an ipsilateral *Horner's syndrome* point to the cavernous sinus as the site of the sixth nerve lesion. The ascending sympathetic fibers leave the carotid artery and join the abducens nerve for a distance of 4 mm within the cavernous sinus. Thus a unilateral abducens nerve lesion associated with an ipsilateral Horner's syndrome (Parkinson syndrome) is of localizing value (Silva et al., 1999). HZO may cause abducens palsy with a Horner's syndrome (Smith et al., 1993). Pituitary adenomas, nasopharyngeal

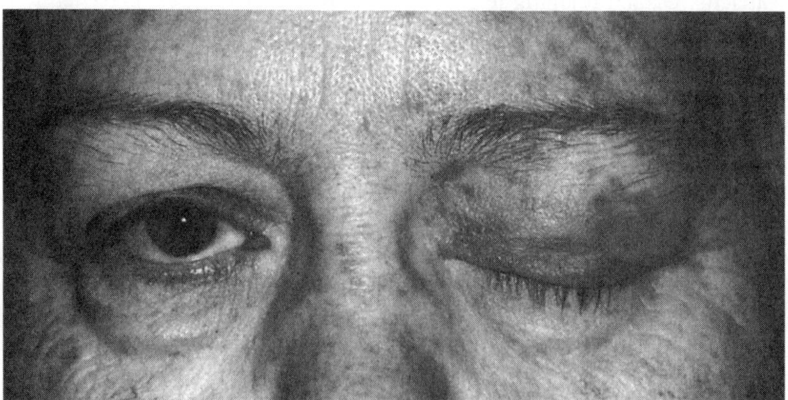

Figure 22–4 Herpes zoster ophthalmicus with a third cranial nerve palsy. A 71 year-old woman developed a left third nerve palsy several weeks after developing pain and vesicles in the distribution of the first division of the left trigeminal nerve. A complete ptosis is evident in this clinical photograph, along with the healing vesicles. [Courtesy of Martin TJ and Corbett JJ (2000). *Requisites in Neuro-ophthalmology*. (Figure 13–4, p. 230), Mosby, St. Louis.]

carcinomas, craniopharyngiomas, and metastases most commonly affect the abducens nerve at the cavernous sinus and superior orbital fissure. Sphenoid sinus carcinoma often causes a spheno-cavernous syndrome, but may also present with an isolated sixth nerve palsy. Carotid-cavernous sinus dural arteriovenous fistulae may present with unilateral or bilateral sixth nerve palsies (Lee et al., 1998). Unilateral, bifrontal, or holocranial headache is a common feature of this condition.

Intracranial Processes

Any process causing *increased intracranial pressure* (e.g., mass lesion, pseudotumor cerebri, venous sinus thrombosis) may cause headache and occasionally patients will refer this pain to the eye. The headache in patients with IIH may often be pulsatile, be of gradually increasing intensity during the day, awakening the patient at night, may be precipitated by changes in posture, may be constant or intermittent, may be unilateral, bilateral, or holocranial, and is often relieved by lumbar puncture (Wall, 1990). In a prospective study of 50 idiopathic pseudotumor cerebri patients, symptoms included headache in 94% and 44% of individuals complained of retrobulbar pain, especially on eye movement (Wall and George, 1991). Patients with increased intracranial pressure often have papilledema and other neurologic findings suggestive of a mass lesion.

Disorders of the intracranial vasculature may be associated with headache and eye pain. Headache may occur with subarachnoid, subdural, epidural, and intracerebral hemorrhage, with transient ischemic attacks (TIAs), and with cerebral infarction. Pain receptors within the walls of large pain-sensitive arteries at the base may be of importance in the headache that occasionally accompanies TIAs and cerebral infarction. The supratentorial vessels and dura are innervated by branches of the ophthalmic division of the trigeminal nerve and intracranial pain is often referred to the forehead, eye, or temple (Feindel et al., 1960). One quarter of patients with strokes in the distribution of the internal or middle cerebral arteries experience headache that is typically in the orbital or frontal region ipsilateral to the infarct (Gorelick et al., 1986). In another study, among five patients with transient monocular blindness, four had ipsilateral frontal or orbital pain (Grindal and Toole, 1974). Although most patients with occipital infarction have no headache at the time of occlusion, some patients with occipital infarction complain of ipsilateral eye pain, perhaps due to injury to the dural sinuses of the tentorium or superficial cerebral veins causing pain referred to the ophthalmic division of the trigeminal nerve (Knox and Cogan, 1962; Russell, 1973). Occipital hemorrhage may also cause ipsilateral eye or head pain (Ropper and Davis, 1980). Unruptured vascular malformations can also cause episodic headache, occasionally mimicking migraine with visual aura.

Spontaneous intracranial hypotension, often due to spontaneous cerebrospinal fluid leak, characteristically causes headache that is severe when the patient is upright and relieved when the patient is recumbent. The headache is usually diffuse but may refer to the eyes. Associated symptoms may include neck stiffness, nausea and vomiting, sixth nerve palsy, blurred vision, photophobia, tinnitus, and vertigo (Schievink et al., 1996).

Trigeminal Neuropathies

Multiple pathologic processes affecting the trigeminal nerve roots, ganglia, ophthalmic division, or distal ophthalmic branches may cause eye pain. In its cisternal course, the preganglionic trigeminal nerve root may be damaged by tumor (meningioma, schwannoma, metastasis, nasopharyngeal carcinoma), diffuse meningeal processes (e.g., granulomatous, infectious, or carcinomatous meningitis), trauma, or aneurysm. Preganglionic trigeminal nerve involvement is suggested by involvement of the neighboring cranial nerves (especially cranial nerves VI, VII, and VIII). Trigeminal nerve damage is manifested by ipsilateral facial pain, paresthesias, numbness, and sensory loss. The corneal reflex is depressed and a trigeminal motor paresis may occur. Some patients with "idiopathic" trigeminal neuralgia have enhancement of the cisternal segment of the trigeminal nerve on MRI studies (Seidel et al., 2000). This enhancement usually resolves as the pain resolves. The trigeminal roots may be involved by extension of pathologic processes (usually acoustic neuroma or meningioma) located in the cerebellopontine angle.

Lesions of the middle cranial fossa (e.g., tumor, varicella virus infection, sarcoidosis, syphilis, tuberculosis, arachnoiditis, trauma, abscess) may directly damage the Gasserian ganglion in Meckel's cave. Pain, often severe and paroxysmal, is the most characteristic finding and may be hemifacial or involve only select divisions of the trigeminal nerve. Sensory loss occurs in the division(s) affected, and unilateral pterygoid and masseter paresis may occur. Other cranial nerves (especially the abducens nerve) may also be affected.

A unilateral or bilateral trigeminal sensory neuropathy may be seen with *Sjögren's syndrome, rheumatoid arthritis, systemic sclerosis, mixed connective tissue disease, systemic lupus erythematosus, Churg–Strauss syndrome, dermatomyositis,* and *sarcoidosis* (Lecky et al., 1987; Hagen et al., 1990; Förster et al., 1996). Facial numbness with or without paresthesias, often associated with facial pain, is most often seen in a maxillary distribution. Occasionally, symptoms are bilateral. The trigeminal sensory neuropathy may be distinguished from other conditions associated with facial numbness by its frequent sparing of the muscles of mastication. The lesion is thought to involve the trigeminal ganglion or proximal part of the main trigeminal divisions and is perhaps related to the capillaries of the trigeminal ganglion being more permeable than the brain capillaries (blood–brain barrier) to abnormal proteins (Lecky et al., 1987).

Raeder's paratrigeminal syndrome is composed of two essential components: unilateral oculosympathetic paresis and evidence of trigeminal involvement on the same side (Mokri, 1982). The former consists of miosis and ptosis but differs from the typical Horner's syndrome in that facial anhidrosis is absent because the sudomotor fibers to the face that travel extracranially with the external carotid artery are spared. The unilateral head, facial, or retro-orbital pain related to trigeminal dysfunction may be associated with evidence of involvement of other cranial nerves (e.g., cranial nerves IV and VI). This syndrome is usually due to lesions in the middle cranial fossa, especially in the region between the trigeminal ganglion and the internal carotid artery, near the petrous apex. It may also be caused by lesions of the Gasserian ganglion. The usual etiologies include tumor, aneurysm, trauma, and infection.

Lesions located at the apex of the temporal bone, especially metastasis, osteitis or leptomeningitis associated with otitis media, may cause damage to the ophthalmic division of the trigeminal nerve and the nearby abducens nerve (*Gradenigo syndrome*) (Davé et al., 1997). Pain and sensory disturbance in the upper part of the face (ophthalmic distribution) are then associated with ipsilateral lateral rectus palsy. Oculosympathetic paresis (without anhidrosis) may also occur ipsilaterally if the lesions extend to involve sympathetic fibers.

As noted above, lesions within the *cavernous sinus* (e.g., tumor, internal carotid artery aneurysm, trauma, carotid–cavernous fistula, infection) may damage the ophthalmic and maxillary divisions of the trigeminal nerve and the abducens, trochlear, and oculomotor nerves. Through the *superior orbital fissure* pass the abducens, trochlear, and oculomotor nerves as well as the ophthalmic division of the trigeminal nerve. Thus, lesions at the superior orbital fissure (e.g., tumor, trauma, aneurysm, infection) may cause complete (external and internal) ophthalmoplegia associated with pain, paresthesias, and sensory loss in the ophthalmic cutaneous distribution.

HZO is caused by reactivation of latent herpes zoster virus in the Gasserian ganglion that typically involves the first division of the trigeminal nerve (ophthalmic division). The nasociliary branch of this nerve innervates intraocular structures, and intraocular inflammation (keratouveitis) can occur when this branch is involved. The risk of keratouveitis is greatest when vesicles are found in the cutaneous distribution of the nasociliary branch on the lateral aspect and the tip of the nose or the medial canthal area of the eye. Cranial neuropathies can also occur with HZO, usually weeks after the skin eruption (Fig. 22–4). Treating HZO with antiviral agents (acyclovir or famcyclovir) early in its course has greatly reduced the ocular morbidity of this potentially blinding disorder (Lavin, 1998).

Post-herpetic neuralgia in a trigeminal distribution most often follows ophthalmic varicella zoster virus infection. This pain occurs more often in older persons, is described as a constant, burning or gnawing pain in the ophthalmic distribution with superimposed paroxysms of stabbing or shock-like pain, and is often associated with ophthalmic distribution hyperpathia (pain from nonpainful stimuli) and allodynia (exaggerated pain from mildly painful stimuli).

The *peripheral branches of the ophthalmic division of the trigeminal nerve* are most often damaged in isolation by tumors or by fractures of the facial bones or skull. Cutaneous carcinomas of the face (e.g., squamous cell carcinoma, basal cell carcinoma) and some nasopharyngeal carcinomas may present with facial dysesthesias or pain in the distribution of any branch of the trigeminal nerve (ten Hove et al., 1997). These reports demonstrate that it is difficult, initially, to differentiate a "benign" trigeminal neuropathy from more serious malignant conditions associated with a poor prognosis.

Patients with trigeminal pain or sensory loss should undergo neuroimaging with attention to the trigeminal nerve along its entire course (e.g., MRI scan of the brain and face with and without contrast).

Head or Eye Pain Induced by the Valsalva Maneuver

Head or eye pain induced by valsalva maneuver or other maneuvers that increase intracranial pressure (e.g., coughing, sneezing, straining, laughing, bending, stooping, weight lifting, etc.) may indicate the presence of intracranial disease, especially processes affecting posterior fossa structures (e.g., Chiari malformation, basilar invagination from *Paget's disease*, posterior fossa tumor) (Symonds, 1956; Rooke, 1968). Cough or exertional headache on rare occasion may also be the presenting feature of cerebral aneurysm, vertebrobasilar disease, or carotid stenosis. We suggest an MRI in all patients with cough or valsalva induced headache. In some patients, particularly those with a carotid/cephalic bruit or vascular risk factors, a MRA or CT angiogram is also warranted. Most patients, however, with *headache or eye pain induced by exertion, cough, or sexual activity* have a benign etiology (Symonds, 1956; Rooke, 1978). These patients complain of short-lasting (less than one minute, but occasionally 30 minutes), sudden bilateral headache precipitated by cough or other activities. Many of these patients respond favorably to indomethacin (Mathew, 1981).

Other Ocular Causes of Eye Pain and Headache

Many patients with bilateral, nonlocalized eye pain or "tiredness" without other head pains ("*eye strain*") may well have an "ocular form" of tension headache as often no etiology for such pain is ever established. Although the importance of refractive error, anisometropia, heterophoria, or heterotropia, or prolonged or "intense" reading or studying in producing this eye pain and headaches in general is overemphasized, these conditions may contribute to eye discomfort, sometimes radiating to the temples or frontal regions, in some individuals (Tomsak, 1991). Patients with headaches should have the benefit of a proper refraction, but corrective measures are unlikely to have a significant effect on most common headaches.

Accommodative amplitude declines steadily with age. This means that even emmetropic individuals will eventually need reading glasses to help them focus at near. However, this process of *presbyopia* is not a significant cause of ocular discomfort or headache. Cameron noted that only 6 of 50 patients with the onset of presbyopia described headache with near tasks, and of these, three improved with bifocals or reading glasses (Cameron, 1976). Occasionally medications with anticholinergic effects induce a pharmacologic pseudopresbyopia, but this tends to cause only symptoms of blurred vision, not pain.

"Asthenopia" literally means "weak vision," but the term is frequently used to describe so-called "eye-strain" headaches that are thought to be the result of uncorrected (or improperly corrected) refractive errors or ocular misalignment. Afflicted patients describe a mild, bilateral, persistent brow ache that occurs when he or she must "strain" to clear a blurred (or possibly diplopic) image, especially with near tasks (Romano, 1975; Cameron, 1976). Such headaches are associated with extended and persistent close visual tasks and do not occur instantaneously with a visual challenge (Vincent et al., 1989). Tilting the head backward to look at a computer screen through bifocals is another "ocular" cause of headache.

Eye-strain headaches have been blamed on refractive errors (hyperopia, myopia, presbyopia) (Daum et al., 1988) and motility disorders (convergence insufficiency and other ocular misalignments). Of these, only uncorrected hyperopia (farsightedness) and convergence insufficiency are likely to cause any significant degree of ocular or cranial discomfort.

Individuals who are *hyperopic* (farsighted) do not have sufficient refractive power in a relaxed state to focus light rays from any plane, due to an eyeball that is too short relative to its optical power. When uncorrected, these subjects must keep their ciliary muscle "turned on" at all times to see clearly, even with distant focus. Attempts to focus at near require enormous effort. This requirement for constant contraction of the ciliary muscle can cause the "asthenopic" brow-and-eye ache that intensifies with efforts to focus on near objects. It is not entirely clear whether the resulting asthenopic discomfort is due to fatigue of the ciliary muscles, traction on the scleral spur, or the action of accessory facial muscles (Cameron, 1976). Interestingly, hyperopic children do not usually experience this fatigue, because their accommodative reserve is so great. Patients may not become symptomatic until they are in their thirties, when waning accommodative reserve creates eye fatigue and blur, and their *latent hyperopia* is discovered by the eye doctor. Brow-ache and frontal headache disappear when the hyperopia is corrected with glasses. Occasionally, overcorrected myopic individuals (see further on) experience similar symptoms because their (too-strong) glasses make them hyperopic.

Subjects with *myopia* (nearsightedness) have an eyeball that is too long for the amount of focusing power in the cornea and lens. These individuals can focus clearly at near with little or no contraction of the ciliary muscle, but have blurry distant vision. Uncorrected myopes do not have problems with ciliary muscle overuse, but they may develop orbicularis muscle fatigue and discomfort from constant squinting.

Astigmatism refers to refractive errors that are not spherically uniform, but differ along a given meridian. Astigmatism can be the result of nonuniformity of the cornea or the lens. The word must sound intimidating, as many patients ascribe all sorts of ills (including headache) to the discovery of their "astigmatism." In truth, some degree of astigmatism is present in virtually everyone, and even a great amount of astigmatism (corrected, uncorrected, or improperly corrected) is not likely to cause significant headache. In a similar manner, anisometropia (a marked difference in the power of the lenses between the two eyes) is not likely to induce headaches.

The relative frequency of eye-strain-induced headache was explored by Cameron, who reviewed 50 patients who were referred to his ophthalmology practice with a chief complaint of headache. Only five patients had symptoms that could be attributed to visual effort and eye strain, and two of these five patients had relief of their discomfort after their refractive error was corrected (Cameron, 1976).

When *convergence insufficiency* is present, there is too little convergence for the required amount of accommodation; therefore patients are exophoric or intermittently exotropic at near. Extra effort is required to maintain single binocular vision at near, which can cause fatigue and asthenopic symptoms or diplopia with extended near tasks (Mahto, 1972). Medications, head injuries, aging, and some neurologic syndromes (such as Parkinson's disease) are associated with convergence insufficiency, but this condition is very common in the normal population as well. Although brow ache and ocular discomfort can occur as a result of convergence insufficiency, these symptoms only occur after a reasonable amount of near effort. Headache or ocular discomfort that occurs instantly upon glancing at a word on a page is nonphysiologic. Reading spectacles with prisms to reduce near effort often correct the visual impairment and aid the eye discomfort in patients with convergence insufficiency.

Convergence spasm is actually a spasm of the near synkinetic triad, with blurred vision from excessive accommodation, miotic pupils, and esotropia from excessive convergence. This uncomfortable condition occurs most often in young, anxious, but otherwise healthy students. It is usually transient, and is more likely to occur in undercorrected hyperopes or overcorrected myopes. In isolation, convergence spasm is not usually associated with systemic diseases (and may be "functional" or deliberate), but it may also be one component of dorsal midbrain syndrome (in which case the pupils are usually large) or other neurologic disorders. Convergence spasm can be distinguished from bilateral sixth nerve palsies by the presence of miotic pupils (as part of the synkinetic near reflex).

Many, and perhaps most, patients with chronic unilateral or bilateral eye pain with a normal ophthalmologic and neuro-ophthalmologic examination end up being classified as idiopathic eye pain. This designation is similar to the diagnosis of "atypical facial pain" or more appropriately facial pain of unknown cause. The pain may be unilateral or bilateral, may be of aching or burning nature, and does not occur in a trigeminal distribution. In all of these patients, an indolent underlying pathologic processes affecting the teeth, sinuses, jaw, and intracranial contents (see further on) must be carefully excluded.

PAIN REFERRED TO THE EYE FROM NONOPHTHALMIC OR NONCRANIAL PATHOLOGIC PROCESSES (SECONDARY EYE PAIN)

Diseases of carotid artery may cause eye pain and headaches. *Carotodynia* refers to pain arising from the region of the cervical carotid artery that frequently radiates to the jaw, face, ear, and head, including the eye on the ipsilateral side. The pain may be dull, throbbing, or stabbing and occur in bouts lasting days to weeks or be chronic. Icepick-like jabs may occur. During episodes the carotid artery may be tender and the pain may be accentuated by swallowing, sneezing, coughing, and neck motion. Carotodynia may be a migraine variant but its existence as a true entity has been questioned by some authors (Biousse and Bousser, 1994). In any patient with such pain, other painful disorders of the carotid artery and neck must be considered. These include carotid dissection, carotid atherosclerosis or aneurysm (including ruptured aneurysm), and giant cell arteritis as well as nonvascular neck diseases, such as *thyroiditis*, tumors, and *mastoiditis*.

Carotid artery dissection presents with the sudden or gradual onset of ipsilateral neck or hemicranial pain, including eye or face pain, often but variably associated with other neurologic findings including an ipsilateral Horner's syndrome, TIA, stroke, anterior ischemic optic neuropathy, subarachnoid hemorrhage, or lower cranial nerve palsies (Mokri et al., 1986; Biousse et al., 1994, 1998). Seventy-four percent of patients with carotid dissection complain of cephalic pain, on the same side as the dissection in 79%, lasting from 1 hour to 30 days with a median of 5 days (Biousse et al., 1994). Biousse et al. state that "the association of a third order Horner's syndrome and orbital and/or ipsilateral head pain or neck pain of acute onset is so characteristic that it should be considered diagnostic of internal carotid artery dissection unless proven otherwise" (Biousse et al., 1998). Ophthalmic division pain may also occur in patients with *high-grade carotid stenosis* or *occlusion* and is often exacerbated by bending or straining (Fisher, 1951). The *ocular ischemic syndrome* is a progressive disorder due to hypoperfusion of the eye that may be associated with transient visual loss and ocular discomfort or frank pain localized to the orbit and upper face that is often decreased when the patient lies down. This syndrome is often associated with a "red" rather than a "quiet" eye. Although usually due to severe atherosclerotic carotid or ophthalmic artery disease, the ocular ischemic syndrome may also occur with giant cell arteritis, carotid artery dissection, cavernous sinus thrombosis, Takayasu's disease, fibromuscular dysplasia, mucormycosis, HZO, myelofibrosis, vasospasm, and following aneurysm repair. Headache may also occur *after carotid endarterectomy* (Pearce, 1976). This headache may be intense, is often throbbing, is located anteriorly over the head, occurs 26–72 hours after surgery, is often accompanied by nausea, and is self limited, lasting days to months. Patients with suspected carotid dissection may require imaging of the carotid in the neck and head (e.g., MRI scan, MRI angiography, catheter carotid angiography).

Giant cell arteritis (GCA) is an important cause of headache in individuals aged 55 or older. The headache with GCA may be unilateral or bilateral, is often temporal but may involve any or all aspects of the cranium, may be of gradual or explosive onset, is usually dull and boring with occasional superimposed icepick-like or lancinating pain, is seldom throbbing, is often worse at night and aggravated by exposure to cold, and may or may not be associated with scalp tenderness. Because of the high-risk of visual loss if left untreated, GCA must be considered as a possible diagnosis in any patient aged 55 years or older with the new onset of any head pain. A serum ESR, C-reactive protein, and temporal artery biopsy should be considered for prompt diagnosis.

TABLE 22–4 "Red Flags" of a Potentially Life-threatening or Vision-threatening Process Causing Eye Pain in a Patient with a Normal Neuro-ophthalmologic and Ophthalmologic Examination..

Any history of malignancy (consider orbital, cavernous sinus, meningeal, or cerebral metastasis)
History of bleeding tendency, leukemia, or patient on anticoagulation (consider orbital or cerebral hemorrhage)
New eye pain or headache in a patient over age 55 (consider giant cell arteritis, tumor)
History of smoking (consider orbital, cavernous sinus, meningeal or cerebral metastasis; consider referred eye or face pain due to lung cancer)
Apoplectic onset of eye pain or excruciatingly severe eye pain in a previously asymptomatic individual ("first and worst" syndrome) (consider hemorrhage, pituitary apoplexy, sphenoid sinusitis, etc.).

Source: From Brazis et al., 2002.

Cervical facet joint damage, usually due to cervical spondylosis, can cause neck pain referred to the ipsilateral temple, forehead, and eye (*cervicogenic headache or eye pain)*. These patients typically have neck pain that is exacerbated by neck movement or pressure over the neck.

Patients with *nonmetastatic lung cancer* may rarely experience "atypical" facial pain as a presenting symptom, during the course of the disease, or upon recurrence of the disease (Broux et al., 1991; Capobianco, 1995). In a review of 10 cases, all complained of severe, aching facial pain typically aural-temporal but occasionally orbital (Capobianco, 1995). The pain was ipsilateral to the lung cancer in all patients. The proposed mechanism for this facial pain is local invasion of the vagus nerve with referred pain by afferent impulses traveling with the visceral pain afferents that synapse with somatic sensory afferents within the descending tract and nucleus of the trigeminal nerve. It behooves clinicians to consider the possibility of lung cancer-related nonmetastatic facial pain in every smoker or former smoker with facial pain of unknown cause.

ORBITAL, SUPERIOR ORBITAL FISSURE, CAVERNOUS SINUS, OR INTRACRANIAL INFILTRATIVE, NEOPLASTIC, OR INFLAMMATORY DISEASE PROCESSES WITH NORMAL OPHTHALMOLOGIC AND NEURO-OPHTHALMOLOGIC EXAM

In many patients presenting with eye pain and a normal ophthalmologic and neuro-ophthalmologic, no etiology for the eye pain is found. Many of the patients may be treated symptomatically and monitored by serial examinations to make sure that no other specific etiology for the pain later presents itself. However, certain "red flags" exist suggesting that the patient may have a potentially vision-threatening or life-threatening process that may be present (e.g., may have orbital malignancy requiring orbital imaging with special techniques to further investigate the cause of the pain). These "red flags" are presented in Table 22–4.

References

Arruga, J, De Rivas, P, Espinet, HL, et al. (1991). Chronic isolated trochlear nerve palsy produced by intracavernous internal carotid artery aneurysm: Report of a case. *J Clin Neuroophthalmol*, 11:104–108.

Benson, WE (1988). Posterior scleritis. *Surv Ophthalmol*, 32(5):297–316.

Biousse, V and Bousser, M-G (1994). The myth of carotidynia. *Neurology*, 44:993–995.

Biousse, V, D'Angelejan-Chatillon, J, Massiou, H, et al. (1994). Head pain in non-traumatic carotid artery dissection: A series of 65 patients. *Cephalgia*, 14:33–36

Biousse, V, Touboul, P-J, D'Anglejan-Chatillon, J, et al. (1998). Ophthalmic manifestations of internal carotid dissection. *Am J Ophthalmol*, 126:565–577.

Brazis, PW, Capobianco, DJ, Chang, F-LF, et al. (1994). Low flow dural arteriovenous shunt: Another cause of "sinister" Tolosa–Hunt syndrome. *Headache*, 34:523–525.

Brazis, PW, Capobianco, DJ, Lee, AG, et al. (2002). The differential diagnosis and evaluation of pain in the "quiet eye." *Neurologist*, 8:82–100.

Brazis, PW and Lee, AG (1996). Optic disk edema with a macular star. *Mayo Clin Proc*, 71:1162–1166.

Brazis, PW, Lee, AG, Stewart, M, et al. (2002). Clinical Review: the differential diagnosis of pain in the quiet eye. *Neurologist*, 8:82–100.

Broux, R, Moonen, G, and Schoenen, J (1991). Unilateral facial pain as the first symptom of lung carcinoma: report of three cases. *Cephalgia*,. 11(Suppl 1):319.

Cameron, ME (1976). Headaches in relation to the eyes. *Med J Aust*, 1(10):292–294.

Capobianco, DJ (1995). Facial pain as a symptom of nonmetastatic lung cancer. *Headache*, 35:581–585.

Cummings, JL, Gittinger, JW (1981). Central dazzle: A thalamic syndrome? *Archives of Neurology*, 38:372–374.

Daum, KM, Good, G, and Tijerina, L (1988). Symptoms in video display terminal operators and the presence of small refractive errors. *J Am Optom Assoc*, 59 (9):691–697.

Davé, AV, Diaz-Marchan, PJ, and Lee, AG (1997). Clinical and magnetic resonance imaging features of Gradenigo syndrome. *Am J Ophthalmol*, 124:568–570.

Dayan, M, Turner, B, and McGhee, C (1996). Acute angle closure glaucoma masquerading as systemic illness. *Br Med J*, 313(7054):413–415.

De Marinis, M, Giraldi, JP, de Feo, A, et al. (1999). Migraine and ocular pain in "glaucoma suspect." *Cephalalgia*, 19(4):243–247.

Eckhardt, LB, McLean, JM, and Goodell, H (1943). Experimental studies on headache. The genesis of pain from the eye. *Proc Assoc Res Nerv Ment Dis*, 23:209–227.

Ederer, F (1986). Migraine and low-tension glaucoma. A case control study. *Invest Ophthalmol Vis Sci*, 27 (4):632–633.

Feindel, W, Penfield, W, and McNaughton, F (1960). The tentorial nerves and localization of intracranial pain in man. *Neurology*, 10:555–563.

Fisher, CM (1951). Occlusion of the internal carotid artery. *Arch Neurol Pschiatr*, 65:346–377.

Förster, C, Brandt, T, Hund, E, et al. (1996). Trigeminal sensory neuropathy in connective tissue disease: Evidence for the site of the lesion. *Neurology*, 46:270–271.

Gerling, J, Jancknecht, P, and Kommerell, G (1998). Orbital pain in optic neuritis and anterior ischemic optic neuropathy. *Neuroophthalmol*, 19:93–99.

Goldberg, RA and Rootman, J (1990). Clinical characteristics of metastatic orbital tumors. *Ophthalmol*, 97:620–624.

Goldberg, RA, Rootman, J, and Cline, RA (1990).Tumors metastatic to the orbit: A changing picture. *Surv Ophthalmol*, 35:1–24.

Gorelick, PB, Hier, DB, Caplan, LR, et al. (1986). Headache in acute cerebrovascular disease. *Neurology*, 36:1445–1450.

Grindal, AB and Toole, JF (1974). Headache and transient ischemic attacks. *Stroke*, 5:603–606.

Gutrecht, JA, Lessell, IM, and Zamani, AA (1990). Central dazzle in trigeminal sensory neuropathy. *Neurology*, 40:722–723.

Hagen, NA, Stevens, JC, and Michet, CJ (1990). Trigeminal sensory neuropathy associated with connective tissue disease. *Neurology*, 40:891–896.

Ischemic Optic Neuropathy Decompression Trial Research Group (IONDT) (1995). Optic nerve decompression for nonarteritic anterior ischemic optic neuropathy (AION) is not effective and may be harmful. *J Am Med Assoc*, 273:625–632.

Ischemic Optic Neuropathy Decompression Trial Research Group (IONDT) (1996). Characteristics of patients with nonarteritic anterior ischemic optic neuropathy eligible for the Ischemic optic neuropathy decompression trial. *Arch Ophthalmol*, 114:1366–1374.

Joseph, A (1999). A tooth for an eye: dental procedures in unrecognized glaucoma. *J R Soc Med*, 92(5):249.

Keane, JR (1996). Cavernous sinus syndrome. Analysis of 151 cases. *Arch Neurol*, 53:967–971.

Knox, DL and Cogan, DG (1962). Eye pain and homonymous hemianopsia. *Am J Ophthalmol*, 54:1091–1093.

Kosmorsky, GS, Hanson, MR, and Tomsak, RL (1988). Carotid- cavernous sinus fistulae presenting as painful ophthlmoplegia without external ocular signs. *J Clin Neuroophthalmol*, 8:131–135.

Lanzino, G, Andreoli, A, Tognetti, F, et al. (1993). Orbital pain and unruptured carotid-posterior communicating artery aneurysms: The role of sensory fibers of the third cranial nerve. *Acta Neurochir*, 120:7–11.

Lavin, PJM (1998). Ocular and facial pain syndromes. In *Neuro-ophthalmology* (ES Rosen, P Eustace, HS Thompson, and WJK Cumming, eds), pp. 23.1–23.18. St Louis, Mosby.

Lecky, BRF, Hughes, RAC, and Murray, NMF (1987). Trigeminal sensory neuropathy. A study of 22 cases. *Brain*, 110:1463–1485.

Lee, AG and Brazis, PW (2003). *Clinical Pathways in Neuro-Ophthalmology. An Evidence-Based Approach* (2nd edn). Theime, NewYork.

Lee, KY, Kim, SM, and Kim, DI. (1998). Isolated bilateral abducens nerve palsy due to carotid cavernous dural arteriovenous fistula. *Yonsei Med J*, 39:283–286.

Mahto, RS (1972). Eye strain from convergence insufficiency. *Br Med J*, 2(813):564–565.

Martin, TJ and Soyka, D (1993) Ocular causes of headache. In *The Headaches*, (J Olesen, P Tfelt-Hansen, and KMA Welch, eds). Raven Press, New York.

Mathew, NT (1981). Indomethicin-responsive headache syndromes. *Headache*, 21:147–150.

McFadzean, RM, Doyle, D, Rampling, R, et al. (1991). Pituitary apoplexy and its effect on *Neurosurgery*, 29:669–675.

Miller, NR (1985). Facial pain and neuralgia. In *Walsh and Hoyt's Clinical Neuro-ophthalmology* (4th edn), Vol. 2, p. 1071. Baltimore, Williams and Wilkins.

Mokri, B (1982). Raeder's paratrigeminal syndrome—Original concept and subsequent deviations. *Arch Neurol*, 39:395–399.

Mokri, B, Sundt, TM, Houser, OW, et al. (1986). Spontaneous dissection of the cervical internal carotid artery. *Ann Neurol*, 19:126–138.

Nussenblatt, RB and Palestine, AG (1989). *Uveitis. Fundamentals and Clinical Practice*. pp. 54–75. Year Book Medical Publishers, Chicago.

Optic Neuritis Study Group. (1991). The clinical profile of optic neuritis: experience of the optic neuritis treatment trial. *Arch Ophthalmol*, 109:1673–1678.

Pearce, J (1976). Headache after carotid endarterectomy. *Br Med J*, 2:85–86.
Phelps, CD and Corbett, JJ (1985) Migraine and low-tension glaucoma. A case-control study. *Invest Ophthalmol Vis Sci*, 26:1105–1108.
Pradalier, A, Hamard, P, Sellem, E, et al. (1998). Migraine and glaucoma: an epidemiologic survey of French ophthalmologists. *Cephalalgia*, 18(2):74–76.
Prasad, P, Subramanya, R, and Upadhyaya, NS (1991) Cluster headache or narrow angle glaucoma? *Indian J Ophthalmol*, 39(4):181–182.
Robinson, R, Toland, J, and Eustace, P (1990). Pituitary apoplexy. A cause for painful third nerve palsy. *Neuroophthalmol*, 10:257–260.
Romano, PE (1975) Pediatric ophthalmic mythology. *Postgrad Med*, 58(4):146–150.
Rooke, E (1968). Benign exertional headache. *Med Clin North Am*, 52:801–808.
Ropper, AH and Davis, KR (1980). Lobar hemorrhage: Acute clinical syndromes in 26 cases. *Ann Neurol*, 8:141–147
Russell, RW (1973). The posterior cerebral circulation. *J R Coll Physicians*, 7:331–346.
Schievink, WI, Meyer, FB, Atkinson, JLD, et al. (1996). Spontaneous spinal cerebrospinal fluid leaks and intracranial hypotension. *J Neurosurgery*, 84:598–605.
Seidel, E, Hansen, C, Urban, PP, et al. (2000). Idiopathic trigeminal sensory neuropathy with gadolinium enhancement in the cisternal segment. *Neurology*, 54:1191–1192.
Selky, AK and Purvin, VA (1994). Isolated trochlear nerve palsy secondary to dural carotid-cavernous sinus fistula. *J Neuroophthalmol*, 14:52–54.
Shindler, KS, Sankar, PS,Volpe, N,J, and Piltz-Seymour, JR (2005). Intermittent headaches as the presenting sign of subacute angle-closure glaucoma. *Neurology*, 65:757–758.
Silva, MN, Saeki, N, Hirai, S, and Yamaura, A (1999). Unusual cranial nerve palsy caused by cavernous sinus aneurysms. Clinical and anatomical considerations reviewed. *Surgical Neurology*, 52:148–149.
Slavin, ML (1987). Isolated trochlear nerve palsy secondary to cavernous sinus meningioma. *Am J Ophthalmol*, 104:433–434.
Smith, EF, Santamarina, L, and Wolintz, AH (1993). Herpes zoster ophthalmicus as a cause of Horner syndrome. *J Clin Neuroophthalmol*, 13:250–253.
Swartz, NG, Beck, RW, Savino, PJ, et al. (1995). Pain in anterior ischemic optic neuropathy. *J Neuroophthalmol*, 15:9–10.
Symonds, C (1956). Cough Headache. *Brain*, 79:557–568.
ten Hove, MW, Glaser, JS, and Schatz, NJ (1997). Occult perineural tumor infiltration of thetrigeminal nerve. Diagnostic considerations. *J Neuroophthalmol*, 17:170 177.
Tomsak, RL (1991). Ophthalmologic aspects of headache. *Med Clin North Am*, 75:693–706.
Vincent, AJP, Spierings, ELH, and Messinger, HB (1989). A controlled study of visual symptoms and eye strain factors in chronic headache. *Headache*, 29:523–527.
Wall, M (1990). The headache profile of idiopathic intracranial hypertension. *Cephalgia*, 10:331–335.
Wall, M and George, D (1991). Idiopathic intracranial hypertension. A prospective study of 50 patients. *Brain*, 114:155–180.
Wang, JJ, Mitchell, P, and Smith, W (1997). Is there an association between migraine headache and open-angle glaucoma? Findings from the Blue Mountain Eye Study. *Ophthalmol*, 104(10):1714–1719.
Watson, NJ, and Kirkby, GR (1989). Acute glaucoma presenting with abdominal symptoms. *Br Med J*, 299:254.
Wright, JE, Sullivan, TJ, Garner, A, et al. (1997). Orbital venous anomalies. *Ophthalmol*, 104:905–913.

23 Disorders of the Mouth and Teeth

Steven B Graff-Radford and Alan C Newman

INTRODUCTION

Orofacial pain is a complex and often puzzling problem that clinicians are faced with on a daily basis. The International Association for the Study of Pain defines pain as "an unpleasant sensory and emotional experience associated with actual or potential tissue damage, or described in terms of such damage" (Mersky, 1986). This definition allows pain to be present without nociception (the recordable neural activity in a delta and c fibers) and encourages the clinician to consider assessing the associated suffering and pain behavior in understanding and treating pain. Before one can treat facial pain it is essential to have an accurate diagnosis. This requires a working knowledge of a classification system. This chapter will describe a comprehensive classification system and address pains that present in the trigeminal nerve distribution.

CLASSIFICATION

The International Headache Society's classification system can be used to describe many orofacial pains (Headache Classification Subcommittee of the International Headache Society, 2004). This classification separates many conditions that may produce facial pain and classifies them independently. Table 23–1 provides an organ-based classification system that simplifies differential diagnosis. The orofacial pains are divided into six categories, which will be reviewed separately.

Extracranial

The eyes (Chapter 20), ears, nose, throat, sinuses (Chapter 22), teeth, lymph glands, and salivary glands may produce pain when noxious stimulation is triggered by infectious, degenerative, edematous, neoplastic, or destructive processes. Although the musculoskeletal system is included in the extracranial structures, it is separated in the classification, as it commonly produces significant chronic pain.

Ear

Pain in the ear is often referred from musculoskeletal structures, such as the temporomandibular joint (TMJ) or muscles of mastication. The teeth may also refer pain to the ear. Pain referred from these structures is described as a dull, achy, or stopped-up sensation. Because the ear is innervated by cranial nerves V, VII, IX, X, and cervical roots C2–3, the source of the referred pain may be difficult to ascertain.

Nose

Pain in the nose may be referred from the teeth, sinuses, or other structures, but it is more likely to be caused by inflammation or local tumor. Referral to an ear, nose, and throat (ENT) specialist is recommended if dental etiology is ruled out.

Throat

Throat pain is usually a local inflammatory reaction secondary to infection; however, other local problems, such as tumor, need to be considered. Other neurologic problems [glossopharyngeal neuralgia, stomatodynia (burning mouth syndrome), and Eagles syndrome] will be included in the discussion of neurogenous pains later in this chapter.

TABLE 23–1 Organ System Classification for Orofacial Pain.

Organ		*Presence*	*Quality*
A	Extracranial	Continuous	Dull
B	Intracranial	Continuous	Variable
C	Psychogenic	Variable	Variable
D	Neurovascular	Intermittent	Throbbing
E	Neuropathic	Intermittent	Sharp, shooting, electric
		Continuous	Burning
F	Musculoskeletal	Continuous	Dull, aching

Sinus and Paranasal Pain

Referred toothache is often due to inflammatory sinus disease. The problem is usually associated with the maxillary sinus, and pain is felt in the maxillary teeth on the involved side. The pain presents as a continuous, dull toothache and the patient may state that the tooth feels extruded. Malaise, fever, and a purulent nasal discharge may accompany the pain. On examination, the sinus may be tender to palpation and the teeth sensitive to percussion. The pain is reduced for the duration of the anesthesia with 4% lidocaine nasal spray or drops. Radiographic sinus examination will demonstrate inflammatory change and is essential in finalizing the diagnosis. Seasonal changes, allergies, and barometric pressure changes may aggravate sinus problems. Sinus disease is classified as either acute or chronic disease. Acute sinusitis often follows an upper respiratory infection or dental disease and can produce nasal mucosal edema, preventing aeration and drainage through the ostia. Nociception will result from the inflammation. Chronic sinus disease usually is not painful. Acute sinusitis should be treated with antibiotics and systemic or topical decongestants. Surgical drainage may be required (see Chapter 20). Almost one-third of migraine sufferers have been given a diagnosis of sinus headache because sinus type symptoms often accompany migraine (Cady and Schreiber, 2002).

Teeth

The most common orofacial pain involves the teeth and their supporting structures. This pain is usually related to dental caries, presenting as a reversible pulpitis. It is characterized by poorly localized pain that may be sensitive to hot or cold stimuli. The reaction to the noxious stimulus (heat or cold) disappears soon after the stimulus is removed. When the carious lesion invades the pulp, an irreversible pulpitis begins. This is characterized by a lingering reaction to noxious stimuli. Periodontitis, which occurs if the microorganisms and inflammatory products invade the periapical area (the area around the root apex) may present with toothache associated with chewing and sensitivity to touch and percussion. Periapical pathology may be observed as an area of increased radiolucency on radiographs. The tooth may have an abnormal response to pulp testing wherein heat, cold, or an electrical stimulus is not perceived. In clinical practice, it is difficult to differentiate reversible and irreversible pulpitis. When the diagnosis is not obvious, careful observation over days or weeks is recommended. Too often endodontic therapy is performed when it is not indicated.

An intermittent pain that is triggered by biting on an offending tooth characterizes cracked-tooth syndrome. Unfortunately the cracks are often difficult to find and do not appear on all X-ray images. The pain is often confused with that of pulpitis or trigeminal neuralgia, resulting in frustration and unnecessary treatment. Thin-cut tomographic images through the tooth's long axis may help define the crack. This study is called a "cracked-tooth survey." Further careful clinical examination, including staining or meticulous bite tests on each tooth cusp, may be useful. Graff-Radford and Gratt used thermography to study cracked teeth and found a difference in cracked-tooth pain and neuropathic facial pain. Patients who have cracked teeth have normal thermograms and patients who have neuropathic pain have asymmetrical thermograms (Graff-Radford et al., 1995). Chronic toothache may be a referred phenomenon. When no obvious local etiology is evident, neuropathic, muscular, or vascular etiologies should be considered (Graff-Radford et al., 1995).

Burning Mouth Syndrome

Burning mouth syndrome is characterized by a burning sensation in one or several oral structures (Tourne and Fricton, 1992). Burning mouth syndrome is more common in women and usually occurs within 3–12 years after menopause (Suarez and Clark, 2006). Causes may be local, systemic, or even psychological. Local factors include contact allergy, denture irritation, oral habits, infection, and possibly reflux esophagitis. Systemic factors include menopause, vitamin and mineral deficiency, diabetes, oral infection, and chemotherapy. Psychogenic factors have often been cited but in an anecdotal fashion. It is essential to rule out a candida infection. Although this may not be obvious to the eye, a swab and culture of the oral mucosa often reveals an incipient fungal infection. Patients with fungal infection respond quickly to antifungal preparations, such as clotrimazole or fluconazole. In the authors' experience, approximately half the patients with burning mouth syndrome have a candida infection. This often follows steroid, antibiotic, or chemotherapy administration. When no systemic or local pathology is identified, the cause is probably neuropathic. Biopsies of the tongue have shown that patients with burning mouth syndrome have a lower density of epithelial nerve fibers than controls (Suarez and Clark, 2006). Topical clonazepam (0.5–1.0 mg three times a day) effectively reduces burning oral pain (Woda et al., 1998). Patients are instructed to suck a tablet for 3 minutes (and then spit it out) three times a day for at least 10 days. Serum concentrations are minimal (3.3 ng/ml) at 1 and 3 hours after application. Woda hypothesized that clonazepam produces a peripheral, not a central, action that disrupts the neuropathologic mechanism. Additional treatments include tricyclic antidepressants, antiepileptic drugs, benzodiazepines, folic acid, and oral rinses.

Intracranial

Intracranial pathology presenting as orofacial pain is exceedingly rare. The pain is usually associated with additional neurologic signs and symptoms. The meninges, cranial nerves, and blood vessels are the intracranial structures that are pain sensitive. Traction, inflammation, distention, or pressure on these structures produces pain referral to distant sites.

Thalamic pain is described as "Unilateral facial pain and dysesthesia attributed to a lesion of the quintothalamic pathway or thalamus. Symptoms may also involve the trunk and limbs of the affected side" (Mersky, 1986). Thalamic infarcts that involve the primary sensory nuclei or damage in other sensory pathways, may lead to the thalamic pain syndrome. The pain quality is moderate to severe, burning or aching, and localized to the contralateral face. The clinical presentation may include hemiplegia and associated allodynia, hyperesthesia, and hyperpathia. Magnetic resonance imaging (MRI) or computed tomography (CT) is used to confirm the diagnosis. Treatment is difficult, but patients respond best to the tricyclic antidepressants or membrane-stabilizing medications (Tables 23–2 and 23–3). Stimulation-produced analgesia, such as acupuncture, transcutaneous electric nerve stimulation, and even deep brain stimulation are options in refractory cases.

Intracranial neoplasms produce pain in approximately 60% of cases. This pain is typically dull, nonpulsatile, and persistent and is aggravated by exertion or postural changes (Bulitt and Tew,

TABLE 23–2 Common Antidepressants Used in Trigeminal Neuropathic Pain.

Medication trade name	*Route*	*Dosage per day*
Amitriptyline	PO	10–150
Desipramine	PO	10–150
Doxepin	PO	10–150
Imipramine	PO	10–150
Nortriptyline	PO	10–150
Trazedone	PO	50–300
Venlafaxine	PO	37.5–225
Duloxetine	PO	30–90

TABLE 23–3 Common Membrane Stabilizers used in Trigeminal Neuropathic Pain.

Trade name	*Dosage (mg/day)*
Baclofen	10–80
Carbamazepine	100–1200
Gabapentin	300–3000
Pregabalin	25–600
Klonopin	0.5–8
Lamotrigine	12.5–100
Pimozide	2–12
Phenytoin	100–400
Topiramate	25–200
Valproic acid	125–2000

1986). Intracranial pathology must be considered when a patient presents with nonodontogenic face pain and other cranial nerve abnormalities. While certain intracranial tumors are more likely than others to produce neurologic problems, they do not all have the same neurologic presentation (Rushton and Rooke, 1962). Tumors that produce facial pain include meningiomas, schwannomas, neurofibromas, acoustic neuromas, and cholesteatomas. Pituitary tumors may result in pain when they erode the sella or place pressure on the Gasserian ganglion owing to cavernous sinus invasion (Cueneo and Rand, 1952). Tumors arising from the trigeminal ganglion produce pain, and those arising from the root do not (Schisano and Olivercrona, 1960). In one study, 16 of 2000 patients with trigeminal neuralgia had brain tumor (Bullitt and Tew, 1986).

Psychogenic

Labeling a disease process psychogenic without clear documented objective criteria is grossly unfair to the patient. Fordyce has pointed out that a patient's pain experiences are often labeled "psychogenic pain" when repeated failures using the biomedical model result in a lengthy medical history (Fordyce and Steger, 1978). Fordyce suggests that the system has not provided adequate diagnosis. Psychogenic pain may be interpreted in many ways. Some consider pain to be psychogenic when the pain behavior is excessive or varies from the physiological sensation or apparent nociceptive cause. A more useful method would use the psychogenic pain label when the emotional and psychological factors are the pain's primary manifestations. The latter alternative requires positive inclusion criteria, and Fordyce divides these into four groups: somatic delusions, somatization disorder, conversion, and depression. Fordyce points out that a psychogenic diagnosis is a philosophical one. The fact that the International Association for the Study of Pain (Mersky, 1986) defines pain as having an emotional component should not allow one to confuse the emotional overlay with a psychogenic etiology.

A better term for pain problems in which no obvious pathology can be determined would be idiopathic, rather than psychogenic or atypical, pain. Further in-depth, systematic, objective study of these disorders needs to be carried out to understand their etiology. An ascribable diagnosis can usually be made if patients whose pain has been described as atypical or idiopathic are evaluated by someone with more experience (Fricton, 1999).

Neurovascular

Pain problems within the neurovascular organ system may not all originate in this system, but they all have the trigeminovascular pathway as the nociceptive mediator (Moskowitz et al., 1988). Neurovascular pains are largely intermittent and involve a complex mechanism that is still not fully understood. Table 23–4 lists the neurovascular pains that may present in the orofacial region.

Migraine, Exertional Headache, and Cough Headache

Although migraine is traditionally considered to present above the oculotragus line, facial migraine is well documented (Lovshin, 1960; Raskin and Prusiner, 1977). Migraine itself is discussed elsewhere in this text.

Lovshin (Lovshin, 1960) was the first to describe facial migraine, which is facial pain that occurs without a headache, a finding that was later confirmed by Raskin (Raskin, 1988). Facial migraine pain is described as dull pain with superimposed throbbing that occurs once to several

TABLE 23–4 Orofacial Pains of Neurovascular Origin.

Migraine
Migraine with aura
Migraine without aura
Exertional migraine
Cluster Headache
Chronic paroxysmal hemicrania
Hemicrania continua
Severe unilateral neuralgiform headache with conjunctival injection and tearing, rhinorrhea and subclinical sweating (SUNCT)

times a week. Each attack lasts minutes to hours. Raskin describes ipsilatertal carotid tenderness, a finding also present when migraine presents in the head. This condition has also been referred to as carotidynia (Raskin and Prusiner, 1977). Raskin believes dental trauma may be a precipitant.

The exertional migraine may also be sub-classified into benign cough headache (BCH) and benign exertional headache. BCH is defined as an intermittent pain, usually bilateral, with severe bursting explosive pain brought on by coughing (Rooke 1968). The pain location is usually in the vertex, occipital, frontal or temporal regions, but as been described as presenting in the tooth (Symonds, 1956; Moncade and Graff-Radford, 1993). This pain is responsive to 25–225 mg/day indomethacin doses. Patients are required to maintain the treatment indefinitely. If decreased the symptoms usually reoccur. When evaluating BCH, Symonds emphasizes the need to rule out intracranial pathology (Symonds, 1956).

Cluster Headache

Cluster headache (Chapter 10) has been called "periodic migrainous neuralgia" when it presents as orofacial pain (Brooke, 1978). Fifty-three percent of Brooke's facial cluster patients had toothache and 47% had jaw pain. Bittar and Graff-Radford described 42 cluster headache patients, 42% of whom received unnecessary dental procedures (Bittar and Graff-Radford, 1992). Cluster headache often presents in the orofacial region, especially in the maxilla. A sphenopaletine ganglion block with local anesthetic is useful as temporary abortive therapy (Torelli and Manzoni, 2004). Occipital nerve blocks can also be used a treatment modality for cluster headaches (Ambrosini and Vandenheede, 2005).

Chronic paroxysmal hemicrania is described as " . . . attacks with largely the same characteristics of pain and associated symptoms and signs as cluster headache, but they are shorter lasting, more frequent, occur mostly in females, and there is absolute effectiveness of indomethacin" (*Cephalalgia*, 2004). Chronic paroxysmal hemicrania may also involve the teeth or present as face pain. The clinical presentation is unchanged, as is the response to indomethacin (Delcanho and Graff-Radford, 1993).

SUNCT syndrome is described as a pain that is associated with short lasting unilateral neuragiform headache attacks with conjunctival injection, tearing, rhinorrhea and subclinical sweating. Sjaastad and co-workers in 1978 first described SUNCT (Sjooscado et al., 1978). Most attacks are reported as moderate to severe, 30 to 120 second pain paroxysms. Pain is usually localized to the eye and may occur in a cluster fashion with some quiet periods. Attack frequency may be up to 30 per day or many per hour (Sjastad, et al., 1989; Sjastad, et al., 1991). Although SUNCT is clinically well identified it is poorly treated. Carbamazepine may be effective in controlling some symptomatology, but not consistently (Sjastad, et al., 1991). Gabapentin may also offer relief in some patients (Graff-Radford, 2000).

Neuropathic

Neuropathic pain suggests that tissue or nerve injury has occurred, with a permanent peripheral nerve and/or central nervous system (CNS) change.

There are two types of neuropathic pain: transient pain and chronic pain. Short-lived pain that follows a stimulus that is potentially tissue-damaging, also referred to as acute pain, is a protective mechanism. Acute pain resolves in an appropriate time period and then normal function is restored. What happens when the stimulus results in chronic pain? Although the injury appears to have healed, nonprotective pain remains. This may be due to central and peripheral nervous system changes (Ren and Dubner, 1999) that may include ongoing

TABLE 23–5 Neuropathic Orofacial Pain.

Intermittent
Trigeminal neuralgia
Glossopharyngeal neuralgia
Nervus intermedius neuralgia
Occipital neuralgia
Continuous
Trigeminal dysesthesia
Trigeminal dysesthesia—sympathetically maintained

peripheral nociception, CNS sensitization, or down-regulation of CNS inhibition.

Clinically, neuropathic pain can be classified as continuous pain and intermittent pain; these subtypes may present simultaneously or independently. Table 23–5 is a clinical classification of neuropathic facial pain.

Intermittent Neuropathic pain

Intermittent neuropathic pain presents clinically as a bright, stimulating, electric, sharp, or burning pain. Examples include trigeminal neuralgia, glossopharyngeal neuralgia, nervus intermedius neuralgia, and occipital neuralgia. These intermittent neuralgias are triggerable, usually by non-noxious stimuli. Vascular nerve compression is the proposed etiology (Fromm and Sessel, 1991). Compression may also be secondary to other structures, including tumors and bony growths (e.g., Eagles Syndrome) (Janetta, 1977; Massey and Massey, 1979).

Trigeminal Neuralgia also called TIC rolerenax candre Trigeminal neuralgia is described as "... a painful unilateral affliction of the face, characterized by brief electric shock-like (lancinating) pain limited to the distribution of one or more divisions of the trigeminal nerve. Pain is commonly evoked by trivial stimuli, including washing, shaving, smoking, talking and brushing the teeth, but may also occur spontaneously. The pain is abrupt in onset and termination may remit for varying periods". Symptomatic trigeminal neuralgia is described as "pain indistinguishable from trigeminal neuralgia, caused by a demonstrable structural lesion." This lesion is usually a tumor, such as an acoustic neuroma, or demyelination, as seen in multiple sclerosis. If tissue or nerve injury is present, continuous trigeminal neuralgia may ensue; this is referred to as traumatic trigeminal neuralgia or trigeminal dysesthesia (Graff-Radford, 2000a) (see Chapter 10).

Ratner and Roberts have proposed that bony cavities found in the alveolar bone are the cause of trigeminal neuralgia and repetitive curettage of these cavities is curative (Ratner et al., 1979; Roberts et al., 1984). Using 15 half-maxillae and 12 half-mandibles from cadavers, Graff-Radford et al. demonstrated that cavities larger than 2 mm in diameter occur throughout normal bone (Graff-Radford et al., 1988). The cavities do not appear to be unique to patients who have trigeminal neuralgia. This sheds doubt on the bony cavity theory and suggests that the curettage may be effective through central mechanisms or peripheral denervation.

Trigeminal neuralgia treatment may be divided into pharmacologic treatment and surgical treatment (Brown, 2005, Burchiel, 1987 and 2005, Janetta, 1996, Jarrahy, 2000, Sindeau, 2002, Sindeau, 2006 and Young, 1999). Table 23–6 outlines the drugs that may be used in pharmacologic treatment Cheshire, 2002; Fromm, 1984; Lechin, 1989 (see Chapter 10).

Less traditional treatments include curettage of the bony cavities as described above. Long-term success rates of 80% have been reported (Ratner et al., 1976; Ratner et al., 1979; Roberts et al., 1984). A study of peripheral streptomycin and lidocaine injections was performed by Sokolovic et al. (1986). Twenty patients were given five injections of 2% lidocaine and 1 g of streptomycin sulfate adjacent to peripheral nerves at 1-month intervals. Sixteen of the patients remained pain-free after 30 months. No side effects were reported and the authors reported no loss of sensation after the local anesthetic wore off. Bittar and Graff-Radford completed a double-blind, placebo-controlled, cross-over study using streptomycin, the results of which were not favorable. They also reported significant swelling associated with the injections (Bittar and Graff-Radford, 1993).

Pretrigeminal Neuralgia Sir Charles Symonds first described pretrigeminal neuralgia (Symonds, 1949). Mitchell later reviewed it (Mitchell, 1980).

TABLE 23–6 Common Membrane Stabilizing Drugs Used in Intermittent Neuralgia Therapy.

Generic	*Trade name*	*Dosage (mg/day)*	*Blood level (Ug/ml)*	*Serum half-life (hours)*
Lioresal	Baclofen	10–80	—	
Carbamazepine	Tegretol (XR)	100–2000	4–12	12–17
Oxcarbazepine	Trileptel	150–2400		12–17
Phenytoin	Dilantin	200–600	10–20	18–24
Valproic acid	Depakote	125–2500	50–100	6–16
Gabapentin	Neurontin	100–5000	—	5–7
Pregabalin	Lyrica	100–600		8–12
Lamotrigine	Lamictal	50–500	2–5	14–59
Klonopin	Clonazepam	0.5–8	—	22–33
Pimozide	Orap	2–12	—	55–154
Topiramate	Topamax	50–1000	—	21

Pretrigeminal neuralgia is an atypical early manifestation of trigeminal neuralgia (Evans et al., 2005). Fromm et al. described 16 patients who initially presented with a dull, continuous toothache in the upper or lower jaw and whose pain changed to classic trigeminal neuralgia (Fromm et al., 1990). In seven cases, the continuous pain was successfully treated with traditional trigeminal neuralgia therapies. The diagnosis of pretrigeminal neuralgia is based on the following criteria: (1) pain is described as a dull toothache; (2) neurologic and dental examinations are normal; (3) CT or MRI scan of the head is normal. The pain of pretrigeminal neuralgia can be interrupted with somatic anesthetic blockade. Merrill and Graff-Radford described 61 patients who were treated for pretrigeminal or trigeminal neuralgia. Of these, 61% had been incorrectly diagnosed and treated with traditional dental therapies (Merrill and Graff-Radford, 1992). The clinician should be aware of pretrigeminal neuralgia before recommending surgery for a patient who has orofacial pain of unclear etiology.

Glossopharyngeal Neuralgia The pain of glossopharyngeal neuralgia is similar in quality and characteristics to that of trigeminal neuralgia, but the pain occurs in the distribution of the glossopharyngeal nerve. It may be confused with Eagles Syndrome (Massey and Massey, 1979), which has a presentation similar to glossopharyngeal neuralgia but is associated with an elongated stylohyoid process that irritates or compresses the glossopharyngeal nerve. Chewing, swallowing, and rotating the head are all triggering factors. Patients may complain of a persistent sore throat. This pain can be decreased with neural blockade. Confirmation of the diagnosis requires a calcified stylohyoid ligament to be demonstrated on radiogram. Treatment is surgical resection of the ligament. Treatment of glossopharyngeal neuralgia is pharmacologic and surgical. Pharmacologic treatment is with membrane stabilizer medications (Table 23–6). Surgical treatment has traditionally been rhizotomy, but now is more commonly microvascular decompression of the nerve. (Graff-Radford et al., 2005) (see Chapter 10).

Nervus Intermedius Neuralgia This pain is described as similar to trigeminal neuralgia but localized to the middle ear. Patients often complain of feeling as though a hot poker is in the ear (Walker, 1966). Treatment is similar to that used for trigeminal neuralgia.

Occipital neuralgia: Occipital neuralgia is pain located in the distribution of the greater and lesser occipital nerves. Pain is described as paroxysmal, sharp electriclike. There is usually an associated trauma at the onset of pain. Graff-Fadford et al have described myofascial trigger points in the splenius cervicus and capitis muscles that may mimic occipital neuralgia and it is suggested that trigger point injections be used to help rule out this possibility (Graff-Radford, et al., 1986).

Surgical neurectomy has been described for occipital neuralgia, but the results are often short lived. Stimulation of the occipital nerves is also beneficial although pharmacologic options should first be exhausted (Johnstone 2006, Weiner 1999).

Continuous Neuropathic Pain

The neuropathic pain that sometimes follows tissue or nerve injury in the trigeminal nerve distribution is called trigeminal dysesthesia. Trigeminal dysesthesia is defined as a continuous pain following complete or partial damage to a peripheral nerve. The pain is described as a continuous, burning numbness and often pulling pain (See Table 23–7).

The trauma that initiates trigeminal dysesthesia is usually quite obvious, for example, wisdom tooth removal or dental implant placement, but trigeminal dysesthesia may occur with minor trauma, such as crown preparation, or following viral infection, such as herpes zoster. The discomfort can be self limiting, depending on nerve regeneration. Campbell stated that approximately 5% of patients who undergo root canal therapy have persistent pain that may be attributed to nerve damage (Campbell et al., 1990). Elies described 17% of patients with mandibular implants who developed persistent sensory change or pain (Ellies and Hawker, 1993; Ellies, 1992). Thermographic studies reveal that all trigeminal dysesthesia patients have abnormal thermograms: some are hot in the pain distribution and some are cold; none are normal. Graff-Radford et al. described a hypothesis for these temperature changes that may be helpful in selecting a treatment (Graff-Radford et al., 1995).

Three peripheral mechanisms may be involved in chronic trigeminal neuropathic pain development: (1) nerve compression, (2) nerve regeneration, and (3) sympathetically maintained pain.

TABLE 23–7 Criteria for Trigeminal Dysesthesia.

History of trauma
Continuous pain
Associated hyperalgesia and allodynia
Temperature change
Block effect (sympathetic versus somatic)

1. Nerve compression. When a peripheral nerve is compressed or injured there is a sustained firing that may be persistent. The closer the damage is to the CNS, the longer the spontaneous neural discharge is. The pain that follows nerve compression can be temporarily relieved with local anesthetic blockade. Following neural trauma, receptor sprouting occurs on the damaged nociceptor, on dorsal horn cells, and on peripheral blood vessels. These receptors may include α-receptors, neuropeptide Y (NPY) receptors and possibly others. Release of trigeminal nucleus substance P, calcitonin gene-related peptide, and other neurotransmitters is increased, which results in further neurogenic inflammation and chronic pain (Bennett and Xie, 1988). When neural inflammation occurs, neuritis ensues. The pain presents as a continuous, dull, burning pain with associated allodynia and hyperalgesia. A neuritis involving the facial nerve (cranial nerve VII) may be present (Bell's palsy). A painful Bell's palsy is usually due to the herpes zoster involving the geniculate ganglion (Ramsay Hunt's syndrome) with facial palsy and a herpes zoster eruption around the ear (Karnes, 1984).

2. Nerve regeneration. Neuroma formation is created by nerve regeneration where the path for regrowth is obstructed. The nerve resprouting and the continuous nerve irritation may result in pain. As in nerve compression, receptor sprouting and neurotransmitter presence increase the pain. Injecting the neuroma with local anesthetic will temporarily block the pain. The sprouting axons fire spontaneously and develop abnormal sensitization to cold, norepinephrine, and mechanical stimulation. This occurs in dorsal root ganglion cells as well as in peripheral terminals. Clinically the neuroma may produce pain only after mechanical stimulation. The pain is aching and burning, with sharp pain volleys.

3. Sympathetically maintained pain. Campbell (et al. (1992) states that the initial trauma to the peripheral nervous system activates nociceptors and results in sprouting of α-adrenergic receptors on the nociceptors. The initial sensory barrage sensitizes the CNS, causing sympathetic afferent activation and increased response to non-noxious stimuli. This causes peripheral norepinephrine release, which activates the peripheral nociceptors and keeps the cycle active. Sympathetic

innervation in the dorsal root ganglia increases with age following neural injury (Roberts and Foglesong, 1988). It is not surprising that the incidence of neuropathic pain increases as we age. Sympathetically maintained pain is aggravated by non-noxious stimuli and can be interrupted temporarily by sympathetic block or α-adrenergic block with phentolamine.

Most orofacial trigeminal dysesthesia occurs in women who are in their fourth decade (Solberg and Graff-Radford, 1988; Vickers et al., 1998;). Continuous dysesthesia is caused by a lesion in the trigeminal nervous system, either peripherally or centrally (Vickers et al., 1998). Sex-based differences are seen in many pain disorders. Although the relationship and role of sex hormones in the generation and perpetuation of central sensitization is not fully understood, it is important (Ren and Dubner, 1999). In a neuropathic pain model using partial sciatic nerve ligation, female rats were more likely than male rats to develop allodynia (Coyle et al., 1995). In studies of ovariectomized female rats, those with estrogen were more likely to develop allodynia after injury than those without estrogen (Coyle et al., 1996).

The therapy for trigeminal dysesthesia is aimed at reducing peripheral nociceptive inputs and simultaneously enhancing CNS pain inhibitory systems (Graff-Radford, 1995b).

Topical Applications Topical therapies have not been well studied. There is some evidence that capsaicin (Zostrix) applied regularly will result in desensitization and pain relief (Scrivani et al., 1999). The recommended dose is five times a day for 5 days, then three times a day for 3 weeks. If the patient cannot withstand the burning produced by the application, the addition of topical local anesthetic, either 4% lidocaine or eutectic mixture of local anaesthetics (EMLA), is useful. Clonidine can be applied to the hyperalgesic region by placing the proprietary subcutaneous delivery patch on the tender area. Alternatively, a 4% gel can be used over a larger area. A neurosensory stent can be used for local intraoral application. An oral impression is taken and an acrylic stent manufactured to cover the painful site. (Graff-Radford, 1995). The topical agent is applied to the gingival surface 24 hours a day.

Topical clonazepam (0.5–1.0 mg three times a day) effectively reduces burning oral pain (Woda et al., 1998). Patients were instructed to suck a tablet for 3 minutes (and then spit it out) three times a day for at least 10 days. Serum concentrations were minimal (3.3 ng/ml) 1 and 3 hours after application. Woda hypothesized that a peripheral, not a central, action disrupted the neuropathologic mechanism.

Procedures Neural blockade is very effective in differentiating sympathetically maintained pain from sympathetically independent pain. It may also be effective in controlling sympathetically maintained pain if it is used repetitively (Elias, 2000). Stellate ganglion blocks, phentolamine infusion, and sphenopalatine blocks are useful in obtaining a chemical sympathetic block. The authors have not observed significant benefit with phentolamine infusion for facial pain. Scrivani, who used 30-mg infusions without benefit, (Scrivani et al., 1999) supports this.

Lidocaine infusion (200 mg over 1 hour) may be used therapeutically for various forms of neuropathic pain (Boas et al., 1982; Rowbotham et al., 1991). Response to intravenous lidocaine may predict which patients will respond to the lidocaine analogue, Mexilatine. Sinnott et al. used an animal model to demonstrate the minimal lidocaine concentration (2.1 μg/ml) that will abolish allodynia (Sinnott et al., 1999). They also describe a ceiling effect. Many animals with experimentally induced allodynia did not obtain persistent relief. They suggest that separate physiological mechanisms, with differing pharmacologies, may account for the variability and postulate that there are different aspects of neuropathic pain.

Pharmacology Antidepressants. Tricyclic antidepressants are effective in many pain problems. Solberg and Graff-Radford have studied the response to amitriptyline in traumatic neuralgia. The effective range is 10–150 mg a day, usually taken in a single dose at bedtime (Solberg and Graff-Radford, 1988). Newer serotonin norepinephrine reuptake inhibitors such as duloxetine actually have a pain indication. Many antidepressants may be used (see Table 23–2).

Membrane stabilizers. These medications include anticonvulsants, lidocaine derivatives, and some muscle relaxants. They have been used for intermittent, sharp electric pains. Table 23–6 summarizes the common medications in this group and their doses.

Behavioral Strategies Before therapy is begun, a behavioral assessment and appropriate testing should be performed. Following the behavioral evaluation, attention is directed to the factors that may impact treatment and determining the most appropriate interventions. Consideration should be given to the following factors: (1) behavioral or operant factors; (2) emotional factors; (3) characterlogical factors; (4) cognitive factors; (5) side effects; (6) medication use; and (7) compliance. Cognitive and behavioral management techniques, such as relaxation, biofeedback and psychotherapeutic and psychopharmacological interventions, may be useful.

Surgery Although not suggested as a therapeutic modality for trigeminal dysesthesia, surgery is an option for trigeminal neuralgia.

Post Herpetic Neuralgia

Post herpetic neuralgia (PHN) is a complex problem whose treatment has frustrated clinicians and patients (Loeser, 1986; Watson and Evans, 1986). Herpes zoster is primarily a disease affecting older people, with some predilection for males (67% males: 33% females to 53% males: 47% females) (Molin, 1969). Herpes zoster localized in the face, including involvement of the facial nerve, occurs in 15%–30% of reported cases, (Molin, 1969). The duration of pain after vesicle outbreak varies, but the pain appears to last longer in older subjects. The number of subjects that go on to PHN (pain after the vesicles have healed) ranges from 14% of males to 25% of females, but almost all are older than 60 years of age (Molin, 1969). No studies to date have suggested that the subset of herpes zoster patients who go on to PHN is predictable. The mechanism whereby the herpetic virus produces the neuralgia condition has not yet been determined. Reports by Head (Head and Campbell, 1900) and Denny-Brown (Denny-Brown and Adams, 1944) reveal that changes occur in the skin and peripheral nerve endings that produce anesthesia or dysesthesia in the dorsal root ganglia characteristic of hemorrhage and lymphocytic infiltration. The adjacent proximal nerves and sensory nerve roots show demyelination and rarely is cell death evident in the spinal cord. There are few controlled studies that assess treatment outcomes in this relentless disease. Watson has described the use of amitriptyline, which has by and large been the treatment of choice (Watson and Evans, 1986). This was confirmed by Max, who showed that amitriptyline, but not lorazepam, was effective in the treatment of PHN (Max et al., 1988). Phenothiazines have been reported to be helpful in the treatment of chronic pain, and Taub reported five case studies in which the combination of amitriptyline and fluphenazine was effective (Taub, 1973). This report included a mix of acute cases (active lesions) and chronic cases (with pain lasting longer than 6 months). Graff-Radford studied the effects of amitriptyline and fluphenazine using a double-blind protocol and found no significant benefit in combining amitriptyline with fluphenazine (Graff-Radford et al., 1988) Recently Pregabalin and Duloxetine have proven beneficial for PHN (Attal, 2006). Sympathetic nerve block is considered by many to be effective in preventing PHN when used in the first 3–6 months following the outbreak of zoster (Elias, 2000). Depending on the effects, between one and six blocks should be performed. There is little purpose in doing more than three blocks if pain relief does not outlast the anesthetic effects. It may be more appropriate to place this category in the autonomic nervous system category, but in some situations sympathetic block does not reduce the pain, which suggests a sympathetically independent pain.

Muskuloskeletal System

The musculoskeletal system is the most common origin of chronic orofacial pain. These disorders may be divided into arthrogenous and muscular (temporomandibular) disorders. The TMJ is different from other body joints. The most recognizable difference between the TMJ and other synovial joints is the TMJ's noninnervated, avascular, fibroconnective tissue articular covering. This is not hyaline in nature, possibly to aid in withstanding twisting, turning, and compressive forces. The fibroconnective tissue covering may also allow for significant remodeling to occur in the TMJ. Another significant difference is its diarthroidal structure. An intracapsular disk divides the joint into upper and lower compartments and provides for the complex hinge and gliding action. The mandible produces a reciprocal effect of one articulation on the other by joining the TMJs. Also interacting in this system is the dental occlusion, which will result in altered forces on the system if it is not in equilibrium. The teeth provide a solid end point to joint movement, unlike any other joint, in which end range of motion is somewhat elastic. Owing to the structure's nature, the intracapsular anatomy can remodel when subjected to extraneous forces. Such remodeling can be brought about through tooth loss, poor dental restoration, macro trauma, and parafunctional habits, such as tooth-clenching and grinding. The remodeling may lead to dysfunction if the tissues are unable to compensate for the abnormal load. In addition, muscular hyperactivity may be initiated to compensate for the lack of equilibrium.

The joint's hinge action allows for about a 25 mm interincisal opening, which occurs primarily in the lower joint space (condylar rotation). The next 20–25 mm requires the disk condyle complex to slide down the temporal eminence, with the disk moving posterior relative to the condyle (translation). Remodeling resulting in a deviation in articular form may interrupt this rhythmic function. The articular tissues are usually characterized by smooth, rounded surfaces until subjected to extraneous forces, which produce remodeling (Solberg et al., 1985). The mechanical interferences that are produced by the remodeling may cause noise as they move over each other. Remodeling is an ongoing process and results in a disease process continuum that begins with soft-tissue change and progresses to involve the bony structures. One might view the process as a failure of the adaptive process to compensate for the extraneous forces exerted on the joint. If there are sufficient joint changes, the articular disk may become displaced (deranged). The usual direction for displacement is anteromedially (Ireland, 1953; Farrar, 1972), although posterior displacement has been reported (Blankestijn and Boering, 1985). The disk displacement may reduce if the individual can manipulate the condyle onto the disk, producing joint noise. This noise is usually heard after the initial 25 mm rotation in the opening movement and again just before the teeth occlude in the closing path. The closing noise is usually much quieter and may be produced by the relocation of the disk in the anterior position. Joint noise occurs in 20%–30% of individuals over 15 years of age (Egermark et al., 1981; Solberg et al., 1979). Sliding of the disk is enabled by the presence of phospholipids, which are protected by hyaluronic acid, which provides lubrication. An overloaded joint can lead to production of reactive oxygen species that causes degradation of hyaluronic acid, allowing the phospholipids to be lysed by phospholipase A2 (Nitzan, 2002). This decrease in lubrication allows the articular surfaces, which are "sticky," to become adherent to each other, promoting derangement.

Pain associated with joint pathology is usually intermittent and associated with function. To confirm the diagnosis of an articular temporomandibular disorder, patients should display at least three of the following four criteria:

1. Limited range of motion (<40 mm);
2. Joint noise (clicking, popping, or crepitus);
3. Tenderness to palpation;
4. Functional pain.

Continuous pain associated with an articular temporomandibular disorder is unusual and usually is produced by associated inflammation or secondary muscle pain. Pain emanating from the ligamentous attachments, the synovium, or the fibrous capsules is usually secondary to infection or trauma to these structures. The differences between synovitis and capsulitis are almost impossible to determine clinically (Bell, 1985).

Articular remodeling is a direct result of adaptive changes that help establish a status quo between joint form and function (Moffett et al., 1964). Osteoarthrosis results from destruction of articular tissues secondary to excessive strain on the remodeling mechanism. The problem is nonpainful and usually only produces mechanical interferences. De Bont has suggested that the degenerative process is due to fatty degeneration and disruption of the collagen fiber network (De Bont et al., 1985). Inflammation of the articular tissue does not occur because of the unvascularized surface. For inflammation to occur, a fundamental arthropathic change, such as the proliferation of inflamed synovial membrane into the articular tissue or the exposure of innervated and vascularized osseous tissue, must occur (De Bont et al., 1985).

Osteoarthrosis is a common condition that progresses with age and affects more women than men (Davis, 1981). Osteoarthrosis is insidious in onset; it is usually not associated with systemic disease, but perhaps initiated through repetitive loading or a variety of factors that occur over a lifetime. The inflammation that occurs in osteoarthritis requires an innervated and vascular surface. This suggests that the adaptive remodeling that continues has been overwhelmed and the tissues below the fibroconnective tissue surface are exposed, allowing the inflammatory process to begin.

Proinflammatory cytokines, such as interleukin-1B (IL-1B), tumor necrosis factor-a, IL-6, and IL-8 are found in joints that have osteoarthritis and internal derangement (Nishimura et al., 2002). It is believed that these proinflammatory cytokines are involved in the pathogenesis of synovitis and joint degeneration. It has been suggested that these chemicals mediate cell–cell interactions that result in the release of tissue-damaging enzymes (Kaneyama et al. 2002).

Bone morphogenetic protein-2 (BMP-2) was studied in patients with internal derangements of the TMJ. On the basis of the results of this study by Suzuki, it was concluded that BMP-2, which induces the formation of bone and cartilage, may be involved in the repair process of internal derangement and/or the pathogenesis of osteoarthritic changes (Kaneyama, 2002). It may be that the proinflammatory cytokines are involved with the tissue destruction of osteoarthritis, which leads to a derangement of the disk, and then BMP-2 becomes involved with the remodeling process.

Muscle Disorders

The disorders that involve muscles may be independent of articular problems but are usually involved when joint dysfunction exists. Their involvement may be mild and produce minimal dysfunction or severe and markedly disabling. When muscle pain problems occur, the treatment may differ depending on the subgroup (defined below).

Myofascial pain syndromes, as classified by the International Association for the Study of Pain Subcommittee on Taxonomy (Mersky, 1986), can be found in any voluntary muscle and are characterized by trigger points, which may cause referred pain and local and referred tenderness (Clark et al., 1981; Moller, 1981). When "active," trigger points are painful to palpation and spontaneously refer pain and autonomic symptoms to remote structures in reproducible patterns characteristic for each muscle (Travell and Simons, 1984). This referred pain is usually the presenting complaint. When "latent," trigger points are still locally tender but do not produce referred phenomena. The pain quality is pressing, tightening, deep, aching, and often poorly circumscribed (Travell and Simons, 1984). It may be associated with swelling, numbness, and stiffness (Ernberg, 1999). Pain, although usually constant, may fluctuate in intensity and shift anatomical sites (Travell and Simons, 1984). Associated symptoms may include autonomic phenomena, most commonly reactive hyperemia or erythema, although photophobia and phonophobia are described (Butler et al., 1975).

The primary complaint for myofascial pain is referred pain. The referral patterns often do not make neurological sense. As an example, pain from a trigger point in the trapezius muscle, which is innervated by cranial nerve XI, may refer to the forehead, which is innervated by cranial nerve V. (Graff-Radford, 1986)

Mens described a hypothesis for muscle pain referral to other deep somatic tissues remote from the site of the original muscle stimulation or lesion (Mens, 1994). He criticizes the convergence-projection pain referral theory by pointing out that there is little convergence in the dorsal horns associated with deep tissues. Mens's hypothesis adds two new components to the convergence-projection theory. First, the convergent connections from deep tissues to dorsal horn neurons are opened only after nociceptive inputs from muscle are activated. The connections that are opened after muscle stimulus are called silent connections. Second, the referral to muscle outside the initially activated site is due to spread of central sensitization to adjacent spinal segments

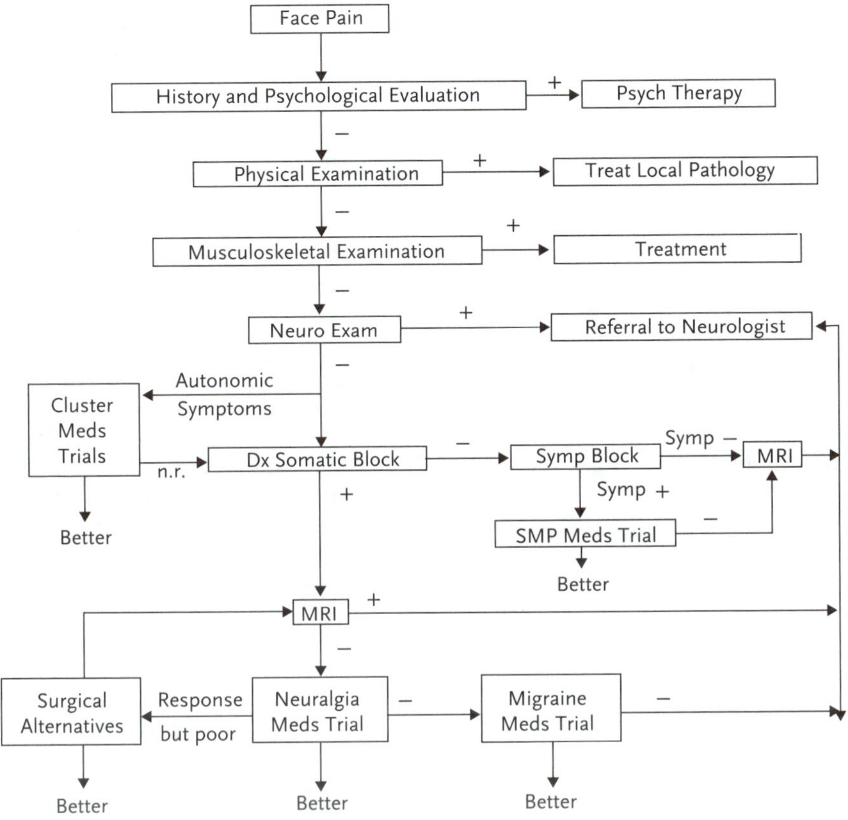

Figure. 23–1 Diagnostic algorithm for facid pain.

(Mens, 1994). The initiating stimulus requires a peripheral inflammatory stimulus. In the animal model described by Mens, the noxious stimulus was bradykinin injected into the muscle. It is unclear what triggers the muscle referral in the clinical setting where there is usually no obvious inflammation-producing incident.

Mens's theory has been used by Simons to discuss a neurophysiological basis for trigger-point pain (Simons, 1994). Simons hypothesizes that neurotransmitters are released in the dorsal horn (trigeminal nucleus) when the tender area in the muscle is palpated, resulting in opening of nociceptive inputs that were previously silent. This causes distant neurons to produce a retrograde referred pain (Simons, 1994). This model accounts for most of the clinical presentation and therapeutic options seen in myofascial pain, but it does not account for initiation of the peripheral tenderness, which must be present to activate the silent connections.

Fields has described a means whereby the CNS may switch on nociception (Fields and Heinricher, 1989). He describes the presence of "on" cells which, when stimulated, may produce activation of trigeminal nucleus nociceptors. Olesen has used Fields's model to describe a hypothesis for tension-type headache (Olesen, 1991). This model describes the interaction of three systems: the vascular system, the supraspinal system, and the myogenic system. The proposed hypothesis suggests that perceived headache pain is facilitated by the CNS, depending on inputs from either muscle or blood vessel. In migraine the inputs are primarily vascular, whereas in tension-type headache the inputs are primarily muscular. This model helps explain why the clinical presentation and therapeutic options in migraine and tension-type headache are often similar, as well as why there is temporary relief with peripheral treatments, such as trigger point injections.

The resultant hyperalgesia or trigger point sensitivity may represent a peripheral sensitization related to serum levels of serotonin (5-HT). Ernberg et al. showed a significant correlation with serum 5-HT and allodynia associated with muscular face pain (Alstergen et al., 1999). When rheumatoid temporomandibuar pain was present, serum 5-HT concentrations correlated with pain. There was no correlation with circulating serum levels of NPY or IL-1B (Alstergen et al., 1999).

Patients who present with facial pain with no obvious etiology should be presumed to have myofascial pain. Myofascial pain can be reproduced by digitally palpating the muscles and confirmed with trigger point injections using 1–2 cc of 1% procaine.

Myofascial pain is treated by enhancing central inhibition with pharmacology or behavioral techniques and simultaneously reducing peripheral inputs with physical therapies, including exercises and trigger-point-specific therapy (Travell and Simons, 1986; Graff-Radford et al., 1987; Davidoff, 1998). Patients must be aware that the goal of therapy is to manage the pain and not to cure it. Patients must also be aware of the role they themselves play in managing the perpetuating factors (Graff-Radford et al., 1987; Davidoff, 1998).

DISCUSSION

Evaluation of orofacial pain must begin with an in-depth medical history, which should include the chief complaint and a narrative history of the complaint, as well as its progression and prior treatment. Not all chronic pain conditions require a psychological evaluation; however, all pain, no matter what its etiology, is subject to behavioral and emotional factors. These behavioral issues should be considered, and a psychological evaluation is suggested when there is any doubt of what part they play. The psychological evaluation is not done to determine whether the pain is psychogenic, but rather to select specific cognitive and behavioral strategies that may be useful in pain management. Once these data are gathered, a neurologic screening examination, TMJ examination, and myofascial palpation should be carried out. At this time, a differential diagnosis can be established and the specific tests outlined above and summarized in Figure 23–1 can be used to narrow the diagnosis. This process permits appropriate diagnosis and effective treatment.

References

Alstergen, P, Ernberg, M, Kopp, S, et al. (1999). TMJ pain in relation to circulating neuropeptide Y, Serotonin, and interleukin—1B in rheumatoid arthritis. *Orofacial Pain*, 13:49–55.

Ambrosini, A, Vandenheede, M, Rossi, P, et al. (2005). Suboccipital injection with a mixture of rapid- and long-acting steroids in cluster headache: a double-blind placebo-controlled study. *Pain*, 118(1–2):92–96. Epub 2005 Oct 3.

Andre', N. (1756). *Traite' sur les maladies de l'urethre*. Delaguette, Paris, pp. 323–343.

Attal, N, Cruccu, G, Haanpaa, M, et al. (2006). EFNS Task Force. EFNS guidelines on pharmacological treatment of neuropathic pain. *Eur J Neurol*, 13(11):1153–1169.

Bell, WE (1985). *Orofacial Pains: Classification, Diagnosis, Management* (3rd edn.). Year Book Medical Publishers, Chicago.

Bennett, GJ and Xie, YK (1988). A peripheral mononeuropathy in rat that produces disorders of pain sensation like those seen in man. *Pain*, 33:87–107.

Bittar, G and Graff-Radford, SB (1992). A Retrospective study of patients with cluster headache. *Oral Med, Oral Path, Oral Surg*, 73:519–525.

Bittar, G and Graff-Radford, SB (1993). The effect of streptomycin/lidocaine block on trigeminal and traumatic neuralgia. *Headache*, 33(3):155–160.

Blankestijn, J and Boering, G (1985). Posterior dislocation of the temporomandibular disk. *Int J Oral Surg*, 14: 437–443.

Boas, RA, Covino, BG, and Shahnarian, A (1982). Analgesic responses to i.v. lignocaine. *Br J Anesth*, 54:501–504.

Brooke, RI (1978). Periodic migrainous neuralgia: a cause of dental pain. *Oral Med*, 46:511–516.

Brown, JA and Pilitsis, JG (2005). Percutaneous balloon compression for the treatment of trigeminal neuralgia: results in 56 patients based on balloon compression pressure monitoring. *Neurosurg Focus*, 18(5):E10.

Bulitt, E, Tew, JM, and Boyd, J (1986). Intracranial tumors with facial pain. *J Neurosurg*, 64:865–871.

Burchiel, KJ (1987). Surgical treatment of trigeminal neuralgia: minor and major operative procedures. In *The Medical and Surgical Management of Trigeminal Neuralgia* (GH Fromm, ed.), pp. 71, 101. Futura Publishing Co., New York.

Burchiel, KJ (2005). Gamma knife and trigeminal neuralgia. *J Neurosurg*, 102(3):431–432.

Butler, JH, Golke, LEA, and Bandt, CL (1975). A descriptive survey of signs and symptoms associated with the myofascial pain dysfunction syndrome. *J Am Dent Assoc*, 90(3):635–639.

Cady, RK and Schreiber, CP (2002). Sinus headache or migraine? Considerations in making a differential diagnosis. *Neurology*, 58(Suppl. 6):S10–14.

Campbell, JN, Meyer, RA, Davis, KD, et al. (1992). Sympathetically mediated pain a unifying hypothesis. In *Hyperalgesia and Allodynia* (WD Willis, ed.), pp. 141–149. Raven Press, New York.

Campbell, Rl, Parks, KW, and Dodds RN (1990). Chronic facial pain associated with endodontic neuropathy. *Oral Surg Oral Med Oral Pathol*, 69:287–290.

Cheshire, WP Jr. (2002). Defining the role for gabapentin in the treatment of trigeminal neuralgia: a retrospective study. *J Pain*, 3(2):137–142.

Clark, GT, Beemsterboer, PL, and Rugh, JD (1981). Nocternal Masseter muscle activity and the symptoms of masticatory dysfunction. *J Oral Rehabil*, 8:279.

Coyle, DE, Sehlhorst, CS, and Mascari C (1995). Female rats are more susceptible to the development of neuropathic pain using the partial sciatic nerve ligation (PSNL) model. *Neurosci Lett*, 186:135–138.

Coyle, DE, Selhorst, CS, and Behbehani, MM (1996). Intact female rats are more susceptive to the development of tactile allodynia than ovariectomized female rats following partial sciatic nerve ligation (PSNL). *Neurosci Lett*, 203:37–40.

Cueneo, HM and Rand, CW (1952). Tumors of the gasserian ganglion. Tumor of the left Gasserian ganglion associated with enlargement of the mandibular nerve. A review of the literature and case report. *J Neurosurg*, 9:423–432.

Davidoff, RA (1998). Trigger points and myofascial pain: toward understanding how they affect headaches. *Cephalalgia*, 18(7):436–438.

Davis, MA (1981). Sex differences in reporting osteoarthritic symptoms: a sociomedical approach. *J Health Soc Behav*, 22:293.

De Bont, LGM, Boering, G, and Liem, RSB (1985). Having a P: Osteoarthritis of the temporomandibular joint: a light microscopic and scanning electron microscopic study of the articular cartilage of the mandibular condyle. *J Oral Maxillofac Surg*, 43:481–488.

Delcanho, RE and Graff-Radford, SB (1993). Chronic Paroxysmal Hemicrania Presenting as Toothache. *J Orofacial Pain*, 7:300–306.

Denny-Brown, D and Adams, R (1944). *Arch Neurol Psychiatry*, 51:216–221.

Egermark-Eriksson, I, Carlsson, GE, and Ingervall, B (1981). Prevalence of mandibular dysfunction and orofacial parafunction in 7-, 11, and 15 year old Swedish children. *Eur J Orthod*, 3:163–172.

Elias, M (2000). Cervical sympathetic and stellate ganglion blocks. *Pain Physician*, 3(3):294–304.

Ellies, LG (1992). Altered sensation following mandibular implant surgery: a retrospective study. *J Prosthet Dent*, 68:664–667.

Ellies, LG and Hawker, PB (1993). The prevalence of altered sensation associated with implant surgery. *Int J Oral Maxillofac Implants*, 8:674–679.

Ernberg, M, Hadenberg-Magnusson, B, Alstergren, P, et al. (1999). Pain, Allodynia, and serum serotonin level in orofacial pain of muscular origin. *J Orofacial Pain*, 13:56–62.

Evans, RW, Graff-Radford, SB, and Bassiur, JP (2005). Pretrigeminal neuralgia. *Headache*, 45(3):242–244

Farrar, WB (1972). Differentiation of temporomandibular joint dysfunction to simplify treatment. *J Prosthet Dent*, 28:629–636.

Fields, HL and Heinricher, M (1989). Brainstem modulation of nociceptor-driven withdrawal reflexes. *Ann NY Acad Sci*, 563;34–44.

Fordyce, WE and Steger, JC (1978). Chronic Pain p125 In *Behavior Medicine Theory and Practice* (DF Pomerteau and JP Brady, eds). Williams and Wilkins, Baltimore.

Fricton, JR (1999). Critical Commentary. A unified concept of idiopathic orofacial pain: clinical Features. *J Orofacial Pain*, 13(3):185–189.

Fromm, GH, Graff-Radford, SB, Terrence, CF, et al. (1990). Can trigeminal neuralgia have a prodrome. *Neurology*, 40:1493–1495.

Fromm, GH and Sessel, BJ (1991). *Trigeminal Neuralgia. Current concepts regarding pathogenesis and treatment.* Butterworth-Heinemann, Boston.

Fromm, GH, Terrence, CF, and Chattha, AS (1984). Baclofen in the treatment of trigeminal neuralgia: double blind study and long term follow up. *Ann Neur*, 15:240–244.

Graff-Radford, SB (1995a). Orofacial Pain. In *Orofacial Pain and Temporomandibular Disorders* (J Fricton and R Dubner, eds), pp. 215–241. Raven Press, New York.

Graff-Radford, SB (1995b). Orofacial Pain of Neurogenous Origin. In *Temporomandibular disorders and Orofacial Pain* (RA Pertes and SG Gross, eds), pp. 329–341. Quintessence, Chicago.

Graff-Radford, SB (2000a). Facial Pain. *Curr Opin Neurol*, 13(3):291–296.

Graff-Radford, SB (2000b). SUNCT syndrome responsive to Gabapentin. *Cephalalgia*, 20(5):515–517.

Graff-Radford, SB, Brechner, T, and Audell, L (1988). McGill Pain Questionnaire changes in postherpetic neuralgia patients undergoing a drug trail (abstr). *Proceedings of the American Pain Society*, p. 69.

Graff-Radford, SB, Jaeger, B, and Reeves, JL (1986). Myofascial pain may present clinically as occipital neuralgia. *Neurosurg*, 19(4):610–613.

Graff-Radford, SB, Ketelaer, MC, Gratt, BM, et al. (1995). Thermographic assessment of neuropathic facial pain. *J Orofacial Pain*, 9:138–146.

Graff-Radford, SB, Newman, A, and Ananda, A (2005). Treatment Options for Glossopharyngeal Neuralgia. *Therapy*, 2(5):733–737.

Graff-Radford, SB, Reeves, JL, and Jaeger, B (1987). Management of headache: the effectiveness of altering factors perpetuating myofascial pain. *Headache*, 27:186–190.

Graff-Radford, SB, Simmons, M, Fox, L, et al. (1988). Are bony cavities exclusively associated with atypical facial pain or trigeminal neuralgia? (abstr). *Proceedings Western USA Pain Society*, 1988.

Head, H and Campbell, AW (1900). The pathology of herpes zoster. *Brain*, 23:353–523.

Ireland, VE (1953). The problem of the clicking jaw. *J Prosthet Dent*, 3:200–212.

Janetta, PJ (1996). Trigeminal neuralgia: treatment by microvascular decompression. In *Neurosurgery* (RH Wilkins and SS Ragachary, eds), pp. 3961–3968. Mc Graw Hill , New York.

Janetta, PJ (1977). Observation on the etiology of trigeminal neuralgia, hemifacial spasm, acoustic nerve dysfunction and glossopharyngeal neuralgia. Definitive microsurgical treatment and results in 117 patients. *Neurochirurgia*, 20:145–154.

Jarrahy, R, Berci, G, and Shahinian, HK (2000). Endoscopic-assisted microvascular decompression of the trigeminal nerve. *Otolaryngol Head Neck Surg*, 123 (3):218–223.

Johnstone, CS and Sundaraj, R (2006). Occipital Nerve Stimulation for the treatment of Occipital Neuralgia-8 case studies. *Pain Med*, 7(5):467.

Kaneyama, K, Segami, N, Nishimura, M, et al. (2002). Importance of proinflammatory cytokines in synovial fluid from 121 joints with Temporomandibular disorders. *British Journal of Oral and Maxillofacial Surgery*, 40:418–423.

Karnes, WE (1984). Diseases of the seventh cranial nerve. In *Peripheral Neuropathy* (2nd edn) (PJ Dyke et al., eds), ch. 55, pp. 1266–1299. Saunders, Philadelphia.

Lechin, F, Van der Dijs, B, Lechin, ME et al. (1989). Pimozide therapy for trigeminal neuralgia. *Arch Neurol*, 46:960–963.

Loeser, JD (1986). Herpes zoster and postherpetic neuralgia. *Pain*, 25:149–164.

Lovshin, LL (1960). Vascular neck pain—a common syndrome seldom recognized: analysis of 100 consecutive cases. *Cleve Clin Q*, 27:5–13.

Massey, EW and Massey, J (1979). Elongated styloid process (Eagles Syndrome) causing hemicrania. *Headache*, 19:339–341.

Max, MB, Schafer, SC, Culnane, M, et al. (1988). Amitriptyline, but not lorazepam, relieves post herpetic neuralgia. *Neurology*, 38:1427–1432.

McGettigan, P and Henry, D (2006). Cardiovascular risk and inhibition of cyclooxygenase: a systematic review of the observational studies of selective and nonselective inhibitors of cyclooxygenase 2. *JAMA*, 296 (13):1633–1644. Epub 2006 Sep, 12.

Mens, S (1994). Referral of Muscle Pain New Aspects. *Pain Forum*, 3(1):1–9.

Merrill, RL and Graff-Radford, SB (1992). Trigeminal Neuralgia: how to rule out the wrong treatment. *JADA*, 123:63–68.

Mersky, H (ed.) (1986). Classification of chronic pain: description of chronic pain syndromes and definition of terms. *Pain*, (Suppl. 3):S1.

Mitchell, RG (1980). Pre trigeminal neuralgia. *Brit Dent J*, 149:167–170.

Moffett, BC, Johnson, LC, McCabe, JB, et al. (1964). Articular remodeling in the adult human temporomandibular joint. *Am J Anat*, 115:119–130.

Molin, L (1969). Aspects of the natural history of herpes zoster. *Act Derm Venereol*, 49:569–583.

Moller, E (1981). The Myogenic factor in headache and facial pain. In *Oral-facial Sensory and Motor Function* (Y Kawamura and R Dubner, eds), p. 225. Quintessence, Tokyo.

Moncada, E and Graff-Radford, SB (1993). Cough headache presenting as toothache. *Headache*, 33:240–243.

Moskowitz, MA, Henrikson, BM, Markowitz, S, et al. (1988). Intra- and extravascular nociceptive mechanisms and the pathogenesis of head pain. In *Basic Mechanisms of Headache* (J Olsen and L Edvinsson, eds) p. 429. Elsevier, Amsterdam.

Nishimura, N, Segami, N, Kaneyama, K, et al. (2002). Proinflammatory cytokines and arthroscopic findings of patients with internal derangement and osterarthritis of the Temporomandibular joint. *Br J Oral Maxillofac Surg*, 40:68–71.

Nitzan, DW and Etsion, I (2002). Adhesive force: the underlying cause of the disc anchorage to the fossa and/or eminence in the temporomandibular joint–a new concept. *Int J Oral Maxillofac Surg*, 31(1):94–99.

Olesen, J (1991). Clinical and pathophysiological observations in migraine and tension type headache explained by integration of vascular, supraspinal and myofascial inputs. *Pain*, 46:125–132.

Raskin, NH (1988). *Headache* (2nd edn). Churchill Livingstone, New York.

Raskin, NH and Prusiner, S (1977). Carotidynia. *Neurol*, 27:43–46.

Ratner, EJ, Person, P, and Kleinman DJ (1976). Oral pathology and trigeminal neuralgia, I Clinical experiences (abstr). *J Dent Res*, 55:B299.

Ratner, EJ, Person, P, Kleinman, DJ, et al. (1979). Jawbone cavities and trigeminal and atypical facial neuralgias. *Oral Surg*, 48:3–20.

Ren, K and Dubner, R (1999). Central nervous system plasticity and persistent pain. *J Orofacial Pain* 13:155–163.

Roberts, WJ and Foglesong, ME (1988). Identification of afferents contributing to sympathetically evoked activity in wide-dynamic-range neurons. *Pain*, 34:305–314.

Roberts, AM, Person, P, Chandran, NB, et al. (1984). Further observations on dental parameters of trigeminal and atypical facial neuralgias. *Oral Surg*, 58:121–129.

Rooke, ED (1968). Benign exertional headache. *Med Clin North Am*, 52(4):801–808.

Rowbotham, MC, Reisner-Keller, LA, and Fields HL (1991). Both intravenous lidocaine and morphine reduce the pain of postherpetic neuralgia. *Neurology*, 41:1024–1028.

Rushton, JG and Rooke, ED (1962). Brain tumor headache. *Headache*, 2:147–152.

Schisano, G and Olivercrona, H (1960). Neuromas of the Gasserian ganglion and trigeminal root. *J Neurosurg*, 17:306.

Scrivani, SJ, Chaudry, A, Maciewicz, RJ, et al. (1999). Chronic Neurogenic facial pain: lack of response to intravenous phentolamine. *J Orofacial Pain*, 13:89–96.

Simons, DG (1994). Neurophysiological basis of pain caused by trigger points. *APS Journal*, 3(1):17–19.

Sindou, M, Howeidy, T, and Acevedo, G (2002). Anatomical observations during microvascular decompression for idiopathic trigeminal neuralgia (with correlations between topography of pain and site of the neurovascular conflict). Prospective study in a series of 579 patients. *Acta Neurochir (Wien)*, 144(1):1–12; discussion 12–3.

Sindou, M, Leston, J, Howeidy, T, et al. (2006). Microvascular decompression for primary Trigeminal Neuralgia (typical or atypical). Long-term effectiveness on pain; prospective study with survival analysis in a consecutive series of 362 patients. *Acta Neurochir (Wien)*, 148(12):1235–1245.

Sjaastad, O, Saunte, C, Salvesen, R, et al. (1989). Short lasting, unilateral neuralgia-form headache attacks with conjunctival injection, tearing, sweating and rhinorrhea. *Cephalalgia*, 9:147–156.

Sjaastad, O, Vhaoj, M, Krusvewski, P, et al. (1991). Short lasting unilateral neuralgia-form headache attacks with conjunctival injection, tearing, etc. (SUNCT):3. Another Norwegian case. *Headache*, 31:175–177.

Sjooscado, Russell D. Hrvni, and Bunaes, U (1978). Multiple neuralgia-form unilateral headache attacks associated with conjunctival injection and tearing and clusters. Noso-logic problem. *Proceedings of the Scandinavian Migraine Society*, p. 31.

Sokolovic, M, Todorovic, L, Stajcic, Z, et al. (1986). Peripheral streptomycin/lidocaine injections in the treatment of idiopathic trigeminal neuralgia. *J Max Fac Surg*, 14:8–9.

Solberg, WK (1986). Masticatory myalgia and its management. *Brit Dent J*, 160:351.

Solberg, WK and Graff-Radford, SB (1988). Orodental Considerations of Facial Pain. *Semin Neurol* 8(4): 318–323, 1988.

Solberg, WK, Hansson, TL, and Nordstrom, BN (1985). The temporomandibular joint in young adults at autopsy: a morphologic classification and evaluation. *J Oral Rehab*, 12:303–321.

Solberg, WK, Woo, MS, and Huston, JB (1979). Prevalence of mandibular dysfunction in young adults. *J Am Dent Assoc*, 98:25–34.

Suarez, P and Clark, GT (2006). Burning mouth syndrome: an update on diagnosis and treatment methods. *J Calif Dent Assoc*, 34(8):611–622.

Symonds, C (1949). Facial pain: Ann Roy Coll Surg Engl, 4:206–212.

Symonds, C (1956). Cough headache. *Brain*, 79:557–568.

Taarnhoj, P (1982). Decompression of the posterior trigeminal root in trigeminal neuralgia: a 30 year follow up review. *J Neurosurg*, 57:14–17.

Taub, A (1973). Relief of post herpetic neuralgia with psychotropic drugs. *J Neurosurg* 39:235–239.

Headache Classification Subcommittee of the International Headache Society (2004). The International Classification of Headache Disorders 2nd Edition. *Cephalalgia*, 24(Suppl. 1):126–130.

Torelli, P and Manzoni, GC (2004). Cluster headache: symptomatic treatment. *Neurol Sci*, 25 (Suppl. 3):S119–122.

Tourne, LPM and Fricton, JR (1992). Burning mouth syndrome: critical review and proposed clinical management. *Oral Surg Oral Med Oral Pathol*, 74:158–167.

Travell, J and Simons, DG (1984). *Myofascial Pain and Dysfunction. The Trigger Point Manual.* Williams and Wilkins, Baltimore.

Vickers RE, Cousins MJ, Walker S, et al. (1998). Analysis of 50 patients with atypical odontalgia. A preliminary report on pharmacologic procedures for diagnosis and treatment. *Oral Surg Oral Med Oral Pathol Oral Radiol Endod*, 85:24–32.

Walker, AE (1966). Neuralgias of the glossopharyngeal, vagus and nervous intermedius nerves. In *Pain* (PR Knighton and PR Dumke, eds), pp. 421–429. Little Brown, Boston.

Watson, PN and Evans, RJ (1986). Postherpetic neuralgia: a review. *Arch Neurol*, 43:836–840.

Weiner, R and Reed, K (1999). Peripheral neruostimulation for control of intractable occipital neuralgia. *Neuromodulation*, 2(3):217–221.

Woda, A, Navez, ML, Picard, P, et al. A possible therapeutic solution for stomatodynia (burning mouth syndrome). *J Orofac Pain*, 12:272–278.

Young, RF, Vermeulen, SS, Grimm P, et al. (1997). Gamma knife radiosurgery for treatment of trigeminal neuralgia. Idiopathic and tumor related. Neurology, 48:608–614.

24 Nasal Disease and Sinus Headache

Stephen D Silberstein, David Dodick, and Thomas O Willcox

Since sinusitis is almost always accompanied by concurrent nasal airway inflammation and, in many cases, is preceded by rhinitis symptoms, we now refer to the disorder as rhinosinusitis. Rhinosinusitis consists of a group of disorders characterized by inflammation of the nasal mucosa and the paranasal sinuses. Rhinosinusitis is increasing in prevalence and incidence, and has been estimated to affect approximately 31 million patients in the United States each year (Moss and Parsons, 1986). It causes significant physical symptoms, negatively affects quality of life, and can substantially impair daily functioning. Rhinosinusitis is commonly divided into acute and chronic forms. Acute rhinosinusitis, a relatively uncommon cause of headache, is because of infection (viral, bacterial, or fungal) of one or more of the paranasal sinuses. In some cases it may have an allergic cause; other patients have idiopathic disease (International Rhinosinusitis Advisory Board, 1997).

Acute bacterial rhinosinusitis infections are much less common today than they were in the preantibiotic era. When they develop, they are frequently the sequela of a viral upper respiratory tract infection. Approximately 0.5%–2% of cases of viral rhinosinusitis develop into bacterial infections (Piccirillo, 2004a). Acute bacterial rhinosinusitis is usually characterized by purulent discharge in the nasal passages and a pain profile that is determined by the site of infection. Other symptoms include nasal congestion, maxillary tooth discomfort, hyposmia or anosmia, cough, facial pain or pressure that is aggravated by bending forward, headache, fever, and malaise. Rhinosinusitis is overdiagnosed as a cause of headache because of the belief that pain on the sinuses must be related to the sinuses. In fact, frontal head pain is more often caused by migraine and tension-type headache. It should not follow that if a patient fails to respond to treatment for migraine and tension-type headache, one should reconsider the diagnosis of rhinosinus disease. Whether nasal obstruction can lead to chronic headache is very controversial (Schønsted-Madsen et al., 1986). Paradoxically, rhinosinus disease also tends to be underdiagnosed, as sphenoid sinus infection is frequently missed (Lew et al., 1983).

Caldwell noted a functional relationship between the ostia of the sinuses and the development of sinusitis (Caldwell, 1893). Hajek and associates emphasized that ostial stenosis is responsible for sinusitis (Hajek, 1926). Hilding and Messerklinger demonstrated that ethmoid sinusitis is frequently a cause of frontal and maxillary rhinosinusitis (Hilding, 1950; Messerklinger, 1978). It was later demonstrated that obstruction of the ostiomeatal complex, the common drainage pathway for the ethmoid, frontal, and maxillary sinuses, is involved in the development of sinus disease (McCaffrey, 1993).

Wolff showed that the sinuses themselves are relatively insensitive to pain (Wolff, 1948). The pain associated with rhinosinusitis comes from engorged and inflamed nasal structures: nasofrontal ducts, turbinates, ostia, and superior nasal spaces. In support of this, Shields et al. found no correlation between pain severity and disease severity by sinus computed tomography (CT) scan (graded by the Lund-McKay, Harvard, or Kennedy staging system) (Shields et al., 2003).

EPIDEMIOLOGY

Rhinosinusitis, which affects more than 31 million people in the United States, resulted in

16 million physician visits in 1985 (Moss and Parsons, 1986); by 1994, the National Health Interview Survey estimated that 35 million people were affected (Agency for Healthcare Policy and Research, 1999). A national health interview survey conducted in the United Sates between 1990 and 1992 found that chronic rhinosinusitis was the second most frequent disease after orthopedic deformities, with an annual average of 33.1 million cases (Collins, 1997). According to data from the National Ambulatory Medical Care Survey, the prevalence of acute rhinosinusitis is increasing, from 0.2% of diagnoses at office visits in 1990 to 0.4% of diagnoses at office visits in 1995 (Agency for Healthcare Policy and Research, 1999). Approximately 0.5% of upper respiratory infections in adults are complicated by rhinosinusitis (Diaz and Bamberger, 1995). As many as 38% of patients seen in adult general medicine clinics with symptoms of rhinosinusitis may have acute bacterial rhinosinusitis. In otolaryngology practices, the prevalence was higher (50%–80%). Although rhinosinusitis is generally more common in children than adults, frontal and sphenoid sinusitis are rare in children. Between 6% and 18% of children in the primary care setting presenting with upper respiratory infections may have acute bacterial rhinosinusitis (Agency for Healthcare Policy and Research, 1999). In the preantibiotic era, the sphenoid sinus was involved in as many as 33% of cases of rhinosinusitis. Today its incidence is approximately 3% (Lew et al., 1983).

In 1996, overall health care expenditures attributable to rhinosinusitis were estimated at $5.8 billion, of which $1.8 billion (30.6%) was for children 12 years or younger. A primary diagnosis of acute or chronic sinusitis accounted for 58.7% of all expenditures ($3.5 billion). Approximately 12% of the costs for asthma, chronic otitis media, and eustachian tube disorders were attributed to diagnosing and treating comorbid sinusitis. Nearly 90% of all expenditures ($5.1 billion) were associated with ambulatory or emergency department services (Ray et al., 1999). It is estimated that more than $200 million is spent annually on cold and sinus prescription products; this does not include over-the-counter medications (Josephson and Gross, 1997).

ANATOMY AND DEVELOPMENT

The ethmoid bone, a T-shaped structure that supports the ethmoid labyrinth, forms the lateral nasal wall. The horizontal limb of the T is formed by the cribriform plate, from which the ethmoid labyrinth is suspended. It has multiple bony septa and the medial projections of the superior and middle turbinates. Lateral to the uncinate process, a secondary projection of the ethmoid bone, is the infundibulum, a recess into which the maxillary sinus drains. The infundibulum drains into the hiatus semilunaris, which in turn drains into the middle meatus, which is located between the uncinate process and the middle turbinate. The frontal sinus drains into the frontal recess, which may drain into the middle meatus or the ethmoidal infundibulum. This region is known as the ostiomeatal complex (maxillary sinus ostium, infundibulum, hiatus semilunaris, middle turbinate, ethmoidal bulla, and frontal ostium) (McCaffrey, 1993). The sphenoidal sinus and posterior

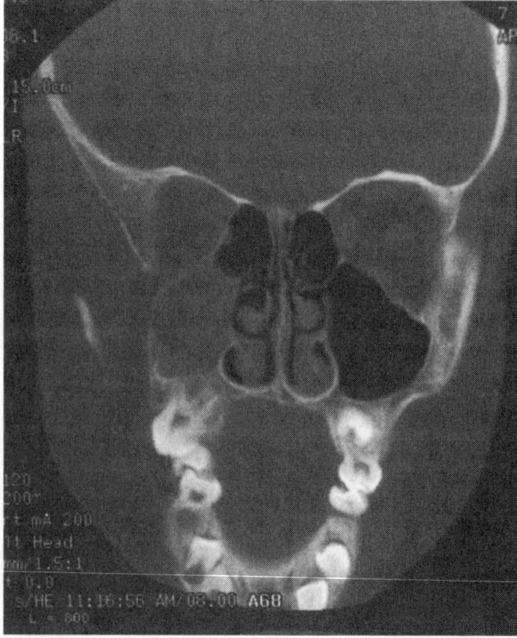

Figure 24–1 Coronol computed tomographic scan of the sinuses, demonstrating normal left-sided anatomy and right maxillary sinus opacification.

ethmoidal cells drain into the sphenoethmoidal recess (Figure 24–1).

The sphenoid sinus is contained within the body of the sphenoid bone deep in the nasal cavity and is divided into two chambers by the intersphenoidal septum. Each sinus communicates with the sphenoethmoidal recess, located medial to the posterior superior aspect of the superior concha. The roof of the sphenoid sinus is related to the middle cranial fossa and the pituitary gland in the sella turcica; laterally are the cavernous sinuses; posteriorly is the clivus and pons; anteriorly the posterior nasal cavity, posterior ethmoid cells, and cribriform plate; and inferiorly the nasopharynx. The cavernous sinus, which is lateral to the sphenoid sinus, contains the internal carotid arteries and the 3rd, 4th, 5th, and 6th cranial nerves. The maxillary division of the 5th nerve may indent the lateral wall of the sphenoid sinus, as may the optic nerve. The sphenoid walls can be extremely thin, and sometimes the sinus cavity is separated from the adjacent structure by just a thin mucosal barrier. Because of the close proximity to the cortical venous system, cranial nerves, and meninges, infection may spread to these structures and present as a central nervous system infection or neurologic catastrophe (Lew et al., 1983; Sofferman, 1983).

The maxillary and ethmoid sinuses, both present at birth, are the most common sites of clinical infection in children. The sphenoid sinuses are present as minute cavities at birth, and it is not until puberty that their main development occurs (Goss, 1959). The frontal sinus begins to develop from the anterior ethmoid sinus at approximately 6 years of age and continues to pneumatize into the late teens. Hypoplasia or aplasia of one or both frontal sinuses has been reported to be between 2% and 20% (Lang, 1989), but true agenesis is rare (Schaefer, 1990). The frontal and sphenoid sinuses become clinically important in the teens and frequently become infected in pansinusitis. Isolated sphenoid sinusitis is rare (Kennedy, 1990b; Reilly, 1990) (Figure 24–2).

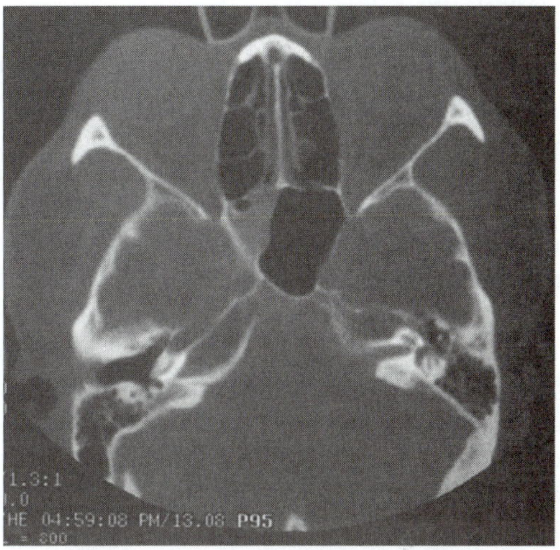

Figure 24–2 Axial computed tomographic scan of the sinuses, demonstrating isolated right sinusitis.

PHYSIOLOGY

The primary functions of the nasal passages are humidification, warming, and removal of particulate material from the inspired air. The paranasal sinuses are air-filled cavities that communicate with the nasal airway. They are lined with pseudostratified-ciliated epithelium, which is covered by a thin layer of mucus. Large inhaled particulate matter passes over this constantly moving ciliated epithelial layer and is deposited there. The cilia and the mucous layer are in constant motion in a predetermined direction. Mucus and debris are transported toward the ostia by the beating of the cilia and are expelled into the nasal airway (Reilly, 1990; Zinreich, 1990; McCaffrey, 1993). This process is termed *mucociliary clearance.*

Bacterial contamination of the sinuses is effectively cleared by mucociliary clearance. If the sinus ostia are obstructed, mucociliary flow is interrupted. Obstruction causes the oxygen tension within the sinus to decrease and the carbon dioxide tension to increase. This anaerobic, high carbon dioxide, stagnant environment can facilitate bacterial growth (McCaffrey, 1993). Unobstructed flow through the sinus ostia and its narrow communicating passage within the ostiomeatal complex is integral to mucociliary clearance and sinus ventilation. Persistent low-grade inflammation in the ethmoid sinus may cause few localizing symptoms but can predispose to recurrent maxillary and frontal rhinosinusitis (Reilly, 1990; McCaffrey, 1993).

For many years, surgical drainage of the sinuses, avoiding the region of the natural ostia, was the treatment of choice for rhinosinusitis. This procedure alleviated the acute infection, but did not prevent re-accumulation of mucus within the sinus. Because the normal mucociliary clearance transports mucus toward the natural ostia, creating a new ostium at a site distant from the natural ostium fails to direct the flow of mucus to the new opening (McCaffrey, 1993).

All sinuses normally contain anaerobic bacteria, and more than one third harbor both anaerobic and aerobic organisms. Ciliary dysfunction and retention of secretions, commonly a result of ostial obstruction, is necessary for bacterial proliferation and the development of sinus infection. Aerobes present in both normal and disease states include the gram-positive streptococci (alpha, beta, and *Streptococcus pneumoniae*) and *Staphylococcus aureus*, and the gram-negative *Moraxella catarrhalis*, *Haemophilus influenzae*, and *Escherichia coli*. Anaerobic organisms include the gram-positive *Peptococcus* and *Propionibacterium* species. The *Bacteroides* and *Fusobacterium* species also play a role in chronic rhinosinusitis (Kennedy, 1990a; Reilly, 1990). *S. pneumoniae*, *H. influenzae*, and *M. catarrhalis* cause most adult cases of acute maxillary rhinosinusitis (VanCauwenberge et al., 1997). Although Staphylococcus aureus is an infrequent cause of maxillary and ethmoid rhinosinusitis, it is the major cause of acute sphenoid and frontal rhinosinusitis. Rhinosinusitis of dental origin is commonly because of mixed anaerobic infection with bacteroides and anaerobic streptococcus (Diaz and Bamberger, 1995).

Systemic diseases that predispose to rhinosinusitis include cystic fibrosis, immune deficiency, bronchiectasis, and the immobile cilia syndrome (Kartagener's syndrome). In one study, patients with recurrent rhinosinusitis were unable to produce secretions with high concentrations of antimicrobial factors in response to cholinergic stimulation (Jeney et al., 1990). In purulent secretions of patients with rhinosinusitis, the concentrations of IgA, IgG, and IgM are decreased (Engquist et al., 1983). Local factors include upper respiratory infection (usually viral), allergic rhinitis, overuse of topical decongestants, hypertrophied adenoids, deviated nasal septum, nasal polyps, tumors, and cigarette smoke (Reilly, 1990). The most common predisposing factor is mucosal inflammation from a viral upper respiratory infection or allergic rhinitis (Diaz and Bamberger, 1995). The sinuses are involved in nearly 90% of viral upper respiratory infections. Eighty-seven percent of patients with a common cold and no previous history of rhinosinusitis had maxillary sinus abnormalities, 65% had ethmoid sinus abnormalities, and 30%–40% had frontal or sphenoid sinus abnormalities on CT. The abnormalities are most likely because of highly viscid secretions in the sinuses. Seventy-seven percent of patients exhibit obstruction of the infundibulum. These abnormalities usually resolve spontaneously, but some patients develop secondary bacterial infections (Gwaltney et al., 1994). Foreign bodies are a common cause of obstruction in children, and 10% of rhinosinus infections are of dental origin (Diaz and Bamberger, 1995). Loss of immunocompetence because of human immunodeficiency virus (HIV) infection, chemotherapy, posttransplant immunosuppression, insulin-dependent diabetes mellitus, and some connective tissue disorders predisposes patients to rhinosinusitis and increases the likelihood of its persistence. Rhinosinusitis is common in the intensive care unit because prolonged supine positioning compromises mucociliary clearance and adds to the problems created by mucosal drying from transnasal supplemental oxygenation and sinus ostial obstruction from nasotracheal or nasogastric tubes. In an intensive care unit, rhinosinusitis occurred in 95.5% of bedridden patients who had a nasogastric or nasotracheal tube in place for at least 1 week (Rouby et al., 1994). Unobstructed flow through the sinus ostia and its narrow communicating passage within the ostiomeatal complex is integral to mucociliary clearance and ventilation. Persistent low-grade inflammation in the ethmoid sinus may cause few localizing symptoms but can predispose to recurrent maxillary and frontal sinus infections (Reilly, 1990; McCaffrey, 1993).

HIV-positive patients who are deficient in both cell-mediated and humoral immunity are more susceptible to bacterial infection. Rhinosinusitis occurs in 75% of those with acquired immunodeficiency syndrome (AIDS) and is often extensive and difficult to treat, especially if the CD4 count is less than 200/mm^3. As in HIV-negative patients, the ethmoid and maxillary sinuses are predominantly involved (Evans, 1998).

DIAGNOSTIC TESTING

Although rhinosinusitis can usually be diagnosed using only clinical judgment, patients with recurrent or complicated sinus disease might require imaging studies. These studies are an absolute requirement for patients who undergo functional endoscopic sinus surgery (Meltzer et al., 2004). In addition, the physical examination may not be helpful, particularly in sphenoid rhinosinusitis. Not all patients are febrile, and sinus tenderness is not always present. Pus is not always seen in sphenoid rhinosinusitis. Kibblewhite and associates found purulent exudate in only 3 of 14 patients (Kibblewhite et al., 1988). Transillumination of the sinuses has low sensitivity and specificity (Stafford, 1990) and routine anterior rhinoscopy performed with a headlight and nasal speculum allows only limited inspection of the anterior nasal cavity.

Standard Radiography

Standard radiographic studies are inadequate to evaluate rhinosinusitis. Although less costly than other imaging measures, they do not provide adequate diagnostic information. They fail to provide information on the patient's anatomy, and they do not evaluate the anterior ethmoid air cells, the upper two thirds of the nasal cavity, or the infundibular, middle meatus, and frontal recess air passages (Zinreich, 1990). They do not show the extent of inflammatory disease and are inadequate to guide surgery (Meltzer et al., 2004).

Neuroimaging

CT has two major roles in rhinosinusitis: to define the anatomy of the sinuses before surgery and to aid in the diagnosis and management of recurrent or chronic rhinosinusitis (Meltzer et al., 2004). CT is the optimal radiographic study to accurately assess the paranasal sinuses for evidence of disease. The mucosa of the normal noninfected sinus approximates the bone so closely that it cannot be visualized on CT. Therefore, any soft tissue seen within a sinus is abnormal (Schatz and Becker, 1984). CT may demonstrate mucosal thickening, sclerosis, clouding, or air-fluid levels. Imaging must be performed in the coronal plane to adequately demonstrate the ethmoid complex. It can reveal the extent of mucosal disease in the ostiomeatal complex. The test–retest reliability of CT in the assessment of chronic rhinosinusitis was high and stable in a prospective series of patients scheduled for endoscopic sinus surgery (Bhattacharyya, 1999). The prevalence of reversible sinus abnormalities on CT in patients with the common cold is high (Gwaltney et al., 1994). This suggests that CT may not be specific for bacterial infections (Diaz and Bamberger, 1995) (Figure 24–3).

Several authors have attempted to use CT, particularly the volume of paranasal sinus inflammatory disease, to stage rhinosinusitis. The most accepted staging system is that of Lund-Mackay. (Lund and Mackay, 1993) No currently available system allows clinicians to show or judge the evolution of this disease or indicate prognosis. Similarly, a meaningful correlation between symptoms and the presence of inflammatory disease within the various sinuses has not been determined to date (Meltzer et al., 2004).

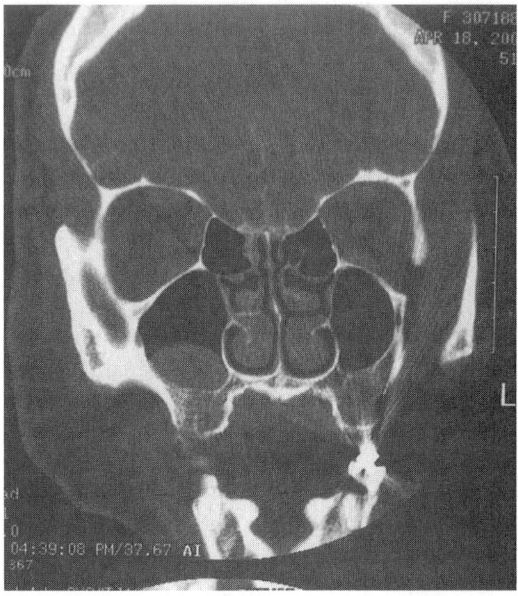

Figure 24–3 Coronal computed tomographic scan of the sinuses, demonstrating normal left-sided anatomy and right maxillary sinus soft tissue. The soft tissue may be mistaken for infection, but it represents a mucous retention cyst.

Unlike CT, magnetic resonance imaging (MRI) does not display the bony anatomy, but it does provide an excellent display of the mucosa. However, the appearance of normal nasal mucosa during the edematous phase of the nasal cycle in MRI scans (T2-weighted images) can resemble pathological changes.

Despite these problems with specificity, MRI is superior to CT in distinguishing between bacterial–viral inflammatory disease and fungal concretions (Zinreich, 1990). Maxillary mucosal thickening of more than 6 mm, complete sinus opacification, and air-fluid levels on neuroimaging correlate to positive sinus cultures (Druce and Siavin, 1991). However, 30%–40% of the normal population will have mucosal thickening on CT evaluation (Havas et al., 1988). The Agency for Health Care Policy and Research (AHCPR) (1999) meta-analysis of six studies showed that sinus radiography has moderate sensitivity (76%) and specificity (79%) compared with sinus puncture in diagnosing acute bacterial rhinosinusitis.

CT or MRI is necessary to definitively diagnose sphenoid rhinosinusitis, because plain X-rays are nondiagnostic in approximately 26% of cases (Goldman et al., 1993). CT scanning is the gold standard for the diagnosis of sphenoid sinus disease; MRI is an adjunct. Lawson and Reino (1997) devised a system to categorize CT findings, which might better define the role of MRI. Type I findings are consistent with inflammatory lesions, such as acute and chronic rhinosinusitis, mucous retention cysts, polyps, and mucoceles, which do not routinely necessitate MRI. In acute rhinosinusitis, an air-fluid level is present within the sinus cavity. With chronic disease, the cavity is partially or totally opacified by hypertrophic mucosa and secretions. A globular opacity partially filling the cavity generally represents a mucous retention cyst or polyp, similar to those present in the other paranasal sinuses. A superior or laterally based "polypoid" mass in the sphenoid sinus may represent such rare entities as an encephalocele or an internal carotid artery aneurysm (Lawson and Reino, 1997) (Figure 24–4).

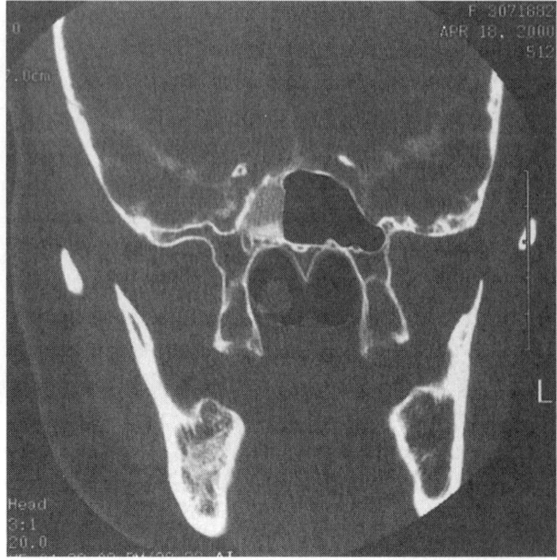

Figure 24–4 Coronal computed tomographic cysternogram of the sinuses, demonstrating contrast enhancement within the right sphenoid sinus secondary to a spontaneous atraumatic encephalocele.

Type II findings include lesions that cause anatomic distortion of a sinus wall (i.e., thinning, expansion, or remodeling). MRI helps to differentiate between mucoceles and benign tumors. A mucocele demonstrates homogenous, low signal intensity in the T1-weighted phase on MRI. A long-standing mucocele produces higher signal intensity in T1-weighted and proton density images because of the concentration of proteinaceous secretions with loss of water. The T2-weighted signal remains high in most lesions until the protein concentration reaches 25%–35%, which causes a decrease, first in the T2-weighted signals, then in the T1-weighted signals. On the other hand, tumors that are highly cellular show intermediate signal intensity in the T1-weighted phase, proton density images, and T2-weighted phase. With increased stromal components, the signal intensity becomes brighter and nonhomogenous in the T2-weighted phase (Lawson and Reino, 1997) (Figure 24–5).

Type III findings consist of total sinus opacification with sclerosis of the surrounding bone. If a mycetoma is suspected, fungal sinusitis may be diagnosed on MRI by the presence of a signal void in the sinus cavity, as opposed to the mixed signal pattern found in the cavity with fibro-osseous disorders (Lawson and Reino, 1997) (Figure 24–6).

Type IV lesions demonstrate evidence of bone erosion. MRI is necessary to obtain information

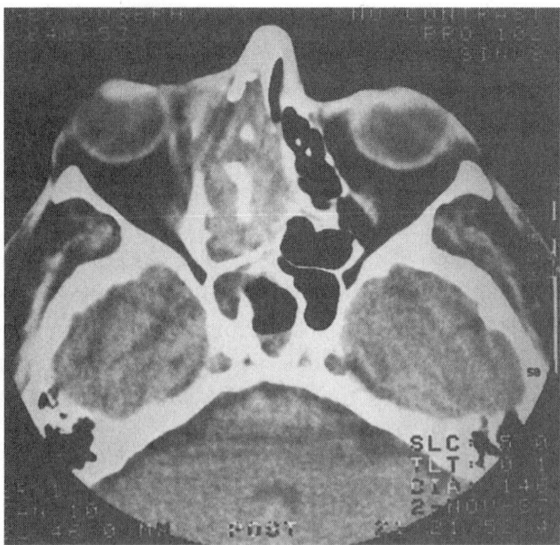

Figure 24–5 Soft-tissue window axial computed tomographic scan of the sinuses, demonstrating a right-sided inverting papilloma that is expanding the ethmoid labyrinth.

about the nature of the lesion and whether extrasinus extension is present. Although most of these lesions are neoplastic, a mucocele may occasionally (7.89% of cases) produce localized areas of bone destruction (Lawson and Reino, 1997) (Figure 24–7).

Type V findings demonstrate perisinus extension. MRI delineates the extent of intracranial and skull base involvement. Bone erosion and extrasinus extension are hallmarks of malignant tumors (Figure 24–8).

Transillumination, Ultrasonography, and Anterior Rhinoscopy

Transillumination of the sinuses has low sensitivity and specificity (Stafford, 1990). Although an A-mode ultrasound scan can demonstrate the presence of fluid or thickened mucosa in a sinus, operator experience plays a significant part, and false-positive examinations are common. Ultrasound scans are usually limited to frontal and antral disease and are most commonly used to follow the response to pharmacotherapy of a rhinosinusitis documented by nasal endoscopy or CT (Williams et al., 1992; Evans, 1994; Fergusen and Mabry, 1997; Wagner, 1996). Studies comparing sinus ultrasonography with puncture or sinus radiography were inconclusive in determining how well ultrasonography identifies patients with

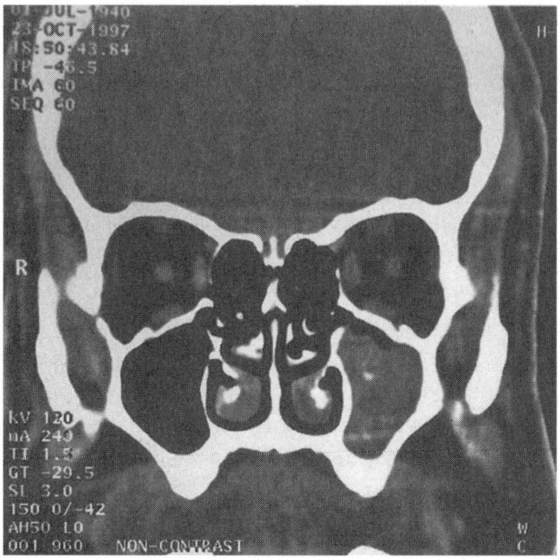

Figure 24–6 Soft-tissue window coronol computed tomographic scan of the sinus, demonstrating an aspergilloma (fungus ball) of the left maxillary antrum. There is heterogeneity of the soft tissue and thickening of the surrounding bone.

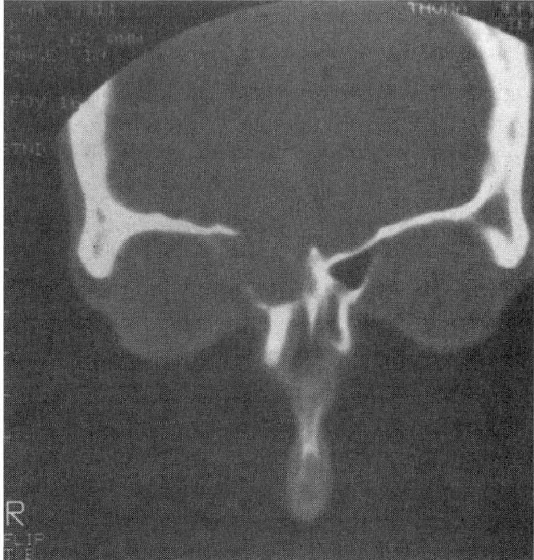

Figure 24–7 Coronal computed tomographic scan of the sinuses, demonstrating a right frontal mucocele with thinning of the floor of the anterior cranial fossa.

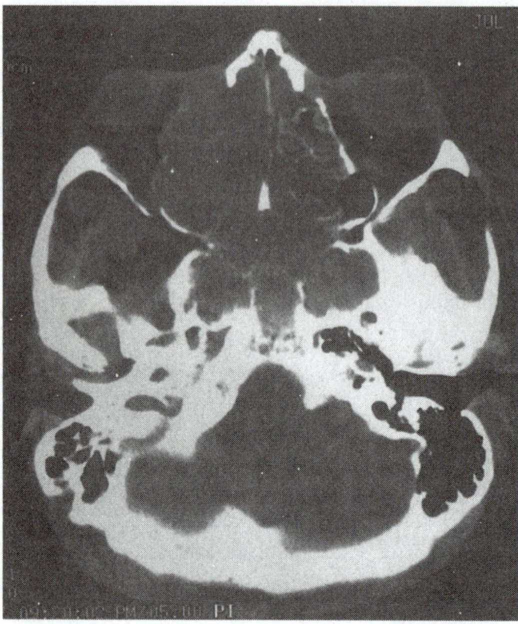

Figure 24–8 Soft-tissue axial window computed tomographic scan of the sinuses, demonstrating a poorly differentiated sinonasal carcinoma that has eroded much of the ethmoid labyrinth. There is also intracranial erosion of the coronal views.

acute bacterial rhinosinusitis. The results of ultrasonography varied substantially, possibly because of differences in patient populations, ultrasonography techniques, or the medical personnel involved in diagnostic testing (Agency for Healthcare Policy and Research, 1999). Ultrasonography has lower sensitivity and specificity than sinus X-rays (Stafford, 1990). Routine anterior rhinoscopy performed with a headlight and nasal speculum allows only limited inspection of the anterior nasal cavity.

Diagnostic Fiberoptic Nasal Endoscopy

Diagnostic endoscopy with a rigid or flexible fiberoptic rhinoscope allows direct visualization of the nasal passages and sinus drainage areas (ostiomeatal complex), and is complementary to CT or MRI. It not only plays an important role in the diagnosis of rhinosinusitis, but can also assist with its treatment. A recent consensus (Meltzer et al., 2004) stated that most clinicians currently believe that: (1) patient symptoms can be an unreliable gauge of disease, (2) endoscopy facilitates proper diagnosis and can detect disease missed on routine history and physical examination or even that missed on imaging studies, (3) discolored drainage (yellow to green) represents a pathologic process draining through the nasal passageways, (4) properly obtained endoscopic cultures are useful in identifying organisms that might be responsible for certain forms of rhinosinusitis, (5) the most important role of endoscopy is in the assessment and treatment of patients with refractory or chronic symptoms and patients who have impending or existing complications of rhinosinusitis, and (6) endoscopy is well tolerated but is not without risk. In contrast to anterior rhinoscopy, endoscopy introduces brilliant illumination into the dark cavities and permits magnified direct visualization of the mucosa, the turbinates, and, in postsurgical patients, the sinus cavities. Nasal endoscopy helps identify erythema, edema, polyps or polypoid swelling, crusting, eosinophilic mucin, and mucopus or frank pus deep in the nasal cavity. The examiner can also identify pus emanating from the middle meatus or sphenoethmoidal recess and in the nasopharynx. Mucosal sinus thickening is frequently present in normal, asymptomatic patients. In these cases, endoscopy should be positive before a diagnosis of rhinosinusitis can be made (Kennedy, 1990b; McCaffrey, 1993). Sphenoid rhinosinusitis is an exception to this generalization.

Patients who have unilateral disease without septal deviation, have severe and disabling symptoms, or are symptomatic and refractory to appropriate empiric therapy are candidates for nasal endoscopy. Endoscopy is also indicated if complications are suspected or if the patient is immunocompromised or has had sinus surgery, trauma, or both (Meltzer et al., 2004). The combination of negative neuroimaging and nasal endoscopy usually, but not always, rules out sinus disease (Zinreich, 1990).

CLINICAL MANIFESTATIONS

In 1996, the American Academy of Otolaryngology—Head and Neck Surgery standardized the terminology for paranasal infections (Benninger et al., 1997). The term *rhinosinusitis* was felt to be more appropriate than sinusitis because rhinitis typically precedes sinusitis, purulent sinusitis without rhinitis is rare, the mucosa of the nose and sinuses are contiguous, and symptoms of nasal obstruction and discharge are prominent in sinusitis (Slavin, 1997). The diagnosis of rhinosinusitis is usually based on symptoms indicating maxillary or frontal sinus involvement. This may occur secondary to, and is frequently a result of, ethmoid disease. Obstruction of the sinus ostia is the usual precursor of sinusitis (Zinreich, 1990).

Rhinosinusitis is divided into four categories based on the temporal course and the signs and symptoms of the disease (Table 24–1) (Lanza and Kennedy, 1997; Meltzer et al., 2004).

Acute rhinosinusitis has a sudden onset and lasts from 1 day to 4 weeks, with complete resolution of the symptoms. *Recurrent acute rhinosinusitis* requires four or more episodes of acute rhinosinusitis, lasting at least 7 days each, in any 1-year period. *Subacute rhinosinusitis* is continuous with acute rhinosinusitis and lasts from 4 to 12 weeks (Lanza and Kennedy, 1997). *Chronic rhinosinusitis* requires that signs or symptoms persist for 12 weeks or longer and may be punctuated by acute infectious episodes.

Most cases of infectious rhinosinusitis that last less than 7 days are viral. Acute bacterial rhinosinusitis in adults most often presents with ≥7 days of purulent anterior rhinorrhea, nasal congestion, postnasal drip, facial or dental pain/pressure, and cough that frequently has a nighttime component.

Facial tenderness and pain, nasal congestion, and purulent nasal discharge are common manifestations of acute rhinosinusitis. Other "classic" signs and symptoms include anosmia, pain upon mastication, and halitosis. An upper respiratory infection or a history of an upper respiratory infection is often present (Stafford, 1990). Although fever is present in approximately 50% of adults and 60% of children, and headache is common, the symptoms of headache, facial pain, and fever are often of minimal value in diagnosing rhinosinusitis. Williams et al. looked at the sensitivity and specificity of individual symptoms in making the diagnosis (Williams et al., 1992). No single item was both sensitive and specific. Maxillary toothache was highly specific (93%) but only 11% of the patients had this symptom. Logistic regression analysis showed five independent predictions of rhinosinusitis: maxillary toothache (odds ratio 2.9), abnormal transillumination (odds ratio 2.7, sensitivity 73%, specificity 54%), poor response to decongestants (odds ratio 2.4), purulent discharge (odds ratio 2.9), and colored nasal discharge (odds ratio 2.2). Headache had an odds ratio of 1.0, with 68% sensitivity and 30% specificity. The low specificity is because of the lack of descriptive features of the headache. Some patients (e.g., those with chronic sphenoid sinusitis) might experience headache as the only symptom of rhinosinusitis. The location of the headache might vary depending on which sinuses are affected. However, headache or facial pain does not generally suggest rhinosinusitis in the absence of other signs and symptoms.

One classification system is based on major and minor clinical criteria. The major symptoms are purulent anterior or posterior nasal discharge, nasal congestion, facial pain or pressure, and fever. Minor symptoms are cough, headache (not otherwise specified), halitosis, and earache (Shapiro and Rachelefsky, 1992). A diagnosis using these criteria requires two major criteria or one major and two minor criteria. However, none of these criteria are both sensitive and specific enough for diagnosis. It has been suggested that highly specific symptoms, such as facial erythema or maxillary toothache, or symptoms that persist for more than 10 days warrant a diagnosis and treatment (International Rhinosinusitis Advisory Board, 1997). The AHCPR evidence report (1999), based on limited evidence, suggested that clinical criteria (i.e., the presence of three or four of the following symptoms: purulent rhinorrhea with unilateral predominance, local pain with unilateral predominance, bilateral purulent rhinorrhea, and the presence of pus in the nasal cavity) may have a diagnostic accuracy similar to that of sinus radiography. Thus, symptoms and signs are only moderately useful in identifying patients who have rhinosinusitis, as determined by the results of sinus aspiration after puncture (Berg and Carenfelt, 1988; Hansen et al., 1995) or by evidence of sinusitis on a sinus radiograph (Axelsson et al., 1970; Williams et al., 1992). The sensitivity, specificity, and predictive values of common symptoms and signs are shown in Table 23–2.

TABLE 24–1 Classification of Adult Rhinosinusitis.

Classification	*Duration*	*Strong history*	*Include in differential*	*Special notes*
Acute	⩽4 weeks	⩾2 major factors, 1 major factor and 2 minor factors, or nasal purulence on examination	1 major factor or ⩾2 minor factors	Fever or facial pain does not constitute a suggestive history in the absence of other nasal signs or symptoms; consider acute bacterial rhinosinusitis if symptoms worsen after 5 days, persist for >10 days, or are out of proportion to those typically associated with viral infection
Subacute	4–12 weeks	Same as chronic	Same as chronic	Complete resolution after effective medical therapy
Recurrent acute	⩾4 episodes per year, with each episode lasting ⩾7–10 days and no intervening signs and symptoms of chronic rhinosinusitis	Same as acute		
Chronic	⩾12 weeks	⩾2 major factors, 1 major factor and 2 minor factors,	1 major factor or ⩾2 minor factors	Facial pain does not constitute a suggestive history in the

(continued)

TABLE 24–2 Various Signs and Symptoms Used to Predict the Presence of Sinusitis

Method of diagnosis of sinusutis and measure of performance	*Purulent nasal discharge*	*Pain on bending forward*	*Maxillary toothache*	*Symptoms after upper respiratory infection*	*Nasal obstruction*	*Pain with chewing*
Bacterial sinusitis on the basis of sinus puncture and a spiratio						
Sensitivity (%)	35	75	66	89	60	—
Specificity (%)	78	77	49	79	22	—
Positive predictive value (%)	62	78	59	83	53	—
Negative predictive value (%)	78	73	56	87	15	—
Sinusitis on the basis of plain sinus radiography						
Sensitivity (%)	61	—	18	70	—	7
Specificity (%)	71	—	93	53	—	86
Positive predictive value (%)	66	—	63	58	—	54
Negative predictivevalue (%)	66	—	64	54	—	53

Source: Adapted from Piccirillo (2004b).

Naranch et al. (2002) compared sinus and systemic tenderness in rhinosinusitis and other disorders. Cutaneous pressures (kg/cm^2) causing pain at 5 sinus and 18 systemic sites were measured. Lower sinus thresholds were found in the rhinosinusitis groups. Sinus and systemic thresholds were both 44% lower in chronic fatigue syndrome subjects than in nonchronic fatigue syndrome subjects, suggesting that systemic hyperalgesia contributes to chronic fatigue syndrome, sinus tenderness, and "rhinosinusitis" complaints.

Children with acute and chronic rhinosinusitis almost always present with purulent nasal discharge, which is not characteristic in adults. Fever is infrequent even with acute rhinosinusitis and is usually associated with complicated acute rhinosinusitis (Muntz and Lusk, 1992).

Maxillary sinusitis pain is most typically located in the cheek, gums, and teeth of the upper jaw. Ethmoid sinusitis pain is generally felt between the eyes. The globe may be tender and eye movement may aggravate pain. Frontal sinusitis pain is felt mainly in the forehead. Ethmoid and maxillary sinusitis are usually associated with rhinitis and are often referred to as rhinosinusitis.

Sphenoid rhinosinusitis is an uncommon infection that accounts for approximately 3% of all cases of acute rhinosinusitis. It is usually accompanied by pansinusitis; less commonly, it occurs alone. In contrast to other paranasal rhinosinus infections, sphenoid rhinosinusitis is frequently misdiagnosed, because the sphenoid sinus is not accessible to direct clinical examination even with the flexible endoscope and is not adequately visualized with routine sinus X-rays (Goldman et al., 1993). Although sphenoid rhinosinusitis is an uncommon cause of headache, it is potentially associated with significant morbidity and mortality and requires early identification and aggressive management (Lew et al., 1983; Kibblewhite et al., 1988; Goldman et al., 1993).

Headache is the most common symptom of acute sphenoid rhinosinusitis and is present in all patients who are able to complain about it. Standing, walking, bending, or coughing aggravates it. It often interferes with sleep and is poorly relieved by narcotics. The location of rhinosinusitis headache is variable: Vertex headache is rare; frontal, occipital, or temporal headache or a combination of these locations is most common. Periorbital pain is common. This is in contrast to the common teaching that retro-orbital or vertex headache is the most common presenting symptom of sphenoid rhinosinusitis (Lew et al., 1983; Kibblewhite et al., 1988; Urquhart et al., 1989; Nordeman and Lucid, 1990; Deans and Welch, 1991; Goldman et al., 1993).

Nausea and vomiting frequently occur during an attack of acute sphenoid rhinosinusitis, but nasal discharge, stuffiness, and postnasal drip are unusual. Fever occurs in more than one half of patients with acute sphenoid rhinosinusitis. Isolated sphenoid rhinosinusitis has been subclassified into four groups (inflammatory, neoplastic, fibro-osseous disorders, and miscellaneous) in a series of 132 cases (Lawson and Reino, 1997). Headache, visual loss, and cranial nerve palsy prevalence was determined in each group. Headache occurred in 98% of the inflammatory lesions, 90% of the benign tumors, and 71% of the malignant tumors. Visual disturbances (blurred vision and loss of visual acuity) were found in 12% of inflammatory lesions, 60% of benign tumors, and 50% of malignant neoplasms. Sixth cranial nerve palsy occurred in 6% of the inflammatory and 50% of the neoplastic cases. Eyelid ptosis (because of third-nerve involvement) occurred in 7.5% of the cases. Other symptoms included cerebrospinal leaks, epistaxis, meningitis, and proptosis. Four patients with fibro-osseous disorder presented with headache.

The diagnosis of acute or chronic rhinosinusitis must be considered in an immunosuppressed patient who has fever, facial pain, swelling and nasal crusting or ulceration. Plain X-rays may exhibit only slight mucosal thickening. Patients who fail to respond to medical treatment should have antral aspiration performed so that the causative organism can be identified and appropriate antibiotic treatment prescribed (Evans, 1998).

Hypertrophic turbinates, atrophic sinus membranes, and nasal passage abnormalities caused by septal deflection may cause headache, but these causes have not been validated by the International Headache Society. Whether nasal obstruction can lead to chronic headache is very controversial (Schønsted-Madsen et al., 1986). Migraine and tension-type headaches are often confused with true sinus headache because of their similar locations. Recurrent episodic pain in the sinus areas is most likely migrainous in nature, with secondary (neurovascular) changes in the sinuses producing local symptoms.

The relationship between headache and subacute and chronic rhinosinus disease is highly controversial (Faleck et al., 1988). Radiographic evidence of sinus disease is very common and does not establish the headache's etiology (Havas et al., 1988). A considerable proportion of adults *not* presenting with symptoms of rhinosinusitis (42.5%, Havas et al., 1988; 15%, Calhoun et al., 1991; 39%, Lloyd et al., 1991) who had CTs for other reasons had coincidental CT findings suggestive of rhinosinusitis (International Rhinosinusitis Advisory Board, 1997). Headache associated with sinus disease is usually continuous, not intermittent. Chronic rhinosinusitis is frequently associated with engorged and swollen nasal mucosa and a purulent or sanguinopurulent nasal discharge. The International Headache Society has not validated chronic rhinosinusitis as a cause of headache or facial pain unless it relapses into an acute stage (Saunte and Soyka, 1993). Patients with rhinosinusitis and headache may not improve following treatment. One patient treated with functional endoscopic surgery for chronic sphenoidal rhinosinusitis continued to have headaches postoperatively despite CT-documented absence of sinus disease (Gilain et al., 1994). This suggests that the headache and rhinosinusitis were coincident unrelated conditions.

Sphenoid rhinosinusitis should be included in the differential diagnosis of acute or subacute headache. It may be mistaken for frontal or ethmoid rhinosinusitis, aseptic meningitis, brain abscess, or septic thrombophlebitis. It can mimic trigeminal neuralgia, migraine, carotid artery aneurysm, or brain tumor (Lew et al., 1983; Kibblewhite et al., 1988; Goldman et al., 1993). Other causes of sphenoid sinus disease include mucoceles and benign and malignant tumors (Lawson and Reino, 1997).

The clinical features of a severe, intractable, new-onset headache that interferes with sleep, increases in severity, has no specific location, and is not relieved by simple analgesics should alert one to the diagnosis of sphenoid rhinosinusitis. Epiphora, pain, or paresthesias in the facial distribution of the 5th nerve and photophobia are suggestive of sphenoid rhinosinusitis (Lew et al., 1983; Turkewitz and Keller, 1987; Kibblewhite et al., 1988; Nordeman and Lucid, 1990; Deans and Welch, 1991; Goldman et al., 1993).

Complications

Sinus infection can result in acute suppurative meningitis, subdural or epidural abscess, and brain abscess. In addition, osteomyelitis and subperiosteal abscess can occur. Infection of the ethmoid and, to a lesser extent, the sphenoid sinuses is responsible for orbital complications, which include edema, orbital cellulitis, and subperiosteal and orbital abscess. Rhinosinusitis thus can be a life-threatening condition and if neglected or mismanaged can lead to intracranial complications (Singh et al., 1995). In a review of patients admitted to the University of Virginia Health Sciences Center with a diagnosis of intracranial suppuration between 1992 and 1997, 15 patients were found who had 22 suppurative intracranial complications of rhinosinusitis. These included epidural abscess (23%), subdural empyema (18%), meningitis (18%), cerebral abscess (14%), superior sagittal sinus thrombosis (9%), cavernous sinus thrombosis (9%), and osteomyelitis (9%). The diagnosis of suppurative intracranial complications of rhinosinusitis requires a high index of suspicion and confirmation by imaging. Patients often present while on a regimen of antibiotics, which may mask or abolish neurologic as well as other symptoms and signs (Gallagher et al., 1998).

A mucocele is a mucus-containing cyst located in the sinuses. These are most common (and benign) in the maxillary sinus (mucus retention cyst). Those located in the frontal, sphenoid, or ethmoid sinus can enlarge and erode into the surrounding structures. A mucopyocele is an infected mucocele (Hilger, 1989).

Sphenoid rhinosinusitis is associated with most major complications, which include bacterial meningitis, cavernous sinus thrombosis, subdural abscess, cortical vein thrombosis, ophthalmoplegia, and pituitary insufficiency (Lew et al., 1983; Sofferman, 1983; Kibblewhite et al., 1988; Goldman et al., 1993). In addition, sphenoid rhinosinusitis can present as an aseptic meningitis because of the presence of a parameningeal focus (Brook et al., 1982). Patients can present with complications of sphenoid rhinosinusitis, including visual loss mimicking optic neuritis, multiple cranial nerve palsies, or papilledema. Sudden onset of neurologic complications, as a result of cavernous sinus thrombosis, can mimic a subarachnoid hemorrhage (Dale and Mackenzie, 1983).

Øktedalen and Lilleas reported on four patients with ethmoid rhinosinusitis who were admitted to an Infectious Disease department with meningitis, sepsis, and orbital cellulitis (Oktedalen and Lilleas, 1992). In Lew's series, 6 of 16 acute cases had meningitis, 5 had cavernous sinus thrombosis, 1 had cortical vein thrombosis, 1 had unilateral ophthalmoplegia, and 1 had orbital cellulitis (Lew et al., 1983). Eight of Kibblewhite's 14 patients had complications on admission (Kibblewhite et al., 1988). None of Goldman's patients had complications (1993). The difference in the complication rate is a result of selection bias: Goldman's patients were retrieved from ER records; Lew's, Kibblewhite's, and Øktedalen and Lilleas's from inpatient records (Lew et al., 1983; Kibblewhite et al., 1988; Oktedalen and Lilleas, 1992; Goldman et al., 1993).

Diagnosis and Differential Diagnosis

The International Headache Society has established new criteria (International Classification of Headache Disorders, ICHD-2) for *Headache attributed to rhinosinusitis* (Headache Classification Committee, 2004) (Table 24–3). To qualify, there must be clinical (purulence in the nasal cavity, nasal obstruction, hyposmia/anosmia and/or fever), nasal endoscopic, CT and/or MRI imaging and/or laboratory evidence of acute or acute-on-chronic rhinosinusitis. Once drainage begins, obstruction is relieved and the headache may begin to abate. These criteria may not be valid for sphenoid rhinosinusitis, however, as purulent discharge is often lacking, and headache may precede sinus drainage.

Although hypertrophic turbinates, atrophic sinus membranes, and nasal passage abnormalities caused by septal deflection may cause headache, these causes have not been validated by the International Headache Society (IHS). Whether nasal obstruction can lead to chronic headache is very controversial (Schønsted-Madsen et al., 1986). Migraine and tension-type headache are often confused with true sinus headache because of their similar locations. Some patients, in addition to all the features of migraine without aura, have head pain in the facial areas, associated congestion of the nose, and headache triggered by weather changes. None of these patients have purulent nasal discharge or the other abnormalities seen in acute rhinosinusitis. Therefore, it is necessary to differentiate headaches caused by rhinosinusitis from so-called "sinus headaches," which are headache attacks fulfilling the criteria of migraine without aura with prominent autonomic symptoms in the nose or migraine without aura triggered by nasal changes.

Table 24–3 Headache Attributed to Rhinosinusitis 11.5.

Diagnostic criteria

A. Frontal headache accompanied by pain in one or more regions of the face, ears, or teeth, and fulfilling criteria C and D
B. Clinical, nasal endoscopic, CT and/or MRI imaging and/or laboratory evidence of acute or acute-on-chronic rhinosinusitis
C. Headache and facial pain develop simultaneously with onset or acute exacerbation of rhinosinusitis
D. Headache and/or facial pain resolve within 7 days after remission or successful treatment of acute or acute-on-chronic rhinosinusitis

In a population-based headache study of 23,564 subjects (Lipton et al., 2002), 4967 individuals called their headache migraine and 3074 individuals had headache that met IHS migraine criteria. Among those with IHS migraine, only 53.4% recognized their headaches as migraine; stress headaches (n = 345) and sinus headaches (n = 365) were the most common erroneous labels reported. People are confused by their headache location. Because the sinuses are close to the eyes, individuals may attribute headaches located in the frontal, supraorbital, or infraorbital region to the sinuses.

In a clinic-based study, headache symptoms, headache-associated disability, and response to therapy among patients with self-described sinus headache were assessed. (Cady and Schreiber,

2002) Patients had to have self-described sinus headaches and at least one migraine symptom: moderate to severe pain, nausea and/or vomiting, photophobia and/or phonophobia, unilateral pain, pain worsening with activity, or pulsating pain. They were excluded if they had a previous migraine diagnosis or exposure to triptans, headaches associated with fever or purulent nasal discharge, or radiographic evidence of a sinus infection.

A selected group of patients with self-described sinus headache had IHS migraine (70%) or migrainous (28%) headache. Most had nasal symptoms, including stuffiness (74%) and runny nose, and 45% said their headaches were precipitated by changes in the weather. Thus, patients who believe they have sinus headache, have no signs or symptoms of rhinosinusitis and have one symptom of migraine, have migraine.

In a prospective, open-label, observational study, 2991 patients aged 18–65 years, with self-described or physician-diagnosed sinus headache, were assigned an ICHD-2 headache diagnosis. (Schreiber et al., 2004) Patients who had a prior migraine diagnosis, prior triptan use, an abnormal sinus X-ray in the preceding 6 months, and who experienced fever or purulent discharge with their typical sinus headache were excluded. Many of the patients reported sinus symptoms, such as sinus pressure (84%), sinus pain (82%), or nasal congestion (63%); most reported IHS migraine symptoms, such as moderate to severe pain (97%), pulsatility (89%), photophobia (79%), nausea (73%), and phonophobia (67%); 29% reported aura and 25% reported vomiting (Figure 24–1). An ICHD-2 diagnosis of migraine or probable migraine was given to 88% of the patients; 8% had episodic tension-type headache and the remaining 4% were categorized as "other" (Levine et al., 2006).

The Sinus, Allergy, and Migraine Headache Study (SAMS) (Eross et al., 2004) investigated 100 consecutive subjects older than 18 who responded to a newspaper advertisement seeking individuals with sinus headache; there were no exclusion criteria. Patients were assigned headache diagnoses according to IHS criteria: 88% were diagnosed with migraine or probable migraine, 3% with headache secondary to rhinosinusitis, 1% with hemicrania continua, 1% with cluster headache, and 9% could not be classified using ICHD-2 criteria. Among those diagnosed with migraine, reasons patients gave for assuming they had sinus headache included: location of pain on the sinuses (98%), pain triggered by changes in the weather (83%), pain associated with rhinorrhea (73%), and the suggestion of this diagnosis by a previous physician (78%); factors cited as triggering sinus headaches also included seasonal variation (73%) and exposure to "allergens" (62%). Of those diagnosed with migraine, 75% reported cranial autonomic symptoms during headaches, with half of the patients experiencing more than one such symptom; the most common features included nasal congestion (56%), eyelid edema (37%), rhinorrhea (25%), conjunctival injection (22%), and lacrimation (19%).

Misdiagnosis of sinus headache for migraine was a result of triggers (weather changes) and symptoms (nasal congestion, rhinorrhea) that were felt to be typical of sinus pathology and pain overlying the paranasal sinuses—"guilt by provocation, location, and association."

Many individuals who believe, either because of self-diagnosis or physician diagnosis, that they suffer from sinus headaches actually have headaches that fulfill ICHD-2 criteria for migraine or probable migraine. Migraine is also the most common diagnosis (58%) in patients complaining of headache and referred for sinus evaluation who are found to show no evidence of rhinosinusitis on CT of the sinuses or endoscopic examination (Perry et al., 2004).

What is the basis of this confusion? Secretion of calcitonin gene-related peptide (CGRP) from trigeminal nerves and vasoactive intestinal peptide (VIP) from parasympathetic nerves is involved in the pathophysiology of migraine and rhinosinusitis. Their levels in human saliva samples can be used as markers of trigeminal and parasympathetic nerve activity. Bellamy et al compared CGRP and VIP levels in the saliva of subjects experiencing noninfectious allergic rhinosinusitis, migraine with sinus symptoms, and no symptoms. Between attacks, baseline salivary levels of CGRP and VIP of allergic rhinosinusitis and migraine subjects were significantly elevated compared with control values. When rhinosinusitis subjects were treated with pseudoephedrine during attacks and obtained symptom relief, the amount of CGRP and VIP returned to baseline. Salivary CGRP and VIP levels during a migraine headache were also significantly reduced within 2 hours after patients were treated with sumatriptan and obtained symptom relief (Bellamy et al., 2006).

The relationship between headache and subacute and chronic rhinosinus disease is highly controversial. Radiographic evidence of sinus disease is very common and does not establish the headache's etiology. (Havas et al., 1988) Headache associated with rhinosinus disease is usually continuous, not intermittent. Chronic rhinosinusitis is frequently associated with engorged and swollen nasal mucosa and a purulent or sanguinopurulent nasal discharge. The IHS has not validated chronic rhinosinusitis as a cause of headache or facial pain unless it relapses into an acute stage (Saunte and Soyka, 1993).

Faleck et al. reported that 10% of 150 children and adolescents who presented with chronic, nonprogressive headache, clinically indistinguishable from "muscle contraction" headache, had radiographic evidence of sinus pathology. None had prominent respiratory symptoms. All improved with treatment directed toward the sinus pathology. Although some had complete sinus opacification, none had endoscopy performed to show active disease in the ostia (Faleck et al., 1988).

Treatment does not improve the headaches of all patients with chronic sphenoid rhinosinusitis. Gilain et al reported a patient treated with functional endoscopic surgery for chronic sphenoidal rhinosinusitis who continued to have headaches postoperatively despite CT-documented absence of sinus disease. (Gilain et al., 1994) This suggests that the headache and rhinosinusitis were coincident, unrelated conditions.

TREATMENT

Acute rhinosinusitis, an inflammatory condition involving the paranasal sinuses as well as the lining of the nasal passages, lasts up to 4 weeks. For the immunocompetent person living in the general community, acute rhinosinusitis is typically believed to be induced by a virus and does not require antibiotics for the first 10–14 days unless complicating features are present, at which point the presumed etiology is bacterial. Chronic rhinosinusitis may have an infectious or noninfectious basis. Underlying disorders that predispose to chronic rhinosinusitis should be identified and treated as part of the treatment of chronic rhinosinusitis (Dykewicz, 2003). Complicating features include severe headache or facial pain, high fever, and impending or actual complications to the eye, lung, or brain. Without complicating features, after 10–14 days of symptoms consistent with rhinosinusitis and objective findings, bacteria are presumed to predominate (Meltzer et al., 2004).

Management goals for the treatment of acute bacterial rhinosinusitis include: (1) treatment of bacterial infection, (2) reduction of ostial swelling, (3) sinus drainage, and (4) maintenance of sinus ostia patency.

Uncomplicated bacterial rhinosinusitis, other than sphenoid rhinosinusitis, should be treated with a broad-spectrum oral antibiotic for 10–14 days. Because nasal culture does not necessarily correlate with sinus pathogens, initial treatment is empiric (Stafford, 1990). Treatment with any antibiotic reduces the rate of clinical failure by one half. A course of inexpensive antibiotic is probably adequate first-line treatment for the patient who has uncomplicated acute bacterial rhinosinusitis (Piccirillo, 2004b). Amoxicillin-clavulanate is considered first-line treatment for the patient with mild to moderate acute bacterial rhinosinusitis who has or has not received antimicrobials in the previous 6 weeks. A patient who has mild symptoms that last longer than 10 days and has not used an antibiotic can use a low dose of amoxicillin-clavulanate. Patients who have used an antibiotic to treat the infection within the previous 6 weeks or those who live in areas of high prevalence of penicillin-resistant *S. pneumoniae* should be given a higher dose of amoxicillin-clavulanate. The quinolones should be reserved for patients who have moderately severe symptoms or have taken an antibiotic in the last 6 weeks (Anon, 2004). Other antibiotics used for this disorder are doxycycline, erythromycin-sulfisoxazole, azithromycin, clarithromycin, telithromycin, and trimethoprim-sulfamethoxazole. More research is needed to understand how the increasing rates of bacterial resistance may affect the choice of antibiotics (Piccirillo, 2004b).

Steam and saline prevent crusting of secretions in the nasal cavity and facilitate mucociliary clearance. Locally active vasoconstrictor agents provide symptomatic relief by shrinking inflamed and swollen nasal mucosa. Their use should be limited to 3–4 days to prevent rebound vasodilation. Oral decongestants should be used if prolonged treatment (longer than 3 days) is necessary. These agents are a-adrenergic agonists that reduce nasal blood flow without the risk of rebound vasodilation (Stafford, 1990).

Antihistamines are not effective in the management of acute rhinosinusitis (Diaz and Bamberger, 1995). Anti-inflammatory topical corticosteroids may help maintain patency of the ostia. One controlled study was performed and showed that intranasal flunisolide spray improved the symptoms of nasal obstruction (Metzger et al., 1993). Treatment failure and recurrent infections are indications to use neuroimaging and endoscopy to search for a source of obstruction. Sinus sampling for culture should be considered. Endoscopic sinus surgery may be necessary to reopen and maintain the patency of the sinus ostia and ostiomeatal complex (Stafford, 1990).

Complications should be treated with high doses of intravenous antibiotics and, if appropriate, surgical drainage of any enclosed space. Methods of prevention include using a humidifier, treating the underlying causes of sinus obstruction (polyps, adenoid hypertrophy, tumors of the nasopharynx, and nasal obstruction from allergic rhinitis), and smoking cessation (Hilger, 1989).

Sphenoid rhinosinusitis without complication may be managed with high-dose intravenous antibiotics and topical and systemic decongestants for 24 hours (Kibblewhite et al., 1988; Goldman et al., 1993). If the fever (if present) and the headache do not start to improve, or if any complications are present or develop, sphenoid sinus drainage is indicated (Druce, 1990). Gilain et al. reviewed 12 cases of isolated sphenoid sinus disease secondary to chronic inflammatory rhinosinusitis in 7 patients, mucoceles in 2, aspergillus lesions in 2, and an isolated polyp in 1. All patients in this series were treated with functional endoscopic sphenoidotomy and improved. All were treated with appropriate postoperative antibiotics, nasal irrigation, oral corticosteroids, and washing and cleaning of the nasal cavity weekly for 4 weeks (Gilain et al., 1994).

Nasal Headache

Many rhinologists believe that septal deformation, especially of traumatic origin, may exert pressure on the sensitive structure of the lateral nasal wall, causing referred pain and "chronic headache." McAuliffe et al. (McAuliffe et al., 1943) studied the sensitivity of the nasal cavities and paranasal sinuses using touch, pressure, and faradic stimulation. The nasal turbinates and sinus ostia were much more sensitive than the mucosal lining of the septum and the paranasal sinuses. Most of the pain elicited was referred pain that was increased in intensity, longer in duration, and referred to larger areas in subjects who had swelling and engorgement of the nasal turbinates and the sinus ostia.

Schønsted-Madsen et al. (1986) followed 444 patients with nasal obstruction, 157 of whom had headache. Treatment consisted of septoplasty, reconstruction of the nasal pyramids, or submucosal conchotomy. The headache was usually localized to the forehead, glabella, or above and around the eyes. Thirty-six patients had constant headaches; 48 had daily headaches, 56 had weekly, and 17 had monthly headache. Fifty-seven patients had mild headache, 66 had moderate headache, and 34 had severe headache. Many of these patients misused analgesics. Eighty percent of the patients who underwent surgery were relieved of nasal obstruction (the primary reason for surgery), and 60% of the patients who underwent surgery were relieved of chronic headache. If the surgery relieved the nasal obstruction, 80% had headache relief; however, if the surgery failed, only 30% had headache relief.

Clerico reported 10 patients who had intractable migraine, tension-type headache, or cluster headache without significant nasal or sinus symptoms. Various intranasal and sinus abnormalities, such as anatomic variation or subclinical inflammation, were found on CT or nasal endoscopy. The patients were treated medically and/or surgically, and all improved (Clerico, 1995). Low and Willatt reported 106 patients who had a submucous resection for a deviated nasal septum. Almost half (47.4%) had recurring headaches preoperatively. Postoperatively, 63.6% had complete or partial relief at follow-up up to 18 months. Although 79.3% had headache relief when evaluated before 1 year, only 46.2% had relief after 1 year (Low and Willatt, 1995).

These studies do not account for the historical relationship between the onset of headache and the development of nasal obstruction, or for the overuse of analgesics or decongestants that may produce daily headache. In addition, any surgical procedure has a powerful placebo effect. It does suggest that a minority of patients with nasal obstruction have headache that is relieved by successful medical or surgical treatment. Because migraine prevalence in the population is approximately 12%, episodic tension-type headache prevalence approximately 90%, and chronic tension-type headache prevalence approximately 3%, these data are difficult to interpret. In addition, these studies had no control group, and only responders were reported in Clerico's study. In controlled trials of medication, the placebo effect can be quite large.

In a retrospective review of operative notes of 170 patients who underwent functional endoscopic sinus surgery, 50 patients (29%) who had a history of chronic headaches were identified. Thirty-seven met the predetermined inclusion criteria for this study: (1) history of chronic headaches, (2) rhinologic cause for these headaches suggested by the presence of contact points as documented by nasal endoscopy and/or CT scans, (3) no other obvious origin or cause of headaches discernible after a thorough evaluation, and (4) surgical intervention that included relief of contact points by inferior, middle, and/or superior turbinoplasty. Following surgery, 29 of the 34 patients in the study group (85%) reported a decrease in headache frequency. However, many patients had severe contact points on CT scan and did not complain of headaches. In fact, most patients with headaches and contact points also had concurrent chronic rhinosinusitis, which served as the primary indication for surgery in this patient population (Parsons and Batra, 1998).

Other open studies (Chow, 1994; Salman and Rebeiz, 1994) and a review (Close and Aviv, 1997) have suggested that headache can be the only clinical presentation of sinus or nasal pathology. These studies do not use IHS criteria for headache or the new diagnostic criteria for rhinosinusitis. With the common involvement of the sinuses on CT with no symptoms of rhinosinusitis, it is very difficult to comment favorably on these open trials.

References

Agency for Health Care Policy and Research (1999). Diagnosis and treatment of acute bacterial rhinosinusitis. Summary. *Evid Rep Technol Assess (Summ)*, 9:1–5.

Anon, JB (2004). Treatment of acute bacterial rhinosinusitis caused by antimicrobial-resistant *Streptococcus pneumoniae*. *Am J Med*, 117(Suppl. 3A):23S–28S.

Axelsson, A, Grebelius, N, Chidekel, N, et al. (1970). The correlation between the radiological examination and the irrigation findings in maxillary sinusitis. *Acta Otolaryngol*, 69:302–306.

Bellamy, JL, Cady, RK, and Durham, PL (2006). Salivary levels of CGRP and VIP in rhinosinusitis and migraine patients. *Headache*, 46:24–33.

Benninger, MS, Anon, J, and Mabry, RL (1997). The medical management of rhinosinusitis (Review). Report of the Rhinosinusitis Task Force Committee Meeting. *Otolaryngol Head Neck Surg*, 117:S41–S49.

Berg, O and Carenfelt, C (1988). Analysis of symptoms and clinical signs in the maxillary sinus empyema. *Acta Otolaryngol*, 105:343–349.

Bhattacharyya, N (1999). Test-retest reliability of computed tomography in the assessment of chronic rhinosinusitis. *Laryngoscope*, 109:1055–1058.

Brook, I, Overturf, GD, Steinberg, EA, et al. (1982). Acute sphenoid sinusitis presenting as aseptic meningitis: a pachymeningitis syndrome. *Int J Pediatr Otorhinolaryngol*, 4:77–81.

Cady, RK and Schreiber, CP (2002). Sinus headache or migraine? Considerations in making a differential diagnosis. *Neurology*, 58:S10–S14.

Caldwell, GW (1893). The accessory sinuses of the nose: an improved method of treatment for suppuration of the maxillary antrum. *NY Med J*, 58:526.

Calhoun, KH, Waggnespack, GA, Simpson, CB, et al. (1991). CT evaluation of the paranasal sinuses in symptomatic and asymptomatic populations. *Otolaryngol Head Neck Surg*, 104:480–483.

Chow, JM (1994). Rhinologic headaches. *Otolaryngol Head Neck Surg*, 111:211–218.

Clerico, DM (1995). Sinus headaches reconsidered: referred cephalgia of rhinologic origin masquerading as refractory primary headaches. *Headache*, 35:185–192.

Close, LG and Aviv, J (1997). Headaches and disease of the nose and paranasal sinuses. *Sem Neurol*, 17:351–354.

Collins, JG (1997). Prevalence of selected chronic conditions. *Vital Health. Stat*, 10(194):1–89.

Dale, BAB and Mackenzie, IJ (1983). The complications of sphenoid sinusitis. *J Laryngol Otol*, 97:661–670.

Deans, JAJ and Welch, AR (1991). Acute isolated sphenoid sinusitis: a disease with complications. *J Laryngol Otol*, 105:1072–1074.

Diaz, I and Bamberger, DM (1995). Acute sinusitis. *Sem Res Inf*, 10:14–20.

Druce, HM (1990). Adjuncts to medical management of sinusitis. *Otolaryngol Head Neck Surg*, 103:880–883.

Druce, HM and Siavin, RG (1991). Sinusitis: a critical need for further study. *J Allergy Clin Immunol*, 88:675–677.

Dykewicz, MS (2003). Allergic disorders: rhinitis and sinusitis. *J Allergy Clin Immunol*, 111:S520–S529

Engquist, S, Lundberg, C, and Venge, P (1983). Effects of drainage in the treatment of acute maxillary sinusitis. *Acta Otolaryngol*, 95:153–159.

Eross, EJ, Dodick, DW, and Eross, MD (2004). The sinus, allergy and migraine study (SAMS). *Headache*, 44:462 (Abstract).

Evans, K (1994). Diagnosis and management of sinusitis. *Br Med J*, 309:1415–1422.

Evans, KL (1998). Recognition and management of sinusitis. *Drugs*, 56:59–71.

Faleck, H, Rothner, AD, Erenberg, G, et al. (1988). Headache and subacute sinusitis in children and adolescents. *Headache*, 28:96–98.

Fergusen, BJ and Mabry, R (1997). Laboratory diagnosis. *Otolaryngol Head Neck Surg*, 117:S12–S26.

Gallagher, RM, Cross, CW, and Phillips, CD (1998). Suppurative intracranial complications of sinusitis. *Laryngoscope*, 108:1635–1642.

Gilain, L, Aidan, D, Coste, A, et al. (1994). Functional endoscopic sinus surgery for isolated sphenoid sinus disease. *Head Neck*, 16:433–437.

Goldman, GE, Fontanarosa, PB, and Anderson, JM (1993). Isolated sphenoid sinusitis. *Am J Emerg Med*, 11:235–238.

Goss, CM (1959). *Gray's Anatomy of the Human Body*. Lea & Febiger, Philadelphia.

Gwaltney, JM, Phillips, CD, Miller, RD, et al. (1994). Computed tomographic study of the common cold. *N Eng J Med*, 330:25–30.

Hajek, M (1926). *Pathology and Treatment of Inflammatory Diseases of the Nasal Accessory Sinuses*. The C.V. Mosby Company, St. Louis.

Hansen, JG, Schmidt, H, Rosborg, J, et al. (1995). Predicting acute maxillary sinusitis in a general practice population. *BMJ*, 311:233–236.

Havas, TE, Motbey, JA, and Gullane, PJ (1988). Prevalence of incidental abnormalities on computed tomographic scans of the paranasal sinuses. *Arch Otolaryngol*, 114:856–859.

Headache Classification Committee (2004). The International Classification of Headache Disorders (2nd Edn). *Cephalalgia*, 24:1–160.

Hilding, AC (1950). Physiologic basis of nasal operations. *Calif Med*, 72:103–107.

Hilger, PA (1989). Diseases of the nose. In *Boie's Fundamentals of Otolaryngology: A Textbook of Ear, Nose, and Throat Disease* (PA Hilger, ed.), pp. 206–248. WB Saunders, Philadelphia.

International Rhinosinusitis Advisory Board (1997). Infectious rhinosinusitis in adults: classification, etiology, and management. *Ear Nose Throat J*, 76: S5–S22.

Jeney, EV, Raphael, GD, Meredith, SD, et al. (1990). Abnormal cholinergic responsiveness in the nasal muscosa of patients with recurrent sinusitis. *J Allergy Clin Immunol*, 86:8–10.

Josephson, GD and Gross, CW (1997). Diagnosis and management of acute and chronic sinusitis. *Comprehensive Therapy*, 23:708–714.

Kennedy, DW (1990a). Overview. *Otolaryngol Head Neck Surg*, 103:847–854.

Kennedy, DW (1990b). Surgical update. *Otolaryngol Head Neck Surg*, 103:884–886.

Kibblewhite, DJ, Cleland, J, and Mintz, DR (1988). Acute sphenoid sinusitis: management strategies. *J Otolaryngol*, 17:159–163.

Lang J, Haas A (1998) The sagittal dimension of the sinus frontalis, its wall thickness, distance from the lamina cribrosa, the depth of the so-called olfactory groove and the ethmoidal canal, *Gegenbaurs Morphol Jahrb*, 134(4):459–469.

Lanza, DC and Kennedy, DW (1997). Adult rhinosinusitis defined. *Otolaryngol Head Neck Surg*, 117:S1–S7

Lawson, W and Reino, AJ (1997). Isolated sphenoid sinus disease: an analysis of 132 cases. *Laryngoscope*, 107:1590–1595.

Levine, HL, Setzen, M, Cady, RK, et al. (2006). An otolaryngology, neurology, allergy, and primary care consensus on diagnosis and treatment of sinus headache. *Otolaryngol Head Neck Surg*, 134:516–523.

Lew, D, Southwick, FS, Montgomery, WW, et al. (1983). Sphenoid sinusitis: a review of 30 cases. *N Engl J Med*, 19:1149–1154.

Lipton, RB, Stewart, WF, and Liberman, JN (2002). Self-awareness of migraine: interpreting the labels that headache sufferers apply to their headaches. *Neurology*, 58:S21–S26.

Lloyd, GA, Lund, VJ, and Scadding, GK (1991). CT of the paranasal sinuses and functional endoscopic surgery: a critical analysis of 100 symptomatic patients. *J Laryngol Otol*, 105:181–185.

Low, WK and Willatt, DJ (1995). Headaches associated with nasal obstruction due to deviated nasal septum. *Headache*, 35:404–406.

Lund, VJ and Mackay, IS (1993). Staging in rhinosinusitus. *Rhinology*, 31:183–184.

McAuliffe, GW, Goodell, H, and Wolff, HG (1943). Experimental studies on headache: pain from the nasal and paranasal structures. *Res Publ Assoc Res Nerv Ment Dis*, 23:185–206.

McCaffrey, TV (1993). Functional endoscopic sinus surgery: an overview. *Mayo Clin Proc*, 68:675–677.

Meltzer, EO, Hamilos, DL, Hadley, JA, et al. (2004). Rhinosinusitis: establishing definitions for clinical research and patient care. *Otolaryngol Head Neck Surg*, 131:S1–S62.

Messerklinger, W (1978). *Endoscopy of the nose*. Urban and Schwartzenberg, Baltimore.

Metzger, EO, Orgel, HA, Backhaus, JW, et al. (1993). Intranasal flunisolide spray as an adjunct to roal antibiotic therapy for sinusitis. *J Allergy Clin Immunol*, 92:812–823.

Moss, AJ and Parsons, VL.(1986). Current estimates from the National Health Interview Survey. United States 1985. Vital Health Stat.10(160):i–iv, 1–182.

Muntz, HR and Lusk, RP (1992). Signs and symptoms of chronic sinusitis. *In Pediatric Sinusitis* (RP Lusk, ed.), pp. 1–6. Raven Press Ltd, New York.

Naranch, K, Park, YJ, Ramirez, MR, et al. (2002). A tender sinus does not always mean rhinosinusitis. *Otolaryngol Head Neck Surg*, 127:387–397.

Nordeman, L and Lucid, E (1990). Sphenoid sinusitis, a cause of debilitating headache. *J Emerg Med*, 8:557–559.

Oktedalen, O and Lilleas, F (1992). Septic complications to sphenoidal sinus infection. *Scand J Infect Dis*, 24:353–356.

Parsons, DS and Batra, PS (1998). Functional endoscopic sinus surgical outcomes for contact point headaches. *Laryngoscope*, 108:696–702.

Perry, BF, Login, IS, and Kountakis, SE (2004). Nonrhinologic headache in a tertiary rhinology practice. *Otolaryngol Head Neck Surg*, 130:449–452.

Piccirillo, JF (2004a). Acute bacterial sinus infections are frequently overdiagnosed. *N Engl J Med*, 351:902–910.

Piccirillo, JF (2004b). Clinical practice. Acute bacterial sinusitis. *N Engl J Med*, 351:902–910.

Ray, NF, Baraniuk, JN, Thamer, M, et al. (1999). Healthcare expenditures for sinusitis in 1996: contributions of asthma, rhinitis, and other airway disorders. *J Allergy Clin Immunol*, 103:408–414.

Reilly, JS (1990). The sinusitis cycle. *Otolaryngol Head Neck Surg*, 103:856–862.

Rouby, J, Laurent, P, Gosnach, M, et al. (1994). Risk factors and clinical relevance of nosocomial maxillary sinusitis in the critically ill. *Am J Resp Crit Care Med*, 150:776–783.

Salman, SD and Rebeiz, EE (1994). Sinusitis and headache. *J Med Libanais*, 42:200–202.

Saunte, C and Soyka, D (1993). Headache related to ear, nose, and sinus disorders. In *The headaches* (J Olesen, P Tfelt-Hansen, KMA Welch, eds), pp. 753–757, Raven Press, New York.

Schaefer SD, Close LG 1990 Endoscopic management of frontal sinus disease. *Laryngoscope*, 100(2 Pt 1):155–160.

Schatz, CJ and Becker, TS (1984). Normal CT anatomy of the paranasal sinuses. *Radiol Clin North Am*, 22:107–118.

Schønsted-Madsen, U, Stoksted, P, Christensen, PH, et al. (1986). Chronic headache related to nasal obstruction. *J Laryngol Otol*, 100:165–170.

Schreiber, CP, Hutchinson, S, Webster, CJ, et al. (2004). Prevalence of migraine in patients with a history of self-reported or physician-diagnosed "sinus" headache. *Arch Intern Med*, 164:1769–1772.

Shapiro, GG and Rachelefsky, GS (1992). Introduction and definition of sinusitis. *J Allergy Clin Immunol*, 90:417–418.

Shields, G, Seikaly, H, LeBoeuf, M, et al. (2003). Correlation between facial pain or headache and computed tomography in rhinosinusitis in Canadian and U.S. subjects. *Laryngoscope*, 113:943–945.

Singh, B, VanDellen, J, Ramjettan, S, (1995). Sinogenic intracranial complications. *J Laryngol Otol*, 109:945–950.

Slavin, RG (1997). Nasal polyps and sinusitis. *JAMA*, 278:1849–1854.

Sofferman, RA (1983). Cavernous sinus thrombophlebitis secondary to sphenoid sinusitis. *Laryngoscope*, 93:797–800.

Stafford, CT (1990). The clinician's view of sinusitis. *Otolaryngol Head Neck Surg*, 103:870–875.

Turkewitz, D and Keller, R (1987). Acute headache in childhood: a case of sphenoid sinusitis. *Pediatr Emerg Care*, 3:155–157.

Urquhart, AC, Fung, G, and McIntosh, WA (1989). Isolated sphenoiditis: a diagnostic problem. *J Laryngol Otol*, 103:526–527.

VanCauwenberge, PB, Ingels, KJ, Bachert, CL, et al. (1997). Microbiology of chronic sinusitis. *Acta Otorhinolaryngol Belg*, 51:239–246.

Wagner, W (1996). Changing diagnostic and treatment strategies for chronic sinusitis. *Cleve Clin J Med*, 63:396–405.

Williams, JW, Simel, DL, Roberts, L, et al. (1992). Clinical evaluation of sinusitis. *Ann Intern Med*, 117:705–710.

Wolff, HG (1948). *Wolff's Headache and Other Head Pain*. Oxford University Press, New York.

Zinreich, SJ (1990). Paranasal sinus imaging. *Otolaryngol Head Neck Surg*, 103:863–869.

25 Cranial Neuralgias and Other Causes of Facial Pain

Todd D Rozen and David J Capobianco

TRIGEMINAL NEURALGIA

Trigeminal neuralgia is a distinctive, painful disorder of the face that is easily evoked by trivial stimuli and undergoes a relapsing, remitting course. There are approximately 15,000 new cases of trigeminal neuralgia per year. It is a disorder of the elderly, and often cause severe disability. It is characterized by brief electric shock-like pain and is limited to one or more divisions of the trigeminal nerve. Patients who have experienced this disorder are often fearful that, while in a pain remission period, the attacks will recur. Trigeminal neuralgia can be treated both medically and surgically. The epidemiology, diagnostic criteria, and pathophysiology of trigeminal neuralgia will be reviewed, and a stepwise approach to treatment will be discussed.

Epidemiology

In 1968, Penman (1968) estimated the annual prevalence of trigeminal neuralgia to be 4.7 per 1 million men and 7.2 per 1 million women. In 1966, Brewis and colleagues found an annual incidence rate of 2.1 cases per 100,000 individuals from only 10 cases reported between 1955 and 1961, in Carlisle, England (Brewis et al., 1966). Three incidence studies have been reported from Rochester, Minnesota. Kurland examined the time period of 1945 through 1956 and found four new cases per 100,000 population per year (Kurland, 1958). Yoshimasu et al. (1972) studied the time period of 1945 through 1969 and found four new cases per 100,000 population per year (5/100,000 women per year and 2.7/100,000 men per year). Katusic et al.'s (1990) study from 1945 through 1984, found 4.3 new cases per 100,000 population per year, with a gender distribution of 5.9 cases per 100,000 population in women and 3.4 new cases per 100,000 population in men. Extrapolating the Rochester, Minnesota data to the United States population suggests an annual incidence of 15,000 new cases per year.

The peak incidence of idiopathic trigeminal neuralgia occurs in the fifth to seventh decade, with 90% of cases beginning after the age of 40. The gender distribution is uneven with a female predominance (1.5 female cases to every 1 male case). The gender ratio varies in different studied populations, from 1.8:1 in the Rochester, Minnesota population to 1.17:1 in a Massachusetts hospitalized population of 526 patients (Rothman and Monson, 1973).

Familial cases of trigeminal neuralgia are very rare but have been reported. Harris (1926) found nine members of the same family with trigeminal neuralgia. Yoshimasu et al. (1972) found 1 of 36 patients with a family history of trigeminal neuralgia. Pollack et al. (1988) identified 33 cases of hereditary trigeminal neuralgia in 699 patients. Katusic et al. (1990) found 4 of 75 patients with a family history of trigeminal neuralgia. In these familial cases, trigeminal neuralgia presented earlier in each successive generation. Duff et al. (1999) identified a family with trigeminal neuralgia and contralateral hemifacial spasm. The transmission of trigeminal neuralgia in this family suggested an autosomal dominant inheritance.

Clinical Characteristics

The pain of trigeminal neuralgia is a sharp, shooting, electric shock-like sensation. It is extremely severe, with usual maximum intensity without latency. The pain typically lasts seconds, although it can last up to 2 minutes. Multiple attacks may occur daily, for weeks or months at a time. Most individuals have short periods of pain-free time in-between spikes of pain, but they may have difficulty detecting this remission and often state that their pain is constant. Others have continuous interictal pain, which is dull, burning, or throbbing in quality. These individuals may have a worse prognosis for successful treatment than those without interictal pain. Szapiro et al. (1985) found that microvascular decompression was less successful in individuals who had a dull ache in between trigeminal neuralgia attacks than in individuals without interictal pain; 95% without paroxysmal pain did well compared to 58% with interictal pain. Jassim (1994) completed a 3-year prospective study of individuals with interictal pain before they underwent radiofrequency (RF) thermocoagulation. He found that these patients continued to have background pain and more side effects after RF than those patients who had pain-free intervals between their trigeminal neuralgia attacks.

Trigeminal neuralgia pain occurs in the distribution of the trigeminal nerve. White and Sweet (1969a) completed a literature review search of 8124 patients and found that 61% had right-sided attacks and 36% had left-sided attacks. Most individuals experience the pain in the maxillary and mandibular divisions of the trigeminal nerve. It occurs much less frequent in the ophthalmic division (Table 25–1). Only 4% of trigeminal neuralgia cases are bilateral, and most of those individuals have underlying multiple sclerosis. Trigeminal neuralgia never spreads across the midline and bilateral cases are never synchronous. Trigeminal neuralgia is a paroxysmal disorder with a relapsing or remitting course. More than 50% of individuals will have at least a 6-month remission during their lifetime and 24% will have a 12-month remission (Rushton and MacDonald, 1957).

TABLE 25–1 Pain Distribution in Trigeminal Neuralgia.

V_1 alone	4%
V_2 alone	17%
V_3 alone	15%
$V_2 + V_3$	32%
$V_1 + V_2$	14%
$V_1 + V_2 + V_3$	17%

Trigeminal neuralgia attacks can be triggered by trivial stimuli. The slightest touch, even the movement of a single fine hair, can trigger a volley of pain, as can cold air, chewing, talking, facial movement, brushing of teeth, and emotional distress. Rare triggers include auditory stimuli, acute infection, and trauma. Touch and vibration appear to trigger more attacks than pinprick. In approximately 50% of trigeminal neuralgia sufferers, attacks can be triggered by non-noxious stimuli touching small areas around the face, nose, and lips. These "trigger zones" can be as small as 1–2 mm in diameter. The pain intensity that is elicited is independent of the trigger zone size. In most patients, the pain will start within the trigger zone, but in 5%–9% of patients the pain occurs outside of it. Most individuals have a refractory period (a time after the stimulation of a trigger zone) during which restimulation will not elicit an attack of trigeminal neuralgia. The length of the refractory period is proportional to the duration and severity of the prior painful attack.

A patient experiencing a trigeminal neuralgia attack typically freezes in place with the hands slowly rising to the area of pain on the face but not touching it. The patient then grimaces or contorts the face in a tic (tic douloureux) and then either remains in this position or cries out in pain.

Diagnosis and Testing

The International Classification of Headache Disorders 2nd Edition (2004) have established diagnostic criteria for classical and symptomatic trigeminal neuralgia (Table 25–2). Classical trigeminal neuralgia is diagnosed by its clinical presentation and an examination that is normal except for the presence of trigger zones. Fifteen to twenty-five percent of individuals exhibit a sensory loss on examination; however, this is hardly ever recognized by the patient. Most physicians feel that one must investigate for symptomatic or secondary trigeminal neuralgia if sensory loss is noted on examination. The most common underlying secondary causes of trigeminal neuralgia include multiple sclerosis, basilar artery aneurysm, neoplasm (epidermoid, acoustic neuroma, meningioma, trigeminal neuroma), arterial or venous compression, syringobulbia, and brainstem infarction. Other authorities believe that sensory

TABLE 25–2 Trigeminal Neuralgia.

13.1.1 Classical Trigeminal Neuralgia

Diagnostic criteria

A. Paroxysmal attacks of pain lasting from a fraction of a second to 2 minutes, affecting one or more divisions of the trigeminal nerve and fulfilling criteria B and C
B. Pain has at least one of the following characteristics
   1. Intense, sharp, superficial or stabbing
   2. Precipitated from trigger areas or by trigger factors
C. Attacks are stereotyped in the individual patient
D. There is no clinically evident neurological deficit
E. Not attributed to another disease

13.1.2 Symptomatic Trigeminal Neuralgia

Diagnostic criteria

A. Paroxysmal attacks of pain lasting from a fraction of a second to 2 minutes, affecting one or more divisions of the trigeminal nerve and fulfilling criteria B and C
B. Pain has at least one of the following characteristics
   1. Intense, sharp, superficial or stabbing
   2. Precipitated from trigger areas or by trigger factors
C. Attacks are stereotyped in the individual patient
D. A causative lesion, other than vascular compression, has been demonstrated by special investigations and/or posterior fossa exploration

loss is not abnormal unless it is marked and progressive. Most who find sensory loss on examination will have the patient undergo neuroimaging, specifically a magnetic resonance imaging (MRI) study to rule out underlying pathologic process. MRI can also visualize neurovascular contacts, while MR angiography (MRA) can establish the true relationship between nerve and vessel. The probability that a surgical procedure, such as microvascular decompression, will be beneficial to the patient is enhanced if MRI/MRA discloses a vascular loop compressing the trigeminal nerve at the root entry zone. Majoie et al. (2000) assessed the diagnostic yield of MRI in patients who had symptoms and signs related to the trigeminal nerve. A normal examination and trigeminal neuralgia symptoms alone were highly correlated with a negative MRI study. Impaired sensation, subjective feelings of facial numbness, other positive neurologic signs and symptoms, progression of symptoms and signs, and symptoms that had been present for less than 1 year correlated with an abnormal MRI. Akimoto et al. (2002) looked at the value of three-dimensional (3D) images reconstructed from two types of high-resolution MR studies (3D-CISS and 3D-FISP) for the visualization of neurovascular contacts in patients with trigeminal neuralgia. Twenty-four individuals underwent preoperative 3D-FISP and 3D-CISS imaging. Three-dimensional reconstruction of nerves and vessels was performed with the use of a volume-rendering method. Surgical findings were correlated with the findings documented on 3D imaging. The authors found that 3D-CISS and 3D-FISP images readily showed the spatial relationship between trigeminal nerve and compressive vessel. The responsible arteries could be identified from the 3D reconstructed images, and this closely simulated the intraoperative findings.

Anderson et al. (2006) assessed the value of high-resolution 3D time-of-flight (TOF) MRA and gadolinium (Gad)-enhanced 3D spoiled gradient-recalled imaging in the visualization of neurovascular compression in patients with trigeminal neuralgia. Forty-eight patients with one-sided trigeminal neuralgia were studied. All patients then underwent microvascular decompression surgery. Results from the neuroimaging studies were compared with interoperative findings. MR angiography in combination with 3D Gad imaging identified surgically verified neurovascular contact in 42 of 46 (91%) symptomatic nerves. The offending vessel was correctly identified in 31 of 41 cases. The authors concluded that double-blind assessment of surgical and neuroradiological findings confirms that neurovascular compression can be visualized with good sensitivity in patients with trigeminal neuralgia by 3D TOF MRA in combination with Gad-enhanced 3D spoiled gradient-recalled sequences.

Trigeminal evoked potentials may also be a valuable diagnostic aid in the search for underlying compressive lesions of the trigeminal nerve. Sundaram et al. (1999) demonstrated abnormal trigeminal evoked potentials in all patients with trigeminal neuralgia resulting from known intracranial mass lesions, suggesting that trigeminal evoked potentials should be considered in the normal workup of patients who have trigeminal neuralgia and negative MRI. If the evoked potential responses are abnormal, then nerve compression is still the most likely cause of the patient's trigeminal neuralgia symptoms. Trigeminal evoked potentials may also be useful to predict recovery of nerve function after pain-relieving techniques, such as microvascular decompression. Leandri et al. (1998) examined 10 trigeminal neuralgia patients who had MRI- and MRA-documented neurovascular contact. Immediate recovery of pre-procedure abnormal trigeminal evoked potentials after decompression suggested recovery of nerve function and a good clinical outcome.

Pathogenesis

The true cause of trigeminal neuralgia is unknown. It is believed that both peripheral and central neuronal dysfunction play an important role. It has been suggested that chronic focal demyelination secondary to irritation of the trigeminal nerve at the root entry zone (usually caused by vascular compression) leads to increased firing rates in trigeminal primary afferents, as well as impairment of the efficacy of the inhibitory mechanisms in the trigeminal brainstem complex, which normally controls this level of activity. This leads to a greater than normal excitability of the trigeminal brainstem complex which then responds to tactile stimuli as it typically would noxious stimuli. Fromm (1991) suggested that in this setting there is increased paroxysmal firing of wide dynamic range (WDR) neurons, which are typically excited by noxious and non-noxious stimuli in the trigeminal nucleus caudalis, as well as hypersensitivity of low threshold mechanoreceptors (LTMs) in the trigeminal nucleus oralis. The LTM neurons become hyperactive and start to fire at rates normally seen with noxious stimuli, resulting in paroxysmal trigeminal neuralgia. Hyperactivity of both LTM and WDR neurons may explain why both noxious and non-noxious stimuli trigger trigeminal neuralgia attacks. Raskin (1988) remarked that several features of trigeminal neuralgia suggest a centrally mediated process. These include the presence of refractory, continued volleys of pain after nerve stimulation and the central action of all medicines that are successful in treating trigeminal neuralgia.

Elevated levels of vasoactive intestinal peptide (VIP) have been found in patients undergoing an attack of trigeminal neuralgia. Zhao et al. (2002) documented raised levels of VIP in blood taken from the external jugular vein of 16 individuals having an attack of trigeminal neuralgia. The authors suggested that VIP maybe playing a role in induction of trigeminal neuralgia attacks by enhancing the effects of substance P in localized neurogenic inflammation. Cranial parasympathetic fibers contain VIP suggesting that there is some parasympathetic activation during trigeminal neuralgia attacks. VIP levels are also elevated during a cluster headache and chronic paroxysmal hemicrania (CPH) both of which are short-lasting headache syndromes marked by severe pain and associated autonomic symptoms (Goadsby and Edvinsson, 1994). Autonomic symptoms, specifically signs of parasympathetic activation are not thought to be part of the trigeminal neuralgia symptom complex. Pareja et al. (2002) evaluated a total of 26 episodes of V-1 distribution trigeminal neuralgia attacks in two female patients. Mild lacrimation without conjunctival injection, rhinorrhea or ptosis was observed, even with long-lasting attacks. As this study suggests a relative lack of autonomic symptoms in trigeminal neuralgia versus cluster headache and CPH it would be interesting to compare VIP levels in these three syndromes. One would expect much higher VIP levels during attacks of cluster headache and CPH than during an attack of trigeminal neuralgia based on the clinical presentation of these distinct disorders.

Finally in a number of reported idiopathic trigeminal neuralgia cases, vessel compression of the trigeminal nerve is noted on either imaging or with surgical evaluation. A recent study looked at the size of the cerebellopontine cistern to see if trigeminal neuralgia patients may be predisposed to nerve/vessel contact because of their cranial anatomy (Rasche, et al., 2006). Twenty-five patients with unilateral trigeminal neuralgia and seventeen controls were studied using a high-resolution 1.5-T MRI of the parapontine region and the trigeminal nerve. The volume of the pontomesencephalic cistern was calculated using a standardized method. In patients with trigeminal neuralgia, the mean difference of the volume of the affected and opposite side was 13%. In all trigeminal neuralgia patients, a significantly smaller volume of the cistern was found on the affected side ($p < 0.01$). Controls did not show this difference in volumes. Thus, the authors have suggested that a smaller cistern may be correlated with the occurrence of neurovascular compression in trigeminal neuralgia patients.

Treatment

Both medical and surgical modalities may be used to treat trigeminal neuralgia. Patients are typically started with drug treatment. Drug therapy for trigeminal neuralgia dates back to the 1600s when purgatives were used, but it was not until the 1940s, when phenytoin was first utilized for trigeminal neuralgia, an effective therapy was available. Other important dates in the history of medical treatment for trigeminal neuralgia are 1962 (carbamazepine), 1976 (clonazepam), and 1980 (baclofen). New treatments are continually being tried for trigeminal neuralgia because most drugs have very low success rates and prevalent side effects. The drugs, which are currently being utilized for the treatment of trigeminal neuralgia, will be discussed separately, with comments on mechanisms of action, pharmacokinetics, dosing strategies, and studies.

Carbamazepine

Carbamazepine is recognized as the best available drug for the tic of trigeminal neuralgia and is the first-line agent used by most physicians. Its proposed mechanism of action is decreasing the response of trigeminal mechanoreceptive neurons to peripheral stimulation. Carbamazepine has several important pharmacokinetic properties that make it unique. Since it causes its own induction of metabolism, a therapeutic level may not be maintained if the patient stays on the same dose of carbamazepine. It is important to allow at least 20 days for metabolism autoinduction to occur before looking at a maintenance dose for carbamazepine. A serum concentration range of 24–43 μmol/l is targeted. The half-life of carbamazepine also changes over time. Initially, it is between 20 and 40 hours, but with chronic dosing it is between 11 and 27 hours. This unrecognized pharmacokinetic change may explain why the drug becomes less effective if a constant dose is maintained. Counteracting these half-life changes by altering dose frequency could lead to less failure with chronic carbamazepine therapy.

To avoid neurotoxicity, carbamazepine should be started at a low dose (100 mg one to two times a day). The dose can be increased by 100–200 mg every 3 days until pain relief is achieved. The usual maintenance dose is between 400 and 800 mg a day; most patients remain on less than 1200 mg a day, although some need a dose of 1500 mg a day or more. If the dose is below 800 mg a day, carbamazepine can be given twice daily, however, a dose that is above 800 mg a day must be given three to four times a day.

Adequately treated trigeminal neuralgia sufferers will not know if they are in an active phase or in remission. Pain-free patients should have their medications tapered to avoid unneeded treatment exposure and to avoid neurotoxicity. It is helpful for patients to maintain pain calendars to demonstrate changes in pain pattern (intensity or frequency). When individuals have been pain-free for 4–6 weeks carbamazepine may be tapered. This should be done slowly, by 100 mg every 3–7 days. If pain paroxysms return, the dose can be increased, but to the smallest pain-relieving level.

Drowsiness is a common initial side effect of carbamazepine; it usually abates after several days. Daytime drowsiness can be minimized by giving larger doses at bedtime. This schedule may have the added benefit of being more therapeutic to the patient, as it provides higher morning drug serum concentrations, and most attacks of trigeminal neuralgia occur in the morning. Other side effects include dizziness, nausea, vomiting, nystagmus, ataxia, and diplopia. Carbamazepine may activate latent psychosis and cause agitation in the elderly. Hematologic side effects occur in 2%–6% of patients and include leukopenia and aplastic anemia. A complete blood count is recommended every 2 weeks for the first 2 months of therapy. In addition, liver and renal function tests should be completed before starting the drug, 2 weeks into dosing, and then at 8–12 week intervals. Leukopenia, which resolves spontaneously in 10% of patients may develop. If this occurs, discontinuation of the drug or blood count monitoring at 2-week intervals is mandatory. Maintaining the same carbamazepine dose for several days will usually alleviate minor central nervous system (CNS) side effects.

Carbamazepine is highly effective. It delivers pain relief in up to 80% of individuals, both initially and short-term. Relief occurs within several hours to several days after starting the drug; 94% of patients experience pain relief within 48 hours (Zakrzewska, 1955a). Over time, however, fewer responders continue to have sustained relief. Taylor et al. (1981) followed patients for 16 years and found that although 69% of patients had initial benefit, carbamazepine was only effective in 56% by the end of the study. Approximately 5%–19% of individuals are carbamazepine-intolerant.

Phenytoin

Phenytoin was the first effective drug for trigeminal neuralgia but is now a second- or third-line agent. Its proposed mechanism of action is depression of the response of spinal trigeminal neurons to maxillary nerve stimulation. Pharmacokinetically, phenytoin follows zero-order kinetics, so a small increase in dosage can lead to a rapid rise in plasma levels and a heightened risk of neurotoxicity.

The starting dose of phenytoin is 200 mg a day. The usual total target dose is between 300 and 500 mg a day given in 3 divided doses. Phenytoin, in its parenteral form, can be utilized as acute therapy for trigeminal neuralgia in the emergency department. Two-hundred-fifty milligrams of phenytoin given intravenously over 5 minutes can abort a trigeminal neuralgia attack immediately and the pain relief may last from 4 hours to 3 days (Raskin, 1988). Studies utilizing fosphenytoin in the same manner have not been undertaken.

Side effects of phenytoin include gum hyperplasia, hirsutism, depression, and impaired memory. Co-administered carbamazepine can raise serum phenytoin concentrations, while phenytoin can decrease the half-life of carbamazepine.

In most individuals, pain improves within 24–48 hours after phenytoin administration. Initial effectiveness is up to 60% (Zakrzewska, 1955a). There is no good comparison data with other medicinal therapies in the literature. Phenytoin's effectiveness decreases over time with less than 30% of patients responding after 2 years.

Baclofen

Baclofen is a γ-aminobutyric acid (GABA) analog that can be used alone or in combination with phenytoin or carbamazepine. Its proposed mechanism of action is suppression of the response of spinal trigeminal neurons to maxillary nerve stimulation. Oral baclofen has rapid gastrointestinal absorption, with peak serum concentrations occurring within 3–8 hours. Baclofen has a very short serum half-life so a multiple daily-dosing regime is required to maintain serum concentrations. Baclofen is excreted via the kidneys.

As monotherapy, baclofen is started at 5–10 mg three times a day. The dose can be increased by 5–10 mg every other day until pain is relieved. The normal maintenance dose is between 50 and 60 mg a day in 4–6 divided doses. The typical maximum tolerated dose is 80 mg a day. Because of baclofen's short half-life, additional doses should be interspersed between previous doses. When a patient is pain-free baclofen must be tapered gradually; hallucinations, anxiety, and seizures may develop if it is tapered too quickly. Baclofen should be tapered by no more than 5–10 mg a week.

When baclofen is combined with other medication, the dosage of each drug needed for pain relief is often lower than what was needed as monotherapy. If baclofen is added to carbamazepine, the carbamazepine dose should be reduced to 600 mg a day and baclofen added at its normal dosing schedule (5–10 mg three times a day, with 5–10 mg increasing increments every other day). If baclofen is added to phenytoin, the phenytoin dose should be reduced to 300 mg a day and baclofen started at its normal dosing schedule.

The most common side effects of baclofen include drowsiness, dizziness, and gastrointestinal discomfort. Approximately 10% of patients cannot tolerate the drug.

Other Agents

Clonazepam Clonazepam was studied by Court and Kase (1976) who found it to be effective in 65% of individuals with trigeminal neuralgia. Sixteen of these patients were carbamazepine nonresponders and, of these, eight did well on clonazepam. Even though a number of patients had good pain relief on clonazepam at a 6–8 mg dose, 85% experienced ataxia or dizziness. Clonazepam should be started at an initial dose of 0.25–0.5 mg three times a day and increased by 0.25–0.5 mg every 3–5 days until pain relief is obtained. The normal therapeutic dosing range is between 1.5 and 8 mg a day. Side effects include drowsiness, fatigue, and dizziness, which can be decreased by dividing the dosing schedule.

Valproic Acid Valproic acid was studied by Peiris et al. (1980), in an open-label study using 600–1200 mg a day. Thirteen of twenty patients had a good response (six became pain-free and three had a greater than 50% reduction in pain). Four responders required combination therapy to achieve pain relief. The initial dose of valproic acid is 250–500 mg a day, increasing by 125–250 mg a week, up to 1500 mg a day, or higher if tolerated. Valproic acid is given two to three times a day. One of valproic acid's problems is that it may take weeks to see a response. Valproic acid in the form of divalproex sodium may be better tolerated.

Lamotrigine Lamotrigine, a sodium channel modulator, is a new oral agent for trigeminal neuralgia. Zakrzewska (1997) studied 14 patients using lamotrigine as an add-on therapy to carbamazepine or phenytoin. Eleven of thirteen patients had better efficacy on lamotrigine than on placebo. Pain relief usually began within 24 hours of finding a therapeutic dose. The normal pain-relieving dose was 400 mg a day. The Zakrzewska study (1997) was a very short trial, lasting for only 2 weeks, so the long-term efficacy of lamotrigine could not be ascertained. Lunardi et al. (1997) utilized lamotrigine as monotherapy for trigeminal neuralgia with a 3–8 months follow-up time. Eleven of fifteen patients had an excellent response on 150 to 250 mg a day. Eight patients became pain-free on lamotrigine. Lamotrigine should be started at 25 mg a day and the dose increased to 25 mg every seventh day, up to 400 mg a day. A faster increase can lead to a drug-induced rash. Individuals respond between 150 and 400 mg a day. Lamotrigine has several benefits compared to carbamazepine and phenytoin. It has a better side-effect profile, and there is no autoinduction of metabolism, so dosing is stable over time. If used in combination with carbamazepine or phenytoin, it does not alter their metabolism. Lamotrigine's major side effect is a drug rash (major drawback—slow dosing schedule) that can evolve into a Stevens–Johnson syndrome. The rash normally starts early in therapy. If a rash appears the drug should be stopped immediately.

Pimozide Pimozide is a dopamine receptor antagonist. In a double-blind, crossover trial, it was more effective than carbamazepine for trigeminal neuralgia. The overall dose is between 4 and 12 mg a day. Pimozide's major drawback is its poor side-effect profile, which includes mental retardation, hand tremor, memory impairment, and parkinsonism. Adverse events are noted in up to 83% of patients (Lechin, et al., 1989). Newer atypical antipsychotics which have shown some success in migraine, have not been studied for trigeminal neuralgia.

Gabapentin Gabapentin is anecdotally effective for trigeminal neuralgia. There are two isolated case reports in the literature of gabapentin monotherapy (Sist, et al., 1997). One of the individuals required 2400 mg a day for pain relief and the other needed 900 mg a day. The onset of pain relief came within 1 week of achieving a therapeutic drug dose. Gabapentin was also shown to be successful for treating multiple sclerosis-induced trigeminal neuralgia (Khan, 1998). Seven patients who had been refractory to treatment were treated with gabapentin. Six of them had complete pain relief, while the seventh had partial pain relief. Pain relief began 3–4 days after beginning therapy and was complete within 2 weeks. Gabapentin maintained its effect through 1 year follow-up

(Khan, 1998). Gabapentin is started at 300 mg a day and increased to 300 mg every other day to every third day until pain relief is achieved. There is probably no top dose of gabapentin, but most limit the dose to 4000–5000 mg a day. Compared to carbamazepine and phenytoin, gabapentin has minimal side effects and is generally better tolerated by older patients.

Oxcarbazepine Oxcarbazepine, a keto derivative of carbamazepine, has recently obtained Food and Drug Administration (FDA) approval for the treatment of epilepsy. It is probably equal or superior to carbamazepine in the treatment of trigeminal neuralgia. Oxcarbazepine has very rapid oral absorption, with maximum blood concentrations occurring within 1 hour of dosing. Farago (1987) treated 13 patients with oxcarbazepine for a mean of 11 months. Treatment resulted in substantial pain reduction or complete pain relief in all patients. In 6 patients, pain relief occurred within 24 hours, and all patients had pain relief by 72 hours. The effective oxcarbazepine dose was 10–20 mg/kg of body weight. Zakrzewska and Patsalos (1989) used oxcarbazepine to treat 6 patients who were refractory to carbamazepine; all had some pain relief within 24 hours of the initial dose. In an open-label trial of oxcarbazepine, 13 of 15 patients who were switched from carbamazepine to oxcarbazepine demonstrated pain reduction, while 10 became pain-free on doses of 900–1800 mg a day (Remillard, 1994). Oxcarbazepine should be started at a dose of 150–300 mg and increased every third day in 150–300 mg increments until there is pain relief (the total dose needed is usually less than 1200 mg a day). Oxcarbazepine's side effect profile appears to be better than carbamazepine's, although the risk of hyponatremia is the same.

Topiramate Topiramate, a novel antiepileptic, was shown to be successful in treating refractory trigeminal neuralgia in multiple-sclerosis patients. In an open-label, consecutive case series, five patients became completely pain-free on topiramate. Four patients had pain relief with 200 mg, while a single patient needed 300 mg. All but one patient were able to discontinue their trigeminal neuralgia medications. Patients remained pain-free on topiramate through 6 month follow-up (Din, et al., 2000). Gilron et al. (2001) completed a pilot study to evaluate the efficacy of topiramate in trigeminal neuralgia using a randomized, double-blind, placebo-controlled, two-period crossover design. Only three patients were in the study. All three patients responded to topiramate in this main study and then entered a subsequent confirmatory study consisting of three topiramate-placebo crossovers. In the main study, topiramate reduced pain by 31%, 42%, and 64% in the three patients ($p = 0.04$). However, topiramate showed no effect in the confirmatory study . Thus, more trials looking at this antiepileptic in prevention of trigeminal neuralgia need to be done.

Triptans Triptans are specific serotonin agonists that modulate neurogenic inflammation, pain processing at the trigeminal nucleus caudalis and also cause vessel constriction. Triptans help alleviate the pain of trigeminal-based head-pain syndromes including migraine and cluster headache. There have been several recent reports looking at the usefulness of triptans for trigeminal neuralgia pain. Kanai et al. (2006) looked at 15 patients with idiopathic trigeminal neuralgia. Each patient was given 1 ml of saline subcutaneously as a placebo, followed 15 minutes later with subcutaneous sumatriptan (3 mg) and this was followed the next day by oral sumatriptan (50 mg twice daily) for 1 week. Pain visual analog scale did not change after saline, but significantly decreased after subcutaneous sumatriptan and after 1 week of oral sumatriptan.

Rules for Medicinal Therapy in Trigeminal Neuralgia

1. Do not overtreat. Look for remissions and taper the drug if the patient has been pain-free for 4–6 weeks, but be alert for recurrences. Pain diaries are useful to document pain-free intervals.
2. Chronic anticonvulsant therapy, especially in an older population, can cause cognitive impairment. Use the smallest pain-relieving dose possible.
3. Many trigeminal neuralgia patients become less responsive to medication with time. Try the drug to its fullest potential, recognize

changes in pharmacokinetics (e.g., changing half-life of carbamazepine over time), and adjust doses accordingly.

4. Minimize medication side effects by carefully titrating doses throughout the day, avoiding peaks and troughs.
5. Aim for monotherapy, but polypharmacy is an acceptable and successful treatment scheme in trigeminal neuralgia.
6. Lamotrigine, gabapentin, topiramate, and oxcarbazepine may be more effective and better tolerated than carbamazepine and phenytoin.

Nonmedicinal Therapy for Trigeminal Neuralgia

A recent trend in pain management has been nonmedicinal alternatives to medical therapy. Acupuncture may have some benefit in trigeminal neuralgia. Shuhan et al. (1991) studied the role of acupuncture in 1500 trigeminal neuralgia patients. The treatment course was 10 days (daily or every other day) and was repeated in 3–5 days if unsuccessful. Most patients required an average of 26 sessions to obtain relief. Five hundred and thirty-nine patients were followed from 1 to 6 years, and 99.2% of them were helped. Approximately 44% had a recurrence of trigeminal neuralgia attacks but the attacks were less severe than they were before therapy. Patients who had a shorter past history of trigeminal neuralgia had the best response. There was no correlation between success of acupuncture and pain distribution or the patient's age or gender. This was not a controlled trial.

Surgical Treatment for Trigeminal Neuralgia

Candidates for surgical therapy for trigeminal neuralgia include patients who have failed medical therapy (which occurs approximately 30% of the time) or patients who initially responded but later became intolerant to medical therapy. Approximately 50% of trigeminal neuralgia sufferers will require surgery (Table 25–3).

Extracranial Peripheral Denervation

Extracranial peripheral denervation previously was the most common surgical technique utilized for trigeminal neuralgia. The goal of this procedure is to interrupt signals from trigeminal peripheral afferents by temporarily or permanently destroying the afferent fibers via chemical, thermal, or traumatic measures. The location of the trigeminal neuralgia pain or trigger zones determines which nerve branch needs to be denervated. Peripheral denervation is performed at the supraorbital notch for ophthalmic division pain, the infraorbital notch for maxillary division pain, and the mental foramen for mandibular division pain. Lidocaine and bupivacaine are used for temporary denervation, while more permanent denervation is achieved with alcohol, freezing, and heating. Cutting or avulsing the nerve via neurectomy is also a surgical treatment option. Extracranial peripheral denervation has many advantages. There is good pain relief, with a 50%–100% success rate. Only a small area of denervation is necessary and there is no risk of corneal denervation or keratitis.

TABLE 25–3 Drug Therapy for Trigeminal Neuralgia.

Medication	*Dose range*	*Time to relief*
Carbamazepine	400–800 mg/day	24–48 hours
Phenytoin	300–500 mg/day	24–48 hours
Baclofen	40–80 mg/day	?
Clonazepam	1.5–8 mg/day	?
Valproic acid	500–1500 mg/day	Weeks
Lamotrigine	150–400 mg/day	24 hours
Pimozide	4–12 mg	?
Gabapentin	900–2400 mg/day	1 week
Oxcarbazepine	900–1800 mg/day	24–72 hours

It is an office procedure and requires only a brief postoperative recovery period. Finally, it enables the patient to appreciate what loss of sensation would mean if a more permanent procedure, such as RF thermocoagulation of the Gasserian ganglion, were to be performed (Zakrzewska, 1955b). A major disadvantage of extracranial peripheral denervation is that it can be a very painful procedure if not performed under sedation and the elderly population who suffer with trigeminal neuralgia are at increased risk of complications with anesthesia. Peripheral denervation only provides short-term pain relief. With lidocaine, pain returns in hours to days; with alcohol it returns in 6–18 months; with freezing 4–14 months; and with neurectomy 20–30 months. Serious complications of peripheral denervation are rare but include skin necrosis and eye hemorrhage if denervation is completed in the ophthalmic division. Extracranial peripheral denervation is now recommended for the elderly patient with a short life expectancy or the patient who needs immediate pain relief and is medically unfit for a more invasive procedure. Extracranial peripheral denervation studies are plagued by methodologic issues, including the use of nonspecific diagnostic criteria, endpoints that are not defined, a length of follow-up that is not documented, and a lack of prospective observations.

Percutaneous Denervation of the Gasserian Ganglion and Retrogasserian Rootlets

This procedure involves partial destruction of the trigeminal nerve with either heat (RF), glycerol, or balloon compression. Under radiographic control a device is inserted into the cheek and directed through the foramen ovale into the area of the Gasserian ganglion and rootlets and the specific denervating agent is then utilized.

RF Thermocoagulation RF thermocoagulation is the most commonly used surgical treatment for trigeminal neuralgia. More than 90% of patients experience relief from the initial procedure. The response is almost always immediate. Pain recurrence rates range from 4%–65% (Zakrzewska, 1955c) and correlate with length of follow up. The longest follow-up study of RF has been 13 years. RF thermocoagulation has less denervation at the initial procedure and one of the lowest recurrence rates of all trigeminal neuralgia surgical procedures (Table 25–4). Side effects of RF thermocoagulation include moderate dysesthesias in 5%–25% of patients, severe dysesthesias in 2%–10%, corneal sensory loss in 20%, and anesthesia dolorosa in 1%–5% (Zakrzewska, 1955c). The minor side effects can be reduced by making the endpoint hypoalgesia rather than analgesia. Major side effects include intracranial hemorrhage, stroke, and infection. Weakness of the muscles of mastication occurs in approximately 53% of individuals (Onofrio, 1975) and is usually temporary and resolves in 3–6 months. RF thermocoagulation has the advantage of being a highly specific procedure that is safe in the elderly and delivers immediate pain relief. It has a very low recurrence rate with low mortality. Disadvantages include cost and the need for a skilled surgeon. The procedure can cause corneal anesthesia if done in the ophthalmic division, and sensory loss can go beyond the area affected by the technique. Anesthesia dolorosa and keratitis may occur.

Glycerol Trigeminal Rhizotomy Glycerol trigeminal rhizotomy is an alternative to RF. Sterile glycerol acts as a mild denervating agent when injected into the Gasserian ganglion. Glycerol rhizotomy is effective in up to 90% of individuals, and 50% experience pain relief within 24 hours. Others

TABLE 25–4 Surgical Procedures for Trigeminal Neuralgia.

1. Peripheral techniques: cause selective trauma to branches of the trigeminal nerve and try to prevent conduction of afferent painful stimuli
2. Gasserian ganglion techniques: are directed at the trigeminal root and try to cause selective damage to A delta and C fibers
3. Posterior fossa surgery: done to restore functional anatomy by removing compressive lesions, typical arteries or veins

may not experience pain relief until 7–10 days after the procedure. Glycerol rhizotomy has a high recurrence rate; 28% of patients experience a recurrence of pain within 1 year and 50% by 2 years (often within 6–12 months). Documented ranges of recurrence rates are 10%–72% (Fujimaki, et al., 1990; Arias, 2000). The procedure has very few side effects, but some form of sensory loss may occur in 26%–71% of patients, but this is less than with RF lesions. Glycerol trigeminal rhizotomy is a highly specific technique that is safe in the elderly and requires no general anesthesia. It is less complicated than RF thermocoagulation. There is incomplete sensory loss and no mortality. Disadvantages include delayed pain relief, which can take up to 10 days. There are many initial failures, since the procedure needs correct needle placement, and it has a fairly high recurrence rate. Glycerol trigeminal rhizotomy is particularly useful for the patient with ophthalmic division pain. Corneal anesthesia and keratitis occur less frequently with glycerol than with RF thermocoagulation.

Percutaneous Balloon Compression Percutaneous balloon compression is a technique that is used infrequently. Under general anesthesia, a Fogarty balloon catheter is inserted through the foramen ovale. The balloon is then inflated, causing compression of the Gasserian ganglion. Initial success rates are high, between 80% and 90%. Approximately 28% of patient, however, will have some recurrence with a mean time to relapse of 6.5 months (Meglio and Cioni, 1989). Problems with the technique (compared with RF and glycerol denervation) include general anesthesia requirements; increased risk of intracranial hemorrhage with large trochar insertion; and, as this is not a selective procedure, the amount of sensory loss is not known until the procedure has been completed. Autonomic dysfunction from balloon inflation can induce bradycardia and hypotension. Thus, cardiac disease is a contraindication to percutaneous balloon compression.

Microvascular Decompression Microvascular decompression (MVD) is based on the theory that trigeminal neuralgia is due to a vascular loop compressing the trigeminal nerve at the root entry zone, leading to focal irritation, demyelination, and subsequent pain. As many as 96% of patients who undergo MVD for trigeminal neuralgia have documented vessel compression of the trigeminal nerve. Hamlyn and King (1992) found that 90% of patients who underwent vascular decompression had vessel compression compared to only 13% of age- and gender-matched nontrigeminal neuralgia cadaver patients. Most vascular loops leading to trigeminal nerve irritation are arterial and arise from the superior cerebellar artery. Venous compression occurs approximately 12%–15% of the time.

Microvascular decompression was initially used by Dandy and perfected by Janetta. It requires a suboccipital retromastoid craniectomy. If a vascular compressive lesion is identified the trigeminal nerve is decompressed by placing synthetic material between the nerve and the compressing vessel. Barker (1996) completed a long-term outcome study of MVD of 1185 patients over a 20-year period and showed that 80% had complete pain relief following the procedure, while 7.6% obtained partial relief. At 10 years, 70% continued to show excellent results, meaning that they had pain relief and no extra medications were needed, while 4% had partial relief. Of patients who did not have complete relief, 34% resumed chronic medication, 20% had an additional ablative procedure, and 22% had an ablative procedure and needed chronic medication. Recurrence rates were minimal, only 1%–6%, and most occurred within the first 2 years. The belief was that if there is no pain relapse within two years of MVD, patients will likely remain pain-free. Konda (2001) documented long-term follow-up data on 281 patients who underwent MVD for trigeminal neuralgia between 1976 and 2000. Patients were followed from 5 to 20 years. Complete pain relief was documented in 96.7%, although only 82.5% were satisfied with the procedure.

Sindou et al. (2006) reported on a series of 362 patients having clear-cut vascular compression and treated with pure MVD without any additional cut or coagulation of the adjacent root fibers. Follow-up was 1–18 years (8-year average). One year after operation, 81.2% of patients were pain free of paroxysmal pain, background pain and required no medication, while 3.6% still had a background of pain but no need for medication, 15.2% failed the procedure. At the 8-year average follow-up pain-free rates were 80% complete, 4.9% with background pain and 15.1% labeled as failures. Kaplan–Meier analysis estimated the probability of total cure at 15 years to be 73.4%.

The advantages of MVD include a long-lasting response, preservation of nerve function, no risk of anesthesia dolorosa, and a low recurrence rate. Factors increasing recurrence rates after MVD include female gender, symptoms present for longer than 8 years, venous compression, lack of immediate postoperative pain relief, less significant vascular contact with the trigeminal nerve, and a history of dull background pain between attacks (Zakrzewska, 1955d). Disadvantages of microvascular decompression include possible mortality and the risks of damaging cranial nerves other than the trigeminal, especially the trochlear nerve. Complications from microvascular decompression include death in 0%–1% of patients (cerebellar hemorrhage and infarction) (Zakrzewska, 1955d), intracranial hemorrhage or stroke in 1%–2%, hearing loss in up to 21% (permanent in 3%–8%), and sensory loss in 5%–31%(10). In most institutions, MVD is carried out if RF thermocoagulation has failed, but others utilize MVD as a first-line therapy for medically refractory trigeminal neuralgia.

What is the role of repeat exploration if the initial MVD procedure has failed to alleviate pain or if pain has recurred? Speculated causes of MVD failure include: incomplete vascular decompression with the initial procedure, recurrence of vascular compression, slippage of the synthetic implant, or scarring of the implant leading to nerve compression. Kureshi and Wilkins (1998) performed repeat exploration in 31 patients, 23 of whom had trigeminal neuralgia and 8 hemifacial spasm. On repeat exploration, they noted that the initial implant was in good position (nondisplaced) in 100% of patients. A new compressive element (artery, scarred implant, bony ridge) was noted in 30% of patients. Postsurgical complication after repeat exploration occurred in 30% of patients, typically involving hearing loss or facial weakness. The authors concluded that repeat exploration in failed MVD is unwarranted because of the lack of finding of any significant compressive lesions on repeat exploration and the relatively high complication rate of the procedure. Instead of repeat exploratory surgery, the patient should be sent for another form of ablative procedure (i.e., RF rhizotomy) or tried again on medications. Jannetta and Bissonette (1985) looked at 51 patients with mild MVD and found persistent arterial or venous compression in 44 patients and scarred implants in 5 patients on repeat exploration. Bederson and Wilson (1989) found no abnormality on repeat exploration in 90% of 20 studied patients, while Cho et al. (1994) in 53 patients found that 23% had arterial loop compression on repeat exploration, 13% had venous compression, and 13% had implant compression. There is no consensus on the role of repeat exploration in failed MVD.

Gamma Knife Radiosurgery Gamma knife radiosurgery, a form of stereotactic radiosurgery, is one of the newest therapeutic techniques for trigeminal neuralgia. The procedure entails the use of a stereotactic head frame, stereotactic imaging of the trigeminal nerve root entry zone, and radiation of the trigeminal nerve, usually 2–4 mm anterior to the brainstem. The normal radiation dose received is 70–80 Gy. The brainstem normally receives less than 20% of the total radiation dosage. Young et al. (1997) examined 51 patients after gamma knife radiosurgery; 49 had idiopathic trigeminal neuralgia, and 2 had multiple sclerosis-induced trigeminal neuralgia. All patients were medical nonresponders, and 22 of them were surgical nonresponders. Thirty-eight of fifty-one patients (74.5%) were completely pain-free after gamma knife radiosurgery. A 50%–90% decrease in facial pain was seen in another 13.7% of patients, while 11.1% failed the procedure. Follow-up was for 6–36 months, with mean follow-up being 16.3 months. Most patients (80.4%) remained pain-free or continued with marked pain reduction. Time to initial pain relief could be quite long, anywhere from 1 to 120 days, with a mean of 14 days. Kondziolka et al. (1996) reported on a five-center study of gamma knife radiosurgery for trigeminal neuralgia. Fifty percent of individuals became pain-free and pain was reduced by 50%–90% in another 34% of patients. Ten percent failed to respond. Overall, 84% of patients felt they had an excellent to good response. Mean follow-up time was 9.2 months. A problem with this study was that different techniques were used in different institutions, which suggests possible inconsistencies in the results of the study. In addition, there was a very short follow-up period. Rogers et al. (2002) assessed the efficacy of gamma knife in 15 patients with multiple sclerosis-induced trigeminal neuralgia. The treatment targeted the ipsilateral trigeminal nerve at its junction with the pons. A 70–90-Gy maximum radiation dose was given. Mean follow-up time was 17 months (6–38 months). Eighty percent (12 out of 15 patients) of the treated patients experienced pain relief with a mean latency to onset of response of 13 days (range 1–61 days). Maximum pain relief occurred after a mean latency of 56 days (range 1–157 days). Five patients had a repeat procedure and all improved. Complications were minimal only involving facial hypesthesias. Two of fifteen patients developed facial symptoms after the initial gamma knife while two of five patients developed facial numbness after a second gamma-knife procedure. The facial hypesthesias were felt to be mild and not bothersome to the patient, and this adverse event only occurred in patients who had complete relief of their trigeminal neuralgia pain.

A recent study has suggested that post gamma-knife pontine enhancement on MRI is a positive prognostic sign for pain relief. Gorgulho et al. (2006) studied 37 patients post gamma knife with brain MRIs. Enhancement on MRI was observed in 21 cases (56.75%) with nerve enhancement in 9, pons enhancement in 4, pons-nerve enhancement in 4, and tumor enhancement in 4. MRIs were unremarkable in 16 cases. Pons enhancement correlated with pain relief ($p = 0.0087$) but not with nerve enhancement ($p = 0.22$).

The advantages of gamma knife radiosurgery in trigeminal neuralgia include a very short procedure time (only 2.5–3 hours), the need for only local anesthesia, and efficacy that is almost equal to more invasive procedures. Overall, there appears to be a low initial complication rate with gamma knife; only 6% of the patients in the Kondziolka et al. (1996) study had complications, only one patient in the Young et al. (1997) study had adverse events while 13% developed side effects in the Rogers et al. (2002) study. A disadvantage of gamma knife radiosurgery versus other surgical techniques for trigeminal neuralgia is a prolonged time latency between procedure and onset of pain relief. Most trigeminal neuralgia patients cannot wait months for pain relief, as the syndrome can be excruciating and disabling. There is also no long-term follow-up data of gamma knife radiosurgery in trigeminal neuralgia. Finally, no one knows what the true delayed radiation complications of gamma knife radiosurgery are (especially in young patients). The proposed mechanism of action of gamma knife radiosurgery for trigeminal neuralgia is inactivating pathologic ephaptic transmission without damaging normal axonal conduction. Gamma knife radiosurgery costs three times more than percutaneous denervation and approximaely 40% less than MVD.

On the Horizon

Electrical Stimulation of the Gasserian Ganglion

Holsheimer (2001) reviewed data from 8 clinical trials involving 267 patients with chronic, intractable trigeminal neuralgia. A small percutaneous stimulation electrode was placed through the foramen ovale to the Gasserian cistern. If a percutaneous test stimulation was successful (at least 50% pain relief) the electrode was internalized and connected to a subcutaneous pulse generator. Of 233 patients with medication-resistant trigeminal neuralgia, 48% had at least a 50% long-term improvement in pain. Eighty-three percent of patients with a positive test stimulation had at least 50% long-term pain relief, and 70% had at least 75% long-term pain improvement. Interestingly, patients with postherpetic-induced trigeminal distribution pain did not do as well, with less than 10% of patients showing significant improvement. It appears that stimulation of the Gasserian ganglion maybe a promising new treatment modality for medication-resistant trigeminal neuralgia.

Botulinum Toxin Injections

Recently botulinum toxin injections have been utilized in the treatment of migraine and hemifacial spasm. At present, there is growing data on the use of botulinum toxin in trigeminal neuralgia. Micheli et al. (2002) documented a case of a 70-year-old man with hemifacial spasm and trigeminal neuralgia secondary to an ectatic basilar artery. Botulinum toxin type A, was injected at five sites in the orbicularis oculi muscle and one site over the buccinator muscle. The patient obtained relief not only from the spasms but also the trigeminal neuralgia pain. Spasms and pain recurred after the botulinum toxin effects wore off. Repeat injections provided recurrent pain relief. Piovesan et al. (2005) treated 13 trigeminal neuralgia patients with botulinum toxin A in an open-label investigation. In all patients visual analog pain scale and surface area of pain were reduced. Most of these patients were able to reduce their preventive medication dosing by more than 50% while 4 of them were able to come off medication completely. Dosing of Botox depended on area injected but ranged from 6 to 9 units.

GLOSSOPHARYNGEAL NEURALGIA

Glossopharyngeal neuralgia is an uncommon facial-pain syndrome that was first described by Weisenburg in 1910 (Weisenburg, 1910). Its incidence is between 0.2% and 1.3% of trigeminal neuralgia (White and Sweet, 1969b). Symptoms typically begin after the sixth decade (Rushton, et al., 1981). Since the pain is felt in the sensory distribution of the glossopharyngeal and vagus nerves, some authors use the term "vagoglossopharyngeal neuralgia" for this disorder. Like trigeminal neuralgia, it may go into remission (Rushton, et al., 1981). Glossopharyngeal neuralgia and trigeminal neuralgia occur in a combined form in 10% of patients.

Glossopharyngeal neuralgia is characterized by paroxysmal pain in the throat, tonsillar fossa, tongue, and ear. The onset is abrupt, and it may persist for several seconds to 1 minute. The attacks of pain are invariably triggered not by chewing, but by swallowing, particularly cold liquids, and, on occasion, by yawning or sneezing. Almost 2% of patients lose consciousness during pain paroxysms, probably due to bradycardia or systole. The physical examination is normal, yet occasionally a trigger zone within the preauricular or postauricular area, the neck, or the external auditory canal is identified. Application of a local anesthetic to the oropharynx has both therapeutic and diagnostic implications (Rushton, et al., 1981).

The evaluation of a patient with glossopharyngeal neuralgia should include an MRI scan with contrast. Secondary glossopharyngeal neuralgia may be due to an oropharyngeal malignancy, a peritonsillar infection, or vascular compression wherein a loop of a posterior fossa vessel compresses the nerve.

Glossopharyngeal neuralgia is treated with anticonvulsant medications, such as carbamazepine, phenytoin, baclofen, and gabapentin. Patients who are refractory to medical therapy can be treated surgically with intracranial sectioning of the glossopharyngeal nerve and the upper rootlets of the vagus nerve. Microvascular decompression of the 9th cranial nerve is also effective (Kondo, 1998). Overall, the number of studies in the literature looking at treatment strategies for glossopharyngeal neuralgia are limited and much less prevalent than studies dealing with trigeminal neuralgia.

CONCLUSION

Trigeminal neuralgia and glossopharyngeal neuralgia are extremely painful conditions that typically afflict an older population. Distinct clinical characteristics guide the diagnosis of these unique syndromes. Treatment involves medication first and then surgical procedures if a patient is refractory to medicinal therapy. Antiepileptic medications are the most effective agents for these disorders.

ATYPICAL FACIAL PAIN

Atypical facial pain includes those types of facial pain that do not represent "typical" or classifiable pain syndromes. The term was introduced by Frazier and Russell, largely to distinguish trigeminal neuralgia from the myriad of other causes of facial pain (Frazier and Russell, 1924). Fay (1932) was the first to postulate that nondescript facial pain not only may be due to an underlying vascular mechanism but in some patients could represent a referred pain syndrome.

The term "atypical facial pain" has been questioned over the years by several experienced clinicians. Rushton et al. (1959) wrote "Danger exists in considering atypical facial pain an entity since this would imply a common cause, and its use would assume that a definite diagnosis has been made." We agree with Raskin (1988) that a preferable term is "facial pain of unknown cause." If "typical" atypical facial pain exists, it should be considered only after facial pain secondary to anatomic and pathophysiologic disturbances have been excluded. An abnormal neurologic examination is not compatible with the diagnosis of atypical facial pain. A complete general and neurologic examination and on occasion consultations with colleagues in otorhinolaryngology, dentistry, and occasionally ophthalmology may be necessary. Appropriate imaging studies may be necessary to exclude nasopharyngeal and sinus neoplasms, structural abnormalities at the skull base, and dental conditions, such as maxillary and/or cryptic mandibular microabscesses. The possibility of squamous cell and basal cell carcinoma of the face should also be considered.

Facial pain as a presenting symptom of nonmetastatic lung carcinoma was suggested initially by Fay (1932), who wrote, "I discovered a lesion in the lung ... the pain being referred to the face. This may be a coincidence but I suspect not." This association was revived in a case report by Des Prez and Freemon (1983). A total of 33 cases have been reported. The clinical features of this underrecognized syndrome have come into sharper focus since the original description by Fay (Capobianco, 1995; Eross, et al., 2003; Abraham et al., 2003). Of the 30 patients for whom smoking habits were reported, nearly all (91%) were either current or former smokers. The pain, often characterized as a severe aching discomfort, was typically located in or around the ear (91%); other locations included the jaw (48%) and temple (38%). In each case, the pain was ipsilateral to the occult lung lesion. An increased erythrocyte sedimentation rate was noted in 73% (11 out of 15) of patients in whom the test was performed. Nearly 66% of patients for whom data were available met the criteria of the clinical triad of (1) a current or former smoker, (2) periauricular pain, and (3) increased erythrocyte sedimentation rate. Additional features that, if present, should raise concern about the possibility of an occult lung lesion include weight loss, new cough or hemoptysis, and digital clubbing. The mechanism of referral of pain from the chest to the ipsilateral ear or face presumably involves either direct tumor invasion or compression of the vagus nerve. The vagus is a mixed nerve containing motor, sensory, and parasympathetic components. General visceral afferents project sensory input from the pharynx, larynx, thorax, and abdomen to the nodose ganglion, which then projects to the nucleus solitarius located in the medulla. The jugular ganglion projects general somatic afferents to the nucleus of the trigeminal nerve. The general somatic afferents carry impulses from the skin of the concha of the external ear through the auricular ramus and dura mater of the posterior fossa via the meningeal ramus. Thus, a lung lesion that infiltrates or compresses the vagus nerve may refer pain to the ear through convergence of general visceral afferents and general somatic afferents in the medulla. This dual territory of vagal innervation provides the anatomic substrate for the brain to perceive nociceptive input from the chest as if it were emanating from the ear or meninges. It behooves clinicians to consider the possibility that facial pain may be related to nonmetastatic lung cancer in every smoker or former smoker with unexplained facial pain or otalgia. All such patients should have chest radiography. If the results are equivocal or negative, computed tomography of the chest should be considered to ensure that an occult lung lesion is not missed. Several cases have been reported recently in which the chest radiograph was normal but chest computed tomography demonstrated an occult lung lesion ipsilateral to the facial pain (Abraham et al., 2003). Computed tomography was performed in these patients because of a clinical profile of smoking with periauricular pain (Abraham et al., 2003). In general, medical management, including opioids, is largely ineffective in alleviating the pain in such cases. The definitive treatment must be directed at the underlying lung lesion.

Patients in whom "typical" atypical facial pain is eventually diagnosed possess the following features, which distinguish this pain disorder from the major facial neuralgias (Campbell, 1988; Solomon and Lipton, 1988, 1990). The pain is steady, generally unilateral (on occasion may become bilateral), and poorly localized yet typically involving the eye, nose, cheek, temple, or jaw. The pain may spread over the area supplied by the cervical roots. The pain is usually described as deep and aching yet is not infrequently characterized graphically as tearing, ripping, crushing, or pulling. Absent are the paroxysms of short duration (1–30 seconds) followed by freedom from pain seen in trigeminal neuralgia. Although the patient reports intense pain, quite often the patient does not appear to be in outward distress. The pain is generally present all day every day and often worsens over time. Absent are the trigger zones characteristic of the neuralgias. Attacks are not precipitated by cold air, cold water in the mouth, swallowing, talking, chewing, shaving, or washing the face. The typical patient is a woman in her 30s or 40s, who is often depressed. The depression does not imply a causal relationship but may reflect the effect of unresolved pain. The pain is not significantly reduced or eliminated by division of the 5th or 9th cranial nerve. Surgical procedures are often performed in vain and only serve to aggravate the underlying problem. Some patients may suffer from a form of migraine involving the face, so-called facial migraine. This diagnosis should be considered if the facial pain is intermittent, throbbing, and associated with nausea, photophobia, and/or phonophobia. A careful search for triggering factors, such as menses, alcohol ingestion, exertion, or changes in the sleep-wake cycle, may provide a useful clue as to a migrainous mechanism. In such situations, a trial with antimigraine medications, both acute and preventive, may prove helpful. Cluster headache, the so-called lower-half form, should also be considered, particularly if the pain is of short duration and associated with ipsilateral autonomic accompaniments (Campbell, 1988).

Many patients with chronic, long-standing atypical facial pain require a multifaceted treatment approach. These patients often have undergone numerous surgical (dental, nasal, or sinus) procedures to no avail. Treatment can include pain-relieving or analgesic medications, antimigraine as well as antineuralgic medications, and nonpharmacologic treatment strategies, including biofeedback and relaxation techniques.

References

Abraham, PJ, Capobianco, DJ, and Cheshire, WP (2003). Facial pain as the presenting symptom of lung carcinoma with normal chest radiograph. *Headache*, 43 (5):499–504.

Akimoto, H, Nagaoka, T, Nariai, T, Takada, Y, Ohno, K, and Yoshino, N (2002). Preoperative evaluation of neurovascular compression in patients with trigeminal neuralgia by use of three-dimensional reconstruction from two types of high-resolution magnetic resonance imaging. *Neurosurgery*, 51(4):956–961; discussion 961–952.

Anderson, VC, Berryhill, PC, Sandquist, MA, Ciaverella, DP, Nesbit, GM, and Burchiel KJ (2006). High-resolution three-dimensional magnetic resonance angiography and three-dimensional spoiled gradient-recalled imaging in the evaluation of neurovascular compression in patients with trigeminal neuralgia: a double-blind pilot study. *Neurosurgery*, 58(4):666–673; discussion 666–673.

Arias, MJ (2000). Percutaneous retrogasserian glycerol rhizotomies for trigeminal neuralgia. A prospective study of 100 cases. *Neurosurgery*, 65:32–36.

Barker, FG 2nd, Jannetta, PJ, Bissonette, DJ, Larkins, MV, and Jho, HD (1996). The long-term outcome of microvascular decompression for trigeminal neuralgia. *N Engl J Med*, 334(17):1077–1083.

Bederson, JB and Wilson, CB (1989). Evaluation of microvascular decompression and partial sensory rhizotomy in 252 cases of trigeminal neuralgia. *J Neurosurg*, 71 (3):359–367.

Brewis, M, Poskanzer, DC, Rolland, C, and Miller, H (1966). Neurological disease in an English city. *Acta Neurol Scand*, 42(Suppl. 24):21–89.

Campbell, JK (1988). Facial pain due to migraine and cluster headache. *Semin Neurol*, 8(4):324–331.

Capobianco, DJ (1995). Facial pain as a symptom of nonmetastatic lung cancer. *Headache*, 35(10):581–585.

Cho, DY, Chang, CG, Wang, YC, Wang, FH, Shen, CC, and Yang, DY (1994). Repeat operations in failed microvascular decompression for trigeminal neuralgia. *Neurosurgery*, 35(4):665–669; discussion 669–670.

Court, JE and Kase, CS (1976). Treatment of tic douloureux with a new anticonvulsant (clonazepam). *J Neurol Neurosurg Psychiatry*, 39(3):297–299.

Des Prez, RD and Freemon, FR (1983). Facial pain associated with lung cancer: a case report. *Headache*, 23 (1):43–44.

Din, MU, Zvartan-Hind, M, Gilari, A, Lisak, R, and Khan, OA (2000). Topiramate relieved refractory trigeminal neuralgia in multiple sclerosis patients. *Neurology*, 54: A60 (Abstract).

Duff, JM, Spinner, RJ, Lindor, NM, Dodick, DW, and Atkinson, JL (1999). Familial trigeminal neuralgia and contralateral hemifacial spasm. *Neurology*, 53 (1):216–218.

Eross, EJ, Dodick, DW, Swanson, JW, and Capobianco, DJ (2003). A review of intractable facial pain secondary to underlying lung neoplasms. *Cephalalgia*, 23(1):2–5.

Farago, F (1987). Trigeminal neuralgia: its treatment with two new carbamazepine analogues. *Eur Neurol*, 26 (2):73–83.

Fay, T (1932). Atypical facial neuralgia, a syndrome of vascular pain. *Ann Otol Rhinol Laryngol* 41:1030–1062.

Frazier, CH and Russell, EC (1924). Neuralgia of the face. An analysis of 754 cases with relation to pain and other sensory phenomena before and after operation. *Arch Neurol Psychiatry*, 11:557–563.

Fromm, GH (1991). Pathophysiology of trigeminal neuralgia. In *Trigeminal Neuralgia: Current Concepts Regarding Pathogenesis and Treatment* (GH, Fromm and

BJ Sessle, eds). pp. 105–130. Butterworth-Heinemann, Boston.

Fujimaki, T, Fukushima, T, and Miyazaki, S (1990). Percutaneous retrogasserian glycerol injection in the management of trigeminal neuralgia: long-term followup results. *J Neurosurg*, 73:212–216.

Gilron, I, Booher, SL, Rowan, JS, and Max, MB (2001). Topiramate in trigeminal neuralgia: a randomized, placebo-controlled multiple crossover pilot study. *Clin Neuropharmacol*, 24(2):109–112.

Goadsby, PJ and Edvinsson, L (1994). Human in vivo evidence for trigeminovascular activation in cluster headache. Neuropeptide changes and effects of acute attacks therapies. *Brain*, 117(Pt 3):427–434.

Gorgulho, A, De Salles, AA, McArthur, D, Agazaryan, N, Medin, P, Solberg, T, et al. (2006). Brainstem and trigeminal nerve changes after radiosurgery for trigeminal pain. *Surg Neurol*, 66(2):127–135; discussion 135.

Hamlyn, PJ and King, TT (1992). Neurovascular compression in trigeminal neuralgia: a clinical and anatomical study. *J Neurosurg*, 76(6):948–954.

Harris, W (1926). Chronic paroxysmal trigeminal neuralgia. In *Neuritis and Neuralgia* (W Harris, ed.). pp. 150–222. Oxford University Press, Oxford (UK).

Headache Classification Subcommittee of the International Headache Society (2004). International classification of headache disorders, 2nd edition. *Cephalalgia*, 24(Suppl. 1):9–160.

Holsheimer, J (2001). Electrical stimulation of the trigeminal tract in chronic, intractable facial neuralgia. *Arch Physiol Biochem*, 109(4):304–308.

Jannetta, PJ and Bissonette, DJ (1985). Management of the failed patient with trigeminal neuralgia. *Clin Neurosurg*, 32:334–347.

Jassim, SA (1994). *Patient's assessment of outcome after radiofrequency thermocoagulation for management of trigeminal neuralgia*. University of London, London.

Kanai, A, Suzuki, A, Osawa, S, and Hoka, S (2006). Sumatriptan alleviates pain in patients with trigeminal neuralgia. *Clin J Pain*, 22(8):677–680.

Katusic, S, Beard, CM, Bergstralh, E, and Kurland, LT (1990). Incidence and clinical features of trigeminal neuralgia, Rochester, Minnesota, 1945–1984. *Ann Neurol*, 27(1):89–95.

Khan, OA (1998). Gabapentin relieves trigeminal neuralgia in multiple sclerosis patients. *Neurology*, 51 (2):611–614.

Kondo, A (1998). Follow-up results of using microvascular decompression for treatment of glossopharyngeal neuralgia. *J Neurosurg*, 88(2):221–225.

Kondo, A (2001). Microvascular decompression surgery for trigeminal neuralgia. *Stereotact Funct Neurosurg*, 77 (1–4):187–189.

Kondziolka, D, Lunsford, LD, Flickinger, JC, Young, RF, Vermeulen, S, Duma, CM, et al. (1996). Stereotactic radiosurgery for trigeminal neuralgia: a multiinstitutional study using the gamma unit. *J Neurosurg*, 84 (6):940–945.

Kureshi, SA and Wilkins, RH (1998). Posterior fossa reexploration for persistent or recurrent trigeminal neuralgia or hemifacial spasm: surgical findings and therapeutic implications. *Neurosurgery*, 43(5):1111–1117.

Kurland, LT (1958). Descriptive epidemiology of selected neurologic and myopathic disorders with particular reference to a survey in Rochester, Minnesota. *J Chronic Dis*, 8(4):378–418.

Leandri, M, Eldridge, P, and Miles, J (1998). Recovery of nerve conduction following microvascular decompression for trigeminal neuralgia. *Neurology*, 51 (6):1641–1646.

Lechin, F, van der Dijs, B, Lechin, ME, Amat, J, Lechin, AE, Cabrera, A, et al. (1989). Pimozide therapy for trigeminal neuralgia. *Arch Neurol*, 46(9):960–963.

Lunardi, G, Leandri, M, Albano, C, Cultrera, S, Fracassi, M, Rubino, V, et al. (1997). Clinical effectiveness of lamotrigine and plasma levels in essential and symptomatic trigeminal neuralgia. *Neurology*, 48 (6):1714–1717.

Majoie, CB, Hulsmans, FJ, Castelijns, JA, Verbeeten, B, Tiren, D, and vanBeek, EJ (2000). Symptoms and signs related to the trigeminal nerve: diagnostic yield of MR imaging. *Radiology*, 209:557–562.

Meglio, M and Cioni, B (1989). Percutaneous procedures for trigeminal neuralgia: microcompression versus radiofrequency thermocoagulation. Personal experience. *Pain*, 38(1):9–16.

Micheli, F, Scorticati, MC, and Raina, G (2002). Beneficial effects of botulinum toxin type a for patients with painful tic convulsif. *Clin Neuropharmacol*, 25 (5):260–262.

Onofrio, BM (1975). Radiofrequency percutaneous Gasserian ganglion lesions. Results in 140 patients with trigeminal pain. *J Neurosurg*, 42(2):132–139.

Pareja, JA, Baron, M, Gili, P, Yanguela, J, Caminero, AB, Dobato, JL, et al. (2002). Objective assessment of autonomic signs during triggered first division trigeminal neuralgia. *Cephalalgia*, 22(4):251–255.

Peiris, JB, Perera, GL, Devendra, SV, and Lionel, ND (1980). Sodium valproate in trigeminal neuralgia. *Med J Aust*, 2(5):278.

Penman, J (1968). Trigeminal neuralgia. In *Handbook of Clinical Neurology: Headaches and Cranial Neuralgias* (PJ Vinker, GW Bruyn, eds). pp. 296–322. North Holland, Amsterdam.

Piovesan, EJ, Teive, HG, Kowacs, PA, Della Coletta, MV, Werneck, LC, and Silberstein, SD (2005). An open study of botulinum-A toxin treatment of trigeminal neuralgia. *Neurology*, 65(8):1306–1308.

Pollack, IF, Jannetta, PJ, and Bissonette, DJ (1988). Bilateral trigeminal neuralgia: a 14-year experience with microvascular decompression. *J Neurosurg*, 68 (4):559–565.

Rasche, D, Kress, B, Stippich, C, Nennig, E, Sartor, K, and Tronnier, VM (2006). Volumetric measurement of the pontomesencephalic cistern in patients with trigeminal neuralgia and healthy controls. *Neurosurgery*, 59 (3):614–620; discussion 614–620.

Raskin, NH (1988). Facial pain. In *Headache* (NH Raskin, ed.). pp. 333–374. Churchill Livingstone, New York.

Remillard, G (1994). Oxcarbazepine and intractable trigeminal neuralgia. *Epilepsia*, 35:28–29.

Rogers, CL, Shetter, AG, Ponce, FA, Fiedler, JA, Smith, KA, and Speiser, BL (2002). Gamma knife radiosurgery for trigeminal neuralgia associated with multiple sclerosis. *J Neurosurg*, 97(Suppl. 5):529–532.

Rothman, KJ and Monson, RR (1973). Epidemiology of trigeminal neuralgia. *J Chronic Dis*, 26(1):1–12.

Rushton, JG and MacDonald, HNA (1957). Trigeminal neuralgia. Special considerations of nonsurgical treatment. *JAMA*, 165:437–440.

Rushton, JG, Gibilisco JA, and Goldstein, NP (1959). Atypical face pain. *JAMA*, 171:545–548.

Rushton, JG, Stevens, JC, and Miller, RH (1981). Glossopharyngeal (vagoglossopharyngeal) neuralgia: a study of 217 cases. *Arch Neurol*, 38(4):201–205.

Shuhan, G, Benren, X, and Yuhuan, Z (1991). Treatment of primary trigeminal neuralgia with acupuncture in 1500 cases. *J Trad Chin Med*, 11:3–6.

Sindou, M, Leston, J, Howeidy, T, Decullier, E, and Chapuis, F (2006). Micro-vascular decompression for primary trigeminal neuralgia (typical or atypical). Long-term effectiveness on pain; prospective study with survival analysis in a consecutive series of 362 patients. *Acta Neurochir (Wien)*, 148(12):1235–1245.

Sist, T, Filadora, V, Miner, M, and Lema, M (1997). Gabapentin for idiopathic trigeminal neuralgia: report of two cases. *Neurology*, 48(5):1467.

Solomon, S and Lipton, RB (1988). Atypical facial pain: a review. *Semin Neurol*, 8(4):332–338.

Solomon, S and Lipton, RB (1990). Facial pain. *Neurol Clin*, 8(4):913–928.

Sundaram, PK, Hegde, AS, Chandramouli, BA, and Das, BS (1999). Trigeminal evoked potentials in patients with symptomatic trigeminal neuralgia due to intracranial mass lesions. *Neurol India*, 47(2):94–97.

Szapiro, J Jr., Sindou, M, and Szapiro, J (1985). Prognostic factors in microvascular decompression for trigeminal neuralgia. *Neurosurgery*, 17(6):920–929.

Taylor, JC, Brauer, S, and Espir, ML (1981). Long-term treatment of trigeminal neuralgia with carbamazepine. *Postgrad Med J*, 57(663):16–18.

Weisenburg, TH (1910). Cerebello-pontine tumor diagnosed for six years as tic douloureux. The symptoms of irritation of the 9th and 12th cranial nerves. *JAMA*, 54:1600–1604.

White, JC and Sweet, WH (1969a). Periodic migrainous neuralgia. In *Pain and The Neurosurgeon. A 40-year Experience* (JC White and WH Sweet, eds). pp. 123–256. Charles C. Thomas, Springfield, Illinois.

White, JC and Sweet, WH (1969b). In *Pain and the Neurosurgeon: a 40-year Experience* (JC White and WH Sweet, eds). pp. 345–434. Charles C. Thomas, Springfield, Illinois.

Yoshimasu, F, Kurland, LT, and Elveback, LR (1972). Tic douloureux in Rochester, Minnesota, 1945–1969. *Neurology*, 22(9):952–956.

Young, RF, Vermeulen, SS, Grimm, P, Blasko, J, and Posewitz, A (1997). Gamma Knife radiosurgery for treatment of trigeminal neuralgia: idiopathic and tumor related. *Neurology*, 48(3):608–614.

Zakrzewska, JM (1955a). Medical management. In *Trigeminal Neuralgia* (JM Zakrzewska, ed.). pp. 80–107. W.B. Saunders Co., London.

Zakrzewska, JM (1955b). Peripheral surgery. In *Trigeminal Neuralgia* (JM Zakrzewska, ed.). pp. 108–123. W.B. Saunders Co., London.

Zakrzewska, JM (1955c). Posterior fossa surgery. In *Trigeminal Neuralgia* (JM Zakrzewska, ed.). pp. 157–168. W.B. Saunders Co., London.

Zakrzewska, JM (1955d). Surgery at the level of the gasserian ganglion. In *Trigeminal Neuralgia* (JM Zakrzewska, ed.). 125–156. W.B. Saunders Co., London.

Zakrzewska, JM and Patsalos, PN (1989). Oxcarbazepine: a new drug in the management of intractable trigeminal neuralgia. *J Neurol Neurosurg Psychiatry* 52 (4):472–476.

Zakrzewska, JM, Chaudhry, Z, Nurmikko, TJ, Patton, DW, and Mullens, EL (1997). Lamotrigine (lamictal) in refractory trigeminal neuralgia: results from a double-blind placebo controlled crossover trial. *Pain* 73 (2):223–230.

Zhao, Y, Jiang, X, and Liu, Y (2002). [Observation of vasoactive intestinal polypeptide in patients with trigeminal neuralgia: a 16-cases report]. *Hua Xi Kou Qiang Yi Xue Za Zhi*, 20(1):33–34, 38.

26 Giant Cell Arteritis and Polymyalgia Rheumatica

Todd J Schwedt, Gene G Hunder, and David W Dodick

Headache is the most common presenting symptom of giant cell (temporal) arteritis (GCA) in an elderly patient (Hollenhorst et al., 1960; Caselli, Daube, et al., 1988). Headache is a prominent symptom in approximately 70% of patients, and the initial symptom in one-third of patients (Caselli, Daube, et al., 1988). The headache itself may be clinically nonspecific, but it generally represents a new symptom in patients who do not have a history of prior headaches, or a different type of headache in patients with a preexisting history of headache. It is characteristically throbbing, continuous, and focally worst in the temporal or, less often, occipital region. Many patients may have swollen, erythematous, and painful superficial temporal arteries (Fig. 26–1). An elevated erythrocyte sedimentation rate (ESR) or C-reactive protein (CRP) can provide a timely diagnosis and guide early treatment, and the diagnosis can be subsequently confirmed with a temporal artery biopsy (TAB). Corticosteroid therapy generally produces symptomatic relief within days. Despite commensurate normalization of the ESR and CRP, active vasculitis probably continues for at least several weeks. GCA can also involve the aortic arch and its branches, resulting in a wide variety of vascular complications; therefore, prompt diagnosis and treatment are imperative.

EPIDEMIOLOGY

Among people 50 years of age and older, GCA has a prevalence of 133 per 100,000 and an annual incidence of 17.4 per 100,000 (Huston et al., 1978). GCA becomes more common with older age, reaching an annual incidence of 29.6 per 100,000 in those 70–79 years old (Huston et al., 1978). GCA affects females to males in a 3:1 ratio (Salvarani et al., 1995, 2004). It is more common in whites, Scandinavians, and British, and in those living at higher latitudes (Liang et al., 1974). A hereditary predisposition to GCA has been suggested by the higher frequency of disease among those with similar ethnicity and by reports of familial aggregation. An association of GCA and polymyalgia rheumatica (PMR) with human leukocyte antigen-DR4 (HLA-DR4) has been identified (Weyand, Hunder, et al., 1994). Autopsy studies showing a GCA prevalence of 1.7% suggest that many patients with GCA never underwent a diagnosis (Ostberg, 1973).

PATHOLOGICAL CONSIDERATIONS

Histopathology

Patients with GCA have damage to the blood vessel wall, which is primarily the result of cellular immune mechanisms. Activated $CD4^+$ T helper cells respond to an antigen, the precise identity of which remains uncertain, that is presented by macrophages (Banks et al., 1983; Shiiki et al., 1989; Wawryk et al., 1991; Weyand, Hicok, et al., 1994). The inflammatory response often appears to be centered around the internal elastic lamina (Wilkinson and Russell, 1972) and results in the formation of multinucleated giant cells that represent the histologic hallmark of GCA (Fig. 26–2). The multinucleated giant cells frequently can be seen to contain elastic fiber fragments (Banks et al., 1983), suggesting the possibility that the specific antigen inciting the inflammatory response may be elastin (Hellman, 1993; Hunder et al., 1993).

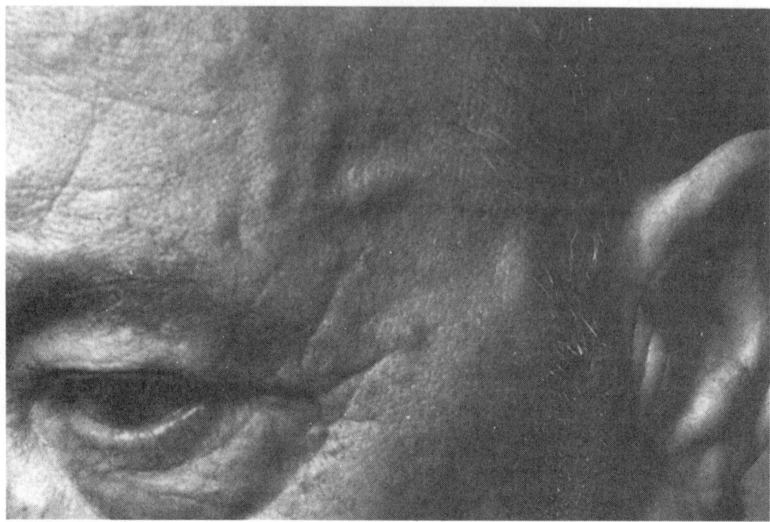

Figure 26–1 Seventy-year-old man with giant cell arteritis. A portion of the anterior branch of the left temporal artery is visibly swollen. It was tender and thickened to palpation.

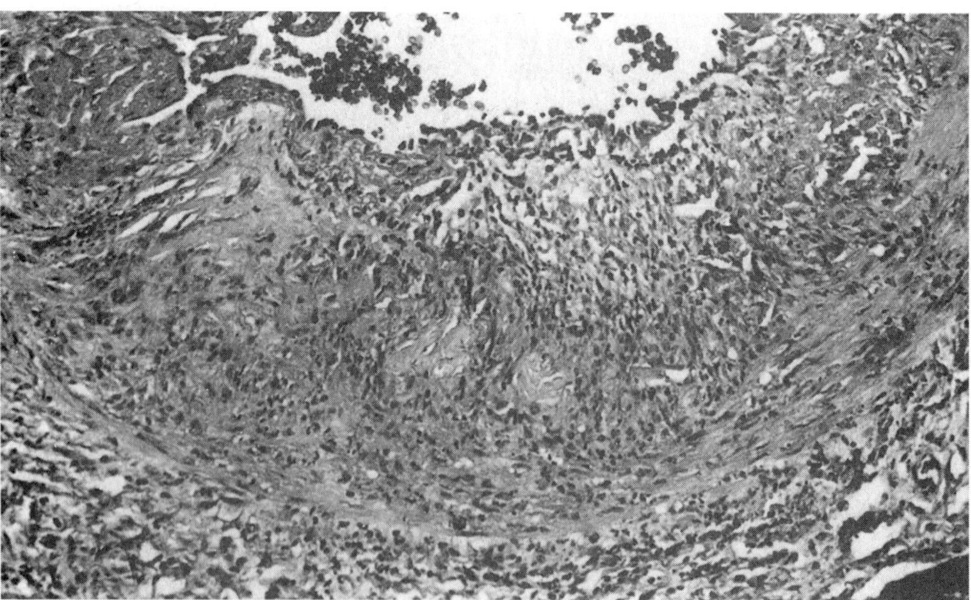

Figure 26–2 Temporal artery biopsy specimen showing active inflammation in all three vascular layers (intima, media, adventitia). The lumen is partially shown, at the top of the figure, and is narrowed. In most temporal artery biopsy specimens with giant cell arteritis, the media, especially the inner media in the region of the internal elastic lamina, is involved to the greatest extent and the intimal and adventitial layers are involved to a lesser degree than in this patient. (Hematoxylin and eosin stain, original × 200).

Vascular Topography

The superficial temporal artery (STA) is involved in almost all patients, hence the term "temporal arteritis." However, GCA is more a disease of the aortic arch (Cardell and Handley, 1951; Heptinstall et al., 1954; Ostberg, 1972; Klein et al., 1975; Evans et al., 1995) and its branches (Fig. 26–3), even though the aortic arch involvement is less than the STA involvement. Aortic arch-derived vessels that are occasionally involved include the coronary arteries (Cardell and Handley, 1951; Ostberg, 1972); the subclavian, axillary, and proximal brachial arteries (Heptinstall et al., 1954; Andrews, 1966; Ostberg, 1972; Pollock et al., 1973; Klein et al., 1975; Howard et al., 1984); and cervicocephalic arteries, including the carotid and vertebral arteries (Cooke et al., 1946; Cardell and Handley, 1951; Heptinstall et al., 1954; Crompton, 1959; Russell, 1959; Whitfield et al., 1963; Hamrin et al., 1965; Andrews, 1966; Bruk, 1967; Ostberg, 1972; Wilkinson and Russell, 1972; Pollock et al., 1973; Mowat and Hazelman, 1974; Klein et al., 1975; Graham et al., 1981; Howard et al., 1984; Evans et al., 1995). In fatal cases of GCA, autopsy studies have shown that the vertebral arteries are involved as frequently as the superficial temporal arteries (Heptinstall et al., 1954; Crompton, 1959; Wilkinson and Russell, 1972). Vertebral arteritis is extracranial, but it may extend intracranially up to 5 mm beyond dural penetration following the internal elastic lamina (Wilkinson and Russell, 1972). Because intracranial arteries lack an internal elastic lamina, GCA does not cause a widespread intracranial cerebral vasculitis, and basilar artery involvement is rare (Heptinstall et al., 1954; Gibb et al., 1985). Intraorbital branches, especially the posterior ciliary and ophthalmic arteries, are commonly affected (Wagener and Hollenhorst, 1958; Crompton, 1959; Wilkinson and Russell, 1972; Barricks et al., 1977). Less often, the descending aorta (Ostberg, 1972; Klein et al., 1975; Evans, Batts, et al., 1994; Evans et al., 1995), mesenteric (Klein et al., 1975), renal (Klein et al., 1975), iliac, and femoral arteries (Cardell and Handley, 1951; Heptinstall et al., 1954; Ostberg, 1972; Klein et al., 1975; Caselli, Hunder, et al., 1988) are affected. Pulmonary arterial involvement also has been described (Heptinstall et al., 1954; Klein et al., 1975).

CRANIOFACIAL PAIN SYNDROMES IN THE GCA PATIENT

Headache

The headache of GCA may have no pathognomonic features, but some qualities can be diagnostically suggestive. The most important feature is that the headache is either a new finding in a patient without a history of headaches or a new headache type in a patient with a history of chronic headaches. Thus GCA should be considered in all patients 50 years of age or older with new-onset headache or with a change in prior headaches. The headache quality is usually described as throbbing, generalized, and continuous. Pain may be constant from onset, intermittent, or may transform from intermittent to constant (Ward et al., 2005). The headaches of GCA may mimic common primary headache disorders. International Headache Society diagnostic criteria for GCA are illustrated in Table 26–1 (Headache Classification Committee of the International Headache Society, 2004). The temples are often focally painful and generally hurt to touch. Patients occasionally describe tender red cords in their temples (Fig. 26–1) or scalp tenderness when combing their hair. Rarely, the headache is predominantly occipital. One-third of patients lack these clinical signs of temporal or occipital artery inflammation. Approximately 5% of patients experience visual scintillations, suggestive of a migraine aura (Caselli, Daube, et al., 1988; Campbell and Caselli, 1991), though not specifically in a fixed temporal relationship with the headache. It is not known what significance these scintillations may have, but they should be viewed as a possible sign of retinal or optic nerve ischemia due to the vasculitis rather than a benign migrainous aura. A very rare cause of headache in the GCA patient is intracerebral hemorrhage, which has been reported (Hollenhorst et al., 1960), but its infrequency suggests that it is probably unrelated to vasculitis.

Other Craniofacial Pain Syndromes

Occipitonuchal pain may result from vasculitic involvement of the occipital arteries, or it may be part of the more generalized proximal limb, spine, and truncal pain that characterizes PMR. PMR

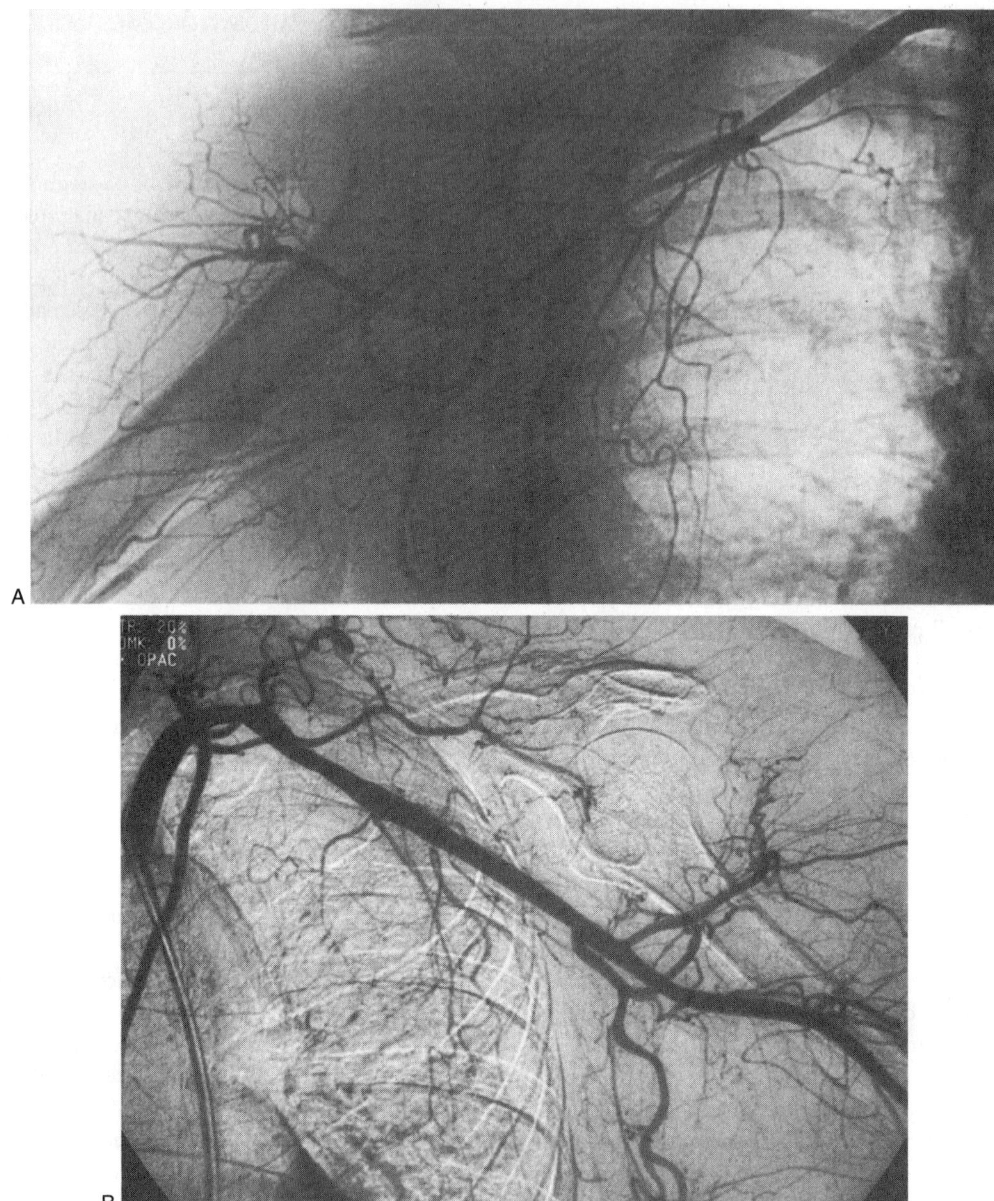

Figure 26–3 Angiogram in a patient with giant cell arteritis and aortic arch syndrome. (*A*) Right subclavian artery and distal vessels. The distal axillary artery tapers progressively and becomes occluded at the axillary–brachial artery junction. The proximal brachial artery fills again via the abundant collateral vessels. (*B*) Left subclavian artery shows a focal smooth-walled, tapered area typical of vasculitis. There are prominent collateral vessels seen distally (shown), which resulted from a more distal severe brachial artery stenosis (not shown).

occurs in approximately 50% of GCA patients, and is the initial symptom in one-fourth of GCA patients (Caselli, Daube, et al., 1988). Ischemia of jaw and tongue muscles can cause jaw and tongue claudication. Jaw claudication occurs in approximately 40% of patients and is the initial symptom in roughly 4% of patients (Caselli, Daube, et al., 1988). Tongue claudication occurs in

Table 26–1 Giant Cell Arteritis—International Headache Society Diagnostic Criteria.

A. Any new persisting headache fulfilling criteria C and D
B. At least one of the following:
   (a) Swollen tender scalp artery with elevated erythrocyte sedimentation rate (ESR) and/or C-reactive protein (CRP)
   (b) Temporal artery biopsy demonstrating giant cell arteritis
C. Headache develops in close temporal relation to other symptoms and signs of giant cell arteritis
D. Headache resolves or greatly improves within 3 days of high-dose steroid treatment

approximately 4% of patients and is rarely the initial symptom (Caselli, Daube, et al., 1988). Rare cranial neuropathic syndromes, which may be a source of discomfort to patients, include transient hemianesthesia of the tongue (Caselli, Daube, et al., 1988), lingual paralysis (Kinmont and McCallum, 1964), and facial pain due to facial artery vasculitis (Das and Laskin, 1966) (which might be mistaken for trigeminal neuralgia). Approximately 15% of patients with GCA have carotodynia (Caselli, Daube, et al., 1988). Presumably, this reflects carotid vasculitis, but angiographic studies of such patients who lack other signs and symptoms of carotid artery disease are lacking.

NEUROLOGIC DISEASE IN THE SETTING OF ACTIVE GCA

The following complications may accompany the headache of GCA, and are important features of the disease that the headache may portend.

CENTRAL NERVOUS SYSTEM COMPLICATIONS

Optic Neuropathy

Optic neuropathy is one of the most feared complications of GCA. Amaurosis fugax occurs in 10%–12% of patients with GCA (Huston et al., 1978; Caselli, Daube, et al., 1988), and permanent loss of vision due to anterior ischemic optic neuropathy (AION) occurs in 8% (Caselli, Daube, et al., 1988) to 23% (Koorey, 1984). Before the advent and widespread use of corticosteroid therapy, however, most series reported that patients with transient loss of vision went on to develop permanent, bilateral loss of vision due to AION (Wagener and Hollenhorst, 1958; Russell, 1959; Hollenhorst et al., 1960; Mowat and Hazelman, 1974). After monocular onset, the second eye became affected within days (Wagener and Hollenhorst, 1958). Prompt diagnosis and effective corticosteroid therapy have drastically reduced the number of patients with permanent loss of vision due to GCA (Hall et al., 1983). AION most often results from vasculitis of the posterior ciliary artery, and occasionally from vasculitis or occlusion of the central retinal artery (Wagener and Hollenhorst, 1958; Hollenhorst et al., 1960). During acute AION, ophthalmoscopy shows sludging of blood in retinal arterioles, which can be orthostatically sensitive (Hollenhorst, 1967). Diagnostically important funduscopic signs of optic nerve swelling may lag behind visual loss and the acute ophthalmoscopic finding of papillary and retinal ischemia by roughly 36 hours (Wagener and Hollenhorst, 1958). Occasionally, however, optic neuropathy is entirely retrobulbar without acute funduscopic changes (Wagener and Hollenhorst, 1958). In acute AION, the optic disk becomes pale with blurred margins due to papilledema (Wagener and Hollenhorst, 1958). As AION evolves, the absolute amount of disk elevation tends to be modest (<3 diopters in most cases), with infrequent areas of disk hemorrhage (Barricks et al., 1977). Optic disk edema resolves within 10 days or so, and is replaced by optic atrophy within 2–4 weeks, even in retrobulbar cases (Wagener and Hollenhorst, 1958). Residual visual field defects are usually altitudinal (Wagener and Hollenhorst, 1958). In patients with central retinal artery occlusion, there may be pallor and edema of the entire retina and optic disk, together with a macular cherry-red spot (Hollenhorst et al., 1960).

Ocular Motility Disorders

Diplopia occurs in approximately 2% (Caselli, Daube, et al., 1988) to 14% (Hollenhorst et al., 1960; Huston et al., 1978) of patients with GCA. It may be static (in cases of oculomotor nerve infarction) or fluctuate daily (similar to myasthenia gravis) (Russell, 1959; Hollenhorst et al., 1960; Hollenhorst, 1967). Any level of the oculomotor apparatus can be involved, including the extraocular muscles (EOMs), nerves (Dimant et al., 1980), and brainstem (Monteiro et al., 1984), but the EOM is the most common site (Russell, 1959; Barricks et al., 1977). Ptosis and miosis may occur together (Horner's syndrome) or separately, as well as in conjunction with other oculomotor disturbances (Dimant et al., 1980; Monteiro et al., 1984).

Cerebrovascular Disease

Clinically, auscultable bruits reflect the topographic distribution of GCA. Carotid bruits occur in 10%–20% of all GCA patients and are often bilateral (Hamrin et al., 1965; Caselli, Daube, 1988). Sixty percent of patients with bilateral carotid bruits also have upper limb bruits or claudication or both (Caselli, Daube, 1988). Approximately 40% of GCA patients who have carotid bruits sustain some type of ischemic eye or brain complication [amaurosis fugax, transient ischemic attack (TIA), permanent visual loss, or stroke], although permanent deficits (permanent visual loss and stroke) do not occur more often than in GCA patients without carotid bruits (Caselli, 1988a). The known propensity of GCA to affect carotid and vertebral arteries should be considered in GCA patients with TIAs and cerebral infarction (Caselli, 1988a; Caselli, 1990), even though atherosclerosis, hypertension, and cardiac disease remain the most important causes of cerebral infarction in elderly patients with or without GCA (Huston et al., 1978). Approximately 4% of GCA patients experience a TIA or stroke at some point during their illness (Caselli, 1988a). A relatively greater proportion of TIAs and cerebral infarctions occur in the vertebrobasilar territory than the carotid territory in the population of GCA patients compared with the general population (Caselli, 1988a). Unfortunately, there are few clinical features that reliably distinguish a vasculitic from an atheromatous cause, although in rare instances atheroembolic material has been observed funduscopically or angiographically in the setting of active GCA (Hollenhorst, 1967; Caselli, 1988a). Lacunar infarction syndromes due to hypertensive small vessel disease would not specifically be expected to result from a cervicocephalic arteritis, but it may be difficult to reliably distinguish a small- from a large-vessel stroke syndrome acutely, or without neuroimaging.

Other Large Artery Involvement

Aortic dissection, aortic aneurysm, and large artery stenosis occur with an increased frequency in patients with GCA. Large artery disease may not be apparent until several years into the course of GCA (Evans et al., 1995). Patients with GCA are approximately 17 times more likely to have thoracic aortic aneurysm and 2.4 times more likely to develop an abdominal aortic aneurysm than those in the general population (Evans et al., 1995). Patients with GCA, who also have hypertension, PMR with a marked acute inflammatory response, aortic insufficiency murmur, hyperlipidemia, and coronary artery disease, have an increased risk of developing aortic aneurysmal disease (Nuenninghoff et al., 2003; Gonzalez-Gay et al., 2004).

Neuro-otologic Disorders

GCA is one of the several vasculitides that can lead to acute auditory nerve infarction, but it is a rare occurrence (Hollenhorst et al., 1960; Caselli, 1988a). Acute unilateral hearing loss is the most suggestive symptom, but we have seen GCA patients with vertigo that resolved with corticosteroid therapy (Caselli, Daube, et al., 1988).

Encephalopathy

The differential diagnosis of encephalopathy in the GCA patient is extensive and can relate to the disease itself, complications of treatment, or unrelated factors. Acute encephalopathy may be caused by GCA itself as a result of cerebral infarction (Cooke et al., 1946; Heptinstall et al., 1954; Russell, 1959; Wilkinson and Russell, 1972; Gibb et al., 1985; Caselli, 1990; Tomer et al., 1992). Cognitive changes may result from thalamic, mesial temporal, and mesencephalic involvement in some cases, and magnetic resonance imaging (MRI) [or computed tomography (CT)] should be performed. Acute encephalopathy is a poor prognostic sign, and many such patients progress to coma and death (Cooke et al., 1946; Heptinstall et al., 1954; Russell, 1959; Wilkinson and Russell, 1972; Gibb et al., 1985). With steroid therapy, some patients may stabilize, and over time can experience some recovery (Caselli, 1990; Tomer et al., 1992). One comatose patient had triphasic waves on the electroencephalogram, and steroid treatment led to complete recovery (Tomer et al., 1992). Recurrent episodes of acute encephalopathy with progressive cognitive impairment can lead to a more chronic multi-infarct dementia due to cervicocephalic arterial involvement by GCA (Caselli, 1990). In our experience, encephalopathy and dementia due to GCA are uncommon (Caselli, Daube, et al., 1988; Caselli, 1990), although earlier literature suggested that they were frequent complications (Vereker, 1952; Paulley and Hughes, 1960). Corticosteroid therapy itself may cause encephalopathy primarily (steroid psychosis) or secondarily. There are numerous potential steroid-related complications, such as metabolic abnormalities and systemic and central nervous system infections (which occur more commonly in immunocompromised hosts). Finally, diseases that are prevalent in the elderly and are unrelated to GCA can cause encephalopathy and dementia, such as degenerative and vascular dementias, chronic subdural hematoma, and sedating medications.

Seizures

Although there is no evidence that GCA directly causes seizures, seizures may complicate the clinical course of any patient who has sustained a cortical infarction, whether or not the underlying mechanism was related to GCA. Seizures may also complicate the clinical course of patients with encephalopathy related primarily or secondarily to steroids, and so there are various reasons seizures may occur in the patient with GCA.

Myelopathy

On rare occasions, GCA may cause acute cervical myelopathy (Cloake, 1951; Brennan and Sandyk, 1982; Gibb et al., 1985; Caselli, Daube, et al., 1988). The vasculitis presumably extends to the anterior spinal artery from the vertebral arteries (Gibb et al., 1985). Myelopathic involvement may presage a fatal outcome (Gibb et al., 1985), although prompt treatment with corticosteroids may permit neurologic stabilization (Caselli, Daube, et al., 1988) and improvement (Brennan and Sandyk, 1982).

PERIPHERAL NERVOUS SYSTEM COMPLICATIONS

Mononeuropathies

GCA occasionally affects large peripheral arteries and their branches (Klein et al., 1975), which can include the nutrient arteries of peripheral nerves (Caselli, Daube, et al., 1988) and result in mononeuropathies or mononeuritis multiplex (Meneely and Bigelow, 1953; Russell, 1959; Warrell et al., 1968; Fryer and Singer, 1971; Massey and Weed, 1978; Dux et al., 1981; Sànchez et al., 1983; Shapiro et al., 1983; Feigal et al., 1985; Caselli, Hunder, et al., 1988). The incidence of acute ischemic mononeuropathies in GCA patients is difficult to estimate, but is probably approximately 2% (Caselli, Hunder, et al., 1988). Prognosis for neurologic recovery with corticosteroid treatment is good, provided that vascular compromise does not lead to loss of the affected limb (Caselli, Hunder, et al., 1988). Essentially, all named peripheral nerves can be involved as ischemic mononeuropathies. Among the spinal nerves, the fifth cervical nerve has been reported by several authors (Fryer and Singer, 1971; Sànchez et al., 1983; Shapiro et al., 1983; Caselli, Hunder, et al., 1988) to be susceptible to GCA. Patients with GCA also can develop mononeuropathies that occur at common compression sites and are unrelated to vasculitis.

For example, approximately 5% have carpal tunnel syndrome (Caselli, Hunder, et al., 1988). In some cases, median nerve compression might be related to PMR-induced wrist synovitis.

Peripheral Neuropathy

Mild abnormalities of nerve conduction studies and electromyography (EMG) are common in elderly patients. Although such findings may suggest a peripheral neuropathy, the relationship of such neuropathies to GCA is uncertain. In other patients, however, antecedent ischemic mononeuropathies may accrue and eventually resemble a "diffuse," severe, peripheral neuropathy (Warrell et al., 1968; Feigal et al., 1985; Caselli, Hunder, et al., 1988). However, this is much less likely to be caused by GCA than by other causes of vasculitis.

Myopathy

GCA does not cause an inflammatory myopathy, although there are rare examples of localized inflammation in muscle (Andrews, 1966). PMR may falsely lead to the clinical suspicion of a myopathy, and steroid therapy commonly causes a mild, noninflammatory myopathy ("steroid myopathy"). In typical cases of PMR without vasculitic involvement of the peripheral nervous system, EMG results are normal (Caselli, Hunder, et al., 1988).

LABORATORY EVALUATION

Blood Tests

When a patient's diagnosis is suspected to be GCA, an ESR should be performed immediately and the results obtained that same day so that steroid therapy may be instituted promptly. Though nonspecific, the combination of headache and an elevated ESR in an elderly patient is highly suspicious for GCA. The ESR is elevated in approximately 97% of patients with GCA who are not taking corticosteroids. The mean value is 85 [standard deviation (SD) 32] mm in 1 hour (Westergren method) (Campbell and Caselli, 1991). Other acute-phase reactant proteins are also increased. The CRP has become increasingly used to monitor disease activity in recent years, and is more sensitive than the ESR in some patients. Other common laboratory abnormalities include a normochromic microcytic anemia (mean hemoglobin value, 11.7 g/dl, SD 1.6) and thrombocytosis (mean platelet count $427 \times 10^3/\mu l$, SD 116×10^3). Mild elevations of serum transaminases and alkaline phosphatase occur in 15% of patients, and elevations of plasma α-2 globulins occur in 72% of patients (Campbell and Caselli, 1991).

Prebiopsy Predictors of GCA

A combination of clinical features, physical examination, and laboratory findings can be helpful in predicting TAB results. Positive likelihood ratios have been associated with headache (1.22, 1.04–1.43), jaw claudication (4.03, 2.38–6.80), temporal artery pain (2.26, 1.14–4.48), any visual symptom (1.30, 1.03–1.65), diplopia (1.99, 1.29–3.07), and weight loss (1.30, 1.13–1.50) (Niederkohr and Levin, 2005). The odds of a positive TAB have consistently been found to be elevated when jaw claudication is present, increasing the odds by nine times in one study (Hayreh et al., 1997). Temporal artery abnormalities on examination (loss of pulse, pain on palpation, nodularity) have also consistently been associated with positive biopsy, increasing the odds by approximately 3 (Gonzalez-Gay et al., 2001). Elevated ESR, CRP, anemia, and thrombocytosis are also predictive. ESR of 47–107 mm/hour has been associated with an odds ratio of 2 (1–4.1, $p = 0.045$), and an ESR greater than 107 mm/hour with an odds ratio of 2.7 (1.2–5.9, $p = 0.011$) (Hayreh et al., 1997). CRP greater than 2.45 mg/dl associates with an odds ratio for positive biopsy of 3.2 (1.2–8.6, $p = 0.021$) (Hayreh et al., 1997). A combination of clinical symptoms, physical examination findings, and laboratory abnormalities are most predictive of a biopsy positive for GCA. For example, a combination of recent-onset headache, jaw claudication, and abnormal temporal artery on examination has a specificity of 94.8% with biopsy as the gold standard (Vilaseca et al., 1987). Logistic regression analysis of 1113 patients who underwent TAB between 1988 and 1997 at the Mayo Clinic in Rochester, Minnesota, yielded the following six predictors: new headache, jaw claudication, scalp tenderness, elevated ESR, ischemic optic neuropathy, and older age. Low scores on this predictive equation were associated with a probability of positive TAB of less than 10%, while high scores were associated with a probability of positive biopsy of more than 80% (Younge et al., 2004).

Temporal Artery Biopsy

The ESR or CRP are essential tests for early diagnosis and help to guide therapy in the acute setting, but GCA is a chronic disease that requires long-term steroid use. Greater diagnostic specificity than that provided solely by these tests is therefore important. Confirmation by TAB should be considered in every patient in whom GCA is suspected. Glucocorticoids can be started before the TAB if necessary, but if this is done, TAB should be performed as soon as possible (preferably within a few days) to avoid steroid-induced histologic suppression or alteration of vasculitis in the TAB specimen that would make diagnostic accuracy more problematic. However, patients may continue to have histologic evidence of GCA on TAB as long as 6 weeks after the institution of steroids, even if there has been clinical resolution of symptoms (Achkar et al., 1994; Evans, Batts, et al., 1994). We recommend a 3–5 cm specimen from the most symptomatic side, and we obtain bilateral specimens if frozen sections are negative (Caselli and Hunder, 1993). If the TAB segment is long and multiple histologic sections are taken, 86% of cases will be correctly diagnosed by unilateral biopsy (Hall and Hunder, 1984). Histologic features include intimal proliferation with luminal stenosis, disruption of the internal elastic lamina by a mononuclear cell infiltrate, invasion and necrosis of the media progressing to panarteritic involvement by mononuclear cells, giant-cell formation with granulomata within the mononuclear cell infiltrate, and, variably, intraluminal thrombosis (Fig. 26–2). Involvement of the affected artery is often patchy (skip lesions) (Hall et al., 1983; Hall and Hunder, 1984).

Aortic Arch and Cerebral Angiography

Aortic arch and cerebral angiography are not routine diagnostic tests for GCA, but some patients with GCA undergo these studies for stroke-related symptoms. In such patients, the vertebral and external carotid arteries (including the STA) may show vasculitic changes of alternating stenotic segments (Caselli, Daube, et al., 1988) or occlusion (Caselli, 1990) (Fig. 26–2). Superficial temporal angiography, however, is less reliable than TAB for establishing a diagnosis. Internal carotid arteries may be occluded (Cull, 1979; Howard et al., 1984; Caselli, Daube, et al., 1988; Caselli, 1990), but they rarely have a characteristic vasculitic pattern. Subclavian, axillary, and proximal brachial arterial involvement produces a characteristic angiographic pattern of vasculitis that consists of long-smooth stenotic segments alternating with nonstenotic segments and tapered occlusions (Heptinstall et al., 1954; Hamrin et al., 1965; Andrews, 1966; Ostberg, 1972; Pollock et al., 1973; Klein et al., 1975; Howard et al., 1984; Evans et al., 1995) (Fig. 26–3).

TREATMENT AND PROGNOSIS

Oral corticosteroids remain the mainstay of treatment. Most patients will require prednisone for 1–2 years, with initial doses of 40–60 mg daily. If a patient presents with an acute neurologic syndrome or rapidly worsening neurologic status, whether it be visual loss, mononeuritis multiplex, or acute encephalopathy, treatment may begin with an intravenous pulse over several days (1000 mg methylprednisolone per day) or with a very high oral dose of steroids (up to 120 mg prednisone), though there is no controlled study that has compared the efficacy and safety of this more aggressive regimen to conventional therapy. The starting dose is then tapered over a few weeks, so that by the end of the first month of therapy most patients are taking approximately 40 mg of prednisone daily. Subsequent reductions by 2.5–5 mg amounts may be made every 1–3 weeks as tolerated. A patient with GCA who has a relapse may require only a modest increment in dose to control the flare in symptoms. By 6 months, approximately half of the patients will have reduced their daily dose to 7.5 mg per day, and three-fourth will have done so by 1 year (Proven et al., 2003). A recent study suggests that initiation of therapy with pulse glucocorticoids may shorten the total length of therapy required and the total dose of oral glucocorticoids needed (Mazlumzadeh et al., 2006).

After the initiation of steroid treatment, the headache usually resolves within days. The ESR may drop within days and become normal in 1 or 2 weeks. Neurologic deficits can improve, but irreversible end-organ infarction may preclude clinically significant gains in some patients. Occasionally, a mild headache may persist for 2–4 weeks without any other clinical or laboratory signs of disease activity. Mild jaw claudication may persist up to several weeks before resolving completely. Neurovascular complications may occur during the initial tapering of corticosteroid dosage, typically approximately 1 month after beginning treatment (Caselli, Daube, et al., 1988), emphasizing the utility of ESR monitoring and the importance of small steroid decrements. Approximately 50% of disease relapses occur during the first month after corticosteroid discontinuation, and 95% occur during the first year (Andersson et al., 1986).

Long-term corticosteroid therapy is often required for the treatment of GCA. The median time to discontinuation of corticosteroids is approximately 22 months (Proven et al., 2003). Approximately 43% of patients with GCA continue on steroid treatment at 5 years and 25% at 9 years after diagnosis (Andersson et al., 1986). Chronic steroid therapy is fraught with complications. Complications occur in approximately 86% of patients and are multiple in approximately 58% (Proven et al., 2003). These include diabetes mellitus, bone fractures (vertebral compression fractures, hip fractures, etc.), gastrointestinal bleeding, steroid myopathy, steroid psychosis, and immunosuppression-related infections. Alternate therapeutic strategies would therefore be of potentially great utility for many patients. However, none have yet been shown to be reliably effective and safe. Some studies have suggested that much lower doses and more rapid tapering schedules are sufficient. One such study advocated initiating treatment with 20 mg of prednisolone daily and tapering it 10 mg daily within 3 months (Lundberg and Hedfors, 1990). Although many patients may respond to this regimen with symptomatic improvement of headache, PMR, and reduction of ESR, a substantial number of patients will experience symptomatic worsening of symptoms (Lundberg and Hedfors, 1990). Headache and PMR, though they are the most common symptoms of GCA, are not the reason these patients are treated with high-dose steroids. Higher doses are required to prevent irreversible ischemic ophthalmologic and neurologic complications. Trials of other immunosuppressant drugs, including azathioprine (De Silva and Hazleman, 1986), methotrexate (Krall et al., 1989), cyclophosphamide (DeVita et al., 1992), and dapsone (Demaziere, 1989), have been attempted for their steroid-sparing effects. Steroid dosages have been successfully lowered in some patients on each of these drugs, but inconsistently. Toxicity can be a significant problem, particularly with dapsone and cyclophosphamide. Azathioprine has no acute effect, and its steroid-sparing effects may not be evident for a year (DeVita et al., 1992). Limited experience suggests that cyclophosphamide may be the most consistently effective immunosuppressant other than corticosteroids (Demaziere, 1989; DeVita et al., 1992; Caselli and Hunder, 1993), and may permit more rapid steroid tapering when instituted after a relapse. However, it is also the most toxic agent.

In summary, GCA is an important neurologic disease that must be familiar to all medical practitioners who work with elderly patients. Although it commonly presents with headache, it is not a disease confined to the province of a headache specialist.

References

Achkar, AA, Lie, JT, Hunder, GG, et al. (1994). How does previous corticosteroid treatment affect the biopsy findings in giant cell (temporal) arteritis? *Ann Intern Med*, 120:987–992.

Andersson, R, Malmvall, BE, and Bengtsson, BA (1986). Long-term corticosteroid treatment in giant cell arteritis. *Acta Med Scand*, 220:465–469.

Andrews, JM (1966). Giant-cell (temporal) arteritis. A disease with variable clinical manifestations. *Neurology*, 16:963–971.

Banks, PM, Cohen, MD, Ginsburg, WW, et al. (1983). Immunohistologic and cytochemical studies of temporal arteritis. *Arthritis Rheum*, 26:1201–1207.

Barricks, ME, Traviesa, DB, Glaser, JS, et al. (1977). Ophthahnoplegia in cranial arteritis. *Brain*, 100:209–221.

Brennan, MJW and Sandyk, R (1982). Reversible quadriplegia in a patient with giant-cell arteritis. *S Afr Med J*, 62:81–82.

Bruk, MI (1967). Articular and vascular manifestations of polymyalgia rheumatica. *Ann Rheum Dis*, 26:103–116.

Calamia, KT and Hunder, GG (1980). Clinical manifestations of giant cell (temporal) arteritis. *Clin Rheum Dis*, 6:389–415.

Campbell, JK and Caselli, RJ (1991). Headache and other craniofacial pain. In WG Bradley, RB Daroff, GM

Fenichel, and CD Marsden (eds), *Neurology in Clinical Practice: Principles of Diagnosis and Management* (pp. 1507–1561). Butterworth-Heinemann, Philadelphia, PA.

Cardell, BS and Hanley, T (1951). A fatal case of giant-cell or temporal arteritis. *J Pathol Bacteriol*, 63:587–597.

Caselli, RJ (1990). Giant cell (temporal) arteritis: A treatable cause of multi-infarct dementia. *Neurology*, 40:753–755.

Caselli, RJ, Daube, JR, Hunder, GG, et al. (1988). Peripheral neuropathic syndromes in giant cell (temporal) arteritis. *Neurology*, 38:685–689.

Caselli, RJ and Hunder, GG (1993). Giant cell (temporal) arteritis and cerebral vasculitis. In RT Johnson and JW Griffin (eds), *Current Therapy in Neurologic Disease*, 4th edn. (pp 196–201). B.C. Decker, Hamilton: ontario, Canada.

Caselli, RJ, Hunder, GG, and Whisnant, JP (1988). Neurologic disease in giant cell (temporal) arteritis. *Neurology*, 38:352–359.

Cloake, PCP (1951). Temporal arteritis. *Proc R Soc Med*, 44:847–852.

Cooke, WT, Cloake, PCP, Govan, ADT, et al. (1946). Temporal arteritis: a generalized vascular disease. *Q J Med*, 15:47–75.

Crompton, MR (1959). The visual changes in temporal (giant-cell) arteritis: Report of a case with autopsy findings. *Brain*, 82:377–390.

Cull, RE (1979). Internal carotid artery occlusion caused by giant cell arteritis. *J Neurol Neurosurg Psychiatry*, 42:1066–1067.

Das, AK and Laskin, DM (1966). Temporal arteritis of the facial artery. *J Oral Surg*, 24:226–232.

De Silva, M and Hazleman, BL (1986). Azathioprine in giant cell arteritis/polymyalgia rheumatica: a double-blind study. *Ann Rheum Dis*, 45:136–138.

Demaziere, A (1989). Dapsone in the long term treatment of temporal arteritis (letter). *Am J Med*, 87:3.

DeVita, S, Tavoni, A, Jeraitano, G, et al. (1992). Treatment of giant cell arteritis with cyclophosphamide pulses (letter). *J Intern Med*, 232:373–375.

Dimant, J, Grob, D, and Brunner, NG (1980). Ophthalmoplegia, ptosis, and miosis in temporal arteritis. *Neurology*, 30:1054–1058.

Dux, S, Pithk, S, and Rosenfeld, JB (1981). Popliteal neuritis complicating temporal arteritis. *Harefuah*, 101:291.

Evans, JM, Batts, KP, and Hunder, GG (1994). Persistent giant cell arteritis despite corticosteroid treatment. *Mayo Clin Proc*, 69:1060–1061.

Evans, JM, Bowles, CA, Bjornsson, J, et al. (1994). Thoracic aneurysm and rupture in giant cell arteritis. *Arthritis Rheum*, 37:1539–1544.

Evans, JM, O'Fallon, MO, and Hunder, GG (1995). Increased incidence of aortic aneurysm and dissection in giant cell (temporal) arteritis. A population based study. *Ann Intern Med*, 122:502–507.

Feigal, DW, Robbins, DL, and Leek, JC (1985). Giant cell arteritis associated with mononeuritis multiplex and complement-activating 19S IgM rheumatoid factor. *Am J Med*, 79:495–500.

Fryer, DG and Singer, RS (1971). Giant-cell arteritis with cervical radiculopathy. *Bull Mason Clin*, 25:143–151.

Gibb, WRG, Urry, PA, and Lees, AJ (1985). Giant cell arteritis with spinal cord infarction and basilar artery thrombosis. *J Neurol Neurosurg Psychiatry*, 48:945–948.

Gonzalez-Gay, MA, Barcia-Porrua, C, Llorca, J, et al. (2001). Biopsy-negative giant cell arteritis: clinical spectrum and predictive factors for positive temporal artery biopsy. *Semin Arthritis Rheum*, 30:249–256.

Gonzalez-Gay, MA, Garcia-Porrua, C, Pineiro, A, et al. (2004). Aortic aneurysm and dissection in patients with biopsy-proven giant cell arteritis from northwestern Spain. *Medicine*, 83:335–341.

Graham, E, Holland, A, Avery, A, et al. (1981). Prognosis in giant-cell arteritis. *Br Med J*, 282:269–271.

Hall, S and Hunder, GG (1984). Is temporal artery biopsy prudent? *Mayo Clin Proc*, 59:793–796.

Hall, S, Persellin, S, Lie, JT, et al. (1983). The therapeutic impact of temporal artery biopsy. *Lancet*, 2:1217–1220.

Hamrin, B, Jonsson, N, and Landberg, T (1965). Involvement of large vessels in polymyalgia arteritica. *Lancet*, 1:1193–1196.

Hayreh, SS, Podhajsky, PA, Raman, R, et al. (1997) Giant cell arteritis:validity and reliability of various diagnostic criteria. *Am J Ophthalmol*, 123:285–296.

Headache Classification Committee of the International Headache Society (2004). International Classification of Headache Disorders II. *Cephalalgia*, 24 (Suppl.):1–151.

Hellman, DB (1993). Immunopathogenesis, diagnosis, and treatment of giant cell arteritis, temporal arteritis, polymyalgia rheumatica, and Takayasu's arteritis. *Curr Opin Rheumatol*, 5:25–32.

Heptinstall, RH, Porter, KA, and Barkley, H (1954). Giant-cell (temporal) arteritis. *J Pathol Bacteriol*, 67:507–519.

Hollenhorst, RW (1967). Effect of posture of retinal ischemia from temporal arteritis. *Arch Ophthalmol*, 78:569–577.

Hollenhorst, RW, Brown, JR, Wagener, HP, et al. (1960). Neurologic aspects of temporal arteritis. *Neurology*, 10:490–498.

Howard, GF III, Ho, SU, Kim, KS, et al. (1984). Bilateral carotid artery occlusion resulting from giant cell arteritis. *Ann Neurol*, 15:204–207.

Hunder, GG, Lie, JT, Goronzy, JJ, et al. (1993). Pathogenesis of giant cell arteritis. *Arthritis Rheum*, 36:757–761.

Huston, KA, Hunder, GG, Lie, JT, et al. (1978). Temporal arteritis. A 25-year epidemiologic, clinical, and pathologic study. *Ann Intern Med*, 88:162–167.

Kinmont, PDC and McCallum, DI (1964). Skin manifestations of giant-cell arteritis. *Br J Dermatol*, 76:299–308.

Klein, RG, Hunder, GG, Stanson, AW, et al. (1975). Large artery involvement in giant cell (temporal) arteritis. *Ann Intern Med*, 83:806–812.

Koorey, DJ (1984). Cranial arteritis. A twenty-year review of cases. *Aust NZ J Med*, 14:143–147.

Krall, PL, Mazenec, DJ, and Wilke, WS (1989). Methotrexate for corticosteroid-resistant polymyalgia rheumatica and giant cell arteritis. *Cleve Clin Med J*, 56:253–257.

Liang, GC, Simkin, PA, Hunder, GG, et al. (1974). Familial aggregation of polymyalgia rheumatica and giant cell arteritis. *Arthritis Rheum*, 17:19–24.

Lundberg, I and Hedfors, E (1990). Restricted dose and duration of corticosteroid treatment in patients with polymyalgia rheumatica and temporal arteritis. *J Rheumatol*, 17:1340–1345.

Massey, EW and Weed, T (1978). Sciatic neuropathy with giant-cell arteritis (letter). *N Engl J Med*, 298:917.

Mazlumzadeh, M, Hunder, GG, Easley, KA, et al. (2006). Treatment of giant cell arteritis using induction therapy with high-dose glucocorticoids:a double-blind, placebo-controlled, randomized prospective clinical trial. *Arthritis Rheum*, 54:3310–3318.

Meneely, JK Jr. and Bigelow, NH (1953). Temporal arteritis. A critical evaluation of this disorder and a report of three cases. *Am J Med*, 14:46–51.

Monteiro, MLR, Coppeto, JR, and Greco, P (1984). Giant cell arteritis of the posterior cerebral circulation presenting with ataxia and ophthalmoplegia. *Arch Ophthalmol*, 102:407–409.

Mowat, AG and Hazleman, BL (1974). Polymyalgia rheumatica-a clinical study with particular reference to arterial disease. *J Rheumatol*, 1:190–202.

Niederkohr, RD, and Levin, LA (2005). Management of the patient with suspected temporal arteritis: a decision-analytic approach. *Ophthalmology*, 112:744–756.

Nuenninghoff, DM, Hunder, GG, Christianson, TJH (2003). Incidence and predictors of large-artery complication (aortic aneurysm, aortic dissection, and/or large-artery stenosis) in patients with giant cell arteritis. *Arthritis Rheum*, 48:3522–3531.

Östberg, G (1972). Morphological changes in the large arteries in polymyalgia arteritica. *Acta Med Scand*, (Suppl) 533:135–164.

Ostberg, G. (1973). On arteritis with special reference to polymyalgia arteritica. *Acta Pathol Microbiol Scand*, 237(Suppl. A):1–59.

Paulley, JW and Hughes, JP (1960). Giant-cell arteritis, or arteritis of the aged. *Br Med J*, 2:1562–1567.

Pollock, M, Blennerhassett, JB, and Clarke, AM (1973). Giant cell arteritis and the subclavian steal syndrome. *Neurology*, 23:653–657.

Proven, A, Sherine, EG, Orces, C, et al. (2003). Glucocorticoid therapy in giant cell arteritis: duration and adverse outcomes. *Arthritis Rheum*, 49:703–708.

Russell, RWR (1959). Giant-cell arteritis. A review of 35 cases. *Q J Med*, 28:471–489.

Salvarani, C, Crowson, CS, O'Fallon, WM, et al. (2004). Reappraisal of the epidemiology of giant cell arteritis in Olmsted County, Minnesota, over a fifty-year period. *Arthritis Rheum*, 51:264–268.

Salvarani, C, Gabriel, SE, O'Fallon, WM, et al. (1995). The incidence of giant cell arteritis in Olmsted County, Minnesota: apparent fluctuations in a cyclic pattern. *Ann Intern Med*, 123:192–194.

Sànchez, MC, Arenillas, JLC, Gutierrez, DA, et al. (1983). Cervical radiculopathy: A rare symptom of giant cell arteritis. *Arthritis Rheum*, 26:207–209.

Shapiro, L, Medsger, TA Jr., and Nicholas, JJ (1983). Brachial plexitis mimicking C5 radiculopathy-a presentation of giant cell arteritis (letter). *J Rheumatol*, 10:670–671.

Shiiki, H, Shimokama, T, and Watanabe, T (1989). Temporal arteritis: cell composition and the possible pathogenetic role of cell mediated immunity. *Hum Pathol*, 20:1057–1064.

Tomer, Y, Neufeld, MY, and Shoenfeld, Y (1992). Coma with triphasic wave pattern in EEG as a complications of temporal arteritis. *Neurology*, 42:439–441.

Vereker, R (1952). The psychiatric aspects of temporal arteritis. *J Ment Sci*, 98:280–286.

Vilaseca, J, Gonzalez, A, Cid, MC, et al. (1987). Clinical usefulness of temporal artery biopsy. *Ann Rheum Dis*, 46:282–285.

Wagener, HP and Hollenhorst, RW (1958). The ocular lesions of temporal arteritis. *Am J Ophthalmol*, 45:617–630.

Ward, TN and Levin, M (2005). Headache in giant cell arteritis and other arteritides. *Neurol Sci*, 26,: S134–S137.

Warrell, DA, Godfrey, S, and Olsen, EGJ (1968). Giant-cell arteritis with peripheral neuropathy. *Lancet*, 1:1010–1013.

Wawryk, SO, Ayberk, H, Boyd, AW, et al. (1991). Analysis of adhesion molecules in the immunopathogenesis of giant cell arteritis. *J Clin Pathol*, 44:497–501.

Weyand, CM, Hicok, KC, Hunder, GG, et al. (1992). The HLA-DRB1 locus as a genetic component in giant cell arteritis. Mapping of a disease-linked sequence motif to the antigen binding side of the HLA-DR molecule. *J Clin Invest*, 90:2355–2361.

Weyand, CM, Hicok, KC, Hunder, GG, et al. (1994). Tissue cytokine patterns in patients with polymyalgia rheumatica and giant cell arteritis. *Ann Intern Med*, 121:484–491.

Weyand, CM, Hunder, NN, Hicok, KC, et al. (1994). HLA-DRB1 alleles in polymyalgia rheumatica, giant cell arteritis, and rheumatoid arthritis. *Arthritis Rheum*, 37:514–520.

Whitfield, AGW, Bateman, M, and Cooke, WT (1963). Temporal arteritis. *Br J Ophthalmol*, 47:555–566.

Wilkinson, IMS and Russell, RWR (1972). Arteries of the head and neck in giant cell arteritis: a pathological study to show the pattern of arterial involvement. *Arch Neurol*, 27:378–391.

Younge, BR, Cook, BE, Bartley, GB, et al. (2004). Initiation of glucocorticoid therapy: before or after temporal artery biopsy? *Mayo Clin Proc*, 79:483–491.

IV Special Topics

27 Headaches in Children

Paul Winner, DO, Andrew D Hershey, and Zhicheng Li

INTRODUCTION

Headache is a frequent symptom in the pediatric population. Acute headaches can often accompany a systemic infection, an organic disorder or other secondary cause. When an acute headache occurs repeatedly or episodically it is often a primary headache with migraine and tension-type headache being the most frequent cause in children and adolescents. A chronic or very frequent headache may be secondary to migraine. Headache disorders can affect the lifestyle of both the child and his or her family resulting in significant disability. This can include time lost from school and parental absence from work, while also affecting the child and parent interaction at home and the child's social interaction with peers. The majority of children and adolescents with headache never consult a physician (Sillanpää et al., 1991).

Although historical references to headaches date back over 6000 years (Rose, 1995), children's headaches have frequently been ignored. In 1873, William Henry Day, a British pediatrician, devoted a chapter in his pediatric textbook to headaches in children (Day, 1873) and in 1921 Comby first published an article on childhood migraine (Comby, 1921). The beginning of the modern era of the study of headaches in children and adolescents start first with Vahlquist who reported his initial criteria for childhood migraine (Vahlquist and Hackzell, 1949). These criteria were the basis for Bille's landmark epidemiology study in 1962 of 9000 schoolchildren (Bille, 1962) that have been followed for 40 years (Bille, 1997). In the last decade, the study of childhood and adolescent headaches has greatly expanded with several texts and multiple manuscripts.

This chapter will discuss some of these recent findings in epidemiology, clinical features, management, and prognosis of headaches in the pediatric population. The genetics, anatomy, pathology, and pathophysiology of pain and migraine will be reviewed.

EPIDEMIOLOGY

Epidemiologic studies of headaches in children and adolescents can include all complaints of headache or can be divided into studies of individual headache types including: (1) migraine headaches, (2) tension-type headaches, and (3) other types of headaches. These studies can be further divided into population-based and specialized clinic-based research. Only a few studies have looked at cluster headaches in children and adolescents.

Epidemiologic studies require a standardized case definition. The 1988 and 2004 criteria of the International Headache Society (IHS), the International Classification of Headache Disorders (ICHD) is the usual foundation for epidemiologic research (Headache Classification Committee of the IHS, 1988; Headache Classification Subcommittee of the IHS, 2004). These criteria provide commonality in the diagnosis of all headache disorders and are intended to serve as the bases for all scientific research in headache medicine, including epidemiology studies. Owing both to the rather recent adoption of these criteria and their incompleteness in recognizing childhood headache disorders, estimates of the prevalence and incidence of primary headache disorders have varied greatly, not only in children and adolescents, but also in adults. Epidemiologic studies of headache in young children are further complicated by the inability of young children to describe their pain or recall features associated with their headaches that may vary considerably from attack to attack.

The epidemiology of a disease can be measured both by incidence and by prevalence. Incidence refers to the rate of onset of new cases of a particular disease in a defined population. Prevalence refers to the frequency with which a specific disorder is seen in the population at a given time. By the age of 3, 3%–8% of children have experienced a headache (Sillanpää, 1976; Zuckerman et al., 1987). By age 5, this increases to 19.5% and by age 7 increases to 37%–51.5% with a further increase in headache prevalence to 57%–82% in 7- to 15-year-olds (Bille, 1962; Deubner, 1977; Sillanpää, 1983; Sillanpää et al., 1991). This increase in headache prevalence occurs in both boys and girls, ages 3–11 with a slightly higher prevalence in boys than girls (Mortimer et al., 1992). In boys, headache prevalence is stable from 7 to 14 years of age and declines thereafter, whereas girls showed an increase in headache prevalence from 7 to 22 years of age (Sillanpää, 1983).

The epidemiology of migraine in children has been more closely examined. At the age of 7, prevalence ranges from 1.2% to 3.2% (males > females), while between 7 and 11 years of age the prevalence ranges from 4% to 11% (males = females) and for adolescents above 11 the prevalence ranges from 8% to 23% (males < females) (Bille, 1962; Sillanpää, 1976, 1983; Mortimer et al., 1992). Many of these studies used clinical-based criteria. With the adoption of ICHD-I in 1988 (Headache Classification Committee of the IHS, 1988) and subsequent revision with ICHD-II in 2004 (Headache Classification Subcommittee of the IHS, 2004), multiple studies have looked at the epidemiology of migraine as well as tension-type headache. Using ICHD-I, Abu-Arafeh and Russell found in a sample of 2165 children between the ages of 5 and 15 that 10.6% had migraine (7.8% had migraine without aura and 2.8% had migraine with aura) and 0.9% had tension-type headache (Abu-Arafeh and Russell, 1994). They noted that this may be an underestimate due to some patients not fulfilling ICHD-I. Additional studies using ICHD-I have found the general range of migraine to be 6.1%–10.6% (Lee and Olness, 1997; Barea et al., 1996; Mavromichalis et al., 1999; Lu et al., 2000; Al Jumah et al., 2002; Ayatollahi et al., 2002; Zwart et al., 2004). In older adolescents (age 15–19 years old), the prevalence appears to be even higher with 28% having migraine (19% with migraine without aura, 9% with migraine with aura) (Split and Neuman, 1999). The use of ICHD-II for epidemiology studies has been less extensive. A study of 12–17 year olds in Bursa found the prevalence of migraine to be 14.5% (Karli et al., 2006).

The incidence of migraine has been evaluated with telephone interviews of more than 10,000 individuals between the ages of 12 and 29 years (Stewart et al., 1992). Based on 392 males and 1018 females with migraine, the estimated age- and sex-specific incidence rates for migraine with and without aura were calculated, where incidence of migraine with aura in males was 6.6/1000 person years, and peaked at 5–6 years of age. The peak incidence of migraine without aura in males was 10/1000 person years and peaked at 10–11 years of age. New cases of migraine were uncommon in men in their 20s. The incidence of migraine with aura in females was 14.1/1000 person years and peaked at 12–13 years of age; the incidence of migraine without aura was 18.9/1000 person years and peaked at 14–17 years of age.

The epidemiology of tension-type headaches in children and adolescents has been less well studied with wide variability in the reported prevalence. The range of reported prevalence varied widely ranging from 0.9% (Abu-Arafeh and Russell, 1994) to 12.1% (Ayatollahi et al., 2002) to 18% (Zwart et al., 2004) to 25.9% (Karli et al., 2006) to 72.8% (Barea et al., 1996). Clearly, further studies that look specifically at the incidence and prevalence of episodic and chronic tension-type headaches in children and adolescents are needed.

The incidence and prevalence of cluster headaches in individuals under the age of 20 has not been well studied. The typical age of onset of cluster headaches occurs in the late 20s, but one series found that 10% of patients were between 10 and 19 years of age (Pearce, 1980).

CLASSIFICATION

Prior to the publication of ICHD-I in 1988, several classifications were used for headaches in children (Vahlquist, 1955; Deubner, 1977; Congdon and Forsythe, 1979; Prensky and Sommer, 1979). These criteria were largely clinically based as was true for the criteria for adult migraine. In order to address this variability in headache diagnosis and to establish a basis for the scientific study of headache, ICHD-I was developed (Headache Classification Committee of the IHS, 1988). Several studies compared the diagnoses of migraine in children utilizing the historical criteria with ICHD-I (Mortimer et al., 1992; Seshia et al., 1994; Maytal et al., 1997; Gherpelli et al., 1998). These studies found that ICHD-I was unable to diagnose a large fraction of children with migraine and these studies, as well as others, suggested revisions to ICHD-I for children and adolescents with migraine (Metsahonkala and Sillanpaa, 1994; Gallai et al., 1995; Hamalainen et al., 1995; Seshia and Wolstein, 1995; Wobel-Bingol et al., 1996; Maytal et al., 1997;Winner et al., 1997; Gherpelli et al., 1998). These suggestions were based on the shorter duration of the migraine attacks in children and the observation that it was either bitemporal or bifrontal in many children.

In 2004, ICHD-II was published and although these criticisms did not result in a change in the criteria, several footnotes were added that recognized the importance of sleep in the duration, the bilateral location in children, the shorter duration—even allowing a reduction to 1 hour with diary confirmation, and the inference of photophobia and phonophobia by parental observation. Although these allowances were an improvement, recent assessments of the criteria demonstrate that there are still deficits (Bigal et al., 2005; Hershey et al., 2005; Lima et al., 2005). These criteria remain the current standard for the diagnosis of migraine, although future tools may assist with this diagnosis.

To date, no studies have addressed the appropriateness and accuracy of other primary headaches (i.e., tension-type headaches or cluster headaches) or secondary headaches in children or adolescents. In addition, much debate exists over the diagnosis of chronic daily headache in adults, although this was identified as a problem with the beginning of clarification in ICHD-II.

EVALUATION

The evaluation of the child or adolescent with headache is the key to appropriate treatment and recent practice parameters have been established for this purpose (Lewis et al., 2002). A properly obtained history will differentiate the various headache types and their etiologies. This interview and evaluation process needs to be developmentally appropriate and may require both collaborative and independent assessment with the child and parent.

The history should begin with details about the headache and headache history. This should not only include the characterization of the headaches in terms of pain quality, severity, frequency, duration, and associated symptoms, but should also include onset triggers or symptoms and impact of the disease including an assessment of disability and quality of life. Response of previous treatments tried, an analysis of the child's and parents' perception of the etiology and a thorough family history is also essential. Due to the potential of the headaches representing a secondary headache, questions that deal with secondary symptoms of increased intracranial pressure or progressive neurologic disease, including ataxia, lethargy, seizures, visual disturbances, focal weakness, personality change, and loss of intellectual abilities need to be included. In addition, the child and parent should be queried about potential comorbid or aggravating features including anxiety, tension, depression and nervousness, school function, previous medical problems, previous medications for both headache and other disorders, and drug and alcohol use, as well as general past medical conditions including early childhood development.

Potentially ominous headache etiologies should be explored if: (1) headache severity has increased dramatically; (2) the headache awakens the child from sleep; or (3) there has been a change in an established headache pattern. Patients with migraine or tension-type headaches should have no symptoms of increased intracranial pressure or progressive neurologic disease.

Following the history, a general physical examination, a thorough neurological examination, and a comprehensive headache examination (Linder, 2005) should be performed. Any abnormality of blood pressure or temperature should be noted. The skin must be closely examined for neurocutaneous abnormalities such as are seen in neurofibromatosis. The skull and neck should be both palpated and auscultated. The sinuses and jaws should be examined for inflammation, tenderness, or temporomandibular joint dysfunction. Most patients with migraine or tension-type headaches have a completely normal physical examination, especially between attacks.

When performing the neurologic examination, one should look carefully for signs of trauma or nuchal rigidity. The head circumference, optic fundi, eye movements, strength, reflexes, and coordination should be recorded. Any abnormality of the neurologic examination requires further investigation, as children and adolescents with migraine and tension-type headaches have normal neurologic examinations between attacks.

LABORATORY TESTS

For primary headaches, laboratory tests are generally not warranted. When a secondary cause or an abnormality in the neurological examination is revealed, further evaluation may be warranted (Lewis et al., 2002).

The diagnosis of structural central nervous system (CNS) disorders has been revolutionized by computed tomography (CT) and magnetic resonance imaging (MRI). Both are safe, rapid, and accurate methods of evaluating the intracranial contents. They are useful in diagnosing congenital malformations, cranial infections, trauma, neoplasms, degenerative disorders, and neurocutaneous and vascular abnormalities. In acute situations, they may be lifesaving. Although MRI incurs greater cost, takes longer, and may require sedation, it can demonstrate lesions not visible on CT including white matter changes, and disorders of the craniospinal junction. Most patients with migraine or tension-type headaches and no symptoms of progressive neurologic disease or increased intracranial pressure and a normal neurologic examination do not require imaging.

SPECIFIC HEADACHE SYNDROMES

As noted above, ICHD-I and ICHD-II separate headaches into primary headaches and secondary headaches. Most recurrent, episodic headaches in children represent primary headaches with migraine being the primary headache that is most frequently brought to a physician's and families' attention. Secondary headaches, on the other hand, are directly attributable to another cause and contribute to acute headaches without a previous history of headaches or an acute change in headaches in patients with a history of primary headaches (Table 27–1). In addition, if the headache type changes or appears to be progressively worsening, additional secondary causes may need to be considered (Table 27–2). This, however, can also include primary headaches that make up the chronic daily headache category and include chronic migraine and chronic tension-type headache.

Table 27–1 Acute Headache.

Acute generalized	*Acute localized*
Systemic infection (ICHD-II 9.2)	Sinusitis (ICHD-II 11.5)
CNS infection (ICHD-II 9.1)	Otitis (ICHD-II 11.4)
Toxins: lead CO_2 (ICHD-II 8)	Ocular abnormality (ICHD-II 11.3)
Postseizure (ICHD-II 1.5.5 or 7.6)	Dental disease (ICHD-II 11.6)
Electrolyte imbalance (ICHD-II 10)	Trauma (ICHD-II 5)
Hypertension (ICHD-II 10.3)	Occipital neuralgia (ICHD-II 13.8)
Hypoglycemia (ICHD-II 10.5)	
Temporomandibular (ICHD-II 11.7)	
Postlumbar puncture (ICHD-II 7.2.1)	Joint dysfunction (ICHD-II)
Trauma (ICHD-II 5)	
Embolic (ICHD-II)	
Vascular thrombosis (ICHD-II 6)	
Hemorrhage (ICHD-II 6)	
Collagen disease (ICHD-II 6.4.1?)	
Exertional (ICHD-II 4.3)	
Shunt malfunction (ICHD-II 7.1.3)	

Abbreviations: CNS, central nervous system.

TABLE 27–2 Chronic Progressive.

Tumor (ICHD-II 7.4)
Pseudotumor, intracranial hypertension (ICHD-II 7.1.1)
Brain abscess (ICHD-II 9.1.4)
Subdural hematoma (ICHD-II 6.2.1)
Hydrocephalus (ICHD-II 7.1.3)

The evaluation of a child with headache in the emergency room is directed toward ruling out organic disease and life-threatening illness and then relieving the pain (Clinical policy for the initial approach to adolescents and adults presenting to the emergency department with a chief complaint of headache. American College of Emergency Physicians, 1996). From 5% to 17% of children seen in an emergency department with headache, this may be a serious, life-threatening disorder. In a study of 696 pediatric emergency room patients with headache (1.3% of total patients seen), 24% were 2–5 years old, 57.6% were 6–12 years old and 18.1% were 13–18 years old (Burton et al., 1997). Of the children with headaches a secondary infectious contribution was most frequently diagnosed with 39% having a concurrent viral illness, 16% diagnosed with sinusitis, and 4.9% diagnosed with streptococcal pharyngitis. In addition, 15.6% of the headaches appeared to be migraine, 6.6% trauma association and felt to represent posttraumatic headaches, and 4.5% had tension-type headaches. Serious conditions included 5.2% of patients with viral meningitis and one case each of shunt malfunction, hydrocephalus, lymphoma, and trauma.

In a separate review of pediatric emergency department headaches, the most common cause (57%) was an upper respiratory tract infection (Lewis and Qureshi, 2000). Migraine without aura was seen in 18% of patients and cause was undetermined in 7%. Serious neurologic problems were noted in 17.5%, including 9% with viral meningitis, 2.6% with brain tumors, 2% with shunt malfunctions, 1.3% with intracranial hemorrhage, 1.3% with postictal headache, and 1.3% with headache secondary to trauma. All children with "serious" problems exhibited neurologic symptoms or clear-cut abnormalities on examination. An organic disorder should be suspected if the headache is accompanied by neurologic symptoms or abnormalities on the neurologic examination. Patients with life-threatening headache may require extensive laboratory testing, including neuroimaging and lumbar puncture.

The treatment of acute headache, in the practitioner's office or in the emergency room, depends on its etiology (primary headache versus secondary headache). If a secondary headache is strongly suspected, treatment should include both the relief of the pain as well as the treatment of the suspected underlying cause. Treatment of pain and associated symptoms should not include medications that alter mental status, change clinical signs, or compound the secondary disorder. Once effective treatment of the secondary cause has been attained, the headache symptoms should resolve. If this does not happen, additional diagnosis must be considered, including the possibility of a primary headache that was exacerbated by a secondary disorder.

MIGRAINE

Migraine is an acute recurrent headache characterized by episodic, periodic, and paroxysmal attacks of pain separated by pain-free intervals. ICHD-II (Headache Classification Subcommittee of the IHS, 2004) has established criteria for the diagnosis of migraine. These criteria include several footnotes that recognize some of the unique features of childhood migraine including a shorter duration with sleep included as part of the duration, the increased incidence of a bilateral location—especially frontal or bitemporal with exclusive occipital headache being of increased concern, and ability to include parental observation of photophobia and phonophobia. Migraine attacks may be precipitated by triggers, but adequate documentation of the role of triggers in the pathogenesis of migraine is not available. The most frequently observed triggers in children include inadequate or altered sleep, skipping meals, stress or concentration, weather changes, bright light, and loud noises. In addition, adolescent girls may begin to have a menstrual pattern with their migraines triggered or increased during their menstrual period. The role of specific food triggers has been called into questions based on the lack of reproducibility of dietary triggers across attacks.

However, if there is a consistent pattern of headaches after particular food items this should be discussed with the patient (Ulrich, Gervil, 1999).

As noted above migraine frequently has a genetic basis. In families of children with migraine, 50%–90% of relatives also have migraine. Whether this disorder is inherited as an autosomal dominant with variable penetrance or is a complex multifactored hereditary disorder has not been determined (Russell, 1996 and Svensson, 1999).

In addition to migraine, many children may also have other periodic syndrome diseases (Table 27–3) (Lanzi et al., 1997). Several of these are included in the ICHD-II, either as migraine variants or in the appendix. This may relate to the underlying hypersensitivity of the nervous system with variable manifestations by age. Frequently, young children with these periodic syndrome components will evolve into migraine patients, suggesting a direct pathophysiological correlation.

TYPES OF MIGRAINE

In this section, we will emphasize issues in children and adolescents with migraine.

Migraine without Aura (ICHD-II 1.1)

Migraine without aura is the most prevalent form of migraine in children and adolescents (Winner et al., 2003). Children may report premonitory features including personality change, irritability, and lethargy. Oftentimes, the child may be unaware of these symptoms with the parent observing the change in their child. This progresses into the typical feature of migraine without aura described in the ICHD-II criteria. For many children sleep is an effective treatment with the child waking up feeling refreshed. Migraines may differ between attacks with a wide variation in the frequency, severity, and duration of migraine among children and adults characterized by the Spectrum study in adults (Lipton et al., 2000, and Kallela, 2001).

Table 27–3 Periodic Syndromes.

- Migraine (ICHD-II, 1.1, 1.2, 1.6)
- Cyclic vomiting (ICHD-II, 1.3.1)
- Abdominal migraine (ICHD-II, 1.3.2)
- Benign paroxysmal vertigo of childhood (ICHD-II, 1.3.3)
- Alternating hemiplegia of childhood (ICHD-II, A1.3.4)
- Benign paroxysmal torticollis (ICHD-II, A1.3.5)
- Motion sickness/car sickness
- Recurrent un-explained fever
- Sleep disturbances
  - —Night terrors
  - —Sleep walking
  - —Sleep talking

Migraine without aura is not usually associated with neurologic symptoms or signs. Migraine associated with transient neurologic disturbances has been called complex or complicated migraine by some authors (Barlow, 1984; Hockaday, 1988). The neurologic deficits are presumed to be secondary to neuronal dysfunction, and the syndromes are described by their vascular territories or neurologic deficits, although there may not be a strict correlation. The ICHD-II includes some of these under migraine with aura and are thought to be due to transient neurological dysfunction. Most resolve spontaneously and leave no sequela. When patients have headaches associated with neurologic symptoms and/or signs, it is important to differentiate "complex" migraine from serious underlying intracranial conditions and neuroimaging with an MRI should be performed. If seizures are suspected, electroencephalography may be useful, although it has little place in routine evaluation of migraine.

Confusional migraine is a disorder that simulates a toxic encephalopathy (Ehyai and Fenichel, 1978; Ferrera and Reicho, 1996; Al-Twaijri and Shevell, 2002). Headache is followed by confusion and a communicative disorder, which may be an expressive or receptive aphasia. Drug abuse is frequently suspected. The neurologic examination shows "confusion" and may or may not show focal features. The evaluation should include toxicology screening, electroencephalogram (EEG), imaging studies, and possibly lumbar puncture to rule out encephalitis. The EEG may show slowing over of the dominant hemisphere. The disorder, which may be the first manifestation of migraine or appear in individuals who have had previous migraine attacks or previous episodes of confusion, usually clears in 6–12 hours. Data concerning the efficacy of preventive measures in these syndromes are not available.

Migraine with Aura (ICHD-II 1.2)

Migraine with aura is less frequent in children and adolescents than migraine without aura. (Gervil, Ulrich, 1999) The aura is visual, sensory, or dysphasic. The visual aura in children is frequently described as brightly colored lights or moving lights like light bulbs going off everywhere. Less frequently the visual aura may be described as distorted images, scotomata, visual field defects, or fortification spectra (Ulrich, Olesen, 2000). This appears to change with development with the adult-type aura developing during adolescence. Sensory aura is usually unilateral and has often been described as worms or bugs crawling up the hand to the arm and finally to the face followed by a numb sensation. Dysphasic aura is the least frequent and has been described as difficulty speaking more than a lack of understanding. This type of aura may explain some of the confusional or complex migraine discussed above.

Hemiplegic migraine (ICHD-II* 1.2.4*—familial, ICHD-II* 1.2.5*—sporadic). True weakness before or during a migraine attack is not classified as a typical migraine with aura, but as a special type of migraine with aura—hemiplegic migraine. This can be further sub-classified based on the familial or sporadic nature of the diagnosis. The headache is often contralateral to the weakness. The patient may have additional aura symptoms with the hemiplegia. In the familial form, three genes have been identified that cause this etiology (Deng, YM, 1995; Dichgans, M, 2005 and Ophoff, 1996). The differential diagnosis of hemiplegic migraine includes thromboembolism, arteriovenous malformation, moyamoya syndrome, mitochondrial disorder, and tumor. Cardiac disease, oral contraceptive use, smoking, or hypercoagulable states may play a contributory role. If a headache is associated with a meningismus, a CT scan followed by a lumbar puncture may be indicated to rule out hemorrhage. Cerebrospinal fluid (CSF) pleocytosis has been reported during some hemiplegic migraine attacks. Some attacks may be precipitated by minor head trauma.

Basilar-type migraine (ICHD-II* 1.2.6*). Basilar-type migraine was first described by Bickerstaff (1962). It is characterized by recurrent attacks aura that originates from the brainstem and includes dysarthria, vertigo, tinnitus, hypacusia, diplopia, bilateral visual symptoms, ataxia, decreased level of consciousness, and bilateral paraethesias. The syndrome affects adolescents more frequently than adults. These symptoms may precede the headache and the patients may also have typical migraine with aura. There has begun to be some evidence that this may be a variant of migraine with aura, without distinction between basilar-type migraine and migraine with aura (Kirchmann et al., 2006). In addition, the historical concern of this representing basilar artery spasm has not been demonstrated and this may represent bihemispherical dysfunction rather than brainstem involvement.

When the aura presents as distorted images bizarre visual illusions, or spatial distortions, Alice-in-Wonderland syndrome may be considered (Golden, 1979; Murray, 1982; Evans and Rolak, 2004). Children may describe micropsia, macropsia, metamorphopsia, or teleopsia before the headache begins. Somatic disturbances, such as dysphasia, dysesthesia, hemiplegia, and speech disturbances, are less frequent. The aura usually lasts 20 minutes and may be followed by a unilateral headache contralateral to the aura or a bilateral headache that is usually described as severe and throbbing. This headache is frequently associated with pallor, anorexia, abdominal pain, photophobia, phonophobia, and nausea and vomiting.

Childhood Periodic Syndromes (ICHD-II 1.3)

ICHD-II includes cyclic vomiting (1.3.1), abdominal migraine (1.3.2), and benign paroxysmal vertigo (1.3.3) within the main criteria, while alternating hemiplegia of childhood (A1.3.4) and benign paroxysmal torticollis (A1.3.5) are included within the appendix. Additional periodic syndromes may include motion sickness, sleep disturbances (sleep walking, sleep talking, and night terrors) and episodes of unexplained fevers. The common features of these disorders are their recurrent, periodic nature and the co-association with migraine or a family history of migraine.

Cyclic vomiting (ICHD-II* 1.3.1*). Cyclic vomiting is a symptom complex that occurs in infants, children, andless commonly, adolescents, and adults. It is characterized by repeated episodes of severe vomiting and dehydration (Li et al., 1998, 1999; Li, 2000; Li and Balint, 2000; Li and Misiewicz, 2003). Between events, these children are healthy. Headache is not usually part of this syndrome. It is necessary to rule out intermittent bowel obstruction and metabolic disease before arriving at the diagnosis of cyclic vomiting. According to several authors, migraine prophylaxis can be effective in decreasing the frequency and severity of attacks. General treatment measures include hydration, antiemetics, and sedation.

Abdominal migraine (ICHD-II 1.3.2). Abdominal migraine or recurrent abdominal pain has been described as recurrent episodes of midline abdominal pain lasting 1–72 hours. Like migraine the pain is moderate to severe and may be associated with anorexia, nausea, vomiting or pallor, but without headache or head pain. It needs to be distinguished from cyclic vomiting which has a predictable nature (Symon and Russell, 1995; Catto-Smith and Ranuh, 2003) and from true migraine in which head pain is present. Gastrointestinal and renal disease needs to be ruled out before this diagnosis can be made. Abdominal migraine and migraine have similar demographic, social, and clinical features with a suggestion that they may have overlapping pathogenesis (Abu-Arafeh and Russell, 1995b). In addition, many of these children evolve into migraine and many of the migraine treatments may also be effective for abdominal migraine (Russell et al., 2002).

Benign paroxysmal vertigo (ICHD-II 1.3.3). Benign paroxysmal vertigo is not uncommon in children and may occur in up to 2.6% of children (Abu-Arafeh and Russell, 1995a). It more commonly affects younger children, who develop sudden unsteadiness and grab on to whatever is near them for stability (Fenichel, 1967). Consciousness is not lost. Nystagmus may be present. Vomiting may or may not occur. The spells last only minutes and afterwards the child is normal and will resume play or want to sleep. The spells usually occur in clusters over days to weeks and then subside. Laboratory evaluation is probably unnecessary in clear-cut cases. In less clear-cut cases, EEG and MRI scanning should be performed.

This disorder evolves into common migraine in later childhood and adolescence (Herraiz et al., 1999; Lindskog et al., 1999). Although antihistamine therapy has been suggested, no definitive therapeutic studies have been performed.

Alternating hemiplegia of childhood (ICHD-II A1.3.4). Alternating hemiplegia consists of attacks of hemiparesis, monoparesis, or quadriparesis, accompanied by decreased tone and occasionally involuntary movements (Rho and Chugani, 1998; Swoboda et al., 2004). The children are normal at the onset of their symptoms. The symptoms are often reversed by sleep. Over time, more attacks occur and the children demonstrate developmental problems. This condition can be related to brainstem dysfunction (Rinalduzzi et al., 2006) or a microvasculature disorder (Auvin et al., 2006). Comparisons have been made with hemiplegic migraine, however there is conflicting evidence for the role of the second gene identified for familial hemiplegic migraine—ATP1A2 (Bassi et al., 2004; Kors et al., 2004). Children with alternating hemiplegia may be helped by topiramate (Di Rosa et al., 2006).

Paroxysmal torticollis (ICHD-II A1.3.5). Paroxysmal torticollis is characterized by attacks of head tilt, vomiting, and ataxia that last from hours to days and are often felt to be benign (Drigo et al., 2000). It usually occurs in younger children. There is often a family history of migraine. This syndrome may evolve into more typical migraine in later years. There has been familial co-association with hemiplegic migraine in small case studies with one observation of common defects in the CACNA1A gene (Giffin et al., 2002). In clear-cut cases, no evaluation is necessary; however, in problematic cases, EEG and MRI may be necessary to evaluate for posterior fossa disease. No studies have shown that specific medications are effective in preventing recurrence of this syndrome.

Retinal Migraine (ICHD-II 1.4)

Retinal migraine is also called ocular or ophthalmic migraine (Grosberg et al., 2006). It is uncommon in children and adolescents. Patients report sudden, momentary monocular blackouts or grayouts or blinding visual disturbances that may or may not be followed by a headache. Examination of the fundus during an attack may disclose retinal vein and artery constriction, and retinal pallor. Some patients suffer visual sequela, presumably due to retinal infarction. Evaluation for hypocoagulable states, embolic sources, and other vascular abnormalities should be carried out.

Chronic Migraine (ICHD-II 1.5.1)

When migraine attacks start to occur frequently (>15 headache days per month), chronic migraine should be considered. Chronic migraine was added to the ICHD-II criteria and the criteria remain somewhat controversial with alternate criteria (Bigal et al., 2006) and modification of the criteria using the ICHD-II appendix (Olesen et al., 2006) have been suggested. Functionally, any child with headaches that have migraine features and having very frequent headaches should be considered having chronic migraine. Evaluation and treatment needs to include an assessment of medication overuse (ICHD-II 8) and contribution of psychosocial or biobehavioral features including adequate sleep, nutrition, and exercise. In adolescent chronic migraine can create significant disability and impact both the child's and parent's quality of life (Hershey, 2003; Wang et al., 2006). Treatment requires a combination of acute therapy, preventative therapy, and biohavioral therapy as outlined below.

Status Migrainosus (ICHD-II 1.5.2)

Status migrainosus or a prolonged migraine (>72 hours) may often contribute to emergency department and inpatient management of migraine. This may be due to inadequate acute therapy or inadequate response to effective acute therapy. Although the prevalence in children is not known, in older adolescents this may be as high as 15% of migraine patients (Split and Neuman, 1999). In the emergency department, prochlorperazine may be effective for status migrainosus (Kabbouche et al., 2001). Dihydroergotamine (DHE) has been demonstrated to be effective in adults with status migrainosus (Silberstein and Young, 1995) and may be effective in children (Linder, 1994).

MANAGEMENT

All patients will require an acute treatment strategy; as well as, benefit potentially from nonpharmacologic measures. The need for preventive treatment is under-recognized and under-utilized. For the patients with disability a combination of acute and preventive therapy alone with nonpharmacologic measures will be needed. Presently, there are no food and drug administration (FDA) approved acute or preventive medications for the treatment of migraine or cluster headache in the pediatric population. Fortunately, the use of medication to treat migraine in children as been studied and we will present selective date to help guide management decisions.

The use of a headache calendar is valuable for determining the frequency and severity of headaches before, during, and after treatment. It may demonstrate patterns of headache not previously suspected. Acute treatment is used to end attacks after they have begun by interfering with the migraine cascade. Preventive treatment is used to decrease the frequency and severity of future attacks. Nonpharmacologic treatment includes: education (of both the patient and their parents), biofeedback, stress reduction, and dietary triggers (Wasiewski and Rothner, 1999).

Acute Treatment

Migraine nonspecific. The mainstay of pharmacologic management of childhood migraine is intermittent oral analgesics (Table 27–4). Acetaminophen, ibuprofen, and naproxen sodium used early in the course of the headache at appropriate doses are frequently effective (Bruni et al., 1991; Graf and Riback, 1995; Hämäläinen et al., 1997). Two medications in combination, such as acetaminophen and ibuprofen, may be helpful. Combination medications, which may include barbiturates or narcotics, play a secondary role if the initial agents fail (Solomon, 1995; Wasiewski and Rothner, 1999). Medications containing barbiturates need to be used with caution in this age group due to the potential for the development of rebound headaches (Medication Overuse Headache). Narcotics should be avoided during the initial stages of treatment, as they may not only exacerbate the nausea and vomiting but tolerance, addiction, and abuse may develop. As a rescue therapy, narcotics can be used very effectively under appropriate medical supervision.

Table 27–4 Migraine Nonspecific Treatment.

Medication	*Dosage*	*Comment*
Acetaminophen[a]	10–15 mg/kg/dose Q 4–6 hours	Available as suppository
Ibuprofen[a]	4–10 mg/kg/dose Q 6–8 hours	No suppository available
Acetaminophen[b] + codeine	0.5–1 mg/kg/dose Q 6–8 hours	No suppository available
Fioricet	1 tab Q 6-hours	Number of tablets should be limited
Antiemetics		
Trimethobenzamide	15–20 mg/kg/day Divide Q 6-hours	100 mg/200 mg suppository
Perchlorperazine[b]	0.4 mg/kg/day Divide Q 6–8 hours	2.5, 5, and 25 mg suppository extrapyramidal reactions

[a] May be used together.

[b] Use with caution.

Antiemetics may be useful, since anorexia, abdominal pain, and vomiting occur in 90% of patients (Jones et al., 1989; Tek et al., 1990). Gastric stasis and nausea and vomiting may preclude the use of oral analgesics. Antiemetics alone may provide substantial relief and sometimes are effective in eliminating all associated symptoms, including pain. These agents may be administered orally, intranasally, rectally, or parenterally. Dystonic reactions may occur and should be anticipated.

Migraine-specific treatment. Commonly utilized treatment include: the triptans, ergot preparations, a combination drug (Midrin), and nonsteroidal anti-inflammatory drugs (NSAIDs) (Table 27–5). (Yuill et al., 1972; Silberstein and Young, 1995). Medications can be administered orally, intranasally, parenterally, and rectally.

The triptan drugs are currently being studied in children and adolescents. They are well-absorbed orally, intranasally, and parenterally. A double-blind, placebo-controlled trial of sumatriptan was conducted at 35 sites with 302 adolescents (Winner et al., 2001). Twenty-five, fifty, and one hundred milligram tablets were tested. All tested doses of sumatriptan were statistically significantly superior to placebo at 180 and 240 minutes, with 74% pain relief at 4 hours. The recurrence rates varied from 18% to 28% with all three doses. No significant adverse events (AEs) were noted in this study.

Sumatriptan nasal spray (NS) was studied in a randomized, double-blind, placebo-controlled study of adolescents whose ages ranged from 12 to 17 years (Rothner et al., 2000). A single attack was treated. In this study, 5, 10, and 20 mg doses were studied. At 1 hour post-dose, headache relief was noted in 56% of patients using 10 mg or 20%, compared with 41% of the placebo group. All three doses were superior to placebo with respect to the cumulative percentage of patients who attained headache relief within 2 hours. When reviewing the pain-free data, the 20 mg dose of sumatriptan NS helped 36% of patients. There was no difference with regard to headache recurrence among the treatment groups compared with the placebo group.

The most common AE was taste disturbance. If this side effect is removed from the calculation, the overall incidence of AEs for the nasal treatment group is similar to the placebo group. No serious AE was reported. The sumatriptan 20 mg NS provided rapid relief and was well tolerated in the adolescent migraine population.

The most recent sumatriptan NS study compared the efficacy and tolerability of 5 and 20 mg versus placebo in the acute treatment of migraine in adolescent subjects. (Winner et al., 1996). In this study, 738 adolescent subjects (mean age: 14 years) with ⩾6-month history of migraine (with or without aura) self-treated a single attack of moderate or severe migraine. Efficacy was based on

TABLE 27–5 Migraine-specific Medication.

Medication	*Dosage*	*Comment*
Midrin/Duradrin[a]	2 caps at onset	>50 kg - max 5 caps
	1 additional cap/hour × 1	<50 kg - max 3 caps
Ergot[a]	2 mg sublingual, may repeat × 1 in 1 hour	>50 kg
Sumatriptan[a]	SQ 0.06–0.1 mg/kg	See protocol
	Oral 25 mg	<50 kg
	Oral 50 mg	>50 kg
	Nasal 5 mg	<50 kg
	Nasal 20 mg	>50 kg
Almotriptan[a]	12.5 mg	>50 kg
Zomitriptan[a]	2.5–5.0 mg	>50 kg
	Nasal 5 mg	
Eletriptan[a]	20, 40 mg	>50 kg
		>50 kg
DHE nasal spray[a]	As directed	>50 kg

Abbreviations: DHE, dihydroergotamine; SQ, subcutaneous.

[a] Not approved by the Food and Drug Administration (FDA) for children below 18 years.

headache relief, sustained relief, pain-free rate, presence/absence of associated symptoms, headache recurrence, and use of rescue medications. Tolerability was based on AEs and vital signs (Winner, Rothner, Wooen, et al., 2004).

Sumatriptan NS 20 mg provided greater headache relief than placebo at 30 minutes (42% versus 33%, respectively; $p = 0.046$), 1 hour (61% versus 52%; $p = 0.087$), and 2 hours (68% versus 58%; $p = 0.025$) post-dose. Sumatriptan NS 20 mg also provided greater sustained headache relief from 1 through 24 hours post-dose ($p = 0.061$) and from 2 through 24 hours post-dose ($p = 0.021$) than placebo. Significant differences ($p < 0.05$) in favor of sumatriptan NS 20 mg over placebo were observed for several secondary efficacy endpoints. In general, sumatriptan NS 5 mg was more effective than placebo but the differences did not reach statistical significance. Both doses of sumatriptan NS were well tolerated. No AEs were serious or led to study withdrawal. The most common event was taste disturbance (2%, placebo; 19%, sumatriptan NS 5 mg; 25%, sumatriptan NS 20 mg) (Winner, Rothner, Wooen, et al., 2004).

A recent study assessed the pooled efficacy and tolerability results of 5 and 20 mg sumatriptan NS versus placebo from two large US randomized, placebo-controlled, double-blind, parallel-group studies in adolescents 12–17 years of age with at least 6-month history of migraine [Study 1 (placebo $n = 130$; 5 mg $n = 127$; 20 mg $n = 117$) and Study 2 (placebo $N = 244$; 5 mg $N = 250$; 20 mg $N = 237$)]. The total pooled population was 1105 (placebo $N = 374$; 5 mg $N = 377$; 20 mg $N = 354$). Subjects in both trials self-treated a single moderate or severe attack. The percentage of subjects with headache relief (moderate/severe pain reduced to mild or none) or pain free (moderate/severe pain reduced to none) were evaluated at 30 minutes, 1 hour, and 2 hours post-dose; as well as sustained relief (relief maintained without rescue or recurrence) from 1 and 2 hours up to 24 hours (Winner, Rothner, Webster, et al., 2004).

The pooled results for sumatriptan NS 20 mg demonstrate significantly greater headache relief compared to placebo at 30 minutes (39% versus 30%, $p = 0.016$), 1 hour (59% versus 48%, $p = 0.007$), and 2 hours (67% versus 57, $p = 0.005$); for sumatriptan NS 5 mg, the study showed significantly greater headache relief compared to placebo at 2 hours (64% versus 57%, $p = 0.037$). Sustained relief from 1 to 24 hours was greater for sumatriptan NS 5 mg (37%, $p = 0.041$) and for sumatriptan NS 20 mg (41%, $p = 0.003$). Sustained relief from

2 to 24 hours was also greater for sumatriptan NS 5 mg (49%, $p = 0.001$) and sumatriptan NS 20 mg (50%, $p = 0.002$) versus placebo (38%). For the pain-free endpoint, the pooled results show a greater efficacy with sumatriptan NS 20 mg compared to placebo at 1 hour (20% versus 14%, $p = 0.034$) and 2 hours (42% versus 28%, $p = 0.001$). The most frequent treatment related AEs for placebo, 5 and 20 mg sumatriptan NS, respectively, were: taste disturbance (2%, 19%, and 26%), nausea (3%, 4%, and 7%), vomiting (1%, 2%, and 4%), and burning/stinging sensation (1%, 1%, and 3%). Infrequent (1%) were pressure/tightness and chest symptoms reported in each of the treatment groups (Winner, Rothner, Webster, et al., 2004). These studies provide evidence of significant headache relief compared to placebo by 30 minutes for sumatriptan NS 20 mg and 2 hours for sumatriptan NS 5 and 20 mg. The results also demonstrate significant sustained headache relief from 1 to 24 hours for sumatriptan NS 5 and 20 mg. Significantly more sumatriptan NS 20 mg subjects were pain free beginning at 1 hour post-dose. Sumatriptan NS is affective and generally well tolerated in the treatment of acute migraine in adolescent subjects (Winner, Rothner, Webster, et al., 2004).

A 5 mg tablet formulation of rizatriptan was evaluated in patients aged 12–17 years in a double-blind, placebo-controlled, parallel-group, single-attack study (Winner et al., 2002). Sixty-six percent of the adolescents had pain relief at 2 hours with this dosage. The headache-free status at 2 hours was 32%. There were no serious AEs. The most common AEs were fatigue, dizziness, somnolence, dry mouth, and nausea. Forty-four percent of adolescent patients on 5 mg of rizatriptan reported no functional disability at 2 hours. Further studies of rizatriptan, zolmitriptan, and naratriptan are being conducted in the pediatric and adolescent population. Adverse effects associated with the triptans include tingling, dizziness, warm/hot sensations, and injection site reactions. Headache recurrence is less of a problem in adolescents than in adults.

Zolmitriptan (Zomig) has been studied in a subgroup of adolescents (12–17 years). The first two migraine subgroups were treated with 2.5 mg and subsequent attacks with 2.5 or 5 mg at each patient's discretion. The overall headache response at 2 hours was 80% (88% and 70% with zolmitriptan, 2.5 and 5 mg, respectively). Treatment was well tolerated (Linder and Dowson, 2000).

Zolmitriptan NS, 5 mg, was studied in a unique placebo, double-blind, cross-over study. Initially all patient received placebo, then if the patient responded to placebo in 15 minutes the study was complete for that particular patient. If the patient continued to have headache pain, the patient would receive a second dose of study drug, which consisted of either another placebo or active drug. This study had an intent-to-treat (ITT) population of 171 and the one hour response was 58.1% for NS versus 43.3% for placebo. One hour pain-free was 27.7% for the NS and 10.2% for placebo. The 2 hours sustained headache relief was 53.4% for the NS and 36.2% for the placebo. With utilizing the placebo lead in protocol for the NS all statistics were significant at the 0.05 level. Unfortunately, at the time of this writing, the FDA and the pharmaceutical company are still in discussion about the rationalization for the lead in placebo, thus no formal recommendation by the FDA has been received (Lewis et al., 2007).

Eletriptan (Relpax) was studied in a multi-center, double-blind, placebo-controlled study comparing the 40 mg with placebo in the adolescent age group, 12–17 years of age. This dose was well tolerated and AE profile was similar to those seen in adults. A total of 274 patients were enrolled in the study. Standard measure of headache response at 2 hours showed a very high placebo response (57%) and a similar response to eletriptan (57%). This study may have been flawed due to the fact that the patients could treat their headache up to 4 hours after the onset of the headache. By contrast there is a significant advantage for eletriptan in headache recurrence (11% versus 25% with a $p = 0.028$). Overall this medication is well tolerated by patients (Winner et al., 2007).

Almotriptan (Axert): In double-blind, placebo-controlled kinetic study was done utilizing almotriptan at a dose of 6.25–12.5–25 mg. In this study there were four co-primary end points utilizing the study drug versus placebo. The co-end points were: pain relief, photophobia, phonophobia and nausea at 2 hours. Pain relief was noted at 2 hours in 55.3% with placebo versus and 71% of patients receiving the 6.25 mg dose; 72.9% in patient receiving the 12.5 mg dose. Both of these are significant at the 0.001 level and 68.7% on the 25 mg which is significant at 0.022 level. Photophobia and phonophobia improved significantly with only 12.5 mg dose. This study was done in a complicated step-down procedure which negated findings of all endpoints were not reached for the 25 mg. Unfortunately this was the case, thus the data in regard to the 12.5 mg dose, which was significant, for pain relief and associated symptoms at 2 hours has to be further investigated by the drug company. At this time the recommended dose for adolescents is 12.5 mg. All three dose levels were well tolerated in the adolescent age group of 12–17. There were no significant AEs or change in any hematological chemical parameters, nor any abnormalities describes in electrocardiogram (ECG) monitoring. Further studies are in progress at this time for almotriptan 12.5 mg versus placebo. Presently none of the triptans are approved for use in pediatric migraine population. The above data supports they are well tolerated in populations studied.

Prescribing considerations for triptans include; but are not limited to, prior evaluation for patients with risk of coronary artery disease, peripheral vascular syndromes or other significant underlying cardiovascular disease. They should not be used if patients are experiencing an atypical headache or hemiplegic migraine. Cases of life-threatening serotonin syndrome have been reported during combined use of selective serotonin reuptake inhibitors/serotonin-norepinephrine reuptake inhibitors (SSRIs/SNRIs) and triptans. Triptans should be used during pregnancy only if potential benefit justifies the potential risk to the fetus. Caution should be exercised when considering administration to a nursing woman (*Physicians' Desk Reference*, 2007).

Ergotamine tartrate remains a useful agent, but the risk of nausea and ergot rebound withdrawal headaches limits its value in patients in the pediatric and adolescent age group. One should generally limit ergot use to no more than twice weekly. Adverse effects include nausea, vomiting, and vasoconstriction. An intranasal formulation of DHE has been approved for adult use. DHE-45, which needs dosage adjustment depending on age, can be used intramuscularly, subcutaneously, or intravenously with a concomitant antiemetic. Children between the ages of 6 and 9 years should receive 0.1 mg per dose, those between the ages of 9 and 12 should receive 0.5 mg per dose, and those between the ages of 12 and 16 should receive 0.75 mg per dose. It may be helpful to bring the child to the office on a day when he or she does not have a migraine and give the child a test dose of DHE to make sure the medication does not cause significant nausea. If nausea occurs, the dose can be lowered. In general, problems can be avoided by lowering the dose, diluting the DHE with 30–60 cc of saline, and administering the solution intravenously over a period of 0.5–1 hour (Linder, 1994). In addition, 20–30 minutes before the administration of DHE, metoclopramide can be given to prevent nausea or vomiting. In addition to preventing nausea, metoclopramide has antidopaminergic effects, which can be helpful in treating migraine. Some children are sensitive to antiemetics, such as metoclopramide, and may develop extrapyramidal side effects, which can be readily reversed with 1 mg/kg of diphenhydramine. Extrapyramidal side effects may also be seen with oral metoclopramide; if this occurs, it usually occurs between the fifth and eighth dose and is readily reversible with diphenhydramine. Phenergan, which, is easily administered and has a rapid onset of efficacy, may be substituted for metoclopramide.

Isometheptene mucate, a sympathomimetic agent that includes acetaminophen and a mild sedative, is useful for adolescents with migraine (Yuill et al., 1972). It is generally better tolerated than the ergots.

NSAIDs, including naproxen, flurbiprofen, and meclofenamate are useful for the acute treatment of migraine (Pradalier et al., 1988; Lewis et al., 1994). The maximal allowable dosage should be utilized at the onset of the attack.

Preventive treatment. Preventive therapy should be considered when individuals have frequent and prolonged attacks that interfere with their ability to function (Table 27–6). Many medications have been used for migraine prevention, including: anticonvulsants, antidepressants, β-blockers, calcium channel blockers, cyproheptadine, and NSAIDs (Diamond and Medina, 1976; Olesen, 1986; Peatfield, 1986; Couch et al., 1976). Recently, the anticonvulsants topiramate and valproate have been successfully utilized in the prophylaxis of

TABLE 27–6 Migraine Preventive Treatment.

Drug	Dosage	Comment
Cyproheptadine	0.25 mg/kg/day 1/3AM-2/3 h.s.	Sedation appetite stimulation
Propranolol	0.6–1.5 mg/kg/day divide 3 doses	[a]Cardiac, vivid dreams depression
Amitriptyline	0.1–2 mg/kg/day h.s.	[a]Cardiac, sedation
Verapamil	4–8 mg/kg/day divide 3 doses	[a]Cardiac, constipation
Depakote	10–30 mg/kg/day divide 2 or 3 doses	Hepatic pancreatic dysfunction, anorexia or weight gain
Topiramate	50–100 mg/day divide 2 doses	Metabolic acidosis, myopia, angle closure glaucoma, oligohidrosis, hyperthermia, weight loss

[a] Standard dosing recommendations.

migraine (Hering and Kuritzky, 1992; Serdaroglu et al., 2002; Winner et al., 2005).

Recent anticonvulsant data regarding the prevention of migraines in children and adolescence are from a randomized, double-blind, placebo-controlled trial evaluating topiramate (Topamax) (Winner et al., 2005). Topiramate has been demonstrated to be effective for migraine prevention in adults. Topiramate has been studied in children meeting proposed IHS classification for diagnosis of pediatric migraine with or without aura ($N = 162$; age range 6–15 years; 52% male, 48% female) were randomized 2:1 to topiramate ($n = 112$) or placebo ($n = 50$). Topiramate was initiated at 15 mg/day and titrated over 8 weeks to a dose approximating 2.0–3.0 mg/kg/day, or their maximum tolerated dose, whichever was less. The maximum dose allowed was 200 mg/day this titration phase was followed by a 12-week maintenance phase. Efficacy was assessed ion the ITT population, defined as subjects who received study medication and had at least one post-baseline efficacy assessment ($n = 108$ for topiramate, $n = 49$ for placebo). The primary efficacy measure was the mean for change in migraine days/month (28 days) between baseline and the entire double-blind phase. Secondary efficacy variables included categorical response rates (>50% and >75% reduction from baseline) (Winner et al., 2005). Topiramate reduced mean monthly migraine days by 2.6 from a baseline of 5.4 days compared to a reduction of 1.9 days for placebo from a baseline of 5.5 days, which approached statistical significance ($p = 0.065$). There was considerable variation of placebo group migraine rates in different age groups. A significantly greater percentage of patients receiving Topiramate (32%) showed greater reduction in mean monthly migraine days than patients receiving placebo (14%, $p = 0.020$). However, the percentage of topiramate treated patients exhibiting a more than 50% reduction in mean of monthly migraine days (55%) was not satisfactory different from that of placebo treated patients (47%). Discontinuation rates due to AEs were in the 6.5% for topiramate and 4.1% for placebo. The most common AEs in the topiramate group were upper respiratory tract infection (19.4% topiramate versus 6.1 placebo), anorexia (13.0% topiramate versus 8.2 placebo), weight decrease (9.3 topiramate versus 6.1% placebo), paresthesia (8.3% topiramate versus 0.0% placebo), and somnolence (8.3 topiramate versus 6.1 placebo). The reported mean dose of topiramate was 109 mg/day at the end of the study (Winner et al., 2005). This preliminary study notes the potential utility if topiramate for the prevention of pediatric migraines, with the target dose being 100 mg daily divided bid. Topiramate was well tolerated in this pediatric population. Further studies are warranted to establish the efficacy of topiramate for the treatment of pediatric migraine (Winner et al., 2005).

Although the other anticonvulsants have been used by clinicians, there are limited studies to support their use. When used in migraine prevention, the antiepileptic doses are usually prescribed (Winner et al., 2001).

Valproate, an anticonvulsant, has been evaluated for efficacy in migraine in adults (Hering and Kuritzky, 1992). Treatment with Valproate significantly reduced the number and severity of migraine attacks. To date, it has not been studied in childhood or adolescent migraine. No correlation was found between valproate levels and the frequency, severity, or duration of migraine attacks. In the adult population, no serious side effects were reported. Hepatic toxicity may occur in younger children; however, this is rare. Reported common side effects include weight gain, tremor, hair loss, and nausea. There is concern regarding Valproate's relationship to polycystic ovaries.

Antidepressant medications are effective in migraine prophylaxis (Gomersall and Stuart, 1973; Moreland et al., 1979) and tricyclic antidepressants are more effective than the newer SSRIs. The selection of the specific antidepressant should be based primarily on whether or not the patient has a sleep disturbance. Patients who initiate and maintain sleep easily are better able to tolerate nonsedating drugs. Patients who have difficulty initiating and maintaining sleep respond better to sedating drugs. The nonsedating antidepressants include protriptyline and desipramine. Sedating antidepressants include amitriptyline, nortriptyline, and imipramine. Patients frequently are intolerant of the anticholinergic side effects, such as dry mouth, blurred vision, urinary retention, and constipation, of antidepressants. These medications should be initiated at low dosages and increased slowly. Cardiac conduction problems can occur with all tricyclic antidepressants and may cause prolongation of the PR, QRS, and QT intervals. Selective SSRIs have not been well studied in migraine in children.

Beta blockers are first-line drugs for migraine prophylaxis (Diamond and Medina, 1976; Ludvigsson, 1974). They also may have anxiolytic effects. Beta blockers that are effective in migraine prophylaxis include propranolol and timolol. Beta blockers are generally well tolerated, but they are contraindicated in patients with bronchospastic disease, diabetes, and Wolff–Parkinson–White syndrome. Side effects include depression, fatigue, sleep disorders, and decreased athletic endurance. Studies utilizing β-blockers in children have had conflicting results. One of three studies found them effective, whereas two found no difference from placebo (Ludvigsson, 1974; Forsythe et al., 1984; Olness et al., 1987).

Calcium entry blockers, including verapamil, diltiazem, flunarazine, nimodipine, and nicardipine, have been useful in the prophylaxis of migraine. Data regarding their efficacy vary. They are not convincingly effective in children. The most common adverse effects are daytime sedation, weight gain, depression, and constipation.

Flunarazine, a drug not available in the United States, has been found to be effective and well-tolerated in three European childhood studies of migraine prophylaxis (Pothmann, 1987; Sorge et al., 1988).

Cyproheptadine is used for migraine prophylaxis in children. However, its use for this purpose has not been supported by medical research, and the drug does not have an approved indication for headache. A nightly dose of 4–12 mg is used. Common side effects include fatigue and weight gain (Peroutka and Allen, 1984; Levinstein, 1991).

NSAIDs are widely prescribed as analgesics and antipyretics (Pradalier et al., 1988). They are valuable in acute and preventive migraine treatment. NSAIDs that have been reported to have prophylactic activity in migraine include aspirin, naproxen, flurbiprofen, ketoprofen, flufenamic acid, and fenoprofen. AEs are relatively common. Gastrointestinal (GI) effects include dyspepsia, heartburn, nausea, vomiting, diarrhea, constipation, abdominal pain, and GI bleeding. Renal effects include decreased glomerular filtration rate and water retention. Both indomethacin and fenoprofen appear to be more nephrotoxic than other NSAIDs.

Nonpharmacologic therapy. Nonpharmacologic preventive measures that may reduce headache frequency include sleep hygiene, diet, and exercise (Powers and Andrasik, 2005). Sleep hygiene can have a significant effect on childhood headaches. A balanced diet, avoiding foods that precipitate migraine, can be useful. Food triggers may affect 5%–15% of patients. Regular exercise, although not well studied, may be beneficial in reducing headache frequency. Studies involving biofeedback have proven it to be as effective as β-blockers (McGrath and Reid, 1995). If stress is a significant contributing feature, counseling, relaxation therapy, and cognitive training have been found to be helpful (Larsson and Melin, 1988).

PROGNOSIS

The short-term prognosis for migraine in children is favorable, with greater than 50% of patients reporting improvement within 6 months of medical intervention, regardless of the treatment method used (Hockaday, 1988; Bille, 1997). The long-term prognosis suggests that two-thirds of children go into remission for 2 or more years through adolescence and early adulthood. Approximately 60% of migraineurs who had adolescent-onset migraines, however, reported ongoing migraine after 30 years of age. Congden and Forsythe (1979) reported that 37 of 108 children (34%) had headache remission (Congdon and Forsythe, 1979). Sillanpää (1994) suggested that the remission rate for those whose onset was before 8 years of age was 22%, and boys were more likely to remit than girls (Sillanpää, 1994). The remission rate for those whose onset was between 8 and 14 years of age was 25%, and girls were more likely to remit than boys, by a ratio of 3:2. The prognosis of childhood migraine is better in boys than in girls but is, at best, variable.

SECONDARY HEADACHE DISORDERS

Chronic Progressive Headaches

Chronic progressive headache implies a pathological process within the cranium (Cohen, 1995). Prominent in this group of disorders are hydrocephalus, brain tumor, pseudotumor cerebri, brain abscess, intracranial hemorrhage, and chronic subdural hematoma. Rare cases include toxic processes, endocrine disturbances, congenital anomalies, degenerative disorders, and metabolic conditions may cause progressive headache. Prompt diagnostic work-up and medical treatment are mandatory.

First and foremost attention should be paid to history. There are suggestions for possible secondary etiology in the presentation of headache. These hints are included in Table 27–7. The basic assumption is that a "good" headache is the one that exists more than 1 year and has been stable in all respects including, but not limited to, pain intensity, quality, duration, frequency, location, manner of onset, response to medication, etc. Secondary etiology should be considered in any headache that is rapidly worsening in one or more respects.

The general and the neurologic examination may (rarely) be normal or may demonstrate papilledema, a sixth cranial nerve palsy, or other focal neurologic signs. When neurologic signs are present, their localization may lead to a specific diagnosis.

Radiological or other lab tests should be ordered to verify a clinical diagnosis but not to create one. If a cranial or intracranial cause is suspected, MRI may be diagnostic. A head CT scan is more practical in emergencies as it is quick and readily available in many medical facilities.

Lumbar puncture becomes an integral part of headache evaluation when a CSF profile can aid the investigation yet history, exam, and noninvasive testing do not suffice for a specific diagnosis and treatment. It is preceded by an imaging study when a mass lesion or increased intracranial pressure is suspected. However, it should be expedited if it is indicated.

Hydrocephalus. Hydrocephalus is a condition in which increased ventricular volume with or without increased pressure is secondary to an obstruction or decreased CSF absorption (Abbott et al., 1991; Cohen, 1995). It may be secondary to a congenital anomaly, such as aqueductal stenosis, or it may develop following bacterial meningitis or intracranial hemorrhage. Symptoms and signs are those of nonlocalized increased intracranial pressure. When the disorder is chronic, macrocephaly may be present. MRI is diagnostic and a diversion procedure, such as a third ventriculostomy or a shunting procedure, is the treatment of choice.

Brain tumors. Brain tumors are the second most frequent type of neoplasm in children and adolescents (Honig and Charney, 1982; Gilles, 1991). About two-third of children with brain tumor experience either chronic or frequent

TABLE 27–7 Headache Alarms in Children.

1. New headache less than 1 year history or headache in less than 5 years age[d,f]
2. Sudden onset and maximally intense immediately[f,i]
3. Headache does not respect sleep—waking up in the middle of the night; headache on awakening, headache not relieved by sleeping[a,b]
4. Radical change or progressive worsening in any aspect in established headaches[d,f,i]
5. Headache with new deficit, facial pain/tenderness, stiff neck/neck pain, vomiting, papilledema, altered mental status or seizure, motor/sensory/cranial nerve/cerebellar deficit.[c,d,f,g,i]
6. Headache triggered or worsened by increasing intracranial pressure maneuvers-cough, squatting, Valsalva maneuver, exertion, etc.[f,g,h]
7. Headache with an fever that is otherwise unexplained[c,e,g]
8. Headache in an immuno-compromised, cancer, ventriculo-peritoneal shunt patient.[c,e]
9. Headache with exclusive and persistent unilaterality.[h]
10. Headache without a familial history.[a,b]

[a] Medina, et al., 2001.

[b] Medina et al., 1997.

[c] Dodick, 2003.

[d] Lewis, et al., 2002.

[e] Newman and Lipton, 1998.

[f] Sobri, et al, 2003.

[g] Dodick, 1997.

[h] Joubert, 2005.

headaches on presentation (The epidemiology of headache among children with brain tumor. Headache in children with brain tumors. The Childhood Brain Tumor Consortium, 1991). The headaches usually are of fair recent onset, progressive in frequency and severity, but temporary plateaus can occur. Typical primary headache semiology and/or good response to acute or preventive medications do not rule out brain tumor or other secondary headache etiologies. A combination of history, exam, and judicious use of accessory tests is the best clinical approach to avoid misdiagnosis.

The pain is secondary to traction on pain-sensitive structures or obstruction of CSF flow with resultant hydrocephalus. The headache is not always localizing. Supratentorial tumors may cause frontal headaches, posterior fossa tumors may cause occipital headache, and hemispheric tumors may cause unilateral pain. Normal activity, such as changing position, defecating, coughing, or exertion, may exacerbate the pain. Although the quality of the pain and its severity are not diagnostic, it frequently is more severe in the morning and associated with and relieved by vomiting. It may awaken them at night. MRI scanning is usually diagnostic. Various treatment modalities, including surgery, radiation, and chemotherapy, singly or in combination, are utilized.

Idiopathic intracranial hypertension (Pseudotumor cerebri). Pseudotumor cerebri is increased intracranial pressure without evidence of an infection, mass lesion, or hydrocephalus (Baker et al., 1989). It has a higher incidence in adolescent females (Gordon, 1997). Patients usually have headache and papilledema, as well as an associated sixth nerve palsy and diplopia. Tinnitus may be present. Visual field testing may reveal an enlarged blind spot. Pseudotumor without papilledema has been reported (Marcelis and Silberstein, 1991). MRI reveals normal to small ventricles. Lumbar puncture demonstrates normal chemistries but elevated pressure 20 cm water in nonobese patients and 25 m water in obese patients (Headache Classification Subcommittee of the IHS, 2004). Headache should improve with removal of CSF via lumbar puncture. The disorder has been associated with a variety of conditions, including obesity, menstrual irregularity, chronic otitis, and various medications. Treatment consists of careful observation, removal of offending agents, diuretic or steroid administration, and repeated lumbar punctures, with removal of sufficient CSF to return the pressure to normal. If vision is threatened, lumbar peritoneal shunt or surgical decompression of the optic nerve may be indicated.

Brain abscess. Brain abscess is rare but may occur in patients with cyanotic congenital heart disease, chronic infections, or immunosuppression secondary to chemotherapy or human immunodeficiency virus (HIV) infection (Tekkok and Erbengi, 1992). There may be single or multiple abscesses. Symptoms include fever, headache, focal weakness, and seizures. Abnormal neurologic signs include papilledema and focal neurologic deficits. MRI is usually diagnostic. Antibiotics and surgical drainage are the treatments of choice.

Subdural hematoma and other intracranial hemorrhage may be secondary to head trauma (accidental or secondary to child abuse), blood dyscrasia, or vascular abnormality, including malformations and aneurysms (Dhellemmes et al., 1985; Roach and Riela, 1995). Again, history is the key to diagnosis. Symptoms include sudden onset or progressive worsening headache, vomiting, and lethargy. The examination may reveal macrocephaly, papilledema, retinal hemorrhages, and focal neurologic abnormalities. If any intracranial bleeding is suspected, emergent CT scan may demonstrate blood. MRI with magnetic resonance angiography (MRA) usually demonstrates the abnormality. Therapies include corticosteroids, surgical drainage, a shunting procedure, and/or interventional neuroradiology procedures, accordingly.

Chronic Nonprogressive Headaches

Chronic nonprogressive headaches are common in adolescents (Solomon et al., 1992; Gladstein et al., 1997). Bille (1962) states that they are three times more common than migraine by age 15. Their etiology is unknown. This category also includes stress-related headaches, headaches caused by conversion reaction, headaches that are depressive equivalents, and headaches related to malingering. This group does not include migraine headaches that are precipitated by stress. The disorder may occur alone or in association with migraine. It may occur episodically, less than 15 times a month, or chronically, more than 15 times a month. These headaches seem to be less common in children under 10–12 years of age and more frequent in adolescents (Akhtar et al., 1998). They affect females more frequently than males. The frequent nonmigrainous headaches described by Bille (1962) are tension-type headaches and occur in 16% of adolescents by 15 years of age.

The clinical features of chronic nonprogressive headaches in adolescents have not been well defined (Gladstein and Holden, 1996). The symptoms seem similar to those noted in adults. The headaches are frequently described as frontal and pressure or band-like. Associated tenderness in the occipital and cervical region may be present. There is no aura. Patients who have both disorders describe the pain as less severe than migraine. Some patients have mild nausea but not vomiting. The pain may be present for the entire day, a portion of the day, or come and go throughout the day. Many adolescents with this disorder continue their usual activities. Few seem bothered by light or noise. The patients frequently describe the headaches in a nonspecific manner and may also describe mild blurred vision, fatigue, and dizziness. Many take medications in excess.

Details concerning school absence, headaches in other family members, alcohol and drug abuse, divorce, parental absence from the home, or the death of a close relative or friend may be important. Some patients have a previous history of recurrent abdominal pain or limb pain for which no cause was found. Some have a history of chronic behavioral difficulties. A noncephalic illness or trauma may precede the chronic headaches. When asked, many adolescents seem to be able to identify aggravating factors, such as fatigue due to erratic sleep patterns and stressful situations at home and at school. The headache also seems to aggravate fatigue, impair concentration, and cause irritability and anxiety. It rarely awakens the patient from sleep. Weather and food do not play important roles. In many patients, physical activity and exercise exacerbate the headache.

The general physical and neurologic examinations are normal. Laboratory testing is generally not needed, but patients frequently have had tests done before consultation or request them. Routine blood counts, sedimentation rates, and metabolic profiles have been nonrevealing. CT scans and MRI scans in these patients show no abnormality or unrelated minor abnormalities. A psychological evaluation or counseling may enable patients to recognize their "stress." Many parents inadvertently perpetuate their children's chronic headaches by providing secondary gain in the form of attention and relief from stress.

If an adolescent has had daily or constant headaches for longer than 8 weeks, no symptoms of increased intracranial pressure or progressive neurologic disease, a normal general physical and neurological examination, an organic etiology is unlikely. A psychological evaluation may lead to the appropriate diagnosis.

Patients with chronic headache pain frequently show a variety of psychological and behavioral symptoms. The psychological factors and learned behavioral patterns often maintain the patient's symptoms. The methodologies used to evaluate such patients differ, but direct and indirect measures, including a headache diary, structured self-report measures, and objective psychological testing, are useful. The evaluation should assess the pain itself, including antecedents, precipitants, and responses; the effects on the patient, including global psychological and social function; and the patient's environment, including family, school, and social factors.

Depression, overt and covert, as well as anxiety has been studied in patients with chronic nonprogressive headaches (Andrasik et al., 1988; Larsson and Melin, 1988). The controlled studies of depression indicate significantly more depressive symptoms in these patients when compared with headache-free controls. In addition, significantly more anxiety is reported. Other concerns include "stress," but what is considered stressful by one individual may seem trivial to another. Precipitants in children and adolescents with chronic headache include genetic predisposition, achievement motivation and fear of failure, somatic preoccupation, and major negative life changes or life events, including divorce, moving, or the death of a close friend or relative.

Acute episodic tension-type headache in a child or teenager does not present a serious management problem unless it becomes chronic or daily and results in altered function. The occasional use of over-the-counter analgesics, including acetaminophen and ibuprofen, either separately or combined, resting in a dark room, applying an ice pack, and avoiding stressful situations is usually sufficient. Daily or frequent use of aspirin, acetaminophen, NSAIDs, caffeine-containing compounds, barbiturate-containing compounds, and narcotic analgesics should be avoided, as they may cause physical side effects and actually perpetuate the headache (Symons, 1998; Limmroth et al., 2002; Lake, 2006). Discontinuation of these compounds is necessary in order to achieve a successful outcome (Vasconcellos et al., 1998; Smith and Stoneman, 2004; Trucco et al., 2005).

Preventive medication is needed when the headache is interfering with daily life and/or school. Anticonvulsants (e.g., topiramate), tricyclic antidepressants (e.g., amitriptyline), β-blockers (e.g., propranolol), calcium channel blockers (e.g., flunarizine—not available in the US), antihistamine (e.g., cyproheptadine), and NSAIDs can be used to mitigate the impairment from chronic headache (Couch et al., 1976; Diamond and Medina, 1976; Olesen, 1986; Peatfield, 1986). Both parents and patients should be educated about their expectation about preventive therapy. Any objective, significant reduction in headache frequency, severity, duration, or total acute medication usage, and/or enhanced responsiveness to acute headache treatment is considered a clinical success.

In addition, psychological interventions are useful, including relaxation training, stress management training, and behavioral contingency management (Richter et al., 1986; Labbe, 1995; Connelly et al., 2006). The treatment may range from self-taught relaxation to computer-based technique to intensive multidisciplinary family intervention programs. Parents should be taught to reinforce normal behaviors. If more serious underlying psychopathology is suspected, a child psychiatry consultation may be needed. Patients may also benefit from physical therapy, daily exercise, sleep regulation, and an improved diet.

OTHER HEADACHES

Mixed headaches (Rothner, 1995b; Gladstein and Holden, 1996) . Pediatric and adolescent patients may have the mixed headache syndrome, which is migraine superimposed on chronic nonprogressive headaches. The combination is not uncommon and requires a combined psychological and pharmacological approach.

Cluster headaches. These are rare in children but approximately 20% cluster headache patients present in 10–19 year of age (Maytal et al., 1992; McNabb and Whitehouse, 1999; Ekbom et al., 2002, Russell, 1997). They consist of severe unilateral pain that lasts 30–45 minutes, is located behind or around the eye, and may be associated with ptosis, miosis, nasal congestion, rhinorrhea, and injection of the conjunctiva. Attacks occur several times a day and frequently awaken the patient. Episodes occur for several weeks or months and then disappear for months to years. Acute treatment includes steroids, ergotamine, oxygen, and triptans (Couch and Ziegler, 1978; Fogan, 1985; Mather et al., 1991; Maytal et al., 1992; Bahra et al., 2000; Van Vliet et al., 2001). Prophylactic medications include lithium, verapamil, melatonin, topiramate, and testosterone in selected patients (Mathew, 1978; Leone et al., 2000; Peres and Rozen, 2001; Rapoport et al., 2003; Stillman, 2006).

Temporal Mandibular Joint (TMJ) dysfunction. This may present with unilateral pain just below the ear (Belfer and Kaban, 1982; Pillemer et al., 1987) that is aggravated by chewing. Headache can be the only symptom for TMJ dysfunction in children and adolescents, with an overall prevalence of 11.4%, 14.2% for girls and 8.7% for boys (Thilander et al., 2002). Signs of this disorder may be found in up to 25% of 5–17 years aged children (Thilander et al., 2002), with a range from 10% to 60% in various age groups of children and adolescents (Ogura et al., 1985; Mohlin et al., 1991; Pahkala and Laine, 1991; Motegi et al., 1992; Keeling et al., 1994; Deng et al., 1995). On examination, patients may have jaw clicking or locking, tenderness over their jaw with limitation of mouth opening. TMJ dysfunction is associated with muscle spasms, fatigue, stress, malocclusion, bruxism, teeth clenching, and excessive gum chewing. A combination of muscle relaxants, anti-inflammatory drugs, and counseling may be beneficial. Major dental surgery and costly therapeutic programs are usually unnecessary.

Occipital neuralgia. This is a pain starting at the upper neck or base of the skull and radiating to the back of the head and the area behind the ears (Hammond and Danta, 1978; Rothner, 1995a; Kondev and Minster, 2003; Dugan et al., 1962) In essence, it is a neuropathy from various causes. The pain may be unilateral or bilateral and it can be elicited by movement, especially hyperextension of the head. It may be seen in athletes or individuals involved in flexion/extension automobile accidents. Physical examination may show tenderness alone the greater occipital nerve, limitation of motion, and decreased sensation over the C2 dermatome. An MRI that focuses on the cervicocranial junction can help rule out a congenital anomaly or other pathological process. Treatment modalities vary, but may include a soft cervical collar, analgesics, muscle relaxants, local injections, and physical therapy. Only rarely is surgery needed. The prognosis is quite good.

Four syndromes that are infrequently seen in pediatric and adolescent medicine are specifically responsive to indomethacin (Mathew, 1981; Moorjani and Rothner, 2001). These include exertional headaches precipitated by sports; cyclic migraine, in which the patient exhibits cycles of migraine headache daily for several weeks followed by 3–4 months without headache; chronic paroxysmal hemicrania, which is characterized by multiple, unilateral, daily bouts of pain that last 5–30 minutes; and hemicrania continua, which occurs in females and is characterized by severe, steady, unilateral, nonparoxysmal hemicrania localized to the frontal part of the head and not associated with nausea and vomiting. Indomethacin can be dramatically helpful in these patients, but close monitoring initially and GI protection may be needed.

References

Abbott, R, Epstein, FJ and Wisoff, JH (1991). Chronic headache associated with a functioning shunt: usefulness of pressure monitoring. *Neurosurgery*, 28 (1):72–76; discussion 76–7.

Abu-Arafeh, I, and Russell, G (1994). Prevalence of headache and migraine in schoolchildren. *BMJ*, 309:765–769.

Abu-Arafeh, I, and Russell, G (1995a). Paroxysmal vertigo as a migraine equivalent in children: a population-based study. *Cephalalgia*, 15(1):22–25; discussion 4.

Abu-Arafeh, I, and Russell, G (1995b). Prevalence and clinical features of abdominal migraine compared with those of migraine headache. *Arch Dis Child*, 72 (5):413–417.

Akhtar, ND, Mannix, LK, O'Neill, KM et al. (1998). Distribution of headache syndromes among children of various ages. *Neurology*, 50(Suppl.):A83.

Al-Twaijri, WA, and Shevell, MI (2002). Pediatric migraine equivalents: occurrence and clinical features in practice. *Pediatr Neurol*, 26(5):365–368.

Al Jumah, M, Awada, A, and Al Azzam, S (2002). Headache syndromes amongst schoolchildren in Riyadh, Saudi Arabia. *Headache*, 42(4):281–286.

Andrasik, F, Kabela, E, Quinn, S, et al. (1988). Psychological functioning of children who have recurrent migraine. *Pain*, 34(1):43–52.

Auvin, S, Joriot-Chekaf, S, Cuvellier, JC et al. (2006). Small vessel abnormalities in alternating hemiplegia of childhood: pathophysiologic implications. *Neurology*, 66(4):499–504.

Ayatollahi, SM, Moradi, F, and Ayatollahi, SA (2002). Prevalences of migraine and tension-type headache in adolescent girls of Shiraz (southern Iran). *Headache*, 42(4):287–290.

Bahra, A, Gawel, MJ, Hardebo, JE, et al. (2000). Oral zolmitriptan is effective in the acute treatment of cluster headache. *Neurology*, 54(9):1832–1839.

Baker, RS, Baumann, RJ, and Buncic, JR, (1989). Idiopathic intracranial hypertension (pseudotumor cerebri) in pediatric patients. *Pediatr Neurol*, 5(1):5–11.

Barea, JM, Tannhauser, M and Rotta, NT (1996). An epidemiologic study of headache among children and adolescents of southern Brazil. *Cephalalgia*, 16:545–549.

Barlow, CF (1984). *Headaches and Migraine in Childhood*. Vol. 91, *Clinics in Develomental Medicine*. Spastics International Medical Publications, London.

Bassi, MT, Bresolin, N, Tonelli, A, et al. (2004). A novel mutation in the ATP1A2 gene causes alternating hemiplegia of childhood. *J Med Genet*, 41(8):621–628.

Belfer, ML and Kaban, LB (1982). Temporomandibular joint dysfunction with facial pain in children. *Pediatrics*, 69(5):564–567.

Bickerstaff, ER (1962). The basilar artery and the migraineepilepsy syndrome. *Proc R Soc Med*, 55:167–169.

Bigal, ME, Rapoport, AM, Tepper, SJ et al. (2005). The classification of chronic daily headache in adolescents—a comparison between the second edition of the international classification of headache disorders and alternative diagnostic criteria. *Headache*, 45 (5):582–589.

Bigal, ME, Tepper, SJ, Sheftell, FD et al. (2006). Field testing alternative criteria for chronic migraine. *Cephalalgia*, 26(4):477–482.

Bille, B (1962). Migraine in school children. *Acta Paediatr*, 51(Suppl. 136):16–151.

Bille, B (1997). A 40-year follow-up of school children with migraine. *Cephalalgia*, 17:488–491.

Bruni, O, Cortesi, F, Guidetti, V et al. (1991). Acetylsalicylic vs acetaminophen in childhood and adolescence acute migraine. In *Juvenile Headache. Int. Congr Ser Excerpta Med.* (V Gallai and V Guidetti, eds.). Elsevier Science Publishers BV, Amsterdam.

Burton, LJ, Quinn, B, Pratt-Cheney, JL et al. (1997). Headache etiology in a pediatric emergency department. *Pediatr Emerg Care*, 13(1):1–4.

Catto-Smith, AG and Ranuh, R (2003). Abdominal migraine and cyclical vomiting. *Semin Pediatr Surg*, 12 (4):254–258.

Clinical policy for the initial approach to adolescents and adults presenting to the emergency department with a chief complaint of headache. American College of Emergency Physicians (1996). *Ann Emerg Med*, 27 (6):821–844.

Cohen, BH (1995). Headaches as a symptom of neurological disease. *Sem Ped Neuro*, 2:144–150.

Comby, J (1921). La migraine chez les enfants. *Arch de Médec des Enfants*, 24:29–49.

Congdon, PJ and Forsythe, WI (1979). Migraine in childhood: a study of 300 children. *Dev Med Child Neurol*, 21:209–216.

Connelly, M, Rapoff, MA, Thompson, N et al. (2006). Headstrong: a pilot study of a CD-ROM intervention for recurrent pediatric headache. *J Pediatr Psychol*, 31 (7):737–747.

Couch, JR Jr. and Ziegler, DK (1978). Prednisone therapy for cluster headache. *Headache*, 18(4):219–221.

Couch, JR, Ziegler, DK, and Hassanein, R (1976). Amitriptyline in the prophylaxis of migraine. Effectiveness and relationship of antimigraine and antidepressant effects. *Neurology*, 26:121–127.

Day, WH (1873). *Essays on Diseases of Children*. J & A Churchill, London.

De Fusco, M, Marconi, R, Silvestri, L et al. (2003). Haploinsufficiency of ATP1A2 encoding the Na^+/K^+ pump alpha2 subunit associated with familial hemiplegic migraine type 2. *Nat Genet*, 33(2):192–196.

Deng, YM, Fu, MK, and Hagg, U (1995). Prevalence of temporomandibular joint dysfunction (TMJD) in Chinese children and adolescents. A cross-sectional epidemiological study. *Eur J Orthod*, 17(4):305–309.

Deubner, DC (1977). An epidemilogic study of migraine and headache in 10–20 year olds. *Headache*, 17:173–180.

Dhellemmes, P, Lejeune, JP, Christiaens, JL et al. (1985). Traumatic extradural hematomas in infancy and childhood. Experience with 144 cases. *J Neurosurg*, 62 (6):861–864.

Di Rosa, G, Spano, M, Pustorino, G, et al. (2006). Alternating hemiplegia of childhood successfully treated with topiramate: 18 months of follow-up. *Neurology*, 66 (1):146.

Diamond, S, and Medina. JL (1976). Double blind study of propranolol for migraine prophylaxis. *Headache*, 16 (1):24–27.

Dichgans, M, Freilinger, T, Eckstein, G et al. (2005). Mutation in the neuronal voltage-gated sodium channel SCN1A in familial hemiplegic migraine. *Lancet*, 366 (9483):371–377.

Dodick, D (1997). Headache as a symptom of ominous disease: what are the warning signals? *Postgrad Med*, 101(5):46–50,55–56,62–64.

Dodick, WD (2003). Diagnosing headache: clinical clues and clinical rules. *Adv Stud Med*, 3(2):87–92.

Drigo, P, Carli, G, and Laverda, AM (2000). Benign paroxysmal torticollis of infancy. *Brain Dev*, 22(3):169–172.

Ehyai, A and Fenichel, GM (1978). The natural history of acute confusional migraine. *Arch Neurol*, 35 (6):368–369.

Ekbom, K, Svensson, DA, Traff, H, et al. (2002). Age at onset and sex ratio in cluster headache: observations over three decades. *Cephalalgia*, 22(2):94–100.

The epidemiology of headache among children with brain tumor. Headache in children with brain tumors. The Childhood Brain Tumor Consortium (1991). *J Neurooncol*, 10(1):31–46.

Evans, RW and Rolak, LA (2004). The Alice in Wonderland syndrome. *Headache*, 44(6):624–625.

Fenichel, GM (1967). Migraine as a cause of benign paroxysmal vertigo of childhood. *J Pediat*, 71:114–115.

Ferrera, PC and Reicho, PR (1996). Acute confusional migraine and trauma-triggered migraine. *Am J Emerg Med*, 14(3):276–278.

Fogan, L (1985). Treatment of cluster headache. A double-blind comparison of oxygen v air inhalation. *Arch Neurol*, 42(4):362–363.

Forsythe, WI, Gillies, D, and Sills, MA (1984). Propanolol ('Inderal') in the treatment of childhood migraine. *Dev Med Child Neurol*, 26(6):737–741.

Gallai, V, Sarchielli, P, Carboni, F, et al. (1995). Applicability of the 1988 IHS criteria to headaches patients under the age of 18 years attending 21 Italian headache clinics. *Headache*, 35:146–153.

Gervil, M, Ulrich, V, Kaprio, J, et al. (1999). The relative role of genetic and environmental factors in migraine without aura. *Neurology*, 53(5):995–999.

Gervil, M, Ulrich, V, Kyvik, KO, et al. (1999). Migraine without aura: a population-based twin study. *Ann Neurol*, 46(4):606–611.

Gherpelli, JLD, Nagae Poetscher, LM, Souza, AMMH, et al. (1998). Migraine in childhood and adolescence. A critical study of the diagnostic criteria and of the influence of age on clinical findings. *Cephalalgia*, 18:333–341.

Giffin, NJ, Benton, S, and Goadsby, PJ (2002). Benign paroxysmal torticollis of infancy: four new cases and linkage to CACNA1A mutation. *Dev Med Child Neurol*, 44(7):490–493.

Gilles, FH (1991). The epidemiology of headache among children with brain tumor. *J NeuroOncol*, 10:31–46.

Gladstein, J and Holden, EW (1996). Chronic daily headache in children and adolescents: a 2-year prospective study. *Headache*, 36:349–351.

Gladstein, J, Holden, EW, Winner, P, et al. (1997). Chronic daily headaches in children and adolescents: current status and recommendations for the future. *Headache*, 37:626–629.

Golden, GS (1979). The Alice in Wonderland syndrome in juvenile migraine. *Pediatrics*, 63(4):517–519.

Gomersall, JD and Stuart, A (1973). Amitriptyline in migraine prophylaxis. *J Neurol Neurosurg Psychiatry*, 36:684–690.

Gordon, K (1997). Pediatric pseudotumor cerebri: descriptive epidemiology. *Can J Neurol Sci*, 24(3):219–221.

Graf, WD and Riback, PS (1995). Pharmacologic treatment of recurrent pediatric headache. *Pediatr Ann*, 24 (9):477–484.

Grayson, S, Neher, JO, Howard, E, et al. (2005). Cinical inquiries. When is neuroimaging warranted for headache? *J Fam Pract*, 54(11):988–991.

Grosberg, BM, Solomon, S, Friedman, DI, et al. (2006). Retinal migraine reappraised. *Cephalalgia*, 26 (11):1275–1286.

Hamalainen, ML, Hoppu, K, and Santavuori, PR (1995). Effect of age on the fulfilment of the IHS criteria for migraine in children at a headache clinic. *Cephalalgia*, 15(5):404–409.

Hämäläinen, ML, Hoppu, K, Valkeila, E, et al. (1997). Ibuprofen or acetaminophen for the acute treatment of migraine in children. *Neurology*, 48:103–107.

Hammond, SR and Danta, G (1978). Occipital neuralgia. *Clin Exp Neurol*, 15:258–270.

Headache Classification Committee of the International Headache Society. Classification and diagnostic criteria for headache disorders, cranial neuralgias and facial pain (1988). *Cephalalgia*, 8(Suppl. 7):1–96.

Headache Classification Subcommittee of the International Headache Society. The International Classification of Headache Disorders (2004). *Cephalagia*, 24 (Suppl. 1):1–160.

Hering, R and Kuritzky, A (1992). Sodium valproate in the prophylactic treatment of migraine: a double-blind study versus placebo. *Cephalalgia*, 12(2):81–84.

Herraiz, C, Calvin, FJ, Tapia, MC, et al. (1999). The migraine: benign paroxysmal vertigo of childhood complex. *Int Tinnitus J*, 5(1):50–52.

Hershey, AD (2003). Chronic daily headaches in children. *Expert Opin Pharmacother*, 4(4):485–491.

Hershey, AD, Winner, P, Kabbouche, MA, et al. (2005). Use of the ICHD-II criteria in the diagnosis of pediatric migraine. *Headache*, 45(10):1288–1297.

Hockaday, JM (1988). Definitions, clinical features, and diagnosis of childhood migraine. In *Migraine in Childhood* (JM Hockaday, ed.), Butterworths, London.

Honig, PJ and Charney, EB (1982). Children with brain tumor headaches. Distinguishing features. *Am J Dis Child*, 136(2):121–124.

Jones, J, Sklar, D, Dougherty, J, et al. (1989). Randomized double-blind trial of intravenous prochlorperazine for the treatment of acute headache. *JAMA*, 261:1174–1176.

Joubert, J (2005). Diagnosing headache. *Aust Fam Physician*, 34(8):621–625.

Kabbouche, MA, Vockell, AL, LeCates, SL, et al. (2001). Tolerability and effectiveness of prochlorperazine for intractable migraine in children. *Pediatrics*, 107(4):E62.

Kallela, M, Wessman, M, and Farkkila, M (2001). Validation of a migraine-specific questionnaire for use in family studies. *Eur J Neurol*, 8(1):61–66.

Kallela, M, Wessman, M, Havanka, H, et al. (2001). Familial migraine with and without aura: clinical characteristics and co-occurrence. *Eur J Neurol*, 8(5):441–449.

Karli, N, Akis, N, Zarifoglu, M, et al. (2006). Headache prevalence in adolescents aged 12 to 17: a student-based epidemiological study in Bursa. *Headache*, 46 (4):649–655.

Keeling, SD, McGorray, S, Wheeler, TT, et al. (1994). Risk factors associated with temporomandibular joint sounds in children 6 to 12 years of age. *Am J Orthod Dentofacial Orthop*, 105(3):279–287.

Kirchmann, M, Thomsen, LL, and Olesen, J (2006). Basilar-type migraine: clinical, epidemiologic, and genetic features. *Neurology*, 66(6):880–886.

Kondev, L and Minster, A (2003). Headache and facial pain in children and adolescents. *Otolaryngol Clin North Am*, 36(6):1153–1170.

Kors, EE, Vanmolkot, KR, Haan, J, et al. (2004). Alternating hemiplegia of childhood: no mutations in the second familial hemiplegic migraine gene ATP1A2. *Neuropediatrics*, 35(5):293–296.

Labbe, E (1995). Treatment of childhood migraine with autogenic training and skin temperature biofeedback: a component analysis. *Headache*, 35:10–13.

Lake, AE 3rd (2006). Medication overuse headache: biobehavioral issues and solutions. *Headache*, 46(Suppl. 3): S88–S97.

Lanzi, G, Zambrino, CA, Balottin, U, et al. (1997). Periodic syndrome and migraine in children and adolescents. *Ital J Neurol*, 18:283–288.

Larsson, B and Melin L, (1988). The psychological treatment of recurrent headache in adolescents—short-term outcome and its prediction. *Headache*, 28 (3):187–195.

Lee, LH and Olness, KN, (1997). Clinical and demographic characteristics of migraine in urban children. *Headache*, 37:269–276.

Leone, M, D'Amico, D, Frediani, F, et al. (2000). Verapamil in the prophylaxis of episodic cluster headache: a double-blind study versus placebo. *Neurology*, 54 (6):1382–1385.

Levinstein, B (1991). A comparative study of cyproheptadine, amitriptyline, and propranolol in the treatment of adolescent migraine. *Cephalagia*, 11:122–123.

Lewis, DW, Ashwal, S, Dahl, G, et al. (2002). Practice parameter: evaluation of children and adolescents with recurrent headaches: report of the Quality Standards Subcommittee of the American Academy of Neurology and the Practice Committee of the Child Neurology Society. *Neurology*, 59(4):490–498.

Lewis, DW and Qureshi, F (2000). Acute headache in children and adolescents presenting to the emergency department. *Headuche*, 40(3):200–203.

Lewis, D, Winner, P, Hershey, AD, et al. (2007). Efficacy of zolmitriptan nasal spray in adolescent migraine: the "Double-Diamond" study. *Pediatrics*, 120(2):390–396.

Lewis, DW, Middlebrook, M, Mehallick, L, et al. (1994). Naproxen for migraine prophylaxis. *Ann Neurol*, 36:542–543.

Li, BU (2000). Cyclic vomiting syndrome. *Curr Treat Options Gastroenterol*, 3(5):395–402.

Li, BU and Balint, JP (2000). Cyclic vomiting syndrome: evolution in our understanding of a brain-gut disorder. *Adv Pediatr*, 47:117–160.

Li, BU and Misiewicz, L (2003). Cyclic vomiting syndrome: a brain-gut disorder. *Gastroenterol Clin North Am*, 32(3):997–1019.

Li, BU, Murray, RD, Heitlinger, LA, et al. (1999). Is cyclic vomiting syndrome related to migraine? *J Pediatr*, 134 (5):567–572.

Li, BU, Murray, RD, Heitlinger, LA, et al. (1998). Heterogeneity of diagnoses presenting as cyclic vomiting. *Pediatrics*, 102(3):583–587.

Lima, MM, Padula, NA, Santos, LC, et al. (2005). Critical analysis of the international classification of headache disorders diagnostic criteria (ICHD I-1988) and (ICHD II-2004), for migraine in children and adolescents. *Cephalalgia*, 25(11):1042–1047.

Limmroth, V, Katsarava, Z, Fritsche, G, et al. (2002). Features of medication overuse headahe following overuse of different acute headache drugs. *Neurology*, 59:1011–1014.

Linder, SL (1994). Treatment of childhood headache wtih dihydroergotamine mesylate. *Headache*, 34:578–580.

Linder, SL (2005). Understanding the comprehensive pediatric headache examination. *Pediatr Ann*, 34 (6):442–446.

Linder, SL and Dowson, AJ (2000). Zolmitriptan provides effective migraine relief in adolescents. *Int J Clin Pract*, 54(7):466–469.

Lindskog, U, Odkvist, L, Noaksson, L, et al. (1999). Benign paroxysmal vertigo in childhood: a long-term follow-up. *Headache*, 39:33–37.

Lipton, RB, Stewart, WF, Cady, R, et al. (2000). Sumatriptan for the range of headaches in migraine sufferers: results of the spectrum study. *Headache*, 40:783–791.

Lu, SR, Fuh, JL, Juang, KD, et al. (2000). Migraine prevalence in adolescents aged 13-15: a student population-based study in Taiwan. *Cephalalgia*, 20(5):479–485.

Ludvigsson, J (1974). Propranolol used in prophylaxis of migraine in children. *Acta Neurol Scand*, 50:109–115.

Marcelis, J and Silberstein, SD (1991). Idiopathic intracranial hypertension without papilledema. *Arch Neurol*, 48(4):392–399.

Mather, PJ, Silberstein, SD, Schulman, EA et al. (1991). The treatment of cluster headache with repetitive intravenous dihydroergotamine. *Headache*, 31 (8):525–532.

Mathew, NT (1978). Clinical subtypes of cluster headache and response to lithium therapy. *Headache*, 18 (1):27–29.

Mathew, NT (1981). Indomethacin responsive headache syndromes. *Headache*, 21(4):147–150.

Mavromichalis, I, Anagnostopoulos, D, Metaxas, N, et al. (1999). Prevalence of migraine in schoolchildren and some clinical comparisons between migraine with and without aura. *Headache*, 39(10):728–736.

Maytal, J, Lipton, RB, Solomon, S, et al. (1992). Childhood onset cluster headaches. *Headache*, 32(6):275–279.

Maytal, J, Young, M, Shechter, A, et al. (1997). Pediatric migraine and the International Headache Society (IHS) criteria. *Neurology*, 48:602–607.

McGrath, PJ and Reid, GJ (1995). Behavioral treatment of pediatric headache. *Pediatr Ann*, 24(9):486–491.

McNabb, S and Whitehouse, W (1999). Cluster headache-like disorder in childhood. *Arch Dis Child*, 81 (6):511–512.

Medina, LS, Pinter, JD, Zurakowski, D, et al. (1997). Children with headache: clinical predictors of surgical space-occupying lesions and the role of neuroimaging. *Radiology*, 202(3):819–824.

Medina, LS, Kuntz, KM, and Pomeroy, S (2001). Children with headache suspected of having a brain tumor: a cost-effectiveness analysis of diagnostic strategies. *Pediatrics*, 108(2):255–263.

Metsahonkala, L and Sillanpaa, M (1994). Migraine in children—an evaluation of the IHS criteria. *Cephalalgia*, 14(4):285–290.

Mohlin, B, Pilley, JR, and Shaw, WC (1991). A survey of craniomandibular disorders in 1000 12-year-olds. Study design and baseline data in a follow-up study. *Eur J Orthod*, 13(2):111–123.

Moorjani, BI and Rothner, AD (2001). Indomethacin-responsive headaches in children and adolescents. *Semin Pediatr Neurol*, 8(1):40–45.

Moreland, TJ, Storli, OV, and Mogstad, TE (1979). Doxepin in the prophylactic treatment of mixed vascular and tension headache. *Headache*, 19:382–383.

Mortimer, MJ, Kay, J, and Jaron, A (1992). Epidemiology of headache and childhood migraine in an urban general practice using ad hoc, Vahlquist and IHS criteria. *Dev Med Child Neurol*, 34:1095–1101.

Motegi, E, Miyazaki, H, Ogura, I, et al. (1992). An orthodontic study of temporomandibular joint disorders. Part 1: epidemiological research in Japanese 6-18 year olds. *Angle Orthod*, 62(4):249–256.

Murray, TJ (1982). The neurology of Alice in Wonderland. *Can J Neurol Sci*, 9(4):453–457.

Newman, LC and Lipton, RB (1998). Emergency department evaluation of headache. *Neurol Clin*, 16 (2):285–303.

Ogura, T, Morinushi, T, Ohno, H, et al. (1985). An epidemiological study of TMJ dysfunction syndrome in adolescents. *J Pedod*, 10(1):22–35.

Olesen, J (1986). Role of calcium entry blockers in the prophylaxis of migraine. *Eur Neurol*, 25(Suppl. 1):72–79.

Olesen, J, Bousser, MG, Diener, HC, et al. (2006). New appendix criteria open for a broader concept of chronic migraine. *Cephalalgia*, 26(6):742–746.

Olness, K, MacDonald, JT, and Uden, DL (1987). Comparison of self-hypnosis and propranolol in the treatment of juvenile classic migraine. *Pediatrics*, 79 (4):593–597.

Ophoff, RA, Terwindt, GM, Vergouwe, MN, et al. (1996). Familial hemiplegic migraine and episodic ataxia type-2 are caused by mutations in the Ca2 + channel gene CACNL1A4. *Cell*, 87:544–552.

Pahkala, R and Laine, T (1991). Variation in function of the masticatory system in 1008 rural children. *J Clin Pediatr Dent*, 16(1):25–30.

Pearce, JM (1980). Chronic migrainous neuralgia: a variant of cluster headache. *Brain*, 103(1):149–159.

Peatfield, RC (1986). Principles in the management of headache. *Practitioner*, 230(1412):125–129.

Peres, MF and Rozen, TD (2001). Melatonin in the preventive treatment of chronic cluster headache. *Cephalalgia*, 21(10):993–995.

Peroutka, SJ and Allen, GS (1984). The calcium antagonist properties of cyproheptadine: implications for antimigraine action. *Neurology*, 34(3):304–309.

Physicians' Desk Reference (2007). (61 edn). Thomson PDR, Montvale, NJ.

Pillemer, FG, Masek, BJ, and Kaban, LB (1987). Temporomandibular joint dysfunction and facial pain in children: an approach to diagnosis and treatment. *Pediatrics*, 80(4):565–570.

Pothmann, R (1987). [Prevention of migraine with flunarizine and acetylsalicylic acid. A double-blind study]. *Monatsschr Kinderheilkd*, 135(9):646–649.

Powers, SW and Andrasik, F (2005). Biobehavioral treatment, disability, and psychological effects of pediatric headache. *Pediatr Ann*, 34(6):461–465.

Pradalier, A, Clapin, A, and Dry, J (1988). Treatment review: non-steroid anti-inflammatory drugs in the treatment and long-term prevention of migraine attacks. *Headache*, 28(8):550–557.

Prensky, AL and Sommer, D (1979). Diagnosis and treatment of migraine in children. *Neurology*, 29:506–510.

Rapoport, AM, Bigal, ME, Tepper, SJ, et al. (2003). Treatment of cluster headache with topiramate: effects and side-effects in five patients. *Cephalalgia*, 23(1):69–70; author reply 70.

Rho, JM and Chugani, HT (1998). Alternating hemiplegia of childhood: insights into its pathophysiology. *J Child Neurol*, 13(1):39–45.

Richter, IL, McGrath, PJ, Humphreys, PJ, et al. (1986). Cognitive and relaxation treatment of paediatric migraine. *Pain*, 25(2):195–203.

Rinalduzzi, S, Valeriani, M, and Vigevano, F (2006). Brainstem dysfunction in alternating hemiplegia of childhood: a neurophysiological study. *Cephalalgia*, 26 (5):511–5119.

Roach, ES and Rielam, AR (1995). *Pediatric Cerebrovascular Disorders* (2nd edn). Futura, New York.

Rose, FC (1995). The history of migraine from mesopotamian to medieval times. *Cephalagia*, S15:1–3.

Rothner, AD (1995a). Miscellaneous headache syndromes in children and adolescents. *Semin Pediatr Neurol*, 2 (2):159–164.

Rothner, AD (1995b). The evaluation of headaches in children and adolescents. *Semin Pediatr Neurol*, 2 (2):109–118.

Rothner, AD, Winner, P, Nett, R, et al. (2000). One-year tolerability and efficacy of sumatriptan nasal spray in adolescents with migraine: results of a multicenter, open-label study. *Clin Ther*, 22(12):1533–1546.

Russell, G, Abu-Arafeh, I, and Symon, DN (2002). Abdominal migraine: evidence for existence and treatment options. *Paediatr Drugs,* 4(1):1–8.

Russell, MB (1997). Genetic epidemiology of migraine and cluster headache. *Cephalalgia,* 17:683–701.

Russell, MB, Iselius, L, and Olesen, J (1996). Migraine without aura and migraine with aura are inherited disorders. *Cephalalgia,* 16:305–309.

Serdaroglu, G, Erhan, E, Tekgul, H, et al. (2002). Sodium valproate prophylaxis in childhood migraine. *Headache,* 42(8):819–822.

Seshia, SS and Wolstein, JR (1995). International Headache Society classification and diagnostic criteria in children: a proposal for revision. *Dev Med Child Neurol,* 37(10):879–882.

Seshia, SS, Wolstin, JR, Adams, C, et al. (1994). International Headache Society criteria and childhood headache. *Dev Med Child Neurol,* 36:419–428.

Silberstein, SD and Young, WB (1995). Safety and efficacy of ergotamine tartrate and dihydroergotamine in the treatment of migraine and status migrainosus. *Neurology,* 45:577–584.

Sillanpää, M (1994). Headache in children. In *Headache Classification and Epidemiology* (J Olesen, ed.), pp. 517–523, Raven Press, New York.

Sillanpää, M (1976). Prevalence of migraine and other headache in Finnish children starting school. *Headache,* 15:288–290.

Sillanpää, M (1983). Changes in the prevalence of migraine and other headaches during the first seven school years. *Headache,* 23:15–19.

Sillanpää, M, Piekkala, P, and Kero, P (1991). Prevalence of headache at preschool age in an unselected child population. *Cephalalgia,* 11:239–242.

Smith, TR and Stoneman, J (2004). Medication overuse headache from antimigraine therapy: clinical features, pathogenesis and management. *Drugs,* 64 (22):2503–2514.

Sobri, M, Lamont, AC, Alias, NA, et al. (2003). Red flags in patients presenting with headache: clinical indications for neuroimaging. *Br J Radiol,* 76(908):532–535.

Solomon, GD (1995). The pharmacology of medications used in treating headache. *Semin Pediatr Neurol,* 2 (2):165–177.

Solomon, S, Lipton, RB, and Newman, LC (1992). Clinical features of chronic daily headache. *Headache,* 32:325–329.

Sorge, F, De Simone, R, Marano, E, et al. (1988). Flunarizine in prophylaxis of childhood migraine. A double-blind, placebo-controlled, crossover study. *Cephalalgia,* 8(1):1–6.

Split, W and Neuman, W (1999). Epidemiology of migraine among students from randomly selected secondary schools in Lodz. *Headache,* 39:494–501.

Stewart, WF, Bigal, ME, Kolodner, K, et al. (2006). Familial risk of migraine: variation by proband age at onset and headache severity. *Neurology,* 66(3):344–348.

Stewart, WF, Lipton, RB, Celentano, DD, et al. (1992). Prevalence of migraine headache in the United States. *JAMA,* 267(1):64–70.

Stillman, MJ (2006). Testosterone replacement therapy for treatment refractory cluster headache. *Headache,* 46 (6):925–933.

Svensson, DA, Larsson, B, Bille, B, et al. (1999). Genetic and environmental influences on recurrent headaches in eight to nine-year-old twins. *Cephalalgia,* 19 (10):866–872.

Swoboda, KJ, Kanavakis, E, Xaidara, A, et al. (2004). Alternating hemiplegia of childhood or familial hemiplegic migraine? A novel ATP1A2 mutation. *Ann Neurol,* 55 (6):884–887.

Symon, DN and Russell, G (1995). The relationship between cyclic vomiting syndrome and abdominal migraine. *J Pediatr Gastroenterol Nutr,* 21(Suppl. 1): S42–S43.

Symons, DNK (1998). Twelve cases of analgesic headache. *Arch Dis Child,* 78:555–556.

Tek, DS, McClellan, DS, Olshaker, JS, et al. (1990). A prospective, double-blind study of metoclopramide hydrochloride for the control of migraine in the emergency department. *Ann Emerg Med,* 19(10):1083–1087.

Tekkok, IH and Erbengi, A (1992). Management of brain abscess in children: review of 130 cases over a period of 21 years. *Childs Nerv Syst,* 8(7):411–416.

Thilander, B, Rubio, G, Pena, L, et al. (2002). Prevalence of temporomandibular dysfunction and its association with malocclusion in children and adolescents: an epidemiologic study related to specified stages of dental development. *Angle Orthod,* 72(2):146–154.

Trucco, M, Meineri, P, and Ruiz, L (2005). Preliminary results of a withdrawal and detoxification therapeutic regimen in patients with probable chronic migraine and probable medication overuse headache. *J Headache Pain,* 6(4):334–337.

Ulrich, V, Gervil, M, Fenger, K, et al. (1999). The prevalence and characteristics of migraine in twins from the general population. *Headache,* 39(3):173–180.

Ulrich, V, Olesen, J, Gervil, M, et al. (2000). Possible risk factors and precipitants for migraine with aura in discordant twin-pairs: a population-based study. *Cephalalgia,* 20(9):821–825.

Vahlquist, B (1955). Migraine in children. *Int Arch Allergy Appl Immunol,* 7(4–6):348–355.

Vahlquist, B and Hackzell, G (1949). Migraine of early onset. A study of thirty one cases in which the disease first appeared between one and four years of age. *Acta Paediatr,* 38:622–636.

Van Vliet, JA, Bahra, A, Martin, V, et al. (2001). Intranasal sumatriptan is effective in the treatment of acute cluster headache: a double-blind, placebo-controlled, crossover study. *Cephalalgia,* 21:270.

Vasconcellos, E, Pina-Garza, JE, Millan, EJ, et al. (1998). Analgesic rebound headache in children and adolescents. *J Child Neurol,* 13(9):443–447.

Wang, SJ, Fuh, JL, Lu, SR, et al. (2006). Chronic daily headache in adolescents: prevalence, impact, and medication overuse. *Neurology,* 66(2):193–197.

Wasiewski, WW and Rothner, AD (1999). Pediatric migraine headache: Diagnosis, evaluation, and management. *Neurologist,* 5:122–134.

Winner, P, Lewis, D, Visser, WH, et al. (2002). Rizatriptan 5 mg for the acute treatment of migraine in adolescents: a randomized, double-blind, placebo-controlled study. *Headache,* 42(1):49–55.

Winner, P, Linder, SL, and Wasiewski, W (2001). Pharmacologic treatment of headache. In *Headache in Children and Adolescents.* (Paul Winner, A David Rothner eds.), pp. 87–115, BC Decker, Hamilton.

Winner, P, Pearlman, EM, Linder, SL, et al. (2005). Topiramate for migraine prevention in children: a randomized, double-blind, placebo-controlled trial. *Headache,* 45(10):1304–1312.

Winner, P, Prensky, A, and Linder, S (1996). Efficacy and safety of oral sumatriptan in adolescent migraines. Paper read at American Association for the Study of Headache, at Chicago, IL

Winner, P, Rothner, AD, Putnam, DG, et al. (2003). Demographic and migraine characteristics of adolescents with migraine: Glaxo Wellcome clinical trials' database. *Headache,* 43(5):451–457.

Winner, P, Rothner, AD, Wooen, J, et al. (2004). Randomized, double-blind, placebo-controlled study of sumatriptan nasal spray in adolescent migraineurs. *Neurology,* 62:A182.

Winner, P, Rothner, A, Webster, C, et al. (2004). Overall efficacy of sumatriptan nasal spray in adolescent migraineurs: pooled results from US placebo-controlled trials. *Headache,* 44:465.

Winner, P, Wasiewski, W, Gladstein, J, et al. (1997). Multicenter prospective evaluation of proposed pediatric migraine revisions to the IHS criteria. *Headache,* 37 (9):545–548.

Winner, P, Linder, S, Lipton, R, et al. (2007). Eletriptan for the acute treatment of migraine in adolescents: results of a double-blind, placebo-controlled trial. *Headache,* 47:511–518.

Wobel-Bingol, C, Wober, C, Wagner-Ennsgraber, C, et al. (1996). IHS criteria and gender: a study on migraine and tension-type headache in children and adolescents. *Cephalalgia,* 16:107–112.

Yuill, GM, Swinburn, WR, and Liversedge, LA (1972). A double-blind crossover trial of isometheptene mucate compound and ergotamine in migraine. *Br J Clin Pract,* 26(2):76–79.

Zuckerman, B, Stevenson, J, and Bailey, V (1987). Stomachaches and headaches in a community sample of preschool children. *Pediatrics,* 79(5):677–682.

Zwart, JA, Dyb, G, Holmen, TL, et al. (2004). The prevalence of migraine and tension-type headaches among adolescents in Norway. The Nord-Trondelag Health Study (Head-HUNT-Youth), a large population-based epidemiological study. *Cephalalgia,* 24(5):373–379.

28 Headaches in Women

Elizabeth Loder and Stephen D Silberstein

OVERVIEW

Headache prevalence and disability are heavily concentrated in women of childbearing age. This is especially true for migraine, where good-quality clinical, epidemiologic, and basic science observations strongly support the view that hormonal factors are an important influence on the phenotypic expression of headache. This chapter examines selected issues of special importance to medical practitioners who evaluate and treat primary headache disorders in women. Many of these are related to the influence of ovarian steroid cycling on the biological mechanisms of headache. Still others have to do with cultural and medical factors that differentially affect females. The emphasis on migraine is inevitable, since that is the headache disorder which has attracted the most clinical and research attention.

MENSTRUATION AND HEADACHE

The connection between the menstrual cycle and headache is most obvious and clinically important for migraine. Girls are more likely to experience the onset of migraine during the year of menarche than at any other time, and menstrual exacerbations are commonly reported (Dalsgaard-Nielsen, 1970). Some women with tension-type headache report that hormonal fluctuations provoke their headaches, but the connection is not as well established as for migraine (Scharff et al., 1995; Fragoso et al., 2003; Holzhammer and Wober, 2006). Prominent menstrual exacerbations of cluster headache are likewise not the rule, although a series of patients with menstrual migraine and cluster-like features has been described (Robbins, 1996; van Vliet et al., 2006).

The International Classification of Headache Disorders-II (ICHD-II) contains new candidate criteria for menstrual migraine (Headache Classification Subcommittee of the International Headache Society, 2004). These define menstrual attacks as those that occur during a 5-day interval of time extending from 2 days before through 3 days after the onset of menses. In pure menstrual migraine without aura, attacks of migraine without aura occur during this interval and at no other time of the month, while in menstrually related migraine without aura, attacks regularly occur during this interval but also at other times of the month. Roughly, 60% of women with migraine experience an attack pattern consistent with menstrually related migraine, while 14% have attacks that are exclusively linked with menses. In some women there is no obvious connection between the menstrual cycle and migraine (Epstein et al., 1975). A wide variety of evidence supports the view that menstrual migraine is triggered by estrogen withdrawal, which produces migraine attacks in susceptible women (Somerville, 1972a, 1975; Silberstein, 1995). Although falling estrogen levels correlate with menstrual susceptibility to migraine, they do not clearly lead to postovulatory headaches (MacGregor et al., 2006).

Since treatment differs, it is important to distinguish between menstrual migraine and premenstrual headaches, which are a somatic symptom in premenstrual or late luteal phase dysphoric disorder or the "premenstrual syndrome" (PMS) as it is sometimes called. In these syndromes, headaches occur in conjunction with, and may be overshadowed by, prominent affective lability, anxiety, fatigue, and other symptoms. Symptoms are relieved by the onset of menstruation, and prophylactic treatment with selective serotonin reuptake inhibitors can be helpful (Pearlstein, 2002; Johnson, 2004; Futterman and Rapkin, 2006). With menstrual migraine, headache is the major symptom and is not reliably relieved by the onset of menstruation. The presence and severity of headache does appear to modulate PMS symptoms in women with migraine, and it has been suggested that because of this overlap the syndromes should not be separated (Facchinetti et al., 1993, 1994; Facchinetti, 1994; Martin et al., 2006).

TREATMENT OF HEADACHES ASSOCIATED WITH THE MENSTRUAL CYCLE

Overview

Recall is an unreliable way to determine a connection between headaches and the menstrual period; hence several cycles of recorded diary information about headaches and the menstrual cycle are recommended to confirm a diagnosis of menstrual-related headache or plan treatment. Attacks of menstrual migraine may differ from nonmenstrual attacks in the same woman. Menstrual attacks are less likely to be associated with aura, and in treatment-seeking women may be longer, more difficult to treat, or more prone to recur (MacGregor and Hackshaw, 2004). In women who have frequent headaches, however, the onset of menstruation is responsible for only a small proportion of attacks overall (Johannes et al., 1995). In the general population, the differences between menstrual and nonmenstrual headaches are much less apparent (Stewart et al., 2000).

Acute Treatment of Menstrual Attacks of Migraine

Drugs that are effective and commonly used for the acute treatment of migraine generally work well for menstrual attacks. These include nonsteroidal anti-inflammatory drugs (NSAIDs), dihydroergotamine (DHE), the triptans, and the combination of aspirin, acetaminophen, and caffeine (AAC) (Silberstein et al., 1999). DHE, a nonselective 5-HT_1 agonist available in parenteral form and as a nasal spray (NS), is effective for the treatment of menstrual migraine (D'Alessandro et al., 1983). Triptans that have been studied also appear to be equally effective for nonmenstrual attacks and the attacks that coincide with menstruation (Solbach and Waymer, 1993; Silberstein et al., 2000, 2002; Loder et al., 2004; Tuchman et al., 2006). If severe menstrual migraine cannot be adequately controlled with NSAIDs, ergots, DHE, or selective 5-HT_1 agonists (triptans), then analgesics combined with opioids, opioids alone, high-dose corticosteroids, major tranquilizers (chlorpromazine, haloperidol, thiothixene, droperidol), or a course of parenteral DHE can be considered (Silberstein and Merriam, 1993). Women with regular, severe menstrual migraines that still respond poorly to treatment are the candidates for preventive therapy (either continuous or short-term) and may respond better to acute therapy for individual attacks when on preventive treatment.

Menstrual Migraine Prevention

Preventive treatment strategies for menstrual migraine are outlined in Table 28–1. Women who are already using preventive medication throughout the month can try increasing the dose perimenstrually, although this strategy has not been validated in clinical trials. Women who do not have reasons to take preventive medication on a daily basis throughout the month often can be treated successfully with short-term prophylaxis, in which a scheduled dose of medication is given daily during the vulnerable portion of the menstrual cycle, often for 5–7 days. Regular periods and a predictable relationship between the attacks and menstruation are essential for this strategy to succeed (Loder, 2004). The use of ovulation predictor kits may help women with irregular cycles time treatment. Since the interval from ovulation to the onset of menstrual bleeding is generally fixed at around 14 days, the expected onset of headache can often be surmised (MacGregor et al., 2005).

It is important to note that trials of short-term prophylaxis have employed widely variable definitions of menstrual migraine and different treatment intervals, making comparisons among treatments difficult (Loder, 2002). Drugs that have been used perimenstrually for short-term prophylaxis include NSAIDs, ergotamine, DHE, methysergide, methergine, the triptans, and

TABLE 28–1 Strategies for the Preventive Treatment of Menstrual Migraine.

Perimenstrual use of standard preventive drugs
Perimenstrual use of nonstandard preventive drugs

- Nonsteroidal anti-inflammatory drugs (NSAIDs)
- Ergotamine and its derivatives
- Triptans
- Magnesium

Hormonal therapy

- Estrogens (with or without androgens or progestin)
- Combined oral contraceptives
- Synthetic androgens (Danazol)
- Antiestrogen (Tamoxifen)
- Medical oophorectomy (GnRH analogs) with or without add-back estrogens

Dopamine agonists (Bromocriptine)

magnesium (Martin, 2004). NSAIDs in adequate doses can be used preventively beginning 1–2 days before the expected onset of headache and continued for the duration of vulnerability. Optimal dose and duration of treatment can be determined through trial and error over several months. The most commonly used NSAID for this purpose is naproxen sodium 550 mg po BID (Sances et al., 1990). If the first NSAID fails, a different NSAID from another chemical class should be tried. NSAIDs are cost-effective and may be useful for other menstrual symptoms such as cramping, making them a natural starting point for short-term prophylaxis.

Ergotamine and DHE can be used prophylactically at the time of menses without significant risk of developing ergot dependence (Edelson, 1985). Ergotamine tartrate, at bedtime or twice a day, is an effective prophylactic agent. Ergotamine, in combination with belladonna and phenobarbital (Bellergal), may be useful in treating other perimenstrual symptoms in addition to headache (Robinson et al., 1977). Ergonovine maleate, an ergot derivative no longer available, provided a 65% improvement in headache severity and duration when given perimenstrually (Gallagher, 1989). Methylergonovine maleate is sometimes used in its place. DHE NS, given every 8 hours for 6 days beginning 3 days before the expected onset of headache, was used in a placebo-controlled double-blind short-term trial for the treatment of menstrual migraine. The mean pain severity rating for DHE NS was lower than placebo for 67.5% of the 40 evaluable patients (Silberstein, 1996).

Newman et al. used oral sumatriptan (25 mg TID) 2–3 days before the expected headache onset and continued for a total of 5 days in an open-label study of 20 women with menstrual migraine (Newman et al., 1998). In 126 sumatriptan-treated cycles, headache was absent in 52.4% of subjects and reduced in severity by 50% or greater in 42%. Breakthrough headaches were rare and significantly reduced in severity compared with the baseline headaches. A 1 mg BID scheduled dose of naratriptan was more effective than placebo for short-term perimenstrual prophylaxis of menstrual migraine (Newman et al., 2001). A loading dose of 10 mg of frovatriptan followed by 2.5 mg BID was also more effective than placebo when used for short-term prophylaxis (Silberstein et al., 2004).

A placebo-controlled double-blind study of 24 women with PMS and migraine has shown that 360 mg of oral magnesium pyrrolidone carboxylic acid decreases the severity of PMS symptoms and the duration and intensity of menstrual migraine attacks that occur before the onset of menstruation (Facchinetti et al., 1991).

There is no evidence that diuretics or vitamins help with menstrual migraine. Diuretics may be helpful for fluid retention and other premenstrual symptoms, but do not have an impact on migraine (Vellacott and O'Brien, 1987; Wang et al., 1995). Pyridoxine has also been studied and appears ineffective (Hagen et al., 1985; Williams et al., 1985). High doses of pyridoxine cause a sensory neuropathy, so this treatment should be discouraged (Umapathi and Chaudhry, 2005). Phytoestrogens have been studied for menstrual migraine prophylaxis, but trial methods make it impossible to reach a conclusion about their efficacy (Burke et al., 2002; Ferrante et al., 2004).

If severe menstrual migraine cannot be controlled with nonhormonal measures, hormonal therapy may be indicated. Successful hormonal or hormonal modulation therapy of menstrual migraine has been reported with estrogens (de Lignieres et al., 1986) (alone or combination with progesterone or testosterone) (Magos et al., 1983), combined OCs, synthetic androgens, estrogen modulators and antagonists (Calton and Burnett, 1984), and medical oophorectomy with gonadotropin releasing hormone (GnRH) analog with or without add-back therapy and prolactin (PRL) release inhibitors (Thomas et al., 1991). Progesterone is probably not effective in the treatment of headache or the symptoms of PMS (Freeman et al., 1995), despite many favorable anecdotal reports (Sachs et al., 2007).

The estradiol cutaneous patch provides a relatively stable plasma estrogen level over the time of application (Judd, 1987; Bidmon, et al., 1990; Stumpf, 1990). Levels are less stable with higher-dose patches. Serum estrogen levels rise within 4 hours of applying the transdermal patch and are proportional to the dose [For patch transdermal therapeutic system (TTS), 25 serum levels are around 23 pg/ml; for TTS 50 $\approx$39 ng/ml; and TTS 100 $\approx$74 pg/ml.].

There appears to be a dose threshold. A study using a 25 patch from 4 days before to 4 days after menstruation showed that it was not as effective as the same regimen with a TTS 100 patch (Pradalier et al., 1994). It has been suggested that a serum estradiol level of at least 60–80 pg/ml is required to prevent estrogen withdrawal migraine (Dennerstein et al., 1978).

Combinations of estrogens and progestins in the form of combination oral contraceptives may be a reasonable approach for some patients who have intractable menstrual migraine, particularly if it is associated with severe dysmenorrhea or other indications for ovulation suppression such as endometriosis. This form of treatment is not appropriate for women of any age who have migraine with aura or women with any form of migraine who are over 35, for whom treatment guidelines discourage the use of exogenous estrogens because of the risk of stroke (Stang et al., 2000; ACOG Committee on Practice Bulletins-Gynecology, 2006). Tamoxifen (Nolvadex) (Powles, 1986; O'Dea and Davis, 1990), a selective estrogen receptor modulator (SERM) that binds to a cytosol estrogen receptor, may be effective for resistant menstrual headaches, although long-term tolerability has not been assessed. A dose of 5–15 mg per day for days 7–14 of the menstrual cycle has provided significant relief of menstrual headache. The effectiveness of other SERMs for the treatment of menstrual headaches has not been studied.

Other methods of suppressing ovulation have been studied for the treatment of PMS. In two placebo-controlled double-blind studies, GnRH analogs were significantly better than placebo in controlling both the behavioral and physical symptoms of PMS (headache, breast fullness and tenderness, bloating, and fatigue) (Freeman et al., 1997; Leather et al., 1999; Sundstrom et al., 1999). Based on this, it seemed plausible that GnRH analog treatment might also be effective in menstrual migraine, and such regimens have been investigated. Since GnRH analogs induce hypogonadism, with many of the same short-term and long-term adverse effects (AEs) as menopause, treatment is usually limited to 6 months unless replacement estrogens are used. It has been suggested that such add-back therapy does not necessarily interfere with effective GnRH agonist treatment, but does prevent bone mineral loss and mitigate some of the other hypoestrogenic effects of such regimens (Studd and Leather, 1996). However, one study suggested that add-back estrogen did attenuate the clinical benefit of a GnRH regimen in PMS (Leather et al., 1999). Guideline cautions about the use of exogenous estrogen in women with migraine should be borne in mind in selecting appropriate candidates for this therapy as well.

Evidence available to date suggests that GnRH agonist administration, alone or with add-back therapy, may be a reasonable treatment for carefully selected patients who have severe, perimenstrual migraine headaches, although results are modest (Holdaway et al., 1991; Murray and Muse, 1997). Martin et al. attempted this treatment in a group of women with refractory migraine who were not selected on the basis of menstrual attacks (Martin et al., 2003). In this group of patients, minimization of hormonal fluctuations alone with GnRH agonist therapy did not produce improvement in headache; the addition of add-back estrogen produced a modest improvement in headache index compared with the addition of placebo.

Another strategy that has been suggested for refractory menstrual headaches is the use of a dopamine receptor agonist, either short-term or continuously. Bromocriptine (Parlodel), a dopamine D2 receptor agonist, is an inhibitor of prolactin release (Hockaday et al., 1976). In an open trial, 24 women with severe, disabling menstrual migraine occurring within 3 days of menstruation were treated with continuous bromocriptine 2.5 mg three times daily. Seventy-five per cent of the women had at least a 25% reduction in headache compared to baseline. Overall headache frequency decreased 72%. None of the patients had less than a 10% increase in headache; three could not tolerate bromocriptine, and three did not benefit (Herzog, 1997).

HEADACHE AND HORMONAL CONTRACEPTION

Combination estrogen–progestin oral contraceptives (COCs) are still the most commonly used form of hormonal contraception, although vaginal and transdermal methods of hormone administration are becoming popular. Traditional COC regimens consist of 21 days of estrogen–progestin pills followed by 7 pill-free or placebo pill days (Petitti, 2003). Thromboembolic complications, including stroke, are reduced with newer, low-estrogen formulations, but the prevalence of breakthrough bleeding is increased and affects tolerability. Progestin-only oral contraceptives are also available, as are implantable and injection progestins.

Some new contraceptive formulations and dosing strategies are available that reduce or eliminate the duration and extent of hormone withdrawal and, perhaps, hormone withdrawal symptoms (Nelson, 2005; Foidart et al., 2006). Although COCs are commonly blamed for worsening of headache, the evidence that this is so is not very strong. The issue is of importance primarily in migraine; COCs or hormonal factors do not have a significant influence on tension-type or cluster headache.

Generally, data from specialty headache clinics show an increased incidence, severity, and refractoriness of migraine in COC users, while studies from contraceptive clinics and in the general population of women show little effect on headache (Loder et al., 2005b). Abrupt estrogen withdrawal during the 7-day placebo or pill-free week is more likely to be the cause of COC-connected headache than are the hormones themselves. Some evidence suggests that attenuating or eliminating this drop in estrogen, either with estrogen supplementation or through the use of continuous dosing regimens, may reduce headache problems (Sulak et al., 1997; Edelman et al., 2006). However, in a recent trial comparing an extended duration transdermal contraceptive with a traditional regimen, headache worsened from baseline in both groups, although the extent of worsening was less in the extended duration group (LaGuardia et al., 2005). A recent Cochrane review concluded that the long-term consequences of additional estrogen exposure with these regimens are unknown (Edelman et al., 2006).

There is some suggestion that COCs can provoke a first migraine attack. Older women and those with a family history of migraine are more likely to experience COC-associated worsening of headache (Loder et al., 2005b). Guidelines from the World Health Organization, American College of Obstetrics and Gynecology, and the International Headache Society discourage the use of estrogen-containing contraceptives in women who have migraine with aura, and urge caution in those who have migraine without aura and are over 35 or have other risk factors for thromboembolic complications such as smoking, obesity, or hypertension (Bousser et al., 2000; Guillebaud, 2001; Stanback and Katz, 2002; ACOG Committee on Practice Bulletins-Gynecology, 2006; Gaffield et al., 2006).

It can be difficult to apply these guidelines to individual patients. Clinical judgment is needed to weigh the risks and benefits of hormonal contraception for a particular woman (Loder et al., 2005a). Progestin-only hormonal contraception may be safer, but may aggravate headache (Harel et al., 1995; Archer et al., 1997).

HEADACHE AND PREGNANCY

A majority of women with migraine report improvement in headache during pregnancy, although headaches rarely remit completely and improvement occurs gradually over the first trimester (Granella et al., 1993, 2000; Sances et al.,

2003). Roughly, a quarter of women with migraine report no change or even worsening of headaches during pregnancy. Women with a history of menstrual attacks and migraine without aura are more likely to improve, and those with tension-type or mixed migraine and tension-type headaches are less likely to improve. Headaches are unlikely to improve if they have not done so by the end of the first trimester, making that a natural point at which to reconsider and perhaps intensify treatment strategies (Lance and Anthony, 1966; Somerville, 1972b; Marcus et al., 1999).

Although the headache of migraine is frequently better with the high, stable estrogen levels of pregnancy, aura may occur more frequently or for the first time during pregnancy (Granella et al., 2000; Ertresvag et al., 2005). The paradox of improvement in headache and worsening of aura during pregnancy or other high-estrogen states is probably best explained by the different effects of estrogen on the underlying causal mechanisms of headache and aura. Most experts believe headache and aura are separate, though linked, processes. High estrogen and progesterone levels appear to facilitate spreading depression, the glial/neuronal phenomenon believed to underlie aura (Sachs et al., 2007). Estrogen also appears to facilitate vasodilation, but progesterone does not (Gupta et al., 2007). Estrogen and progesterone are antinociceptive at high levels, which may explain why women have elevated pain thresholds during late pregnancy (Whipple et al., 1990). Antinociception involves somatic as well as visceral noxious stimuli. Hormone-simulated pregnancy involves spinal κ and δ-opioid receptors (Dawson-Basoa and Gintzler, 1998) and descending noradrenergic pathways that terminate on spinal α2-adrenergic receptors (Liu and Gintzler, 1999). Gestational antinociception requires their coincident activation, i.e., the effect of blocking either κ or δ receptors is the same as blocking both (Dawson-Basoa and Gintzler, 1998).

Preconception Advice for Women with Headache

Like all women of childbearing age, women with pre-existing headache problems who are attempting pregnancy should be advised to take a daily multivitamin supplement containing at least 400 μg (0.4 mg) of folic acid, to reduce the risk of neural tube defects in any pregnancy that might occur (Czeizel and Dudas, 1992). Some medications typically used to treat headache, such as divalproex sodium and barbiturates, interfere with folate metabolism (Alsdorf and Wyszynski, 2005).

When pregnancy is desired, medication discontinuation should be attempted before conception. There is no reason to believe that long medication-free intervals are needed; women can attempt pregnancy as soon as medications have been stopped. If medication elimination is not possible, drugs least likely to cause pregnancy problems should be chosen and used in the lowest effective dose (Mannix et al., 2002).

In women undergoing infertility treatment, migraine may be triggered by estrogen withdrawal following drug-induced hypothalamic–pituitary–-ovarian axis down-regulation (Amir et al., 2005). Several case reports have suggested that clomiphene, a drug used in some infertility regimens, might increase the risk of migrainous infarction (Ertresvag et al., 2005; Parra et al., 2006).

In general, evidence is reassuring about pregnancy outcomes in women with migraine. A comparison of pregnancy results in 450 migraineurs compared with 136 nonmigrainous controls did not find an increased risk of birth defects or pregnancy complications, although it was probably underpowered to detect anything other than a large increase in risk (Wainscott et al., 1978). A retrospective evaluation of a Danish database suggested a possible increased risk for low birth weight in babies born to women with migraine, but could not adjust for confounding factors (Olesen et al., 2000). A retrospective case–control study suggested that severe maternal migraine during pregnancy might be associated with congenital limb deficiencies. The authors reported an odds ratio of 2.5 (95% confidence interval 1.1–5.8) for maternal migraine at any time during the second or third trimester in pregnancies complicated by limb deficiencies compared with unaffected pregnancies. The methods used to ascertain migraine and associated medication use were of questionable accuracy, however, and further study is needed (Banhidy et al., 2006a). Results from this same database of over 38,000 deliveries showed that mean gestational age and birth weight in babies born to women with migraine did not differ from the general population, and the proportion of low birth weight and preterm births were the same. (Banhidy et al., 2006b)

Migraine appears to be associated with an increased risk of several maternal pregnancy complications. A large population-based study found that women with migraine were more likely to have been diagnosed with gestational hypertension, even after taking into account age and number of pregnancies (Scher et al., 2005). The risk of preeclampsia in migraineurs appears to increase in proportion to disease severity, and preeclampsia may appear earlier and be more severe in women with migraine (Moore and Redman, 1983; Rubin and McCabe, 1984; Marcoux et al., 1992; Adeney et al., 2005; Facchinetti et al., 2005; Adeney and Williams, 2006). Preeclampsia is the leading cause of maternal morbidity and mortality in developed countries (Noris et al., 2005). This suggests that pregnant women with migraine should be carefully monitored for the development of preeclampsia. Headaches that mimic migraine can be an early feature of the disorder, and a high index of suspicion is necessary to distinguish these from a woman's typical migraine attacks.

Good-quality evidence supports the use of magnesium in preeclampsia to prevent seizures (Altman et al., 2002). Interestingly, parenteral magnesium in the doses typically used for preeclampsia and eclampsia also has shown efficacy in migraine treatment, and is well tolerated (Ramadan et al., 1989; Seelig, 1993; Welch and Ramadan, 1995; Rozen, 2003). Magnesium is, therefore, a treatment to consider in situations where it is difficult to distinguish between the headache of preeclampsia and the headache of migraine, or where the two conditions may overlap. Magnesium supplementation, as a method of prophylaxis of migraine in pregnancy, may also be reasonable. Delivery is the definitive treatment for preeclampsia and eclampsia, and headache and other symptoms should disappear within a week.

Migraine is a risk factor for pregnancy-related stroke. In a recent study that examined 2850 pregnancy-related discharges which included a diagnosis of stroke, migraine was the medical condition most strongly associated with stroke, with an odds ratio of 16.9 (9.7–29.5). The risk was highest in women over the age of 35. Ergot derivatives such as bromocriptine and methylergonovine, which may be used in the immediate postpartum period, have been implicated as possible causes of postpartum stroke and reversible cerebral vasoconstriction syndromes, as have other sympathomimetic or vasoconstrictor drugs such as triptans (Raroque et al., 1993; Iffy et al., 1998; Granier et al., 1999; Witlin et al., 2000; Sato et al., 2004; Campos and Yamamoto, 2006). Women with migraine may be more susceptible to this complication, so it is prudent to minimize the use of such drugs in postpartum women with migraine.

Treatment of Headache in Pregnancy Since there is a good chance that migraine will improve by the end of the first trimester, many women are motivated to rely on nonpharmacologic treatment strategies including ice, massage, and biofeedback. Biofeedback is an effective treatment for headaches in pregnancy, but as it requires patient training it is probably most effective if training is commenced before pregnancy (Marcus et al., 1995; Scharff et al., 1996). For pregnant women with migraine who continue to have severe, intractable headaches, especially if they are associated with nausea, vomiting, and possible dehydration, treatment of some sort is usually necessary. These symptoms are not only disruptive for the patient but also at some point they pose a risk to the mother and fetus, which outweighs the potential risk of medications used to treat migraine.

The major concern in managing the pregnant migraineur is the effect of medication on the fetus and, unfortunately, limited information is available. The authors of one study concluded that "inadequate information is available for pregnant women and their physicians to determine whether the benefits exceed the teratogenic risks for most drug treatments introduced in the past 20 years" (Lo and Friedman, 2002).

Methods of Assessing the Pregnancy Risks of Drugs There are a number of methods available to help judge the risk of drugs during pregnancy. The United States Food and Drug Administration (FDA) pregnancy risk rating system, used in the pregnancy portion of FDA-approved product labels, is probably the most familiar, accessible, and commonly used method of assessing risk. This system assigns drugs to one of five categories (A, B, C, D, or X) that are intended to provide "therapeutic guidance" by weighing the risks and benefits of the drug (Pregnancy categories for prescription drugs, 1982). The current labeling system has been criticized as confusing and oversimplified. Forty percent of drugs do not have a pregnancy category listed (Boothby and Doering, 2001). In 1996, the FDA established a task force to advise it on revamping the rating system, but 10 years later little progress has been made.

The Teratogen Information Service (TERIS) classification is an online, automated database of teratogen information, which classifies drugs in one of seven risk categories: "none," "minimal," "small," "moderate," "high," "undetermined," and "unlikely." These categories are meant to assess teratogenic risk, rather than (as with the FDA categories) to balance harms and benefits. Agreement between TERIS and FDA ratings is no greater than would be expected by chance alone, and there are inconsistencies among other rating systems as well (Friedman et al., 1990; Addis et al., 2000). Rather than relying on a single method of risk determination, such as the FDA classification, it is advisable to look for a synthesis of information from multiple sources (Friedman et al., 1990).

The Pregnancy Risks of Selected Medications Used to Treat Headache Triptans, which are serotonin agonists acting at 1B and 1D receptor subtypes, are widely used to treat acute attacks of headache and are very effective. Information on pregnancy risks is most extensive for sumatriptan, the first marketed drug in the class. All triptans, including sumatriptan, are currently rated as FDA pregnancy class C, which means that "safety in human pregnancy has not been determined" and that "potential benefits should justify potential risks" if a decision is made to use the drug during pregnancy.

Information from multiple sources shows no signal of teratogenicity from sumatriptan use in pregnancy (Fox and Spierings, 2000; Loder, 2003). Unlike ergots, sumatriptan does not appear to increase uterine contractions or affect uterine blood flow in animal studies (Feniuk et al., 1989). Despite this reassuring information, caution is still advisable because, although the data are sufficient to exclude a large increase in risk for a single birth defect, it is likely that there will never be adequate information to rule out a small increase in risk for common birth defects or a modest increase in risk for rare birth defects. Information available for other drugs in this class is inadequate to generate meaningful risk estimates (Fiore et al., 2005).

Ergotamine and other ergot-related drugs such as methysergide are contraindicated in pregnancy, based on the evidence that ergots decrease uterine blood flow may be linked to fetal hypoxia and growth retardation and increase uterine muscle tone. A number of case reports also suggest an association of ergotamine with specific birth defects (Raymond, 1995; Hosking, 1996; Smets et al., 2004; Acs et al., 2006).

In the absence of controlled studies or other sources of information, the risk of many other migraine drugs during pregnancy is largely speculative. Drugs with a longer record of use are preferred when drug treatment of migraine in pregnancy is necessary, on the theory that the longer a drug has been in use the better the chance that any signal of teratogenicity will have emerged. These include medications such as nonspecific narcotic analgesics, acetaminophen, or NSAIDs or sedating phenothiazines.

Acute Treatment of Headache in Pregnancy Acute treatment, often referred to as symptomatic treatment, is aimed at reducing the severity and duration of symptoms in an individual headache attack. NSAIDs, acetaminophen (alone or with an opioid), or an opioid alone can be used during pregnancy. Aspirin in low intermittent doses is unlikely to be a significant teratogenic risk, but large or frequent doses, especially if given near term, may be associated with maternal and fetal bleeding, since aspirin irreversibly inhibits platelet activity and may interfere with closure of the ductus arteriosus when used in late pregnancy. It is probably best to avoid aspirin, indomethacin, and other very potent inhibitors of prostaglandin synthesis during pregnancy, unless there is a definite therapeutic need for them other than headache (Needs and Brooks, 1985). Less potent NSAIDs, such as ibuprofen, may be taken safely for pain during early or mid-pregnancy. However, their use should be limited during later pregnancy because some NSAIDs may affect closure of the fetal ductus arteriosus (Hermes-DeSantis and Clyman, 2006).

Barbiturate-containing drugs are probably best avoided or strictly limited during pregnancy, in part because experience shows that these drugs are frequently associated with overuse or abuse syndromes; neonatal withdrawal from butalbital used during pregnancy has been described (Ostrea, 1982). In addition, there are concerns that in utero exposure to barbiturate medications may have long-term neurodevelopmental effects (Reinisch et al., 1995; Holmes et al., 2005).

The pregnancy risks of complementary, herbal, and other "natural" treatments are even less well studied than those of pharmaceutical products. Such products are not necessarily safer than commercially produced pharmaceutical products, and their purity is not subject to the same strict government oversight. In the case of feverfew, for example, an herbal treatment often promoted for the treatment of migraine, preliminary studies in rats suggest possible teratogenicity and it has been suggested that a full reproductive study is warranted (Yao et al., 2006). Specific advice to patients to avoid such treatments may protect them against the advice they receive elsewhere. One study showed that 82% of health food store clerks asked to recommend a treatment for migraine and nausea did so, and that 5% of recommendations were for products specifically contraindicated in pregnancy, while most others were for products whose safety in pregnancy has not been well studied (Buckner et al., 2005).

The associated symptoms of migraine, such as nausea and vomiting, can be as disabling as the headache pain itself, and may be especially troublesome during pregnancy, which by itself can be an important cause of nausea and vomiting. Metoclopramide, which decreases gastric atony and enhances absorption of coadministered medications, is extremely useful in migraine treatment (Allena et al., 2005). Mild nausea can also be treated with phosphorylated carbohydrate solution (emetrol) or doxylamine succinate and vitamin B6 (pyridoxine). A recent study concluded that, within its sample size and at modest doses, there was no indication of a teratogenic effect of vitamin B6 (Shrim et al., 2006; Thaver et al., 2006). Another study reached a similar conclusion about ondansetron, making that another reasonable choice for nausea treatment, although it is not known to have a beneficial effect on headache (Einarson et al., 2004). Combination therapy may be more effective than single-drug therapy in treating nausea. A recent study compared the combination of pyridoxine and metoclopramide with prochlorperazine and promethazine, and found the combination more effective (Bsat et al., 2003). More severe nausea may require the use of injections or suppositories.

In the United States, trimethobenzamide, chlorpromazine, prochlorperazine, and promethazine are available orally, parenterally, and by suppository, and all their usage can be considered. Corticosteroids are sometimes helpful for prolonged attacks of migraine. Some experts prefer prednisone in preference to dexamethasone in preganancy, because the latter crosses the placenta more readily. There is evidence that that first trimester corticosteroid exposure is not a major teratogenic risk (Crowther and Harding, 2003; Leung et al., 2003; Gur et al., 2004).

PREVENTIVE TREATMENT OF HEADACHE IN PREGNANCY

Increased frequency and severity of migraine associated with nausea and vomiting may justify the use of daily prophylactic, or preventive, medication to reduce the frequency and severity of headache attacks. The threshold for initiation of preventive treatment of migraine is much higher than for nonpregnant patients, and it is used only when absolutely necessary, typically when frequent and particularly incapacitating headaches occur, are unresponsive to symptomatic therapy and may result in dehydration and fetal distress. The risks and treatment alternatives should be thoroughly discussed with the patient and her partner.

The β-adrenergic blocker, propranolol, is generally recommended as a first-line choice for migraine prophylaxis in pregnancy, based on the reassuring experience with its use in pregnant women with hypertension. It is not suspected of being a teratogen, but AEs, including intrauterine growth retardation, have been reported (Pruyn et al., 1979; Redmond, 1982; Cissoko et al., 2005). Other preventive drugs can be considered if propranolol is ineffective, contraindicated, or when the patient has a coexistent illness that requires treatment and a drug exists that might provide dual benefit. The pregnancy categories of selected treatment alternatives are listed in Table 28–2.

Biofeedback-assisted relaxation has also been studied as a preventive treatment for migraine during pregnancy. Its efficacy is similar to that of pharmacologic therapy. Its major drawbacks are cost and time; it is often not covered by insurance (Marcus et al., 1995; Scharff et al., 1996; Sandor and Afra, 2005).

Table 28–2 Pregnancy Risk Ratings and Lactation Compatibility of Selected Drugs Used in Headache Treatment.

	Pregnancy risk		
Acute medications	*FDA*[a]	*TERIS*[b]	*Breast-feeding*[c]
DHE	X	Minimal	Not listed
Ergotamine	X	Minimal	Caution
Sumatriptan	C	Unlikely	Compatible
Almotriptan, eletriptan, frovatriptan, naratriptan, rizatriptan, zolmitriptan	C	Undetermined	Not listed
Acetaminophen	B	None	Compatible
Aspirin	C[d]	Minimal	Caution
Caffeine (moderate intake)	B	None	Compatible
Ibuprofen	B[d]	Minimal	Compatible
Naproxen	B[d]	Undetermined	Compatible
Butorphanol	B[e]	Undetermined	Compatible
Lidocaine	B	None (local)	Compatible
Barbiturates	C[e]	Unlikely	Caution
Preventive medications			
Amitriptyline	C	Unlikely	Concern
Atenolol	D	Undetermined	Caution
Magnesium	B	Unlikely	Compatible
Propranolol and timolol	C[f]	Undetermined	Compatible
Valproic acid	D	Moderate	Caution
Topiramate	C	Undetermined	Not listed
Antiemetics/miscellaneous			
Doylamine and vitamin B6	A	None	Compatible
Emetrol	B	Undetermined	Not listed
Metoclopramide	B	Unlikely	Concern
Prednisone	C[g]	None–minimal	Compatible
Promethazine	C	None	Compatible

[a] US FDA risk categories: A, controlled human studies show no risk; B, no evidence of risk in humans, but there are no controlled human studies; C, risk to humans has not been ruled out; D, positive evidence of risk to humans from human and/or animal studies; X, contraindicated in pregnancy.

[b] Teratogen information service risk categories: none; unlikely; minimal; small; moderate; high; undetermined.

[c] American Academy of Pediatrics Drugs and Breastfeeding Categories: concern (effects unknown, but may be of concern); caution (drugs that have been associated with significant effects on some nursing infants and should be given with caution); usually compatible.

[d] D in third trimester.

[e] D if prolonged or at term.

[f] Second/third trimester.

[g] First trimester.

LACTATION

Like other women, those with headache should be encouraged to breast-feed their infants. The effects of lactation on migraine are not entirely clear. One large case series showed no significant effect on headache, while another suggested that lactation might have a positive effect on migraine (Wall, 1992; Sances et al., 2003). Any positive effect of lactation on migraine would likely be mediated through ovulation suppression, which is very sensitive to the regularity of nursing. In any case, several effective headache treatments are compatible with breast-feeding, so women do not have to choose between headache treatment and nursing. The American Academy of Pediatrics (AAP) Committee on Drugs has published a list of commonly used drugs and categorized them according to their effects on lactation into several categories: effects unknown but may be of concern; use with caution or usually compatible (American Academy of Pediatrics Committee on Drugs, 2001). An addendum to this list was recently published (Ressel, 2002).

The AAP considers several triptans to be compatible with breast-feeding (American Academy of Pediatrics Committee on Drugs, 2001). When adjusted for weight, the infant dose of sumatriptan has been calculated to be only 0.5% of the oral maternal dose (Wojnar-Horton et al., 1996). Nursing frequency and the time between maternal ingestion of the drug and nursing probably also influence drug levels in milk. Infant exposure may be further reduced by timing breast-feeding for just before a medication dose, or pumping and discarding milk following a dose.

Drugs safe for use in pregnancy are not necessarily safe for use during breastfeeding. For example, metoclopramide has an FDA pregnancy category rating of B, but an AAP lactation rating of "caution" because it is highly concentrated in breast milk. Divalproex is compatible with nursing, but contraindicated in pregnancy. It is ideal when migraine treatment is needed during pregnancy to select regimens that also are compatible with nursing. This minimizes the chance that drug transitions will be overlooked during the hectic postdelivery period.

Propranolol can be used during pregnancy and continued during breast-feeding. The migraineur who is breastfeeding should avoid bromocriptine, ergotamine, and lithium, and use benzodiazepines, antidepressants, and neuroleptics cautiously. Acetaminophen is compatible with breast-feeding and is preferred to aspirin. Moderate caffeine use is compatible with breast-feeding. However, accumulation may occur in infants whose mothers use excessive amounts. Intermittent use of opioids is probably safe, but can cause infant sedation and is not preferred if there are other effective alternatives. Barbiturates also can cause infant sedation and are not a first-line choice for headache treatment in nursing women. Table 28–2 lists the compatibility of selected headache medications with breast-feeding.

POSTPARTUM HEADACHES

Postpartum headache is common. Most studies suggest that it occurs in a quarter to a third of women in the general obstetrical population during the 6 weeks after delivery, and in about half of women with a prior history of headache (see Table 28–3).

The differential diagnosis of postpartum headaches includes all of the disorders that cause headache outside and during pregnancy, but the risk of several dangerous causes of headache is increased. These include cerebral venous thrombosis, preeclampsia and eclampsia, intracranial hemorrhage and low-volume headache syndromes related to the use of epidural anesthesia during delivery. For this reason, a diagnosis of benign headache cannot be assumed in patients with postpartum headache, even those prone to benign headaches before delivery.

Treatment of postpartum headache depends on the diagnosis. Even if migraine is diagnosed, ergotamine and its derivatives should be avoided because they have been implicated as possible causes of postpartum stroke and postpartum reversible cerebral vasoconstriction syndromes (Raroque et al., 1993; Iffy et al., 1998; Granier et al., 1999; Sato et al., 2004; Campos and Yamamoto, 2006; Calabrese et al., 2007). Other case reports suggest that sympathomimetic or cerebral vasoconstrictor drugs such as sumatriptan can also be dangerous if used to treat postdural puncture headache (Oliver and White, 2002). Until the uncertainties about the dangers of these medications are resolved, it is best to avoid the use of

Table 28–3 The Prevalence of Postpartum Headache and Migraine in Selected Studies.

Author, year	*Population*	*Prevalence*	*Comment*
Goldszmidt et al., 2005	General obstetrical population	39% reported headache or neck pain within a week of delivery; 75% were primary headaches	Prospective cohort study of almost a thousand women, using structured interview and ICHD criteria
Saurel-Cubizolles et al., 2000	General obstetrical population	1/3 of women reported headache	A longitudinal study that interviewed women after delivery and again at 5 and 12 months postpartum
Grove, 1973	General obstetrical population excluding women who had received epidural analgesia $n = 187$	23%	Mostly on 1st and 2nd postpartum days
Stein et al., 1984	General obstetrical population	39%	Most headaches occurred between the 4th and 6th postpartum day
Benhamou et al., 1995	Women who had epidurals without known dural puncture (mailed survey to 1198 women)	12%	Survey response rate was only 41%; response rate was too low in women who did not have epidurals to draw meaningful conclusions
Marcus et al., 1999	49 women with headache	67% reported postpartum headaches no different from second trimester headaches	A previous study by the same group of 30 women was too small for statistical analysis (Scharff et al., 1997)
Granella et al., 1993	Women with migraine attending a headache clinic	5% reported migraine began for the first-time postpartum	A retrospective study, thus subject to problems of recall bias and limitations in recall
Sances et al., 2003	Women with migraine attending an obstetrical clinic	34% experienced migraine recurrence within the 1st postpartum week, and 55.3% within the 1st four postpartum weeks	

these drugs in patients with postpartum headache. As with headaches that occur during pregnancy, opioids, hydration and sedating antinausea medications are generally safe treatment choices. Nonoral routes of administration are preferred.

Headache and Menopause Migraine prevalence and disability decrease with advancing age in both men and women (Goldstein and Chen, 1982). In women, much of this improvement is popularly attributed to menopause and the cessation of ovarian steroid hormone cycles. The actual effect of menopause on headache varies from woman to woman. Significant, troublesome exacerbation of headache, especially migraine, during the perimenopause (the period of time leading up to menopause, marked by missed and irregular periods) is common (Wang et al., 2003; Gracia et al., 2005; Moloney et al., 2006). Many studies do not distinguish between women who are perimenopausal and those who are postmenopausal, perhaps accounting for variable observations of regression, worsening, or no change in headache with menopause. The preponderance of evidence does suggest, however, that natural menopause ultimately has a beneficial effect on migraine severity once it is well established (Epstein et al., 1975; Edelson, 1985; Neri et al., 1993; Mattsson, 2003). Some evidence suggests that abrupt surgical menopause may worsen migraine (Neri et al., 1993). Evidence is less clear about the effect of menopause on other headache types. Neri found that 70% of women with tension-type headache reported no change or worsening in headache once menopause was established (Neri et al., 1993).

Menopause is the permanent cessation of menstruation, and is diagnosed when 12 continuous months have passed without a menstrual period (Gracia et al., 2005). Sex steroid hormone levels are low and gonadotropin levels are elevated once menopause is achieved, but estrogen secretion is actually elevated throughout the menstrual cycle during some phases of the perimenopause. The hypothalamic–pituitary axis becomes increasingly insensitive to estrogen during the perimenopause, so ovarian hypofunction alone does not account for all symptoms of the menopausal transition (Weiss et al., 2004). Menstrual cycles become irregular, often shortening in duration, and breakthrough bleeding may occur. The luteal phase of the cycle is often shortened or inadequate and ovulation does not reliably occur, although pregnancy remains a possibility (Weiss, 2001a, 2001b; Gracia and Freeman, 2004).

Exogenous estrogen alone [estrogen replacement therapy (ERT)] or in combination with progestins [hormone replacement therapy (HRT)] have been popular methods of relieving estrogen deprivation symptoms and preventing osteoporosis. Since the publication of the Women's Health Initiative trial results showing that estrogen increases the risk of stroke and cardiovascular complications, however, enthusiasm for these regimens has declined precipitously (Prentice et al., 2006). Some women continue to need them, however, to relieve intolerable vasomotor symptoms or preserve bone mass; the lowest effective dose and duration of therapy is preferred (Mattsson et al., 2004; Tamborini and Ruiz, 2004).

A number of investigators have studied the association between various HRT and ERT regimens and migraine, although none has investigated HRT or ERT specifically as a treatment for migraine. In general, continuous rather than interrupted, and transdermal rather than oral, regimens cause the least worsening of pre-existing migraine (Nand et al., 1998; Nappi et al., 2001; Facchinetti et al., 2002). Estrogen replacement therapy does not appear to have an effect on tension-type or cluster headache (Nappi et al., 2001; van Vliet et al., 2006).

Headache management can be difficult in women who require hormonal replacement therapy for menopausal symptoms but develop headaches as a result of the therapy. Empirical strategies that can be considered include reducing the dose of estrogen or changing the type of estrogen from a conjugated estrogen to pure estradiol, to synthetic ethinyl estradiol, or to a pure estrone. In a controlled double-blind crossover trial of menopausal women, Aylward et al. found that oral estropipate decreased the frequency and intensity of headache, whereas ethinyl estradiol increased the headache (Aylward et al., 1974). Interrupted regimens are no longer common; when they were, Kudrow reported a 58% improvement in headache control when women were switched to a reduced, continuous dose of estrogen (Kudrow, 1975). Other investigators have suggested that parenteral estrogen or testosterone supplementation might be helpful. Greenblatt and Bruneteau (1974) studied postmenopausal women with oral-estrogen-induced headaches, and found that their headaches could be improved by switching from oral to parenteral estrogens (estradiol) and adding androgens (testosterone) (Greenblatt and Bruneteau, 1974).

Progestins, used to prevent endometrial hyperplasia, may aggravate headache in addition to other symptoms of PMS, particularly if used cyclically; but it is not clear whether the dose makes a difference. Nand studied three HRT regimens with the same dose of estrogen but varying doses of medroxyprogesterone, and did not find any differences in headache complaints related to the dose. He noted that headache and other side-effects declined over the first 3 months of use (Nand et al., 1998). Nonetheless, giving a lower dose of a progestin and avoiding interrupted regimens have been advocated to help control headaches that worsen on HRT. Another strategy is to change the type of progestin. One study suggested that norethisterone might be associated with less worsening of headache (Rosano et al., 2000; Facchinetti et al., 2002). For women with a uterus who have intolerable central nervous system symptoms with progestins, an estrogen-only regimen may be used in conjunction with regular testing to exclude endometrial proliferation.

Physical and Sexual Abuse Girls and women are more likely than males to experience physical and sexual abuse (Anderson et al., 1993; Kellogg and American Academy of Pediatrics Committee on Child Abuse and Neglect, 2005). Evidence links a number of chronic physical conditions, including headache, to abuse (Romans et al., 2002; Tietjen, et al., 2007). Childhood abuse or neglect may predispose to the development of chronic pain problems in adulthood, and the extent of exposure is linked in a dose–response relationship with the development of somatic symptoms, including headache (Yucel et al., 2002; Graham-Bermann and Seng, 2005). It is good practice to ask about abuse when taking a headache history.

References

ACOG Committee on Practice Bulletins-Gynecology (2006). ACOG practice bulletin. No. 73: use of hormonal contraception in women with coexisting medical conditions. *Obstet Gynecol*, 107(6):1453–1472.

Acs, N, Banhidy, F, Puho, E, and Czeizel, AE (2006). A possible dose-dependent teratogenic effect of ergotamine. *Reprod Toxicol*, 22(3):551–552.

Addis, A, Sharabi, S, and Bonati, M (2000). Risk classification systems for drug use during pregnancy: are they a reliable source of information? *Drug saf*, 23 (3):245–253.

Adeney, KL and Williams, MA (2006). Migraine headaches and preeclampsia: an epidemiologic review. *Headache*, 46(5):794–803.

Adeney, KL, Williams, MA, Miller, RS, et al. (2005). Risk of preeclampsia in relation to maternal history of migraine headaches. *J Matern F Neonatal Med*, 18(3):167–172.

Allena, M, Magis, D, and Schoenen, J (2005). A trial of metoclopramide vs sumatriptan for the emergency department treatment of migraines. *Neurology*, 65 (8):1339–1340; author reply 1339–1340.

Alsdorf, R and Wyszynski, DF (2005). Teratogenicity of sodium valproate. *Expert Opin Drug Saf*, 4(2):345–353.

Altman, D, Carroli, G, Duley, L, et al. (2002). Do women with pre-eclampsia, and their babies, benefit from magnesium sulphate? the magpie trial: a randomised placebo-controlled trial. *Lancet*, 359(9321):1877–1890.

American Academy of Pediatrics Committee on Drugs. (2001). Transfer of drugs and other chemicals into human milk. *Pediatrics*, 108(3):776–789.

Amir, BY, Yaacov, B Guy, B, et al. (2005). Headaches in women undergoing in vitro fertilization and embryo-transfer treatment. *Headache*, 45(3):215–219.

Anderson, J, Martin, J, Mullen, P, et al. (1993). Prevalence of childhood sexual abuse experiences in a community sample of women. *J Am Acad Child Adolesc Psychiatry*, 32(5), 911–919.

Archer, B, Irwin, D, Jensen, K, et al. (1997). Depot medroxyprogesterone. management of side-effects commonly associated with its contraceptive use. *J Nurse Midwifery*, 42(2):104–111.

Aylward, M, Holly, F, and Parker, RJ (1974). An evaluation of clinical response to piperazine oestrone sulphate ('harmogen') in menopause patients. *Curr Med Res Opin*, 2(7):417–423.

Banhidy, F, Acs, N, Horvath-Puho, E, et al. (2006a). Maternal severe migraine and risk of congenital limb deficiencies. *Birth Defects Res A Clin Mol Teratol*, 76 (8):592–601.

Banhidy, F, Acs, N, Horvath-Puho, E, et al. (2006b). Pregnancy complications and delivery outcomes in pregnant women with severe migraine. *Eur J Obstet Gynecol Reprod Biol* [Epub ahead of print].

Benhamou, D, Hamza, J, and Ducot, B (1995). Post partum headache after epidural analgesia without dural puncture. *Int J Obstet Anesth*, 4(1):17–20.

Bidmon, HJ, Pitts, JD, Solomon, HF, et al. (1990). Estradiol distribution and penetration in rat skin after topical application, studied by high resolution autoradiography. *Histochemistry*, 95(1):43–54.

Boothby, LA and Doering, PL (2001). FDA labeling system for drugs in pregnancy. *Ann Pharmacother*, 35 (11):1485–1489.

Bousser, MG, Conard, J, Kittner, S, et al. (2000). Recommendations on the risk of ischaemic stroke associated with use of combined oral contraceptives and hormone replacement therapy in women with migraine. the international headache society task force on combined oral contraceptives & hormone replacement therapy. *Cephalalgia*, 20(3):155–156.

Bsat, FA, Hoffman, DE, and Seubert, DE (2003). Comparison of three outpatient regimens in the management of nausea and vomiting in pregnancy. *J Perinatol*, 23 (7):531–535.

Buckner, KD, Chavez, ML, Raney, EC, et al. (2005). Health food stores' recommendations for nausea and migraines during pregnancy. *Ann Pharmacother*, 39 (2):274–279.

Burke, BE, Olson, RD, and Cusack, BJ (2002). Randomized, controlled trial of phytoestrogen in the prophylactic treatment of menstrual migraine. *Biochem Pharmacother*, 56(6):283–288.

Calabrese, LH, Dodick, DW, Schwedt, TJ, et al. (2007). Narrative review: reversible cerebral vasoconstriction syndromes. *Ann Intern Med* 146(1):34–44.

Calton, GJ and Burnett, JW (1984). Danazol and migraine. *New Engl J Med*, 310(11):721–722.

Campos, CR and Yamamoto, FI (2006). Intracerebral hemorrhage in postpartum cerebral angiopathy associated with the use of isometheptene. *Int J Gynaecol Obstet*, 95(2):151–152.

Cissoko, H, Jonville-Bera, AP, Swortfiguer, D, et al. (2005). Neonatal outcome after exposure to beta adrenergic blockers late in pregnancy. [Exposition aux betabloquants en fin de grossesse] *Archives de Pediatrie*, 12 (5):543–547.

Crowther, CA and Harding, J. (2003). Repeat doses of prenatal corticosteroids for women at risk of preterm birth for preventing neonatal respiratory disease. *Cochrane Database Syst Rev*, (3):CD003935.

Czeizel, AE and Dudas, I. (1992). Prevention of the first occurrence of neural-tube defects by periconceptional vitamin supplementation. *New Engl J Med*, 327(26), 1832–1835.

D'Alessandro, R, Gamberini, G, Lozito, A, et al. (1983). Menstrual migraine: intermittent prophylaxis with a timed-release pharmacological formulation of dihydroergotamine. *Cephalalgia*, 3(Suppl. 1):156–158.

Dalsgaard-Nielsen, T (1970). Some aspects of the epidemiology of migraine in denmark. *Headache*, 10 (1):14–23.

Dawson-Basoa, M, and Gintzler, AR (1998). Gestational and ovarian sex steroid antinociception: synergy between spinal kappa and delta opioid systems. *Brain Res*, 794:61–67

de Lignieres, B, Vincens, M, Mauvais-Jarvis, P, et al. (1986). Prevention of menstrual migraine by percutaneous oestradiol. *Br Med J*, 293(6561):1540.

Dennerstein, L, Wood, C, Hudson, B, et al. (1978). Clinical features and plasma hormone levels after surgical menopause. *Aust N Z J Obstet Gynaecol*, 18 (3):202–205.

Edelman, A, Gallo, MF, Nichols, MD, et al. (2006). Continuous versus cyclic use of combined oral contraceptives for contraception: systematic cochrane review of randomized controlled trials. *Hum Reprod*, 21 (3):573–578.

Edelson, RN (1985). Menstrual migraine and other hormonal aspects of migraine. *Headache*, 25(7):376–379.

Einarson, A, Maltepe, C, Navioz, Y, et al. (2004). The safety of ondansetron for nausea and vomiting of pregnancy: a prospective comparative study. *BJOG*, 111(9):940–943.

Epstein, MT, Hockaday, JM, and Hockaday, TD (1975). Migraine and reproductive hormones throughout the menstrual cycle. *Lancet*, 1(7906):543–548.

Ertresvag, JM, Zwart, JA, Helde, G, et al. (2005). Headache and transient focal neurological symptoms during pregnancy, a prospective cohort. *Acta Neurol Scand*, 111(4):233–237.

Facchinetti, F (1994). The premenstrual syndrome belongs in the diagnostic criteria for menstrual migraine. *Cephalalgia*, 14(6):413–414.

Facchinetti, F, Allais, G, D'Amico, R, et al. (2005). The relationship between headache and preeclampsia: a case-control study. *Eur J Obstet Gynecol Reprod Biol*, 121(2):143–148.

Facchinetti, F, Fioroni, L, Martignoni, E, et al. (1994). Changes of opioid modulation of the hypothalamo-pituitary-adrenal axis in patients with severe premenstrual syndrome. *Psychosom Med*, 56(5):418–422.

Facchinetti, F, Nappi, RE, Tirelli, A, et al. (2002). Hormone supplementation differently affects migraine in postmenopausal women. *Headache*, 42(9):924–929.

Facchinetti, F, Neri, I, Martignoni, E, et al. (1993). The association of menstrual migraine with the premenstrual syndrome. *Cephalalgia*, 13(6):422–425.

Facchinetti, F, Sances, G, Borella, P, et al. (1991). Magnesium prophylaxis of menstrual migraine: effects on intracellular magnesium. *Headache*, 31(5):298–301.

Feniuk, W, Humphrey, PP, and Perren, MJ (1989). GR43175 does not share the complex pharmacology of the ergots. *Cephalalgia*, 9 (Suppl. 9):35–39.

Ferrante, F, Fusco, E, Calabresi, P, et al. (2004). Phytooestrogens in the prophylaxis of menstrual migraine. *Clin Neuropharmacol*, 27(3):137–140.

Fiore, M Shields, KE, Santanello, N, et al. (2005). Exposure to rizatriptan during pregnancy: post-marketing experience up to 30 June 2004. *Cephalalgia*, 25(9):685–688.

Foidart, JM Sulak, PJ, Schellschmidt, I, et al. (2006). The use of an oral contraceptive containing ethinylestradiol and drospirenone in an extended regimen over 126 days. *Contraception*, 73(1):34–40.

Fox, AW and Spierings, EL (2000). Sumatriptan and pregnancy outcome. *Headache*, 40(10):860–861.

Fragoso, YD, Carvalho, R, Ferrero, F, et al. (2003). Crying as a precipitating factor for migraine and tension-type headache. *Sao Paulo Med J*, 121(1):31–33.

Freeman, EW, Rickels, K, Sondheimer, SJ, et al. (1995). A double-blind trial of oral progesterone, alprazolam, and placebo in treatment of severe premenstrual syndrome. *JAMA*, 274(1):51–57.

Freeman, EW, Sondheimer, SJ, and Rickels, K (1997). Gonadotropin-releasing hormone agonist in the treatment of premenstrual symptoms with and without ongoing dysphoria: a controlled study. *Psychopharmacol Bull* 33(2):303–309.

Friedman, JM, Little, BB, Brent, RL, et al. (1990). Potential human teratogenicity of frequently prescribed drugs. *Obstet Gynecol*, 75(4):594–599.

Futterman, LA, and Rapkin, AJ (2006). Diagnosis of premenstrual disorders. *J Reprod Med*, 51(4 Suppl.):349–358.

Gaffield, ME, Curtis, KM, Mohllajee, AP, et al. (2006). Medical eligibility criteria for new contraceptive methods: combined hormonal patch, combined hormonal vaginal ring and the etonogestrel implant. *Contraception*, 73(2):134–144.

Gallagher, RM (1989). Menstrual migraine and intermittent ergonovine therapy. *Headache*, 29(6):366–367.

Goldstein, M and Chen, TC (1982). The epidemiology of disabling headache. *Adv Neurol*, 33:377–390.

Goldszmidt, E, Kern, R, Chaput, A, et al. (2005). The incidence and etiology of postpartum headaches: a prospective cohort study. *Can J Anaesth*, 52 (9):971–977.

Gracia, CR and Freeman, EW (2004). Acute consequences of the menopausal transition: the rise of common menopausal symptoms. *Endocrinol Metab Clin North Am*, 33(4):675–689.

Gracia, CR, Sammel, MD, Freeman, EW, et al. (2005). Defining menopause status: creation of a new definition to identify the early changes of the menopausal transition. *Menopause*, 12(2):128–135.

Graham-Bermann, SA and Seng, J (2005). Violence exposure and traumatic stress symptoms as additional predictors of health problems in high-risk children. *J Pediatr*, 146(3):349–354.

Granella, F, Sances, G, Pucci, E, et al. (2000). Migraine with aura and reproductive life events: a case control study. *Cephalalgia*, 20(8):701–707.

Granella, F, Sances, G, Zanferrari, C, et al. (1993). Migraine without aura and reproductive life events: a clinical epidemiological study in 1300 women. *Headache*, 33(7):385–389.

Granier, I Garcia, E, Geissler, A, et al. (1999). Postpartum cerebral angiopathy associated with the administration of sumatriptan and dihydroergotamine—a case report. *Intensive Care Med*, 25(5):532–534.

Greenblatt, RB and Bruneteau, DW (1974). Menopausal headaches—psychogenic or metabolic? *J Am Geriatr Soc*, 22(4):186–190.

Grove, LH (1973). Backache, headache and bladder dysfunction after delivery. *Br J Anaesth*, 45 (11):1147–1149.

Guillebaud, J (2001). Medical-eligibility criteria for contraceptive use. *Lancet*, 357(9266):1378–1379.

Gupta, S, Villalón, CM, Mehrotra, S, et al. (2007). Female sex hormones and rat dural vasodilatation to CGRP, periarterial electrical stimulation and capsaicin. *Headache*, 47(2):225–235.

Gur, C, Diav-Citrin, O, Shechtman, S, Arnon, J, & Ornoy, A. (2004). Pregnancy outcome after first trimester exposure to corticosteroids: a prospective controlled study. *Reprod Toxicol*, 18(1):93–101.

Hagen, I, Nesheim, BI, and Tuntland, T (1985). No effect of vitamin B-6 against premenstrual tension. A controlled clinical study. *Acta Obstet Gynecol Scand*, 64 (8):667–670.

Harel, Z, Biro, FM, and Kollar, LM (1995). Depo-provera in adolescents: effects of early second injection or prior oral contraception. *J Adolesc Health*, 16(5):379–384.

Headache Classification Subcommittee of the International Headache Society (2004). The international classification of headache disorders: 2nd edition. *Cephalalgia*, 24(Suppl. 1):9–160.

Hermes-DeSantis, ER and Clyman, RI (2006). Patent ductus arteriosus: Pathophysiology and management. *J Perinatol*, 26 (Suppl. 1):S14–S18; discussion S22–S23.

Herzog, AG (1997). Continuous bromocriptine therapy in menstrual migraine. *Neurology*, 48(1):101–102.

Hockaday, JM, Peet, KM, and Hockaday, TD (1976). Bromocriptine in migraine. *Headache*, 16(3):109–114.

Holdaway, IM, Parr, CE, and France, J (1991). Treatment of a patient with severe menstrual migraine using the depot LHRH analogue zoladex. *Aust NZ J Obstet Gynaecol*, 31(2):164–165.

Holmes, LB, Coull, BA, Dorfman, J, et al. (2005). The correlation of deficits in IQ with midface and digit hypoplasia in children exposed in utero to anticonvulsant drugs. *J Perinatol*, 146(1):118–122.

Holzhammer, J and Wober, C (2006). Non-alimentary trigger factors of migraine and tension-type headache. [Nichtalimentare Triggerfaktoren bei Migrane und Kopfschmerz vom Spannungstyp] *Schmerz*, 20 (3):226–237.

Hosking, SP (1996). Ergotamine use in pregnancy. *Aust NZ J Obstet Gynaecol*, 36(2):159–160.

Iffy, L, Zito, GE, Jakobovits, AA, et al. (1998). Postpartum intracranial haemorrhage in normotensive users of bromocriptine for ablactation. *Pharmacoepidemiol Drug Saf*, 7(3), 167–171.

Johannes, CB, Linet, MS, Stewart, WF, et al. (1995). Relationship of headache to phase of the menstrual cycle among young women: a daily diary study. *Neurology*, 45(6):1076–1082.

Johnson, SR (2004). Premenstrual syndrome, premenstrual dysphoric disorder, and beyond: a clinical primer for practitioners. *Obstet Gynecol*, 104(4):845–859.

Judd, H (1987). Efficacy of transdermal estradiol. *Am J Obstet Gynecol*, 156(5):1326–1331.

Kellogg, N and American Academy of Pediatrics Committee on Child Abuse and Neglect. (2005). The evaluation of sexual abuse in children. *Pediatrics*, 116(2):506–512.

Kudrow, L (1975). The relationship of headache frequency to hormone use in migraine. *Headache*, 15(1):36–40.

LaGuardia, KD, Fisher, AC, Bainbridge, JD, et al. (2005). Suppression of estrogen-withdrawal headache with extended transdermal contraception. *Fertil Steril*, 83 (6):1875–1877.

Lance, JW and Anthony, M (1966). Some clinical aspects of migraine. A prospective survey of 500 patients. *Arch Neurol*, 15(4), 356–361.

Leather, AT, Studd, JW, Watson, NR, et al. (1999). The treatment of severe premenstrual syndrome with goserelin with and without 'add-back' estrogen therapy: a placebo-controlled study. *Gynecol Endocrinol*, 13 (1):48–55.

Leung, TN, Lam, PM, Ng, PC, et al. (2003). Repeated courses of antenatal corticosteroids: is it justified? *Acta Obstet Gynecol Scand*, 82(7):589–596.

Liu, NJ and Gintzler, AR (1999). Gestational and ovarian sex steroid antinociception: relevance of uterine afferent and spinal α2-noradrenergic activity. *Pain*, 83:359–368.

Lo, WY and Friedman, JM (2002). Teratogenicity of recently introduced medications in human pregnancy. *Obstet Gynecol*, 100(3):465–473.

Loder, E (2002). Prophylaxis of menstrual migraine with triptans: problems and possibilities. *Neurology*, 59 (11):1677–1681

Loder, E (2003). Safety of sumatriptan in pregnancy: a review of the data so far. *CNS Drugs*, 17(1):1–7.

Loder, E (2004). Menstrual migraine: timing is everything. *Neurology*, 63(2):202–203.

Loder, E, Silberstein, SD, Abu-Shakra, S, et al. (2004). Efficacy and tolerability of oral zolmitriptan in menstrually associated migraine: a randomized, prospective, parallel-group, double-blind, placebo-controlled study. *Headache*, 44(2):120–130.

Loder, EW, Buse, DC, and Golub, JR (2005a). Headache and combination estrogen-progestin oral contraceptives: integrating evidence, guidelines, and clinical practice. *Headache*, 45(3):224–231.

Loder, EW, Buse, DC, and Golub, JR (2005b). Headache as a side effect of combination estrogen-progestin oral contraceptives: a systematic review. *Am J Obstet Gynecol*, 193(3 Pt 1):636–649.

MacGregor, EA, Frith, A, Ellis, J, et al. (2005). Predicting menstrual migraine with a home-use fertility monitor. *Neurology*, 64(3):561–563.

MacGregor, EA, Frith, A, Ellis, J, et al. (2006). Incidence of migraine relative to menstrual cycle phases of rising and falling estrogen. *Neurology*, 67(12):2154–2158.

MacGregor, EA and Hackshaw, A (2004). Prevalence of migraine on each day of the natural menstrual cycle. *Neurology*, 63(2):351–353.

Magos, AL, Zilkha, KJ, and Studd, JW (1983). Treatment of menstrual migraine by oestradiol implants. *J Neurol Neurosurg Psychiatry*, 46(11):1044–1046.

Mannix, LK, Diamond, M, and Loder, E (2002). Women and headache: a treatment approach based on life stages. *Cleve Clin J Med*, 69(6):488–500.

Marcoux, S, Berube, S, Brisson, J, et al. (1992). History of migraine and risk of pregnancy-induced hypertension. *Epidemiology*, 3(1):53–56.

Marcus, DA, Scharff, L, and Turk, DC (1995). Nonpharmacological management of headaches during pregnancy. *Psychiatr Med*, 57(6):527–535.

Marcus, DA, Scharff, L, and Turk, D (1999). Longitudinal prospective study of headache during pregnancy and postpartum. *Headache*, 39(9):625–632.

Martin, VT (2004). Menstrual migraine: a review of prophylactic therapies. *Curr Pain Headache Rep*, 8(3):229–237.

Martin, V, Wernke, S, Mandell, K, et al. (2003). Medical oophorectomy with and without estrogen add-back therapy in the prevention of migraine headache. *Headache*, 43(4):309–321.

Martin, VT, Wernke, S, Mandell, K, et al. (2006). Symptoms of premenstrual syndrome and their association with migraine headache. *Headache*, 46(1):125–137.

Mattsson, P (2003). Hormonal factors in migraine: a population-based study of women aged 40 to 74 years. *Headache*, 43(1):27–35.

Mattsson, LA, Skouby, SO, Heikkinen, J, et al. (2004). A low-dose start in hormone replacement therapy provides a beneficial bleeding profile and few side-effects: randomized comparison with a conventional-dose regimen. *Climacteric*, 7(1):59–69.

Moloney, MF, Strickland, OL, DeRossett, SE, et al. (2006). The experiences of midlife women with migraines. *J Nurs Scholarsh*, 38(3):278–285.

Moore, MP and Redman, CW (1983). Case-control study of severe pre-eclampsia of early onset. *Br Med J (Clinical research ed.)*, 287(6392):580–583.

Murray, SC and Muse, KN (1997). Effective treatment of severe menstrual migraine headaches with gonadotropin-releasing hormone agonist and "add-back" therapy. *Fertil Steril*, 67(2):390–393.

Nand, SL, Webster, MA, Baber, R, et al. (1998). Menopausal symptom control and side-effects on continuous estrone sulfate and three doses of medroxyprogesterone acetate. Ogen/Provera study group. *Climacteric*, 1(3):211–218.

Nappi, RE, Cagnacci, A, Granella, F, et al. (2001). Course of primary headaches during hormone replacement therapy. *Maturitas*, 38(2):157–163.

Needs, CJ and Brooks, PM (1985). Antirheumatic medication in pregnancy. *Br J Rheumatol*, 24(3):282–290.

Nelson, AL (2005). Extended-cycle oral contraception: a new option for routine use. *Treat Endocrinol*, 4(3):139–145.

Neri, I, Granella, F, Nappi, R, et al. (1993). Characteristics of headache at menopause: a clinico-epidemiologic study. *Maturitas*, 17(1):31–37.

Newman, LC, Lipton, RB, Lay, CL, et al. (1998). A pilot study of oral sumatriptan as intermittent prophylaxis of menstruation-related migraine. *Neurology*, 51 (1):307–309.

Newman, L, Mannix, LK, Landy, S, et al. (2001). Naratriptan as short-term prophylaxis of menstrually associated migraine: a randomized, double-blind, placebo-controlled study. *Headache*, 41(3):248–256.

Noris, M, Perico, N, and Remuzzi, G. (2005). Mechanisms of disease: pre-eclampsia. *Nat Clin Pract Nephrol*, 1 (2):98–114; quiz 120.

O'Dea, JP and Davis, EH (1990). Tamoxifen in the treatment of menstrual migraine. *Neurology*, 40 (9):1470–1471.

Olesen, C, Steffensen, FH, Sorensen, HT, et al. (2000). Pregnancy outcome following prescription for sumatriptan. *Headache*, 40(1):20–24.

Oliver, CD and White, SA (2002). Unexplained fitting in three parturients suffering from postdural puncture headache. *Br J Anaesth*, 89(5):782–785.

Ostrea, EM Jr. (1982). Neonatal withdrawal from intrauterine exposure to butalbital. *Am J Obstet Gynecol*, 143(5):597–598.

Parra, J, Brocalero-Camacho, A, Sancho, J, et al. (2006). Migrainous infarction and clomiphene citrate. [Infarto migranoso y citrato de clomifeno] *Revista de neurologia*, 42(9):572–574.

Pearlstein, T (2002). Selective serotonin reuptake inhibitors for premenstrual dysphoric disorder: the emerging gold standard? *Drugs*, *62*(13), 1869–1885.

Petitti, DB (2003). Clinical practice. combination estrogen-progestin oral contraceptives. *N Engl J Med*, 349 (15):1443–1450.

Powles, T (1986). Prevention of migrainous headaches by tamoxifen. *Lancet*, ii:1334.

Pradalier, A, Vincent, D, Beaulieu, PH, et al. (1994). Correlation between estradiol plasma level and therapeutic effect on menstrual migraine. In *New Advances in Headache Research* (F Rose, ed.), pp. 129–130, 131. Smith-Gordon, London.

Pregnancy categories for prescription drugs. (1982). *FDA Drug Bull*, 12(3):24–25.

Prentice, RL, Langer, RD, Stefanick, ML, et al. (2006). Combined analysis of women's health initiative observational and clinical trial data on postmenopausal hormone treatment and cardiovascular disease. *Am J Epidemiol*, 163(7):589–599.

Pruyn, SC, Phelan, JP, Buchanan, GC (1979). Long-term propranolol therapy in pregnancy: maternal and fetal outcome. *Am J Obstet Gynecol*, 135(4):485–489.

Ramadan, NM, Halvorson, H, Vande-Linde, A, et al. (1989). Low brain magnesium in migraine. *Headache*, 29(9):590–593.

Raroque, HG Jr, Tesfa, G, and Purdy, P (1993). Postpartum cerebral angiopathy. is there a role for sympathomimetic drugs? *Stroke*, 24(12):2108–2110.

Raymond, GV (1995). Teratogen update: ergot and ergotamine. *Teratology*, 51(5):344–347.

Redmond, GP (1982). Propranolol and fetal growth retardation. *Semin Perinatol*, 6(2):142–147.

Reinisch, JM, Sanders, SA, Mortensen, EL, et al. (1995). In utero exposure to phenobarbital and intelligence deficits in adult men. *JAMA*, 274(19):1518–1525.

Ressel, G (2002). AAP updates statement for transfer of drugs and other chemicals into breast milk. american academy of pediatrics. *Am Fam Physician*, 65 (5):979–980.

Robinson, K, Huntington, KM, and Wallace, MG (1977). Treatment of the premenstrual syndrome. *Br J Obstet Gynaecol*, 84(10):784–788.

Robbins, L (1996). Menstrual migraine with features of cluster headache. A report of 10 cases. *Headache*, 36 (3):166–167.

Romans, S, Belaise, C, Martin, J, et al. (2002). Childhood abuse and later medical disorders in women. an epidemiological study. *Psychother Psychosom*, 71 (3):141–150.

Rosano, GM, Sarais, C, Zoncu, S, et al. (2000). The relative effects of progesterone and progestins in hormone replacement therapy. *Hum Reprod*, 15 (Suppl 1):60–73.

Rozen, TD (2003). Aborting a prolonged migrainous aura with intravenous prochlorperazine and magnesium sulfate. *Headache*, 43(8):901–903.

Rubin, PC, and McCabe, R (1984). Postpartum migraine and severe pre-eclampsia. *Lancet*, 2(8397):285–286.

Sachs, M, Pape, HC, Speckmann, EJ, et al. (2007). The effect of estrogen and progesterone on spreading depression in rat neocortical tissues. *Neuromuscul Disord*, 25(1):27–34.

Sances, G, Granella, F, Nappi, RE, et al. (2003). Course of migraine during pregnancy and postpartum: a prospective study. *Cephalalgia*, 23(3):197–205.

Sances, G, Martignoni, E, Fioroni, L, et al. (1990). Naproxen sodium in menstrual migraine prophylaxis: a double-blind placebo controlled study. *Headache*, 30 (11):705–709.

Sandor, PS and Afra, J (2005). Nonpharmacologic treatment of migraine. *Curr Pain Headache Rep*, 9 (3):202–205.

Sato, S, Shimizu, M, Endo, K, et al. (2004). Postpartum cerebral angiopathy—a case report the vasculopathy associated with co-administration of two vasoconstrictives, methylergometrine maleate and sumatriptan. *Rinsho shinkeigaku*, 44(2):96–101.

Saurel-Cubizolles, MJ, Romito, P, Lelong, N, et al. (2000). Women's health after childbirth: a longitudinal study in France and Italy. *BJOG*, 107(10):1202–1209.

Scharff, L, Turk, DC, and Marcus, DA (1995). Triggers of headache episodes and coping responses of headache diagnostic groups. *Headache*, 35(7):397–403.

Scharff, L, Marcus, DA, and Turk, DC (1996). Maintenance of effects in the nonmedical treatment of headaches during pregnancy. *Headache*, 36(5):285–290.

Scharff, L, Marcus, DA, and Turk, DC (1997). Headache during pregnancy and in the postpartum: a prospective study. *Headache*, 37(4):203–210.

Scher, AI, Terwindt, GM, Picavet, HS, et al. (2005). Cardiovascular risk factors and migraine: the GEM population-based study. *Neurology*, 64(4):614–620.

Seelig, MS (1993). Interrelationship of magnesium and estrogen in cardiovascular and bone disorders, eclampsia, migraine and premenstrual syndrome. *J Am Coll Nutr*, 12(4):442–458.

Shrim, A, Boskovic, R, Maltepe, C, et al. (2006). Pregnancy outcome following use of large doses of vitamin B6 in the first trimester. *J Obstet Gynaecol*, 26(8):749–751.

Silberstein, SD (1995). Migraine and women. the link between headache and hormones. *Postgrad Med*, 97 (4):147–153.

Silberstein, S (1996). DHE-45 in the prophylaxis of menstrually related migraine. *Cephalalgia*, 16:371.

Silberstein, SD (1995). Migraine and women. the link between headache and hormones. *Postgrad Med*, 97 (4):147–153.

Silberstein, SD, Armellino, JJ, Hoffman, HD, et al. (1999). Treatment of menstruation-associated migraine with the nonprescription combination of acetaminophen, aspirin, and caffeine: results from three randomized, placebo-controlled studies. *Clin Ther*, 21(3):475–491.

Silberstein, SD, Elkind, AH, Schreiber, C, et al. (2004). A randomized trial of frovatriptan for the intermittent prevention of menstrual migraine. *Neurology*, 63 (2):261–269.

Silberstein, SD, Massiou, H, Le Jeunne, C, et al. (2000). Rizatriptan in the treatment of menstrual migraine. *Obstet Gynecol*, 96(2):237–242.

Silberstein, SD, Massiou, H, McCarroll, KA, et al. (2002). Further evaluation of rizatriptan in menstrual migraine: retrospective analysis of long-term data. *Headache*, 42(9):917–923.

Silberstein, SD and Merriam, GR (1993). Sex hormones and headache. *J Pain Symptom Manage*, 8(2):98–114.

Smets, K, Zecic, A, and Willems, J (2004). Ergotamine as a possible cause of mobius sequence: additional clinical observation. *J Child Neurol* 19(5):398.

Solbach, MP and Waymer, RS (1993). Treatment of menstruation-associated migraine headache with subcutaneous sumatriptan. *Obstet Gynecol*, 82(5):769–772.

Somerville, BW (1972a). The role of estradiol withdrawal in the etiology of menstrual migraine. *Neurology*, 22 (4):355–365.

Somerville, BW (1972b). A study of migraine in pregnancy. *Neurology*, 22(8):824–828.

Somerville, BW (1975). Estrogen-withdrawal migraine. II. attempted prophylaxis by continuous estradiol administration. *Neurology*, 25(3):245–250.

Stanback, J and Katz, K (2002). Methodological quality of WHO medical eligibility criteria for contraceptive use. *Contraception*, 66(1):1–5.

Stang, A, Schwingl, P, and Rivera, R (2000). New contraceptive eligibility checklists for provision of combined oral contraceptives and depot-medroxyprogesterone acetate in community-based programmes. *Bull World Health Organ*, 78(8):1015–1023.

Stein, G, Morton, J, Marsh, A, et al. (1984). Headaches after childbirth. *Acta Neurol Scand*, 69(2):74–79.

Stewart, WF, Lipton, RB, Chee, E, et al. (2000). Menstrual cycle and headache in a population sample of migraineurs. *Neurology*, 55(10):1517–1523.

Studd, J and Leather, AT (1996). The need for add-back with gonadotrophin-releasing hormone agonist therapy. *Br J Obstet Gynaecol*, 103 (Suppl.) 14:1–4.

Stumpf, PG (1990). Pharmacokinetics of estrogen. *Obstet Gynecol*, 75(4 Suppl), 9S–14S; discussion 15S–17S.

Sulak, PJ, Cressman, BE, Waldrop, E, et al. (1997). Extending the duration of active oral contraceptive pills to manage hormone withdrawal symptoms. *Obstet Gynecol*, 89(2):179–183.

Sundstrom, I, Nyberg, S, Bixo, M, et al. (1999). Treatment of premenstrual syndrome with gonadotropin-releasing hormone agonist in a low dose regimen. *Acta Obstet Gynecol Scand*, 78(10):891–899.

Tamborini, A and Ruiz, JC (2004). Current role of hormone replacement therapy in the prevention of postmenopausal osteoporosis: gynecologic point of view. [Place actuelle du traitement hormonal substitutif dans la prevention de l'osteoporose postmenopausique : le point de vue du gynecologue] *Rev Med Interne*, 25(Suppl 5):S580–S587.

Thaver, D, Saeed, MA, and Bhutta, ZA (2006). Pyridoxine (vitamin B6) supplementation in pregnancy. *Cochrane Database Syst Rev*, (2):CD000179.

Thomas, EJ, Okuda, KJ, and Thomas, NM (1991). The combination of a depot gonadotrophin releasing hormone agonist and cyclical hormone replacement therapy for dysfunctional uterine bleeding. *Br J Obstet Gynaecol*, 98(11):1155–1159.

Tietjen, GE, Brandes, JL, Digre, KB, et al. (2007). High prevalence of somatic symptoms and depression in women with disabling chronic headache. *Neurology*, 68:134–140.

Tuchman, M, Hee, A, Emeribe, U, et al. (2006). Efficacy and tolerability of zolmitriptan oral tablet in the acute treatment of menstrual migraine. *CNS drugs*, 20 (12):1019–1026.

Umapathi, T and Chaudhry, V (2005). Toxic neuropathy. *Curr Opin Neurobiol*, 18(5):574–580.

van Vliet, JA, Favier, I, Helmerhorst, FM, et al. (2006). Cluster headache in women: relation with menstruation, use of oral contraceptives, pregnancy, and menopause. *J Neurol Neurosurg Psychiatry*, 77 (5):690–692.

Vellacott, ID and O'Brien, PM (1987). Effect of spironolactone on premenstrual syndrome symptoms. *J Reprod Med*, 32(6):429–434.

Wainscott, G, Sullivan, FM, Volans, GN, et al. (1978). The outcome of pregnancy in women suffering from migraine. *Postgrad Med J*, 54(628):98–102.

Wall, VR (1992). Breastfeeding and migraine headaches. *J Hum Lact*, 8(4):209–212.

Wang, M, Hammarback, S, Lindhe, BA, et al. (1995). Treatment of premenstrual syndrome by spironolactone: a double-blind, placebo-controlled study. *Acta Obstet Gynecol Scand*, 74(10):803–808.

Wang, SJ, Fuh, JL, Lu, SR, et al. (2003). Migraine prevalence during menopausal transition. *Headache*, 43 (5):470–478.

Weiss, G (2001a). Clinical implications of perimenopausal steroid changes. *Climacteric*, 4(2):93–94.

Weiss, G (2001b). Menstrual irregularities and the perimenopause. *J Soc Gynecol Investig*, 8(1 Suppl Proceedings):S65–S66.

Weiss, G, Skurnick, JH, Goldsmith, LT, et al. (2004). Menopause and hypothalamic-pituitary sensitivity to estrogen. *JAMA*, 292(24):2991–2996.

Welch, KM and Ramadan, NM (1995). Mitochondria, magnesium and migraine. *J Neurol Sci*, 134(1–2):9–14.
Whipple, B, Josimovich, JB, and Komisaruk, BR (1990). Sensory thresholds during the antepartum, intrapartum and postpartum periods. *Int J Nurs Stud*, 27:213–221.
Williams, MJ, Harris, RI, and Dean, BC (1985). Controlled trial of pyridoxine in the premenstrual syndrome. *J Int Med Res*, 13(3):174–179.
Witlin, AG, Mattar, F, and Sibai, BM (2000). Postpartum stroke: a twenty-year experience. *Am J Obstet Gynecol*, 183(1):83–88.
Wojnar-Horton, RE, Hackett, LP, Yapp, P, et al. (1996). Distribution and excretion of sumatriptan in human milk. *Br J Clin Pharmacol*, 41(3):217–221.
Yao, M, Ritchie, HE, and Brown-Woodman, PD (2006). A reproductive screening test of feverfew: is a full reproductive study warranted? *Reprod Toxicol*, 22 (4):688–693.
Yucel, B, Ozyalcin, S, Sertel, HO, et al. (2002). Childhood traumatic events and dissociative experiences in patients with chronic headache and low back pain. *Clin J Pain*, 18(6):394–401.

29 Headaches in the Elderly

Jerry W Swanson, David J Capobianco, and Stefan Evers

INTRODUCTION

Before considering the issue of headaches in the elderly, one must first consider how the term elderly is defined. One dictionary definition of elderly is: rather old; being past middle age (from: Merriam Webster Online, accessed November 12, 2006). Another whimsical definition is based on the term middle age: The definition of "middle age" always involves adding 15 years to your own age, until such time as you cannot avoid defining yourself as middle aged, at which time the definition of "older" becomes . . . your own age +15 (Anonymous).

These definitions reflect the fact that age grouping is a social convention rather than a biologically founded one. In 1980, the United Nations defined 60 years as the time of transition to the aging sector of the population (McFayden, 1990). In industrialized countries, age-based criteria for usual retirement (usually 65 years) has become regarded as the beginning of old age. Although we often discuss the elderly as though they represent a homogenous portion of the population, one of the results of gerontologic research is that heterogeneity increases with age. This finding should not be unexpected since the entry into this segment of the population is in the 60s and this population contains individuals who may differ from one another by 40 or more years in age. In addition, it is well known that biological changes that are associated with the development of health problems vary considerably across this age group.

Nevertheless, the chronologic grouping is useful in considering the size of this segment of the population. For instance, in the United States, the population over the age of 65 years now totals over 34 million and by 2030 it is estimated that there will be 80 million persons over age 65, which will account for nearly 20% of the population (Giddens et al., 2003.). Further, those who are over 75 years now number greater than 13 million (Giddens et al., 2003). These increasing numbers of older persons are the result of an increase in life expectancy; this increase is due to a large number of factors but primarily because of successful efforts in controlling the spread of infectious diseases and premature deaths among infants and children. Given the increasing percentage of the elderly in the population as well as the absolute numbers of elderly, this group will make up a substantial number of individuals seeking care for a variety of conditions, including headache.

OVERVIEW OF EPIDEMIOLOGY OF HEADACHES IN THE ELDERLY

Headache prevalence varies as a function of age. While the studies of headache in the older population are not numerous, they generally point to an overall reduction of headaches in this segment of the population. For example, migraine prevalence peaks at approximately 40 years and thereafter declines until after age 60 years when the prevalence is 2.5% in men and 7.5% in women (Lipton et al., 2001).

In a community survey in Italy, the 1-year prevalence rates of headache in individuals older than 65 years were 62.5% in women and 36.6% for men. These rates declined steadily with advancing age from 56.7% from ages 65–74 to 26.1% for ages 85–96 (Prencipe et al., 2001).

In a headache survey in the region of Vitória, Espírito Santo, Brazil, headache prevalence was 35% for individuals over the age of 55 years, a decline when compared to younger individuals (Domingues et al., 2004).

A population survey in San Marino showed a decline in headache prevalence in both men and women aged 61 years and older compared to younger adults (D'Alessandro et al., 1988). The prevalence rate continued to decrease in men and women older than age 71 years.

In a population survey of individuals older than 75 years in Wales, Waters (1974) reported that 21% of men and 55% of women had recurrent headaches. In a more recent survey of headache in North Staffordshire, UK, individuals 66 years and older had a 3-month prevalence in 40.6% in men and a 49.7% 3-month prevalence in women (Boardman et al., 2003), which were lower than in younger age groups.

In a community-based study in East Boston, MA of nearly 4000 persons aged 65 years and older, 53% of women and 36% of men described headache in the previous year. (Cook et al., 1989) In this study, the prevalence of headache declined with advancing age. Of note, women had a higher prevalence of frequent headache and there was less of a decline in prevalence of frequent headache with age compared to overall headache prevalence. In fact, 17% of individuals had headache at least several times per month.

In another study of prevalence of health symptoms, headache ranked as the 10th most common symptom among elderly women and the 14th most common symptom among elderly men (Hale et al., 1986).

In comparison to these studies, a population survey of individuals 65 years and older on Kinmen Island, China found 21% of men and 51% of women had at least one headache episode (Wang et al. 1997).

These studies illustrate that despite the relative decline of headache with advancing age, the high representation of the elderly in the population and the substantial prevalence of headache in this population result in a significant number of the elderly who suffer from headaches.

PRIMARY HEADACHE DISORDERS

Migraine

While it is clear that the prevalence of migraine decreases with age, the new onset of migraine and other primary headache disorders in the elderly are relatively uncommon. For example, in the community survey in Italy, 16.9% of those with headache had onset at 65 years and older. Of these, 80.6% were diagnosed with tension-type headaches and 4.2% had migraine headaches, and 15.3% had symptomatic (secondary) headaches (Prencipe et al., 2001). As noted above, a large population-based survey in the US. showed that migraine declines such that after age 60 years, the prevalence is 2.5% in men and 7.5% in women (Lipton et al. 2001). In the US and European diagnostic guidelines, brain imaging is required when establishing the diagnosis for the first time after the age of 40 years (Germany) or 45 years (US), even if the features are typical and the neurological examination is normal.

The clinical features of migraine in the elderly are often different than seen in younger patients. Pain is more commonly bilateral and more diffuse than restricted to one area of the head (e.g., temporal, frontal). Photophobia, phonophobia, and nausea, and vomiting occur less frequently than in younger individuals (Martins et al., 2006). Conversely, vegetative symptoms associated with migraine attacks such as pallor and dry mouth occur more commonly in the elderly (Martins et al., 2006). These changes in features may lead to a misdiagnosis of tension-type headaches.

While migraine visual aura may become less common or cease in some individuals, one population-based study of women aged 40–74 years showed no significant change in the prevalence, frequency or duration over this age span (Mattsson et al., 2000). Migraine aura may occur for the first time in middle-aged or elderly patients and as in younger adults, the aura is invariably visual followed by somotosensory as the next most common type of aura symptom. These symptoms may raise concern about focal brain ischemia (transient ischemic attacks) or less commonly focal seizures. Fisher (1980) called attention to migraine aura in older individuals and coined the term "late-life migrainous accompaniments." He outlined the key diagnostic features, which are listed in Table 29–1. A careful history may be all that is needed to confirm the diagnosis, especially if the attacks have recurred over years and the examination is normal. On the other hand, recent

TABLE 29–1 Key Diagnostic Features of Late-life Migrainous Accompaniments.

1. Scintillations or other visual display in the spell; next in order, paresthesias, aphasia, dysarthria, and paralysis
2. Buildup of scintillations (does not occur in cerebrovascular disease)
3. March of paresthesias (does not occur in cerebrovascular disease)
4. Progression from one accompaniment to another, often with a delay
5. Occurrence of two or more similar spells (helps exclude embolism)
6. Headache in the spell
7. Episodes last 15–25 minutes
8. Characteristic midlife flurry of migrainous accompaniments
9. Generally benign course
10. Normal angiography (excludes thrombosis)
11. Exclusion of cerebral thrombosis, embolism and dissection, epilepsy, thrombocythemia, polycythemia, and thrombotic thrombocytopenia

Source: Fisher (1980).

onset of symptoms may require an extensive evaluation to exclude other conditions.

Treatment of Migraine in the Elderly

Treatment of migraine, as well as other primary headache disorders, provides some challenges in older patients that are not usually present in younger patients. While no medications are specifically contraindicated on the basis of advanced age, several issues related to medications require consideration when prescribing pharmacologic agents.

As adults age, there is a slow increase in the variation between individuals with regard to the doses of medication necessary to result in a specific effect. This results from changes in pharmacokinetics and pharmacodynamics (Oates, 2006).

Pharmacokinetic changes occur because of changes in body composition and the function of drug-eliminating organs. The decrease in lean body mass, total-body water, and serum albumin, combined with a rise in percentage of body fat, changes distribution of drugs in a way that is dependent on their lipid solubility and protein binding. The clearance of several drugs declines in older persons. Kidney function decreases at a variable pace, often to approximately 50% of that in early adulthood. In addition, hepatic blood flow and metabolism are decreased in elderly individuals, but there is substantial interindividual variation. Activities of hepatic cytochrome P450 enzymes tend to decline, but conjugation function is relatively maintained. The elimination half-lives of pharmacologic agents are often longer as a result of the greater apparent volumes of distribution of lipid-soluble drugs and/or reductions of kidney or metabolic clearance (Oates, 2006).

Alterations in pharmacodynamics are also significant aspects in management of medications in the elderly. Drugs that depress the central nervous system yield greater impacts at any particular plasma concentration. Despite a reduction of dose to account for age-related pharmacokinetic alterations, physiological changes and loss of homeostatic flexibility can lead to an increase in undesirable side-effects (Oates, 2006). For instance, β-adrenergic blockers may cause lethargy and confusion. Treatment with tricyclic antidepressants is more likely to be sedating in the elderly and confusion and urinary retention can occur. Nonsteroidal anti-inflammatory agents are more likely to result in renal dysfunction related to a reduction in creatinine clearance. Because of these factors, when medications are instituted, they should be started in small dosages and advanced slowly with careful monitoring for side-effects.

The elderly also tend to have more coexistent medical conditions than younger headache sufferers. These may contraindicate some medications. For example, β-adrenergic blockers may worsen depression and congestive heart failure. Verapamil may worsen congestive heart failure. Topiramate may worsen any tendency toward cognitive dysfunction. Divalproex sodium may worsen hepatic function. Uncontrolled hypertension, ischemic cerebrovascular disease, and coronary disease are contraindications for the use of triptans, ergotamine, and dihydroergotamine.

Because of coexistent conditions, older patients often are on more drugs than their younger counterparts. This increases the risk for drug interactions and adverse events. Polypharmacy should be avoided as much as possible. In addition to efficacy, agents need to be selected based on their potential interaction with other drugs.

Despite the above challenges, care providers should not develop a nihilistic attitude regarding the treatment of migraine headaches. Treatment should be customized for each patient, addressing both the needs for treatment of headache and comorbid conditions which may alter choices of therapy. When starting medications, especially prophylactic agents, begin with a low dose and slowly titrate the dose upward to a therapeutic target. Avoid polypharmacy which increases the likelihood of adverse events. Finally, carefully consider nonpharmacologic approaches to therapy (Lake, 2001).

Tension-type Headache

The 1-year period prevalence of episodic tension-type headache in a large US community survey in individuals aged 60–65 years of age was 25.6% for men and 27.1% for women compared to the peak prevalence of 42.3% in men and 46.9% for women, which were observed in the 30–39-year-old group. The 1-year period prevalence for chronic tension-type headaches was found to be 1.5% in men and 2.7% in women aged 60 years and older compared to an overall 1-year period prevalence of 1.4% in men and 2.8% in women (Schwartz et al., 1998). Tension-type headache may begin in the elderly not infrequently, as noted in the community survey in Italy, where 16.9% of those with headache had onset at 65 years and older and of these, 80.6% were diagnosed with tension-type headaches (Prencipe et al., 2001).

Since the tension-type headache phenotype can be due to a variety of secondary headaches and because secondary causes for headache are more common in the elderly, the diagnosis should be made only after careful assessment and secondary causes have been excluded. Treatment of tension-type headaches is outlined in Chapter 10.

Cluster Headache

The data regarding cluster headache prevalence in the elderly is sparse. The lifetime prevalence of cluster headache has been estimated to range from 95 to 279/1,00,000 (Tonon et al., 2002; Torelli et al., 2005; Ekbom et al., 2006). In the Parma study, only 2 of 15 patients were reported as having cluster attacks after the age of 60 (Torelli et al., 2005). Clinic-based studies suggest that while cluster headache typically begins in the 20s, onset may occur after the age of 60 years in up to 10% of patients (Silberstein and Young, 1998). One study suggests that the length of remission phases increases over time from a mean of 1.1 years to a mean of 3.5 years (Igarashi and Sakai, 1996).

While cluster headache usually begins in early to mid-life (mean onset approximately 30 years), occasional elderly patients have been described with new onset cluster headache (Torelli et al., 2005). The oldest age of onset reported is a 91-year-old woman (Seidler et al., 2006); accordingly, the clinician should be open to considering a new diagnosis of this disorder in the elderly if secondary causes are excluded. Little information is available with respect to the natural history of cluster headaches. Evidence indicates that the episodic and chronic forms of the disorder are often relatively stable and that the disorder can be continue throughout life. Nevertheless, clinical experience and a single prospective study clearly demonstrate that some patients will enter a lasting remission phase with increasing age (Manzoni et al., 1981).

Treatment of cluster headache can be challenging and is well-outlined in Chapter 13 of this volume. Special issues with respect to the pharmacologic agents in the elderly are outlined under migraine. Corticosteroids, which play an important role in transitional prophylaxis, should be used with care in the elderly because of the high prevalence of osteoporosis.

Chronic Daily Headache

Chronic daily headache 1-year prevalence in individuals over the age of 65 years has been reported to be 3.9% in a study from China (Wang et al., 2000) with the prevalence of chronic migraine of 1.6% and chronic tension-type headache of 2.7%. Twenty-five percent were identified as overusing acute headache medications.

In a study of individuals older than 65 years in Italy, the overall prevalence of chronic daily 4.4% in a study from Italy (Prencipe et al., 2001). In the Italian study, the prevalence of chronic migraine was 1.6% and chronic tension-type headache was 1.6%. In the Italian study, acute headache medication overuse was reported in 37.5% of patients with chronic daily headache of which 69.2% had transformed migraine and 23.8% had chronic tension-type headache.

In a population-based study of chronic daily headache in Spain (Castillo et al., 1999), the prevalence of chronic daily headache was 11.5% of women and 0.5% of men greater than 60 years of age. In fact chronic daily headache had its second highest prevalence in women of this age group in this study.

In a population-based study in Norway the prevalence of chronic headache (>14 days per month) was determined for three age groups 60 years and older (Hagen et al., 2000). The prevalence for ages 60–69 years was 3.2% in women and 1.9% in men, for the ages 70–79 years was 2.4% of women and 2.4% of men and in those aged 80 years and older it was 2.3% in women and 2.6% in men. Chronic tension-type headache and chronic migraine headache were not separately reported in these age groups.

Finally, in a population-based study in France, the prevalence of chronic daily headache at ages greater than 65 years was approximately 3% in women and just over 2% in men (Lanteri-Minet et al., 2003).

These studies, while showing some variation in prevalence, clearly demonstrate that chronic daily headache remains a substantial problem in the elderly.

As with younger age groups, chronic daily headache in elderly patients falls primarily into two groups: chronic migraine (or the similar disorder transformed migraine) without or with acute headache medication overuse and chronic tension-type headaches without or with acute headache medication overuse. These challenging disorders are considered in detail in Chapter 12. Clearly when acute headache medication overuse is present, it must be aggressively addressed both to reduce headache frequency and severity and to prevent potential side-effects/toxicity from the chronic use of analgesics and other medications in this age group.

Hypnic Headache

Hypnic headache is a rare headache disorder that was first described by Raskin (1988). He noted, "Over the past ten years six patients have been encountered with a curious sleep-related ('hypnic') headache syndrome, which is clinically distinct from the cluster headache syndrome, yet also occurs with clockwork regularity and appears to be remarkably responsive to the administration of lithium." Raskin's report emphasized that this is a disorder seen in the elderly; subsequent reports have shown that while the elderly are mainly afflicted, younger individuals may develop hypnic headaches, too. There are no epidemiologic studies of hypnic headache but this diagnosis represented one headache diagnosis for every 1400 patients evaluated for headache at one institution (Dodick et al., 1998).

Since Raskin's initial description, there have been approximately 100 cases reported in the literature with a review by Evers and Goadsby (2003) finding a mean onset of age of 63 ± 11 years (range 38–83 years). Women are more commonly affected than men. It has also, been termed "alarm clock" headache due to its occurrence at the same time during sleep. Hypnic headache may be either bilateral (in about 60%) or unilateral. Duration usually ranges from minutes to 3 hours with occasional episodes reported to last up to 6 hours (Evers and Goadsby, 2003). Pain severity is usually moderate with perhaps 20% reporting some severe attacks and an even smaller number describing mild attacks. The frequency of attacks varies from occasional attacks to a near nightly occurrence. Uncommonly, attacks occur during daytime naps (Evers, 2003). The International Headache Society now has criteria for the diagnosis of hypnic headaches, which are outlined in Table 29–2 (Headache Classification Subcommittee of the International Headache Society, 2004).

Reflecting the rarity of the disorder, the natural history is not completely known. In Evers' and Goadsby's (2003) review, only 12 of the 71 individuals were noted to have had a spontaneous remission.

A single case of hypnic headache associated with a posterior fossa meningioma has been reported. The headaches remitted after resection of the tumor (Peatfield and Mendoza, 2003). It is advisable to undertake neuroimaging in patients who present with this headache pattern to help exclude secondary headache disorders.

Many patients have been reported to have coexistent or preexistent primary headache disorders such as migraine and tension-type headache (De Simone et al., 2006).

Table 29–2 Hypnic Headache.

Diagnostic criteria

A. Dull headache fulfilling criteria B–D
B. Develops only during sleep, and awakens patient
C. At least two of the following characteristics:
   Occurs >15 times per month.
   Lasts 15 minutes after waking.
   First occurs after age of 50 years.
D. No autonomic symptoms and no more than one of nausea, photophobia or phonophobia
E. Not attributed to another disorder

Source: Headache Classification Subcommittee of the International Headache Society (2004), 51.

Polysomnography has been done in some patients and a review of the literature found 20 recorded attacks (De Simone et al., 2006). Of these, 15 (75%) arose during rapid eye movement (REM) sleep with two attacks arising during stage 2 and 3 attacks during stage 3 non-REM sleep. Sleep-disordered breathing was found in 7 of 23 patients undergoing polysomnography, but only one attack was definitely time-related to significant hypoxia (De Simone et al., 2006).

The pathophysiology of hypnic headache is unknown. There is speculation that hypnic headache is a REM sleep-related disorder resulting from dysfunction of the brainstem neural network that regulates sleep-wake rhythms. In support of this is experimental data of a substantial decrease of dorsal raphe nucleus activity during REM phases of sleep. Along with the periaqueductal gray, the dorsal raphe nucleus also plays a role in antinociception. An impairment of these areas that are involved in regulation of sleep-wake cycles and pain processing might account for the headache arising during sleep (De Simone et al., 2006). The report by many patients that the onset of headache occurs at the same time during the night raises the question whether the attacks are controlled by a time-related process, perhaps in the suprachiasmatic nuclei of the hypothalamus. These nuclei have connections with the periaqueductal gray. The function of the hypothalamic-pineal axis, and in particular, the suprachiasmatic nuclei is diminished in advanced age and melatonin secretion is decreased. One might speculate that the reduction of melatonin may predispose certain patients to headache. (Evers and Goadsby, 2003).

A variety of treatments for acute treatment of hypnic headache have been utilized. Aspirin and ergotamine have been helpful in some cases. Sumatriptan via injection has usually been ineffective (Evers and Goadsby 2003). Rizatriptan has been reported to be acutely effective in a single case (Schurks et al., 2006).

Many medications have been utilized for prophylaxis (Evers and Goadsby 2003). As observed by Raskin (1988), lithium is usually effective (in a dose of 300–600 mg at bedtime). Tolerability of this agent can be problematic, though. Indomethacin in a dose of 75 mg at bedtime is effective in some patients. Caffeine 40–60 mg at bedtime can also be effective. There have been single or small numbers of cases reporting verapamil, melatonin, gabapentin, prednisone, pizotifen, and acetazolamide as sometimes effective (Evers and Goadsby, 2003). There are also recent cases reported to respond to topiramate (Guido and Specchio, 2006) or pregabalin (Ulrich et al., 2006).

Other Primary Headache Disorders

In addition to those already outlined, there are several other primary headache disorders. These include the trigeminal autonomic cephalalgias as well as other disorders. Of these, SUNCT (short-lasting unilateral neuralgiform headache attacks with conjunctival injection and tearing) and SUNA (short-lasting unilateral neuralgiform headache attacks with autonomic features) have been noted to occur not infrequently after the age of 50 years. In a report of 43 cases of SUNCT and 9 cases of SUNA, Cohen et al. (2006) noted that the average age was over age 50 years with the oldest patient in the series 87 years old. There is the report of one patient who presented at age 88 years with new onset SUNCT (The differential diagnosis of these disorders and their treatment are outlined in Chapter 13.

SECONDARY HEADACHES

Secondary headaches account for a higher proportion of new onset headaches in the elderly than in younger individuals. For example, the Italian study, 15.3% had symptomatic (secondary) headaches (Prencipe et al., 2001). Clinic-based experience also confirms that secondary headaches make up a higher proportion of elderly who present with new headache (Solomon et al., 1990). The differential diagnosis of secondary headaches is broad and includes medication-induced headaches, space-occupying lesions, central nervous system (CNS) infections, cerebrovascular disease, giant cell arteritis, disorders affecting cranial structures (e.g., acute angle closure glaucoma) and can be a manifestation of angina. Accordingly, the clinician must approach each elderly individual with recent onset or worsening headaches as potentially having a secondary cause for their symptomatology. Secondary headaches are considered in several other chapters in this book; only a select group, which has particular relevance to the elderly, is reviewed here.

Headaches Associated with Vascular Disorders

While cerebrovascular disorders occur in over a wide range of ages, stroke is more common in the elderly. Both cerebral ischemia and hemorrhage may be preceded or accompanied by headache. Accordingly, the possibility of a cerebrovascular cause must be given careful consideration in older patients with new onset headaches. Please see Chapter 16 for additional details.

Giant cell arteritis is a disorder that rarely occurs before age 50 years and becomes increasingly common with increasing age. It needs to be considered in every patient aged 50 and older with new onset headaches. This disorder is discussed in detail in Chapter 25.

Headaches Associated with Intracranial Disease

Malignant brain tumors occur more common in the elderly than in younger patients with a relative risk in the United States of 3.86 for those individuals greater than 65 years of age compared to individuals 20–65 years of age (Deorah et al., 2006). In addition, meningiomas, which account for approximately 25% of all intracranial neoplasms in the US, have increasing prevalence with increasing age; the risk continues to rise in the elderly beyond age 85 years (Claus et al., 2005). Another major source of intracranial tumors is metastases from systemic cancers. Headache is a frequent presenting complaint of brain tumors (Forsyth and Posner, 1993) although it is usually not the only symptom (Vázquez-Barquero et al., 1994) and often there are abnormalities on neurologic examination. Patients with a previous history of primary headaches such as tension-type headaches or migraine headaches may present with headaches of similar phenotype (Forsyth and Posner, 1993) as a result of an intracranial neoplasm. Accordingly, it is paramount that the physicians have a high index of suspicion for possible intracranial tumors in elderly patients who present with new or different headaches. A low threshold for obtaining neuroimaging should be maintained.

Subdural hematomas can present acutely or subacutely. While usually a result of head trauma, this may be trivial and not recalled by the elderly patient. In the elderly, these are more likely to present in a chronic fashion over weeks to months often with headache, focal neurologic symptoms and cognitive changes (Roger et al., 2006). Once again, a high index of suspicion must be maintained so that the diagnosis is not overlooked.

Headaches Associated with Disorders of the Neck, Head, and Cranial Structures

Criteria for the diagnosis of cervicogenic headache are outlined by the International Headache Society (Headache Classification Subcommittee of the International Headache Society, 2004). Associated notes in the criteria indicate that cervical spondylosis and osteochondritis are NOT accepted as valid causes of cervicogenic headache. Accordingly, it is prudent not to attribute headaches to these conditions, which are not infrequently present in the elderly. While some cervical pathology may be responsible for headaches, experts note the controversy in the literature surrounding the diagnosis of this entity (Bogduk, 2004). Please see Chapter 20 for additional information.

Acute angle closure glaucoma is more common over the age of 50 years (Foster, 2002). Acute glaucoma typically presents with severe pain, nausea with or without vomiting, photophobia, visual halos, redness, and reduced vision.

Signs on examination include conjunctival injection, hazy cornea, fixed and mid-dilated pupil, and markedly elevated intraocular pressure (Lewis and Fourman, 1998). In the elderly, the presentation may be atypical with headache, malaise, and nausea and vomiting with the typical symptoms overshadowed by these (Gandhewar and Kamath, 2005). To further complicate matters, there is the syndrome of subacute angle-closure glaucoma (Lewis and Fourman 1998; Shindler et al., 2005). Patients with this disorder have mild to moderate intermittent symptoms with episodes manifested by blurred vision, facial pain or headache, and often nausea and/or vomiting. The episodes usually last 1–4 hours and can occur at any time of day. Affected individuals have no symptoms between attacks with an eye that is white and normal in appearance. It is of paramount importance that these diagnoses be carefully considered and patients for whom there is a high index of suspicion for these disorders be appropriately referred for gonioscopy, which is critical for diagnosis. If these disorders remain undiagnosed they can lead to permanent ocular damage with permanent visual loss. See Chapter 21 for additional information.

Headaches Associated with Disorders of Homeostasis

A variety of homeostatic disorders have been linked to headache. Some of these are more likely to be seen in the elderly than in other age groups.

Sleep apnea has been linked to headaches. These are typically present on awakening and are bilateral with few associated features. They resolve within 30 minutes and cease with effective treatment of sleep apnea (Headache Classification Subcommittee of the International Headache Society, 2004).

Cardiac cephalalgia is headache that is associated with myocardial ischemia. Six percent of 150 consecutive patients had head pain on at least some occasions with angina, but typically not as an isolated symptom (Sampson and Cheitlin, 1971). Rarely, headache is the only symptom related to myocardial ischemia. It typically occurs in the context of exertion or other activities that provoke angina. Accordingly it is an uncommon cause of exertional headache (Vernay et al., 1989; Lipton et al., 1997). The diagnosis is usually confirmed by a positive cardiac stress test, which shows evidence of cardiac ischemia at a time coincident with development of the headache and with resolution of the headaches after successful treatment of the cardiac ischemia. The mechanism of cardiac cephalalgia is likely secondary to convergence of sympathetic or vagal afferent input and convergence of Lissauer's tract with upper cervical root input (to explain posterior headache) or with the pars caudalis of the trigeminal nucleus and tract (to explain anterior headache) (Grace et al., 1997).

Headache associated with dialysis occurs following hemodialysis, typically resolving within 72 hours of dialysis. Sometimes this is associated with obtundation or coma. There is some evidence to suggest a low serum magnesium, perhaps coupled with a high serum sodium predisposes to dialysis headache although other factors may well play a role (Goksel et al., 2006).

Headaches Associated with a Substance or its Withdrawal

The elderly often have multiple medical problems and accordingly are taking many pharmacologic agents. Many medications are associated with the development of headaches. Table 29–3, although not exhaustive, lists several medications that can be associated with headaches. In addition, both caffeine and alcohol can be associated with their consumption or withdrawal and accordingly, their use should be determined in all patients. Headaches associated with medication use may be nonspecific but sometimes have characteristics associated with migraine.

Treatment primarily involves tapering and withdrawal of potentially offending agents when this is feasible. Sometimes the presumed offending agent is necessary for treatment of a significant medical problem and no alternatives are available. Treatment may necessitate addition of a medication to manage the headaches.

Trigeminal neuralgia, which has a high prevalence in the elderly, is not addressed in this chapter since this is rarely confused diagnostically with other headache disorders. Please see Chapter 24 for information on this topic and other cranial neuralgias.

Table 29–3 Partial List of Medications Associated with Headache.

- Antibiotics
  Tetracyclines, trimethoprim-sulfamethoxazole, metronidazole, nitrofurantoin, rifampin, isoniazid, griseofulvin
- Antiplatelet agent
  Dipyridamole
- Bronchodilators
  Aminophylline, theophylline, pseudoephedrine
- Cardiovascular
  Vasodilators (nitrates, nicotinic acid) Antihypertensives (nifedipine, methyldopa, reserpine, hydralazine, some calcium antagonists) Antiarrhythmics (quinidine, digoxin)
- CNS
  Sedatives (alcohol, barbiturates, benzodiazepines) Stimulants (caffeine, methylphenidate) Antiparkinsonians (amantadine, levodopa, bromocriptine) Antidepressants [trazodone and selective serotonin reuptake inhibitors (SSRIs)]
- Endocrinologic
  Octreotide
- Gastrointestinal
  Cimetidine, omeprazole, ondansetron, ranitidine
- Hematologic or oncologic
  Erythropoietin, tamoxifen
- Hemorheologic
  Pentoxifylline
- Immunosuppressant
  Cyclosporine, sirolimus, everolimus
- Immunologic
  Interferons, immunoglobulins, alemtuzumab
- Nonsteroidal antiinflammatory drugs (NSAIDs)
  Indomethacin, diclofenac, piroxicam
- Reproductive
  Estrogens, selective inhibitors of cyclic guanosine monophosphate (cGMP)-specific phosphodiesterase type 5 (PDE5)

Source: SD Silberstein, DJ Capobianco, and DW Dodick (2003). Migraine in special populations. Neurology, 60 (Suppl. 2):S50–S57; Headache Classification Subcommittee of the International Headache Society (2004), 144.

References

Boardman, HF, Thomas, E, Croft, PR, et al. (2003). Epidemiology of headache in an English district. *Cephalalgia,* 23:129–137.

Bogduk, N (2004). The neck and headaches. *Neurol Clin,* 22:151–171.

Castillo, J, Munoz, P, Guitera, V, et al. (1999). Epidemiology of chronic daily headache in the general population. *Headache,* 39:190–196.

Claus, EB,Bondy, ML, Schildkraut, JM, et al. (2005). Epidemiology of intracranial meningioma. *Neurosurgery,* 57:1088–1095.

Cohen, AS, Matharu, MS, and Goadsby, PJ (2006). Short-lasting unilateral neuralgiform headache attacks with conjunctival injection and tearing (SUNCT) or cranial autonomic features (SUNA)—a prospective clinical study of SUNCT and SUNA. *Brain,* 129:2746–2760.

Cook, NR, Evans, DA, Funkenstein, HH, et al. (1989). Correlates of headache in a population-based cohort of elderly. *Arch Neurol,* 46:1338–1344.

D'Alessandro, R, Benassi, G, Lenzi, PL, et al. (1988). Epidemiology of headache in the Republic of San Marino. *J Neurol Neurosurg Psychiatr,* 51:21–27.

Deorah, S, Lynch, CF, Sibenaller, ZA, et al. (2006). Trends in brain cancer incidence and survival in the United States: Surveillance, Epidemiology, and End Results Program, 1973 to 2001. *Neurosurg Focus,* 20:E1.

De Simone, R, Marano, E, Ranieri, A, et al. (2006). Hypnic headache: an update. *Neurol Sci,* 27(Suppl. 2): S144–S148.

Dodick, DW, Mosek, AC, and Campbell, JK (1998). The hypnic ("alarm clock") headache syndrome. *Cephalalgia,* 18:152–156.

Domingues, RB, Kuster, GW, Dutra, LA, et al. (2004) Headache epidemiology in Vitória, Espírito Santo. *Arq Neuropsiquiatr,* 62:588–591.

Ekbom, K, Svensson, DA, Pedersen, NL, et al. (2006). Lifetime prevalence and concordance risk of cluster headache in the Swedish twin population. *Neurology,* 67:798–803.

Evers, S and Goadsby, PJ (2003). Hypnic headache: clinical features, pathophysiology, and treatment. *Neurology,* 60:905–909.

Fisher, CM (1980). Late-life migraine accompaniments as a cause of unexplained transient ischemic attacks. *Can J Neurol Sci,* 7:9–17.

Forsyth, PA and Posner, JB (1993). Headaches in patients with brain tumors: a study of 111 patients. *Neurology,* 43:1678–1683.

Foster, PJ (2002). The epidemiology of primary angle closure and associated glaucomatous optic neuropathy. *Semin Ophthalmol,* 17:50–58.

Gandhewar, RR and Kamath, GG (2005). Acute glaucoma presentations in the elderly. *Emerg Med J,* 22:306–307.

Giddens, A, Duneier, M, and Appelbaum, RP (2003). *Introduction to Sociology.* WW. Norton Company, New York.

Goksel, BK, Torun, D, Karaca, S, et al. (2006). Is low blood magnesium level associated with hemodialysis headache? *Headache*, 46:40–45.

Grace, A, Horgan, J, Breathnach, K, et al. (1997). Anginal headache and its basis. *Cephalalgia*, 17:195–196.

Guido, N and Specchio, LM (2006). Successful treatment of hypnic headache with topiramate: a case report. *Headache*, 46:1205–1206.

Hagen, K, Zwart, J-A, Vatten, L, et al. (2000). Prevalence of migraine and nonmigrainous headache—head-HUNT, a large population-based study. *Cephalalgia*, 20:900–906.

Hale, WE, Perkins, LL, May, FE, et al. (1986). Symptom prevalence in the elderly. An evaluation of age, sex, disease, and medication use. *J Am Geriatr Soc*, 34:333–340.

Headache Classification Subcommittee of the International Headache Society (2004). *Cephalalgia*, 24 (Suppl. 1):1–160.

Igarashi, H and Sakai, F (1996). Natural history of cluster history. *Cephalalgia*, 16:390–391. Abstract.

Lake, AE (2001). Behavioral and nonpharmacologic treatments of headache. *Med Clin North Am*, 85:1055–1075.

Lanteri-Minet, M, Auray, JP, El Hasnaoui, A, et al. (2003). Prevalence and description of chronic daily headache in the general population in France. *Pain*, 102:143–149.

Lewis, J, and Fourman, S (1998). Subacute angle-closure glaucoma as a cause of headache in the presence of a white eye. *Headache*, 38:684–686.

Lipton, RB, Lowenkopf, T, Bajwa, ZH, et al. (1997). Cardiac cephalgia: a treatable form of exertional headache. *Neurology*, 49:813–816.

Lipton, RB, Stewart, WF, Diamond, S et al. (2001). Prevalence and burden of migraine in the United States: data from the American Migraine Study II. *Headache*, 41:646–657.

Manzoni, GC, Terzano, MG, Moretti, G, et al. (1981). Clinical observations in 76 cluster headache cases. *Eur Neurol*, 20:88–94.

Martins, KM, Bordini, CA, Bigal, ME, et al. (2006). Migraine in the Elderly: a comparison with migraine in young adults. *Headache*, 46:312–316.

Mattsson, P, Svärdsudd, K, Lundberg, PO, et al. (2000). The prevalence of migraine in women aged 40-74 years: a population-based study. *Cephalalgia*, 20:893–899.

McFayden, D (1990). International demographic trends. In RL Kane, JG Evans, and D McFayden (eds) *Improving the Health of Older People: A World View* (pp. 19–29). New York: Oxford University Press.

Oates, JA (2006). The science of drug therapy. In *Goodman & Gilman's The Pharmacological Basis of Therapeutics* (11th edn.), Chapter 5. (LL Brunton, KL Parker, ILO Buxton, and DK Blumenthal, eds.). Access Medicine/ McGraw-Hill. Available: http://www.accessmedicine.com/content.aspx?aID=950923 [November 14, 2006].

Peatfield, RC and Mendoza, ND (2003). Posterior fossa meningioma presenting as hypnic headache. *Headache*, 43:1007–1008.

Prencipe, M, Casini, AR, Ferretti, C, et al. (2001). Prevalence of headache in an elderly population: attack frequency, disability, and use of medication. *J Neurol Neurosurg Psychiatr*, 70:377–381.

Raskin, NH (1988). The hypnic headache syndrome. *Headache*, 28:534–536.

Roger, EP, Butler, J, and Benzel, EC (2006). Neurosurgery in the elderly: brain tumors and subdural hematomas. *Clin Geriatr Med*, 22:623–644.

Sampson, JJ and Cheitlin, MD (1971), Pathophysiology and differential diagnosis of Cardiac Pain. *Prog Cardiovacular Dis*, 13:507–531.

Schurks, M, Kastrup, O, and Diener, HC (2006). Triptan responsive hypnic headache? *Eur J Neurol*, 13:666–667.

Schwartz, BS, Stewart, WF, Simon, D.et al. (1998). Epidemiology of tension-type headache. *JAMA*, 279:381–383.

Seidler, S, Marthol, H, Pawlowski, M, et al. (2006). Cluster headache in a ninety one year old woman. *Headache*, 46:179–180.

Shindler, KS, Sankar, PS, Volpe, NJ, et al. (2005). Intermittent headaches as the presenting sign of subacute angle-closure glaucoma. *Neurology*, 65:757–758

Silberstein, SD and Young, WB (1998). Headache. In MSJ Pathy (ed.), *Principles and Practice of Geriatric Medicine* (3rd edn., pp. 733–746). New York: John Wiley and Sons.

Solomon, GD, Kunkel, RS Jr., and Frame, J (1990). Demographics of headache in elderly patients. *Headache*, 30:273–276.

Tonon, C, Guttmann, S, Volpini, M et al. (2002). Prevalence and incidence of cluster headache in the Republic of San Marino. *Neurology*, 58:1407–1409.

Torelli, P, Beghi, E, and Manzoni, GC (2005). Cluster headache prevalence in the Italian general population. *Neurology*, 64:469–474.

Ulrich, K, Gunreben, B, Lang, E et al. (2006). Pregabalin in the therapy of hypnic headache. *Cephalalgia*, 26:1031–1032.

Vázquez-Barquero, A, Ibánez, FJ, Herrera, S et al. (1994). Isolated headache as the presenting clinical manifestation of intracranial tumors: a prospective study. *Cephalalgia*, 14:270–272.

Vernay, D., Deffond, D, Fraysse, P et al. (1989). Walk headache: an unusual manifestation of ischemic heart disease. *Headache*, 29:350–351.

Vikelis, M, Xifaras, M, and Mitsikostas, DD (2005). SUNCT syndrome in the elderly. *Cephalalgia*, 25:1091–1092.

Wang, SJ, Liu, HC, Fuh, JL, et al. (1997). Prevalence of headaches in a Chinese elderly population in Kinmen: age and gender effect and cross-cultural comparisons. *Neurology*, 49:195–200.

Wang, SJ, Fuh, JL, Lu, SR, et al. (2000). Chronic daily headache in Chinese elderly: prevalence, risk factors, and biannual follow-up. *Neurology*, 54:314–319.

Waters, WE (1974). The Pontypridd headache survey. *Headache*, 14:81–90.

30 Behavioral Management of Headache

Kenneth A Holroyd, Donald B Penzien, Jeanetta C Rains, Gay L Lipchik, and Dawn C Buse

HAROLD WOLFF'S VISION

Like many pioneers, Harold G Wolff, MD, is honored but ignored. He is justifiably honored for his groundbreaking formulation of scientific (i.e., testable) hypotheses about the pathophysiology of migraine and tension headache and for his experimental work that established the study of benign headache as a legitimate scientific enterprise. At the same time, the thesis of over two decades of Wolff's work—that to truly understand psychophysiological disorders such as headache we need to understand how psychosocial and physiological variables interact to induce headache episodes—is ignored (Wolff, 1948; Wolff and Wolff, 1948; Wolff, 1953; Simmons and Wolff, 1954). Toward this end, Wolff pioneered innovative methods of observing psychological and physiological responses as people coped with naturalistic stressors, or with cleverly designed laboratory stressors. He also vigorously pursued efforts to integrate knowledge from the social and medical sciences that would be necessary to this understanding. The monograph *Social Science and Medicine* (co-authored with Dr. Leo Simmons) states Wolff's thesis concisely: "In our opinion . . . it is the joint province of both social and physical (medical) scientists to work on the central linkage, namely, how specified stresses work to evoke particular (psychophysiological) reaction patterns" (pp. 144–145; Simmons and Wolff, 1954). Wolff's focus on psychophysiology—the interaction of psychological and physiological variables—in generating headaches and his emphasis on the integration of relevant knowledge from the social and medical sciences would place him in the mainstream of behavioral medicine today.

Preparation of this chapter was supported in part by National Institutes of Health (NIH) (NINDS 32374).

OVERVIEW OF BEHAVIORAL INTERVENTIONS

Self-management refers to the active involvement of the individual in the management of his or her chronic disease, and is specifically defined as "the individual's ability to manage the symptoms, treatments, physical and psychosocial consequences and lifestyle changes inherent in living with a chronic condition" (Barlow et al., 2002). As depicted in Fig. 30–1, the effective self-management of chronic headache disorders requires that the individual: (1) self-monitor headache-relevant information (e.g., early headache warning signs, headache triggers, acute medication use, and medication response), (2) possess specific behavioral headache management skills as well as general problem solving skills, and (3) possess the motivation and confidence (self-efficacy) necessary to effectively adapt and use these skills in daily life. Chronic disease self-management models embody active patient/healthcare provider collaboration, with considerable responsibility on the part of patients to manage their own disorders (Holroyd and Creer, 1986). With counsel from the healthcare provider, the patient assumes the lion's share of the responsibility to (1) engage in daily health promotion and behaviors that prevent or limit exacerbations of his/her disease or disorder, and (2) enact predetermined medication and behavioral treatment strategies when symptoms do occur.

Self-management interventions designed to help individuals manage chronic disorders such as arthritis, asthma, diabetes, and low back pain

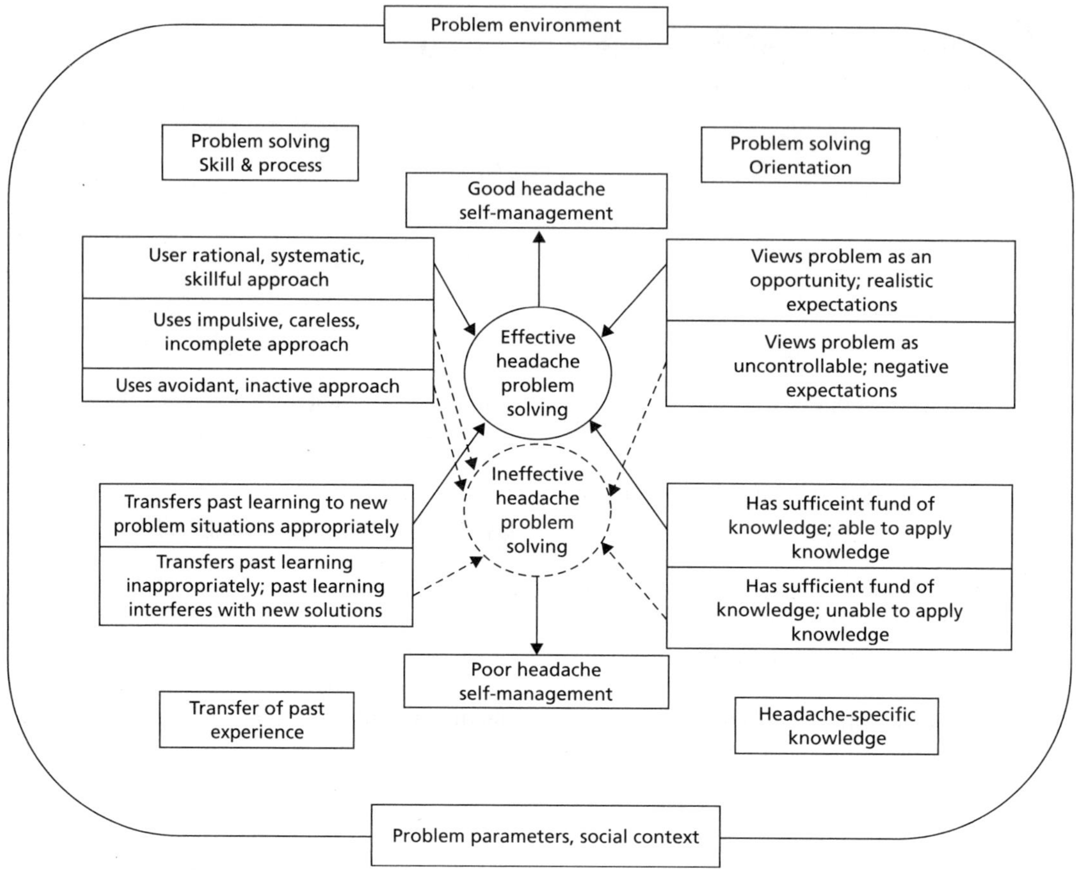

Figure 30–1 Expectances, knowledge, and problem-solving skills required for effective self-management of chronic headaches. (Adapted from Hills-Briggs, 2003.)

have proven effective in reducing symptoms, disability, and, in some cases, medical costs (Von Korff et al., 1997; Lorig et al., 2001; Lorig and Holman, 2003; Holman and Lorig, 2004; Newman et al., 2004). Unfortunately, the application of self-management interventions in the headache disorders has lagged behind applications with other chronic disorders (Penzien et al., 2004).

Behavioral Interventions

Behavior therapies are well suited as a treatment option for headache sufferers who have at least one of the following characteristics: (1) preference for nonpharmacologic interventions; (2) poor tolerance of pharmacologic treatment; (3) medical contraindications for pharmacologic treatments; (4) inadequate response to pharmacologic treatment; (5) pregnancy, planned pregnancy, or nursing; (6) history of excessive use of analgesic or other acute medications; and (7) life stress, deficient coping skills or comorbid psychological disorder that aggravate headache problems or disability. The long-term goals of behavior therapy include: reduced frequency and severity of headaches, reduced headache-related disability and affective distress, reduced reliance on poorly tolerated or unwanted pharmacotherapies, and enhanced personal control of headaches. Behavioral interventions specifically targeting the modifiable risk factors for the progression of migraine from episodic to chronic and daily progression are likely to prove fruitful (Lipton and Pan, 2004; Bigal and Lipton, 2006).

The three behavioral interventions described below each provide a different set of skills for managing headaches and headache-related disability and are best used in the context of self-management training as described earlier. Although these treatments attempt to influence both the frequency and the severity of headaches, they emphasize the *prevention* of headache episodes.

Relaxation Training

Relaxation training is a basic skill and an introduction to the use of behavioral headache self-management that should probably be included in all self-management programs. Relaxation skills (Bernstein et al., 2000) enable headache sufferers to exert control over specific headache-related physiological responses and to lower physiological and mental arousal. Patients are instructed to practice a graduated hierarchy of relaxation techniques (diaphragmatic breathing, progressive muscle relaxation, relaxation imagery, meditation) initially for 20–30 minutes per day; then they are able to master increasingly brief relaxation techniques (cue controlled relaxation, self-control relaxation), to relax briefly (e.g., for 30 seconds) throughout the day, and whenever they notice mental or bodily signs of tension, or signs signaling headache onset.

Cognitive-behavior Therapy

Cognitive-behavior therapy provides an overall framework not only for teaching skills for both managing and coping with headaches but also for addressing the comorbid psychological problems commonly seen in the headache clinic setting. Cognitive-behavior therapy addresses the cognitive, affective, and behavioral factors that influence headaches and increase headache-related disability (Holroyd et al., 1998; Lipchik et al., 2002). Patients monitor the circumstances in which their headaches occur or worsen and the thoughts and feelings surrounding these headaches. Once stressful or high-disability situations are identified, dysfunctional cognitions are identified and challenged. Cognitive targets are stress-, pain-, or disability-generating *thoughts* (e.g., "Catastrophizing") and the *beliefs* that help generate these thoughts (e.g., "I'm unable to tolerate pain and *must* have immediate relief"). The goal is to teach patients to "catch" and challenge these thoughts, thus managing headache-related stress, reducing disability, and enhancing positive coping efforts. Cognitive problem-solving skills also help patients address environmental sources of stress or reinforcements for disability, as well as barriers to the effective application of behavioral headache management skills (where these are potentially changeable). Problem-solving skills also help patients solve problems that will inevitably be encountered as they attempt to integrate newly learned headache management skills into their unique daily routine.

Biofeedback Training

The incorporation of biofeedback training into a self-management program is likely to depend on headache diagnosis, patient interest, and available resources. Thermal (hand warming) feedback—feedback of skin temperature from a finger—and electromyographic (EMG) feedback—feedback of electrical activity from muscles of the scalp, neck, and sometimes the upper body—are the most commonly used biofeedback modalities, although electroencephalographic ("neurofeedback") biofeedback with the goal of teaching self-regulation of cortical excitability has received recent attention (Schwartz and Andrasik, 2003). Patients are instructed to use a home biofeedback training device or to practice the self-regulation skills they are learning during clinic-based biofeedback training sessions for approximately 20–30 minutes per day. As they master physiological self-regulation skills, they are encouraged to integrate their use of self-regulation skills into their daily routine in the same manner as described earlier for relaxation skills.

Behavioral Treatment Formats

Behavioral treatment for headache can be administered individually or in a group, and in a clinic-based, limited-contact, and, possibly, even without face-to-face contact with a behavioral clinician via telephone, the Internet, or mass media.

Clinic-based Treatment

Clinic-based treatments typically involve 6–12 weekly sessions, 45–60 minutes long for individual treatment, and 60–120 minutes for a group. Although this format provides more healthcare provider time and attention and allows the provider greater observation of the patient than does a limited therapist contact format, it is more costly in regard to clinician time and patient travel. Descriptions of clinic-based treatments are available in Blanchard and Andrasik (1985) for individual treatment, and Scharff and Marcus (1994) for group treatment.

Limited-contact Treatment

The limited therapist contact treatments have employed the therapy components adapted from the standard clinic-based behavioral treatments described earlier, but the intervention typically involves only three to four monthly treatment sessions. Clinic visits introduce headache management skills and address problems encountered in acquiring or using these skills. Patient manuals and audio recordings typically guide the learning and refinement of skills that are practiced at home, with clinician assistance via phone calls. Lipchik et al., (2002) and Blanchard and Andrasik (1985) provide detailed descriptions of limited-contact treatment.

Nonprofessional Administered Treatment

The self-management literature has emphasized the use of groups led by trained nonprofessional leaders who suffer from a chronic disorder. Well-established training and certification programs have been established for lay leaders, and detailed guides for conducting lay-led but professionally supervised self-management groups for chronic disorders such as arthritis, asthma, diabetes, and chronic back pain have been established (e.g., http://patienteducation.stanford.edu). Recently, lay-led group education or self-management groups have also been evaluated for the management of migraine (Merelle et al., 2006, in press; Rothrock et al., 2006).

No Contact Treatment

No contact treatment refers here to programs that are designed to enable individuals to acquire and successfully use behavioral headache management skills without either clinic visits or face-to-face instruction from a behavioral clinician. Learning at home or at the workplace, community library, or other setting may be supervised by a behavioral clinician via the telephone or via the Internet. Alternately, the need for supervision by a "live" behavioral clinician might be eliminated by building the clinicians functions into the home study program (Nicholson et al., 2005). In medical settings, no contact treatment has the potential to dramatically increase access to behavioral treatment by enabling even healthcare providers without access to a behaviorally trained clinician to include behavioral treatment in the medical management of headaches.

EFFICACY OF BEHAVIORAL TREATMENTS

Since the mid-twentieth century, behavioral headache research literature has grown, matured scientifically, and had a substantive impact on contemporary headache management. The past three decades have amassed a considerable evidence base addressing behavioral headache treatments. Behavioral headache research productivity has continued to grow in both number and breadth of studies. Publication trends show greater proportions of controlled than uncontrolled trials, and assessment of a broadening range of behavioral and functional variables pertinent to average headache sufferer (Rains et al., 2005).

A number of meta-analytic reviews of the behavioral literature have been published using varying study inclusion/exclusion criteria. Whereas the majority of these reviews have included evidence from all the available treatment studies regardless of experimental design or publication status, the most recent meta-analyses have selectively summarized only well-designed and reported randomized and controlled trials. The sections that follow summarize these reviews and compare the findings derived from the differing review methodologies. Meta-analyses are described for the migraine, tension-type headache (TTH), and limited-contact therapy format literatures.

Behavioral Treatments for Migraine

With support from the Agency for Healthcare Research and Quality (AHRQ), Goslin and colleagues (1999) employed conservative study inclusion criteria to produce a comprehensive meta-analysis of the behavioral literature. Their literature search identified 355 articles describing behavioral and physical treatments for migraine, of which 70 reported controlled trials of behavioral migraine treatments for adults. Thirty-nine trials met all of their stringent design and data requirements, and those trials in turn yielded 60 treatment groups [e.g., relaxation training, temperature biofeedback, cognitive-behavioral therapy (stress-management training), wait list control]. Outcome data were calculated using two metrics: summary effect size estimates and mean percentage headache improvement from pretreatment to posttreatment. The behavioral treatments yielded 32%–49% reductions in migraine versus 5% reduction for no-treatment controls (Fig. 30–2). The effect size estimates indicated that relaxation training, thermal biofeedback combined with relaxation, EMG biofeedback, and cognitive-behavioral therapy all were statistically more effective than wait list control.

Based upon the evidence provided by the AHRQ meta-analysis, the *U.S. Headache Consortium* (a multidisciplinary assemblage of seven professional practice organizations; Silberstein, 2000) made the following recommendations pertaining to behavioral interventions for migraine: (1) relaxation training, thermal biofeedback combined with relaxation training, EMG biofeedback, and cognitive-behavioral therapy may be considered as treatment options for the prevention of migraine (Grade A Evidence), and (2) behavioral therapy may be combined with preventive drug therapy to achieve added clinical improvement for migraine (Grade B Evidence) (Campbell et al., 1999). Focused upon the management of migraine by the primary care practitioner, the

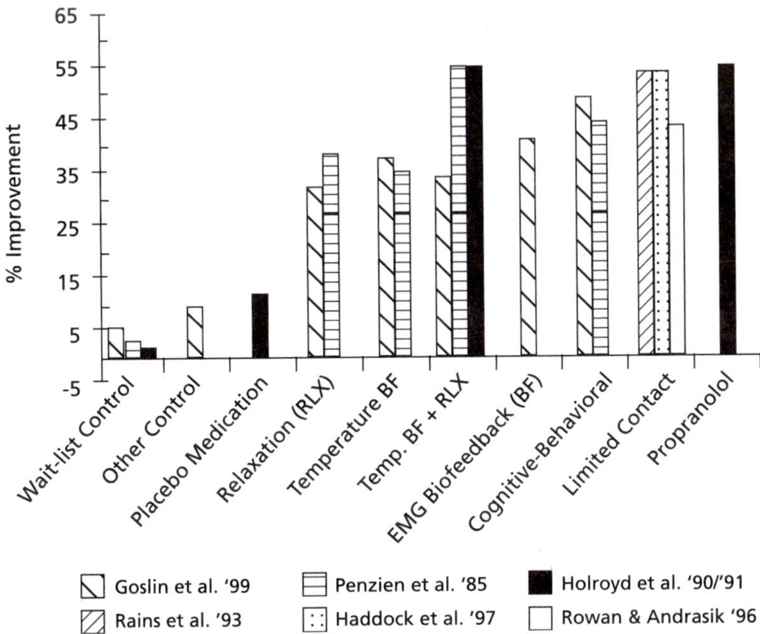

Figure 30–2 Outcome scores of various meta-analyses of behavioral and pharmacological treatments for migraine: Percent improvement scores by treatment condition. BF, biofeedback training; RLX, relaxation training.

guideline is available online in its entirety (http://www.aan.com/).

Unlike the AHRQ-sponsored meta-analysis (1999), which employed highly selective study inclusion criteria, all of the earlier meta-analyses were maximally inclusive of the available evidence (Blanchard et al., 1980; Blanchard and Andrasik, 1982; Penzien, Holroyd, Holm, et al., 1985; Holroyd and Penzien, 1990). Despite their differing study inclusion criteria, the findings of the earlier meta-analyses closely paralleled the AHRQ review, indicating that behavioral treatments for migraine headache are effective (35%–55% improvement) and more effective than control conditions (Fig. 30–2).

The most recent meta-analysis of behavioral headache therapies examined trials of biofeedback training for migraine (Nestoriuc and Martin, 2007). Their literature search identified 86 outcome studies, of which 55 met inclusion criteria. Biofeedback therapies overall yielded a medium effect size ($d = 0.58$, 95% CI = 0.52, 0.64), were more effective than control conditions, and proved stable over an average follow-up of 17 months. Moderator analyses revealed that biofeedback in combination with home training was more effective than therapies without home training. There was no substantial relationship between study validity ratings and treatment effects, and intention-to-treat analysis showed that treatment effects remained stable when drop-outs were considered nonresponders.

Behavioral Versus Pharmacologic Therapies

While comparative efficacy of pharmacologic versus behavioral therapies for migraine has only rarely been assessed in head-to-head studies, meta-analytic comparisons have shown similar levels of improvement in migraine with propranolol (32 trials) and combined relaxation and biofeedback training (35 trials) (Holroyd and Penzien, 1990; Holroyd et al., 1991). By comparison, only a 12% average improvement was achieved with placebo medication (see Fig. 30–2). While similar meta-analytic comparisons of behavioral interventions with other preventive drug therapies are not available, there is little to suggest that findings would differ. Direct comparisons of preventive medications have given no indication that there are differences in effectiveness in the general samples of migraine sufferer typically included in clinical trials. Thus, preventive pharmacologic and behavioral therapies appear to be similarly viable interventions for migraine patients.

Behavioral Treatments for TTH

McCrory and colleagues (2001) reported a meta-analysis of behavioral treatments for TTH that employed the methodology closely paralleling the AHRQ-sponsored behavioral migraine review (Goslin et al., 1999). Like the latter review, McCrory and colleagues' employed conservative study inclusion criteria to produce their meta-analysis and selectively included only randomized, controlled trials. Their literature search identified 107 articles describing behavioral treatments for TTH. The 35 randomized and controlled trials that met the stringent study inclusion criteria yielded 77 treatment groups (e.g., relaxation training, EMG biofeedback, cognitive-behavioral therapy, wait list control). For comparison, outcome data from the three extant controlled trials evaluating amitriptyline for TTH (commonly prescribed for prophylaxis) was similarly extracted. As for the AHRQ migraine review (Goslin et al., 1999), outcome data were calculated using summary effect size estimates and average improvement from pretreatment to posttreatment. Behavioral treatments yielded 37%–50% reduction in headache versus 2% reduction for wait list, and 9% for other controls (Fig. 30–3). The effect size estimates indicated that statistically all of the behavioral interventions were more effective than wait list control.

The review by McCrory and colleagues (2001) is the only meta-analysis of TTH literature date to employ highly selective study inclusion criteria (similar to Goslin et al. for migraine). Other meta-analyses of this literature were maximally inclusive of the available evidence (Blanchard et al., 1980; Holroyd and Penzien, 1986; Bogaards and terKuile, 1994). Despite their differing study inclusion criteria, the findings of the earlier meta-analyses closely paralleled those of McCrory and colleagues' (2001), indicating that behavioral treatments for TTH are efficacious (35%–55% headache improvement) and more effective than

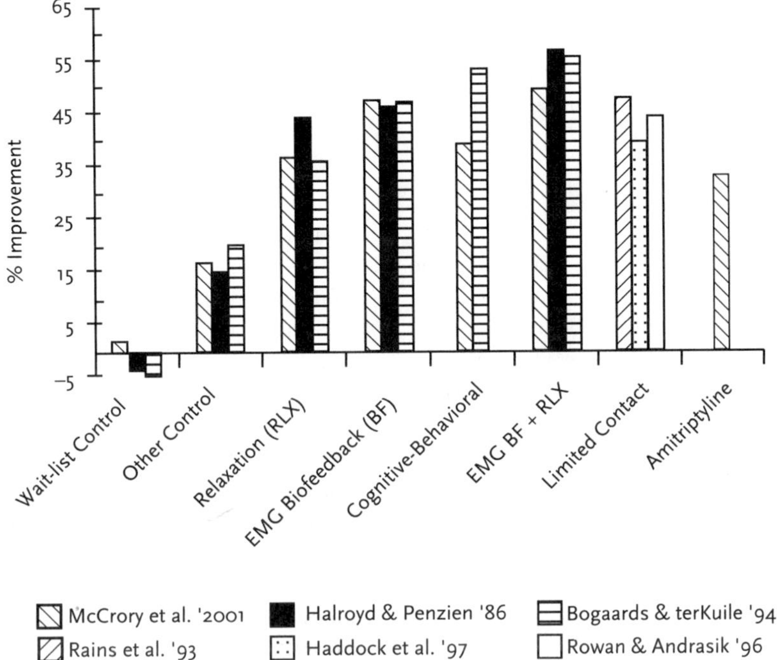

Figure 30–3 Outcome scores of various meta-analyses of behavioral and pharmacological treatments for tension-type headache: percent improvement scores by treatment condition. RLX, relaxation training.

control conditions (see Fig. 30–2). The three controlled trials of amitriptyline for TTH reviewed by McCrory et al. (2001) have yielded, on average, a 33% reduction in headache activity, which is on the low end of the range achieved by behavioral therapies.

Limited-contact Treatment

Limited-contact and clinic-based treatment formats have yielded similar outcomes when compared directly (Jurish et al., 1983; Teders et al., 1984; Richardson and McGrath, 1989) or compared via meta-analysis. Haddock and colleagues (1997) published the most comprehensive meta-analytic review of the limited-contact treatment literature to date. Their literature search yielded 20 randomized controlled trials examining patients with migraine and TTH. Limited-contact interventions averaged three clinic visits versus nine visits for clinic-based interventions. Analyses of standardized effect size scores revealed limited-contact treatment to be more effective than control conditions, and equivalent or superior to clinic-based treatment. Likewise, analyses of the percentage of patients showing clinically meaningful improvements revealed that limited-contact treatment was similar to clinic-based treatment for patients with migraine (53% versus 52%) and TTH (40% versus 42%). The findings of Haddock and colleagues (1997) were consistent with the earlier meta-analyses literature by Rowan and Andrasik (1996) and by Rains et al. (1993) (see Figs. 30–2 and 30–3).

Group Treatment

Although the effectiveness of the same behavioral intervention administered individually and in a group have not been directly compared in the treatment of recurrent headache disorders, there is no indication that these two treatment formats differ in effectiveness. A meta-analysis of 10 studies where behavioral treatments were administered in a group treatment format reported a 53% reduction in headache activity (Rains et al., 1993)—a level of improvement similar to that reported when the same behavioral interventions are individually administered. Where patient flow is adequate, group rather than individual administration of treatment thus allows the cost of treatment to be reduced and health professionals' time to be efficiently used.

Treatment Administered by Nonprofessionals

Two randomized trials have examined the effectiveness of headache education or behavioral treatment of migraine administered by nonprofessionals. In the first trial (Rothrock et al., 2006), 100 consecutive patients at a regional neurology-based headache clinic were randomized to medical treatment by a headache specialist with or without receiving headache education classes. Three 90-minute headache education classes (didactic instruction about migraines and migraine treatment, plus opportunity for discussion and problem solving) were coled by two trained lay volunteers with migraine. At a 6-month evaluation, medical management plus headache education was associated with significantly greater reductions than medical management alone in headache frequency (43% versus 0%) and functionally incapacitating headache frequency (43% versus 23%) per month. The headache education class also was associated significantly with fewer total patient calls (54 versus 244) and fewer unscheduled headache clinic or emergency department visits (25 versus 50) than medical management alone. In addition, acute therapy use tended to be lower (5.3 versus 15.6 days/month), analgesic overuse less frequent (0% versus 36% of patients), and adherence with preventive medication higher (96% versus 59% of patients) in the headache education condition.

In the second trial, Merelle and colleagues (in press) randomized 129 migraine sufferers to seven home-based small group behavioral treatment sessions or to wait list control. The 2-hour behavioral treatment sessions were led by nonprofessionals with migraine who had previously completed the behavioral migraine management program and received additional training as leaders. The behavioral migraine management program included self-monitoring of migraines (identification of migraine triggers, premonitory symptoms) and cognitive-behavioral (relaxation and stress reduction) skills for managing migraines. While the nonprofessional-led behavioral migraine management groups successfully increased participants' confidence in their ability to manage their migraines (self-efficacy), the modest 21% reduction in attack frequency observed with behavioral migraine management was smaller than that typically observed when behavioral clinicians have administered similar treatments, and only marginally ($p < 0.07$) differed from the 6% reduction observed in the wait list control group.

Similar problems to those encountered in the Merelle et al. (in press) study have also been encountered when behavioral interventions for headache have been administered by school nurses or physical education instructors, rather than behaviorally trained clinicians (see below). Behavioral treatments may be more difficult than headache education classes for nonprofessionals to administer effectively, because they require not only greater tailoring of treatment elements to the needs of individual participants but also effective problem-solving assistance when difficulties are encountered in learning and using relaxation and cognitive-behavioral stress management skills. However, both nonprofessional-led headache classes and nonprofessional-administered behavioral treatment deserve additional research attention. Future efforts to effectively train nonprofessional "tutors," and to develop effective headache education classes and behavioral treatments that can be administered by nonprofessionals, should draw on the larger body of relevant work on the self-management of chronic disease (e.g., Lorig et al, 2001; Lorig and Holman, 2003; Holman and Lorig, 2004; Newman et al., 2004).

No-contact Treatment

Telephone-administered Treatment Three small studies with children or adolescents have reported positive results with behavioral programs in which home learning is supervised by telephone (McGrath et al., 1992; Connelly et al., 2005; Cottrell et al., in press). In the best controlled of these studies ($n = 87$; age 11–18), McGrath and colleagues (1992) compared multicomponent behavioral programs for migraine (education, relaxation training, stress management, pain coping strategies, assertiveness, problem-solving) provided in either an 8-week therapist-administered format, or an 8-week home study format. The home study program included a workbook and audiotapes, with supervision provided via weekly telephone calls. Home study proved as effective as therapist-administered treatment (66% versus 44% of adolescents showing significant migraine reductions, respectively), and both programs were more effective than a one-session control condition that included weekly phone calls.

Cottrell and colleagues (in press) randomized adolescents ($n = 30$; mean age = 14 years) to either an 8-week telephone-supervised home study program similar to that of McGrath and colleagues (1992), but tailored for migraine (e.g., thermal biofeedback was added), or to "treatment as usual" with "triptan" therapy. Adolescents expressed a preference for the telephone-administered format over clinic treatment, were able to successfully perform behavioral migraine management skills when observed, and exhibited improvements in migraine comparable to those observed in clinic-based behavioral treatment and triptan therapy. A third study (Connelly et al., 2005) used an interactive computer-administered home study program that included education, relaxation training, challenging stressful thoughts, problem-solving, and pain-coping strategies. The program was contained on a compact disc (CD), rather than the traditional workbooks and audiotapes used in the two previous studies. Children with migraine ($n = 37$, age range 7–12 years) were randomized to receive the CD plus drug therapy (preventive and abortive medications), or to receive drug therapy alone. Both groups received weekly phone contacts. Children receiving the computer-administered program were more likely to show clinically significant ($\geqslant 50\%$) reductions in migraine than the children who received drug therapy alone.

Internet-administered Treatment Efforts to teach headache management skills via the Internet have been only modestly effective and have been plagued by high drop-out rates (Schneider et al., 1999; Strom et al., 2000; Andersson et al., 2003; Devineni and Blanchard, 2005; Hicks et al., 2006). In the best designed study to date, Devineni and Blanchard (2005) enrolled 156 participants from around the world who reported a medical diagnosis of either migraine or TTH in a 4-week online behavioral treatment program. Almost 40% of treatment completers recorded significant reductions in headache activity, but more than 40% of participants also dropped out. Drop-outs reported less severe headaches, less improvement, and fewer years of computer experience. Much of what was said about telephone-administered treatment can be repeated for Internet-administered treatment, though evidence for the effectiveness of Internet treatment is more limited.

Mass Media–administered Treatment A novel public health intervention in the Netherlands used mass media to teach behavioral skills (de Bruin-Kofman et al., 1997). Approximately 15,000 participants purchased home study materials that presented relaxation and cognitive behavioral skills for managing headaches. Each skill was demonstrated in 1 of 10 television programs; 10 radio programs presented solutions to problems encountered by participants. Outcome was assessed in only a small subsample ($n = 271$), but the 164 participants who completed the program evaluation recorded, on average, a 50% reduction in headache frequency and a reduction of about 4.5 days of lost work for more than 4 months. The strong public interest in this program, and preliminary positive outcome data, raise the possibility that these skills can be effectively taught via mass media.

Although the formats for administering behavioral treatment reviewed earlier are unlikely to be suitable for all patients, they offer promising cost-effective alternatives to clinic-based behavioral treatment. Additional information is needed about the patients most likely to benefit from each intervention strategy as well as about the optimal designs for these interventions. Data on long-term outcomes including negative "side effects" of these interventions are needed. For example, it is important that "failure" in no-contact behavioral treatment does not discourage individuals from seeking conventional medical or psychological treatment. Hopefully, these formative studies will encourage continued innovation in the use of communications technologies in the teaching of behavioral headache management skills.

Maintenance of Improvements

It is relatively well established that improvements in migraine and TTH achieved with psychological treatments tend to be maintained, at least for the 3- to 9-month follow-up periods that have most frequently been evaluated. For example, improvements reported at such short-term follow-up evaluations have been larger than the improvements observed at posttreatment evaluations in 65 patient samples included in two meta-analytic reviews (Penzien, Holroyd, Holm, et al., 1985; Holroyd and Penzien, 1986). Long-term follow-up (greater than 1 year) results also have been positive, but are less definitive because a significant proportion of patients typically are lost to follow-up over longer follow-up periods. However, at least 45% reductions in headache activity also have been reported in 14 of 15 studies that used daily headache recordings to assess improvement in 1–3 years after psychological treatment and in three studies that assessed improvement in 5–7 years after treatment (Blanchard, 1987, 1992; Gauthier and Carrier, 1991).

Combining Behavioral and Drug Therapy

Although research on this topic remains limited, evidence of the benefits of combined drug and behavioral therapy continues to grow.

Migraine

The most recent randomized trial of combined therapy examined behavioral migraine management and preventive (β-blocker) therapies in 232 migraine sufferers experiencing at least 3 (mean = 6) migraines with disability per month, despite "optimal" acute therapy (Holroyd et al., 2006). It can be seen in Fig. 30–4 that the combination therapy yielded significantly higher response rate (⩾50% reduction in migraines) than either behavioral or preventive drug therapy alone. On quality-of-life measures, the combined therapy and behavior therapy alone produced similar improvements that were larger than that observed with preventive drug therapy alone.

Earlier studies that evaluated the combination of preventive (β-blocker) therapy and (thermal)

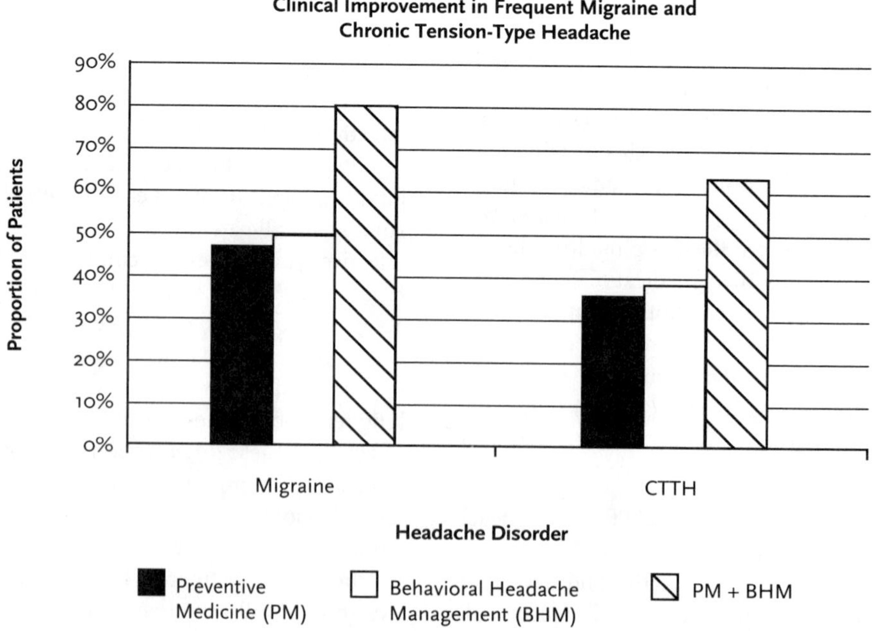

Figure 30–4 Results from two recent trials examining the effectiveness of combined behavioral and preventive drug therapy for migraine (left) and chronic tension-type headache (right). CTTH, chronic tension-type headache.

biofeedback training also found the combined treatment highly effective in managing recurrent migraines (yielding more than a 70% reduction on average; Mathew, 1981; Holroyd et al., 1995), although the benefits of combined therapy relative to preventive drug therapy were not evaluated or unclear in previous trials. Trials that examine the separate and combined effects of behavioral and prophylactic drug therapies for both frequent episodic migraine and for chronic migraine are needed.

In developing an algorithm for combining preventive drug and behavioral therapies in clinical practice, we have argued that if migraines are frequent or severe, or psychological problems complicate treatment, conjoint behavior and drug therapy should be considered (Holroyd et al., 1998). If migraines are less frequent and not complicated by psychological problems, behavioral and drug therapies may be equally viable treatment alternatives for many patients. In the latter case, patient preference, treatment costs, and presence of medication contraindications (e.g., possibility of pregnancy, breastfeeding) might then influence the treatment modality chosen.

Tension-type Headache

The treatment of chronic TTH trial (Holroyd et al., 2001; Holroyd and Labus, 2005) examined the benefits of combined (cognitive) behavior therapy and preventive (tricyclic antidepressant) medication in 203 patients with chronic (mean 26 headache days per month) TTH, extending results from earlier trials (Holroyd et al., 1991). It can be seen in Fig. 30–4 that the combination therapy yielded significantly higher response rate ($\geqslant$50% reduction in headache activity) than either behavioral or preventive drug therapy alone.

An earlier study (Reich and Gottesman, 1993) raises the possibility that combined behavioral and drug therapy for chronic TTHs may improve short-term outcomes, but undermine long-term outcomes with behavior therapy, a phenomenon observed in the treatment of both anxiety disorders and insomnia. In this study, the combination of preventive (tricyclic antidepressant) medication and EMG biofeedback training yielded better results initially than did EMG biofeedback training alone; however, beginning at month 8, this difference disappeared; and after the tapering of antidepressant medication at month 16, the combined treatment fared more poorly than did biofeedback training alone. The authors of early study (Bruhn et al., 1979) found EMG biofeedback to be more effective than drug therapy (an individualized combination of antidepressant medication, analgesics, muscle relaxants, sedatives plus physical therapy as judged appropriate), and also noted that "Drug therapy and physical therapy reinforce a tendency to dependent behavior . . . but biofeedback educates the patient to control his own well being" (p. 36).

COMPLICATIONS AND COMORBIDITIES OF HEADACHE DISORDERS

This section addresses the use of behavioral intervention in the management of medication-overuse headache and in the management of the mood, anxiety, and sleep disorder that frequently accompany headache disorders.

Medication-overuse Headache

It is essential that behavioral clinicians appreciate the risk of analgesic or medication-overuse headaches (MOHs; i.e., *rebound headache*), which can result when headache-prone patients overuse symptomatic headache drugs causing a refractory headache condition (Headache Classification Subcommittee, 2004). MOHs are notably refractory to both pharmacological (e.g., Kudrow, 1982; Mathew et al., 1990) and nonpharmacological therapies (Michultka et al., 1989). For example, one retrospective review of patient records (Michultka et al., 1989) found that less than a third of "high medication consumption" patients achieved clinically significant reductions in headache activity (50% or greater reduction in headache activity) after behavioral treatment, while more than half of the patients with the same primary headache diagnosis using lower levels of medication showed this level of improvement.

Management

Protocols for withdrawal of overused medications are now well established (Boes et al., 2006), and many but not all patients will revert to an episodic headache pattern after discontinuation of medication overuse. Unfortunately, available evidence indicates that relapse rates among MOH patients who have successfully withdrawn from medication overuse can be greater than 30% within 1 year (Bigal et al., 2004; Katsarava et al, 2005; Lake, 2006), with the relapse rate increasing over time (Katsarava et al., 2005). MOH often is further complicated by the presence of a psychiatric [both Axis I clinical syndromes and Axis II personality disorders in Diagnostic and Statistical Manual of Mental Disorders IV (DSM-IV) terms] disorder (Atasoy et al., 2005; Radat et al., 2005; Lake, 2006). For example, Atasoy and colleagues (2005) observed a psychiatric disorder in 68% of MOH patients with prior episodic TTH and in 54% of MOH patients with prior episodic migraine, but only 39% of chronic TTH patients *without* MOH.

Several clinical series (e.g., Baumgartner, et al., 1989; Diener et al., 1989; Blanchard et al., 1992; Mathew et al., 1990) have documented the benefits of analgesic and abortive medication withdrawal combined with pharmacological and behavioral therapy. For example, Baumgartner and colleagues (1989) reported, at a 17-month follow-up evaluation, medication withdrawal accompanied by prophylactic pharmacotherapy and relaxation training produced significant reductions in headache activity in 61% of patients who had been using high levels (35–40 doses per week) of medication. Grazzi and colleagues (2002) observed that a combination of pharmacologic (inpatient medication withdrawal plus preventive medication) and behavioral (biofeedback-assisted relaxation training) treatment was more efficacious than pharmacologic therapy alone in the long-term (3-year) management of MOH. The Grazzi study requires replication, but suggests that behavioral treatment may improve long-term outcomes for patients with MOH.

Mood and Anxiety Disorders

Population data indicate that most mood and anxiety disorders are comorbid with migraine (see Chapter 9 this volume, Hamelsky and Lipton, 2006 and Penzien et al., 2006 for reviews). Although similar population data are limited for TTH, mood and anxiety disorders appear comorbid with chronic (but not episodic) TTH (see Chapter 11 this volume and Heckman and Holroyd, 2006 for reviews). Probably because of selection factors, mood and anxiety disorders are reported at higher rates in clinical samples than in population samples, and in headache subspecialty settings than primary care, with the highest rates reported in regional headache centers. In clinical settings, mood and anxiety disorders also have been reported more frequently in chronic than in episodic migraine or TTH and when medication overuse is present (Juang et al., 2000; Heckman and Holroyd, 2006). It is important to identify and manage mood and anxiety disorders if only because they further impair the daily functioning and quality-of-life of individuals already burdened with a headache disorder (Holroyd et al., 2000; Lipton et al., 2000; Lanteri-Minet et al., 2005; Baskin et al., 2006; Strine et al., 2006).

Screening

There are a number of approaches to screening for mood and anxiety disorders in the medical setting, so an effective strategy can be selected that best fits an individual practice or clinic setting. For example, standardized screening instruments can be administered to all new patients, or only to patients who screen positive on "red flag" questions incorporated into a typical headache interview. The most widely used screening instrument is probably the Primary Care Evaluation of Mental Disorders, available as both a clinician-structured interview (Spitzer et al., 1994) and as a patient-completed questionnaire (Patient Health Questionnaire; Spitzer et al., 1999). These instruments were designed (and validated) for use in medical settings and can be used to screen for multiple psychiatric disorders or for a single disorder. A positive screening result should, of course, be followed by a careful diagnostic workup, and clinicians should be aware of the overlap of somatic symptoms associated with headache, depression, and anxiety disorders in order to avoid inappropriate or incorrect psychiatric diagnoses. The reader is referred to the detailed review by Maizels and colleagues (2006) for a full discussion of screening.

Management

Integrating cognitive-behavioral treatment (CBT) for headaches with CBT for mood or anxiety disorders offers a logically consistent approach to the management of headaches and co-occurring mood or anxiety disorders (Lake et al., 2005; Lipchik et al., 2006). CBT treatments for mood and anxiety disorders are outlined in Table 30–1.

A large literature attests to the effectiveness of CBT for the primary mood and anxiety disorders. CBT consistently produces outcomes that equal (and often exceed) those of pharmacotherapy for depression as well as anxiety disorders, including panic disorder (Gould et al., 1995), generalized anxiety disorder (Gould, et al., 1997), obsessive-compulsive disorder (Kobak et al., 1998; Franklin and Foa, 2002; Sousa et al., 2006), and posttraumatic stress disorder (Foa, 2000). Improvements may be maintained longer with CBT than with pharmacotherapy (Brown and Barlow, 1995; Gould et al., 1997), as CBT has been found to be of value in preventing relapse in the long-term treatment of both mood and anxiety disorders (Otto et al., 2005; Ball et al., 2006). Thus CBT is a first-line treatment for mild to moderately severe unipolar depression (American Psychiatric Association, 2000), and for anxiety disorders, including panic disorder, generalized anxiety disorder, and obsessive-compulsive disorder (Royal Australian and New Zealand College of Psychiatrists, 2003; Sheehan and Mao, 2003; Cloos, 2005).

Sleep Disorders

Although epidemiological studies are lacking, in the headache clinic, the prevalence of a wide range of sleep disorders, including insomnia, sleep apnea, circadian phase abnormalities, narcolepsy, periodic limb movements and fibrositis, appears to be elevated (Rains and Poceta, 2006). However, insomnia is by far the most prevalent, observed in 38% to more than 60% of headache patients (Maizels and Burchette, 2004; Kelman and Rains, 2005), and more prevalent in chronic than in episodic headache (Rothrock et al., 1996).

Screening

The mnemonic *REST* is a useful prompt for four key questions to screen for the presence of a sleep disorder: the *restorative* nature of the patient's sleep, *excessive* daytime sleepiness, tiredness or fatigue, the presence of habitual *snoring*, and whether the *total* sleep time is sufficient. Regular morning headache has been associated with a number of sleep disorders, suggesting that patients exhibiting this headache pattern should be queried about sleep.

Sleep apnea is suggested by symptoms (e.g., snoring, witnessed apnea, waking gasping, nocturia, night sweats, hypersomnia > insomnia), the presence of risk factors (e.g., overweight/obese, craniofacial features that narrow the airway, alcohol/sedatives/hypnotics, smoking) or commonly associated disorders (e.g., hypertension, Type II diabetes, neuromuscular disorders) (Young et al., 2002; Tishler et al., 2003). Standardized questionnaires (Devine et al., 2005) and prediction equations (Harding, 2001) are available to assist in quantifying the risk for sleep disorders such as

TABLE 30–1 Behavioral Treatment Interventions for Psychiatric Comorbidities.

Treatment (rationale)	*Indication*	*Instructions*
Relaxation and breathing retraining [*skills to gain voluntary control over and reduce the symptoms of anxiety (dizziness, shortness of breath, increased heart rate, chest tightness, tingling)*]	High physiological or emotional arousal associated with anxiety disorders	Abdominal breathing to slow rate of respiration and reduce arousal—typically taught before other relaxation techniques Progressive relaxation training to reduce physical tension (may be facilitated by EMG or other forms of biofeedback) Autogenic training to establish calm mental state Guided imagery to deepen relaxation or to evoke a quick relaxation response, or to provide a brief respite from an anxiety-producing situation

Abbreviation: EMG, electromyography.

sleep apnea, restless leg syndrome, and insomnia. The addition of a sleep assessment to the headache diary (Rains and Poceta, 2006) also can be helpful in assessing sleep problems.

Management of Insomnia

Integrating behavioral interventions for headaches with behavioral interventions for insomnia offers a therapeutically consistent approach to the management of headaches and co-occurring insomnia. Both interventions share techniques including daily self-monitoring, progressive relaxation training, behavior modification, and cognitive therapy (Rains and Poceta, 2006). Behavioral and cognitive-behavioral interventions for insomnia are described in Table 30–2 (see also Morin, 1993; Perlis et al., 2005).

Sleep hygiene education alone, the most widely recognized and used insomnia intervention, is relatively ineffective (Morgenthaler et al., 2006). Behavioral treatments for insomnia have demonstrated efficacy comparable or superior to hypnotic medications in the short term (Smith et al., 2002) and long term (Morin et al., 1994; Murtagh and Greenwood, 1995) in the treatment of primary insomnia, as well as insomnia secondary to a wide range of medical and psychiatric conditions (Smith et al., 2005). Owing to efficacy, durability of treatment effects, and lack of side-effects, behavioral treatment is the preferred approach to chronic insomnia (Morgenthaler et al., 2006). Behavioral interventions (Morin, 1993; Perlis et al., 2005) can be administered alone or in combination with pharmacologic treatments.

A brief behavioral insomnia intervention with demonstrated efficacy in the primary care setting is also appropriate for headache clinic setting. This two-session intervention uses simplified stimulus control, sleep restriction, and sleep hygiene interventions (Edinger and Sampson, 2003): (1) eliminate sleep-incompatible activities (television watching, reading, planning, and worrying) in the bed and bedroom; (2) avoid all daytime napping, and (3) follow a consistent sleep–wake schedule by adhering to agreed-upon bed and rising times (bed and rising times were negotiated after determining the average sleep time that the patient reported during the 2-week sleep-log monitoring). Each participant selects his or her standard bed and rising time subject to the requirement that the interval between these two times equals his or her pretreatment average sleep time + 30 minutes.

In the only randomized controlled trial of behavioral sleep modification in the headache clinic, Calhoun and Ford (in press) randomized patients with transformed migraine to headache therapy plus either a brief behavioral sleep intervention similar to that described earlier for insomnia or a sham intervention (e.g., consistent meals, acupressure as instructed, range of motion exercises) for insomnia. The behavioral intervention yielded significant improvements over the sham intervention in headache frequency (28.1% versus − 3.0%) and intensity (39.4% versus 12.1%), with 35% of the treatment group reverting to episodic headache by the sixth week of treatment compared to none of the control group. Notably, improvements in headache were proportionate to the number of sleep behaviors changed.

BEHAVIORAL ADHERENCE FACILITATION FOR DRUG THERAPIES

Nonadherence undermines the effectiveness of abortive and prophylactic therapies for headache, and behavioral strategies may improve adherence. Literature demonstrates that 11% of all headache prescriptions were never filled (Gallagher and Kunkel, 2003), 25%–50% of patients are noncompliant with various prophylactic medications (Fitzpatrick and Hopkins, 1983; Packard and Brown, 1986; Mulleners et al., 1998), and 70% do not use abortive medications (ergotamine) optimally (Holroyd et al., 1989). Likewise, misuse or overuse of triptans and other symptomatic medication can seriously aggravate primary headache disorders, and is associated with treatment failure (Ottervanger et al., 1996; Cupini and Calabresi, 2005). For migraineurs, self-reported reasons for delaying acute treatments include concerns over side-effects, medication overuse, dependency or addiction, waiting to see if the headache was migraine or severe migraine, medication cost, prescriber cautions, and insurance-imposed limits (Foley et al., 2005). The general

TABLE 30–2 Behavioral Treatment Strategies Suggested for Insomnia Based on Symptoms.

Treatment (rationale)	*Indication*	*Instructions*
Relaxation Training (*skills to gain voluntary control over and reduce the state of hypervigilance that is incompatible w/sleep*)	High physiologic, cognitive, or emotional arousal	Progressive relaxation training to reduce physical tension (may be facilitated by EMG or other forms of biofeedback) Autogenic training to establish calm mental state and deter intrusive and arousing thoughts
Stimulus Control (*based on operant conditioning principles and reinforces associations between the "state of sleepiness" and the sleep environment*)	Difficulty falling asleep or staying sleep	1. Go to bed only when sleepy 2. If unable to fall asleep 10–20 minutes (*without watching clock, 10–20 minutes is equal to repositioning twice to try to fall asleep*), leave the bedroom. Return only when sleepy again 3. Use the bed and bedroom for sleep only 4. Set alarm and rise daily at a regular time—do not snooze 5. Do not nap during the day
Sleep Restriction* [*maximizes homeostatic "sleep drive" by restricting the time in bed to approximately the actual sleep time (based on sleep diary)*]	Excessive time spent in bed not sleeping; frequent awakenings	1. Use the sleep diary to determine: "time in bed" and "actual sleep time" 2. Restrict "time in bed" to approximately the average number of hours of "actual sleep time" per night. (Prescribe specific bed/wake times) 3. As diary demonstrates actual sleep time is 85% of time in bed, increase by 15–30 minute increments 4. Keep a fixed wake time, regardless of the actual sleep duration. (*short nights are expected and increase sleep drive on subsequent night*) 5. If sleeping <85% time in bed for 10 days, restrict time in bed further by 15–30 minutes increments

(continued)

Table 30–2 (continued)

Treatment (rationale)	*Indication*	*Instructions*
Cognitive Therapy *(to identify, challenge, and replace irrational beliefs and fears about sleep and sleep loss, which provoke anxiety and perpetuate insomnia)*	Racing, obsessive thoughts at bedtime; unrealistic expectations; catastrophizing or ruminative worry about sleep	1. Patients may be asked to self-monitor or solicit beliefs and fears about sleep *(or questionnaire (Edinger, 2001)* 2. Identify anxiety-provoking insomnia-perpetuating cognitions 3. Cognitive techniques are taught to challenge dysfunctional beliefs and restructure rational statements that the patient will apply when the dysfunctional thought or emotional state occurs
Sleep Hygiene Education *(basic sleep-promoting behaviors and avoiding activities not conducive to sleep)*	Any of the above or poor sleep habits	1. Avoid daytime naps 2. Eliminate stimulants (caffeine, nicotine, etc.) 3. Maintain a regular bed/wake schedule 7 days per week 4. Dark, quiet, comfortable sleep environment 5. Avoid alcohol 6. Regular exercise (avoid exercising 5 hours before bed) 7. Use the bed only for sleep and sex (behaviors conducive to sleep)

Abbreviations: EMG, electromyography.

*Restriction may initially create a modestly increased sleep loss or sleep deprivation and daytime sleepiness; though this deprivation heightens sleep drive to facilitate sleep at night, it may also result in daytime sleepiness. Patients should be warned about this, especially if often engaged in hazardous activities. Over successive weeks, the sleepiness will remit as the time in bed is gradually increased and the individual's maximum efficient sleep time is achieved.

medical literature suggests a decline in adherence with multiple medications, more frequent or complex medication dosing regimens, higher medication costs, side-effects, psychiatric comorbidity, as well as psychological factors (e.g., low internal locus of control, self-efficacy; Rains et al., 2006).

Risks for nonadherence should be considered in headache treatment planning and evaluated over time as a variable potentially impacting treatment outcome. Patients may be assessed with respect of their "readiness for change" and their active participation enlisted in the adherence-monitoring process (Rains et al., 2006). Behavioral and social learning principles enhance prescribing practices with: use of simplified regimens, fixed-dose combinations, or unit-of-use packaging when possible; stimulus control strategies (e.g., day-of-the-week pill box, electronic calendars/palm pilots/cell phones, environmental cues like meals, personalized internal cues for abortive medications); communication skills such as active listening, enlisting patient in treatment planning process, soliciting/trouble-shooting potential barriers to adherence, supplementing verbal instructions with written materials, requesting patients restate recommendations back to the provider; and medication contracts. Screening and management of psychiatric comorbidities can also improve adherence.

Dedicated behavioral interventions can facilitate the use of prescribed medications. Holroyd and colleagues (1989) improved adherence with ergotamine. Patients randomized to an adherence-enhancing group participated in a one-half hour education session, and received three brief phone calls to identify and remedy problems with medication use and were provided a self-management workbook to assist the patient in monitoring and identifying adherence problems, improve decision-making, and correct adherence problems. Patients receiving the adherence intervention attempted to abort 70% of migraine attacks and showed clinically significant reductions in headache activity (40% improvement at post treatment). In contrast, the control group who received standard medication management attempted to abort only approximately 40% of their migraines and showed smaller reductions in migraine activity (26% improvement at posttreatment).

OLDER ADULTS AND CHILDREN

Older Adults

Although the prevalence of headaches tends to decrease with age (Lipton, et al., 1994), it has been estimated that recurrent headaches are a significant problem for approximately 17% of individuals above the age of 65 (Cook et al., 1989). Standard pharmacological treatment of headaches in the older adult can be problematic both due to side-effects and the possibility of drug interactions, since patients are likely to be using multiple medications for other medical conditions. Behavioral interventions are attractive for older adults, since they do not pose either of these challenges. Tailoring behavioral interventions to target the special needs of older patients can significantly enhance treatment efficacy. Prospective studies evaluating interventions adapted for elderly patients have reported positive results with CBT, relaxation training, and biofeedback training for both migraine and TTH (e.g., Arena et al. 1988, 1991; Kabela et al., 1989; Nicholson and Blanchard, 1993; Mosley et al., 1995).

In an exemplary study, Mosley and colleagues (1995) found CBT combined with relaxation training to be more effective than relaxation training alone in elderly headache patients (aged 60–78 years), with 64% of CBT participants achieving clinically significant improvement. To facilitate learning of headache management skills among their elderly patients, Mosely and colleagues provided supplementary audiotapes and written materials designed to assist patients in practicing and learning skills, allowed ample time to practice elementary skills before more advanced skills were introduced, and provided weekly phone contacts to answer questions and identify problems. These findings suggest that relatively simple adjustments in standard behavioral treatment procedures can enhance the application of behavioral interventions for older headache sufferers.

Children and Adolescents

Epidemiology and Impact

Headaches occur in close to 70% of children, with epidemiological surveys suggesting that 1%–3%

of 7-year-olds and 4%–11% of 7–11-year-olds suffer from migraine (Sillanpaa, 1983; Linet et al, 1989). The female-to-male sex ratio increases from approximately age 12–42 and probably approaches 2–1 by late adolescence. Although good data on the prevalence of pediatric TTH are lacking, Bille (1962) reported that 15% of children aged 7–15 experienced nonmigrainous headaches by age 15—the majority of which were probably TTH.

Headache is often underdiagnosed and untreated in children and adolescents, and has many potential negative consequences that may include educational impairment, anxiety, depression, and reduced quality of life (Karwautz et al., 1999; Powers et al., 2003; Grazzi et al., 2004). Childood headache has been found to predict headache, physcial, and psychological problems in adulthod (Bille, 1997; Fearon and Hotopf, 2001). Therefore, beyond its obvious immediate benefit, successful treatment of headaches in children and adolescents may have the potential to prevent development of chronic headache problems in adulthood (Bille, 1997).

Migraine

Although evidence about the effectiveness of behavioral interventions with children and adolescents is more limited than for adults, published studies raise the possibility that behavioral treatments may be more effective with children and adolescents than with adults (Blanchard and Andrasik, 1982; Blanchard, 1992; Hermann et al., 1995; Holroyd, 2002; Trautmann et al., 2006). A recent meta-analysis of 22 studies by Trautmann and colleagues (2006) examined the effectiveness of the primary behavioral interventions (relaxation, biofeedback and cognitive-behavior therapy) for pediatric headache (migraine as well as TTH). In the analysis of clinically significant change (16 studies, 22 treatment groups, 587 patients), behavioral treatment was associated with a large treatment effect (Effect size (ES) = 0.87), corresponding to clinically significant improvement in 70% of children who received behavior therapy, but in only 30% of control group children. Improvements with behavior therapy also were stable at 1-year follow-up.

Our (K.A.H.) unpublished analysis of 25 clinic studies evaluating behavioral treatments for migraine is presented in Figure 30–5, where the proportion of children showing clinically significant (⩾50%) improvements in migraine with each of the treatments is displayed. It can be seen that each of the behavioral interventions has been significantly more effective than control conditions (odds ratios from approximately 7–20), and that behavioral interventions containing thermal biofeedback training have been more effective than relaxation or CBT interventions alone (odds ratios 2.5).

The comparative effectiveness of preventive drug and behavioral therapies in the management of migraine in children and adolescents has been addressed in just two studies—both of which favored behavioral treatment. In the first study (Olness et al., 1987), combined relaxation and self-hypnosis training yielded significantly better results than propranolol in children aged 6–12 years with migraine with aura. In fact, only relaxation/self-hypnosis produced better results than placebo. Similar findings were reported by Sartory et al. (1998), who compared the efficacy of metoprolol and two behavioral treatments (stress management plus either relaxation training or cephalic vasomotor biofeedback) in children with migraine aged 8–16 years. Combined

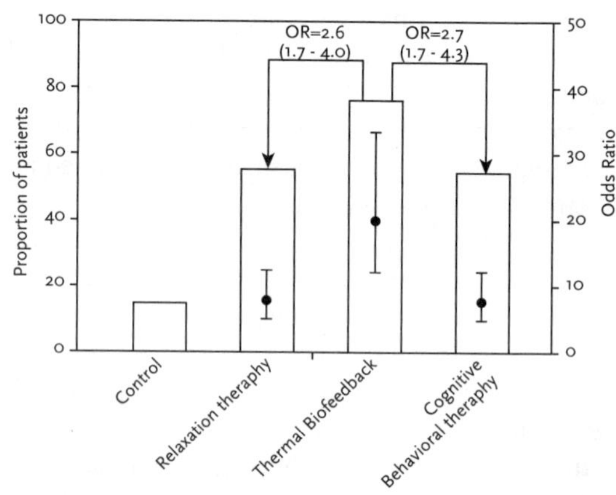

Figure 30–5 Proportion of participants clinically improved (>50% reduction in migraine activity) from 25 trials of behavioral treatments for pediatric migraine (left axis). Odds ratios (right axis) and 95% confidence intervals (bars) for comparison with wait list control. OR, odds ratio.

relaxation/stress-management training yielded the best outcomes (>50% improvement in 80% of patients), while metoprolol yielded the poorest outcomes (>50% improvement in 42% of patients).

Tension-type Headache

Although behavioral interventions have seldom been evaluated in young children with TTH, there are some encouraging data with adolescents. For example, in a reanalysis of data from three early studies, Larsson and Melin (1988) concluded that therapist-administered relaxation training produced larger improvements (63% reduction in headache) in adolescents with episodic tension headache than a pseudotherapy control treatment. Several other recent studies have shown that EMG biofeedback training has yielded quite positive results with TTH (e.g., Grazzi et al., 1990; Bussone et al., 1998). More information is needed about the effectiveness of behavioral interventions for both episodic and chronic TTH, and about the relative effectiveness of drug and behavioral interventions with TTH.

School-based Behavioral Interventions

School-based group relaxation training—at least when administered by a behaviorally trained clinician—appears effective in managing migraines for many adolescents. Larsson and colleagues have taught relaxation skills for the management of headaches in secondary schools in Uppsala, Sweden, for 20 years. In a summary of seven relaxation training trials conducted in the school setting ($n = 228$, age 10–18 years), Larsson and colleagues (2005) reported that clinically significant ($\geqslant 50\%$) improvements in migraine were obtained in about half of students who participated in a 6- to 10-session, therapist-administered, group relaxation training program. Follow-up data indicated that improvements were maintained for at least 6–10 months. Unfortunately, neither a relaxation training program conducted by a school nurse nor a self-help relaxation training program that included a relaxation manual and audiotapes of relaxation instructions proved effective (only approximately 15% of students improved; Larsson et al., 2005). The latter finding was echoed by Passchier and colleagues (1990) who found the relaxation training conducted by school gym instructors to be similarly ineffective. Methods of teaching school personnel the clinical skills necessary to effectively administer relaxation training will be needed if behavioral headache management programs are to be offered to the large number adolescents with recurrent headaches in the school setting.

WOMEN: BEHAVIORAL ISSUES AND INTERVENTIONS

It is sometimes suggested that headaches associated with hormonal changes, or aggravated by hormonal preparations, may be more resistant to behavioral interventions than other types of headaches; however, data do not support this assumption (Gauthier et al., 1991; Holroyd and Lipchik, 2000). The limited body of research on the effectiveness of behavioral treatments for headaches related to the female hormonal cycle, pregnancy, and postpartum or during lactation has yielded conflicting results.

Menstrually Related Migraine

Only a few studies have evaluated the effectiveness of behavioral treatments specifically for menstrually related migraine (MRM), and they have yielded conflicting results. The lack of a standard definition of MRM until recently has made it difficult to interpret results and compare results across studies (Holroyd and Lipchik, 2000; Blanchard and Kim, 2005). The findings of the study by Blanchard and Kim (2005) highlight the impact of the definition of MRM. The researchers examined the outcome of behavioral interventions (thermal biofeedback with autogenic training or progressive muscle relaxation training) for patients with menstrually related headache using three differing sets of diagnostic criteria for MRM, and outcomes differed depending upon the diagnostic criteria employed. The revised International Headache Soceity classification (Headache Classification Subcommittee, 2004) delineates the formal criteria for "pure menstrual migraine" and "MRM without aura" in the appendix, which should help alleviate this lack of clarity in future research.

Pregnancy

Behavioral approaches are excellent options for managing headaches during conception and pregnancy, postpartum, and lactation (Pfaffenrath and Rehm, 1998; Marcus, 2007). Behavioral headache interventions benefit patients of childbearing age by limiting the potential en vitro exposure to medication. The majority of pregnancies are unplanned in the United States (Rosenberg et al., 1995), and the majority of women do not know that they are pregnant until several weeks into the pregnancy. Successful self-management of headache during pregnancy may help limit the use of medication and improve quality of life for the sufferer. Although migraine typically improves during pregnancy (55%–80% of women report improvement; Bousser et al. 1993; Silberstein 1997), migraine frequency and severity also can remain stable or worsen during pregnancy (especially in migraine with aura; Bousser et al. 1993; Marcus et al., 1999; Sances et al., 2003). As behavioral self-management skills take time to master, they should be introduced as early as possible to patients who are considering pregnancy.

Data on the efficacy of behavioral approaches for headache management for pregnant and postpartum/lactating migraineurs are limited. Furthermore, attack frequency often decreases spontaneously during the second and third trimesters, making causal interpretation difficult in uncontrolled studies. In the single controlled study to date, Marcus et al., (1995) randomized pregnant migraineurs to a behavioral intervention (education, relaxation training, thermal biofeedback training, and physical therapy exercises) or a pseudotherapy control condition (educational plus biofeedback training to decrease finger temperature). The interventions were initiated during the second trimester and completed before delivery. The behavioral intervention yielded substantially larger reductions in headache activity (81% versus 33% reduction) and a greater number of patients with clinically significant improvements (73% versus 29% of participants) relative to the control condition. The improvements with treatment were maintained throughout the perinatal period and at 3- and 6-month follow-up evaluations (Scharff, et al., 1996). Interestingly, no differences were observed among the women who did or did not breastfeed, suggesting that breastfeeding had no effect on the maintenance of benefits. Despite the small scale of this study, these findings help to confirm that behavioral interventions provide a viable option for pregnant migraineurs.

FUTURE DIRECTIONS

More than three decades of research has produced reasonably effective behavioral treatments for migraine and TTH; yet this has had little impact on the care of the typical headache patient. Thus, there is a need to address the financial, educational, cultural, and system barriers to the integration of behavioral interventions into headache care, as well as gaps in the evidence base and limitations of current behavioral treatments that may contribute to this problem. Given our evolving healthcare environment that continues to challenge providers to reduce costs, this doubtless will prove a difficult task. Hopefully, the clinical trials guidelines for behavioral headache research recently developed by the American Headache Society (Penzien et al., 2005) will serve as a catalyst for innovative, high-quality research that, in turn, will generate innovative behavioral strategies for improving headache care while optimizing healthcare resource utilization.

We recently have articulated 10 critical needs and research priorities for future behavioral headache research (Penzien et al., 2005), which are summarized in Table 30–3. In addition to the domains listed in Table 30–3, there are other important areas of research including the interaction of behavioral and environmental factors with genetics in influencing the onset and progression of headache disorders, behavioral treatment of elderly headache patients, culturally sensitive care, and cost-benefit analysis of innovative delivery systems for behavioral treatments. We hope that researchers will be inspired to tackle these problems and that funding support will be available. Behavioral headache researchers are confronted by large challenges, but also by unprecedented opportunities.

Table 30–3 Unmet Needs and Priorities for Behavioral Headache Research.

Replication and extension	Much research examining behavioral factors and behavioral therapies for headache merits replication using updated standards and more rigorous methodology (e.g., current diagnostic criteria, larger samples, improved reporting)
Access and barriers to implementation	Behavioral treatments are *not* readily accessible to many (most) headache sufferers (including children); research is needed to articulate the barriers to broader application of established behavioral therapies
Referral and treatment algorithms	Algorithms for optimizing the utilization of behavioral headache therapies should be developed and validated; this includes algorithms for identifying candidates for behavioral headache therapy as well as for optimally matching patients to specific forms of behavioral headache therapy or specific combinations of behavioral plus medication therapies
Compliance facilitation	Many (most) headache sufferers fail to optimally use medication, yet few studies address treatment compliance; researchers should evaluate efficacy and effectiveness of behavioral strategies targeting compliance facilitation
Self-management model	A comprehensive self-management training model for chronic headache (paralleling successful self-management applications for other chronic diseases) merits further development
Behavioral intervention within medical practice	The majority of headache sufferers receive treatment within the physician's office setting, but behavioral headache self-management principles are not well integrated into routine medical practice; research should develop and evaluate strategies for efficiently integrating behavioral interventions within medical practice
Psychiatric comorbidities and targets for intervention	Psychological/psychiatric conditions comorbid with headache often remain unrecognized and poorly managed; research should evaluate the strategies for screening and managing psychiatric disorders that impede headache treatment
Prevention of disease progression	Development of strategies to prevent progression of headache from episodic to "chronic daily" through risk factor modification, preventive drug therapies, and early use of acute therapies is an important focus for future investigation. Behavioral research and interventions targeting modifiable risk factors for disease progression are needed
Therapeutic mechanisms	Therapeutic mechanisms of behavioral headache treatments are poorly articulated; research isolating the essential and active components of behavioral treatments would prove worthwhile
Innovative treatment formats and information technologies	Continued development of novel formats is needed for the delivery of behavioral headache interventions (i.e., alternatives to standard, time-intensive clinic-based therapies); emerging technologies show promise for facilitating behavioral assessment and intervention for headache

References

American Psychiatric Association (2000). Diagnostic and Statistical Manual of Mental Disorders. American Psychiatric Press, Washington, DC.

Andersson, G, Lundstom, P, and Strom, L (2003). A controlled trial of self-help treatment of recurrent headache conducted via the Internet. *Headache,* 43:353–361.

Arena, JG, Hannah, SL, Bruno, GM, et al. (1991). Electromyographic biofeedback training for tension headache in the elderly: a prospective study. *Biofeedback Self Reg,* 35:187–195.

Arena, JG, Hightower, NE, and Chong, GC (1988). Relaxation therapy for tension headache in the elderly: a prospective study. *Psychol Aging,* 3(1):96.

Atasoy, HT, Atasoy, N, Unal, AE, et al. (2005). Psychiatric comorbidity in medication overuse headache patients

with pre-existing headache type of episodic tension-type headache. *Eur J Pain*, 9(3):285–291.
Ball, JR, Mitchell, PB, Corry, JC, et al. (2006). A randomized controlled trial of cognitive therapy for bipolar disorder: focus on long-term change. *J Clin Psychiatry*, 67:277–286.
Barlow, J, Wright, C, Sheasby, J, et al. (2002). Self-management approaches for people with chronic conditions: a review. *Patient Educ Couns*, 48:177–187.
Baskin, SM, Lipchik, GL, and Smitherman, TA (2006). Mood and anxiety disorders in chronic headache. *Headache*, 46(Suppl. 3):S76–S87.
Baumgartner, C, Wessely, P, Bingol, C, et al. (1989). Longterm prognosis of analgesic withdrawal in patients with drug-induced headaches. *Headache*, 29 (8):510–514.
Bernstein, DA, Borkovec, TD, and Hazlett-Stevens, H (2000). *New Directions in Progressive Relaxation Training: A Guidebook for Helping Professions*. Praeger Publishers, Westport, CT.
Bigal, ME and Lipton, RB (2006). Modifiable risk factors for migraine progression. *Headache*, 46(9):1334–1343.
Bigal, ME, Rapoport, AM, Sheftell, FD, et al. (2004). Transformed migraine and medication overuse in a tertiary headache centre–Clinical characteristics and treatment outcomes. *Cephalalgia*, 24(6):483–490.
Bille, B (1962). Migraine in school children. *Acta Paediatr Scand*, 51:1–151.
Bille, B (1997). A 40-year follow-up of school children with migraine. *Cephalalgia*, 17:488–491.
Blanchard, EB (1987). Long-term effects of behavioral treatment of chronic headache. *Behav Ther*, 23:375–385.
Blanchard, EB (1992). Psychological treatment of benign headache disorders. *J Consul Clin Psychol*, 60:537–551.
Blanchard, EB and Andrasik, F (1982). Psychological assessment and treatment of headache: recent developments and emerging issues. *J Consult Clin Psychol*, 50 (6): 859–879.
Blanchard, EB and Andrasik, F (1985). *Management of Chronic Headaches: A Psychological Approach*. Pergamon Press, Elmsford, NY.
Blanchard, EB, Andrasik, F, Ahles, TA, et al. (1980). Migraine and tension-type headache: a meta-analytic review. *Behav Ther*, 11:613–631.
Blanchard, EB and Kim, M (2005). The effect of the definition of menstrually-related headache on the response to biofeedback treatment. *Appl Psychophysiol Biofeedback*, 30(1):53–63.
Blanchard EB, Taylor AE, Dentinger MP (1992). Preliminary results from the self-regulatory treatment of high-medication-consumption headache, Biofeedback Self Regul 17:179–202.
Boes, CJ, Black, DF, and Dodick, DW (2006). Pathophysiology and management of transformed migraine and medication overuse headache. *Semin Neurol*, 26 (2):232–241.
Bogaards, MC and terKuile, MM (1994). Treatment of recurrent tension headache: a meta-analytic review. *Clin J Pain*, 10:174–190.
Bousser, MG, Ratinahirana, H, and Darbois, X (1993). Migraine and pregnancy: a prospective study of 703 women after delivery. *Neurology*, 40:437.
Brown, TA and Barlow, DH (1995). Long-term outcome in cognitive-behavioral treatment of panic disorder: clinical predictors and alternative strategies for assessment. *J Consult Clin Psychol*, 63:754–765.
Bruhn, P, Olesen, J, and Melgaard, B (1979). Controlled trial of EMG feedback in muscle contraction headache. *Ann Neurol*, 6:34–36.
Bussone, G, Grazzi, L, D'Amico, D, et al. (1998). Biofeedback-assisted relaxation training for pediatric tension-type headache: a controlled study. *Cephalagia*, 18:464–467.
Calhoun, AH and Ford, S (in press). Behavioral sleep modifications may revert transformed migraine to episodic migraine. *Headache*.
Campbell, JK, Penzien, DB, and Wall, EM (1999). *Evidence-based Guidelines for Migraine Headache: Behavioral and Physical Treatments*. Prepared for the US Headache Consortium. Available : http://www.aan.com/professionals/practice/pdfs/gl0089.pdf. Accessed March, 2007.
Cloos, JM (2005). The treatment of panic disorder. *Curr Opin Psychiatry*, 18:45–50.
Connelly, M, Rapoff, M, Thompson, N, et al. (2005). Headstrong: A pilot study of a CD-ROM Intervention for recurrent pediatric headache. *J Pediatr Psychol*, 31 (7):737–747.
Cook, NR, Evans, DA, Funkenstein, H, et al. (1989). Correlates of headache in a population-based cohort of elderly. *Arch Neurol*, 46:1338–1344.
Cottrell, C, Drew, J, Holroyd, K, et al. (in press). Feasibility of telephone administered behavioral treatment for adolescent migraine. *Headache*.
Cupini, LM and Calabresi, P (2005). Medication-overuse headache: pathophysiological insights. *J Headache Pain*, 6(4):199–202.
de Bruin-Kofman, AT, van de Wiel, H, Groenman, NH, et al. (1997). Effects of a mass media behavioral treatment for chronic headache: a pilot study. *Headache*, 37:415–420.
Devine, EB, Hakim, Z, and Green, J (2005). A systematic review of patient-reported outcome instruments measuring sleep dysfunction in adults. *Pharmacoeconomics*, 23 (9):889–912.
Devineni, T and Blanchard, EB (2005). A randomized controlled trial of an Internet-based treatment for chronic headache. *Behav Res Ther*, 43:277–292.
Diener, HC, Dichgans, J, Scholz, E, et al. (1989). Analgesic-induced chronic headache: long-term results of withdrawal therapy. *J Neurol*, 236:9–14.
Edinger, JD and Sampson, WS (2003). A primary care "friendly" cognitive behavioral insomnia therapy. *Sleep*, 2:177–182.
Edinger JD, Wohlgemuth WK. Psychometric comparisons of the standard and abbreviated DBAS-10 versions of the dysfunctional beliefs and attitudes about sleep questionnaire. Sleep Med 2001;2(6):493–500.
Fearon, P and Hotopf, M (2001). Relation between headache in childhood and physical and psychiatric

symptoms in adulthood: national birth cohort study. *BMJ*, 322(7295):1145.
Fitzpatrick, RM and Hopkins, AP (1983). Effects of referral to a specialist for headache. *J R Soc Med*, 76(2):112–115.
Foa, EB (2000). Psychosocial treatment of posttraumatic stress disorder. *J Clin Psychiatry*, 61(Suppl. 5):43–48.
Foley, KA, Cady, R, Martin, V, et al. (2005). Treating early versus treating mild: timing of migraine prescription medications among patients with diagnosed migraine. *Headache*, 45(5):538–545.
Franklin, ME and Foa, EB (2002). Cognitive behavioral treatments for obsessive compulsive disorder. In *A Guide to Treatments that Work* (2nd edn) (PE Nathan and JM Gorman, eds). pp. 367–386. Oxford University Press, New York.
Gallagher, RM and Kunkel, R (2003). Migraine medication attributes important for patient compliance: concerns about side effects may delay treatment. *Headache*, 43:36–43.
Gauthier, JG and Carrier, S (1991). Long-term effects of biofeedback on migraine headache: a prospective follow-up study. *Headache*, 31(9):605–612.
Gauthier, JG, Fournier A, and Roberge, C (1991). The differential effects of biofeedback in the treatment of menstrual and non-menstrual migraine. *Headache*, 31:82–90.
Goslin, RE, Gray, RN, McCrory, DC, et al. (1999). *Behavioral and physical treatments for migraine headache. Technical review* 2.2. Prepared for the Agency for Health Care Policy and Research under Contract No. 290–94–2025. National Technical Information Service: NTIS Accession No. PB99–127946.
Gould, RA, Otto, MW, and Pollack, MH (1995). A meta-analysis of treatment outcome for panic disorder. *Clin Psychol Rev*, 15:819–844.
Gould, RA, Otto, MW, Pollack, MH, et al. (1997). Cognitive behavioral and pharmacological treatment of generalized anxiety disorder: a preliminary meta-analysis. *Behav Ther*, 28:285–305.
Grazzi, L, Andrasik, F, D'Amico, D, et al. (2002). Behavioral and pharmacologic treatment of transformed migraine with analgesic overuse: outcome at 3 years. *Headache*, 42(6):483–490.
Grazzi, L, D'Amico, D, Usai, S, et al. (2004). Disability in young patients suffering from primary headaches. *Neurol Sci*, 25:111–112.
Grazzi, I, Leone, F, Frediani, F, et al. (1990). A therapeutic alternative for tension headache in children: treatment and 1-year follow-up results. *Biofeedback Self Reg*, 15 (1):1–6.
Haddock, CK, Rowan, AB, Andrasik, F, et al. (1997). Home-based behavioral treatments for chronic benign headache: a meta-analysis of controlled trials. *Cephalalgia*, 17(2):113–118.
Hamelsky, SW and Lipton, RB (2006). Psychiatric comorbidity of migraine. *Headache*, 46(9):1327–33.
Harding, S (2001). Prediction formulae for sleep-disordered breathing. *Curr Opin Pulm Med*, 7(6):381–385.
Headache Classification Subcommittee of the International Headache Society (2004). The international classification of headache disorders 2nd edition. *Cephalalgia*, 24(Suppl. 1):1–160.
Heckman, BD and Holroyd, KA (2006). Tension-type headache and psychiatric comorbidity. *Curr Pain Headache Rep*, 10(6):439–447.
Hermann, C, Kim, M, and Blanchard, EB (1995). Behavioral and prophylactic pharmacological intervention studies of pediatric migraine: an exploratory meta-analysis. *Pain*, 60:239–255.
Hicks, C, von Baeyer, C, and McGrath, P (2006). Online psychological treatment for pediatric recurrent pain: a randomized evaluation. *J Pediatr Psychol*, 31 (7):1–13.
Hills-Briggs, F (2003). Problem solving in diabetes self-management: a model of chronic illness self-management behavior. *Ann Behav Med*, 25(3):182–193.
Holman, H and Lorig, K (2004). Patient self-management: a key to effectiveness and efficiency in care of chronic disease. *Public Health Rep*, 119(3):239–243.
Holroyd, KA (2002). Assessment and psychological treatment of recurrent headache disorders. *J Consult Clin Psychol*, 70:656–677.
Holroyd, K, Cottrell, C, O'Donnell, F, et al. (2006). Does preventive medication, behavioral migraine management or their combination add to optimal acute therapy in the management of frequent migraines: the TSM trial. *Headache*, 46:835.
Holroyd, KA and Creer, TL (eds) (1986). *Self-management of Chronic Disease: Handbook of Clinical Interventions and Research*. Academic Press, Orlando, FL 29–58.
Holroyd, KA, Cordingley, GE, Pingel, JD, et al. (1989). Enhancing the effectiveness of abortive therapy: a controlled evaluation of self-management training. *Headache*, 29(3):148–153.
Holroyd, KA, France, JL, Cordingley, GE, et al. (1995). Enhancing the effectiveness of relaxation/thermal biofeedback training with propranolol HCI *J Consult Clin Psychol*, 63:327–330.
Holroyd, KA and Labus, J (2005). Treatment of chronic tension-type headache: moderators of response to drug and behavior therapy. *J Pain*, 6:S54.
Holroyd, KA and Lipchik, GL (2000). Sex differences in recurrent headache disorders. In *Sex, Gender and Pain: from the Benchtop to the Clinic* (RB Fillingim, ed.), pp. 251–279. IASP Press, Seattle.
Holroyd, KA, Lipchik, GL, and Penzien, DB (1998). Psychological management of recurrent headache disorders: Empirical basis for clinical practice. In *Empirically Supported Therapies: Best Practice in Professional Psychology* (KS Dobson and KD Craig, eds), pp. 187–236. Sage Publications, Thousand Oaks, CA.
Holroyd, KA, Nash, JM, Pingel, JD, et al. (1991). A comparison of pharmacological (amitriptyline HCL) and nonpharmacological (cognitive-behavioral) therapies for chronic tension headaches. *J Consult Clin Psychol*, 59(3):387–393.
Holroyd, KA, O'Donnell, FJ, Stensland, M, et al. (2001). Management of chronic tension-type headache with tricyclic antidepressant medication, stress

management therapy, and their combination: A randomized controlled trial. *JAMA*, 285:2208–2215.

Holroyd, KA and Penzien, DB (1986). Client variables and the behavioral treatment of recurrent tension headache: A meta-analytic review. *J Behav Med*, 9:515–536.

Holroyd, KA and Penzien, DB (1990). Pharmacological vs. nonpharmacological prophylaxis of recurrent migraine headache: A meta-analytic review of clinical trials. *Pain*, 42:1–13.

Holroyd, KA, Penzien, DB, and Cordingley, GA (1991). Propranolol in the prevention of recurrent migraine: A meta-analytic review. *Headache*, 31:333–340.

Holroyd, K, Stensland, M, Lipchik, G, et al. (2000). Psychosocial correlates and impact of chronic tension-type headaches. *Headache*, 40:3–16.

Juang, K, Wang, S, and Fuh, J (2000). Comorbidity of depressive and anxiety disorders in chronic daily headache and its subtypes. *Headache*, 40(10):818–823.

Jurish, SE, Blanchard, EB, Andrasik, F, et al. (1983). Home- versus clinic-based treatment of vascular headache. *J Consult Clin Psychol*, 51:743–751.

Kabela, E, Blanchard, EB, Appelbaum, KA, et al. (1989). Self-regulatory treatment of headache in the elderly. *Biofeedback Self Reg*, 14(3):219–228.

Karwautz, A, Wober, C, Lang, T, et al. (1999). Psychosocial factors in children and adolescents with migraine and tension-type headache: a controlled study and review of the literature. *Cephalalgia*, 19:32–43.

Katsarava, Z, Muessig, M, Dzagnidze, A, et al. (2005). Medication overuse headache: rates and predictors for relapse in a 4-year prospective study. *Cephalalgia*, 25(1):12–15.

Kelman, L and Rains, JC (2005). Headache and sleep: examination of sleep patterns and complaints in a large clinical sample of migraineurs. *Headache*, 45 (7):904–910.

Kobak KA, Greist, JH, Jefferson, JW, et al. (1998). Behavioral versus pharmacological treatments of obsessive compulsive disorder: a meta-analysis. *Psychopharmacol*, 136:205–216.

Kudrow, L (1982). Paradoxical effects of frequent analgesic use. In *Advances in Neurology: Headache: Physiopathological and Clinical Concepts Vol.* 33 (M Critchley, AP Friedman, S Gorini, et al., eds), pp. 336–341. Raven Press, New York.

Lake, AE 3rd (2006). Medication overuse headache: biobehavioral issues and solutions. *Headache*, 46(Suppl. 3): S88–S97.

Lake, AE, Rains JC, Penzien, DB, et al. (2005). Headache and psychiatric comorbidity: historical context, clinical implications, and research relevance. *Headache*, 45, 493–506.

Lanteri-Minet, M, Radat, F, Chautard, MH et al. (2005). Anxiety and depression associated with migraine: influence on migraine subjects' disability and quality of life, and acute migraine management. *Pain*, 118:319–326.

Larsson, B, Carlsson, J, Fichtel, A, et al. (2005). Relaxation treatment of adolescent headache sufferers: results from a school-based replication series. *Headache*, 45 (6):692–704.

Larsson, B and Melin, L (1988). The psychological treatment of recurrent headache in adolescents—Short-term outcome and its prediction. *Headache*, 28:187–195.

Linet, MS, Stewart, WF, Celentano, DD, et al. (1989). An epidemiologic study of headache among adolescents and young adults. *JAMA*, 261:2211–2216.

Lipchik, GL, Holroyd, KA, and Nash, JM (2002). Cognitive-behavioral management of recurrent headache disorders: a minimal-therapist contact approach. In *Psychological Approaches to Pain Management* (2nd ed.) (DC Turk and RS Gatchel, eds), pp. 356–389. Guilford, New York.

Lipchik, GL, Smitherman, T, Penzien, DB, et al. (2006). Basic principles and techniques of behavioral therapy for comorbid psychiatric disorders in headache patients. *Headache*, 46(Suppl. 3), S119–S132

Lipton, RB, Hamelsky, SW, Kolodner, K, et al. (2000). Migraine, quality of life, and depression: a population based study. *Neurology*, 55:629–635.

Lipton, RB and Pan, J (2004). Is migraine a progressive disease? *JAMA*, 291(4):493–494.

Lipton, RB, Silberstein, SD, and Stewart, WF (1994). An update on the epidemiology of migraine. *Headache*, 34:319–328.

Lorig, K and Holman, H (2003). Self-management education: history, definition, outcomes, and mechanisms. *Ann Behav Med*, 26(1):1–7.

Lorig, KR, Sobel, DS, Ritter, PL, et al. (2001). Effect of a self-management program on patients with chronic disease. *Eff Clin Pract*, 4:256–262.

Maizels, M and Burchette, R (2004). Somatic symptoms in headache patients: the influence of headache diagnosis, frequency, and comorbidity. *Headache*, 44:983–993.

Maizels, M, Smitherman, TA, and Penzien, DB (2006). A review of screening tools for psychiatric comorbidity in headache patients. *Headache*, 46(Suppl. 3): S98–S109.

Marcus, DA (2007). Headache in pregnancy. *Curr Treat Options Neurol*, 9(1):23–30.

Marcus, DA, Scharff, L, and Turk, DC (1995). Nonpharmacological management of headache during pregnancy. *Psychosom Med*, 57:527–535.

Marcus, DA, Scharff, L, and Turk, DC (1999). Longitudinal prospective study of headache during pregnancy and postpartum. *Headache*, 39(9):625–632.

Mathew, NT (1981). Prophylaxis of migraine and mixed headache: a randomized controlled study. *Headache*, 21(3):105–109.

Mathew, NT, Kurman, R, and Perez, F (1990). Drug induced refractory headache: clinical features and management. *Headache*, 30:634–638.

McCrory, DC, Penzien, DB, Hasselblad, V, et al. (2001). *Evidence Report: Behavioral and Physical Treatments for Tension-type and Cervicogenic Headache.* Foundation for Chiropractic Education and Research. Des Moines, IA, Product No. 2085.

McGrath, PJ, Humphreys, P, Keene, D, et al. (1992). The efficacy and efficiency of a self-administered treatment for adolescent migraine. *Pain*, 49(3):321–324.

Merelle, SY, Sorbi, MJ, and Passchier, J (2006). The preliminary effectiveness of migraine lay trainers in a home-based behavioral management training. *Patient Educ Couns*, 61(2):307–311.

Merelle, SY, Sorbi, MJ, et al. (in press). Migraine patients as trainers of their fellow-patients in non-pharmacological preventive attack management: short-term effects of a randomized controlled trial. *Cephalalgia*.

Michultka, DM, Blanchard, EB, Appelbaum, KA, et al. (1989). The refractory headache patient: II. High medication consumption (analgesic rebound) headache. *Behav Res Ther*, 27:411–420.

Morgenthaler, T, Kramer, M, Alessi, C, et al. (2006). American Academy of Sleep Medicine. Practice parameters for the psychological and behavioral treatment of insomnia: an update. An American academy of sleep medicine report. *Sleep*, 129(11):1415–1419.

Morin, CM (1993). *Insomnia: Psychological Assessment and Management*. Guilford Press, New York.

Morin, CM, Culbert, JP, and Schwartz, SM (1994). Nonpharmacological interventions for insomnia: a meta-analysis of treatment efficacy. *Am J Psychiatry*, 151(8):1172–1180.

Mosley, TH, Grotheus, CA, and Meeks, WM (1995). Treatment of tension headache in the elderly: a controlled evaluation of relaxation training and relaxation combined with cognitive-behavior therapy. *J Clin Geropsychol*, 1:175–188.

Mulleners, WM, Whitmarsh, TE, and Steiner, TJ (1998). Noncompliance may render migraine prophylaxis useless, but once-daily regimens are better. *Cephalalgia*, 18(1):52–56.

Murtagh, DR and Greenwood, KM (1995). Identifying effective psychological treatments for insomnia: a meta-analysis. *J Consult Clin Psychol*, 63(1):79–89.

Nestoriuc, Y and Martin, A (2007). Efficacy of biofeedback for migraine: a meta-analysis. *Pain*, 128(1–2):111–127.

Newman, S, Steed, L, and Mulligan, K (2004). Self-management interventions for chronic illness. *Lancet*, 364:1523–1537.

Nicholson, NL and Blanchard, EB (1993). A controlled evaluation of behavioral treatment of chronic headache in the elderly. *Behav Ther*, 24(3):67–76.

Nicholson, R, Nash, J, and Andrasik, F (2005). A self-administered behavioral intervention using tailored messages for migraine. *Headache*, 45:1124–1139.

Olness, K, MacDonald, JT, and Uden, DL (1987). Comparison of self-hypnosis and propranolol in the treatment of juvenile migraine. *Pediatrics*, 79:593–597.

Ottervanger, JP, Valkenburg, HA, Grobbee, DE, et al. (1996). Pattern of sumatriptan use and overuse in general practice. *Eur J Clin Pharmacol*, 50(5):353–355.

Packard, RC and Brown, F (1986). Multiple headaches in a case of multiple personality disorder. *Headache*, 26 (2):99–102.

Passchier, J, van den Bree, MBM, Emmen, HH, et al. (1990). Relaxation training in school classes does not reduce headache complaints. *Headache*, 30:660–664.

Penzien, DB, Andrasik, F, Freidenberg, BM, et al. (2005). Guidelines for trials of behavioral treatments for recurrent headache. *Headache*, 45:S109–S131.

Penzien, DB, Holroyd, KA, Holm, JE, et al. (1985). Behavioral management of migraine: results from five-dozen group outcome studies. *Headache*, 25:162.

Penzien, DB, Peatfield, RC, and Lipchik, GL (2006). Headache in patients with co-morbid psychiatric disease. In *The Headaches* (3rd edn) (J Olesen et al., eds), pp. 1117–1124. Lippincott, Williams, & Wilkins, Philadelphia.

Penzien, DB, Rains, JC, Lipchik, GL, et al. (2004). Behavioral interventions for tension-type headache: overview of current therapies and recommendation for a self-management model for chronic headache. *Curr Pain Headache Rep*, 8:489–499.

Penzien, DB, Rains, JC, Lipchik, GL, et al. (2005). Future directions in behavioral headache research: applications for an evolving healthcare environment. *Headache*, 45:526–534.

Perlis, ML, Jungquist, C, Smith, MT, et al. (2005). *Cognitive Behavioral Treatment of Insomnia*. Springer, New York.

Pfaffenrath, V and Rehm, M (1998). Migraine in pregnancy: what are the safest treatment options? *Drug Saf*, 19 (5):383–388.

Powers, SW, Patton, SR, Hommel, KA, et al. (2003). Quality of life in childhood migraines: clinical impact and comparison to other chronic illness. *Pediatr*, 112:1–5.

Radat, F, Creac'h, C, and Swendsen, JD (2005). Psychiatric comorbidity in the evolution of migraine to medication overuse headache. *Cephalalgia*, 25:519–522.

Rains, JC, Lipchik, GA, and Penzien, DB (2006). Behavioral facilitation of medical treatment for headache—Part I: review of headache treatment compliance. *Headache*, 46(9):1387–1394.

Rains, JC, Penzien, DB, and Holroyd, KA (1993). Meta-analysis of alternative behavioral treatments for recurrent headache. *Headache*, 33:279–280.

Rains, JC, Penzien, DB, McCrory, DC, et al. (2005). Behavioral headache treatment: history, review of the empirical literature, and methodological critique. *Headache*, 45, S91–S108.

Rains, JC, Penzien, DB, and Lipchik, GA (2006). Behavioral facilitation of medical treatment for headache—Part II: theoretical models and behavioral strategies for improving adherence. *Headache*, 46(9):1395–1403.

Rains, JC and Poceta, JS (2006). Headache and sleep disorders: review and clinical implications for headache management. *Headache*, 46(9):1344–1361.

Reich, BA and Gottesman, M (1993). Biofeedback and psychotherapy in the treatment of muscle contraction/tension-type headache. In *Headache: Diagnosis and Treatment* (CD Tollison and RS Kunkel, eds), pp. 167–183. Williams and Wilkins, Baltimore.

Richardson, GM and McGrath, PJ (1989). Cognitive-behavioral therapy for migraine headaches: a minimal-therapist-contact approach versus a clinic-based approach. *Headache*, 29:352–357.

Rosenberg, MJ, Waugh, MS, and Long, S (1995). Unintended pregnancies and use, misuse and discontinuation of oral contraceptives. *J Reprod Med*, 40(5):355–360.

Rothrock, J, Parada, V, Sims, C, et al. (2006). The impact of intensive patient education on clinical outcome in a clinic-based migraine population. *Headache*, 46:726–731.

Rothrock, J, Patel, M, Lyden, P, et al. (1996). Demographic and clinical characteristics of patients with episodic migraine versus chronic daily headache. *Cephalalgia*, 16(1):44–49.

Rowan, AB and Andrasik, F (1996). Efficacy and cost-effectiveness of minimal therapist contact treatments for chronic headache: a review. *Behav Ther*, 27:207–234.

Royal Australian and New Zealand College of Psychiatrists (2003). Australian and New Zealand clinical practice guidelines for the treatment of panic disorder and agoraphobia. *Aust N Z J Psychiatry*, 37:641–656.

Sances, G, Granella, F, Nappi, RE, et al. (2003). Course of migraine during pregnancy and postpartum: a prospective study. *Cephalalgia*, 23(3):197–205.

Sartory, G, Muller, B, Metsch, J, et al. (1998). A comparison of psychological and pharmacological treatment of pediatric migraine. *Behav Res Ther*, 36(12):1155–1170.

Scharff, L and Marcus, DA (1994). Interdisciplinary outpatient group treatment of intractable headache. *Headache*, 34:73–78.

Scharff L, Marcus D, Turk D (1996). Maintenance of effects in the nonmedical treatment of headache during pregnancy, Headache 36:285–290.

Schneider, WJ, Furth, PA, Blalock, TH, et al. (1999). A pilot study of a headache program in the workplace. *J Occup Environ Med*, 41:868–871.

Schwartz, MS and Andrasik, F (2003). *Biofeedback: A Practitioner's Guide* (3rd edn.). Guilford Press, New York.

Sheehan, DV and Mao, CG (2003). Paroxetine treatment of generalized anxiety disorder. *Psychopharmacol Bull*, 37(Suppl. 1):64–75.

Silberstein, SD (1997). Migraine and pregnancy. In *Neurologic Clinics: Advances in Headache*. Vol. 15 (NT Mathew, ed.), pp. 209–231. WB Saunders, Philadelphia. 209–231.

Silberstein, SD (2000). Practice parameter: evidence-based guidelines for migraine headache (an evidence-based review): report of the Quality Standards Subcommittee of the American Academy of Neurology. *Neurology*, 55 (6):754–762.

Sillanpaa M (1983). Prevalence of headache in prepuberty. *Headache*, 23(1):10–14.

Sillanpää, M and Anttila, P (1996). Increasing prevalence of headache in 7-year-old schoolchildren. *Headache*, 36:466–470.

Simmons, LW and Wolff, HG (1954). *Social Science in Medicine*. Russell Sage Foundation, New York.

Smith, MT, Huang, MI, and Manber, R (2005). Cognitive behavior therapy for chronic insomnia occurring within the context of medical and psychiatric disorders. *Clin Psychol Rev*. 25(5):559–592.

Smith, MT, Perlis, ML, Park, A, et al. (2002). Comparative meta-analysis of pharmacotherapy and behavior therapy for persistent insomnia. *Am J Psychiatry*, 159 (1):5–11.

Sousa, MB, Isolan, LR, Oliveira, RR, et al. (2006). A randomized clinical trial of cognitive-behavioral group therapy and sertraline in the treatment of obsessive-compulsive disorder. *J Clin Psychiatry*, 67:1133–1139.

Spitzer, AL, Kroenke, K, and Williams, JBW (1999). Validation and utility of a self-report version of the PRIME-MD: the PHQ primary care study. *JAMA*, 282:1737–1744.

Spitzer, RL, Williams, JBW, Kroenke, K, et al. (1994). Utility of a new procedure for diagnosing mental disorders in primary care: the PRIME MD 1000 study. *JAMA*, 272:1749–1756.

Strine, T, Chapman, D, and Balluz, L (2006). Population-based US study of severe headaches in adults: psychological distress and comorbidities. *Headache*, 46:223–232.

Strom, L, Peterson, R, and Andersson, G (2000). A controlled trial of self-help treatment of recurrent headache conducted via the Internet. *J Consult Clin Psychol*, 68:722–727.

Teders, SJ, Blanchard, EB, Andrasik, F, et al. (1984). Relaxation training for tension headache: comparative efficacy and cost-effectiveness of a minimal therapist contact versus a therapist delivered procedure. *Behav Ther*, 15:59–70.

Tishler, PV, Larkin, EK, and Schluchter, MD (2003). Redline S Incidence of sleep-disordered breathing in an urban adult population: the relative importance of risk factors in the development of sleep-disordered breathing. *JAMA*, 289(17):2230–2237.

Trautmann, E, Lackschewitz, H, and Kroner-Herwig, B (2006). Psychological treatment of recurrent headache in children and adolescents—A meta-analysis. *Cephalalgia*, 26(12):1411–1426.

Von Korff, M, Gruman, J, Schaefer, J, et al. (1997). Collaborative management of chronic illness. *Ann Int Med*, 127(12):1097–1102.

Wolff, HG (1948). *Headache and Other Head Pain* (1st edn). Oxford University Press, New York.

Wolff, HG (1953). *Stress and Disease*. Charles C Thomas: Springfield, IL

Wolff, HG and Wolff, S (1948). *Pain*. Charles C Thomas: Springfield, IL

Young, T, Shahar, E, Nieto, FJ, et al. (2002). Predictors of sleep-disordered breathing in community-dwelling adults: The Sleep Heart Health Study. *Arch Intern Med*, 162(8):893–900.

31 Emergency Headache, Including Thunderclap Headache

David W Dodick, Eelco FM Wijdicks, and Anne Ducros

Each minute, approximately six patients visit an emergency department (ED) in the United States with a chief complaint of headache. This results in approximately 300,000 visits annually and makes headache the fifth most common complaint seen in US EDs (American College of Emergency Physicians, 2002). The minority of these patients have a secondary cause for headache, and an even smaller number have a grave and potentially catastrophic cause for headache, such as meningitis or subarachnoid hemorrhage (SAH). The majority of patients presenting to the ED have a primary headache disorder, such as migraine, and while only 10% of those presenting to the ED with headache are "repeat customers," more than 50% of headache visits to the ED are comprised of patients who seek care for headache in the ED on a repeated basis (Blumenthal et al., 2003). Therefore, the task of distinguishing primary from secondary headaches can be daunting for physicians, especially because headache characteristics often lack specificity, "repeat customers" are not immune to serious secondary headaches, and associated symptoms may be subtle or absent. The evaluation of headache patients in the ED must therefore be at once focused, but comprehensive enough so as to not overlook a serious cause. The top priority is thus to establish a precise etiologic diagnosis and to distinguish between primary headaches, benign secondary headaches—such as headache due to influenza—and serious secondary headaches requiring emergent investigations and treatment (SAH, meningitis, intracranial hypertension). The crucial part of the diagnostic procedure is the interview which is further completed by the physical examination. This clinical evaluation determines the management, that is, administration of specific acute headache treatments usually conducted on an outpatient basis for primary headaches, investigations if needed followed by treatment on an outpatient basis for benign secondary headaches, and finally, emergent investigations and treatment in the hospital setting for secondary headaches with serious underlying causes. The treatment of secondary headaches requires the treatment of the underlying cause, for example, embolisation or surgery of a ruptured intracranial aneurysm, antibiotics for bacterial meningitis or steroids in temporal arteritis. It is useful to administrate a symptomatic treatment to patients suffering from acute unusual headaches. However, physicians should be aware that headaches might be alleviated even when they are symptomatic of a serious cause. A good response to the treatment employed should not be a reason for postponing etiologic investigations.

DIAGNOSIS OF HEADACHE IN THE EMERGENCY ROOM

Obtaining a Detailed History of Present and Previous Headaches

The first step of the diagnosis procedure is to obtain a history from the patient by interview. The vast majority of sinister headaches that present to the ED are those that present acutely, either hyperacute within seconds to minutes, or subacute and progressive within days to weeks. The clinician must ask the questions as patients often do not volunteer information that may be important in making the diagnosis. For example, while the onset of headache is one of the most important features, patients seldom volunteer the time to peak onset of the headache and they certainly do not come in complaining of a thunderclap headache (TCH). Therefore, clinicians cannot rely on patients to provide them with all of the important clinical information they need to generate a differential diagnosis. The interview may be very difficult when patients are suffering from intense headaches. Obtaining additional data from the patient's family or friends is often useful. The history should actively solicit the clinical features that are most characteristic of those serious disorders which may present with headache (Table 31–1). When the patient and the physician do not speak the same language, and if there is no available translator, severe headaches should be considered and investigated as potential secondary headaches symptomatic of a serious cause: a cerebral computed tomography (CT) scan and a cerebrospinal fluid (CSF) analysis are mandatory.

Mode of Onset and Time Course of the Actual Headache

The first two questions to ask to the patients are the following:

(1) When did your actual headache start? (acute or chronic headache) and
(2) Have you ever had this same type of headache before? (unusual headache or a new attack of a known headache pattern).

Table 31–1 Historical Features of Secondary Headaches.

1. Presence of systemic symptoms such as fever, night sweats, chills, recent weight loss
2. History of risk factors for secondary headache such as systemic cancer, human immunodeficiency virus (HIV), or use of immunosuppressive drugs or immunodeficiency
3. Neurological signs or symptoms (excluding migraine aura)
4. Onset of headache is hyperacute (onset to peak within seconds or minutes)
5. Age greater than 50, especially in the absence of a prior history of headache
6. Headache is precipitated by valsalva, exacerbated by assuming upright posture, or progressive over days, weeks, or months

Based on the responses to these two questions, three different situations arise. First, the patient is able to say that he has already suffered from several similar headaches since months or years. In such cases, a primary headache disorder is the most likely cause and the description of headache characteristics will help to make a precise diagnosis. Second, the patient denies a previous headache history and reports having headaches for the first time in his life. In such cases, a secondary headache has to be excluded and investigations have to be performed. Finally, the patient reports a history of definite primary headaches but states that his acute headache is different from his usual headaches attacks. In such cases, a secondary headache has to be suspected and investigations are noteworthy. In both latter cases of acute unusual headaches, additionnal questions have to be asked: (1) how did the headache begin? (sudden or progressive onset) and (2) how has the pain changed since its onset? (improvement, worsening or stability). Unusual severe headaches with a sudden onset (TCHs) may reveal a wide range of serious conditions including mainly vascular disorders such as SAH. Unusual progressive headaches are the mode of presentation of multiple conditions including intracranial hypertension, meningitis or meningoencephalitis, local cranial disorders, and temporal arteritis.

Characteristics of Headache That May Help to Sort Patients Requiring Investigations

The intensity of the pain does not help to distinguish between a primary and a secondary headache. Nevertheless any sudden and severe headache (TCH) must be regarded as secondary and further explored in the ED. It is important to consider the concordance between the intensity of the pain described by the patient and the consequences of the pain on his attitude (e.g., does he require bed rest?, does he experience difficulties in expressing himself?). The type and the location of pain are not specific for a peculiar atiology.

The circumstances preceeding the onset of a headache may sometimes guide the physician to an immediate diagnosis: cranial trauma (hemorrhage or cerebral contusion), medication or drugs recently taken, recent dural puncture causing CSF hypotension, fever associated with general disease, etc. However, the circumstances surrounding onset can also be misleading: an exertional headache can be benign but also a symptom of a SAH, a headache after lumbar puncture (LP) is generally caused by a low CSF pressure but can sometimes reveal a cerebral venous thrombosis (Benzon et al., 2003).

The patient's medical history may guide the diagnosis: cardiovascular disease and hypertension (strokes), postpartum or previous history of venous thrombosis of the lower limbs (cerebral venous thrombosis), cancer (cranial metastases), known human immunodeficiency virus (HIV) seropositivity (cerebral toxoplasmosis), anxiety and depression (decompensation with tension type headache), and consumption of psychotropic drugs can all affect headache diagnosis.

Associated Symptoms

Any recent and unusual headache associated with a neurological symptom, such as consciousness impairement, epileptic seizures or focal signs, should always be assumed to be due to an intracranial lesion until proven otherwise. A headache with deterioration of health or claudication of the jaw in a patient of more than 60 years of age should immediately point to a possible diagnosis of temporal arteritis. On the other hand, nausea, vomiting, photophobia and phonophobia are nonspecific symptoms that may be part of a meningeal syndrome but are also associated with migraine. The absence of any associated symptom does not eliminate a secondary headache and should not postpone the initiation of investigations if the headache is recent, unusual, and persistent.

Physical Examination

The first step is to assess blood pressure, pulse rate, and the body temperature. An elevated blood pressure is often the consequence and not the cause of a severe head pain. Headache associated with fever immediately points to an infectious disorder. The skin has to be examined in all febrile headache patients suspected of bacterial meningitis in order to search for purpuric lesions. The rest of the clinical examination should include a neurological as well as a local (head an neck) physical examination. Any abnormality in either the neurological or physical examination indicates the need for further evaluation. On the other hand, a strictly normal clinical examination does not eliminate the possibility of a serious cause and should not preclude investigations.

The first step of neurologic examination is to assess the state of consciousness and to search for a meningeal syndrome. Then, the physician should check for a focal neurological deficit that the interview could have possibly missed. Eyelids and pupils are crucial areas to be examined. A painful Horner's sign points to a dissection of the homolateral internal carotid artery. Headaches associated with a unilateral mydriasis or a complete third cranial nerve paralysis points to an aneurysm of the posterior communicating artery or the termination of the internal carotid artery compressing the third nerve. Patients have to be checked for a static or kinetic cerebellar syndrome that may be overlooked in a patient lying down with severe headaches, vomiting, and reluctant to move. Moreover, the visual field has also to be carefully ascertained even in patients who do not complain of visual troubles. Indeed, a right-handed patient with a right occipital lesion may have a left-sided homonymous hemianopia and complain only about headaches because he is anosognosic of the visual deficit. Finally, a fundoscopic examination will search for papillary edema indicating intracranial hypertension or for hypertensive retinopathy possibly indicating hypertensive encephalopathy.

The local cranial examination should include inspection for redness of the eyes, exophtalmy or swelling of the eyelids, palpation of the temporal arteries, of the eyeballs, and of the cranial sinuses to search for an unusual sensitivity to pressure and, finally, auscultation for cervical or cranial bruits. It is also important to palpate the cervical and chewing muscles which are very often contracted and painful in the case of a tension-type headache.

To Identify Headache Emergencies and Urgencies

The golden rule is to consider all recent and unusual headaches as secondary to an organic cerebral cause and to perform adequate investigations.

In all patients with an acute brutal headache (TCH) and in all patients with an acute progressive and persistent headache, investigations have to be started in the emergency room (Table 31–1). Hospitalization is necessary when a serious underlying cause is rapidly found and has to be treated, but is also often necessary when the first investigations have not permitted a firm diagnosis and additional investigations are required. When a benign secondary headache is obvious after the clinical interview and examination (e.g., headache due to influenza), the patient can be managed as an outpatient. Finally, primary headaches or idiopathic facial neuralgias may show acute exacerbations with intractable pain and an impossibility to eat or drink with a risk of dehydratation. These are pain urgencies that may require hospitalization for a few days to give a parenteral treatment.

Strategy of the Diagnostic Evaluations in the ED

The use of diagnostic testing must be guided by clinical suspicion and differential diagnosis. The usual blood examinations are seldom conclusive, except for an increased erythrocyte sedimentation rate, which indicates temporal arteritis or an infectious state. Any recent headache which is unusual and persistent, whether of sudden or progressive onset, requires two basic examinations to be carried out in a systematic way: a CT scan without contrast injection and a LP.

CT Scan

A cerebral CT scan is the first investigation to perform. Images have to be carefully examined for the presence of abnormal hyperdensities indicating blood either in the subarachnoid spaces or in the cerebral or cerebellar parenchyma, for dilatation of the ventricules indicating hydrocephalus, for a localized hypodensity (ischemia) or a localized mass effect indicating an expansive lesion (tumor, abscess, infarct with oedema). Those abnormalitis will then have to be further investigated later by CT scan with injection or better with an magnetic resonance imaging (MRI). If there is a possibility of acute sinusitis, a scan of the sinuses is the procedure of choice. A normal CT scan does not preclude an organic cause: 5%–10% of SAHs, 30%–50% of cerebral venous thrombosis, most cervical arterial dissections with isolated headaches and local signs, and the vast majority of meningitis present with a normal CT scan and require futher investigations.

Lumbar Puncture

An LP should be performed in all patients with unusual and persistent headaches irrespective of whether the onset was sudden (TCH) or progressive. Analysing the CSF is the only way to diagnose a meningitis. Moreover, the LP permits to diagnose a SAH in the 5% of patients who have a normal CT scan. Measurement of white and red blood cell counts, protein, glucose, opening pressure, and inspection for xanthochromia should be performed. Since visual inspection for xanthochromia is associated with a high rate of false negative interpretation, perhaps up to 50% of samples, spectrophotometry should be performed when available. Spectrophotometry also helps to overcome the problem of false positives which may occur when CSF is not promptly centrifuged and examined, and with traumatic taps. Analysis for bilirubin by spectrophotometry has a sensitivity which nears 100% when LP is performed 12 hours to 2 weeks after SAH (Vermeulen et al., 1989). In headache patients, the LP has to be performed after brain imaging (CT scan or MRI) to rule out a contraindication, that is, a space occupiying lesion with mass effect and risk of brain herniation. Rarely, an LP may be indicated without previous brain imaging when the patient is highly supected of a bacterial meningitis and has a normal consciousness and no focal neurological signs. It is essential to measure the CSF pressure. Intracranial hypertension with normal CT scan requires a check for a cerebral venous thrombosis or a dural fistula.

Cervical and Transcranial Ultrasound Examination

This examination must be conducted when the clinical picture is in favor of a carotid or a vertebral artery dissection. Echography can visualize a hematoma in the arterial wall and cervical and transcranial duplex scanning evaluate the hemodynamic repercussion. However, both examinations can be strictly normal when the dissection affects an intracranial portion of the artery or when the hematoma does not produce a significant arterial stenosis. In such cases, investigations have to be continued with an MRI (cervical and cranial axial sequences with Fat Sat) and a cervical and cerebral MR angiography (MRA).

Magnetic Resonance Imaging

MRI is much more sensitive than CT scan for a number of disorders that may be revealed by isolated headaches. A cerebral MRI has to be performed in all patients with an unusual severe and persitent headache even after a normal CT scan and a normal or near normal LP. Indeed, several conditions revealed by an acute headache may present with a normal CT scan and a normal LP. A large number of sequences are necessary: diffusion weighted sequences (acute ischemic lesions), fluid attenuated inversion recovery (FLAIR) (small cortical subarchnoid hemorrage, pituitary necrosis, posterior leukoencephalopathy), Fat Sat axial cervical and cerebral sequences (arterial dissection), T1 and T2* weighted sequences as well as MR veinography (cerebral venous thrombosis). T1 weighted sequences with gadolimium enhancement are needed to search for a pachymeningeal enhancement when an idiopathic low CSF pressure syndrome is suspected. MRA may disclose an arterial aneurysm, a dissection, or segmental spasms consistent with cerebral vasoconstriction syndromes. If a MR apparatus is not available, a CT veinography and angiography are helpful.

Conventional Cerebral Angiography

This is indicated in the event of acute headaches in only two cases. First, all patients with a SAH must have a conventional angiogram in order to serach for a ruptured aneurysm (85% of the cases). Second, a conventional angiogram may be discussed in some patients with a TCH, if all preceeding investigations are normal and the headaches persit or worsen. Indeed MRA or CT angiography (CTA) may sometimes be insufficient to formally exclude a cerebral venous thrombosis, an arterial dissection especially a vertebral dissection, or a cerebral vasoconstriction syndrome.

MANAGEMENT OF TCH IN THE ED

A TCH is a severe and explosive headache that is maximal in intensity at or within 60 seconds of onset. Every TCH has to be considered as symptomatic of an organic cause and immediately investigated in order to avoid potentially catastrophic consequences. Indeed, 30%–80% of the TCHs reveal an underlying disorder, the most frequent being vascular disorders. The location and the type of TCHs are not specific of a peculiar cause. Duration may range according to the various causes from some minutes to several days. A TCH may be unique or be recurrent over a few days. It may start spontaneously or be triggered by Valsalva maneuvers, physical effort or sexual intercourse. While the term *thunderclap* was initially used to refer to the headache associated with an unruptured intracranial aneurysm, the clinical presentation of numerous other disorders may be similar or identical (Table 31–2) (Schwedt et al., 2006). These disorders may either be vascular or based on intracranial hypotension, infection, or space occupying lesions. When all investigations (including CT, CSF analysis, MRI, MRA and veinography, cervical ultrasound, and transcranial Doppler examination) are normal and no definitive etiology can be found, some rare primary headache disorders may be considered.

The first cause to search for is a SAH. Unenhanced brain CT, is almost without exception the first diagnostic study performed in all patients with TCH because of the extremely high sensitivity (98%) and specificity (>98%) for SAH within the first 12 hours following the onset of headache if interpreted by trained neuroradiologists (Wardlaw and White, 2000). The sensitivity of CT for the detection of SAH declines with increasing duration from hemorrhage onset with less than 90% yield after day 1 decreasing to 50% 5 days after hemorrhage (van Gijn and van Dongen, 1982). CSF evaluation is thus required in all patients who present with TCH and have normal CT scans. Patients with a SAH have to be hospitalized to undergo a conventional angiogram. In 85% of cases a ruptured aneurysm is the cause, and the definitive treatment requires a neurosurgical intervention or in intra-arterial embolisation. Other intracranial hemorrhages account for 5%–10% of the TCHs. Isolated headaches are frequent in

Table 31–2 Disorders That May Present with Thunderclap Headache.

Secondary
Vascular
Reversible cerebral vasoconstriction syndromes
Subarachnoid hemorrhage
Unruptured intracranial aneurysm
Cerebral venous sinus thrombosis
Cervical artery dissection
Acute hypertensive crisis
Ischemic stroke
Intraparenchymal, subdural, extradural hemorrhage
Pituitary apoplexy
Other
Secondary cough, sexual, and exertional headache (Chiari type 1)
Spontaneous intracranial hypotension
Third ventricle colloid cyst
Primary
Benign cough, sexual, and exertional headache
Primary thunderclap headache

cerebellar or intraventricular hemorrhages that mimic a SAH. They are rare but possible in some supratentorial parenchymal hematomas especially right frontal or temporal hematomas in right-handed persons. Finally, a TCH exceptionally reveals a subdural hematoma. CT scan easily diagnoses of these cerebral hemorrhages. Ischemic infarcts with the same topography may also be revealed by isolated brutal headaches. The initial CT scan may be normal, MRI being much more sensitive (diffusion). Patients diagnosed with cerebellar infarcts or hemorrhages have to be hospitalized in intensive care units close to a neurosurgery department because they may deteriorate acutely if a compression of the fourth ventricle provokes an acute hydrocephalus and a brain herniation. Numerous other vascular disorders may present with isolated TCHs including approximately 5% of cervical or intracranial artery dissections, 2%–3% of cerebral venous thrombosis, some pituitary necrosis, rare cases of temporal arteritis, the majority of reversible cerebral vasoconstriction syndromes (RCVSs) (also known as reversible or benign cerebral angiopathy), and some cases of unruptured aneurysms. In all these causes, CT scan and LP may be normal implicating that a MRI with MRA and magnetic resonance venography (MRV) is mandatory. The choice of MR sequences may sometimes be guided by clinical index suspicion (e.g., a unilateral persistent TCH with cervical pain points to a cervical dissection); however, clinical practice demonstrates that it is often impossible to predict the final diagnosis on the basis of clinical features.

An isolated TCH may also reveal a nonvascular condition: acute blocked sinusitis, parenchymal or intraventricular tumors with hydrocephalus (colloid cyst of the third ventricle), some meningitis, and some cases of low CSF pressure syndrome. Indeed, approximately 15% of cases of idiopathic low CSF pressure syndromes are revealed by a TCH. Diagnosis is made on the postural character of the headache (alleviated by lying down) and the typical MRI features (meningeal enhancement, cranio-caudal displacement of the brain structures, subdural collections). If bed rest during a few days does not improve the headache, an autologous epidural blood-patch may represent the treatment of choice.

SECONDARY CAUSES OF TCH

Subarachnoid Hemorrhage

SAH is the most common etiology for secondary TCH and must be the focus of the initial evaluation. Initial misdiagnosis and rebleeding often leads to devastating neurological morbidity and mortality. Approximately 11%–25% of patients presenting with TCH may have SAH (Linn et al., 1994; Landtblom et al., 2002). A prospective, hospital-based study of sudden onset headache found that 11% of patients had SAH (Landtblom et al., 2002). In a community-based prospective study of 148 patients with TCH, 37 (25%) were found to be secondary to SAH (Linn et al., 1994).

Rupture of an intracranial saccular aneurysm is the most common cause of SAH, accounting for approximately 85% of cases (van Gijn and Rinkel, 2001). Pretruncal nonaneurysmal SAH accounts for an additional 10% while a variety of miscellaneous conditions, such as transmural arterial dissection, arteriovenous malformation, dural arteriovenous fistula, mycotic aneurysm and cocaine abuse, may present with SAH (van Gijn and Rinkel, 2001).

Headache is the most common symptom in SAH. A community-based, prospective study demonstrated that 70% of patients with SAH present with headache alone, without loss of consciousness or focal neurological symptoms (Linn et al., 1994). In contrast, less than half of the patients presented with isolated headache in a hospital-based study (Ferro et al., 1991). Headaches may peak at onset or within minutes (Linn et al., 1998). However, while distinctively less common, up to 18% of headaches may have a more gradual and progressive onset, over several hours or days. The headache associated with primary TCH, which has a benign prognosis, is indistinguishable from the headache associated with SAH. Therefore, there are no clinical features of the headache that are characteristic of SAH, though the headache associated with SAH invariably lasts longer than 2 hours and often persists for several days. Although physical exertion or sexual intercourse may precede SAH, SAH may occur without any provocation (Pascual et al., 1996).

Loss of consciousness occurs in one-third of patients with SAH (Vermeulen et al., 1984; Linn et al., 1994). Other associated clinical features include seizures (6%–9%), delirium (16%), stroke (caused by intracerebral hematoma), visual disturbances (due to subhyaloid hemorrhage), nausea, vomiting, dizziness, neck stiffness, and photophobia (Hasan et al., 1993; Pinto et al., 1996; Caeiro et al., 2005).

Physical examination is usually of little help in the evaluation of the suspected SAH patient (Ramirez-Lassepas et al., 1997). Subhyaloid retinal hemorrhages occur in 20%–40% of patients, usually in those with altered levels of consciousness. Although the presence of subhyaloid hemorrhage is a useful finding, detection through an undilated pupil in an agitated patient with photophobia may be difficult (Keane, 1979; Pfausler et al., 1996).

CT of the brain without contrast is the first diagnostic test in the evaluation of suspected SAH. Head CT has a sensitivity that nears 100% within the first 12 hours of SAH but then decreases to approximately 50% by 1 week (van der Wee et al., 1995; Sames et al., 1996; Sidman et al., 1996; Morgenstern et al., 1998; Edlow and Caplan, 2000). If the CT is negative, LP must be performed. In addition to routine CSF studies including cell counts and visual inspection for xanthochromia, analysis by spectrophotometry should also be performed if available. In contrast to the declining yield of CT over time, spectrophotometry is more sensitive after the first 12 hours of hemorrhage. When CSF is collected at least 12 hours after SAH, spectrophotometry has sensitivity greater than 95% (Vermeulen et al., 1989). Patients with SAH should undergo conventional angiography in search of a ruptured aneurysm.

Despite recent advances in the treatment of patients with SAH, overall outcome remains poor (Tolias and Choksey, 1996; Hop et al., 1997). Approximately 10% of patients die before reaching a hospital, case fatality is approximately 50% overall, and one-third of survivors remain dependent (Linn et al., 1994; Schievink et al., 1995).

Intraparenchymal, Subdural, and Extradural Hemorrhages

Approximately 50% of patients with intraparenchymal hemorrhage have headache at onset, especially those with cerebellar or lobar hematoma (Gorelick et al., 1986; Jorgensen et al., 1994; Melo et al., 1996; van Gijn, 1997). Sudden onset headache occurs in approximately 2%–6% of patients with intraparenchymal hematoma. Clinical presentations of cerebellar hemorrhage and SAH may be similar because of the prominent headache and the relative paucity of focal neurological deficits. Vomiting and vertigo may be early symptoms of cerebellar hematoma, while most patients have a slightly impaired level of consciousness and about a half have cerebellar or brainstem signs (van der Hoop et al., 1988; Mathew et al., 1995). Chronic subdural hematomas may present with sudden onset headache (Kotwica and Brzezinski,

1985; Linn et al., 1999). Subdural hematoma is usually associated with trauma, although the trauma may seem trivial and forgotten (Wintzen,1980). Anticoagulation (AC) is associated with 25% of patients with subdural hematoma and in these patients, acute headache followed by a rapidly decreasing level of consciousness is associated with a poor outcome (Wintzen,1980; Wintzen and Tijssen, 1982).

Spontaneous retroclival hematoma is a rare cause of TCH. Retroclival hematoma is usually a rare manifestation of severe head and neck injuries which result in atlanto-axial dislocation (Orrison et al., 1986; Kurosu et al., 1990). Spontaneous hemorrhage, although even more rare, can occur, and may be secondary to dural-based arteriovenous fistulae and meningeal tumors (Tomaras et al., 1995).

Two patients with spontaneous hemorrhage have been reported in the literature, both of whom presented with a TCH on normal neurologic examinations and cerebral angiography (Tomaras et al., 1995; Schievink et al., 2001). CSF analysis and MRI were essential in establishing the proper diagnosis. Although the optimal radiologic approach for the diagnosis of a spontaneous retroclival hematoma has not been clearly established, MRI with gadolinium and cerebral angiography with selective external carotid artery injection have been recommended (Schievink et al., 2001).

Ischemic Stroke

TCH has been reported as a presenting feature of ischemic stroke. Headaches occur in approximately 25% of patients with stroke, one-half developing before the onset of other stroke manifestations (Ferro et al., 1995). In patients with a history of a primary headache disorder, headaches occurring at the time of ischemic stroke often resemble their usual headaches. In patients without such a history, a throbbing headache ipsilateral to the stroke is most common (Vestergaard et al., 1993). Appearance of headache with ischemic stroke is dependent upon the severity, location, and duration of ischemia as well as risk factors including a history of migraine, patient age, and genetic background (Bousset and Welch, 2005). Headache is more common with large ischemic stroke, in the territory of the posterior circulation, in patients with a history of migraine, and those of a younger age (Ferro et al., 1995; Tentschert et al., 2005). Although most patients with stroke-related headaches do not present with TCH, three such patients have been reported in the literature and one case of TCH as the primary clinical feature of embolic bilateral cerebellar infarcts has been seen by the authors (Landtblom et al., 2002; Schwedt and Dodick, 2006). Initial studies for SAH are often nondiagnostic in patients with recent strokes, providing further evidence for the necessity of MRI in patients with TCH.

Reversible Cerebral Vasoconstriction Syndromes

RCVSs comprise a group of disorders characterized by TCH, sometimes associated with neurological symptoms and signs, and reversible vasoconstriction of the cerebral arteries. These syndromes have been given various eponymic or syndromic labels, including Call–Fleming syndrome (Call et al., 1988; Singhal et al., 2002), benign angiopathy of the central nervous system (Calabrese et al., 1993), postpartum angiopathy (Bogousslavsky et al., 1989), TCH with reversible vasospasm (Day and Raskin, 1986; Slivka and Philbrook, 1995; Dodick et al., 1999), migrainous vasospasm or migraine angiitis (Serdaru et al., 1984; Solomon et al., 1990; Gomez et al., 1991; Jackson et al., 1993), and drug-induced cerebral arteritis or angiopathy (Henry et al., 1984; Le Coz et al., 1988; Raroque et al., 1993). In general, these disorders have been poorly characterized, likely share a common underlying pathophysiology, and may be confused with cerebral vasculitis because of the overlapping angiographic features. RCVSs have been reported to occur in various clinical settings (Table 31–3), and although the pathophysiology is not clearly understood, a disturbance in the control of cerebral vascular tone is likely (Calabrese et al., 2007). This alteration in vascular tone may be spontaneous or evoked by various exogenous or endogenous factors. Sympathomimetic and serotonergic drugs and tumors (Henry et al., 1984; Le Coz et al., 1988; Raroque et al.,1993; Nighoghossian et al., 1994; Nighoghossian et al., 1998; Razavi et al., 1999; Singhal et al., 2002; Noskin et al., 2006), endocrine factors, direct or neurosurgical trauma (Suwanwela and Suwanwela, 1972; Hyde-Rowan et al., 1983; LeRoux et al., 1991;

Table 31–3 Conditions Associated with Cerebral Vasoconstriction Syndromes.

Pregnancy and puerperium

Early puerperium, late pregnancy, eclampsia, preeclampsia, and delayed postpartum eclampsia

Drugs and blood products

Phenylpropanolamine, pseudoephedrine, ergotamine tartrate, methergine, bromocryptine, lisuride, selective serotonin reuptake inhibitors, sumatriptan, isometheptine, cocaine, ecstasy, amphetamine derivatives, marijuana, lysergic acid diethylamide, tacrolimus (FK-506), cyclophosphamide, erythropoetin, intravenous immune globulin, red blood cell transfusions

Miscellaneous

Acute hypertension, hypercalcemia, porphyria, pheochromocytoma, bronchial carcinoid tumor, head trauma, spinal subdural hematoma, carotid endarterectomy, neurosurgical procedures

Spontaneous and exertion

Spontaneous, physical exertion, sexual intercourse

Source: Adapted from Calabrese et al. (2007).

Lopez-Valdes et al., 1997; Schaafsma et al., 2002; Singhal et al., 2002 ; Yap et al., 2003), and uncontrolled hypertension (Kontos et al., 1978; Goldstein et al., 1991) have all been implicated. Because vascular tone and caliber is dependent on vascular receptor activity and sensitivity, a spontaneous or evoked central sympathetic response may underlie the alteration and reversible nature of RCVS, in addition to the severe and acute headache seen with these disorders.

As with primary TCH, the headache associated with RCVS may be occipital or diffuse, severe and throbbing, and associated with nausea, emesis, and photosensitivity. It can recur spontaneously while the patient is at rest or can be precipitated by exertion or the Valsalva maneuver. Neurological symptoms and signs, including transient or permanent visual defects, hemiplegia, dysarthria, aphasia, numbness, or ataxia, can occur secondary to ischemia in brain regions that are tenuously supplied by a severely constricted artery. Transient hypertension, which at times can be marked, is not uncommon. Generalized seizures may occur during the acute period, but epilepsy does not ensue. Major ischemic or hemorrhagic stroke, progressive brain edema, and even stroke-related death from progressive or severe, sustained cerebral vasoconstriction have been described (Buckle et al., 1964; Geraghty et al., 1991; Sturm and Macdonell, 2000; Hajj-Ali et al., 2002; Singhal, 2002a, 2002b; Lu et al., 2004).

The diagnosis of RCVS should be considered in patients who present with a TCH without evidence of SAH (Table 31–4). RCVS should also be considered in patients with cryptogenic stroke, particularly in those with severe-onset headache or TCH and symmetrical brain infarctions or edema. The initial evaluation should uniformly include an unenhanced brain CT and if necessary LP to exclude SAH. If the results of the CSF examination are benign, additional brain and neurovascular imaging to assess for other causes of severe headache, including cerebral venous sinus thrombosis (CVST), arterial dissection, unruptured saccular aneurysms, and RCVS, should be done. MRI, MRA, and CTA of the brain and cerebral blood

Table 31–4 Cardinal Features of Reversible Cerebral Vasoconstriction Syndromes.

Severe, acute headache, with or without additional neurologic signs or symptoms

No evidence for aneurysmal subarachnoid hemorrhage

Transfemoral or CT/MR angiography documenting multifocal segmental cerebral artery vasoconstriction

Normal or near-normal CSF protein (<80 %mg, WBC <10 per mm^3, normal glucose)

Angiographic reversibility within 12 weeks after onset

Source: Adapted from Calabrese et al. (2007).

Abbreviations: CSF, cerebrospinal fluid; CT, computed tomography; MRI, magnetic resonance imaging; WBC, white blood cells.

vessels are appropriate first-line imaging techniques to evaluate for RCVS; however, conventional catheter-based angiography is still the gold standard.

The results of brain MRI are frequently normal in RCVS but can reveal evidence of infarction, particularly in arterial "watershed" and "border-zone" regions. Changes consistent with the posterior reversible encephalopathy syndrome (PRES) have also been reported (Dodick et al., 2003; Singhal, 2004; Doss-Esper et al., 2005). The relationship between RCVS and hypertensive encephalopathy, and PRES is unclear. PRES is characterized by reversible gray and white matter edema on MRI that often occur in the setting of hypertensive encephalopathy but have also been described in patients with presentations typical of RCVS (Dodick et al., 2003; Singhal, 2004; Doss-Esper et al., 2005). It is possible therefore that RCVS may occur as a cause of posterior reversible leukoencephalopathy, due to ischemia or cerebral edema, and as a consequence of hypertension in posterior reversible leukoencephalopathy when cerebral autoregulation is overwhelmed by massive increases in arterial and cerebral perfusion pressure. The coexistence of posterior reversible leukoencephalopathy and RCVS suggests that a disturbance in cerebral arterial tone is the pathophysiologic basis of both syndromes.

The characteristic angiographic findings in RCVS are alternating areas of arterial constriction and dilatation, often called "beading," in multiple vascular beds. Alternating areas of constriction and normal vascular caliber, rather than areas of dilatation, can also be seen. These findings may be seen in the large and medium cerebral arteries that constitute the anterior circulation (internal carotid and middle, and anterior cerebral arteries) and the posterior circulation (vertebral, basilar, posterior cerebral, superior cerebellar, anterior inferior cerebellar, and posterior inferior cerebellar arteries) (Hajj-Ali et al., 2002; Singhal, 2002a; Lu et al., 2004). It is important to remember that these findings, although highly characteristic, are not specific for RCVS and cannot be differentiated from the angiographic abnormalities seen with cerebral vasculitis (Calabrese et al., 1997). However, the clinical presentation and MRI are helpful in distinguishing RCVS from primary angiitis of the central nervous system (PACNS) (Table 31–5). In addition, analysis of CSF is critical to help differentiate RCVS from cerebral vasculitis. In RCVS, the CSF is generally normal or near normal. In Singhal's systematic review of 152 patients reported as having reversible cerebral vasoconstriction without aneurysmal SAH, 95% of patients had CSF cell counts less than 10 per mm^3 and protein levels below 80 %mg(Singhal, 2002a). The most specific evidence for RCVS is the demonstration of complete or near-complete reversibility of vasoconstriction within 3 months. Although serial direct or indirect MRA or CTA is the method of choice for documenting reversibility of vasoconstriction, transcranial Doppler

Table 31–5 Clinical and Imaging Features that Distinguish Reversible Cerebral Vasoconstriction Syndrome (RCVS) from Primary Angiitis of the Central Nervous System (PACNS).

Variable	*RCVS*	*PACNS*
Onset	Acute (seconds–minutes)	Subacute or chronic
Headache	Sudden (thunderclap)	Insidious, progressive
CSF	Normal, near-normal	Abnormal in >95%
CT/MRI	Normal, PRES, watershed infarction	Cortical and subcortical infarctions, diffuse white matter hyperintensities
Angiography	Multiple stenosis, reversible	Cut-off, luminal irregularities, often irreversible

Source: Adapted from Calabrese et al. (2007).

Abbreviations: CSF, cerebrospinal fluid; CT, computed tomography; MRI, magnetic resonance imaging; PRES, posterior reversible encephalopathy syndrome.

ultrasonography can be used to monitor the progression or resolution of vasoconstriction on the basis of the measurement of flow velocities.

Treatment for RCVS is guided by anecdotal observations at this point. Resolution of clinical and angiographic features have been reported without treatment. Rapid resolution in severe cases have also been reported after treatment with calcium-channel blockers (Dodick, 2003; Lu et al., 2004) brief courses of glucocorticoids (Hajj-Ali et al., 2002) and magnesium sulfate (Singhal, 2004). Although there are no features which predict a negative outcome, stroke has been reported to occur in up to 54% of patients within days to weeks after onset. Therefore, when vasoconstriction is identified, even in the absence of neurological symptoms, a short course of treatment, usually with calcium-channel blockers, is recommended.

Nimodipine or verapamil has been used successfully and should be considered as first-line therapy (Hajj-Ali et al., 2002; Dodick, 2003; Lu et al., 2004). Calcium-channel blockers should be administered with caution because of the risk for watershed infarction in cerebral regions that may be tenuously perfused by a severely constricted cerebral artery. In patients whose cerebral perfusion appears compromised, high-dose glucocorticoids, which have been shown to reverse experimentally induced vasoconstriction, have been reported to be effective (Chen et al., 2002).

Sentinel Headache from Unruptured Intracranial Aneurysm and Warning Leaks

Sentinel headaches are clinically similar to the headaches that occur with SAH. They develop rapidly, reach maximal intensity within minutes, and may persist for hours or days. These headaches may be due to direct activation of vascular sensory afferents that occurs during stretch of the aneurysm wall or are secondary to SAH that has simply gone undetected and are in the true sense, "warning leaks." Approximately 10%–43% of patients with aneurysmal SAH have a history of a sentinel headache or "warning leak" that occurs days or weeks before aneurysm rupture (Polmear, 2003).

Unfortunately, while this group would benefit most from intervention before rebleeding occurs, these patients make up a large proportion of the 25%–50% of patients with SAH that are misdiagnosed before rupture (Edlow and Caplan, 2000). Misdiagnosis occurs not only because of a failure of physicians to recognize the variable clinical presentations of SAH, but also because of a lack of knowledge regarding the limitations of CT when performed days after the hemorrhage, and failure to perform and interpret CSF tests correctly (Edlow and Caplan, 2000).

The sensitivity of MRA for the detection of intracranial aneurysms depends on the size of the aneurysm, but ranges from 69% to 100% (Sato et al., 2005). When aneurysms are 6 mm or larger, the sensitivity of MRA is greater than 95%. CTA, which has been studied less extensively in regard to its value in the diagnosis of intracranial aneurysm, is thought to have a detection rate of 85%–98% (van Gelder, 2003).

Cerebral Venous Sinus Thrombosis

Headache is a prominent symptom in 75%–95% of patients with CVST (de Bruijn et al., 1996, 2001; Agostini, 2004; Cumurciuc et al., 2005; Terazzi et al., 2005). Although headache is most often accompanied by other symptoms and signs of CVST including seizures, papilledema, altered consciousness, and focal neurological symptoms or signs, 15%–30% of patients present with headache alone. While the majority of headaches are progressive, TCH is the presenting and major clinical feature in 2%–10% of patients with CVST (de Bruijn et al., 1996; Cumurciuc et al., 2005). The headaches of CVST are persistent and may be worsened by Valsalva maneuver or recumbency. CVST is more common in the puerperium and often presents with TCH (Cantu and Barinagarrementeria, 1993). Headache in CVST may be caused by distention of pain-sensitive dural venous sinuses, increased intracranial pressure, or associated ischemic or hemorrhagic stroke (Gladstone et al., 2005).

The initial unenhanced head CT and LP may not disclose evidence of CVST. In patients with normal neurologic examinations, brain CT is normal in approximately 25% of patients with CVST. In those with focal neurologic deficits, CT abnormalities are found in approximately 90% (Rao et al., 1981; Chiras et al., 1985). CT abnormalities may include venous infarcts, cerebral edema, or hyperdensity within the occluded sinus. However, subtle findings on CT may be easily missed or misinterpreted. For example, thrombus in a cerebral vein may be mistaken for SAH (Widjaja et al., 2003). Abnormalities detected by LP that support a diagnosis of CVST are present in only a fraction of patients. Approximately one-half of patients have a combination of elevated red blood cell count, protein, opening pressure, and lymphocytic pleocytosis (Bousser et al., 1985; Barinagarrementeria et al., 1992). MRI will often be sufficient for the diagnosis, but in cases where there is a high index of suspicion and MRI is interpreted to be normal, MRV may be necessary. In a recent study, the sensitivity of T2 susceptibility-weighted (T2SW) and T1-weighted spin-echo image (T1SE) sequences to detect clot in the sinuses or veins is 71%–90% between day 1 and day 3. Thrombosed cortical veins, even in the absence of visible occlusion on MRV, were detected more frequently with T2SW (97%) and T1SE (78%) than with FLAIR or diffusion weighted MRI (<40%) (Idbaih et al., 2006).

Prompt diagnosis is crucial. Results from the International Study on Cerebral Vein and Dural Sinus Thrombosis (ISCVT) including 624 patients with CVST occurring between May 1998 and May 2001, demonstrated a mortality rate of 4.3% (27 patients) during the acute phase and 3.4% (21 patients) within 30 days from symptom onset (Canhao et al., 2005). The main causes of acute death were neurologic, the most frequent mechanism being transtentorial herniation. The prognosis of elderly patients is considerably worse than that of younger patients (Ferro et al., 2005). Only 49% of elderly patients made a complete recovery (versus 82% in younger patients), whereas 27% died and 22% were dependent at the end of follow-up (versus 7% and 2% respectively in younger patients). Elderly patients were more likely to harbor an underlying carcinoma, experience thrombotic events during follow-up, and less likely to experience severe headache. Unlike in younger patients, isolated intracranial hypertension is less common while alterations in consciousness or alertness were more common.

The treatment of CVST includes the use of anticoagulants such as dose-adjusted intravenous heparin or body weight-adjusted subcutaneous low-molecular-weight heparin (LMWH), thrombolysis, and symptomatic therapy including control of seizures and elevated intracranial pressure. Recent guidelines from the European Federation of Neurological Sciences (EFNS) for the treatment of cerebral venous and sinus thrombosis were recently published (Einhäupl et al., 2006). Patients with CVST without contraindications for AC should be treated either with body weight-adjusted subcutaneous LMWH or dose-adjusted intravenous heparin. Concomitant intracranial hemorrhage related to CVST is not a contraindication for heparin therapy. The optimal duration of oral AC after the acute phase is unclear. Oral AC may be given for 3 months if CVST was secondary to a transient risk factor, for 6–12 months in patients with idiopathic CVST and in those with "mild" hereditary thrombophilia. Indefinite AC should be considered in patients with two or more episodes of CVST and in those with one episode of CVST and "severe" hereditary thrombophilia. There is insufficient evidence to support the use of either systemic or local thrombolysis in patients with CVST. If patients deteriorate despite adequate AC and other causes of deterioration have been ruled out, thrombolysis may be a therapeutic option in selected cases, possibly in those without intracranial hemorrhage.

Cervical Artery Dissection

Headache is the most frequent symptom in patients presenting with cervical artery dissection. Headache and/or neck pain is reported by 60%–95% of patients with carotid artery dissections and in approximately 70% of patients with vertebral artery dissections (Silbert et al., 1995). The headaches may be acute, developing in less than 24 hours, progressive over 24 hours, or thunderclap in approximately 20% of patients (Mitsias and Ramadan, 1992). Headache or neck pain as the only symptom of carotid dissection occurs in approximately 8% of patients (Arnold et al., 2006). According to International Headache Society (IHS) diagnostic criteria, headaches secondary to cervical artery dissection must be ipsilateral to the dissected artery (Headache Classification Committee of the International Headache Society, 2004). The headache of carotid artery dissection is invariably ipsilateral to the dissection and most often involves the neck, jaw, face, ear, periorbital, and frontal or temporal region. The headache of vertebral artery dissection is often located in the occipital-nuchal region. However, with both types of dissection, headaches may less commonly be more diffuse and bilateral (Biousse et al., 1994). Neck pain accompanies head pain in one-half of patients with vertebral artery dissection and one-quarter of patients with carotid artery dissection (Silbert et al., 1995). Although it is relatively uncommon for patients with cervical artery dissection to present with headache or neck pain in the absence of other neurologic symptoms and signs, headache may precede neurologic manifestations. In such cases, the median duration from onset of headache to onset of other neurologic manifestations is 4 days with carotid dissection and 14.5 hours with vertebral dissection (Silbert et al., 1995). Associated neurologic symptoms and signs include amaurosis fugax, Horner's syndrome, pulsatile tinnitus, dysgeusia, diplopia, or other stroke manifestations.

The potential for cervical artery dissection to present with headache as an isolated clinical symptom illustrates the need for vascular imaging of the cervical carotid and vertebral arteries in patients presenting with TCH when other intracranial causes have been excluded. In addition, patients presenting with new onset headache or neck pain which is different or unique, must also be imaged appropriately with ultrasound, CTA, MRA, conventional angiography, or MRI of the neck with a fat saturation protocol.

Acute Hypertension

Approximately 20% of patients with hypertensive crises have associated headaches. TCH may be the presenting feature of an acute hypertensive crisis and PRES (Zampaglione et al., 1996; Tang-Wai et al., 2001; Dodick et al., 2003b). The head pain associated with acute hypertensive crises may be the direct result of increased pressure stimulating the sensory afferents that innervate the larger intracranial arteries (Spierings, 2002). Acute hypertensive headaches are often located in the posterior head, likely because of the greater density of sensory afferents from C-2 that supply the posterior circulation. During hypertensive crises, manifestations other than headache are usually present including dizziness, dyspnea, chest pain, psychomotor agitation, focal neurologic deficits, and epistaxis (Zampaglione et al., 1996). Hypertensive emergencies may be associated with end-organ damage including stroke, acute pulmonary edema, and hypertensive encephalopathy.

PRES is a subacute neurological syndrome characterized by headache, seizures, visual impairment, often but not always in the setting of extreme hypertension. The headache of PRES is generally either thunderclap or a severe headache of rapid onset. Patients may have associated nausea and vomiting, altered mental status, and focal neurologic signs (Healton et al., 1982; Hinchey et al., 1996; Stott et al., 2005). PRES may also occur in the setting of disorders other than hypertension including eclampsia, thrombotic thrombocytopenic purpura/hemolytic uremic syndrome, and cyclosporine neurotoxicity (Stott et al., 2005). The disorder can also occur in normotensive individuals when systemic arterial blood pressure is not considered excessively high. Although neurologic deficits are reversible in the majority of patients with PRES, a small percentage may have permanent clinical sequelae due to infarction or hemorrhage (Schwartz, 2002).

Acute hypertensive crises and PRES may be easily overlooked in a patient presenting with TCH where hypertension may be considered part of a stress response to the pain of the headache. However, MRI may show evidence of edema involving the posterior white matter and cortex, often involving the parietal and occipital lobes, and potentially involving the basal ganglia, brainstem, and cerebellum (Schwartz, 2002). Since early imaging abnormalities are secondary to vasogenic edema, as opposed to ischemia or infarction, prompt diagnosis is essential in order to treat while the condition is maximally reversible (Schwartz et al., 1992).

Pituitary Apoplexy

Pituitary apoplexy refers to hemorrhage or infarction of the pituitary gland usually in the setting of a pituitary adenoma. Although pituitary apoplexy is a rarely encountered condition in the clinical setting, autopsy evidence of infarction of more than 25% of the pituitary gland is found in 1%–3% of the population (Reid et al., 1985).

Apoplexy may occur in association with pregnancy, general anesthesia, bromocriptine therapy, and pituitary irradiation, but most often occurs in patients with no known history of a pituitary tumor (Mohr and Hardy, 1982). There is a wide variation in the severity of clinical manifestations in patients with pituitary apoplexy. This ranges from relatively mild symptoms, to adrenal crisis, coma, and sudden death. Patients with pituitary apoplexy most commonly present with a combination of acute headache, nausea, decreased visual acuity, ophthalmoplegia, and reduction in visual fields (Randeva et al., 1999). Headache, usually of sudden and severe onset, is the most common presenting symptom and may be the predominant presenting feature (Randeva et al., 1999). Cases of pituitary apoplexy in patients presenting with TCH and normal physical examinations, CT scans, and CSF studies have been reported (Embil et al., 1997; Dodick and Wijdicks, 1998). Since pituitary tumors are isodense to normal brain tissue on CT, they may be easily overlooked if MRI is not also performed.

NON-VASCULAR CAUSES OF TCH

Spontaneous Intracranial Hypotension

Spontaneous intracranial hypotension (SIH) usually presents as a positional headache that occurs or worsens with a sitting or standing posture and is relieved in recumbency. However, approximately 15% of patients with SIH present with TCH (Schievink et al., 2001; Mokri, 2003; Ferrante and Savino, 2005). SIH is often preceded by minor trauma such as trivial falls, lifting, coughing, and sports activities. Headaches are most often bilateral, in the frontal, fronto-occipital, holocephalic, or occipital regions, and may or may not be throbbing (Mokri, 2003). Headaches are usually accompanied by other features of SIH including nausea, vomiting, neck stiffness or pain, auditory muffling, tinnitus, dizziness, diplopia, visual blurring, interscapular pain, or upper extremity radicular pain.

In patients with SIH, headache and neck pain may be mistaken for SAH. Evaluation for suspected SAH, including brain CT and LP, may provide supporting evidence for SIH but would most often be non-diagnostic unless an opening pressure is obtained and found to be low or unobtainable. CSF is generally clear and colorless, protein concentration is normal or modestly elevated (usually <100 mg/dl), erythrocyte count may be normal or elevated, a lymphocytic pleocytosis up to 50 cells/mm^3 is common, and glucose, cytology, and microbiology are normal (Mokri, 2004). Brain MRI with gadolinium typically reveals one or more features of SIH including diffuse pachymeningeal gadolinium enhancement, cerebellar tonsillar descent, crowding of the posterior fossa, reduction in the pre-pontine space, descent of the optic chiasm, and subdural hematoma. In a significant minority of cases however, MRI with gadolinium may be normal. MRI of the spine may reveal extra-arachnoid CSF collection, pachymeningeal thickening and enhancement, or dilated epidural venous plexus. Nuclear cisternography, CT myelography, or MR myelography may be necessary to confirm the presence and location of the CSF leak.

Third Ventricle Colloid Cyst

Colloid cysts of the third ventricle may present with TCH. Such tumors account for 0.5% of intracranial tumors, affect men more often than women, and are most often diagnosed between the third and fifth decades of life. Headache, the most common symptom of a third ventricular colloid cyst, is reported by 68%–100% of diagnosed patients. The headache typically begins abruptly, may resolve in seconds or last up to 24 hours (Kelly, 1951). Headaches are most commonly located in the bilateral frontal, fronto-parietal or fronto-occipital regions (Michels and Rutz, 1982). The pain is typically severe and may be relieved by recumbency. One-half of patients have associated nausea and vomiting. Loss of consciousness, alterations in cognition, seizures, coma, and death can occur (Young and Silberstein, 1997).

Chiari Type 1 Malformation

Chiari type 1 malformations may present with recurrent short-lasting TCH provoked by cough, straining, or Valsalva. Diagnosis may be made on CT scan, but cerebral MRI with sagittal sequences is more sensitive.

PRIMARY CAUSES OF TCHs

Cough, Exertional, and Sexual Headache

Patients who present with acute onset of severe headache that is precipitated repeatedly by cough, physical exertion, or sexual activity may be classified as having primary cough, exertional, or sexual headache, if all diagnostic studies are negative for a secondary cause. Primary cough headache is precipitated by coughing, straining, or Valsalva, has sudden onset, and a duration of 1 second to 30 minutes (Headache Classification Committee of the International Headache Society, 2004). The most common secondary cause for primary cough headache is Chiari type 1 malformation. Primary exertional headache may be brought on by any form of exercise, must be pulsating, and lasts from 5 minutes to 48 hours (Headache Classification Committee of the International Headache Society, 2004). SAH, intracranial metastases, and sinusitis may present with exertional headache (Pascual et al., 1996). Primary sexual headaches are divided into those that occur before and with orgasm. The orgasmic headaches are often thunderclap (Headache Classification Committee of the International Headache Society, 2004). While SAH is of paramount concern in these patients, especially as the syndrome begins, a growing number of cases of orgasmic TCH associated with reversible cerebral vasoconstriction have been described. Therefore, unless a stereotyped pattern of headaches associated with orgasm have occurred over a long time, a detailed evaluation for SAH and RCVS is important in this group of patients.

Primary TCH

Primary thunderclap headache (PTCH) is a diagnosis of exclusion which can be made only after exhaustive evaluation has failed to disclose an underlying cause. The International Classification of Headache Disorders (ICHD-2) has defined PTCH as a headache that is severe, sudden in onset, reaching maximum intensity in less than 1 minute, that lasts from 1 hour to 10 days. (Table 31–6) (Headache Classification Committee of the International Headache Society, 2004). Although the headache may recur within the first week after onset, it should not recur regularly over subsequent weeks or months. Normal CSF evaluation and brain imaging are also required. Vascular imaging should now be part of the evaluation since a substantial proportion of these patients may have a reversible cerebral vasoconstriction syndrome.

Table 31–6 International Headache Society Diagnostic Criteria for Primary Thunderclap Headache.

A. Severe head pain fulfilling criteria B and C
B. Both of the following characteristics:
   1. Sudden onset, reaching maximum intensity in less than 1 minute
   2. Lasting from 1 hour to 10 days
C. Does not recur regularly over subsequent weeks or months
D. Not attributed to another disorder (normal CSF and normal brain imaging are required)

Abbreviation: CSF, cerebrospinal fluid.

References

Agostini, E (2004). Headache in cerebral venous thrombosis. *Neurol Sci*, 25:S206–S210.

American College of Emergency Physicians (2002). Clinical policy: critical issues in the evaluation and management of patients presenting to the emergency department with acute headache. *Ann Emerg Med*, 39:108–122.

Arnold, M, Cumurciuc, R, Stapf, C, et al. (2006). Pain as the only symptom of cervical artery dissection. *J Neurol Neurosurg Psychiatry*, 77:1021–1024.

Barinagarrementeria, F, Cantu, C, and Arredondo, H (1992). Aseptic cerebral venous thrombosis: proposed prognostic scale. *J Stroke Cerebrovasc Dis*, 2:34–39.

Biousse, V, D'Anglejan-Chatillon, J, Massiou, H, et al. (1994). Head pain in non-traumatic carotid artery dissection: a series of 65 patients. *Cephalalgia*, 14:33–36.

Blumenthal, HJ, Weisz, MA, Kelly, KM, et al. (2003). Treatment of primary headache in the emergency department. *Headache*, 43:1026–1031.

Bogousslavsky, J, Despland, PA, Regli, F, et al. (1989). Postpartum cerebral angiopathy: reversible vasoconstriction assessed by transcranial Doppler ultrasounds. *Eur Neurol*, 29:102–105.

Bousser, MG, Chiras, J, Sauron, B, et al. (1985). Cerebral venous thrombosis: a review of 38 cases. *Stroke*, 16:199–213.

Bousset, MG and Welch, KMA (2005). Relation between migraine and stroke. *Lancet Neurol*, 4:533–542.

Buckle, RM, Duboulay, G, and Smith, B (1964). Death due to cerebral vasoplasm. *J Neurol Neurosurg Psychiatry*, 27:440–444.

Caeiro, L, Menger, C, Ferro, JM, et al. (2005). Delirium in acute subarachnoid haemorrhage. *Cerebrovasc Dis*, 19 (1):31–38.

Calabrese, LH, Dodick, DW, Schwedt, TJ, et al. (2007). Reversible cerebral vasoconstriction syndromes. *Ann Intern Med*, 146:34–44.

Calabrese, LH, Duna, GF, and Lie, JT (1997). Vasculitis in the central nervous system. *Arthritis Rheum*, 40:1189–1201.

Calabrese, LH, Gragg, LA, and Furlan, AJ (1993). Benign angiopathy: a distinct subset of angiographically defined primary angiitis of the central nervous system. *J Rheumatol*, 20:2046–2050.

Call, GK, Fleming, MC, Sealfon, S, et al. (1988). Reversible cerebral segmental vasoconstriction. *Stroke*, 19:1159–1170.

Canhao, P, Ferro, JM, Lindgren, AG, et al. (2005). Causes and predictors of death in cerebral venous thrombosis. *Stroke*, 36:1720–1725.

Cantu, C and Barinagarrementeria, F (1993). Cerebral venous thrombosis associated with pregnancy and peurperium. Review of 67 cases. *Stroke*, 24:1880–1884.

Chen, D, Nishizawa, S, Yokota, N, et al. (2002). High-dose methylprednisolone prevents vasospasm after subarachnoid hemorrhage through inhibition of protein kinase C activation. *Neurol Res*, 24:215–222.

Chiras, J, Bousser, MG, Medler, JF, et al. (1985). CT in cerebral thrombophlebitis. *Neuroradiology*, 27:145–154.

Cumurciuc, R, Crassard, I, Sarov, M, et al. (2005). Headache as the only neurological sign of cerebral venous thrombosis: a series of 17 cases. *J Neurol Neurosurg Psychiatry*, 76:1084–1087.

Day, JW and Raskin, NH (1986). Thunderclap headache: symptom of unruptured cerebral aneurysm. *Lancet*, 2:1247–1248.

de Bruijn, SF, de Haan, RJ, Stam, J, et al. (2001). Clinical features and prognostic factors of cerebral venous sinus thrombosis in a prospective series of 59 patients. *J Neurol Neurosurg Psychiatry*, 70:105–108.

de Bruijn, SF, Stam, J, and Kappelle, LJ (1996). Thunderclap headache as the first symptom of cerebral venous sinus thrombosis. CVST study group. *Lancet*, 348:1623–1625.

Dodick, DW (2003). Reversible segmental cerebral vasoconstriction (Call-Fleming syndrome): the role of calcium antagonists [Editorial]. *Cephalalgia*, 23:163–165.

Dodick, DW and Wijdicks, EFM (1998). Pituitary apoplexy presenting as thunderclap headache. *Neurology*, 50:1510–1511.

Dodick, DW, Brown, RD Jr., Britton, JW, et al. (1999). Nonaneurysmal thunderclap headache with diffuse, multifocal, segmental, and reversible vasospasm. *Cephalalgia*, 19:118–123.

Dodick, DW, Eross, EJ, Drazkowski, JF, et al. (2003a). Thunderclap headache associated with reversible vasospasm and posterior leukoencephalopathy syndrome [Letter]. *Cephalalgia*, 23:994–997.

Doss-Esper, CE, Singhal, AB, Smith, MS, et al. (2005). Reversible posterior leukoencephalopathy, cerebral vasoconstriction, and strokes after intravenous immune globulin therapy in guillain-barre syndrome. *J Neuroimaging*, 15:188–192.

Edlow, JA and Caplan, LR (2000). Avoiding pitfalls in the diagnosis of subarachnoid hemorrhage. *N Engl J Med*, 342:29–36.

Einhäupl, K, Bousser, MG, de Bruijn, SF, et al. (2006). EFNS guideline on the treatment of cerebral venous and sinus thrombosis. *Eur J Neurol*, 13:553–559.

Embil, JM, Matthias, K, and Kinnear, R (1997). A blinding headache. *Lancet*, 350:182.

Ferrante, E and Savino, A (2005). Thunderclap headache caused by spontaneous intracranial hypotension. *Neurol Sci*, 26:S155–S157.

Ferro, J, Canhao, P, Bousser, MG, *et.al.* (2005). Causes and predictors of death in cerebral venous thrombosis. *Stroke*, 36:1927–1932.

Ferro, JM, Lopes, J, and Melo, TP (1991). Investigation into the causes of delayed diagnosis of subarachnoid hemorrhage. *Cerebrovasc Dis*, 1:160–164.

Ferro, JM, Melo, TP, Oliveira, V, et al. (1995). A multivariate study of headache associated with ischemic stroke. *Headache*, 35:315–319.

Geraghty, JJ, Hoch, DB, Robert, ME, et al. (1991). Fatal puerperal cerebral vasospasm and stroke in a young woman. *Neurology*, 41:1145–1147.

Gladstone, JP, Dodick, DW, and Evans, R (2005). The young woman with postpartum "thunderclap" headache. *Headache*, 45:70–74.

Goldstein, M, Wright, J, and Churg, J (1991). *Vasuclitis and Hypertension*. Ikagu-Schoin, New York.

Gomez, CR, Gomez, SM, Puricelli, MS, et al. (1991). Transcranial Doppler in reversible migrainous vasospasm causing cerebellar infarction: report of a case. *Angiology*, 42:152–156.

Gorelick, PB, Hier, DB, Caplan, LR,et al. (1986). Headache in acutecerebrovasculardisease. *Neurology*, 36(11):1445–1450.

Hajj-Ali, RA, Furlan, A, Abou-Chebel, A, et al. (2002). Benign angiopathy of the central nervous system: cohort of 16 patients with clinical course and long-term followup. *Arthritis Rheum*, 47:662–669.

Hasan, D, Schonck, RS, Avezaat, CJ, et al. (1993). Epileptic seizures after subarachnoid hemorrhage. *Ann Neurol*, 33(3):286–291.

Headache Classification Committee of the International Headache Society (2004). The international classification of headache disorders. *Cephalalgia*, 24 (Supp. 1):1–151.

Healton, E, Burst, J, Feinfield, D, et al. (1982). Hypertensive encephalopathy and the neurologic manifestations of malignant hypertension. *Neurology*, 32:127–132.

Henry, PY, Larre, P, Aupy, M, et al. (1984). Reversible cerebral arteriopathy associated with the administration of ergot derivatives. *Cephalalgia*, 4:171–178.

Hinchey, J, Chaves, C, Appignani, B, et al. (1996). A reversible posterior leukoencephalopathy syndrome. *N Engl J Med*, 334:494–500.

Hop, JW, Rinkel, GJ, Algra, A, et al. (1997). Case-fatality rates and functional outcome after subarachnoid hemorrhage: a systematic review. *Stroke*, 28(3):660–664.

Hyde-Rowan, MD, Roessmann, U, and Brodkey, JS (1983). Vasospasm following transsphenoidal tumor removal associated with the arterial changes of oral contraception. *Surg Neurol*, 20:120–124.

Idbaih, A, Boukobza, M, Crassard, I, et al. (2006). MRI of clot in cerebral venous thrombosis: high diagnostic value of susceptibility-weighted images. *Stroke*, 37:991–995.

Jackson, M, Lennox, G, Jaspan, T, et al. (1993). Migraine angiitis precipitated by sex headache and leading to watershed infarction. *Cephalalgia*, 13:427–430.

Jorgensen, HS, Jespersen, HF, Nakayama, H, et al. (1994). Headache in stroke: the Copenhagen stroke study. *Neurology*, 44(10):1793–1797.

Keane, JR (1979). Retinal hemorrhages: its significance in 100 patients with acute encephalopathy of unknown cause. *Arch Neurol*, 36:691–694.

Kelly, R (1951). Colloid cysts of the third ventricle; analysis of twenty-nine cases. *Brain*, 74(1):23–65.

Kontos, HA, Wei, EP, Navari, RM, et al. (1978). Responses of cerebral arteries and arterioles to acute hypotension and hypertension. *Am J Physiol*, 234:H371–H383.

Kotwica, Z and Brzezinski, J (1985). Chronic subdural hematoma presenting as spontaneous subarachnoid hemorrhage. Report of six cases. *J Neurosurg*, 63 (5):691–692.

Kurosu, A, Amano, K, Kubo, O, et al. (1990). Clivus epidural hematoma. *J Neurosurg*, 72:660–662.

Landtblom, AM, Fridriksson, S, Boivie, J, et al. (2002). Sudden onset headache: a prospective study of features, incidence and causes. *Cephalalgia*, 22:354–360.

Le Coz, P, Woimant, F, Rougemont, D, et al. (1988). [Benign cerebral angiopathies and phenylpropanolamine]. *Rev Neurol (Paris)*, 144:295–300.

LeRoux, PD, Haglund, MM, Mayberg, MR, et al. (1991). Symptomatic cerebral vasospasm following tumor resection: report of two cases. *Surg Neurol*, 36:25–31.

Linn, FH, Rinkel, GJ, Algra, A, et al. (1998). Headache characteristics in subarachnoid haemorrhage and benign thunderclap headache. *J Neurol Neurosurg Psychiatry*, 65(5):791–793.

Linn, FH, Rinkel, GJ, and van Gijn, J (1999). Acute severe headache: a subarachnoidal hemorrhage? *Ned Tijdschr Geneeskd*, 143(11):545–550.

Linn, FH, Wijdicks, EF, van der Graaf, Y, et al. (1994). Prospective study of sentinel headache in aneurysmal subarachnoid haemorrhage. *Lancet*, 344 (8922):590–593.

Lopez-Valdes, E, Chang, HM, Pessin, MS, et al. (1997). Cerebral vasoconstriction after carotid surgery. *Neurology*, 49:303–304.

Lu, SR, Liao, YC, Fuh, JL, et al. (2004). Nimodipine for treatment of primary thunderclap headache. *Neurology*, 62:1414–416.

Mathew, P, Teasdale, G, Bannan, A, et al. (1995). Neurosurgical management of cerebellar haematoma and infarct. *J Neurol Neurosurg Psychiatry*, 59(3):287–292.

Melo, TP, Pinto, AN, and Ferro, JM (1996). Headache in intracerebral hematomas. *Neurology*, 47(2):494–500.

Michels, LG and Rutz, D (1982). Colloid cysts of the third ventricle. A radiologic-pathologic correlation. *Arch Neurol*, 39(10):640–643.

Mitsias, P and Ramadan, NM (1992). Headache in ischemic cerebrovascular disease. Part I: clinical features. *Cephalalagia*, 12:269–274.

Mohr, G and Hardy, J (1982). Hemorrhage, necrosis, and apoplexy in pituitary adenomas. *Surg Neurol*, 18:181–189.

Mokri, B (2003). Headaches caused by decreased intracranial pressure: diagnosis and management. *Curr Opin Neurol*, 16:319–326.

Mokri, B (2004). Low cerebrospinal fluid pressure syndromes. *Neurol Clin N Am*, 22:55–74.

Morgenstern, LB, Luna-Gonzales, H, Huber, JC Jr., et al. (1998). Worst headache and subarachnoid hemorrhage: prospective, modern computed tomography and spinal fluid analysis. *Ann Emerg Med*, 32:297–304.

Nighoghossian, N, Derex, L, and Trouillas, P (1998). Multiple intracerebral hemorrhages and vasospasm following antimigrainous drug abuse. *Headache*, 38:478–480.

Nighoghossian, N, Trouillas, P, Loire, R, et al. (1994). Catecholamine syndrome, carcinoid lung tumor and stroke [Letter]. *Eur Neurol*, 34:288–289.

Noskin, O, Jafarimojarrad, E, Libman, RB, et al. (2006). Diffuse cerebral vasoconstriction (Call-Fleming syndrome) and stroke associated with antidepressants. *Neurology*, 67:159–160.

Orrison, WW, Rogde, S, Kinard, RE, et al. (1986). Clivus epidural hematoma: a case report. *Neurosurgery*, 18:194–196.

Pascual, J, Iglesias, F, Oterino, A, et al. (1996). Cough, exertional, and sexual headaches: an analysis of 72 benign and symptomatic cases. *Neurology*, 46 (6):1520–1524.

Pfausler, B, Belcl, R, Metzler, R, et al. (1996). Terson's syndrome in spontaneous subarachnoid hemorrhage: a prospective study in 60 consecutive patients. *J Neurosurg*, 85(3):392–394.

Pinto, AN, Canhao, P, and Ferro, JM (1996). Seizures at the onset of subarachnoid haemorrhage. *J Neurol*, 243 (2):161–164.

Polmear, A (2003). Sentinel headaches in aneurysmal subarachnoid haemorrhage: what is the true incidence? A systematic review. *Cephalalgia*, 23:935–941.

Ramirez-Lassepas, M, Espinosa, CE, Cicero, JJ, et al. (1997). Predictors of intracranial pathologic findings in patients who seek emergency care because of headache. *Arch Neurol*, 54(12):1506–1509.

Randeva, HS, Schoebel, J, Byrne, J, et al. (1999). Classical pituitary apoplexy: clinical features, management and outcome. *Clin Endocrinol*, 51:181–188.

Rao, KCVG, Knipp, HC, and Wagner, EJ (1981). CT findings in cerebral sinus and venous thrombosis. *Radiology*, 140:391–398.

Raroque, HG Jr., Tesfa, G, and Purdy, P (1993). Postpartum cerebral angiopathy. Is there a role for sympathomimetic drugs? *Stroke*, 24:2108–2110.

Razavi, M, Bendixen, B, Maley, JE, et al. (1999). CNS pseudovasculitis in a patient with pheochromocytoma. *Neurology*, 52:1088–1090.

Reid, RL, Quigley, ME, and Yen, SSC (1985). Pituitary apoplexy: a review. *Arch Neurol*, 42:712–719.

Sames, TA, Storrow, AB, Finkelstein, JA, et al. (1996). Sensitivity of new-generation computed tomography in subarachnoid hemorrhage. *Acad Emerg Med*, 3:16–20.

Sato, M, Nakano, M, sasanuma, J, et al. (2005). Preoperative cerebral aneurysm assessment by three-dimensional magnetic resonance angiography: feasibility of surgery without conventional catheter angiography. *Neurosurgery*, 56:903–912.

Schaafsma, A, Veen, L, and Vos, JP (2002). Three cases of hyperperfusion syndrome identified by daily transcranial Doppler investigation after carotid surgery. *Eur J Vasc Endovasc Surg*, 23:17–22.

Schievink, WI, Thompson, RC, Loh, CT, et al. (2001). Spontaneous retroclival hematoma presenting as thunderclap headache. *J Neurosurg*, 95:522–524.

Schievink, WI, Wijdicks, EF, Meyer, FB, et al. (2001). Spontaneous intracranial hypotension mimicking aneurysmal subarachnoid hemorrhage. *Neurosurgery*, 48:513–517.

Schievink, WI, Wijdicks, EF, Parisi, JE, et al. (1995). Sudden death from aneurysmal subarachnoid hemorrhage. *Neurology*, 45(5):871–874.

Schwartz, RB (2002). Hyperperfusion encephalopathies: hypertensive encephalopathy and related conditions. *Neurologist*, 8:22–34.

Schwartz, RB, Jones, KM, Kalina, P, et al. (1992). Hypertensive encephalopathy: findings on CT, MR imaging, and SPECT imaging in 14 cases. *AJR Am J Roentgenol*, 159:379–383.

Schwedt, TJ and Dodick, DW (2006). Thunderclap stroke: embolic cerebellar infarcts presenting as thunderclap headache. *Headache*, 46:520–522.

Schwedt, TJ, Matharu, MS, and Dodick, DW (2006). Thunderclap headache. *Lancet Neurol*, 5:621–631.

Serdaru, M, Chiras, J, Cujas, M, et al. (1984). Isolated benign cerebral vasculitis or migrainous vasospasm? *J Neurol Neurosurg Psychiatry*, 47:73–76.

Sidman, R, Connolly, E, and Lemke, T (1996). Subarachnoid hemorrhage diagnosis: lumbar puncture is still needed when the computed tomography scan is normal. *Acad Emerg Med*, 3:827–831.

Silbert, PL, Mokri, B, and Schievink, WI (1995). Headache and neck pain in spontaneous internal carotid and vertebral artery dissections. *Neurology*, 45:1517–1522.

Singhal, AB (2002a). Cerebral vasoconstriction without subarachnoid blood: associated conditions, clinical and neuroimaging characteristics. *Ann Neurol*, (Suppl.):59–60.

Singhal, AB (2002b). Thunderclap headache, reversible cerebral arterial vasoconstriction, and unruptured aneurysms [Letter]. *J Neurol Neurosurg Psychiatry*, 73:96.

Singhal, AB (2004). Postpartum angiopathy with reversible posterior leukoencephalopathy. *Arch Neurol*, 61:411–416.

Singhal, AB, Caviness, VS, Begleiter, AF, et al. (2002). Cerebral vasoconstriction and stroke after use of serotonergic drugs. *Neurology*, 58:130–133.

Slivka, A and Philbrook, B (1995). Clinical and angiographic features of thunderclap headache. *Headache*, 35:1–6.

Solomon, S, Lipton, RB, and Harris, PY (1990). Arterial stenosis in migraine: spasm or arteriopathy? *Headache*, 30:52–61.

Spierings, ELH (2002). Acute and chronic hypertensive headache and hypertensive encephalopathy. *Cephalalgia*, 22:313–316.

Stott, VL, Hurrell, MA, and Anderson, TJ (2005). Reversible posterior leukoencephalopathy syndrome: a misnomer reviewed. *Inter Med J*, 35:83–90.

Sturm, JW and Macdonell, RA (2000). Recurrent thunderclap headache associated with reversible intracerebral vasospasm causing stroke. *Cephalalgia*, 20:132–135.

Suwanwela, C and Suwanwela, N (1972). Intracranial arterial narrowing and spasm in acute head injury. *J Neurosurg*, 36:314–323.

Tang-Wai, DF, Phan, TG, and Wijdicks, EFM (2001). Hypertensive encephalopathy presenting with thunderclap headache. *Headache*, 41:198–200.

Tentschert, S, Wimmer, R, Greisenegger, WL, et al. (2005). Headache at stroke onset in 2196 patients with ischemic stroke or transient ischemic attack. *Stroke*, 36:e1–e3.

Terazzi, E, Mittino, D, Ruda, R, et al. (2005). Cerebral venous thrombosis: a retrospective multicentre study of 48 patients. *Neurol Sci*, 25:311–315.

Tolias, CM and Choksey, MS (1996). Will increased awareness among physicians of the significance of sudden agonizing headache affect the outcome of subarachnoid hemorrhage? Coventry and Warwickshire Study: audit of subarachnoid hemorrhage (establishing historical controls), hypothesis, campaign layout, and cost estimation. *Stroke*, 27(5):807–812.

Tomaras, C, Horowitz, BL, and Harper, RL (1995). Spontaneous clivus hematoma: case report and literature review. *Neurosurgery*, 37:123–124.

van der Hoop, RG, Vermeulen, M, and van Gijn, J (1988). Cerebellar hemorrhage: diagnosis and treatment. *Surg Neurol*, 29(1):6–10.

van der Wee, N, Rinkel, GJ, Hasan, D, et al. (1995). Detection of subarachnoid haemorrhage on early CT: is lumbar puncture still needed after a negative scan? *J Neurol Neurosurg Psychiatry*, 58:357–359.

Van Gelder, JM (2003). Computed tomographic angiography for detecting cerebral aneurysms: implications of aneurysm size distribution for the sensitivity, specificity, and likelihood ratios. *Neurosurgery*, 53:597–606.

van Gijn, J (1997). Slip-ups in diagnosis of subarachnoid haemorrhage. *Lancet*, 349(9064):1492.

van Gijn, J and Rinkel, GJ (2001). Subarachnoid haemorrhage: diagnosis, causes and management. *Brain*, 124 (Pt 2):249–278.

van Gijn, J and van Dongen, KJ (1982). The time course of aneurysmal hemorrhage on computed tomograms. *Neuroradiology*, 23:153–156.

Vermeulen, M, Hasan, D, Blijenberg, BG, et al. (1989). Xanthochromia after subarachnoid haemorrhage needs no revisitation. *J Neurol Neurosurg Psychiatry*, 52:826–828.

Vermeulen, M, Lindsay, KW, Murray, GD, et al. (1984). Antifibrinolytic treatment in subarachnoid hemorrhage. *N Engl J Med*, 311(7):432–437.

Vestergaard, K, Andersen, G, Nielsen, MI, et al. (1993). Headache in stroke. *Stroke*, 24:1621–1624.

Wardlaw, JM and White, PM (2000). The detection and management of unruptured intracranial aneurysms. *Brain*, 123:205–221.

Widjaja, E, Romanowski, CAJ, Dinanan, AR, et al. (2003). Thunderclap headache: presentation of intracranial sinus thrombosis? *Clinl Radiol*, 58:648–652.

Wintzen, AR and Tijssen, JG (1982). Subdural hematoma and oral anticoagulant therapy. *Arch Neurol*, 39 (2):69–72.

Wintzen, AR (1980). The clinical course of subdural haematoma. A retrospective study of aetiological, chronological and pathological features in 212 patients and a proposed classification. *Brain*, 103 (4):855–867.

Yap, CK, Ismail, A, and Tan, SG (2003). Can the byssus of green-lipped mussel Perna viridis (Linnaeus) from the west coast of Peninsular Malaysia be a biomonitoring organ for Cd, Pb and Zn? Field and laboratory studies. *Environ Int*, 29:521–528.

Young, WB and Silberstein, SD (1997). Paroxysmal headache caused by colloid cyst of the third ventricle: case report and review of the literature. *Headache*, 37 (1):15–20.

Zampaglione, B, Pascale, C, Marchisio, M, et al. (1996). Hypertensive urgencies and emergencies. Prevalence and clinical presentation. *Hypertension*, 27:144–147.

32 Peripheral Procedures: Nerve Blocks, Peripheral Neurostimulation, and Botulinum Neurotoxin Injections

Avi Ashkenazi, Morris Levin, and David W Dodick

INTRODUCTION

Many patients with chronic headaches do not respond optimally to pharmacotherapy (Silberstein and Goadsby, 2002). Efficacy of currently available preventive medications is limited, and their use is associated with potentially disabling side-effects, such as fatigue, drowsiness, weight gain, and cognitive impairment. The triptans, which are effective for migraine and cluster headache (CH), have greatly improved acute headache treatment (Ferrari et al., 2001). However, some patients do not respond to or have adverse events associated with the use of these agents, and they are contraindicated in patients with cardiovascular, cerebrovascular, and peripheral vascular disease, as well as in those with hemiplegic or basilar migraine.

Peripheral nerve blocks have long been used to treat headaches (Wolff, 1948, pp. 182, 465, 526, and 538). These procedures offer patients a potential for rapid relief from headache and associated symptoms. They are generally safe, and are relatively easy to perform in the office. Although many clinicians report positive results from cranial and cervical nerve blocks, few rigorous studies on their efficacy for headaches have been performed. More recently, peripheral nerve stimulation has emerged as a potential treatment modality for some headache patients. Botulinum neurotoxin (BoNT), a potent muscle relaxant, has been studied extensively as a preventive headache treatment, though the data are conflicting at present. Its advantages are a long duration of action and high tolerability. Basic science studies show that the toxin affects the release of neurotransmitters involved in pain transmission, such as calcitonin gene-related peptide (CGRP) and substance P, which supports the rationale for its use in headache patients (Ishikawa et al., 2000; Welch et al., 2000; Dolly, 2003; Cui et al., 2004).

In this chapter, we will review the current data on the efficacy, tolerability, and safety of these peripheral procedures in the treatment of headaches.

NERVE BLOCKS FOR HEADACHE—BACKGROUND

Peripheral anesthetic techniques have been popu. lar headache treatments for many years. Harold Wolff, in the first edition of this book (Wolff, 1948, pp. 182, 465, 526, and 538), commented in several chapters on the usefulness (or lack of usefulness) of superficial injections of procaine in migraine, histamine induced-, and posttraumatic headaches. The general technique of nerve block is relatively easy to learn, side-effects (when it is performed carefully) are minimal, and every practitioner who includes head and neck local anesthetic (LA) procedures in his or her practice has seen numerous successes. However, there is scant evidence for the efficacy of nerve blocks in headache disorders. In general, nerve blocks have not been studied against placebo/sham controls, although one comparative study (Gale et al., 2002) did compare pericranial nerve blocks with cognitive therapy. The results were not striking and the numbers of subjects in each group who completed the study were very low. In addition, classification of headache type was not clear, which is a common problem in interpreting data in this area. It has been established that injections for pain carry a significant placebo effect (de Craen et al., 2000), hence controlled studies of nerve blocks are needed. It will also be necessary to standardize and reproduce the exact techniques of the procedures.

Peripheral nerve blockade to suppress pain is based upon the ability of LAs to selectively block sensory fibers in mixed nerves at relatively low concentrations. The duration of the block depends on the dose and the pharmacokinetic properties of the particular LA(s), but a longer than expected duration of all or some benefits has been a common observation. The mechanism for this is unclear.

Various nerves have been explored as potential targets for blockade in headache disorders. In this section, we will discuss those with either evidence of efficacy or a strong suspicion of usefulness, and we will provide specific techniques with illustrations. The techniques of some nerve blocks are easily learned and can be performed in the office. Others are more involved and require careful training and special equipment. The pharmacologic properties of LAs, as well as commonly used adjunct medications, will be discussed first, particularly regarding potential deleterious effects (which should be clearly specified in informed consent discussions).

Peripheral Nerve Blockade—General Considerations

LAs are weak bases and are available as salts to promote stability and solubility. They all have hydrophilic as well as lipophilic components, properties that make them absorbable and allow them to cross nerve membranes, respectively. They are divided into ester and amide categories. Esters tend to be more allergenic and have relatively short durations of action. The amides, which include the agents most commonly used in local neural blockade (lidocaine, mepivacaine, bupivacaine, and prilocaine), are generally hypoallergenic and well tolerated. All LAs inhibit neural activity by interfering with sodium and potassium currents, thus preventing depolarization. Although specific mechanisms are not yet completely understood, it seems that LAs diffuse into neurons and bind to voltage-gated sodium channels, altering their function. Potassium leak currents are altered as well. Their diffusion across nerve membranes is related to myelin thickness. Thus LAs tend to diffuse much better into C fibers than into A fibers, sparing motor function at the dosages employed in clinical practice.

All LAs are eventually absorbed systemically, and adverse effects will depend on the amount that is used. The most severe effects relate to the occurrence of seizures or loss of consciousness when systemic levels are high. Amide LAs are metabolized by the hepatic cytochrome P-450 3A4 enzyme system. A number of pharmacologic agents (including antiarrhythmics, antibiotics, antiepileptics, calcium channel blockers, β blockers, and antidepressants) can inhibit this system, but, in general, doses used in peripheral nerve blockade are not of concern as long as intravascular injection is avoided. Other adverse effects include local infection, nerve damage with neuroma formation, hematoma (particularly in patients with a bleeding diathesis), and local injury to adjacent structures, depending upon the site of injection.

When injecting, it is essential to understand the sometimes complex anatomy of the area in question, including the individual patient's specific features (e.g., skull defects, local infection, previous surgery). When injecting, one must always pull back the plunger of the syringe to ensure that the needle is not intravascular. This is not entirely reliable when using small gauge needles (30 and smaller) or if back pressure is applied too suddenly. Skin injection tends to distort anatomy, so it is important to ascertain markers carefully or even mark the skin appropriately. Since LAs tend to diffuse well throughout the dermis, multiple injection sites are often unnecessary. Patients should wait in the office until the effects of the anesthetic are apparent [sensation testing should reveal an area of anesthesia corresponding to the usual distribution of the nerve(s) injected]. If further anesthesia is performed, inserting the needle through already anesthetized skin is ideal.

A number of LA agents, including bupivacaine, lidocaine, mepivacaine, and prilocaine, have been used to treat head pain. The latter three have similar potency (approximately one-fourth that of bupivacaine) and a mid-range duration of action. Of these, lidocaine in the 1% solution, with an onset of action at approximately 4–8 minutes after injection and duration of approximately 1–2 hours, is the most common choice. Bupivacaine in the 0.25%–0.50% solution is often chosen for its more prolonged action, with the onset in approximately 8–12 minutes and duration between 4 and 8 hours. Many choose to combine lidocaine with bupivacaine, and some add a corticosteroid medication (although this has no proven benefit). Corticosteroid choices include triamcinolone (Kenalog) or methylprednisolone (Depo-medrol).

Greater Occipital Nerve Block

The greater occipital nerve (GON) is the primary branch of the C_2 root and innervates the scalp from the level of the external occipital protuberance to the vertex. It is located approximately one-third of the distance on a line from the external occipital protuberance to the center of the mastoid (Fig. 32–1). It is adjacent to the occipital artery and can be located by palpating for this artery. Injecting approximately 2 cm lateral to the external occipital protuberance is another useful approximation of the location of the GON (although in some patients this may prove more rostral than ideal). Approximately 2–4 cc of bupivacaine or lidocaine, or a mixture of the two, injected in the area of the GON should be sufficient to anesthetize this nerve.

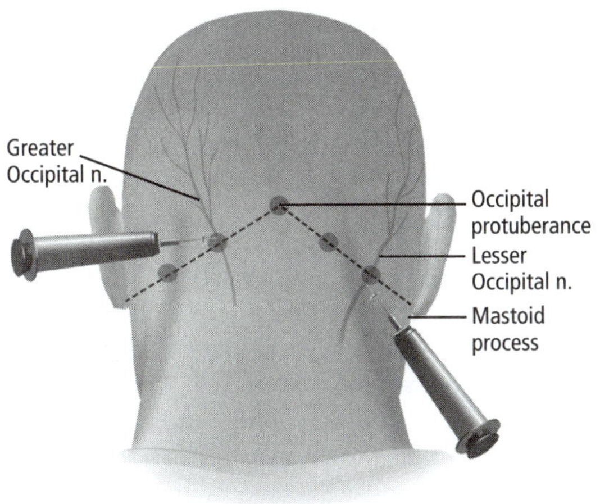

Figure 32–1 Greater and lesser occipital nerve blocks.

Traditionally, the two conditions commonly treated with GON blocks have been occipital neuralgia (aka "neuritis") and so-called cervicogenic headache (both discussed elsewhere). These two entities have been controversial and definitions overlap, but a number of observational studies have shown that many patients are responsive to GON blocks. Occipital neuralgia is defined by the International Classification of Headache Disorders 2nd edition (ICHD-2) (Headache Classification Committee, 2004) as (1) stabbing, with or without aching, pain roughly in the distribution of the GON; (2) tenderness over the nerve; and (3) reduction of pain by blockade of the GON.

GON block was particularly effective in patients with cervicogenic headache in a study of 52 patients with either cervicogenic, migraine, or tension-type headache (TTH) (Bovim and Sand, 1992). In a study of 100 patients diagnosed with cervicogenic headache, repeated GON blocks produced improvement in all subjects (Rothbart et al., 2000). A retrospective study of 184 patients with occipital neuralgia (diagnosed by response to GON block) showed long-lasting improvement after GON steroid injections with a mean of 31 days of relief (Anthony, 1992).

Reports of GON block in migraine have been generally positive, although, as stated earlier, controlled studies have not really been done. In a recent study of 19 patients with acute migraine and allodynia, headache was relieved in 17 and allodynia decreased in all patients (Ashkenazi and Young, 2005). Another study of 25 migraine patients found that 60% of the subjects had significant improvement of migraine pain within 5 minutes of injection (Cook et al., 2006). Long-lasting relief was seen in 26 of 54 migraine patients who received a unilateral GON block with lidocaine and methylprednisolone (Afridi et al., 2006). A recent comparative study of the benefits of GON block in chronic daily headache (CDH) was positive (Ashkenazi et al., 2006).

Chronic TTH (CTTH) seems not to respond to GON block (Leinisch-Dahlke et al., 2005). A small retrospective study of chronic posttraumatic headache patients found that 8 of 10 patients treated with GON block had a good response (Hecht, 2004).

GON blockade has been shown to be effective in the acute, and perhaps preventive, treatment of

CH. In a study of 14 CH patients treated with GON block, 4 had a good response and 5 had a moderate response (Peres et al., 2002). In a double-blind, placebo-controlled study of GON block ipsilateral to the pain side in CH patients, Ambrosini et al. (2005) found that 80% of the treated group responded and none in the placebo (saline injection) group improved. Most patients maintained the effect for at least 4 weeks. Afridi et al. (2006) found that 12 of 22 CH patients responded to GON block, and the response generally lasted for weeks. In the same study, tenderness around the GON seemed to be predictive of a good response to GON block in both migraine and CH patients, although the degree of anesthesia produced was not.

Several unusual adverse effects of GON block have been reported, including local alopecia (Shields et al., 2004) and Cushing's syndrome (Lavin and Workman, 2001).

Lesser Occipital Nerve Block

The lesser occipital nerve (LON) is primarily derived from the cervical plexus (C_2, C_3) and supplies the inferior scalp and upper neck skin. This nerve can be blockaded by injecting approximately 3–5 cc of bupivacaine or lidocaine, or a mixture of the two, two-thirds of the way to the mastoid on the same line used for GON block (Fig. 32–1).

Data supporting the use of LON do not exist, but it is noteworthy that many reports of successful trigger point injection therapy have involved patients who were injected in the region of the LON, begging the question of whether LON blockade was the decisive event. Trigger point injections are not discussed in this chapter due to the lack of reproducible evidence for their usefulness (Silberstein and Goadsby, 2002).

Auriculotemporal Nerve Block

The auriculotemporal nerve (ATN), a branch of the mandibular division of the trigeminal nerve, supplies sensation over the ear and temporalis muscle. Blockade can be done by injecting approximately 3–5 cc of bupivacaine or lidocaine, or a mixture, superior to the posterior portion of the zygoma just anterior to the ear (Fig. 32–2). If this block is successful, anesthesia is obtained over the temporal fossa. Again, evidence for the effectiveness of ATN blockade in any headache disorder is lacking, although selected patients have benefited. The observation that many patients with primary headache disorders complain particularly of temporal pain is important. Interestingly, the ATN block is a component of the so-called circumferential block of the scalp, which involves GON, ATN, and supraorbital/supratrochlear blocks, which, when done bilaterally, essentially anesthetize the entire scalp.

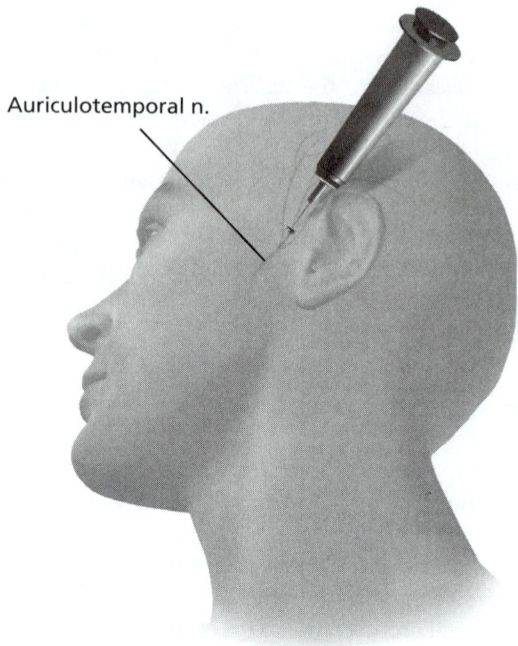

Figure 32–2 Auriculotemporal nerve block.

Supraorbital and Supratrochlear Nerve Blocks

These branches of the ophthalmic division of the trigeminal nerve pass through the orbit above the orbital ridge and are easily accessible to neural blockade (Fig. 32–3). The supratrochlear nerve is blocked by inserting the needle just above the eyebrow over its medial border and injecting approximately 1–2 cc of bupivacaine or lidocaine or a mixture. To anesthetize the supraorbital nerve (SON), which runs approximately 2 cm lateral to the supratrochlear nerve, the needle can be advanced through the same puncture that was used

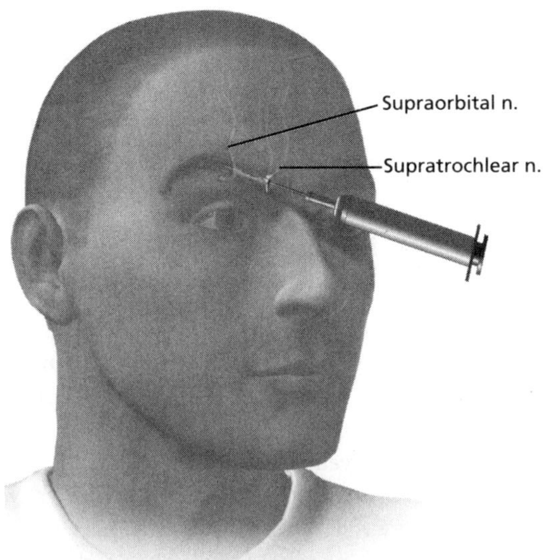

Figure 32–3 Supraorbital and supratrochlear nerve blocks.

for the supratrochlear nerve, and again 1–2 cc of anesthetic can be injected.

Supraorbital neuralgia is defined by the ICHD-2 (Headache Classification Committee, 2004) as (1) pain in the distribution of the SON, (2) tenderness over the nerve in the supraorbital notch, and (3) abolition of pain by blockade or ablation of the SON. The nerve is prone to traumatic injury due to its location, and headaches after frontal trauma with pain localized to this area should raise a high level of suspicion for the diagnosis, which can then be confirmed (and treated) with SON block (Sjaastad et al., 1999).

In a study of SON and/or GON blockade in 29 patients with migraine, 25 patients (85%) had a favorable response. However, this report did not include the data for those who received only SON blocks (Caputi and Firetto, 1997).

Sphenopalatine Ganglion

The sphenopalatine ganglion (also called the pterygopalatine ganglion) contains sensory fibers that contribute to the maxillary branch of the trigeminal nerve, as well as both parasympathetic and sympathetic fibers. Anesthesia of the sphenopalatine ganglion can be done via transcutaneous or intra-oral injection, but topical application of LA to the mucosa overlying it in the lateral wall of the nasal cavity is easier and poses less risk. The procedure is done with the patient supine, with the tip of the nose pointed at the ceiling and the head turned slightly to the side of the block (Fig. 32–4). A long, cotton-tipped applicator is saturated with 4% lidocaine and applied to the lateral posterior wall of the nasal cavity. This is repeated until pain relief is obtained.

Because cocaine applied to the sphenopalatine ganglion region is known to abort a CH attack, LAs have been proposed as a less addictive alternative. Results have been generally positive (Kittrelle et al., 1985; Hardebo and Elner, 1987; Costa et al., 2000), although in one study of 30 male patients with CH results were mostly negative (Robbins, 1995). This seems a reasonable alternative for CH patients, who can learn to do this technique themselves, particularly if they are relatively resistant to other prophylactic and abortive therapies.

Other Sites of Neural Blockade

Other nerves that can be blocked include the glossopharyngeal nerve, as it passes near the styloid process, and the infraorbital nerve. There are clear risks involving instrumentation near the glossopharyngeal nerve since the carotid artery and jugular vein are in very close proximity. Therefore,

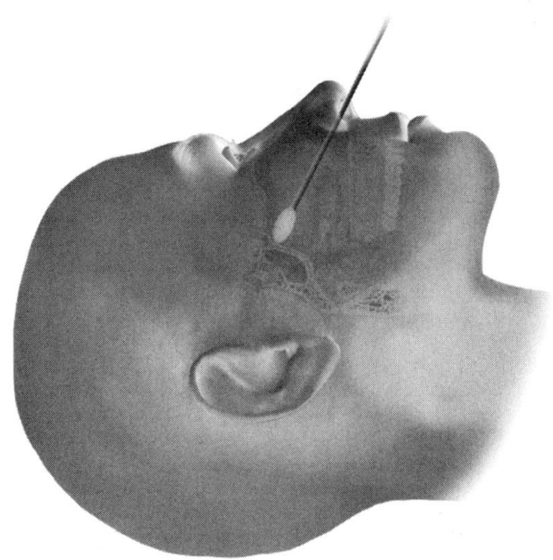

Figure 32–4 Sphenopalatine ganglion block.

this nerve is rarely seen as a convenient target, even in cases of severe glossopharyngeal neuralgia. Infraorbital nerve blockade (IONB) has rarely been reported as effective in headache conditions, although it is recommended in cases of suspected infraorbital neuralgia. It has also been proposed as the treatment for maxillary branch trigeminal neuralgia (TN), and a report of three cases of intractable TN successfully treated with IONB was encouraging (Goto et al., 1999).

Like other joints, cervical joints are known to be potential sources of pain, and for this reason investigators have explored the upper cervical joints as a source of headache. Cervical facet injections and lower cervical intramuscular injections have been proposed for the treatment of headache, with a putative mechanism of neural blockade of mid and lower cervical roots (Mellick and Mellick, 2003), but clear evidence of efficacy is lacking to date. Headache occurs upon noxious stimulation of the atlanto-occipital joint, the lateral atlanto-axial joint, the C_2–C_3 zygapophysial joints, and the C_2–C_3 intervertebral disc. Cervical joints can be anesthetized by either intra-articular injections or blockade of the nerves that innervate the joint. In one study, relief of headache in 20 out of 34 patients with headache occurred after intra-articular injections of LA into the lateral atlanto-axial joint (Aprill et al., 2002). Unfortunately, headache-specific diagnoses in this study are not available and the injections were not blinded.

The third cervical root has been proposed as a target in some headaches, generally those thought to be caused by "whiplash" or other cervical injury or pathology (Bogduk and Marsland, 1986). In one series of 100 patients with neck pain after whiplash injury, 27% experienced headache relief after blockade of the C_2–C_3 facet joint with either lidocaine 2% or bupivacaine 0.5%, and of those for whom headache was the predominant symptom ($n = 40$), 53% experienced relief of headache (Lord et al., 1994). The most common facet joints targeted in clinical practice are the C_2–C_3 joints, followed by the C_3–C_4 joints. Facet joints below C_4 are not commonly injected. These procedures, unlike the other block procedures described earlier, require a specialized fluoroscopic procedure room to ascertain proper placement of the injection needle and a practitioner skilled and experienced with performing these injections.

Because cervical facet joint blockade, and even facet rhizotomies, are performed in headache specialty and pain-clinics across North America, randomized placebo-controlled trials involving patients with accurate headache diagnoses according to ICHD-2 criteria are needed.

Mechanisms

Many centers continue to use peripheral neural blockade as acute and prophylactic treatment of various types of headaches. The mechanism by which the procedure works is not clear. Migraine and CH are believed to be centrally mediated primary headache syndromes, and it is unclear how blocking cervical roots or trigeminal nerve branches affects these processes. The mechanism in acute relief may stem from a reduction in afferent tone, which serves to reduce activity at the first synapse of the nociceptive pathway that governs head and facial pain in the trigeminal nucleus caudalis (TNC) and cervical dorsal horn. There is good evidence that convergence between the cervical and trigeminal systems happens at this level and that changes in one component can modulate the other (Piovesan et al., 2001; Bartsch and Goadsby, 2002, 2003; Busch et al., 2006). But how might long-term improvement result from anesthesia that lasts, at most, 12 hours? Perhaps, there is a physiological explanation for the clinically observed benefit to "breaking a pain cycle," possibly related to a "winding-down" of central sensitization, when incoming traffic via cervical or trigeminal afferents is temporarily reduced or blocked.

When therapeutic anesthetic blocks are used for headaches thought to stem from cervical, occipital, or trigeminal nerve injury or dysfunction, such as posttraumatic damage or vascular compression, mechanisms for pain relief are more transparent. A peripheral neuropathic pain phenomenon is theoretically being ameliorated. However, most peripheral neuropathic pain conditions of the head and neck seem to involve a degree of central sensitization, and peripheral blockade should not help unless, again, it affects a modulatory synaptic change. The prolonged benefits of peripheral blocks are just as difficult to explain as they are in primary headaches. It is possible, as seen with occipital nerve stimulation (ONS), that manipulation of peripheral afferent activity through anesthetic blockade affects central descending pain-modulating circuits. It is also possible that if some of the nociceptors from C_2 and the trigeminal nerve that are accessible under the skin, innervate dura mater, arachnoid mater, and meningeal blood vessels by way of bony penetration through the skull (Burstein R, personal communication), then blockade of these nociceptors may diminish afferent traffic directly into second-order nociception-specific neurons within TNC. Certainly, these procedures have proven helpful for many patients with otherwise intractable pain, and they deserve further careful study in appropriate populations in a controlled fashion.

PERIPHERAL NEUROSTIMULATION

Neurostimulation has long been used in the treatment of pain (Weiner, 2003; Birknes et al., 2006). Data from recent studies suggest that peripheral neurostimulation (PNS) may be effective in the treatment of chronic headache. It has been shown in animal studies that electrical stimulation of the Gasserian ganglion induces structural changes in CGRP-positive perivascular nerve terminals in the dura matter (Knyihar-Csillik et al., 1995). In earlier clinical studies, the methods used for neurostimulation in humans were transcutaneous or percutaneous electrical nerve stimulation (TENS/PENS) (Farina et al., 1986; Ghoname et al., 1999; Ahmed et al., 2000; Allais et al., 2003). More recently, PNS was performed using implanted subcutaneous electrodes (Popeney and Alo, 2003; Matharu et al., 2004; Rodrigo-Royo et al., 2005; Schwedt et al., 2006; Weiner, 2006).

Neurostimulation Using TENS/PENS

In an uncontrolled study, Farina et al. examined the efficacy of TENS in 60 patients with cervicogenic headache, occipital neuralgia, and "muscle contraction" or mixed headache (Farina et al., 1986). TENS electrodes were applied to cervical tender points. TENS treatment was effective in decreasing headache severity and frequency in the three headache groups. In an open study of 60 women with transformed migraine (TM), Allais et al. examined the effect of TENS, laser therapy, and acupuncture on headache (Allais et al., 2003). TENS electrodes were applied to the frontal, temporal, and occipital areas, and to the dorsal aspect of the hand. Patients underwent 10 treatment sessions, each lasting 30 minutes. TENS therapy resulted in a significant decrease in the number of headache days per month, an effect that lasted for 3 months.

PENS is performed by using acupuncture-like needles that are inserted to a depth of 1–3 cm subcutaneously at specific points. Ahmed et al. showed that PENS was more effective than a sham procedure (needles inserted, but no electrical stimulation delivered) in decreasing pain scores of 30 patients with TTH, migraine, or posttraumatic headache (Ahmed et al., 2000). Ghoname et al. used a similar technique to study the effect of PENS on five patients with postelectroconvulsive therapy (ECT) headache (Ghoname et al., 1999). PENS was delivered at the temporal, occipital, cervical, and upper thoracic areas bilaterally. All patients responded favorably to treatment, with either elimination of or marked improvement in ECT-associated headache.

Neurostimulation Using Implantable Electrodes

Neurostimulation of the Greater Occipital and Upper Cervical Nerves

In animal studies, stimulation of the GON has been shown to increase metabolic activity in the TNC as well as in the upper cervical dorsal horn (Goadsby et al., 1997). The same neural sites are activated after mechanical or electrical stimulation of trigeminally innervated structures, such as the superior sagittal sinus (Goadsby and Zagami, 1991). These observations suggest that there is a convergence of sensory input from cervical and trigeminal afferents at the level of the second-order afferent neurons in the TNC. In support of this hypothesis, Bartsch and Goadsby, using a rat model of cranial nociception, demonstrated that some dorsal horn neurons at the C_2 level respond to stimulation of both the dura and the GON (Bartsch and Goadsby, 2002). Moreover, stimulation of the GON has a facilitatory effect on C_2 neuronal response to dural stimulation.

The efficacy of stimulation of the GON or upper cervical nerves on headache was evaluated in a number of studies (Popeney and Alo, 2003; Matharu et al., 2004; Rodrigo-Royo et al., 2005; Schwedt et al., 2006; Weiner, 2006). In an uncontrolled study, Popeney and Aló evaluated the effect of PNS in the upper cervical (C_1–C_3) distribution on head pain and disability in 25 patients with TM (Popeney and Alo, 2003) who had been refractory to multiple pharmacotherapies before PNS. Under fluoroscopic guidance, electrodes were placed subcutaneously at the posterior cervical area and were connected to an implantable pulse generator. Neurostimulation was either intermittent or continuous. The average number of days with headache decreased from 25 per month at baseline to 13 per month after PNS, and average headache severity (on an 11-point verbal scale) decreased from 9 to 6. Disability, as measured by migraine disability assessment (MIDAS) scores, decreased 89%. Complications of the procedure included electrode migration [9 patients (36%)] and infection [1 patient (4%)]. In a similar study, Rodrigo-Royo et al. reported that four patients with cervicogenic headache who had undergone PNS in the C_1–C_3 distribution had a significant improvement in headache severity and disability (Rodrigo-Royo et al., 2005). Schwedt et al., reported on 15 patients with medically intractable chronic migraine ($n = 8$), CH ($n = 3$), hemicrania continua (HC) ($n = 2$), and posttraumatic headache ($n = 2$) who underwent implantation of permanent stimulating electrodes over the GON (Schwedt et al., 2007). Eight patients underwent bilateral lead placement and seven had unilateral lead placement. Patients were evaluated before and 5–42 months (mean 19 months) after implantation. All six mean headache measures improved significantly from baseline. Headache frequency per 90 days improved by 25 days from a baseline of 89 days; headache severity (0–10) improved 2.4 points from a baseline of 7.1 points; migraine disability as measured by MIDAS improved 70 points from a baseline of 179 points and headache impact test-6 (HIT-6) scores improved 11 points from a baseline of 71 points; Beck Depression Inventory II scores improved 8 points from a baseline of 20 points; and the mean subjective percent change in pain was 52%. Most patients (60%) required lead revision within 1 year. One patient required generator revision. Occipital Nerve Stimulation (ONS) may be effective in some patients with intractable headache. Surgical revisions may be commonly required. In two patients, a man with chronic CH (CCH) and a woman with HC, despite significant improvement in their headache frequency and severity, cranial autonomic features in the absence of pain continued to occur (Schwedt et al., 2006).

Matharu et al. studied the effect of sub-occipital stimulation on head pain in eight patients with CDH fulfilling the International Headache Society (IHS) criteria for chronic migraine (Matharu et al., 2004). The stimulating electrodes were implanted in the vicinity of the GON, at the level of C_1. Four patients had an excellent response, with complete headache suppression; two had a "very good" response, with suppression of headache most of the time; and two had a "good" response, with headache severity decreased 50%–75%. All patients maintained the response to treatment throughout a follow-up period averaging 18 months. Three patients had electrode lead migration, necessitating revision, and one had an abdominal hematoma at the site of generator implantation. Positron emission tomography (PET) studies showed significant changes in regional cerebral blood flow (rCBF) in the dorsal rostral pons, anterior cingulate gyrus, and cuneus, which correlated with pain scores.

Two studies recently reported on the efficacy and tolerability of ONS in patients with refractory CCH. Burns et al. reported on eight patients with medically intractable CCH who underwent bilateral implantation of stimulating electrodes and were followed-up for a median of 20 months (range 6–27) (Burns et al., 2007). Six of eight patients reported responses that were sufficiently meaningful for them to recommend the treatment to similarly affected patients with CCH. Two patients noticed a substantial improvement (90% and 95%) in their attacks; three patients noticed a moderate improvement (40%, 60%, and 20%–80%); and one reported mild improvement (25%). Improvements occurred in both frequency and severity of attacks. These changes took place over weeks or months, although attacks returned in days when the device malfunctioned (e.g., with battery depletion). Adverse events of concern were lead migrations in one patient and battery depletion requiring replacement in four. The authors concluded that ONS appears to offer a safe and effective treatment option in CH, which could begin a new era of neurostimulation therapy for primary headache syndromes.

Magis et al. also recently reported on eight patients with drug-resistant CCH, who underwent implantation of a suboccipital neurostimulator ipsilateral to the CH attacks (Magis et al., 2007). Of these eight patients, two were pain-free after a follow-up of 16 and 22 months and, similar to the findings from the study by Schwedt et al., one patient continued to experience autonomic attacks in the absence of pain. Three patients had a 90% reduction in attack frequency, and two patients, one of whom had had the implant for only 3 months, had improvement of approximately 40%. Mean follow-up was 15.1 months (range 3–22 months). In this study, the intensity of attacks decreased earlier than the attack frequency during ONS. All but one patient were able to substantially reduce their preventive drug treatment. Similar to the study by Burns et al., interruption of ONS (switching off the stimulator or battery failure) was followed within days by recurrence and increase of attacks. Cephalic and extracephalic pain thresholds were not altered during the course of treatment. There were no serious adverse events. The authors concluded that ONS could be an effective treatment for drug-resistant CCH, which is safer and less invasive than hypothalamic stimulation. The delay of 2 months or more between implantation and significant clinical improvement suggested that the procedure acts via slow neuromodulatory processes at the level of upper brain stem or diencephalic centers.

In summary, current data suggest that GON stimulation may be effective in the treatment of chronic and drug-resistant migraine and CH, and possibly other headache types including HC and posttraumatic headache. However, these data are derived from uncontrolled studies, and should therefore be viewed with reservation. Several prospective sham-controlled studies on the effect of GON stimulation on chronic migraine are currently ongoing, and the results of these studies will help clarify the role of this treatment modality for chronic migraine.

Vagal Nerve Stimulation

Few studies have evaluated the effect of vagal nerve stimulation (VNS) on headaches (Sadler et al., 2002; Hord et al., 2003; Mauskop, 2005).

Hord et al. examined retrospectively the effect of VNS on head pain in four epileptic patients who had concomitant migraine (Hord et al., 2003). Headache frequency and intensity before and after VNS implantation were compared. All four patients reported on reduction in headache frequency and severity after VNS implantation, one of them experiencing complete headache relief. Improvement in headache was reported to start 1–3 months after VNS implantation. Sadler et al. reported on a 42-year-old man with intractable seizures and migraine (Sadler et al., 2002). After VNS implantation, the patient experienced a dramatic decrease in migraine attack frequency, with prolonged periods of time when he was headache-free. Mauskop reported on the effect of VNS on head pain and related symptoms in six patients with chronic refractory headaches (four with migraine and two with CH) (Mauskop, 2005). Two of the four migraine patients, as well as the two CH patients, experienced significant improvement in headaches after VNS. One migraine patient could not tolerate VNS due to nausea, and another patient experienced only temporary headache relief.

Data from these studies suggest a possible positive effect of VNS on migraine and CH. However, the studies were not controlled and the number of patients was small.

Therefore, until controlled prospective studies are published, no conclusion can be made regarding the effect of VNS on patients with these disorders.

BOTULINUM NEUROTOXIN

BoNT is a potent toxin produced by the anaerobic bacterium, *Clostridium botulinum* (Brin, 1997; Turton et al., 2002). BoNT causes dose-dependent muscle relaxation by blocking acetylcholine release from nerve terminals at the neuromuscular junction. Human intoxication by BoNT results in botulism—an acute, potentially fatal muscle paralysis (Shapiro et al., 1998). When given in minute doses, however, the toxin is effective in the treatment of dystonia and other disorders associated with increased muscle tone (Jankovic and Brin, 1991; Jankovic and Brin, 1997). The analgesic effect of BoNT has long been observed anecdotally when given to patients with dystonia and other disorders. More recently, controlled studies have been conducted to investigate this effect of the toxin and to assess its role in the treatment of headaches [for reviews see Dodick (2003), Ashkenazi and Silberstein (2004)].

Structure and Preparations

BoNT belongs to the clostridial neurotoxin family and exists as seven antigenically distinct serotypes (A–G) (Turton et al., 2002). The toxin is noncovalently linked to nontoxic proteins. In its purified form, it is an approximately 150-kDa polypeptide that consists of two subunits, a light chain and a heavy chain, linked by a disulfide bond (Fig. 32–5). The light chain acts as a zinc-dependent endopeptidase. The heavy chain contains two domains. One, in the C-terminal (H_C), is the ganglioside-binding domain, which has a key role in the toxin's binding to the target cell membrane and its internalization. The other, in the N-terminal (H_N), is the translocation domain that promotes penetration of the light chain through the endosomal membrane into the cytosol.

BoNT type A (BoNT-A) is the most widely used serotype in clinical practice. It is available in the USA as Botox (Allergan, CA) and in Europe as Dysport (Ipsen, UK). Although these two preparations contain the same serotype, they differ in potency and in antigenicity (Brin, 1997; Silberstein, 2001). More recently, BoNT type B (BoNT-B) became available for clinical use in the USA (Myobloc, Elan Pharmaceuticals, CA) and in Europe (NeuroBloc, Elan Pharmaceuticals, CA).

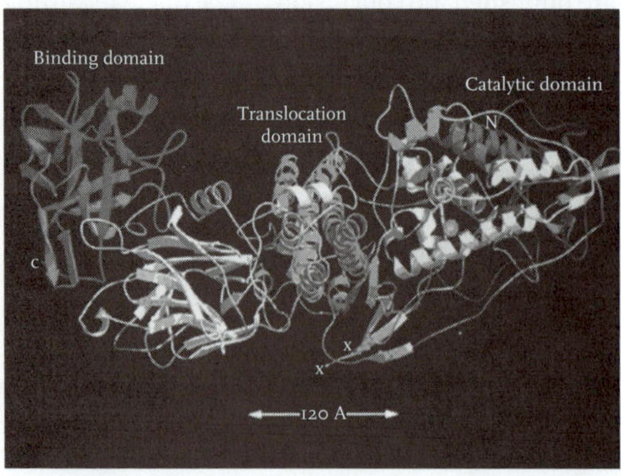

Figure 32–5 Molecular structure of botulinum neurotoxin (BoNT).

Immunology

Since BoNT is a protein of nonhuman origin, it may evoke antibody formation (Brin, 1997; Critchfield, 2002). Once neutralizing antibodies are present, the efficacy of the toxin is lost (Borodic et al., 1996). The reported prevalence of treatment resistance due to antibody formation is variable and depends on the assay used for antibody detection, the patient population, and the treatment protocol. When using an older preparation, treatment resistance to BoNT was estimated to occur in 5%–10% of patients with cervical dystonia (Dauer et al., 1998). Factors that increase the risk for antibody formation include higher doses and short intervals between treatments (Greene et al., 1994; Jankovic and Schwartz, 1995; Zuber et al., 1995). With the new formulation and the relatively low doses used in the treatment of headache, this complication is less likely to occur. Recommendations for minimizing immunoresistance include using the lowest effective dose at the longest possible intervals and avoiding booster injections (Brin, 1997). When resistance to one BoNT serotype develops, switching to a different serotype may restore the therapeutic response (Borodic et al., 1996). This response, however, may be only temporary. In a recent study, 10 patients with antibody-mediated therapeutic failure to BoNT-A were given BoNT-B (NeuroBloc). After an initial response, six patients developed secondary therapeutic failure with documented antibodies to BoNT-B (Dressler et al., 2003).

A new low molecular weight BoNT-A has recently been developed and shown to be effective in an animal model (Sakamoto et al., 2003). This novel toxin may be less immunogenic than the conventional BoNT-A.

Mechanisms of Action

BoNT affects the nervous system through a multistage process that results in the blocking of neurotransmitter release (Brin, 1997; Aoki, 2001;

Turton et al., 2002). The toxin binds to the target nerve terminal through its H_C domain, and is subsequently internalized into an intracellular vesicle. The disulfide bond is then cleaved, and the light chain undergoes translocation to the cytosol. In the final stage, the light chain cleaves one or more proteins involved in neurotransmitter release. The type of protein that is cleaved depends on the toxin serotype. BoNT-A cleaves a synaptosomal-associated protein of 25 kDa (SNAP-25), whereas BoNT-B attacks a vesicle-associated membrane protein (VAMP), also called synaptobrevin. In both cases, the result is the prevention of synaptic vesicle fusion with the plasma membrane and, thus, of neurotransmitter release.

The neuromuscular junction is BoNT's best studied site of action. By interfering with acetylcholine release from the presynaptic axon terminal at this site, BoNT causes a dose-dependent and reversible muscle relaxation. Axonal sprouting, which occurs after BoNT entrance into the cell, causes termination of the toxin effect in 2–6 months. BoNT may also act via afferent mechanisms (Giladi, 1997). In animal models, BoNT was shown to reduce spindle afferent discharges, suggesting a direct effect on gamma motor nerve endings (Filippi et al., 1993). It also caused atrophy of both intrafusal and extrafusal muscle fibers when injected into rats (Rosales et al., 1996).

There is increasing evidence that BoNT affects the central nervous system (CNS) (Hallett, 2000). Earlier animal studies suggested retrograde transport of the toxin into the CNS (Wiegand and Wellhoner, 1977). More recently, however, it was shown that only breakdown products of the toxin were transported in a retrograde manner (Aoki, 1998). Janicki and Habermann found that BoNT inhibits the release of methionine-enkephalin-like material in the rat striatum in vitro (Janicki and Habermann, 1983). However, little evidence currently exists for the penetration of functional toxin into the CNS in humans. The central effects of BoNT are more likely to result from CNS neuroplasticity, induced by alterations in afferent input (Byrnes et al., 1998; Gilio et al., 2000).

Antinociceptive Effects

The analgesic effect of BoNT has long been recognized while used for other indications (Borodic et al., 2001; Gobel et al., 2001; Arezzo, 2002). Often the toxin's analgesic effect occurs earlier and lasts longer than its effect on muscular hyperactivity (Brin, 1997). Pain reduction may also be observed in the absence of weakness. Cui et al. showed that pretreating with BoNT-A inhibited the delayed nociceptive response, as assessed by reduced pain behavior, in rats injected with formalin (Cui et al., 2004). BoNT-A also reduced formalin-evoked glutamate release from primary afferent nerve terminals in this study. These effects were achieved at doses that did not cause muscle weakness. Lew et al. studied the analgesic effect of BoNT-B, given in three different doses, on 122 patients with idiopathic cervical dystonia (Lew et al., 1997). Using the Toronto Western Spasmodic Torticollis Rating Scale pain score, 61%–83% of patients treated with BoNT-B were responders, and the response was dose-dependent. In contrast, a study of healthy volunteers showed that BoNT-A, injected intradermally, reduced the neurogenic flare induced by electrical stimulation, but had little effect on acute pain and allodynia (Kramer et al., 2003). This model is of acute, rather than chronic, pain and may have little relevance to the disorders associated with sensitization.

The analgesic effect of BoNT cannot be explained solely by the reduction of muscle tone induced by the toxin. Smuts et al. injected ten migraine patients with BoNT-A and found no correlation between the decrease in migraine frequency and the denervation pattern in the corrugator muscles, as measured by the amplitude of the compound muscle action potential after injection (Smuts et al., 2004). Moreover, several studies showed little or no direct effect of BoNT on cutaneous nociception (Blersch et al., 2002; Kramer et al., 2003). Other mechanisms must be involved, but their exact nature remains speculative. Several theories have been proposed (Arezzo, 2002): (1) evidence exists that BoNT affects the release of neurotransmitters, other than acetylcholine, that are involved in pain transmission (Dolly, 2003). The toxin has been shown to inhibit the release of substance P in vitro and of glutamate in vivo (Ishikawa et al., 2000; Welch et al., 2000; Cui et al., 2004). The toxin also decreases the release of calcitonin-gene-related peptide (CGRP) from afferent trigeminal nerve terminals (Durham et al., 2004). (2) Via its effect on muscle spindle activity, BoNT can indirectly disrupt the muscle pain associated with abnormal muscle contraction. Since the spindle afferents have important supraspinal projections, the change in their firing pattern caused by BoNT may also cause changes in sensory processing at higher levels of the nervous system. (3) By decreasing prolonged muscle contraction, BoNT may reduce the release of various substances that sensitize muscle nociceptors.

BoNT-A for the Treatment of Migraine

The beneficial effect of BoNT-A in migraine treatment was first noted by patients who were given the toxin for the treatment of facial wrinkles (Binder et al., 2000). Since then, a number of studies have been conducted to examine the efficacy of BoNT-A in migraine therapy (Table 32–1).

Efficacy and Tolerability

Open Label and Noncontrolled Studies Binder et al. conducted an open-label study to examine the efficacy of BoNT-A for migraine treatment (Binder et al., 2000). Treatment protocols were individualized. Of the 77 patients, 51% reported complete relief from migraine symptoms for a mean duration of 4.1 months. Thirty eight percent reported a partial response (more than 50% reduction in headache frequency or severity), with a mean duration of 2.7 months.

Behmand et al. evaluated the efficacy of BoNT-A on migraine, when injected to the corrugator muscles (Behmand et al., 2003). Twenty nine patients were given 25 units at each side to a total of 50 units. At 2 months after treatment, 16 patients (55%) had complete elimination of headaches and 8 (28%) had significant improvement. Eross and Dodick evaluated the effect of BoNT-A (25–100 units) on reducing disability in 54 patients with episodic or chronic migraine (Eross and Dodick, 2002). Using the MIDAS questionnaire, they found that 58% of patients experienced a decrease in migraine-associated disability. This effect of BoNT-A was more pronounced in patients with episodic migraine than in those with chronic migraine (75% versus 53%).

Several other retrospective studies have suggested that BoNT-A may be effective in migraine prevention (Mauskop and Basdeo, 2000; Smuts and Barnard, 2000; Mathew et al., 2002). Results of the above studies should be viewed with reservation due to the lack of a control group, the retrospective design of some studies, and the small size of the studies' samples.

Randomized Controlled Studies

Silberstein et al. examined the efficacy of BoNT-A for migraine prevention in a randomized, double-blind, vehicle-controlled study. The study included 123 patients with episodic migraine (Silberstein et al., 2000). BoNT-A was given into the frontalis, temporalis, and glabellar muscles for a total dose of either 25 or 75 units. Three months after treatment, BoNT-A at the 25-unit dose caused a reduction in migraine frequency of 1.9 attacks/month (versus 1.0 attacks/month for placebo). BoNT-A at this dose also decreased migraine severity and migraine-associated vomiting. The 75-unit dose was not significantly more effective than placebo. BoNT was well tolerated, with transient side-effects that included blepharoptosis, diplopia, and injection site weakness.

Brin et al. examined the effect of BoNT-A on 56 migraine patients (Brin et al., 2000). BoNT was injected into the frontalis and/or temporalis muscles. BoNT-A reduced migraine attack frequency by 1.8 attacks/month, mean headache severity by 4.0 points, and mean headache duration by 15.2 hours (the corresponding values for placebo were 0.2 attacks/month, 0.2 headache severity points, and 5.6 hours). The maximal effect of BoNT was observed at week 12 after treatment.

Barrientos and Chana examined prospectively the efficacy and safety of BoNT-A in the prophylactic treatment of migraine (Barrientos and Chana, 2003). Thirty patients with IHS-defined episodic migraine were randomized to receive either placebo or BoNT-A (50 units), injected at six sites. BoNT-A treatment resulted in a significantly greater decrease in migraine attack frequency at 3 months compared with placebo (−3.1 versus −0.5 attacks/month) BoNT-A therapy was safe and well tolerated.

Table 32–1 Studies of Botulinum Neurotoxin (BoNT) for Migraine Prevention.

Study design	*Diagnosis (n)*	*Patients with medication overuse*	*Injection paradigm*	*BoNT serotype, preparation, and total dose (units)*	*Results*	*Reference*
Prospective, double blind, randomized placebo-controlled	EM (123)	Excluded	Fixed site	Type A (Botox), 25 U or 75 U, single treatment session	25 U: significant reduction in migraine frequency 75 U: no significant efficacy	Silberstein et al., 2000
Prospective, double blind, randomized placebo-controlled	Migraine (type not specified) (56)	Not specified	Fixed site	Type A (Botox), dose variable	Significant reduction in migraine frequency, severity, and duration	Brin et al., 2000
Prospective, placebo-controlled randomized	Migraine (type not specified) (30)	Not specified	Not specified	Type A (Botox), 50 U	Significant reduction in migraine attack frequency	Barrientos and Chana, 2003
Prospective, double blind, randomized placebo-controlled	Migraine (type not specified) (32)	Not specified	Not specified	Type A (Botox), 100 U per session × 2 sessions = 200 U	Significant reduction in migraine-related disability and in consumption of acute-pain medications; no change in number of days with headache	Relja et al., 2003
Prospective, double-blind, randomized placebo-controlled	EM (60)	Excluded	Fixed site	Type A (Botox), 100 U or 16 U, single treatment session	Primary end-point (≥50% reduction in migraine frequency) not met. Accompanying symptom reduction score improved in 16 U group more than in placebo group	Evers et al., 2004

(continued)

Table 32–1 (continued)

Study design	*Diagnosis (n)*	*Patients with medication overuse*	*Injection paradigm*	*BoNT serotype, preparation, and total dose (units)*	*Results*	*Reference*
Prospective, open label	Migraine (type not specified) (77)	Not specified	Fixed site	Type A (Botox), dose variable	Complete elimination of headaches in 51% of patients, significant improvement in additional 38%	Binder et al. 2000
Prospective, open label	Migraine (type not specified) (29)	Not specified	Fixed site	Type A (Botox), 50 U; single treatment session	Complete elimination of headaches in 55% of patients, significant improvement in additional 28%	Behmand et al., 2002
Prospective, open label	Migraine (episodic or chronic) (54)	Not specified	Fixed site	Type A (Botox), 25 U; Additional 25–75 U to cervical paraspinal muscles if required for pain	Improvement (more than 50% reduction) in disability in 58% of patients	Eross and Dodick, 2002
Prospective, open label	EM (21)	Not specified	Fixed site	Type B, 5000 U	Significant reduction in headache frequency and severity	Lake et al., 2003

Abbreviations: EM, episodic migraine; n, number of patients.

Relja and Klepac evaluated the effect of BoNT-A treatment on 32 migraineurs (Relja and Klepac, 2003). Two treatments, at a dose of 100 units each, were given at 3-month intervals. At 6 months after treatment, patients who received BoNT-A significantly decreased their use of triptans. Although total number of days with headache was not reduced after BoNT-A injections, the character of the pain changed to a moderate, non-throbbing headache that was responsive to simple analgesics.

Evers et al. evaluated the effect of BoNT-A in 60 patients with episodic migraine (Evers et al., 2004). BoNT-A was given to the frontalis, temporalis, and cervical muscles (total dose 100 units—group A) or to the frontalis and temporalis muscles alone (total dose 16 units, group B). Group C received placebo injections. At 3 months after treatment, the rate of patients who had 50% or more than 50% reduction in migraine attack frequency (the primary end-point of the study) was not significantly different among the three groups (30% in groups A and B, and 25% in group C). There was, however, a significant difference in the sum score of reduction in accompanying symptoms between group B (BoNT-A 16 units) and group C (placebo) (29% versus 5%). Adverse events were mild and transient.

In summary, current data show a moderate beneficial effect of BoNT-A in the treatment of episodic migraine. Further studies are needed to identify the subgroup of patients who would benefit the most from this treatment.

BoNT-A for the Treatment of CDH

The treatment of CDH is challenging. Many of these patients overuse analgesics and suffer from psychiatric comorbidity (Dodick, 2006). The effect of BoNT in patients with CDH has recently been evaluated in several well-designed studies (Table 32–2). (Ondo et al., 2004; Dodick et al., 2005; Mathew et al., 2005; Silberstein et al., 2005).

Efficacy and Tolerability in Randomized Placebo Controlled Studies

Ondo et al. examined the effect of BoNT-A injections on patients with CDH (Ondo et al., 2004). Sixty patients (14 with chronic migraine and 46 with CTTH) were randomized to receive either BoNT-A (200 units), injected in a "follow-the-pain" approach, or placebo. The number of headache-free days in the BoNT-A group improved significantly from week 8–12. Also, patients' "global impression" improved significantly in the BoNT-A group. However, the primary end-point of the study (number of headache-free days at week 12 compared with baseline) was not met. BoNT-A was well tolerated.

Mathew et al. examined the efficacy of BoNT-A in the prophylactic treatment of CDH in a large study of 355 patients, all of whom had a history of migraine or probable migraine (Mathew et al., 2005). All the patients were initially given placebo injections and, based on subsequent data from their headache diaries, were classified as either placebo responders or placebo nonresponders. Patients were then randomized to receive either BoNT-A, using a follow-the-pain approach at a dose range of 105–260 units every 3 months for a total of three treatment cycles, or placebo. At 6 months after enrollment, the differences between the BoNT-A and the placebo groups in the increase in mean number of headache-free days per 30 days (the primary end-point) was not significant (6.7 versus 5.2 days in placebo nonresponders and 12.1 versus 10.5 days in placebo responders). However, significantly more patients in the BoNT-A group experienced 50% or more decrease in headache days 6 months after enrollment (40.3% versus 25.3%, respectively). Also, the mean decrease from baseline in headache frequency was significantly greater in the BoNT-A group compared with the placebo group (−7.1 versus −3.7 headaches/month). BoNT-A treatment was well tolerated. A subgroup analysis of data from this study, for patients who did not use concurrent headache-preventive drug, (64% of the entire study population) was done by Dodick et al. (Dodick et al., 2005). They found that, in this subgroup, BoNT-A was significantly superior to placebo in reducing the mean frequency of headaches per month after two treatment cycles (−7.8 versus −4.5). BoNT-A treatment was also associated with a significantly greater increase in the number of headache-free days per month compared with placebo (10 versus 6.7 days/month).

TABLE 32–2 Studies of Botulinum Neurotoxin (BoNT) for Chronic Daily Headache (CDH) prevention.

Study design	*Diagnosis (n)*	*Patients with medication overuse*	*Injection paradigm*	*BoNT serotype, preparation and total dose (units)*	*Results*	*Reference*
Prospective, double-blind, randomized placebo-controlled	CM (14) CTTH (46)	Included	Follow the pain	Type A (Botox), 200 U	Primary end-point (change in the number of headache-free days) not met. Patients' "global impression" improved with BoNT-A	Ondo et al., 2004
Prospective, double-blind, randomized placebo-controlled	CDH (355) (most patients probably had TM)	Included	Follow the pain	Type A (Botox), 105–260 U	Primary end-point (change in the number of headache-free days) not met. More patients with BoNT-A had 50% or more decrease in headache frequency at 6 months, compared with placebo.	Mathew et al., 2005
Prospective, double-blind, randomized, placebo-controlled	228 (a subgroup of patients who were not on other preventive	Included	Follow the pain	Type A (Botox), 105–260 U	BoNT-A superior to placebo in reducing the mean frequency of headaches per month. BoNT-A also	Dodick et al.,2005

(continued)

TABLE 32–2 (continued)

Study design	*Diagnosis (n)*	*Patients with medication overuse*	*Injection paradigm*	*BoNT serotype, preparation and total dose (units)*	*Results*	*Reference*
	drugs, from the study by Mathew et al.)				associated with a greater increase in the number of headache-free days per month, compared with placebo.	
Prospective, double-blind, randomized placebo-controlled	TM (375) CTTH (89) NDPH (16) Other or not classified CDH (222)	Included	Fixed site	Type A (Botox), 225, 150, or 75 U	Primary end-point (change in the number of headache-free days) not met. BoNT-A slightly superior to placebo in decreasing total headache frequency and migraine headache frequency.	Silberstein et al., 2005
Prospective, open label	TM (36)	Not specified	Follow the pain	Type B, 5000 U	Improvement in 66% of patients	Opida, 2002

Abbreviations: CDH, chronic daily headache; CM, chronic migraine; CTTH, chronic tension-type headache; n, number of patients; NDPH, new daily persistent headache;TM, transformed migraine.

Silberstein et al. examined the prophylactic effect of BoNT-A in 702 patients with CDH (the majority of whom had TM) (Silberstein et al., 2005). Patients were treated with BoNT-A (at doses of 225, 150, or 75 units, given at fixed predetermined sites) or with placebo. Three treatment sessions were given at 3-month intervals. The mean change from baseline in the number of headache-free days per month (the study primary end-point) did not differ significantly among the patient groups. BoNT-A, at doses of 150 and 225 units, was slightly superior to placebo with regard to the decrease in total headache frequency and migraine headache frequency. The sample of this study consisted of patients with long-standing CDH (average duration—13.7 years), 42% of whom were overusing acute pain mediations.

In summary, the results of these studies are conflicting but suggest that BoNT-A may be effective in the treatment of CDH and, specifically, chronic migraine. However, definitive conclusions must await the results of two large pivotal phase III international multicenter trials on the use of BoNT-A for the treatment of CDH in migraineurs, which are currently underway.

BoNT-A for the Treatment of TTH

TTH has been associated with increased pericranial muscle tone, although the significance of this finding in the pathogenesis of the disease has been debated (Jensen and Olesen, 2000). Since BoNT has muscle relaxation effect, it has been speculated that the toxin may be effective in the treatment of TTH. Early results from small, open-label studies and a small controlled study suggested that BoNT may alleviate TTH pain (Zwart et al., 1994; Wheeler, 1998; Smuts et al., 1999). However, controlled clinical studies conducted subsequently failed to confirm this (Table 32–3). (Rollnik et al., 2000; Schmitt et al., 2001; Padberg et al., 2004; Schulte-Mattler and Krack, 2004; Silberstein et al., 2006).

Efficacy and Tolerability in Randomized Placebo Controlled Studies

Rollnik et al. examined the effect of BoNT-A in 21 patients with TTH (Rollnik et al., 2000). The majority of patients had episodic (rather than chronic) TTH and had not responded to headache-preventive medications before the time of study. Patients were given BoNT-A (Dysport), injected to the frontalis, occipitalis, and temporalis muscles bilaterally at a total dose of 200 units, or placebo. At 4, 8, and 12 weeks after injections, there were no significant differences between the two groups regarding the change in headache severity, headache frequency, or analgesic use.

Schmitt et al. evaluated the effect of BoNT-A (Botox), given to the frontalis and temporalis muscles at a total dose of 20 units, versus placebo in 60 patients with CTTH (Schmitt et al., 2001). The study sample included patients with long-standing disease, many of whom overused acute pain medications. At 4 and 8 weeks after treatment, there was no significant between-group difference regarding headache severity, use of analgesics, or headache-free days. Patients in the BoNT-A group, however, had a significantly greater improvement in affective scores, as measured using the West-Haven-Yale Multidimensional Pain Inventory, compared with the placebo-treated group.

Padberg et al. randomly assigned 40 patients with CTTH to receive a single treatment of either BoNT-A (Botox, 1 unit/kg, up to 100 units) or placebo (Padberg et al., 2004). Patients with medication overuse were excluded. Injection sites were individualized; that is, BoNT was given to muscles with increased tone or tenderness, as judged by the injecting physician. BoNT-A did not differ from placebo with regard to changes in headache severity, mean number of headache days, or patients' assessment of improvement after treatment. In a larger study, Schulte-Mattler and Krack examined the effect of BoNT-A (Dysport) versus placebo in 112 patients with CTTH (Schulte-Mattler and Krack, 2004). Patients with analgesic overuse were excluded. BoNT-A was given at a high dose (500 units) to pericranial and cervical muscles bilaterally, according to a standardized protocol. Neither the primary end-point of the study (the change in the area under the headache curve 11 weeks after treatment) nor any of the secondary end-points were met.

Recently, Silberstein et al. evaluated the efficacy of BoNT-A (Botox) in the treatment of 300 patients with CTTH (Silberstein et al., 2006). A single treatment of BoNT-A or placebo was given. BoNT-A was given at five different doses (50–150

Table 32–3 Studies of Botulinum Neurotoxin (BoNT) for Tension-type Headache (TTH) Prevention

Study design	*Diagnosis (n)*	*Patients with medication overuse*	*Injection paradigm*	*BoNT serotype, preparation and total dose (units)*	*Results*	*Reference*
Prospective, double-blind, randomized placebo-controlled	CTTH (37)	Excluded	Fixed site	Type-A (Botox), 100 U	Significantly greater improvement in headache severity and in the number of headache-free days at 4 months with BoNT-A compared with placebo	Smuts et al., 1999
Prospective, double-blind, randomized placebo-controlled	ETTH (16) CTTH (5)	Excluded	Fixed site	Type-A (Dysport), 200 U	No significant differences between BoNT-A and placebo in change in headache frequency, headache severity, or use of analgesics	Rollnick et al., 2000
Prospective, double-blind, randomized placebo-controlled	CTTH (60)	Included	Fixed site	Type-A (Botox), 20 U	No significant between-group difference regarding headache severity, use of analgesics, or headache-free days. Affective scores improved after BoNT-A treatment	Shmitt et al., 2001
Prospective, double-blind, randomized, placebo-controlled	CTTH (40)	Excluded	Individualized according to sites of muscle tenderness	Type-A (Botox), 1 U/kg , up to 100 U	No significant differences between BoNT-A and placebo in any of the outcome measures	Pedberg et al., 2004

(continued)

Table 32–3 (continued)

Study design	*Diagnosis (n)*	*Patients with medication overuse*	*Injection paradigm*	*BoNT serotype, preparation and total dose (units)*	*Results*	*Reference*
Prospective, double-blind, randomized, placebo-controlled	CTTH (112)	Excluded	Fixed site	Type-A (Dysport), 500 U	None of the study end-point met	Schulte-Matter and krack, 2004
Prospective, double-blind randomized, placebo-controlled	CTTH (300)	Excluded	Fixed site	Type-A (Botox), 50–150 U	Mean change in the number of headache-free days/month slightly greater in the BoNT-A 150 U group compared with placebo, (4.5 vs. 2.8 days). In three of the BoNT-A groups, more patients had 50% or more decrease in TTH days/moth compared with placebo.	Silberstein et al., 2006

Abbreviations: ETTH, episodic tension-type headache; CTTH, chronic tension-type headache; n, number of patients.

units) to 3–5 pericranial and cervical muscles bilaterally, in a fixed-site paradigm. The mean change from baseline in the number of headache-free days per month was somewhat greater in the BoNT-A 150 U group compared with placebo (4.5 versus 2.8 days). Also, in three of the BoNT-A treated groups, more patients experienced 50% or more decrease in TTH days/month at 3 months after injection, compared with placebo. There were no significant differences in headache severity among the study groups. Overall, the therapeutic gain of BoNT-A over placebo in this study was small. BoNT-A was safe and well tolerated.

In summary, current data have failed to demonstrate a significant therapeutic effect of BoNT-A in patients with CTTH. In most studies, BoNT-A was not significantly superior to placebo with regards to primary or secondary end-points, using either the follow-the-pain or fixed-site injection strategy.

Safety

With clinical experience of more than two decades, BoNT-A has proved to be a remarkably safe drug. Based on animal studies, the lethal dose in humans is estimated at approximately 3000 units (Brin, 1997). The doses used for headache treatment are therefore unlikely to be toxic. An antitoxin is available in the event of accidental overdose (Scott, 1988). BoNT should be used with caution for patients with neuromuscular junction diseases (e.g., myasthenia gravis). It is contraindicated for patients who take aminoglycosides, which interfere with neuromuscular transmission (Argov and Mastaglia, 1979). Since there is little data on the safety of BoNT in pregnant and lactating women, it is not recommended for use in these circumstances.

BoNT-B for Headaches

Clinical experience with BoNT-B is far less extensive than that with BoNT-A. Few preliminary studies assessing its efficacy in headache treatment exist. Lake and Saper conducted an open-label study on the efficacy of BoNT-B in the treatment of 21 patients with IHS-defined migraine (Lake and Saper, 2003). Patients were given a total of 5000 units of BoNT-B, injected into 11 sites. They were evaluated at baseline and 4 months after treatment. Mean monthly headache frequency declined from 7.7 preinjection to 4.6 at 4 months after treatment. Significant improvement also occurred in headache intensity, sleep, MIDAS scores, and overall treatment satisfaction. Adverse events were transient and mild. In another open-label study, Opida examined the effect of BoNT-B on headache in 36 patients with TM (Opida, 2002). Patients were given 5000 units of BoNT-B, injected to three or more muscles in a follow-the-pain approach. Twenty-four patients (66%) reported improvement in headache severity as assessed by the numeric rating scale. Headache frequency was also reduced. Adverse events were mild, and included dry mouth and transient pain at the injection site.

BoNT-B may be effective in migraine treatment, but clinical experience is still limited. Currently, it may be considered for patients who develop antibody-mediated resistance to BoNT-A. Larger clinical trials may better define the role of BoNT-B in headache prevention.

BONT for Headache: Administration and Patient Selection It should be noted that the optimal approach for the administration of BoNT to headache patients has not been established. There is currently no evidence for a dose–response effect of the toxin on headache. Moreover, no injection paradigm (standardized fixed-site, follow-the-pain, or mixed) was found to be superior to others. Better patient selection is a key to improving results of BoNT treatment for headache. Factors to be considered include: (1) the use of concurrent preventive medications: there are data suggesting that patients who do not use concurrent headache preventive drugs may respond better to BoNT treatment (Dodick et al., 2005). This needs to be further studied. (2) Pain medication overuse: data from one retrospective study suggested that patients who do not overuse pain medications may benefit more from BoNT treatment than those who do (Tepper et al., 2004). Prospective studies, however, did not confirm these results. (3) Disease duration: Eross et al. found that disease duration of more than 30 years adversely affected outcome after BoNT-A treatment in 61 migraine patients (Eross et al., 2005). (4) Headache characteristics: Jakubowski et al. found, in a sample of 63 migraineurs, that most patients (74%) who improved after BoNT-A treatment (responders) described their headache as a pressure from outside or a head-crushing feeling (imploding headache) or as a feeling of eye-popping (ocular headache) (Jakubowski et al., 2006). Conversely, 92% of nonresponders described their headache as a pressure building up from inside (exploding headache). These data, if validated in larger patient populations, may help select the migraine patients who would best respond to BoNT treatment.

SUMMARY

Despite the paucity of data from controlled studies, peripheral nerve blocks are a viable treatment option for selected groups of headache patients. These procedures are worth considering for patients who have local tenderness at the nerve site or intractable headaches. GON block, the most widely used procedure, is safe and relatively easy to perform in the office. Adverse effects are few and infrequent. The procedure can result in rapid relief of pain and allodynia, an effect that may last for several weeks. Further studies are needed to establish the efficacy of nerve blocks in different headache disorders and to find the optimal drug combination to use for this purpose. The judicious use of facet joint blockade for patients with refractory cervicogenic headache may be indicated, but randomized placebo-controlled studies are desperately needed in patients with chronic headaches. Peripheral nerve stimulation, using implantable electrodes close to the GON, is a promising technique that has the potential for providing long-term pain relief for a selected group of patients. Results of ongoing studies will hopefully clarify the role of this technique and headache subtypes that are most suitable for this treatment modality. BoNT-A appears to have a role in headache prevention for selected patients with chronic migraine, but definitive conclusions will await the results of ongoing randomized, placebo-controlled clinical trials in migraine sufferers with CDH. However, based on current data, the toxin cannot be recommended for patients with CTTH.

References

Afridi, SK, Shields, KG, Bhola, R, et al. (2006). Greater occipital nerve injection in primary headache syndromes—prolonged effects from a single injection. *Pain*, 122:126–129.

Ahmed, HE, White, PF, Craig, WF, et al. (2000). Use of percutaneous electrical nerve stimulation (PENS) in the short-term management of headache. *Headache*, 40:311–315.

Allais, G, De, LC, Quirico, PE, et al. (2003). Non-pharmacological approaches to chronic headaches: transcutaneous electrical nerve stimulation, lasertherapy and acupuncture in transformed migraine treatment. *Neurol Sci*, 24(Suppl. 2):S138–S142.

Ambrosini, A, Vandenheede, M, Rossi, P, et al. (2005). Suboccipital injection with a mixture of rapid- and long-acting steroids in cluster headache: a double-blind placebo-controlled study. *Pain*, 118:92–96.

Anthony, M (1992). Headache and the greater occipital nerve. *Clin Neurol Neurosurg*, 94:297–301.

Aoki, KR (2001). Pharmacology and immunology of botulinum toxin serotypes. *J Neurol*, 248:3–10.

Aoki, R (1998). The development of BOTOX—its history and pharmacology. *Pain Digest*, 8:337–341.

Aprill, C, Axinn, MJ, and Bogduk, N (2002). Occipital headaches stemming from the lateral atlanto-axial (C1-2) joint. *Cephalalgia*, 22:15–22.

Arezzo, JC (2002). Possible mechanisms for the efects of botulinum toxin on pain. *Clin J Pain*, 18:S125–S132.

Argov, Z and Mastaglia, FL (1979). Disorders of neuromuscular transmission caused by drugs. *N Engl J Med*, 301:409–413.

Ashkenazi, A and Silberstein, SD (2004). Botulinum toxin and other new approaches to migraine therapy. *Annu Rev Med*, 55:505–518.

Ashkenazi, A, Silberstein, SD, and Shaw, JW (2006). Greater occipital nerve block for chronic daily headache using local anesthetics with or without corticosteroids—a randomized single-blind study. *Neurology*, 66:A223 (Abstract).

Ashkenazi, A and Young, WB (2005). The effects of greater occipital nerve block and trigger point injection on brush allodynia and pain in migraine. *Headache*, 45:350–354.

Barrientos, N and Chana, P (2003). Botulinum toxin type A in prophylactic treatment of migraine headaches: a preliminary study. *J Headache Pain*, 4:146–151.

Bartsch, T and Goadsby, PJ (2002). Stimulation of the greater occipital nerve induces increased central excitability of dural afferent input. *Brain*, 125:1496–1509.

Bartsch, T and Goadsby, PJ (2003). Increased responses in trigeminocervical nociceptive neurons to cervical input after stimulation of the dura mater. *Brain*, 126:1801–1813.

Behmand, RA, Tucker, T, and Guyuron, B (2003). Single-site botulinum toxin type A injection for elimination of migraine trigger points. *Headache*, 43:1085–1089.

Binder, WJ, Brin, MF, Blitzer, A, et al. (2000). Botulinum toxin type A (Botox) for treatment of migraine headaches: an open-label study. *Otolaryngol Head Neck Surg*, 123:669–676.

Birknes, JK, Sharan, A, and Rezai, AR (2006). Treatment of chronic pain with neurostimulation. *Prog Neurol Surg*, 19:197–207.

Blersch, W, Schulte-Mattler, WJ, Przywara, S, et al. (2002). Botulinum toxin A and the cutaneous nociception in humans: a prospective, double-blind, placebo-controlled, randomized study. *J Neurol Sci*, 205:59–63.

Bogduk, N and Marsland, A (1986). On the concept of third occipital headache. *J Neurol Neurosurg Psychiatry*, 49:775–780.

Borodic, G, Johnson, E, Goodnough, M, et al. (1996). Botulinum toxin therapy, immunologic resistance, and problems with available materials. *Neurology*, 46:26–29.

Borodic, GE, Acquadro, M, and Johnson, EA (2001). Botulinum toxin therapy for pain and inflammatory disorders: mechanisms and therapeutic effects. *Expert Opin Investig Drugs*, 10:1531–1544.

Bovim, G and Sand, T (1992). Cervicogenic headache, migraine without aura and tension-type headache. Diagnostic blockade of greater occipital and supra-orbital nerves. *Pain*, 51:43–48.

Brin, MF (1997). Botulinum toxin: chemistry, pharmacology, toxicity, and immunology. *Muscle Nerve*, 20: S146–S168.

Brin, MF, Swope, DM, O'Brien, et al. (2000). Botox for migraine: double-blind, placebo-controlled, region-specific evaluation. *Cephalalgia*, 20:421–422. (Abstract).

Burns, B, Watkins, L, and Goadsby, PJ (2007). Treatment of medically intractable cluster headache by occipital nerve stimulation: long-term follow-up of eight patients. *Lancet*, 369:1099–1106.

Busch, V, Jakob, W, Juergens, T, et al. (2006). Functional connectivity between trigeminal and occipital nerves revealed by occipital nerve blockade and nociceptive blink reflexes. *Cephalalgia*, 26:50–55.

Byrnes, ML, Thickbroom, GW, Wilson, SA, et al. (1998). The corticomotor representation of upper limb muscles in writer's cramp and changes following botulinum toxin injection. *Brain*, 121:977–988.

Caputi, CA and Firetto, V (1997). Therapeutic blockade of greater occipital and supraorbital nerves in migraine patients. *Headache*, 37:174–179.

Cook, BL, Malik, SN, Shaw, JW, et al. (2006). Greater occipital nerve (GON) block successfully treats migraine within five minutes. *Neurology*, 66:A42 (Abstract).

Costa, A, Pucci, E, Antonaci, F, et al. (2000). The effect of intranasal cocaine and lidocaine on nitroglycerin induced attacks in cluster headache. Cephalalgia 20:85–91.

Critchfield, J (2002). Considering the immune response to botulinum toxin. *Clin J Pain*, 18:S133–S141.

Cui, M, Khanijou, S, Rubino, J, et al. (2004). Subcutaneous administration of botulinum toxin A reduces formalin-induced pain. *Pain*, 107:125–133.

Dauer, Wt, Burke, RE, Greene, P, et al. (1998). Current concepts on the clinical features, aetiology and management of idiopathic cervical dystonia. *Brain*, 121:547–560.

de Craen, AJ, Tijssen, JG, de, GJ, et al. (2000). Placebo effect in the acute treatment of migraine: subcutaneous placebos are better than oral placebos. *J Neurol*, 247:183–188.

Dodick, DW (2003). Botulinum neurotoxin for the treatment of migraine and other primary headache disorders: from bench to bedside. *Headache*, 43(Suppl. 1): S25–S33.

Dodick, DW (2006). Clinical practice. Chronic daily headache. *N Engl J Med*, 354:158–165.

Dodick, DW, Mauskop, A, Elkind, AH, et al. (2005). Botulinum toxin type A for the prophylaxis of chronic daily headache: subgroup analysis of patients not receiving other prophylactic medications: a randomized double-blind, placebo-controlled study. *Headache*, 45:315–324.

Dolly, O (2003). Synaptic transmission: inhibition of neurotransmitter release by botulinum toxins. *Headache*, 43(Suppl. 1):S16–S24.

Dressler, D, Bigalke, H, and Benecke, R (2003). Botulinum toxin type B in antibody-induced botulinum toxin type A therapy failure. *J Neurol*, 250:967–969.

Durham, PL, Cady, R, and Cady, R (2004). Regulation of calcitonin gene-related peptide secretion from trigeminal nerve cells by botulinum toxin type A: implications for migraine therapy. *Headache*, 44:35–42.

Eross, EJ and Dodick, DW (2002). The effects of botulinum toxin type A on disability in episodic and chronic migraine. *Neurology*, 58(7):A497 (Abstract).

Eross, EJ, Gladstone, JP, Lewis, S, et al. (2005). Duration of migraine is a predictor for response to botulinum toxin type A. *Headache*, 45:308–314.

Evers, S, Vollmer-Haase, J, Schwaag, S, et al. (2004). Botulinum toxin A in the prophylactic treatment of migraine—a randomized, double-blind, placebo-controlled study. *Cephalalgia*, 24:838–843.

Farina, S, Granella, F, Malferrari, G, et al. (1986). Headache and cervical spine disorders: classification and treatment with transcutaneous electrical nerve stimulation. *Headache*, 26:431–433.

Ferrari, MD, Roon, KI, Lipton, RB, et al. (2001). Oral triptans (serotonin $5\text{-HT}_{1B/1D}$ agonists) in acute migraine treatment: a metaanalysis of 53 trials. *Lancet*, 358:1668–1675.

Filippi, GM, Errico, P, Santarelli, R, et al. (1993). Botulinum A toxin effects on rat jaw muscle spindles. *Acta Otolaryngol*, 113:400–404.

Gale, G, Nussbaum, D, Rothbart, P, et al. (2002). A randomized treatment study to compare the efficacy of repeated nerve blocks with cognitive therapy for control of chronic head and neck pain. *Pain Res Manag*, 7:185–189.

Ghoname, EA, Craig, WF, and White, PF (1999). Use of percutaneous electrical nerve stimulation (PENS) for treating ECT-induced headaches. *Headache*, 39:502–505.

Giladi, N (1997). The mechanism of action of botulinum toxin type A in focal dystonia is most probably through its dual effect on efferent (motor) and afferent pathways at the injection site. *J Neurol Sci*, 152:123–135.
Gilio, F, Currà, A, Lorenzano, C, et al. (2000). Effects of botulinum toxin type A on intracortical inhibition in patients with dystonia. *Ann Neurol*, 48:20–26.
Goadsby, PJ, Hoskin, KL, and Knight, YE (1997). Stimulation of the greater occipital nerve increases metabolic activity in the trigeminal nucleus caudalis and cervial dorsal horn of the cat. *Pain*, 73:23–28.
Goadsby, PJ and Zagami, AS (1991). Stimulation of the superior sagittal sinus increases metabolic activity and blood flow in certain regions of the brainstem and upper cervical spinal cord of the cat. *Brain*, 114:1001–1011.
Gobel, H, Heinze, A, Kuhn, KH, et al. (2001). Botulinum toxin A in the treatment of headache syndromes and pericranial pain syndromes. *Pain*, 91:195–199.
Goto, F, Ishizaki, K, Yoshikawa, D, et al. (1999). The long lasting effects of peripheral nerve blocks for trigeminal neuralgia using high concentration of tetracaine dissolved in bupivacaine. *Pain*, 79:101–103.
Greene, P, Fahn, S, and Diamond, B (1994). Development of resistance to botulinum toxin type A in patients with torticollis. *Mov Disord*, 9:213–217.
Hallett, M (2000). How does botulinum toxin work? *Ann Neurol*, 48:7–8.
Hardebo, JE and Elner, A (1987). Nerves and vessels in the pterygopalatine fossa and symptoms of cluster headache. *Headache*, 27:528–532.
Headache Classification Committee (2004). The International Classification of Headache Disorders, 2nd edition. *Cephalalgia*, 24:1–160.
Hecht, JS (2004). Occipital nerve blocks in postconcussive headaches: a retrospective review and report of ten patients. *J Head Trauma Rehabil*, 19:58–71.
Hord, ED, Evans, MS, Mueed, S, et al. (2003). The effect of vagus nerve stimulation on migraines. *J Pain*, 4:530–534.
Ishikawa, H, Mitsui, Y, Yoshitomi, T, et al. (2000). Presynaptic effects of botulinum toxin type A on the neuronally evoked response of albino and pigmented rabbit iris sphincter and dilator muscles. *Jpn J Ophthalmol*, 44:106–109.
Jakubowski, M, McAllister, PJ, Bajwa, ZH, et al. (2006). Exploding vs. imploding headache in migraine prophylaxis with Botulinum Toxin A. *Pain*, 24:1872–6623.
Janicki, PK and Habermann, E (1983). Tetanus and botulinum toxins inhibit, and black widow spider venom stimultes the release of methionine-enkephalin-like material in vitro. *J Neurochem*, 41:395–402.
Jankovic, J and Brin, ME (1997). Botulinum toxin: historical perspective and potential new indications. *Muscle Nerve*, 20:S129–S145.
Jankovic, J and Brin, MF (1991). Therapeutic uses of botulinum toxin. *N Engl J Med*, 324:1186–1194.
Jankovic, J and Schwartz, K (1995). Response and immunoresistance to botulinum toxin i njections. *Neurology*, 45:1743–1746.
Jensen, R and Olesen, J (2000). Tension-type headache: an update on mechanisms and treatment. *Curr Opin Neurol*, 13:285–289.
Kittrelle, JP, Grouse, DS, and Seybold, ME (1985). Cluster headache. Local anesthetic abortive agents. *Arch Neurol*, 42:496–498.
Knyihar-Csillik, E, Tajti, J, Mohtasham, S, et al. (1995). Electrical stimulation of the Gasserian ganglion induces structural alterations of calcitonin gene-related peptide-immunoreactive perivascular sensory nerve terminals in the rat cerebral dura mater: a possible model of migraine headache. *Neurosci Lett*, 184:189–192.
Kramer, HH, Angerer, C, Erbguth, F, et al. (2003). Botulinum toxin A reduces neurogenic flare but has almost no effect on pain and hyperalgesia in human skin. *J Neurol*, 250:188–193.
Lake, AE and Saper, JR (2003). Botulinum toxin Type B for migraine prophylaxis: a 4-month open-label prospective outcome study. *Neurology*, 60:A322 (Abstract).
Lavin, PJ and Workman, R (2001). Cushing syndrome induced by serial occipital nerve blocks containing corticosteroids. *Headache*, 41:902–904.
Leinisch-Dahlke, E, Jurgens, T, Bogdahn, U, et al. (2005). Greater occipital nerve block is ineffective in chronic tension type headache. *Cephalalgia*, 25:704–708.
Lew, MF, Adornato, BT, Duane, D, et al. (1997). Botulinum toxin type B: a double-blind, placebo-controlled, safety and efficacy study in cervical dystonia. *Neurology*, 49:701–707.
Lord, S, Barnsley, L, Wallis, B, et al. (1994). Third occipital headache: a prevalence study. *J Neurol Neurosurg Psychiatry*, 57:1187.
Magis, D, Allena, M, Bolla, M, et al. (2007). Occipital nerve stimulation for drug-resistant chronic cluster headache: a prospective pilot study. *Lancet Neurol*, 6:314–321.
Matharu, MS, Bartsch, T, Ward, N, et al. (2004). Central neuromodulation in chronic migraine patients with suboccipital stimulators: a PET study. *Brain*, 127:220–230.
Mathew, NT, Frishberg, BM, Gawel, M, et al. (2005). Botulinum toxin type A (BOTOX) for the prophylactic treatment of chronic daily headache: a randomized, double-blind, Placebo-Controlled Trial. *Headache*, 45:293–307.
Mathew, NT, Kailasam, J, and Meadors, L (2002). "Disease modification" in chronic migraine with botulinum toxin type A: long-term experience. *Headache*, 42:454–S107 (Abstract).
Mauskop, A (2005). Vagus nerve stimulation relieves chronic refractory migraine and cluster headaches. *Cephalalgia*, 25:82–86.
Mauskop, A and Basdeo, R (2000). Botulinum toxin A is an effective prophylactic therapy for migraines. *Cephalalgia*, 20:422 (Abstract).

Mellick, GA and Mellick, LB (2003). Regional head and face pain relief following lower cervical intramuscular anesthetic injection. *Headache*, 43:1109–1111.

Ondo, WG, Vuong, KD, and Derman, HS (2004). Botulinum toxin A for chronic daily headache: a randomized, placebo-controlled, parallel design study. *Cephalalgia*, 24:60–65.

Opida, C (2002). Open-label study of Myobloc (botulinum toxin type b) in the treatment of patients with transformed migraine headaches. *J Pain*, 3:10 (Abstract).

Padberg, M, de Bruijn, SF, de Haan, RJ, et al. (2004). Treatment of chronic tension-type headache with botulinum toxin: a double-blind, placebo-controlled clinical trial. *Cephalalgia*, 24:675–680.

Peres, MF, Stiles, MA, Siow, HC, et al. (2002). Greater occipital nerve blockade for cluster headache. *Cephalalgia*, 22:520–522.

Piovesan, EJ, Kowacs, PA, Tatsui, CE, et al. (2001). Referred pain after painful stimulation of the greater occipital nerve in humans: evidence of convergence of cervical afferences on trigeminal nuclei. *Cephalalgia*, 21:107–109.

Popeney, CA and Alo, KM (2003). Peripheral neurostimulation for the treatment of chronic, disabling transformed migraine. *Headache*, 43:369–375.

Relja, MA and Klepac, N (2003). Botulinum toxin Type-A reduces acute medication (triptans)use in migraine patients. *Neurology*, 60:A321 (Abstract).

Robbins, L (1995). Intranasal lidocaine for cluster headache. Headache 35:83–84.

Rodrigo-Royo, MD, Azcona, JM, Quero, J, et al. (2005). Peripheral neurostimulation in the management of cervicogenic headache: four case reports. *Neuromodulation*, 8:241–248.

Rollnik, JD, Tanneberger, O, Schubert, M, et al. (2000). Treatment of tension-type headache with botulinum toxin type A: a double-blind, placebo-controlled study. *Headache*, 40:300–305.

Rosales, RL, Arimura, K, Takenaga, S, et al. (1996). Extrafusal and intrafusal muscle effects in experimental botulinum toxin-A injection. *Muscle Nerve*, 19:488–496.

Rothbart, P, Fiedler, K, Gale, GD, et al. (2000). A descriptive study of 100 patients undergoing palliative nerve blocks for chronc intractable headache and neck ache. *Pain Res Manag*, 5:243–248.

Sadler, RM, Purdy, RA, and Rahey, S (2002). Vagal nerve stimulation aborts migraine in patient with intractable epilepsy. *Cephalalgia*, 22:482–484.

Sakamoto, T, Asanuma, K, Kaji, R, et al. (2003). Development of a new low molecular weight botulinum type A neurotoxin preparation for treating muscle hyperactivity. *Neurology*, 60:A466 (Abstract).

Schmitt, WJ, Slowey, E, Fravi, N, et al. (2001). Effect of Botulinum toxin A injections in the treatment of chronic tension-type headache: a double-blind, placebo-controlled trial. *Headache*, 41:658–664.

Schulte-Mattler, WJ and Krack P (2004). Treatment of chronic tension-type headache with botulinum toxin A: a randomized, double-blind, placebo-controlled multicenter study. *Pain*, 109:110–114.

Schwedt, TJ, Dodick, DW, Hentz, J, et al. (2007). Occipital nerve stimulation for chronic headache—long-term safety and efficacy. *Cephalalgia*, 27:153–157.

Schwedt, TJ, Dodick, DW, Trentman, TL, et al. (2006). Occipital nerve stimulation for chronic cluster headache and hemicrania continua: pain relief and persistence of autonomic features. *Cephalalgia*, 26:1025–1027.

Scott, AB (1988). Antitoxin reduces botulinum side effects. *Eye*, 2:29–32.

Shapiro, RL, Hatheway, C, and Swerdlow, DL (1998). Botulism in the United States: a clinical and epidemiologic review. *Ann Int Med*, 129:221–228.

Shields, KG, Levy, MJ, and Goadsby, PJ (2004). Alopecia and cutaneous atrophy after greater occipital nerve infiltration with corticosteroid. *Neurology*, 63:2193–2194.

Silberstein, SD (2001). Review of botulinum toxin type A and its clinical applications in migraine headache. *Exp Opin Pharmacother*, 2:1649–1654.

Silberstein, SD and Goadsby, PJ (2002). Migraine: preventive treatment. *Cephalalgia*, 22:491–512.

Silberstein, SD, Gobel, H, Jensen, R, et al. (2006). Botulinum toxin type A in the prophylactic treatment of chronic tension-type headache: a multicentre, double-blind, randomized, placebo-controlled, parallel-group study. *Cephalalgia*, 26:790–800.

Silberstein, SD, Mathew, N, Saper, J, et al. (2000). Botulinum toxin type A as a migraine preventive treatment. *Headache*, 40:445–450.

Silberstein, SD, Stark, SR, Lucas, SM, et al. (2005). Botulinum toxin type A for the prophylactic treatment of chronic daily headache: a randomized, double-blind, placebo-controlled trial. *Mayo Clin Proc*, 80:1126–1137.

Sjaastad, O, Stolt-Nielsen, A, Pareja, JA, et al. (1999). Supraorbital neuralgia. On the clinical manifestations and a possible therapeutic approach. *Headache*, 39:204–212.

Smuts, JA, Baker, MK, Smuts, M, et al. (1999). Prophylactic treatment of chronic tension-type headache using botulinum toxin type A. *Eur J Neurol*, 6:99–102.

Smuts, JA and Barnard, PW (2000). Botulinum toxin type A in the treatment of headache syndromes: a clinical report on 79 patients. *Cephalalgia*, 20:332 (Abstract).

Smuts, JA, Schultz, D, and Barnard, A (2004). Mechanism of action of botulinum toxin type A in migraine prevention: a pilot study. *Headache*, 44:801–805.

Tepper SJ, Bigal ME, Sheftell FD, Rapoport AM (2004). Botulinum neurotoxin type A in the preventive treatment of refractory headache: a review of 100 consecutive cases. *Headache*, 44:794–800.

Turton, K, Chaddock, JA, and Acharya, KR (2002). Botulinum and tetanus neurotoxins: structure, function and therapeutic utility. *Trends Biochem Sci*, 27:552–558.

Weiner, RL (2003). Peripheral nerve neurostimulation. *Neurosurg Clin N Am*, 14:401–408.

Weiner, RL (2006). Occipital neurostimulation (ONS) for treatment of intractable headache disorders. *Pain Med,* 7(Suppl. 1):S137–S139.

Welch, MJ, Purkiss, JR, and Foster, KA (2000). Sensitivity of embryonic rat dorsal root ganglia neurons to *Clostridium botulinum* neurotoxins. *Toxicon,* 38:245–258.

Wheeler, AH (1998). Botulinum Toxin A, adjunctive therapy for refractory headaches associated with pericranial muscle tension. *Headache,* 38:468–471.

Wiegand, H and Wellhoner, HH (1977). The action of botulinum A neurotoxin on the inhibition by antidromic stimulation of the lumbar monosynaptic reflex. *Naunyn Schmiedebergs Arch Pharmacol,* 298:235–238.

Wolff, HG (1948). *Wolff's Headache and Other Head Pain.* Oxford University Press, New York.

Zuber, M, Sebald, M, Bathien, N, et al. (1995). Botulinum antibodies in dystonic patients treated with type A botulinum toxin: Frequency and significance. *Neurology,* 43:1715–1718.

Zwart, JA, Bovim, G, Sand, T, et al. (1994). Tension headache: botulinum toxin paralysis of temporal muscles. *Headache,* 34:458–462.

33 Turning Treatment Failure into Treatment Success

Richard B Lipton, Joel R Saper, and Stephen D Silberstein

INTRODUCTION

Although headache disorders are very common, managing headache patients, particularly those with chronic daily headaches, can be difficult (Mathew, 1982, 1991; Pascual et al., 1995; Lipton et al., 2003). Most patients respond well to treatment, but some patients seem intractable, and a smaller group truly are intractable. Patients who do not respond as expected, or announce at their first visit that nothing will work, can be challenging. It is important to identify the reason or reasons why these patients have not responded to treatment.

Herein, we summarize some common reasons for headache-treatment failure, grouping them into five broad categories (Table 33–1). When evaluating treatment-refractory patients, we find it helpful to consider the following categories: the diagnosis is incomplete or incorrect, exacerbating factors have been missed, pharmacotherapy is inadequate, nonpharmacologic treatment is inadequate, and other factors resulting in treatment failure. This chapter is organized around these five reasons for treatment failure, with an emphasis on opportunities to improve patient outcomes.

Reason 1: The Diagnosis is Incorrect or Incomplete

Inaccurate diagnosis is probably the most common reason for treatment failure. When a patient is not responding to treatment, it is always important to revisit the issue of diagnosis. Major diagnostic issues include the following: a secondary headache disorder is undiagnosed, a primary headache disorder is misdiagnosed, or two or more headache disorders exist. Repeating the history and focusing on all the headache types that are present is an important first step. Looking for red flags by history or on examination may help identify previously undetected or newly arising secondary disorders. We will consider these three forms of diagnostic difficulty one at a time.

Secondary Disorders Go Undiagnosed

Many patients with intractable headache live with the fear that the doctor has "missed something." Clinicians who care for patients with difficult-to-manage headaches often share that concern. While diagnostic vigilance is important, it is equally important to be confident that the diagnosis is correct and to relieve the patient's anxiety. Medication misuse with rebound headache is probably the single most common secondary disorder that causes intractability (Mathew, 1982, 1991; Saper, 1987, 1989). Other less common secondary causes of intractable headache are summarized in Table 33–2. When a patient is not responding, a secondary disorder may have arisen in the context of a primary disorder. Sometimes more than one secondary disorder is present. Detection of many of these disorders requires a systematic approach to the headache history and physical examination as well as a high index of suspicion.

Clues Based on Headache History

The temporal profile of the headache and its onset, as well as the nature and the circumstances of that onset, are crucial for diagnosis. The temporal profile of a headache can provide important etiologic clues. For example,

- Headache of very abrupt onset may suggest a subarachnoid hemorrhage (Linn et al., 1998), pituitary apoplexy (Dodick and Wijdicks, 1998), or other intracranial catastrophes

TABLE 33–1 Possible Reasons Leading to Treatment Failure.

1. **The diagnosis is incomplete or incorrect**
   A secondary headache disorder goes undiagnosed
   A primary headache disorder is misdiagnosed
   The number of headache disorders is not clear
2. **Important exacerbating factors have been missed**
   Acute headache medication or caffeine overuse
   Hormonal triggers
   Dietary or lifestyle triggers
   Psychosocial factors
   Other medications
3. **Pharmacotherapy has been inadequate**
   Ineffective drug
   Excessive initial doses
   Inadequate final doses
   Inadequate duration of treatment
   Combination therapy required
   Poor absorption
   Noncompliance
4. **Nonpharmacologic treatment has been inadequate**
   Physical medicine
   Cognitive behavioral therapy
5. **Other factors**
   Unrealistic expectations
   Comorbid and concomitant conditions
   Inpatient treatment required

(Forsyth and Posner, 1993). These disorders rarely cause chronic headache, but can result in intractability of a single ongoing headache attack. They are of particular concern in patients presenting to the emergency department. Rapid-onset headache also can be acute-onset migraine.

- Sphenoid sinusitis may cause intractable headache of subacute onset and may be missed radiologically unless special views are ordered (Lawson and Reino, 1997).
- Headache onset after age 55 suggests an organic disorder, such as a mass lesion or giant cell arteritis (Edmeads, 1997). Giant cell arteritis is an important preventable cause of blindness in the elderly.

Concurrent events and headache triggers may give clues to headache diagnosis and help the clinician identify causes of intractability:

- Headaches that occur postpartum may be due to cortical vein or dural sinus thrombosis (Ameri and Bousser, 1992). Although often associated with increased intracranial pressure and papilledema, these features need not be present.
- Headache that begins or worsens upon standing suggests a "low cerebrospinal fluid (CSF) pressure" headache (from a spontaneous CSF leak, a previous lumbar puncture, or an epidural block) (Lay et al., 1997).
- Headaches triggered by straining, coughing, or sneezing suggest a hindbrain malformation, occipitocervical junction disorder, or increased intracranial pressure (Sands et al., 1991).
- A headache associated with fever or systemic symptoms suggests an infectious etiology.
- Headaches that are worse on awakening suggest sleep apnea, increased intracranial pressure, or medication withdrawal (Lay et al., 1997).
- Pain that increases with neck flexion or extension suggests an occipitocervical junction disorder or a systemic medical illness (Edmeads, 2001).
- A headache associated with exercise may be an anginal equivalent, a rare disorder sometimes termed cardiac cephalalgia (Lipton et al., 1997).
- Skin rashes or lesions suggest Lyme disease, herpes zoster, sarcoidosis, collagen vascular disease, or other systemic illness (Marks and Rapoport, 1997).
- In patients with HIV, or risk factors for HIV, opportunistic infections, including toxoplasmosis and cryptococcal meningitis, should be considered (Evers et al., 2000).
- A diagnosis of posttraumatic headache may lead to additional treatment, including trigger point injections and facet joint and cervical nerve blocks (Solomon, 2001).
- Postictal headaches might be of special importance, because migraine and epilepsy

Table 33–2 Secondary Headaches that Mimic Chronic Benign Headache Syndromes.

Headache associated with vascular disorders

Cerebrovascular disease, including carotid artery dissection and arteriovenous malformation
Arteritis, including giant cell arteritis

Headache associated with nonvascular intracranial disorders

Low CSF pressure syndrome (spontaneous or posttraumatic CSF "leak")
High CSF pressure without papilledema
Intracranial: Lyme disease, human immunodeficiency virus, encephalitis, fungal meningitis

Headache associated with substances or their withdrawal

Overuse of acute headache medications (rebound or toxic drug overuse syndromes)

Headache associated with cranium, neck, eyes, ears, nose, sinuses, teeth, mouth, or other facial or cranial structures

Otolaryngologic disease, including chronic sphenoid sinusitis (or other sinus disease)
Nasopharyngeal disorders, including carcinoma
Disorders of the trigeminal nerve, including dental and oral disease, jaw pathology
Subacute angle closure glaucoma, optic neuritis, and other ocular disorders
Occipitocervical disease, including Arnold–Chiari Malformation Type I; upper cervical joint, root, or nerve (neuralgic) syndromes

Headache associated with noncephalic infection, metabolic or systemic disturbances

Hepatitis, renal disease, B_{12} deficiency, anemia, exposure to carbon monoxide and other toxins
Hormonal disturbances/endocrinologic disease (estrogen, thyroid disease, hyperprolactinemia, etc.)
Vasculitis/rheumatic/connective tissue disorders

Miscellania

Mediastinal and thoracic processes, including angina, mass lesions, superior vena cava syndrome

occur together with more than twice the frequency that would be expected by chance (Andermann and Andermann, 1987).

- A history of recent root canals, tooth extractions, or oral infections raises the spectre of intracranial infection, including brain abscess (Graff-Radford, 2001).
- If the pain is periorbital, one must consider ocular disturbances, such as subacute angle closure glaucoma, or infection, particularly if ocular redness or tearing occurs (Martin and Soyka, 1993).
- Nasal blockage, drainage, pus, or pressure may suggest sinus disease (Cady and Schreiber, 2002). Nasopharyngeal carcinoma can produce chronic head and face pain and can be identified by detailed, expert examination of the nasopharynx or by neuroimaging (Wenig, 1999).

Clues Based on the Physical Examination

The physical examination should focus on the systems that are important in headache provocation, such as eyes, ears, neck, and other systems with trigeminal innervation. Occipitocervical pain on palpation and movement, submandibular pain (indicating styloid process factors, lymph nodes, carotid artery tenderness masses), disc margin clarity, visual function, eye movement, oral cavity health, and pain and discomfort in the temporomandibular joint area may provide diagnostic clues (Burstein et al., 2000).

Diagnostic testing should follow the clues: Many patients with intractable headache have had multiple neuroimaging procedures. The strategies for investigation of secondary headaches are described in detail in Chapter 5. If prior studies are negative and the history points in this direction, studies targeted to suspected sites of pathology, including the occipitocervical junction, sella tursica, sphenoid sinus, and nasopharyngeal regions, occasionally yield results (Mokri et al., 1979; Frishberg, 1994; Evans, 1996). If the patient is truly intractable, a lumbar puncture may help identify inflammatory or infectious changes that could indicate aseptic or chronic meningitis (including seronegative Lyme disease) (Scelsa et al., 1995), as well as idiopathic intracranial hypertension (without papilledema) (Silberstein and Marcelis, 1990). Neuroimaging does not obviate the utility of lumbar puncture in these circumstances, although the yield is low (Wang et al., 1998). Cisternography or CT myelography is indicated when low CSF pressure is the most likely diagnosis. In such cases, lumbar puncture should be avoided, since it can worsen intracranial hypotension. Obesity and pulsatile tinnitus are risk factors for idiopathic intracranial hypertension (Wang et al., 1998).

Primary Headache is Misdiagnosed

If the wrong primary headache disorder is diagnosed, proper treatment is unlikely. Herein, we will review some primary headache disorders that may be missed or misdiagnosed in clinical practice. All these disorders are described in detail in other chapters. *Hemicrania continua* (Sjaastad and Spierings, 1984; Newman et al., 1994), characterized by chronic, unilateral pain, is commonly mistaken for transformed or chronic migraine (Silberstein et al., 1994; Silberstein and Lipton, 2001). Chronic unilateral pain with superimposed painful exacerbations may be present in both hemicrania continua and chronic migraine. The pain of hemicrania continua rarely remits at all, and the painful exacerbations are often associated with ipsilateral autonomic features, such as conjunctival injection, lacrimation, and ptosis (Sjaastad and Spierings, 1984; Newman et al., 1994; Peres et al., 2001). Most chronic migraine patients have days when they are free of pain, and exacerbations are more typically accompanied by nausea, photophobia, and phonophobia (Silberstein et al., 1994; Silberstein and Lipton, 2001). In addition, patients with hemicrania continua usually do not have an antecedent history of episodic migraine; whereas chronic migraine attacks increase in frequency over time.

If the headaches are longstanding, the patient may not be able to describe their onset. Though pain fluctuates in hemicrania continua, it does not usually have the morning and end-of-dosing-interval exacerbation pattern typical of chronic migraine. It is advisable to offer patients with unilateral chronic daily headache a therapeutic trial with indomethacin prior to other intervention (see Chapter 13).

Paroxysmal hemicrania. Paroxysmal hemicrania is often mistaken for cluster headache (Sjaastad and Dale, 1976; Price and Posner, 1978; Headache Classification Committee of the International Headache Society, 1988; Newman and Lipton, 1997). Both disorders are trigeminal autonomic cephalgias. They are characterized by short-lived, unilateral attacks of pain in the distribution of the first division of the trigeminal nerve with ipsilateral autonomic features (Sjaastad and Dale, 1976; Headache Classification Committee of the International Headache Society, 1988). Both have episodic and chronic forms (Newman and Lipton, 1997). The episodic forms are characterized by frequent attacks of headache over weeks or months, followed by long pain-free remission periods. The chronic forms include frequent headaches for a year or more. While cluster headache shows a male preponderance, the paroxysmal hemicranias show a female preponderance. Cluster attacks last 30–90 minutes and occur 1–5 times daily; paroxysmal hemicrania attacks are shorter (typically 2–30 minutes), and the attack frequency is greater (often five or more attacks per day) (Sjaastad and Dale, 1976; Headache Classification Committee of the International Headache Society, 1988). A prompt response to indomethacin typically confirms the diagnosis (Price and Posner, 1978). In atypical patients, a trial of indomethacin may be warranted when conventional treatment for cluster headaches or trigeminal neuralgia fails (Newman and Lipton, 1997). When headache is controlled, the dose can generally be lowered and headache control is maintained. Responses to indomethacin are usually very clear and easy to evaluate in paroxysmal hemicrania, but may take up to 2 weeks to develop fully.

Hypnic headache. The hypnic headache syndrome is a primary headache disorder of the elderly and usually occurs in individuals over the age of 60 (Newman et al., 1990; Dodick et al., 1998). It is characterized by short-lived attacks (typically 30 minutes) of nocturnal head pain that awaken the patient at a consistent time each night, usually from rapid eye movement sleep. Hypnic headache pain is usually bilateral, throbbing, or diffuse, and it lacks the intense, unilateral, orbital, and periorbital knife-like quality of cluster headache, as well as its autonomic features. Unilateral headache does not exclude the diagnosis. The hypnic headache syndrome responds promptly to an evening dose of lithium carbonate 300 mg or to slow-release lithium. If lithium is unsuccessful, melatonin, caffeine, or 120 mg of verapamil at night may be useful. A recent study/series suggests that unilateral hypnic headache is more common than previously believed (Rasmussen et al., 1992).

Two or More Headache Disorders May be Present

Diagnostic mistakes may occur when two or more headache disorders coexist (Rasmussen et al., 1992). Patients sometimes mix the features of two distinct disorders, creating historical confusion. For example, a patient with migraine beginning after head injury may have components of posttraumatic headache disorder. When a patient with an established headache disorder develops a new headache type, caution is advisable. Sometimes it is difficult to distinguish an intracranial catastrophe from an unusually severe migraine. A superimposed infectious or metabolic process may not be recognized. Intractable bouts of headache in established migraine sufferers, similar to but worse than their preexisting headache, may be due to aseptic meningitis or intracerebral or subarachnoid hemorrhage. Sometimes the disorders co-occur by coincidence alone. For example, a person with migraine may develop a brain tumor. Sometimes one headache disorder may lead to another. For example, migraine may predispose to medication overuse headache. Sometimes headache disorders occur together with greater-than-chance frequency, as in the well-known cluster-tic syndrome.

Exacerbating Factors May Have Been Missed

Migraine attacks may be triggered by a number of factors; still other factors may exacerbate the disease. Factors leading to intractability included medication overuse (prescription or over-the-counter analgesics, butalbital, ergotamine, and triptans), caffeine overuse, dietary or lifestyle triggers, hormonal triggers, psychosocial factors, or the use of other medications that trigger headaches, such as nitroglycerine. Medication overuse is sometimes the cause of a secondary headache disorder and sometimes an exacerbating factor for a primary disorder. In the search for exacerbating factors, we begin by asking about factors the patient may have identified and then probe for common and uncommon exacerbating factors, especially those that are subject to modification or intervention.

Medication overuse and withdrawal is probably the most common cause of intractability (Saper and Jones, 1986; Rapoport et al., 1996). A careful medication history, focusing on both prescription and over-the-counter medication, as well as vitamins, herbs, and natural products, is therefore essential. When asked what medications they are taking, many patients report only prescription medications. Some patients are embarrassed about medication misuse and fear that the physician will judge them harshly. It is therefore important to ask about prescription and over-the-counter medication use in an open, nonjudgmental manner. It is helpful to normalize medication-taking by saying, "Many patients find they need to take something everyday; how often do you take pain relievers?" Excessive use of agents that contain caffeine, opioids, barbiturates, ergots, and triptans produce increased headache frequency and significantly attenuate the effectiveness of both acute and preventive treatments. Caffeine overuse (including the dietary intake) can be an important cause of intractability (Mathew, 1982, 1991; Rapoport et al., 1996). Vitamin A and D overuse may cause headaches. The treatment of medication overuse is described in detail in Chapter 13.

Some patients may have *hormonal factors* that contribute to intractability (Silberstein, 2001). The effects of hormones on headache differ widely from person to person. Falling estrogen levels are a common headache trigger, contributing to migraine exacerbations during menses and during the perimenopausal period. Like endogenous hormones, exogenous hormones (contraceptives and hormone replacement therapy) have effects that vary widely from individual to individual. Historical clues should be sought to determine the influence of hormones on patients who are taking them. If historical evidence suggests that exogenous hormones contributed to intractability, they should probably be modified or even eliminated. However, we can often control headaches despite hormone therapy. Sometimes hormonal therapy, particularly continuous estrogen, improves headache control (Chapter 28).

Dietary or lifestyle factors may play a significant role in headache (Marks and Rapoport, 1997). Stressful life events, such as divorce, separation, death, and problems with children, are risk factors for chronic daily headache (Stewart et al., 2001). Alcohol use, especially red wine, may trigger headaches (Nicolodi and Sicuteri, 1999). Sleep apnea is common in middle-aged obese men and may cause morning headache (Poceta and Dalessio, 1995). Depression or anxiety may present with difficulty in falling asleep or staying asleep, or with early morning awakening. Careful questioning about possible stressors may uncover a source of conflict or a psychologic component to the headache, which can lead to intractability in some patients, especially those with very frequent headaches. Some dietary factors, including aspartame, may trigger headache (Blumenthal and Vance, 1997; Newman and Lipton, 2001).

Occupational and environmental factors may cause or aggravate the headache. Environmental exposures to carbon monoxide, solvents, or other environmental contaminants may trigger headaches (Hampson and Hampson, 2002). Workers in munitions factories may develop nitroglycerine headaches or have migraine triggered (Van Gelderen and Saxena, 1996). Taking certain medications may contribute to headache. Table 33–3 summarizes some of the medications that may cause headache.

Patent foramen ovale (PFO) has emerged as an important factor in migraine (Chapter 17). PFOs are more common in migraine, particularly migraine with aura, sufferers than in the general population. Open studies suggest dramatic reductions in attack frequency following closure. A randomized controlled trial suggests benefit of closure on secondary but not primary endpoints. In the setting of PFO, either particulate matter or biochemical mediators may bypass the lungs and reach the brain to trigger headache. If well-designed studies are positive, PFOs may represent an important endogenous trigger and closure may emerge as an important avenue of treatment.

Pharmacotherapy May be Inadequate

Assuming the diagnosis or diagnoses are correct and remediable exacerbating factors have been addressed, inadequate pharmacotherapy is a

Table 33–3 Selected Medications Reported to Cause Headaches.

Amantadine	Monoamine oxidase inhibitors
Calcium-channel blockers	Nonsteroidal antiinflammatory agents
Caffeine	Nitrates
Corticosteroids	Nicotinic acid
Cyclophosphamide	Phenothiazines
Dipyridamole	Ranitidine
Estrogens	Sympathomimetic agents
Ethanol	Tamoxifen
Hydralazine	Theophyllines (thioxanthines)
Indomethacin	Tetracyclines
L-Dopa	Trimethoprim

major factor in treatment failure. Migraine pharmacotherapy is traditionally divided into acute and preventive approaches (see Chapter X) (Silberstein and Rosenberg, 2000). Acute treatment medication is given with the attack. The goals of acute treatment are to relieve pain and restore function. Preventive treatment is taken on a daily basis, whether or not headache is present. Its goal is to reduce the frequency of attacks. Everyone with migraine needs acute treatment (Silberstein and Rosenberg, 2000). Perhaps 40% of migraine sufferers need preventive treatment (Lipton et al., 2007). In addition, short-term prevention has recently emerged as a proven strategy, particularly for menstrual migraine (see Chapter XX). Inadequate pharmacotherapy may result from failure to use the required strategies (acute, preventive, short-term preventive), inappropriate treatment choice, failure to use combination treatment, or problems with the dose and duration of treatment. Sometimes, patients do not absorb or rapidly metabolize drugs or do not follow directions. Medications appropriate for the patient's diagnosis or diagnoses should be carefully reviewed. It is important to determine the dosage and duration of treatment with prior therapies.

Several common issues may lead to treatment failure in the acute management of migraine. One important issue is the failure to use stratified care in selecting the initial therapy. A randomized trial supports the U.S. Headache Consortium Guidelines in their recommendation for stratified care (Lipton and Silberstein, 2001). That strategy is based on the selection of initial therapy on the basis of patient characteristics, including headache-related disability, at the time of presentation.

When patients report that acute treatment is unsuccessful, it is important to understand what they mean. (1) Was there no response or an incomplete response to treatment? (2) Did treatment response take too long? (3) Did the headache respond well initially but then recur? (4) Did the treatment cause too many side effects? By understanding the type of treatment failure, corrective strategies can be developed.

Early treatment while pain is mild makes treatment more effective (Cady et al., 2000). Recent evidence demonstrates that acute migraine treatment works best if given early in the course of the headache, while pain is still mild. Aspirin plus metoclopramide, ergotamine, and several triptans produce higher pain-free rates if they are given while pain is mild (Cady et al., 2000). Once allodynia and central sensitization develop, treatment is much less likely to work (Wenig, 1999). For that reason, early treatment is an important approach to making acute treatment more successful. Caution is required to avoid the development of medication overuse.

Another option is to change the route of administration. Migraine-related gastric paresis may delay or prevent the absorption of oral medication. Nasal sprays and injections therefore provide important, underused treatment alternatives. It is sometimes useful to escalate the dose or to switch drugs. When switching drugs, it is helpful to consider the difficulty the patient had with the original drug. For example, if tolerability or headache recurrence are the problems, almotriptan, naratriptan, and frovatriptan are important options. If efficacy or speed of onset is the issue, rizatriptan or eletriptan may be helpful; nonoral therapy may also be needed (Ferrari et al., 2001). Some patients require acute combination therapy to get relief. Combining triptans with nonsteroidal antiinflammatory agents is a common strategy that has proven effective (see Chapter 11). A sumatriptan and naproxen combination is now available as a single drug.

Common reasons for preventive treatment failure include incorrect dosing strategies and premature discontinuation. Preventive treatment may be ineffective if the patient is overusing acute medications ("rebounding").

Preventive medications must be given at an adequate dose for an adequate length of time. It is best to start preventive agents at a low dose and then gradually increase the dose until therapeutic effects, treatment-limiting side effects, or the ceiling dose for the agent in question is reached. At least one month is required to evaluate the success or failure of a treatment. Further increases beyond the ceiling dose may be necessary if there is a partial response at the ceiling dose without side effects but the headaches remain disabling. Some patients may take appropriate doses of a drug but not achieve the necessary blood levels for response owing to difficulty with absorption.

Rational polytherapy. Although monotherapy is usually recommended, rational combination therapy is sometimes necessary, especially in the setting of comorbid illness. Antidepressants are usually a rational choice for the depressed or anxious migraine sufferer, but the addition of an antiepileptic medication (divalproex sodium), a beta-blocker, or a calcium-channel blocker may be useful. For the patient with truly refractory headache and refractory depression, a monoamine oxidase inhibitor is sometimes the only effective treatment option. Methysergide, alone or in combination with a calcium-channel blocker, may help control refractory headache, particularly refractory chronic cluster headache. Selection of preventive medications has been reviewed elsewhere (Silberstein and Goadsby, 2002).

Noncompliance with treatment. Noncompliance with prescribed preventive medication or misuse of acute treatment is common. Because migraine attacks are episodic, the patient's motivation to treat may diminish between attacks. Patients may not understand that sustained treatment is necessary to achieve therapeutic success (Holroyd, 2001). Unanticipated side effects may lead patients to discontinue treatment. Compliance may improve if the patient understands the need for long-term treatment and anticipates the process of dose adjustment (Weeks, 1995). Compliance is improved if the patient can see that the degree of disability caused by the headache outweighs the disadvantages of prophylactic drugs. Ideally, after an explanation of the options, the patient will suggest or opt for preventive treatment rather than have the doctor make the decision. Side effects may be better tolerated if the patient knows that they may ameliorate over time (Holroyd et al., 2001). If rebound headaches were present during previous therapeutic trials, it may be necessary to retry unsuccessful but incorrectly used treatments. When treatment trials are repeated, it is well worth explaining the reasons for returning to a previously used drug. Noncompliance with nonpharmacologic treatment can render treatment unsuccessful. If patients do not avoid known provoking factors, poor headache control will result (Holroyd et al., 2001).

Nonpharmacologic Treatment May be Inadequate

Patients who are tense sometimes need physical medicine or behavioral interventions. Patients with occipital tenderness and trigger points often do not get relief from their headache disorder until they are given a nerve block or trigger point injection (Davidoff, 1998). Patients with intractable headache disorders sometimes are relieved by trigger point injections into tender areas, using a combination of a local anesthetic and a depocorticosteroid. Occasional occipital nerve and facet joint blocks are useful, generally when there are concomitant physical signs, such as a sensory abnormality over the C_2 distribution on the back of the head. Physical therapy is often a useful adjunct for these patients. Patients who are tense and anxious and have trouble coping with their daily existence can have trouble getting their headaches under control. Cognitive training helps them decrease the stress they impose on themselves and may improve their headaches (Weeks, 1995; Holroyd et al., 2001). In intractable headache patients, it is useful to separate pain and ability to function. If pain does not improve, behavioral strategies should focus on optimizing function.

Other Reasons for Treatment Failure

Treatment may fail if the patient has unrealistic expectations, comorbid conditions that complicate therapy, or when inpatient treatment is required but not offered. As patients improve, their expectations may escalate and they may forget how bad they were. The patient who has a chronic daily headache may complain a year later that he is no better—he is having two attacks a month that respond promptly to acute treatment. Headache diaries can be used to remind patients about their previous headache pattern. Modulating expectations can be difficult. Patients should not tolerate pain and disability needlessly. But it may not be realistic to expect a treatment regimen to give perfect headache control with no side effects.

Patients with comorbid or concomitant medical or neurologic illness are often more difficult to treat. Comorbid diseases occur in migraineurs with a greater frequency than would be expected by chance. Migraine is comorbid with depression, anxiety, affective disorders, stroke, and epilepsy (Breslau, 1994; Lipton et al., 1994; Tzourio, 1995). These disorders can impose therapeutic challenges and limit treatment options. Concomitant diseases occur together with chance frequency; common concomitant diseases that limit options in migraine treatment include asthma (beta blockers), ulcers and gastritis (nonsteroidal antiinflammatory drugs), and vascular disease and uncontrolled hypertension (triptans, ergot alkaloids). Concomitant obesity may limit the utilization of many prophylactic drugs. A restricted therapeutic armamentarium can severely compromise treatment. Patients with major comorbid psychiatric disorders may require ongoing care with a mental health professional appropriate to the disorder. Psychiatric problems often abate as headache comes under control.

Inpatient care: When outpatient treatment fails and patients have continuing and severe pain and disability, more aggressive treatment interventions may be required (see Chapter 13). Inpatient-level treatment should be reserved for people who require the intense interventions and around-the-clock monitoring that can only be provided in an inpatient setting. Aggressive parenteral treatment to "break" the headache cycle and/or maintain the patient in reasonable comfort during detoxification (if necessary) represents the initial step. Rehydration and careful monitoring are often required. Attendant medical and psychological issues must be addressed, and pharmacologic and nonpharmacologic maintenance treatment can be started.

CONCLUSIONS

In this chapter, we have presented the most common categories of treatment failure in the patients who consult in headache subspecialty centers. The vast majority of refractory headache patients has a biologically determined problem that has either been misdiagnosed, mistreated, or is simply very difficult to treat. Persistence in treating these patients can be very rewarding. U.S. headache subspecialty centers use a team approach to patient management that can help reduce the burden of caring for difficult patients. Nurses, fellows, physician assistants, and psychologists can help support and educate the patient, answer questions, and manage patients. Available inpatient programs provide an important option for carefully selected patients.

References

Ameri, A and Bousser, MG (1992). Cerebral venous thrombosis. *Neurol Clin,* 10:87–111.

Andermann, E and Andermann FA (1987). Migraine-epilepsy relationships: epidemiological and genetic aspects. In *Migraine and Epilepsy* (FA Andermann and E Lugaresi, eds), pp. 281–291. Butterworths, Boston.

Blumenthal, HJ and Vance, DA (1997). Chewing gum headaches. *Headache,* 37:665–666.

Breslau, N, Davis, GC, Schultz LR, et al. (1994). Joint 1994 Wolff Award Presentation. Migraine and major depression: a longitudinal study. *Headache,* 34:387–393.

Burstein, R, Cutrer, MF, and Yarnitsky, D (2000). The development of cutaneous allodynia during a migraine attack: clinical evidence for the sequential recruitment of spinal and supraspinal nociceptive neurons in migraine. *Brain,* 123:1703–1709.

Cady, RK and Schreiber, CP (2002). Sinus headache or migraine? Considerations in making a differential diagnosis. *Neurology,* 58(Suppl. 6):10–14.

Cady, RK, Sheftell, R, Lipton, RB, et al. (2000). Effect of early intervention with sumatriptan on migraine pain: retrospective analyses of data from three clinical trials. *Clin Ther,* 22:1035–1048.

Davidoff, RA (1998). Trigger points and myofascial pain: toward understanding how they affect headaches. *Cephalalgia,* 8:436–448.

Dodick, DW, Mosek, AC, and Campbell, JK (1998). The hypnic ("alarm clock") headache syndrome. *Cephalalgia,* 18:52–56.

Dodick, DW and Wijdicks, EF (1998). Pituitary apoplexy presenting as a thunderclap headache. *Neurology,* 50:510–511.

Edmeads, J (1997). Headaches in older people. How are they different in this age-group? *Postgrad Med,* 101:91–94.

Edmeads, JG (2001). Disorders of the neck: cervicogenic headache. In *Wolff's Headache and Other Head Pain* (SD Silberstein, RB Lipton, and DJ Dalessio, eds), pp. 447–458. Oxford University Press, New York.

Evans, RW (1996). Diagnostic testing for the evaluation of headaches. *Neurologic Clinics,* 14:1–26.

Evers, S, Wibbeke, B, Reichelt, D, et al. (2000). The impact of HIV infection on primary headache. Unexpected findings from retrospective, cross-sectional, and prospective analyses. *Pain,* 85:191–200.

Ferrari, MD, Roon, KI, Lipton, RB, et al. (2001). Oral triptans (serotonin 5-HT(1B/1D) agonists) in acute migraine treatment: a meta-analysis of 53 trials. *Lancet,* 358:1668–1675.

Forsyth, PA and Posner, JB (1993). Headaches in patients with brain tumours: a study of 111 patients. *Neurology,* 43:1678–1683.

Frishberg, BM (1994). The utility of neuroimaging in the evaluation of headache in patients with normal neurologic examinations. *Neurology,* 44:1191–1197.

Graff-Radford, S (2001). Disorders of the mouth and teeth. In *Wolff's Headache and Other Head Pain* (SD Silberstein, RB Lipton, DJ Dalessio, eds), pp. 475–493. Oxford University Press, New York.

Hampson, NB and Hampson, LA (2002). Characteristics of headache associated with acute carbon monoxide poisoning. *Headache,* 42:220–223.

Headache Classification Committee of the International Headache Society (1998). Classification and diagnostic criteria for headache disorders, cranial neuralgias and facial pain. *Cephalalgia,* 8(Suppl. 7):1–96.

Holroyd, KA (2001). Learning from our treatment failures. *Appl Psychophysiol Biofeedback,* 26:319–323.

Holroyd, KA, Penzien, DB, and Lipchik, GL (2001). Behavioral management of headache. In *Wolff's Headache and Other Head Pain* (SD Silberstein, RB Lipton, DJ Dalessio, eds), pp. 562–598. Oxford University Press, New York.

Lake, AE, Saper, JR, Madden, SF, et al. (1993). Comprehensive inpatient treatment for intractable migraine: a prospective long-term outcome study. *Headache,* 33:55–62.

Lawson, W and Reino, AJ (1997). Isolated sphenoid sinus disease: an analysis of 132 cases. *Laryngoscope,* 107:1590–1595.

Lay, CL, Campbell, JK, and Mokri, B (1997). Low cerebrospinal fluid pressure headache. In *Blue Books of Practical Neurology: Headache* (P Goadsby and SD Silberstein, eds), pp. 355–368. Butterworth-Heinemann, Boston.

Linn, FH, Rinkel, GJ, Algra, A, et al. (1998). Headache characteristics in subarachnoid hemorrhage and benign thunderclap headache. *J Neurol Neurosurg Psychiatry,* 65:791–793.

Lipton, RB, Bigal, ME, Diamond, M, et al. (2007). Migraine prevalence, disease burden and the need for preventive therapy. *Neurology,* 68:343–349.

Lipton, RB, Lowenkopf, T, Bajwa, ZH, et al. (1997). Cardiac cephalgia: a treatable form of exertional headache. *Neurology,* 49:813–816.

Lipton, RB and Silberstein, SD (2001). The role of headache-related disability in migraine management: implications for headache treatment guidelines. *Neurology,* 56(Suppl. 1):35–42.

Lipton, RB, Silberstein, SD, Saper, JR, et al. (2003).Why headache treatment fails. *Neurology,* 60:1064–1070.

Marks, DR and Rapoport, AM (1997). Practical evaluation and diagnosis of headache. *Semin Neurol,* 7:307–312.

Martin, TJ and Soyka, D (1993). Ocular causes of headache. In *The Headaches* (J Olesen, P Tfelt-Hansen, and KMA Welch, eds), p. 748. Raven Press, New York.

Mathew, NT (1991). Chronic daily headache: clinical features and natural history. In *Headache and Depression: Serotonin Pathways as a Common Clue* (G Nappi, G Bono, and G Sandrini, eds), pp. 49–59. Raven Press, New York.

Mathew, NT, Stubits, E, and Nigam, MP (1982). Transformation of episodic migraine into daily headache: analysis of factors. *Headache,* 22:66–68.

Mokri, B, Sundt, T, and Houser, W (1979). Spontaneous internal carotid dissection, hemicrania, and Horner's Syndrome. *Arch Neurol,* 36:677–680.

Newman, LC and Lipton, RB (1997). Paroxysmal hemicranias. In *Headache* (PJ Goadsby, SD Silberstein, eds), pp. 243–254. Butterworth-Heinemann, London.

Newman, LC and Lipton, RB (2001). Migraine MLT-down: an unusual presentation of migraine in patients with aspartame-triggered headaches. *Headache,* 41:899–901.

Newman, LC, Lipton, RB, and Solomon, S (1990). The hypnic headache syndrome. *Headache,* 40:1904–1905.

Newman, LC, Lipton, RB, Solomon, S (1994). Hemicrania continua: 10 new cases and a literature review. *Neurology,* 44:2111–2114.

Nicolodi, M and Sicuteri, F (1999). Wine and migraine: compatibility or incompatibility? *Drugs Exp Clin Res,* 25:147–153.

Pascual, J, Combarros, O, Leno, C, et al. (1995). Distribution of headache by diagnosis as the reason for neurologic consultation. *Med Clin,* 104:161–164.

Peres, MFP, Silberstein, SD, Nahmias, S, et al. (2001). Hemicrania continua is not that rare. *Neurology,* 57:948–951.

Poceta, JS and Dalessio, DJ (1995). Identification and treatment of sleep apnea in patients with chronic headache. *Headache,* 35:586–589.

Price, RW and Posner, JB (1978). Chronic paroxysmal hemicrania: a disabling headache syndrome responding to indomethacin. *Ann Neurol,* 3:183–184.

Rapoport, A, Stang, P, Gutterman, DL, et al. (1996). Analgesic rebound headache in clinical practice: data from a physician survey. *Headache,* 36:14–19.

Rasmussen, BK, Jensen, R, Schroll, M, et al. (1992). Interrelations between migraine and tension-type headache in the general population. *Arch Neurol,* 49:914–918.

Sands, GH, Newman, LC, and Lipton, RB (1991). Cough, exertion and other miscellaneous headaches. *Med Clin North Am,* 75:733–748.

Saper, JR (1987). Ergotamine dependency—a review. *Headache,* 27:435–438.

Saper, JR (1989). Chronic headache syndromes. *Neurol Clin,* 7:387–412.

Saper, JR and Jones, JM (1986). Ergotamine tartrate dependency: features and possible mechanisms. *Clin Neuropharmacol,* 9:244–256.

Scelsa, SN, Lipton, RB, Sander, H, et al. (1995). Headache characteristics in hospitalized patients with Lyme disease. *Headache,* 35:125–130.

Silberstein, S and Marcelis, J (1990). Pseudotumor cerebri without papilledema. *Headache,* 30:304–305.

Silberstein, SD (2001). Headache and female hormones: what you need to know. *Curr Opin Neurol,* 14:323–333.
Silberstein, SD and Goadsby, PJ (2002). Migraine: preventive treatment. *Cephalalgia,* 42:491–512.
Silberstein, SD and Lipton, RB (2001). Chronic daily headache, including transformed migraine, chronic tension-type headache, and medication overuse. In *Wolff's Headache and Other Head Pain* (SD Silberstein, RB Lipton, DJ Dalessio, eds), pp. 247–282. Oxford University Press, New York.
Silberstein, SD, Lipton, RB, Solomon, S, et al. (1994). Classification of daily and near-daily headaches: proposed revisions to the IHS criteria. *Headache,* 34:1–7.
Silberstein, SD and Rosenberg, J (2000). Multispecialty consensus on diagnosis and treatment of headache. *Neurology,* 54:1553.
Sjastaad, O and Dale, I (1976). A new (?) clinical headache entity "chronic paroxysmal hemicrania" 2. *Acta Neurol Scand,* 54:140–159.
Sjastaad, O and Spierings, EHL (1984). "Hemicrania Continua." Another headache absolutely responsive to indomethacin. *Cephalalgia,* 4:65–70.
Solomon, S (2001). Posttraumatic headache. *Med Clin North Am,* 85:987–996.
Stewart, WF, Scher, AI, and Lipton, RB (2001). Stressful life events and risk of chronic daily headache: results from the frequent headache epidemiology study. *Cephalalgia,* 21:279. Abstract.
Van Gelderen, EM and Saxena, PR (1996). Nitroglycerin-induced headache. *Cephalalgia,* 16:405.
Wang, SJ, Silberstein, SD, Patterson, S, et al. (1998). Idiopathic intracranial hypertension without papilledema: a case-control study in a headache center. *Neurology,* 51:245–249.
Weeks, R (1995). The difficult headache patient calls for a multifaceted approach. *Neurol Rev,* 3:15–16.
Wenig, BM (1999). Nasopharyngeal carcinoma. *Ann Diagn Pathol,* 3:374–385.

34 Communication in the Care of the Headache Patient

Steven R Hahn

INTRODUCTION

The Importance of Communication Skills

Communication skills are an acknowledged core competency of medicine. All physicians and healthcare providers need to be and feel competent in talking with patients in order to function. Although this truth has always been evident, it has only been in the last decades that a robust pedagogy on medical communication has developed, accompanied by empirical research on the determinants of effective communication, and the allocation of sufficient curricular hours in undergraduate medical education. Milestones in the evolution of concern about effective communication were reached when medical licensure and specialty certification procedures made a commitment to evaluating this competency with performance-based assessment of communication skills using structured evaluation criteria (Duffy et al., 2004). The use of the most rigorous evaluation methodologies (encounters with standardized patients using structured evaluations), for high-stakes certification exams is a process that is still in its infancy. At the same time, the establishment of communications curricula and allocation of training time and resources is very heterogeneous across graduate education programs and has not yet become an established concept in continuing medical education.

Current Practice and Opportunities

Ample research has demonstrated that the quality and content of medical communication is related to outcomes of care (Cox et al., 2004; Roter and Hall, 2006a). However, by their own assessment, physicians' communication skills are not equal to the challenges of clinical communication (Mueller et al., 2006), and empirical studies of actual communication practices commonly demonstrate deficiencies (Roter et al., 1997; Roter and Hall, 2006a, 2006b, 2006d), a finding that has been recently been extended to migraine care (Hahn et al., 2007; Lipton et al., 2007). The evidence also suggests that across a spectrum of clinical experience, communication skills can be improved; studies of interventions to improve communication skills have produced positive outcomes using a variety of strategies (Roter and Hall, 2006c).

The Goal of This Chapter

The purpose of this chapter is to provide an aide to the goal of continued improvement of the communication and interpersonal skills employed by physicians in the care of all patients, including those with headache. To accomplish this goal the chapter has four objectives each of which will be discussed with reference to headache specific research where available:

- Define and discuss the concept of "patient-centered medical care" as the bio-psycho-social model put to action.
- Identify the latent barriers to the acquisition and application of patient-centered communication and interpersonal skills presented by the still predominantly doctor-centered and biomedical focused orientation of contemporary medical education and medical care.
- Present the principal components of patient-centered care; the general architecture of a patient-centered encounter and principal strategies of patient-centered communication.

- Illustrate the application of patient-centered communication and interpersonal skills in the management of specific clinical challenges including:
  - Assessment of impairment
  - Assessment of adherence to treatment
  - Motivational interventions to enhance adherence to medications and life style change
  - Assessment and intervention with family systems.

Studying and Learning from When Things Go Wrong

Despite the recent focus on communication skills in medical training, for the most part physicians learn to communicate with patients by applying their existing communication practices to medical content; they learn the framework of the medical history (i.e., chief complaint, history of present illness, review of systems etc.) and observe and emulate the communication patterns of their teachers. For the most part, these patterns of communication are effective when the assumptions that underlie medical encounters are met. It is when expectations are violated that typical communication skills are insufficient and outcomes suffer. The underlying structure of medical communication and opportunities to improve it are most apparent with patients whose presentations, agendas and personalities deviate from the expected and the normal. For that reason this chapter will draw upon lessons learned in difficult patient care situations where comorbid mental disorders, somatization and family conflict may play an important role.

PATIENT-CENTERED CARE AND THE BIOPSYCHOSOCIAL MODEL

Doctor-centered versus Patient-centered Communication

The biomedical model focuses on a core task of medicine, the diagnosis and treatment of disease. This agenda is sufficiently dominant that in many instances clinician's feel that there is nothing more. We distinguish herein between doctor and patient-centered interviewing and begin by illustrating the differences with two interviews of a composite patient, Michele Ramsey, a 25-year-old woman making an initial visit to a neurologist, self-referred, for headaches. A typical initial interview is recorded in the column of Table 34–1 labeled "doctor-centered interview."

Deficiencies in Doctor-centered Communication and the Biomedical Model

This encounter demonstrates an informed discussion of the elements required to make a syndromal diagnosis of migraine headache. It also exemplifies the communication style of the typical "migraine history" as demonstrated in the American Migraine Communication Study (AMCS) which performed a socio-linguistic analysis of encounters between 14 primary care physicians (PCPs) , 8 neurologists, 6 nurse practitioner/physician assistants (NP/PAs), and 60 of their patients with migraine. The average migraine discussion lasted 12 ± 5.6 minutes, during which clinicians asked an average of 13 questions 91% of which were closed-ended and focused on headache symptoms, triggers, severity and other syndromal features. The result was a doctor-centered, biomedically focused dialog which in this case seems to move seamlessly through the content necessary to make the diagnosis, evaluate and treat the patient's problem. However, the AMCS also demonstrated that after these encounters half of physicians and practitioners were not aligned with their patients on the severity of headaches or headache-related impairment; impairment was only addressed in 10% of encounters and then not very effectively; and most (80%) of subjects who met accepted criteria for preventive medication did not receive it, and in half of the encounters with prevention candidates impairment was not even discussed.

How should we understand these inadequacies and how should we remedy them? In the AMCS a single open-ended question posed by the research associate during post-visit interviews opened a world of discourse that was strikingly absent in the dialog between patients and practitioners. That question, "Tell me, in your own words, how your migraines affect your daily life?" epitomizes a

Table 34–1 Doctor-centered and Patient-centered Interview.

Doctor-centered interview	*Patient-centered interview*
Doctor: Good morning Ms. Ramsey. I'm Dr. Carlton. How can I help you? Patient: Well, I've been having headaches. Doctor: How long have you been having these headaches for? Patient: I got the first one almost a year, maybe 10 months ago. Doctor: You've never had them before? Patient: I think I had one like this when I was 16. Doctor: How many have you had? Patient: About ten. Doctor: How many have you had in the last 3 months? Patient: About half of them, I seem to get one with every other period, and then sometimes in between. I've had two in the last month, I think only one the month before. Doctor: How long do the headaches last? Patient: I usually have to sleep before they go away. If I'm lucky I'm ok when I wake up; but it usually gets parts of two days, sometimes three. Doctor: How severe would you say the headache pain is on a scale of 1–10? Patient: I assume 10 is bad pain? Well, childbirth before the epidural was pretty intense, and they say kidney stones are the worst, so leaving room for those, I've got to give the headaches an 8. Doctor: Where do you feel the pain? Patient: It's usually on the left, in the forehead, the side of my head and down my neck. Doctor: What's the pain like? Patient: It starts out steady, but then it starts to throb; and I get really sensitive. Doctor: What do you mean by sensitive? Do loud noises bother you? Patient: Noises are not so bad . . . Doctor: Do you feel nauseous? Patient: No. . . . Doctor? Doctor: Yes?	Doctor: Good morning Ms. Ramsey, I'm Dr. Carlton. It's a pleasure to meet you. Patient: I'm pleased to meet you too. Dr. Renfrew suggested I come and see you about my headaches. Doctor: Headaches, yes. You know Dr. Renfrew? Patient: Yes, I'm doing data entry and analysis on his chronic pain study. Doctor: Oh, yes; that's an interesting study. Tell me more about what you do. Patient: Well I'm a grad student, health care MBA so I'm working as a research associate and I'm carrying a couple of teaching sections as well. Doctor: Sounds very busy. Patient: That's just the half of it. Doctor: Oh? We should definitely get to your headaches, but it sounds like the "other half" of what's keeping you busy might be important to hear about too. Is there anything else? Patient: Nothing else. I mean I am here because of my headaches, but my life *is* pretty complicated right now. Doctor: We'll see if we can't put it all together before we're done. Why don't you tell me about your headaches? Patient: Well, the pain is very intense, very severe, throbbing. The headaches last from the time I get them until I go to bed, and if I'm lucky it's gone by morning. I feel sick to my stomach, I can't deal with bright lights, which makes working impossible, and noises don't help so much either but their not so bad. And I've been getting them more frequently—that's why I asked Dr. Renfrew, or actually he noticed I was having trouble, and suggested I see you. Doctor: Well coming in sounds like good idea. Tell me more about getting them more frequently? Patient: I think I had one headache like these when I was 16, then not again until almost a year, actually 10 months ago and I've probably

(continued)

Table 34–1 (continued)

Doctor-centered interview	Patient-centered interview
Patient: You asked about noises? Doctor: Yes. Patient: They don't bother me that much, but I absolutely cannot take strong lights. Doctor: OK. You mentioned that your periods seem to set them off, have you noticed anything else? Patient: I think the ones I get that aren't with my period may be more likely when I don't get enough sleep. Doctor: What about alcohol, other foods, stress? Patient: I gave up alcohol because I thought it might be part of the problem. The stress is there all the time. The headaches are what's stressful. Doctor: Yes, I can understand that. Do you think the stress makes them worse? Patient: I don't know, more the other way around. Doctor: You're working? Patient: Grad student. Healthcare MBA. I'm carrying a few teaching sections and I have a job doing data entry and analysis on a chronic pain management program. Doctor: Sounds like a lot. What medications have you tried? Patient: It *is* a lot. I've used all the over the counter medications, and I had some prescriptions for NSAIDs left over from an old ankle sprain. I think that they've all helped some, enough to help me get to sleep, but not enough to make the headache go away without going to sleep. Doctor: Well, I think we can do better than that. You have migraine headaches, and there are medications, triptans, that should help better. Patient: That's what I thought, that's what Dr. Renfrew, the PI on the chronic pain study thought too. He gave me your name. Doctor: Well, it sounds like you need to make sure you get enough sleep since that's one of the things you *can* control that triggers your	had 10 or twelve since then, but more frequently in the last three months—maybe half of them, I had two in the last month, so about two a month maybe a little less—I think I get them with my period, but in between too, especially if I haven't been getting enough sleep. Doctor: Have you noticed any other things that set off the headaches, any "triggers" like alcohol or particular foods? Patient: I gave up red wine because I thought it might be factor; I don't think it made any difference. Nothing else though. Doctor: What's the story with your sleep? Patient: Well, I have an 18-month-old, Peter, he has trouble sleeping a couple of times per week, and I'm up late every night trying to get things done so I don't have much reserve. Doctor: This is part of the "other half of the story?" Patient: Yes, well my husband Adam started his last year in orthopedics and his call schedule has been brutal. So when the baby is up I am too. I suppose that not sleeping has something to do with migraines, if that's what these are. But the truth is, the headaches are more stressful than the "stress" if you know what I mean. When I get a headache I can't function at work, and it is all I can do take care of Peter. There's no way Adam can get home. My Mom helps but I hate to ask her, my Dad's older and has CHF, and the best the NSAIDs I've tried can do is let me get to sleep. Doctor: I think we can do better than NSAIDs, in fact, we can see how you feel about taking medicine to prevent the headaches as well as better medicines to treat them when they start. But your life situation does seem extremely difficult and stressful. Probably for you and for Adam too. Patient: Everyone says you can't anticipate what having a child does to your life and they're right. But I love it, and, don't worry, I'm not depressed and the only thing that I get anxious about is whether I'm going to have another

(continued)

Table 34–1 (continued)

Doctor-centered interview	*Patient-centered interview*
headaches. And let's talk about taking one of the triptans. Patient: I don't know about the sleep, but tell me about the triptan. Doctor: Well, do the best you can. Patient: Sure. Doctor: Now let me tell you about the triptans. They are medications that work specifically with migraine headaches to stop attacks. . . . *The conversation continues with a presentation of how to use triptans and arrangements for a follow-up visit.*	headache—I can't even make plans now. Adam's upset, worried, more upset than worried. But we're ok. It's just that these headaches they're not just a straw, they're a whole bale of straw breaking the camel's back. I assume you mean a daily medication when you talk about prevention? I hate the idea of having to take medicine everyday, but frankly, I am willing to try almost anything. Doctor: OK. I don't want to understate the role that sleep deprivation might be playing in your migraine problem, but I can see how it seems there aren't too many degrees of freedom to change your sleep habits. We can also take a look at other lifestyle issues that might decrease your headache frequency and help you avoid daily preventive medication. Do you want to talk about that now, or do you want to talk about medications? Patient: Let's talk meds. Doctor: OK, tell me what you know about migraine medications; triptans, preventives? Patient: Well I know that the triptans are specifically for migraine, and . . . *The conversation continues with a presentation of how to use triptans and arrangements for a follow-up visit.*

patient-centered question in two ways: first, it is a directed open-ended question which "directs" the patient to an area of inquiry, but leaves the form and content of the response open to the patient. Second, it opens a topic of discussion that transcends the focus of the biomedical model and invites the patient to provide information in which they are the expert; their own experience of their illness.

Patients' responses to this single question revealed types of information that has been demonstrated to dramatically change clinicians' appreciation of the need for migraine-specific and preventive medication. In a quasi-experimental study 125 neurologists and PCPs with self-identified interest in headache first watched an interview focusing on syndromal biomedical information and were asked to rate headache severity, select a treatment strategy, and indicate whether follow up consultation was indicated. They then observed a continuation of the interview containing questions about headache-related disability and repeated their assessment of the patient. A dramatic and significant increase in the proportion of physicians who rated the patient's headaches as severe, and requiring migraine specific treatment and follow up consultation was observed (Holmes et al., 2001). A similar change in physicians' perceptions and clinical response has been documented more informally when similar ratings were performed by physicians first after watching a doctor-patient encounter recorded during the AMCS and then the same patient's response to the open-ended question about headache-related impairment.

A Definition of Patient-centered Care

Patient-centered care has been characterized as having three dimensions articulated by Mead (Mead et al., 2002) and elaborated here:

1. Use of a bio-psychosocial paradigm that
   (a) Includes attention to the patient's psychological well being as well as to their physical well-being;
   (b) Incorporates an understanding of the reciprocal causal relationships between physical illness and psychological and emotional forces;
   (c) Includes consideration of the patient's social milieu as an important factor determining physical and emotional health status and health related behaviors.
2. Involving the patient in decision making and activating the patient in self-care by
   (a) Sharing power in decision making by giving consideration to the patient's preferences and assessments of the value of the outcomes and the burdens of treatments;
   (b) Activating the patient to adher to treatments and engage in health promoting behavior.
3. Attending to the interpersonal dimension of the doctor–patient relationship with the objective of building a therapeutic alliance that includes an appreciation of the patient as a human being and the practitioner as an important person in their lives.

Patient-centered communication is talk that supports these agendas and goals of care. There are a variety of different patterns of discourse and clinical skills that characterize patient-centered communication and which reliably distinguish a patient-centered communication style from so called "doctor-centered" communication. A patient-centered discourse with Ms. Ramsey is illustrated in Table 34–1, along side of the previously discussed doctor-centered interview.

General Features of Patient-centered Communication

There are several general characteristics that distinguish patient-centered from doctor-centered discourse. Many are evident in the example given.

- *The greeting.* In the patient-centered interview the greeting is more personal and given due attention. The agenda for the visit is not the very first order of business. In the interview presented here, the physician postpones addressing the biomedical agenda for only a few seconds, but that is long enough to hear something unique and personal about the patient's social connection to the doctor. This exchange adds substantially to the relationship between doctor and patient and contributes positively to the therapeutic alliance.
- *Question structure.* Many of the doctor's questions take the form, "tell me about [it]?" where the [it] is something important or striking that the patient said in her last statement. This approach is explicitly patient-centered, focusing the dialog on a thread that the patient has introduced yet still guiding the course of the dialog. The physician also uses "directive open-ended questions," for example, "tell me about your headaches?" and elicits in response to just three such questions the same amount of information that required 10–11 questions in the doctor-centered interview.
- *Content.* The physician covers the same symptom syndrome and medical history in the course of the patient-centered interview. Indeed, he learns about the absence of mood and anxiety disorders; important comorbidities that have to be assessed in migraine. However, he also explicitly includes consideration of the patient's social circumstances and psychological state. Even before exploring "the other half of the story" fully he signals his interest, facilitating the patient's subsequent discussion of social and personal information. Our understanding of the consequences of the patient's headache-related functional impairment is palpably more compelling than in the doctor-centered interview. We also learn much more about the patient's sleep deprivation and appreciate the patient's own thoughts about the potential for change. Most importantly, the physician has heard what he needs to know, that is, that preventives should be considered and that the

patient is willing but ambivalent about daily medication.

- *Response to emotional content.* In the patient-centered interview the physician explicitly validates the magnitude of the stress the patient is experiencing by reflecting back what he has heard. He also validates its importance by the attention he gives to the socially stressful and emotionally difficult circumstances. The physician's informed response to the patient's explication of her sleep problem was also much more supportive than the seemingly obvious though ultimately gratuitous advice to get more sleep given in the doctor-centered intervention.
- *Decision making.* By honoring the importance of the patient's experience of her illness and obtaining a better understanding of the patient's perspective, the patient-centered physician was able to reach a well aligned perspective on the potential for changing sleep patterns. Without fully accepting the patient's current opinion, he was still able to avoid an unwittingly authoritarian and simplistic intervention based on his knowledge of the importance of sleep deprivation as a trigger. The physician empowered the patient to help choose whether to focus on non-pharmacological treatments, respecting her ambivalence about daily medication; or to first focus on acute and preventive medications to treat her migraines.
- *Patient education.* At the end of the interview we got a glimpse of the patient-centered approach to patient education which is predicated on the assumption that the content taught should be tailored to the patient's current understanding. Instead of beginning with "the triptan speech" or the "preventive medication speech" the physician "centers" his education on the patient by asking her to talk about what she already knows about these medications.

The end result of the patient-centered interaction is a few moments of care that attend to symptoms and disease features but go beyond to build a positive relationship in which power for decisions can be shared, the psychosocial factors that have a direct impact on migraine can be revealed, and a process of education can begin that is predicated on the patient's current understanding. In current medical practice it is within the bounds of statistical normalcy and even de facto standards of adequate care to treat patients like Ms. Ramsey without knowing that she is a working mother caring for an 18-month-old baby with a sleep problem and a husband who has limited availability because of his call schedule as a surgical resident. But once you've heard her story, it becomes hard to imagine how you could take care of Ms. Ramsey without knowing who she is in this way. The need for this orientation is particularly acute in a condition such as migraine where the reciprocal relationship between the disease and social functioning is so profound that clinical misjudgments such as failure to use preventives when indicated can be directly tied to communication patterns that exclude this data.

THE ARCHITECTURE OF THE MEDICAL INTERVIEW

The Three Functions of the Medical Interview

The structure of a medical interview is driven by the tasks that must be accomplished. These have been described as consisting of three functions served by communication during the medical encounter. The categories of the "three function model" of the medical interview are: (1) gathering data; (2) educating and counseling; and (3) building a relationship (Cohen-Cole, 1991). The sequence or stages of the medical interview can be understood in terms of these functions. The broad stages of the interview as described in models of patient-centered communication [adapted from Smith (Smith et al., 2000)] are:

1. Greeting and setting the stage for the interview;
2. The chief complaint, eliciting and negotiating the agenda;
3. Data gathering and medical history
   - (a) Open-ended questioning, progressively focused
   - (b) Closed-ended, doctor-centered questioning
4. Patient education and counseling.

Setting the Stage for the Interview

Greeting and Introducing

The first step of the interview focuses principally on the goal of building a relationship. Welcoming the patient, greeting them by name and introducing oneself demonstrate concern and respect. It may be more acceptable to "get down to business" quickly in a medical encounter than in other types of social interactions, but failure to attend to this task can damage the doctor–patient relationship immediately if the physician is perceived to be cold, uncaring, or disrespectful. Merely perfunctory attention to introductions may produce a deficiency in trust and confidence in the physician that translates into a lack of confidence in the physician's explanations and recommendations which results in poor adherence to treatment and low patient satisfaction.

Addressing language barriers. A truly engaged greeting and introductions begin to build a safe environment for discussion of emotionally difficult, stigmatizing, and technically complex information. Barriers to communication must also be addressed to "set the stage" for the work of the medical encounter. One of the most important considerations is the ability to communicate with the patient in a language in which they are fluent. If the clinician does not have adequate fluency in an appropriate language a trained medical translator or interpreter, *not a family member or friend,* should be preemptively offered. By interpreter we wish to indicate an individual who can explain or "interpret" the meaning of words and customs of communication and behavior in the context of the patient's culture where as translation refers to the specific linguistic process.

In addition to providing more accurate and informed interpretation, a second reason that a family member or friend should not be used as in interpreter is the need to ensure privacy, including if not especially privacy with regards to other family members. If the translator is a member of the family system, important categories of information may be precluded from discussion. For example, if marital discord or sexual issues are playing a role in the patient's problem and the translator is a child or the spouse this information will be unavailable or distorted.

Identifying Concerns and Negotiating the Agenda

The next phase of the interview begins the process of identifying the focus and content of the work that the doctor and patient will be doing. The usually unexamined assumption about the nature of this stage of the interview is based on the biomedical paradigm which defines the process of care as the task of making a diagnosis and formulating a treatment plan. The most commonly used term for the initial phase of the interview, the "chief complaint," is consistent with these assumptions: A "complaint" is strictly speaking, a statement about a problem, but in this context the expectation is that it will be a symptom, for example, headache. In truth, the reasons that patients see doctors can be grouped into three categories: (1) diagnosis and prognosis; (2) relief of symptoms and treatment of known chronic disease; and (3) adjudication of the sick-role (Lazare et al., 1975; Barsky, 1981). Patients may be concerned about the diagnostic or prognostic significance of a symptom but not need or desire treatment for the symptom or its cause. Similarly, patients may only wish to obtain symptom relief and not be concerned about diagnosis or prognosis, either because they already believe they know the cause of their symptom or do not care.

Adjudication of the sick role covers a broader spectrum of agendas ranging from the bureaucratic such as medication prior authorization, to regulatory, for example, notes to employers regarding missed days or fitness to return to work, or entitlements such as requests for home health aids, visiting nurse services, or disability (Lazare et al., 1975; Barsky, 1981). The most complex and challenging form of adjudicating the sick-role occurs when patients with somatoform symptoms present with a need to have the physician establish that they are entitled to the sick-role and therefore to special consideration or different treatment in the context of their family and social systems.

Perhaps the most fundamental truth about patients' agendas is that they are hoping that the physician can do something for them. Therefore, beginning this phase of the interview with the directive open-ended question, "How can I help you?" offers the patient an opportunity to bring up any agenda, request or concern. It also puts the patient's agenda in the context of anticipated help from the physician. Furthermore it leaves open the possibility that the patient may have more than one agenda for the doctor and the visit.

For that reason, we recommend that the physician ask the patient if he or she has other agendas or requests before engaging in further discussion of what appears to be the "chief" request. It may even be worthwhile asking about each of the three domains of patient agenda explicitly. For example, asking: "Is there anything else bothering you?" to screen for other symptoms in need of relief; "Do you have any other concerns?" to screen for diagnostic or prognostic agendas; and, "Do you have any forms or prescriptions that we need to deal with today?" to screen for sick-role related issues. It is important to coach the patient to present additional items succinctly by cutting off elaboration on the issues mentioned, assuring the patient that each concern will be explored as appropriate. Eliciting all the patient's agendas will also set the stage for "negotiating the visit agenda." The physician should mention any additional issues that he or she wishes to address, and then decide with the patient which of all the potential agenda items will be addressed on the current visit and which subsequently or by other providers. Knowing the visit agenda at the outset is the best way to insure intelligent management of time during the visit. In deciding upon the agenda the physician can state the fact that time is limited explicitly, setting as the reason that a decision has to be made about what to address today. This process is also the most effective way to avoid so called "door knob" complaints that come up just as you are opening the door for the patient to leave.

Taking the History

Directed Open-ended Questions Followed by Closed Ended Questions

The patient-centered history begins with open-ended inquiry about the complaints, concerns, and requests elicited at the outset. "Tell me about your headaches?" is the perfect opener. As mentioned above, the directive open-ended question will typically produce as much information as a series of closed-ended questions about specific headache features. It will also give the patient opportunities at the outset to indicate the extent to which diagnostic concerns, relief of symptoms, and sick-role issues may be important in understanding the patient's problem. After asking appropriate open-ended questions about the presenting problem the physician can ask closed-ended questions to fill in any gaps in the data needed for diagnosis and evaluation.

Addressing the Patient's Experience: Functional Impairment

The biomedical model puts an emphasis on the characteristics of symptoms needed to make a diagnosis. Evaluation of the patient's problem also requires understanding the impact of the patient's medical problems on their functioning and the impact of both symptom and functional impairment on how the patient feels including assessment of clinical mood or anxiety disorder. In the domain of headaches, the single open-ended question, "How do your headaches affect your daily life?" will open the world of the patient's experience of their illness for observation. Probing for role-specific functional impairment should be considered for domains of activity not spontaneously mentioned such as work, family, recreational activities.

Though decisions about management require information about headache-related functional impairment, it was addressed in 10% of migraine encounters in the baseline assessment of communication done in the AMCS. When functional impairment was addressed a robust open-ended question was generally not used. Headache-related functional impairment should be understood in the context of the patient's social systems, particularly work/school and family. It is important for the clinician to screen for problems generated by headache-related impairment that might prompt additional intervention. For example, are family members or individuals in the work place adequately understanding and supportive? Do they need to be educated about the impairment associated with migraine attack? If the patient is indeed adhering to treatment do they need additional validation from the physician either at home or at work? Does the patient need any coaching in how to explain the nature of their problem to others? Is the patient adequately concerned about the consequences of their impairment? Disturbing answers to any of these questions might be good reason to consider counseling or patient and/or family education. Finally, in those circumstances where headache is serving as the foundation of a sick-role coping strategy, discovery that functional impairment is out of proportion to the magnitude of the headache problem will be the most direct way of detecting that problem.

Addressing the Patient's Experience: Mood and Anxiety

Asking patients how they feel is an important indication of concern about their well-being and contributes to an emotionally positive therapeutic alliance. Physician responsiveness to patients' emotional state is associated with higher patient satisfaction (DiMatteo et al., 1980, 1986), reduction in psychological distress (Roter et al., 1995), and symptom resolution (Buller and Buller, 1987). It is also critical to the important clinical task of assessing possible mood and anxiety disorders. Approximately one quarter of primary care patients have clinically significant mood disorders and about a fifth (91%) have anxiety disorders (Spitzer et al., 1994). The prevalence of both conditions is higher in certain headache conditions, especially migraine and chronic daily headache. It is important to realize that affect during the interview is an unreliable indicator of depressed mood. Physicians who do not use a systematic screen will only detect 30% of the clinically significant depression in their practices (Spitzer et al., 1994). Substantial research has demonstrated that no more than two questions, codified in the "PHQ-2," need be asked as an initial screen to detect clinically significant depression: (1) have you been bothered a lot in the last month by feeling sad, down, or depressed? (2) have you been bothered a lot in the last month by a loss of interest or pleasure in your daily activities? (Kroenke et al., 2003) This combination of questions is very sensitive to the presence of depression and patients who answer "no" to both are very unlikely to be depressed. Those who endorse either item should be further evaluated for depression. The "PHQ-9" is a useful clinical tool for diagnosing and assessing the severity of mood disorders and can be used as a patient self-report instrument or presented as a structured interview (Spitzer et al., 1999). Anxiety disorders, although frequently comorbid with depression, make an independent contribution to functional impairment and requires explicit attention when present. Generalized anxiety disorder can be reliably detected and assessed using a seven item screen (Spitzer et al., 2006; Kroenke et al., 2007).

Doctor-centered Dialog

Although patient-centered open-ended questions focused on core symptoms will usually yield most of the information required for the history of the presenting concern, specific items of information are often necessary to clarify symptom syndromes, the timing of symptoms, etc. Closed-ended, doctor-centered interviewing is the most efficient strategy for obtaining this information. Intervals of doctor-centered closed-ended dialog may be required at various times during the history. Therefore it is helpful to mark the transition between the patient-centered and the physician-centered phases of dialog by identifying the categories of information being solicited, and mark a return to patient-centered dialog by indicating that the doctor-centered agenda has been satisfied. Closed-ended doctor-centered dialog is often the most efficient way of addressing such categories of important information as allergies, past surgeries etc. However, as discussed below, closed-ended questions are not a good way to initiate discussion about current medication use.

Educating the Patient About Treatment and Disease: "Ask Tell Ask"

The third function of the medical interview is to instruct that patient about proposed treatments and help them adhere to recommendations. This task will be guided in part by our understanding of the determinants of adherence behavior, specifically the factors that enhance patients' motivation to follow the treatment, the barriers to adherence, and the ways in which we can help patient's change their motivation to change their behaviors. These factors will be addressed below in the discussion of communication. Here we will first consider a basic strategy for the process of patient education that has been called "Ask-Tell-Ask" (Back et al., 2005) that is based on the predicate that at minimum, education is most effective when it is based upon knowledge of what the patient already knows. In the case of patient education about disease and treatment it is not only a question of knowledge, both known, missing and mistaken; it is also important to understand patients' beliefs, attitudes and feelings about the disease and its treatment. Steven Covey's principle, "seek first to understand" is a better characterization of what the clinician needs to know, specifically to understand the patients understanding and experience of illness and treatment. Empirical study of actual doctor-patient communication reveals that this exploration rarely takes place before the standard "migraine speech" or "triptan speech" is delivered (AMCS I).

The first ask. Patients' understanding of their illness and its treatment is like a partially completed jigsaw puzzle. If the bottom left hand corner has been assembled, it will not be helpful to talk about a piece that belongs in the upper right. If a piece has been misplaced it will interfere with completing the puzzle. An open-ended question about the patient's understanding of their illness, medication, etc. will reveal three things:

1. What the patient knows that is correct;
2. The key piece of missing information;
3. The patient's misunderstandings and incorrect beliefs.

Each of the open-ended questions in Table 34–2 which are based upon factors that influence adherence to treatment can serve as the "first ask" of this process.

The tell. When the patient has revealed what they know, what they don't know and their mistaken beliefs and misconceptions, they can then be provided targeted information that reflects the unique landscape of their current understanding.

1. Reinforce and validate what the patient already knows, and avoid wasting time.
2. Provide the next piece of information the patient needs to have.
3. Correct the patient's misunderstandings and mistaken beliefs.

A presentation of information based upon the knowledge revealed by the "first ask" will be radically different from a "migraine speech" or a "how to take triptans speech" based upon an a priori "syllabus."

The second ask. The second ask has three purposes:

1. Assess how much and what part of the "tell" the patient understood and absorbed.
2. Assess the impact of the new information on the patient's attitudes, motivation, and stage of readiness for change.
3. Continue the ask-tell-ask process in an iterative fashion in progression toward the goal of the dialog.

Negotiating a Plan

The closing stages of the interview focus on establishing the patient's understanding of recommendations, a task best accomplished by employing the "second ask" of the ask tell ask sequence to have them restate their understanding of the proposed treatment. After establishing that the patient does understand the proposed treatment it is important to assess the patient's commitment to following the recommendations. It is important to create a nonjudgmental environment that will permit the patient to express any reservations or ask any questions. This is not easy because patients will be reluctant to express disagreement with the physician and may be concerned that asking questions, even informational questions, may be perceived as challenging the physician's authority. In assessing commitment it is important to realize that patients fall into three broad categories of attitudes toward accepting recommendations to take medications (described in greater detail in discussion of the "Therapeutic Decision Model" below): patients who

1. Will take medication simply because the physician tells them it is what they need;
2. Are disinclined to take any medication, perhaps preferring "natural remedies";
3. Will initiate treatment if they understand the recommendation and will formulate an independent judgment of the efficacy and tolerability of their prescription.

TABLE 34–2 Stages of Readiness for Change.

Stage	*Psychology*	*Goal of intervention*	*Strategy*
Pre-contemplation	Lack of concern: ignorance or denial	Raise concern	Educate or address denial
Contemplation	Ambivalence	Shift ambivalence toward action	Address decision balance: re address pros of change; address cons of change
Preparation/ decision/ determination	Commitment	Transform commitment to action	Identify quit or change date
Action	Acquiring new skills and resources	Enhance resources	Provide resources
Maintenance	Integrate skills into new lifestyle habits	Identify barriers to integration	Problem solving around barriers
Relapse	Shame and loss of hope and self-efficacy	Destigmatize, restore hope and self-efficacy	Pre-emptive destimatization, identify residual ambivalence

COMMUNICATION ABOUT MEDICATION USE AND ADHERENCE

The Problem of Nonadherence

Patients do not benefit from medications they do not take. Less than optimal adherence to medication is the rule not the exception across all diseases and medication types, including short term medications for symptomatic conditions. A large number of studies have converged on the conclusion that the average patient on chronic daily medication takes between two-thirds and three-quarters of doses (Haynes, 2001; DiMatteo, 2004). A few studies demonstrate similar findings in migraine. Using a variety of metrics based on surreptitious electronic monitoring of bottle cap openings Mulleners studied adherence to preventive medications in 38 subjects with migraine (Mulleners et al., 1998). The least stringent measure of adherence, the number of times the cap was opened per day, suggested an overall adherence rate of 66% with a range of 54% for three times per day medications and 80% for once daily meds. When calibrated as bottle cap opened "on schedule," rates ranged from only 30% for TID to 66% for once daily medications. Acute medications are also vulnerable to nonadherence. A mailed questionnaire survey study of 1160 migraineurs revealed that two-thirds (67%) delayed or avoided using prescription medications because of concerns about adverse effects and they did so in one-third of the average of 12 headaches that were treated (Gallagher and Kunkel, 2003). Another study of 690 patients receiving a prescription for rizatriptan or other non-triptan abortive revealed a similar pattern of avoidance and delay of treatment in 49% of subjects (Foley et al., 2005). An interventional study employing self-management support demonstrated baseline adherence to ergotamine/caffeine abortive treatment in 40% of attacks which improved to 70% with the intervention. Nonadherence can also take the form of overuse as demonstrated in a study in the Netherlands that detected daily to 10 times per week use of sumatriptan in a minority of patients (Ottervanger et al., 1996).

Communication to Address Nonadherence

Management of nonadherence poses three challenges: (1) detecting nonadherence; (2) assessing motivational deficits and barriers to adherence; and (3) enhancing motivation and lowering barriers to adherence.

Detecting Nonadherence: A Four Step Strategy

Ample research demonstrates that normally honest people will conceal nonadherence from their healthcare providers despite understanding that misinformation may lead to poor decisions. Many observations support the conclusion that patients will go to great lengths to conceal nonadherence, presumably because they want to preserve their healthcare provider's good opinion of them even at the cost of providing misinformation about their actual medication use (Mazze et al., 1984; Simmons et al., 2000; Burnier et al., 2001).

A communication strategy designed to overcome patients' predisposition to conceal has been proposed that is based upon two hypotheses: first, that "normalizing" and "universalizing" nonadherence can lower the stigma of revealing this socially undesirable behavior. Second, that patients who feel that they are active participants in making decisions about medication use that will be based upon the information that they give about their adherence, are more likely to reveal nonadherence than are patients who feel that they are passively reporting socially undesirable behavior and then being judged by their physician. The four steps of this process are:

1. *Ask an open-ended question about medication use.* Specifically ask, "Tell me how you are taking your medications?" The patient's response will reveal the state of their understanding of their regimen and their ability to keep their medications organized. Follow up with questions about strategies used at home to organize and remember medications such as lists, pill organizers, or a family member. Arrange to have access to the family member (in person or by phone) or other mnemonic at subsequent visits. The objective of this step is to reveal the patient's understanding of their regimen.
2. *Reverse the judgmental environment by normalizing and universalizing nonadherence.* Patient's need to be proactively reassured that you know that barriers to adherence, both motivational and practical, are real and therefore some degree of nonadherence would be "normal." Also, that such barriers are ubiquitous and therefore some degree of nonadherence is the rule rather than the exception. The objective of this step is to create a nonjudgmental environment. Our assumption is that this requires an active resetting of patient perception and expectation, not merely the absence of judgmental language.
3. *Make the patient an active participant in the decision about medications and the role of self-reported adherence behavior explicit in that decision.* If the patient is asked to help solve the problem of inadequate treatment outcome by examining how much medicine has actually been applied to the problem before making a decision about changing dose or class, they will understand that their responsibility in decision making is to provide accurate information about adherence. For example, in a patient on preventive medication who is still having frequent headaches the clinician might say,

> "We have a problem to solve. You are still having frequent headaches. That means that your body is not getting enough or effective enough medication. Before we increase the dose of medication, or change to another, we need to make sure that you've actually been able to take the amount we've talked about because prescribing too much medicine, or switching to a different, second-choice medicine before giving this one a good trial would be poor choices to make."

This kind of statement can help make the importance of accurate information about adherence as compelling as the need to give the impression of being a good patient. The objective of this step is to create a collaborative problem-solving process and relationship rather than a judgmental and authoritarian one.

4. *Ask about actual adherence only after setting the stage.* After creating a nonjudgmental collaborative decision making environment the stage is set to actually ask about nonadherence. The key to this step is to make sure it is the last one so that a premature declaration of adherence does not present doctor and patient with the additional challenge of confessing to a "cover-up" on top of nonadherence. There are several strategies that can be employed. One,

building upon the example provided for step 3 above would be to allow a confession of nonadherence without ever actually having to say so in so many words:

"So, should we base our decision on your experience with the medicine up until now, or should we observe you for a while longer to make sure we've given this medicine and dose a good trial?"

Alternatives include asking "Have you missed any doses of medicine in the last week?" This question has been shown to have a sensitivity of about 50% and very good specificity even without the three preceding steps of the four step strategy (Gilbert et al., 1980; Haynes et al., 1980; Stewart, 1987; Cramer et al., 1989; Stephenson et al., 1993). Asking about "forgetting" will typically increase the sensitivity because "forgetting" seems to be more acceptable than "skipping" and certainly more acceptable than "choosing not to take." Finally, it is important to know that adherence improves significantly during the week before a visit (Cramer et al., 1990), so a question about skipping or forgetting that leaves the temporal frame work unstated can allow patients to claim adherence based upon their most recent performance. A question that explicitly refers to a broader time frame will be more revealing. Similarly, when drug levels or rapidly responsive physical parameters such as heart rate or blood pressure are being employed as indices of adherence, it is important to remember that good results can be produced with short term adherence (e.g., less than a day with β blockers or five half-lives with drug levels). Correspondingly, poor results with rapidly responsive parameters may be due to nonadherence as recently as the day of the visit.

Assessing Barriers to Adherence

By the time nonadherence has been detected the clinician may have some sense of which barriers have been affecting adherence. Knowledge of the epidemiology of barriers to adherence will be helpful in efficient screening for those that are relevant. The most general model for understanding the determinants of adherence, the "health beliefs model," proposes that there are five domains to consider:

1. The perceived threat of the illness;
2. The perceived benefit of the treatment;
3. The burden of the treatment;
4. Skills and knowledge required to adhere to the treatment;
5. Social and material support for adherence.

Further elaborations of the theoretical model of adherence behavior have focused on specific elements within these five domains to find points of influence that drive patient behavior. Models include the *Information, Motivation, and Behavioral Skills (IMB)* model, the *"Therapeutic Decision Model"* and the *Stages of Readiness for Change* model. This last model provides a theoretical foundation for motivational interviewing. The stages of readiness for change model identifies six stages, each with its own unique psychological characteristics, that determine which stage-specific motivational interventions will be most successful in moving patients on to the next stage. For "precontemplative" patients who are either unaware that they have a problem or in denial about it, the stage-specific strategy is to raise concern where there was none by correcting ignorance or addressing denial. With the "contemplative" patient who has entered the "yes, but . . ." stage, the task is to shift ambivalence by addressing the pros and cons of adhering or not. Patients who have taken action and are entering the "maintenance" phase need help integrating new behaviors into their lifestyle and daily routine. The stages, their unique psychology, the stage-specific goal of intervention, and the stage-specific strategy that can accomplish the goal are outlined in Table 34–2. Stage of change-specific interventions have been successful in changing patient behavior (Prochaska et al., 1994; Prochaska and Velicer, 1997). This model is applicable to enhancing adherence to medications but is also particularly useful in helping patients with life style changes that may be important in managing headaches.

These models of adherence behavior give guidance to communication about adherence. Specifically, open-ended questions can be used to address the domains of concern identified by the health belief model and its iterations. Table 34–3 illustrates examples of open-ended

Table 34–3 Open-Ended Questions in Adherence Dialog.

Model	*Factor*	*Question*
Information, motivation, behavioral skill	Information	Tell me what you understand about what's going wrong when you get a migraine?
		Tell me what you understand about how the triptan will work?
		Tell me what you understand about how to use the triptan?
		What is your understanding about side effects with this medicine?
		What is your understanding of whether these medications can cause addiction or dependency?
	Motivation	Tell me how concerned you are about preventing migraines compared to treating them after they start?
		What thoughts do you have about beginning an exercise routine?
		What concerns do you have about side effects with this medicine?
		What concerns do you have about taking a daily medicine to prevent migraines?
	Behavioral skills	What strategies do you have for making sure you have access to your triptan when a headache starts?
		How do you decide when to take a triptan?
		Show me how you use the injection?
Therapeutic decision model	Patient testing	How do you think you will make up your mind whether this medicine is working for you?
		Which of these side effects do you think you'll be able to live with, which not?
	Collaborative decision making	How should we work together to monitor the way this medicine is working?
		What has your experience with patient education materials like pamphlets or take home videos been?
	Concordance on attitudes toward treatments	How do you feel about taking medicines for problems like this in general?
		What do you think about non-drug treatments to prevent frequent migraines?
	Effect of patient experience	You've had experience with triptans before; let's talk about that and how you feel about using them.
		You said your mother had migraines; what have you learned from her about dealing with them?
Stages of readiness for change	Pre-contemplative	How concerned are you about the need to decrease the frequency of your migraines?
		What thoughts do you have about getting more sleep?
		How do you feel about getting more regular exercise?

(continued)

TABLE 34–3 (continued)

Model	Factor	Question
	Contemplative	What would be the down side of taking daily medicine to decrease the frequency of your headaches? What do you like about staying up the way you do? What will the challenges be in trying to increase your exercise?
	Maintenance	How can you build the daily medicine into your routine so you don't forget it? What kind of schedule can you really sustain for getting to bed? How will you protect the time you plan to exercise if your work begins to pile up?

questions that can elicit patients' experiences and beliefs regarding the dimensions of illness experience that are identified by the adherence models presented here.

ASSESSING THE FAMILY AND SOCIAL CONTEXT OF ILLNESS: THE GENOGRAM-BASED INTERVIEW

Illness in a Family and Social Context

All illness occurs in the context of the patient's family and social system which influence the nature of impairment associated with headache, the social supports available to the patient, and may be the source of additional social burdens. In some instances family-related sick-role issues can play a defining part in the patient's headache experience. For these reasons, an efficient strategy for talking to patients about their family that can be flexibly applied depending upon the magnitude of the role that family issues are playing is a valuable aid to clinical practice (Hahn, 2002b).

Conducting the Genogram-Based Interview

A genogram-based interview addresses family structure and function in the context of medical and psychiatric illness. It is conducted by drawing a genogram—a graphic representation of the patient's family that uses the iconography of a family tree—while talking to the patient about their family. An example based upon the patient interviewed in Table 34–1 is presented in Figure 34–1. Drawing the genogram with the patient looking on sends a powerful message about interest in the patient as a person and is an invitation to discuss concerns about the family and its interaction with the illness. When there are no family problems the genogram is a quick snap shot of the patient's life that can contribute to the therapeutic relationship and provide a structure for assessing the family medical history.

Screening for Family-systems Problems

Identifying the Unusual

When a genogram is drawn, striking features such as divorce, step-parenting, and unusual composition are revealed. An open-ended question about those features will quickly establish whether they require attention. Patients who discern the physician's intention often volunteer the "real problem" after the first question is asked. The screen for family issues can be completed by asking about family members' reactions to the patient's headaches or vice versa.

The Family Life Cycle

The concept of the "family life cycle" provides a framework for understanding families as they evolve over time; "launching" individuals to form new families, that move through stages driven by biological and social forces. These stages, outlined in Table 34–4, can be characterized by the tasks that must be accomplished in each. Families usually experience dysfunction because they are

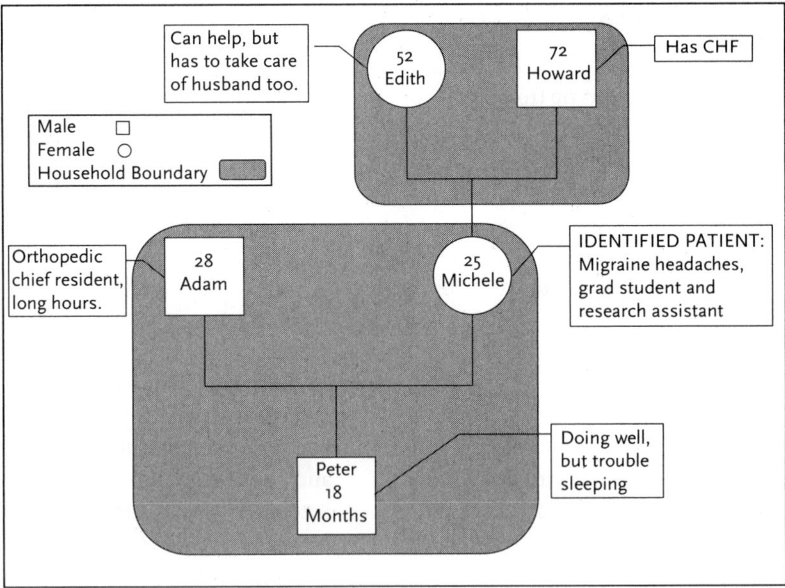

Figure 34–1 Genogram of Michele Ramsey's family.

having problems with these stage-specific tasks. Therefore, open-ended questions about the stage-specific tasks will usually take the interview to the source of difficulty. In families without problems, this screening process takes a few moments and doctor and patient can move on to other agendas. If significant problems are discovered, the physician can take four steps the first of which—identification of the family issues—will have just been accomplished.

Four-step Family Assessment and Intervention in Medical Practice

Step 1. Identify the family problem; encourage the patient to tell his or her story and "bring the pain into the room."
Step 2. Reframe attention to the family problem by identifying it as "just as painful, impairing, and worthy of attention as the headache" or other physical problem(s).
Step 3. "Empathically witness" the patient's struggle to deal with their problem: "I am so impressed with how you are doing despite everything—headache and family issues included—that they have to deal with." Empathic witnessing based upon a deep understanding of the patient's circumstances is powerfully therapeutic.
Step 4. Refer the patient for counseling when significant problems are encountered. Restate the family problems as questions to be answered, and suggest "counseling" as the best strategy for answering that question. When mood and anxiety disorders are discovered they require evaluation and treatment by the primary headache physician with referral to a psychiatrist as needed.

Family Assessment and Intervention with Somatizing Patients and the Sick Role

The four stage family assessment and intervention is useful for addressing family systems with most patients but virtually essential when headache has become the foundation of a somatoform sick-role strategy (Hahn, 2002a) When patient's and their families need the sick-role as a coping strategy, they become refractory to treatment because getting better means giving up the sick-role. Estimates of the prevalence of this problem will vary depending on definition of somatization and demographics however the prevalence of clinically significant somatization in primary care populations ranges from 4% to 18% averaging 8% (Spitzer et al., 1994). Reframing and referring for therapy with hope for the evolution of better coping strategies over time is a desirable remedy.

Table 34–4 Stages of the Family Life Cycle.

Life cycle stage	*Dominant theme*	*Transitional task*
The single young adult	Separating from family of origin	Differentiation from family of origin Developing intimate relationships with peers Establishing career and financial independence
Forming a committed relationship	Commitment to a new family	Formation of a committed relationship Forming and changing relationships with both families of origin
The family with young children	Adjusting to new family members	Adjusting the relationship to make time and space for children Negotiating parenting responsibilities Adjusting relationships with extended families to incorporate parenting and grandparenting
The family with adolescents	Increasing flexibility of boundaries to allow for children's independence	Adjusting boundaries to allow children to move in and out of the family more freely Attending to midlife relationship and career issues Adjusting to aging parent's needs and role
Launching children	Accepting exits and entries into the system	Adjusting committed relationship to absence of children in the household Adjusting relationships with children to their independence and adult status Including new in-laws and becoming grandparents Adjusting to aging or dying parents' needs and role
The family later in life	Adjusting to age and new roles	Maintaining functional status, developing new social and familial roles Supporting central role of middle generation Integrating the elderly into family life Dealing with loss of parents, spouse, peers; life review and integration

SUMMARY

Patient-centered care framed by the patient's psycho-social context will provide the best possible care to patients with headache and other medical problems. A perspective that recognizes the reciprocal relationship between physical symptoms and seemingly unrelated psycho-social problems and mental disorders will allow the patient and clinician to address the multiple causes and sustaining forces in the headache experience. Successful patient-centered care incorporates patients as positive actors in health care decisions; both decisions made in the dialog of the doctor-patient interaction, and perhaps more importantly, the decisions that they will make about adhering to treatment after the consultation is over and they are living with their illness in their own social milieu.

Patient-centered care requires specific communication skills that may seem superfluous or counter-intuitive when medicine is guided by a narrow biomedical paradigm. The patient-centered communication skills enumerated in this discussion will help support patient-centered care. Specifically, the objective of "seeking first to understand" by using ask-tell-ask dialog sequences that begin and end with open-ended questions that guide the information presented in the "tells" sandwiched between, is the essence of patient-centered communication. The application of this strategy in obtaining the medical history, supplemented by closed-ended questions to complete assessment, will optimize efficiency and ensure that the patient's perspective is included in the physician's understanding. In educating patients about their illness and treatment, the same strategy will help guarantee that patient's understanding is in alignment with the physician's, or that differences of opinion or belief are exposed so that they can be addressed. These patterns of communication will bring aspects of patients' adherence into consideration that will require knowledge of explanatory models of adherence behavior such as the health beliefs-based and stages of change models which have been presented here. Similarly, clinicians who with to understand patients' headache experience in the context of their family and social system will need to understand how the sick role interacts with the takes and dynamics of the family life-cycle. The skills, models, and vocabulary presented are intended as a basic tool-kit and framework for learning and teaching optimum communication skills in the care of headache patients.

References

Back, AL, Arnold, RM, Baile, WF, et al. (2005). Approaching difficult communication tasks in oncology. *CA Cancer J Clin,* 55:164–177.

Barsky, AJ, III (1981). Hidden reasons some patients visit doctors. *Ann Intern Med,* 94:492–498.

Buller, MK and Buller, DB (1987). Physicians' communication style and patient satisfaction. *J Health Soc Behav,* 28:375–388.

Burnier, M, Schneider, MP, Chiolero, A, et al. (2001). Electronic compliance monitoring in resistant hypertension: the basis for rational therapeutic decisions. *J Hypertens,* 19:335–341.

Cohen-Cole, S (1991). *The Medical Interview: The Three Function Approach.* Mosby: St. Louis, MO.

Cox, K, Sevenson, F, Britten, N, et al. (2004). *A Systematic Review of Communication Between Patients and Health Care Professionals About Medicine-Taking and Prescribing.* Medicines Partnership: London.

Cramer, JA, Mattson, RH, Prevey, ML, et al. (1989). How often is medication taken as prescribed? A novel assessment technique. *J Am Med Assoc,* 261:3273–3277.

Cramer, JA, Scheyer, RD, and Mattson, RH (1990). Compliance declines between clinic visits. *Arch Intern Med,* 150:1509–1510.

DiMatteo, MR (2004). Variations in patients' adherence to medical recommendations: a quantitative review of 50 years of research. *Med Care,* 42:200–209.

DiMatteo, MR, Hays, RD, and Prince, LM (1986). Relationship of physicians' nonverbal communication skill to patient satisfaction, appointment noncompliance, and physician workload. *Health Psychol,* 5:581–594.

DiMatteo, MR, Taranta, A, Friedman, HS, et al. (1980). Predicting patient satisfaction from physicians' nonverbal communication skills. *Med Care,* 18:376–387.

Duffy, FD, Gordon, GH, Whelan, G, et al. (2004). Assessing competence in communication and interpersonal skills: the Kalamazoo II report. *Acad Med,* 79:495–507.

Foley, KA, Cady, R, Martin, V, et al. (2005). Treating early versus treating mild: timing of migraine prescription medications among patients with diagnosed migraine. *Headache,* 45:538–545.

Gallagher, RM and Kunkel, R (2003). Migraine medication attributes important for patient compliance: concerns about side effects may delay treatment. *Headache,* 43:36–43.

Gilbert, JR, Evans, CE, Haynes, RB, et al. (1980). Predicting compliance with a regimen of digoxin therapy in family practice. *Can Med Assoc J,* 123:119–122.

Hahn, SR (2002a). Caring for patients experienced as difficult. In *Twenty Common Problems in Behavioral Health* (FV deGruy III, WP Dickson, EW Staton, eds), ed.). pp. 259–286, McGraw Hill: New York.

Hahn, SR (2002b). Family assessment in primary care. In *Behavioral Medicine: A Primary Care Handbook* (2nd edn) (MD Feldman and J Christensen, eds), pp. 59–75, MGraw Hill, Appleton & Lange: Stamford, CT.

Hahn, SR, Cady, RK, Nelson, MR, et al. (2007). Improving healthcare professional-patient communication to promote more effective assessment of migraine impairment during and between attacks: results of the American Migraine Communication Study (AMCS) Phase II. In *Diamond Headache Clinic's 20th Annual Practicing Physician's Approach to the Difficult Headache Patient; February 13–17, 2007.* Rancho Mirage, CA.

Haynes, RB (2001). Improving patient adherence: state of the art, with special focus on medication taking for cardiovascular disorders. In *Patient Compliance in Health Care Research: American Heart Association Monograph Series.* (Burkey LE, Okene IS eds) pp. 3–21, Futura Publishing Co: Armonk, NY.

Haynes, RB, Taylor, DW, Sackett, DL, et al. (1980). Can simple clinical measurements detect patient noncompliance? *Hypertension,* 2:757–764.

Holmes, WF, MacGregor, EA, Sawyer, JP, et al. (2001). Information about migraine disability influences physicians' perceptions of illness severity and treatment needs. *Headache,* 41:343–350.

Kroenke, K, Spitzer, RL, and Williams, JB (2003). The Patient Health Questionnaire-2: validity of a two-item depression screener. *Med Care,* 41:1284–1292.

Kroenke, K, Spitzer, RL, Williams, JB, et al. (2007). Anxiety disorders in primary care: prevalence, impairment, comorbidity, and detection. *Ann Intern Med,* 146:317–325.

Lazare, A, Eisenthal, S, and Wasserman, L (1975). The customer approach to patienthood. Attending to patient requests in a walk-in clinic. *Arch Gen Psychiatry,* 32:553–558.

Lipton, RB, Hahn, SR, Cady, RK, et al. (2007). In office discussion of migraine: results from the American Migraine Communication Study. Unpublished work.

Mazze, RS, Shamoon, H, Pasmantier, R, et al. (1984). Reliability of blood glucose monitoring by patients with diabetes mellitus. *Am J Med,* 77:211–217.

Mead, N, Bower, P, and Hann, M (2002). The impact of general practitioners' patient-centredness on patients' post-consultation satisfaction and enablement. *Soc Sci Med,* 55:283–299.

Mueller, PS, Barrier, PA, Call, et al. (2006). Views of new internal medicine faculty of their preparedness and competence in physician-patient communication. *BMC Med Educ,* 6:30.

Mulleners, WM, Whitmarsh, TE, and Steiner, TJ (1998). Noncompliance may render migraine prophylaxis useless, but once-daily regimens are better. *Cephalalgia,* 18:52–56.

Ottervanger, JP, Valkenburg, HA, Grobbee, DE, et al. (1996). Pattern of sumatriptan use and overuse in general practice. *Eur J Clin Pharmacol,* 50:353–355.

Prochaska, JO and Velicer, WF (1997). The transtheoretical model of health behavior change. *Am J Health Promot,* 12:38–48.

Prochaska, JO, Velicer, WF, Rossi, JS, et al. (1994). Stages of change and decisional balance for 12 problem behaviors. *Health Psychol,* 13:39–46.

Roter, DL and Hall, JA (2006a). Consequences of talk: the relationship between talk and outcomes. In *Doctors Talking with Patients/Patients Talking with Doctors: Improving Commununication in Medical Visits* (2nd edn), pp. 143–164. Praeger: Westport, CT.

Roter, DL and Hall, JA (2006b). Giving and withholding information: the special case of informative talk in the medical visit. In *Doctors Talking with Patients/Patients Talking with Doctors: Improving Commununication in Medical Visits* (2nd edn), pp. 127–140. Praeger: Westport, CT.

Roter, DL and Hall, JA (2006c). Improving talk through interventions. In *Doctors Talking with Patients/Patients Talking with Doctors: Improving Commununication in Medical Visits* (2nd edn), pp. 163–181. Praeger: Westport, CT.

Roter, DL and Hall, JA (2006d). The anatomy of a medical visit. In *Doctors Talking with Patients/patients Talking with Doctors: Improving Commununication in Medical Visits* (2nd edn), pp. 109–125. Praeger: Westport, CT.

Roter, DL, Hall, JA, Kern, DE, et al. (1995). Improving physicians' interviewing skills and reducing patients' emotional distress. A randomized clinical trial. *Arch Intern Med,* 155:1877–1884.

Roter, DL, Stewart, M, Putnam, SM, et al. (1997). Communication patterns of primary care physicians. *J Am Med Assoc,* 277:350–356.

Simmons, MS, Nides, MA, Rand, CS, et al. (2000). Unpredictability of deception in compliance with physician-prescribed bronchodilator inhaler use in a clinical trial. *Chest,* 118:290–295.

Smith, RC, Marshall-Dorsey, AA, Osborn, GG, et al. (2000). Evidence-based guidelines for teaching patient-centered interviewing. *Patient Educ Couns,* 39:27–36.

Spitzer, RL, Kroenke, K, and Williams, JB (1999). Validation and utility of a self-report version of PRIME-MD: the PHQ primary care study. Primary Care Evaluation of Mental Disorders. Patient Health Questionnaire. *J Am Med Assoc,* 282:1737–1744.

Spitzer, RL, Kroenke, K, Williams, JB, et al. (2006). A brief measure for assessing generalized anxiety disorder: the GAD-7. *Arch Intern Med,* 166: 1092–1097.

Spitzer, RL, Williams, JB, Kroenke, K, et al. (1994). Utility of a new procedure for diagnosing mental disorders in primary care. The PRIME-MD 1000 study. *J Am Med Assoc,* 272:1749–1756.

Stephenson, BJ, Rowe, BH, Haynes, RB, et al. (1993). The rational clinical examination. Is this patient taking the treatment as prescribed? *J Am Med Assoc,* 269:2779–2781.

Stewart, M (1987). The validity of an interview to assess a patient's drug taking. *Am J Prev Med,* 3:95–100.

Index

Note: Page numbers in *italics* refers to figures and tables